Chronic Illness Care

Editors
Timothy P. Daaleman
Department of Family Medicine
University of North Carolina
CHAPEL HILL, NC, USA

Margaret R. Helton
Department of Family Medicine
University of North Carolina
CHAPEL HILL, NC, USA

ISBN 978-3-031-29170-8   ISBN 978-3-031-29171-5 (eBook)
https://doi.org/10.1007/978-3-031-29171-5

© The Editor(s) (if applicable) and The Author(s), under exclusive license to Springer Nature Switzerland AG 2023
This work is subject to copyright. All rights are solely and exclusively licensed by the Publisher, whether the whole or part of the material is concerned, specifically the rights of translation, reprinting, reuse of illustrations, recitation, broadcasting, reproduction on microfilms or in any other physical way, and transmission or information storage and retrieval, electronic adaptation, computer software, or by similar or dissimilar methodology now known or hereafter developed.
The use of general descriptive names, registered names, trademarks, service marks, etc. in this publication does not imply, even in the absence of a specific statement, that such names are exempt from the relevant protective laws and regulations and therefore free for general use.
The publisher, the authors, and the editors are safe to assume that the advice and information in this book are believed to be true and accurate at the date of publication. Neither the publisher nor the authors or the editors give a warranty, expressed or implied, with respect to the material contained herein or for any errors or omissions that may have been made. The publisher remains neutral with regard to jurisdictional claims in published maps and institutional affiliations.

This Springer imprint is published by the registered company Springer Nature Switzerland AG
The registered company address is: Gewerbestrasse 11, 6330 Cham, Switzerland

Introduction

Chronic diseases are conditions that last for 1 year or more, are not prevented by vaccines or cured by medication, do not spontaneously resolve, and have long-lasting and significant effects on a person's quality of life [1]. The World Health Organization refers to chronic diseases as noncommunicable diseases (NCDs) and reports that NCDs—prior to the COVID-19 pandemic—were responsible for 71% of all deaths globally, primarily due to cardiovascular diseases, cancers, chronic respiratory diseases, and diabetes [2]. Multiple chronic conditions (MCCs) are generally defined as the co-occurrence of two or more chronic physical or mental health conditions and may be synonymous with the term multimorbidity [3]. MCCs can be inclusive of additional factors that contribute to overall disease burden, including functional impairment and social determinants of health, such as food insecurity and experiencing homelessness.

Whether termed chronic disease or illness, NCD, or MCCs, there is a physical, emotional, economic, and social toll for patients and caregivers with this lived experience. Although chronic disease is often associated with older age, persons of all age groups are impacted. More than 15 million of deaths attributed to chronic disease occur between the ages of 30 and 69 years, and the majority are estimated to occur in low- and middle-income countries [2]. Both individual behavioral factors (e.g., tobacco use, diet, physical activity) and larger social forces, such as poverty and urbanization, increase the risk of chronic disease. In addition, there is growing research examining the adverse effects of loneliness or social isolation on chronic disease outcomes [4, 5].

Chronic illness care is the coordinated, comprehensive, and sustained response to these diseases and associated conditions—from initial diagnosis to the end of life—by a range of health care professionals, formal and informal caregivers, and health care and community-based systems [6]. In the United States, individuals with MCCs account for a large share of health service utilization and associated costs: 93% of Medicare spending; 83% of prescription drug costs; 71% of all health care spending; 70% of acute hospital stays; and 64% of outpatient visits [3]. The costs of Social Security and Medicare are expected to grow faster than the gross domestic product due to the aging US population, which will result in projected financing shortfalls for these programs [7].

The COVID-19 pandemic was caused by the severe acute respiratory syndrome coronavirus 2 (SARS-CoV-2) resulting in a range of respiratory and associated symptoms, morbidities, and sequelae that has permanently altered the landscape of chronic disease [8–10]. Beyond the enormous personal and societal losses, the impact of COVID-19 on those with chronic disease has been particularly profound [8, 9, 11]. Most adults hospitalized for COVID-19 had preexisting chronic conditions, and these individuals remain at a greater risk for contracting the virus, experiencing greater disease severity, and are more likely to have had needed health services delayed or interrupted, subsequently reducing providers' and health care systems' capacities to prevent or mitigate disease [8, 12]. The repeated waves of community spread and the associated mitigation efforts, including isolation recommendations, have disrupted lives and created social and economic hardships.

COVID-19 has also laid bare many of the root causes of health inequities and structural racism [9]. Populations with low socioeconomic status and those self-identifying as African-American, Hispanic, and Native American have been adversely impacted by a disproportionate burden of disease [8]. Race and ethnicity are historically associated with social determinants of health, which are defined as the conditions in which "people are born, grow, work, live, and age," reflecting larger forces and systems that impact the conditions of daily life [13, 14]. The pandemic era has widened health disparities, the systematic, disproportionate differences in social determinants that negatively impacts less advantaged groups [8, 9, 15].

The experience of chronic disease has changed and many assumptions about providing health care and associated services for chronically ill patients have been challenged by COVID-19 [8–10, 12]. Fallout from the pandemic has resulted in decreases in preventive services and chronic disease management [8]. For example, cancer screenings declined during the pandemic and modeling estimates project that delays in screening and treatment for breast and colorectal cancer may result in approximately 10,000 preventable deaths in the United States [16, 17]. In addition, substantial ground has been lost in chronic care due to interruptions in immunizations and deferred treatment for mental health and substance use disorders [8].

Health care providers and systems adapted to COVID-19-associated disruptions in services, such as those due to social and physical distancing, staff reductions, and practice closures, with telehealth, which expanded the scope of practice for non-physician providers, and by temporarily removing many organizational, policy, and fiscal roadblocks, particularly around reimbursement [8, 9]. Unfortunately, these adaptive changes have not addressed a fundamental problem; contemporary approaches, systems, and policies of health care do not support optimal care for chronically ill patients, particularly for marginalized populations [9].

The second edition of *Chronic Illness Care: Principles and Practice* responds to this fundamental problem by providing a comprehensive and organized body of information regarding chronic illness care [18]. The first edition of the textbook recognized that improving the health status and promoting the quality of life for individuals with chronic conditions necessitated change on many levels, as well as a paradigm shift regarding care approaches to providing care [19]. The second edition is still organized using a social-ecological framework, which is derived from systems theory and looks at the interdependent influences between individuals and their larger environment [20]. This framework considers multiple domains across several levels of influence and provides a grounding to the book (Fig. 1). Different sections of the book aggregate individual chapters, presenting key principles and concepts, as well as evidence and examples that illustrate and support these ideas.

The new edition incorporates the impact that health inequities exposed by the COVID-19 pandemic has on chronic illness care and outcomes. The book starts with chapters that focus on individual factors that influence chronic disease, which may be considered fixed (e.g., genetics) or behavioral (e.g., tobacco use, physical activity, substance use disorders). This section also includes a chapter on chronic disease self-management. Part II addresses the role of others in an individual's experience of chronic disease and acknowledges formal and informal social networks and support systems, including family, friends, and peers. Content covers areas from the usually supportive role of family and other caregivers to the negative influence of domestic violence, abuse, and neglect. This section recognizes the role of community support from patient navigators, peers, and agencies and organizations as emerging stakeholders in the management of chronic disease.

Introduction

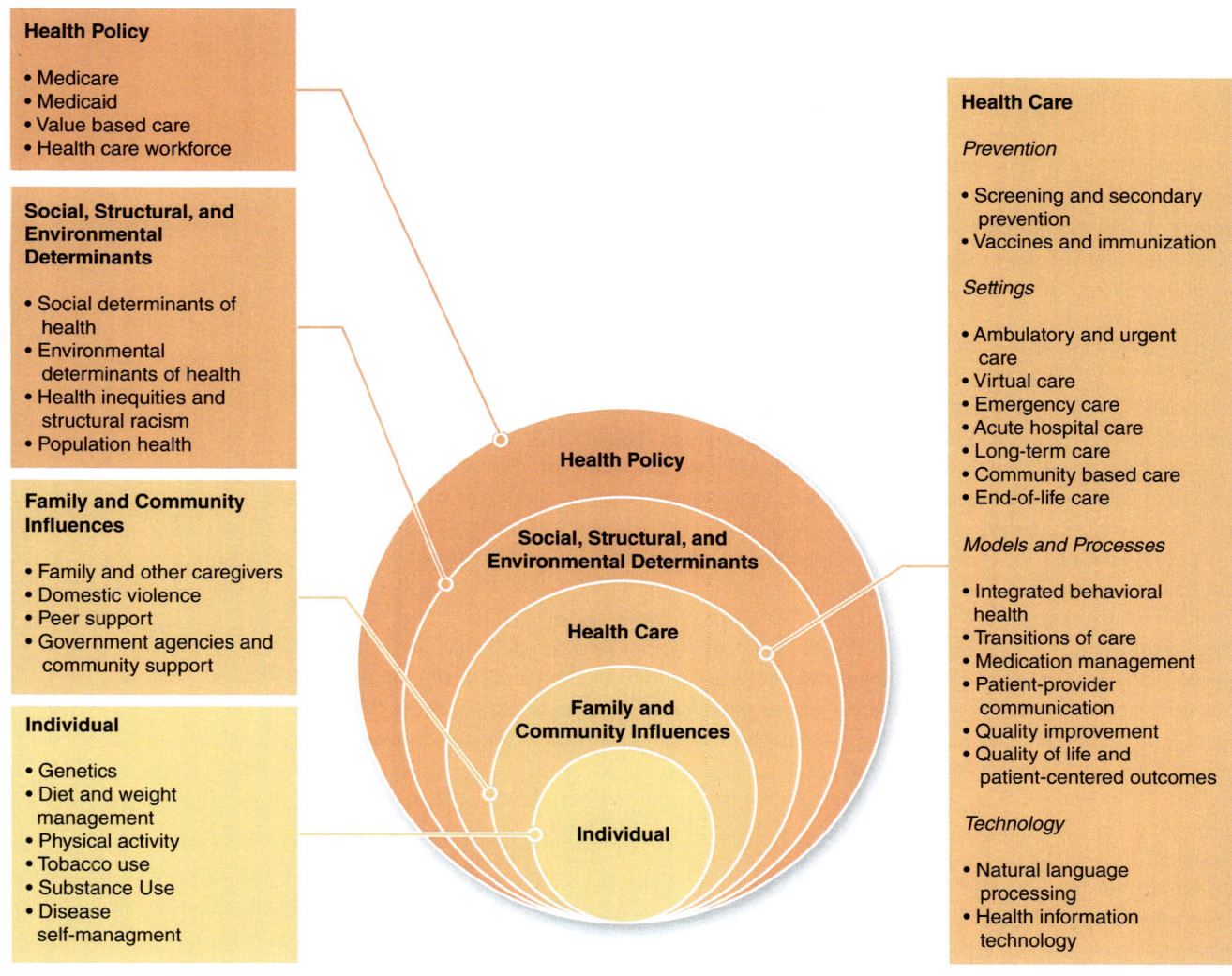

Fig. 1 A Socio-Ecologic Framework for Chronic Illness Care

The principles and practices that are foundational to providing chronic care is the largest section and occupies a central place in the book. Part III does not focus on the medical diagnosis and treatment of specific chronic diseases, due to the rapid pace of research and scholarship that informs and changes practice, and the ready dissemination of clinical information via information technology and other electronic sources. Rather, chapters in this section cover key principles that form foundations of care provision in health care settings where chronic care is provided, including outpatient and inpatient settings, the emergency department, nursing homes, rehabilitation centers, and community-based care. There are information needs that are common to chronic care providers across these settings, and this section includes chapters on secondary prevention, medication management, patient–provider communication, and end-of-life care.

COVID-19 has led to additional chapters on vaccines and immunizations, virtual care, and on care of patients with COVID-associated chronic conditions. Chapters that provide approaches to caring for chronically ill patients with unique needs and challenges (e.g., children and adolescents, older adults) have been expanded to include adults with persistent mental health disorders, cancer survivors, and military veterans. Care of vulnerable populations, including persons experiencing homelessness, incarcerated persons, and the LGBTQ community have also been added.

As the paradigm for chronic illness care changes, the organizational structures for delivering health care services are also undergoing transformation. The Chronic Care Model, which identifies key health care system elements that promote quality chronic illness care, helps to frame Part IV [21]. Chapters in this section cover key concepts and models that are primarily located in outpatient settings, including integrated behavioral health care, population health, transitions of care, quality improvement, and the use of health information technology. Content specific to natural language processing and machine learning, as well as patient-centered outcomes, have been added to this section.

Part V recognizes that social and environmental factors affect chronic illness, whether through a cumulative exposure to unclean air or water, or through health behaviors that are mediated by social interactions. This section closes with a chapter on health inequities and structural racism as background to understand how historical and social determinants have adversely influenced the health of disadvantaged populations. Local, state, and national regulations and laws, including policies regarding the allocation of resources and access to health care services, are components of the policy environment in which chronically ill patients live and receive their health care. These are critical issues that require ongoing examination and improvement if a viable and sustainable health care system is to meet the needs of chronically ill patients. Chapters in this section include the major US federal programs influencing chronic care delivery (i.e., Medicare and Medicaid), and an understanding of the health care work force that is needed to provide care.

This textbook responds to the fundamental problems of chronic illness care that have been called out by the COVID-19 pandemic [9]. By providing new ways of thinking about chronic illness care, it can be a useful resource to the physicians, nurses, social workers, pharmacists, policy-makers, educators, and others who are committed to the care of persons with chronic illness.

References

1. National Center for Chronic Disease Prevention and Health Promotion. About chronic diseases. Atlanta: Centers for Disease Control and Prevention; 2022. https://www.cdc.gov/chronicdisease/about/index.htm.
2. World Health Organization. Noncommunicable diseases, fact sheets. World Health Organization;2021.https://www.who.int/news-room/fact-sheets/detail/noncommunicable-diseases.
3. Bierman AS, Wang J, O'Malley PG, Moss DK. Transforming care for people with multiple chronic conditions: Agency for Healthcare Research and Quality's research agenda. Health Serv Res. 2021;56 Suppl 1(Suppl 1):973–9.

4. Hajek A, Kretzler B, König HH. Multimorbidity, loneliness, and social isolation. a systematic review. Int J Environ Res Public Health. 2020;17(22):8688.
5. Liu X, Yu HJ, Gao Y, Zhou J, Zhou M, Wan L, et al. Combined association of multiple chronic diseases and social isolation with the functional disability after stroke in elderly patients: a multicenter cross-sectional study in China. BMC Geriatr. 2021;21(1):495.
6. Martin CM. Chronic disease and illness care. Can Fam Physician. 2007;53(12):2086–91.
7. Trustees of the Federal Old-Age and Survivors Insurance and Federal Disability Insurance Trust Funds. The 2022 annual report of the Board of Trustees of the Federal Old-Age and Survivors Insurance and Federal Disability Insurance Trust Funds Washington, DC; 2022. p. 1–275. https://www.ssa.gov/oact/TR/2022/tr2022.pdf.
8. Hacker KA, Briss PA, Richardson L, Wright J, Petersen R. COVID-19 and chronic disease: the impact now and in the future. Prevent Chron Dis [Internet]. 2021;18:E62. https://www.cdc.gov/pcd/issues/2021/21_0086.htm.
9. Chin MH. Uncomfortable truths—What Covid-19 has revealed about chronic-disease care in America. N Engl J Med. 2021;385(18):1633–6.
10. Murphy SL, Kochanek KD, Xu J, Arias E. Mortality in the United States, 2020. NCHS Data Brief. 2021;427:1–8.
11. Islam N, Jdanov DA, Shkolnikov VM, et al. Effects of COVID-19 pandemic on life expectancy and premature mortality in 2020: time series analysis in 37 countries. BMJ [Internet]. 2021;375:e66768 p. https://doi.org/10.1136/bmj-2021-066768.
12. Riley KE, et al. Managing medicare beneficiaries with chronic conditions during the COVID-19 pandemic. New York: Commonwealth Fund; 2021. https://doi.org/10.26099/j3c3-7p61.
13. WHO. Social determinants of health report by the Secretariat. World Health Organization 132nd Session 2012;7.3.
14. CDC. Social determinants of health: know what affects health. Centers for Disease Control and Prevention. 2017.
15. Braveman P. Health disparities and health equity: concepts and measurement. Annu Rev Public Health. 2006;27:167–94.
16. London JW, Fazio-Eynullayeva E, Palchuk MB, et al. Effects of the COVID-19 pandemic on cancer related patient encounters. JCO Clin Cancer Inform. 2020;4(4):657–65.
17. Sharpless NE. COVID-19 and cancer. Science. 2020;368(6497):1290.
18. US Department of Health and Human Services. Multiple chronic conditions—a strategic framework: optimum health and quality of life for individuals with multiple chronic conditions. Washington, DC: US Department of Health and Human Services; 2010.
19. Daaleman TP, Helton MR. Preface: introduction to chronic illness care. In: Daaleman TP, Helton MR, editors. Chronic illness care, principles and practice. Cham: Springer; 2018. p. vii–ix.
20. National Center for Injury Prevention and Control, Division of Violence Prevention. The social-ecological model: a framework for prevention. Atlanta: Centers for Disease Control and Prevention. 2022. https://www.cdc.gov/violenceprevention/about/social-ecologicalmodel.html.
21. Coleman K, Austin BT, Brach C, Wagner EH. Evidence on the chronic care model in the new millenium. Health Aff (Millwood). 2009;28(1):75–85.

School of Medicine
University of North Carolina at Chapel Hill
Chapel Hill, NC, USA

Timothy P. Daaleman, DO, MPH
Margaret R. Helton, MD

Contents

Part I Individual Influences on Chronic Illness

1. **Genetic Contributions and Personalized Medicine** 3
   J. Kevin Hicks

2. **Obesity and Chronic Disease** 19
   Debbie Phipps and Margaret R. Helton

3. **Promoting Physical Activity** 29
   Nailah Adams Morancie, Catherine Ellis, Alyssa Heinrich, and Justin Lee

4. **Tobacco Use and Dependence** 41
   Kimberly A. Shoenbill, M. Justin Byron, Ashley A. Weiner, and Adam O. Goldstein

5. **Chronic Disease Self-Management** 61
   Liza Straub and Maria Thekkekandam

6. **Alcohol and Drug Use Disorders** 71
   Michael H. Baca-Atlas, Stefani N. Baca-Atlas, and Kelly Bossenbroek Fedoriw

Part II Family, Social, and Community Support

7. **Family and Other Caregivers** 87
   Alexandra Targan and Caroline Collins Roberts

8. **Domestic Violence, Abuse, and Neglect** 99
   Samantha Schilling and Adam Zolotor

9. **Peer Support** 113
   Edwin B. Fisher, Patrick Y. Tang, Muchieh Coufal, Yuexing Liu,
   Samantha L. Luu, Megan Evans, and Weiping Jia

10. **Government Agencies and Community Organizations** 129
    Sherry Shackelford Hay and Marni Gwyther Holder

Part III Providing Chronic Illness Care

11. **Screening and Secondary Prevention** 145
    Erik Butler and Katrina Donahue

12. **Vaccines and Immunization** 155
    Zachary J. Pettigrew, Min Kim, and Sylvia Becker-Dreps

13. **Medication Management and Treatment Adherence** 181
    Emily M. Hawes and Kimberly A. Sanders

14	**Patient-Provider Communication and Interactions** 195	

Kelly Lacy Smith and Jennifer Martini

15 Ambulatory Primary Care and Urgent Care 209
Clark Denniston and LeRon Jackson

16 Virtual Care 221
Vinay Reddy and Amir Barzin

17 Acute Hospital Care 231
Amir Barzin, Yee Lam, and Matthew Zeitler

18 Emergency Care 245
Ryan M. Finn, Mary Mulcare, and Christina Shenvi

19 Post-Acute and Long-Term Care 255
Karen Halpert and Margaret R. Helton

20 Home- and Community-Based Care 269
Amy C. Denham and Christine E. Kistler

21 End-of-Life Care 285
Margaret R. Helton and Jenny T. van der Steen

22 Special Population: Children and Adolescents 301
Morgan A. McEachern, Ashley Rietz, and Cristy Page

23 Special Population: Older Adults 311
Collin Burks and Mallory McClester Brown

24 Special Population: Adults with Intellectual and Developmental Disabilities . . . 321
Victoria L. Boggiano and Timothy P. Daaleman

**25 Special Population: Adults with Severe and Persistent
Mental Health Disorders** 335
Kathleen Barnhouse, Sandra Clark, and Jessica Waters Davis

26 Special Population: LGBTQ Community 347
Julie M. Austen, Rita Lahlou, and Modjulie Moore

27 Special Population: Care of Incarcerated Persons 359
Rachel Sandler Silva and Evan Ashkin

28 Special Population: Care of Immigrants and Refugees 371
Martha C. Carlough and Rana Alkhaldi

29 Special Population: COVID-Associated Chronic Conditions 381
John M. Baratta and Louise King

30 Special Population: Care of Cancer Survivors 395
Bogda Koczwara

31 Special Populations: Care of Military Veterans 407
Shawn Kane

32 Special Populations: Care of Persons Experiencing Homelessness 417
Richard Moore II and Timothy P. Daaleman

Part IV Organizational Frameworks for Chronic Illness Care

33 Integrated Behavioral Health Care 431
Linda Myerholtz, Nathaniel A. Sowa, and Brianna Lombardi

34 Transitions of Care 447
Catherine L. Coe, Mallory McClester Brown, and Christine E. Kistler

35 Population Health 459
Amy N. Prentice, Rayhaan Adams, Deborah S. Porterfield,
and Timothy P. Daaleman

**36 Artificial Intelligence, Machine Learning, and
Natural Language Processing** 469
Kimberly A. Shoenbill, Suranga N. Kasturi, and Eneida A. Mendonca

37 Health Information Technology 481
Carlton Moore

38 Quality Improvement 497
Dana Neutze and Brian Wiggs

39 Quality of Life and Patient-Centered Outcomes 511
Maria Gabriela Castro and Margaret C. Wang

Part V Social and Environmental Determinants of Chronic Illness

40 Social Determinants of Health 527
Robert L. Ferrer

41 Environmental Determinants of Health 547
Michelle Del Rio and Jacqueline MacDonald Gibson

42 Health Inequities and Structural Racism 567
Dana Iglesias and Alexa Mieses Malchuk

Part VI Health Policy and Chronic Illness Care

43 Medicare 583
Jonathan Oberlander

44 Medicaid 597
Pam Silberman and Ciara Zachary

45 Value-Based Care 607
Mark Gwynne

46 Health Care Workforce 619
Erin Fraher, Bruce Fried, and Brianna Lombardi

Index 633

Contributors

Rayhaan Adams Department of Family Medicine, University of North Carolina at Chapel Hill, Chapel Hill, NC, USA

Rana Alkhaldi Department of Family Medicine, University of North Carolina at Chapel Hill, Chapel Hill, NC, USA

Evan Ashkin Department of Family Medicine, University of North Carolina at Chapel Hill, Chapel Hill, NC, USA

Julie M. Austen Frank Porter Graham Child Development Institute, University of North Carolina at Chapel Hill, Chapel Hill, NC, USA

Michael H. Baca-Atlas Department of Family Medicine, University of North Carolina at Chapel Hill, Chapel Hill, NC, USA

Stefani N. Baca-Atlas University of North Carolina at Chapel Hill School of Social Work, Chapel Hill, NC, USA

John M. Baratta, MD, MBA Department of Physical Medicine and Rehabilitation, University of North Carolina at Chapel Hill, Chapel Hill, NC, USA

Kathleen Barnhouse Department of Family Medicine, University of North Carolina at Chapel Hill, Chapel Hill, NC, USA

Amir Barzin Department of Family Medicine, University of North Carolina at Chapel Hill, Chapel Hill, NC, USA

Sylvia Becker-Dreps Department of Family Medicine, University of North Carolina at Chapel Hill, Chapel Hill, NC, USA

Victoria L. Boggiano Department of Family Medicine, University of North Carolina at Chapel Hill, School of Medicine, Chapel Hill, NC, USA

Collin Burks Division of Geriatrics, Duke University, Durham, NC, USA

Erik Butler Department of Family Medicine, University of North Carolina at Chapel Hill, Chapel Hill, NC, USA

M. Justin Byron Department of Family Medicine, University of North Carolina at Chapel Hill, Chapel Hill, NC, USA

Martha C. Carlough Department of Family Medicine, University of North Carolina at Chapel Hill, Chapel Hill, NC, USA

Maria Gabriela Castro Department of Family Medicine, University of North Carolina at Chapel Hill, Chapel Hill, NC, USA

Sandra Clark Department of Family Medicine, University of North Carolina at Chapel Hill, Chapel Hill, NC, USA

Department of Psychiatry, University of North Carolina at Chapel Hill, Chapel Hill, NC, USA

Catherine L. Coe Department of Family Medicine, University of North Carolina at Chapel Hill, Chapel Hill, NC, USA

Muchieh Coufal Peers for Progress, Department of Health Behavior, Gillings School of Global Public Health, University of North Carolina-Chapel Hill, Chapel Hill, NC, USA

Asian Center for Health Education, Plano, TX, USA

Timothy P. Daaleman Department of Family Medicine, University of North Carolina at Chapel Hill, School of Medicine, Chapel Hill, NC, USA

Jessica Waters Davis Department of Family Medicine, University of North Carolina at Chapel Hill, Chapel Hill, NC, USA

Department of Psychiatry, University of North Carolina at Chapel Hill, Chapel Hill, NC, USA

Amy C. Denham Department of Family Medicine, University of North Carolina at Chapel Hill School of Medicine, Chapel Hill, NC, USA

Clark Denniston, MD Department of Family Medicine, University of North Carolina at Chapel Hill, Chapel Hill, NC, USA

Katrina Donahue Department of Family Medicine, University of North Carolina at Chapel Hill, Chapel Hill, NC, USA

Catherine Ellis Departments of Family Medicine and Orthopedics, University of North Carolina at Chapel Hill, Chapel Hill, NC, USA

Megan Evans Department of Psychiatry, Yale University, New Haven, CT, USA

Kelly Bossenbroek Fedoriw Department of Family Medicine, University of North Carolina at Chapel Hill, Chapel Hill, NC, USA

Robert L. Ferrer Family and Community Medicine, UT Health San Antonio, San Antonio, TX, USA

Ryan M. Finn Rayus Radiology, Mayo Clinic and University of Minnesota, Minneapolis, MN, USA

Edwin B. Fisher Peers for Progress, Department of Health Behavior, Gillings School of Global Public Health, University of North Carolina at Chapel Hill, Chapel Hill, NC, USA

Erin Fraher Department of Family Medicine, University of North Carolina at Chapel Hill, Chapel Hill, NC, USA

Cecil G. Sheps Center for Health Services Research, University of North Carolina at Chapel Hill, Chapel Hill, USA

Bruce Fried Department of Health Policy and Management, University of North Carolina at Chapel Hill, Chapel Hill, NC, USA

Jacqueline MacDonald Gibson Department of Civil, Construction, and Environmental Engineering, North Carolina State University, Raleigh, USA

Adam O. Goldstein Lineberger Comprehensive Cancer Center, University of North Carolina Health Care System, Chapel Hill, NC, USA

Department of Family Medicine, University of North Carolina at Chapel Hill, Chapel Hill, NC, USA

Mark Gwynne Department of Family Medicine, University of North Carolina at Chapel Hill, Chapel Hill, NC, USA

Karen Halpert Department of Family Medicine, University of North Carolina at Chapel Hill, Chapel Hill, NC, USA

Emily M. Hawes Department of Family Medicine, University of North Carolina at Chapel Hill School of Medicine, Chapel Hill, NC, USA

University of North Carolina Eshelman School of Pharmacy, Chapel Hill, NC, USA

Sherry Shackelford Hay Department of Family Medicine, University of North Carolina at Chapel Hill, Chapel Hill, NC, USA

Alyssa Heinrich Department of Family Medicine, University of North Carolina at Chapel Hill, Chapel Hill, NC, USA

Margaret R. Helton Department of Family Medicine, University of North Carolina at Chapel Hill, Chapel Hill, NC, USA

J. Kevin Hicks Department of Individualized Cancer Management, Moffitt Cancer Center, Tampa, FL, USA

Marni Gwyther Holder Department of Family Medicine, University of North Carolina at Chapel Hill, Chapel Hill, NC, USA

Dana Iglesias Department of Family Medicine, University of North Carolina at Chapel Hill, Chapel Hill, NC, USA

LeRon Jackson Department of Family Medicine, University of North Carolina at Chapel Hill, Chapel Hill, NC, USA

Weiping Jia Shanghai Jiaotong University Affiliated Sixth People's Hospital and Shanghai Diabetes Institute, Shanghai, China

Shawn Kane Department of Family Medicine, University of North Carolina at Chapel Hill, Chapel Hill, NC, USA

Suranga N. Kasturi Black Dog Institute, University of New South Wales, Sydney, NSW, Australia

Center for Biomedical Informatics, Regenstrief Institute, Indianapolis, IN, USA

Min Kim Division of Infectious Diseases, Department of Medicine, University of North Carolina at Chapel Hill, Chapel Hill, NC, USA

Louise King, MD Department of Medicine, University of North Carolina, Chapel Hill, NC, USA

Christine E. Kistler Department of Family Medicine, University of North Carolina School of Medicine, Chapel Hill, NC, USA

Bogda Koczwara Flinders University and Flinders Medical Centre, Adelaide, SA, Australia

Rita Lahlou Department of Family Medicine, University of North Carolina at Chapel Hill, Chapel Hill, NC, USA

Yee Lam Department of Family Medicine, University of North Carolina at Chapel Hill, Chapel Hill, NC, USA

Justin Lee Department of Family Medicine, University of North Carolina at Chapel Hill, Chapel Hill, NC, USA

Yuexing Liu Shanghai Jiaotong University Affiliated Sixth People's Hospital and Shanghai Diabetes Institute, Shanghai, China

Brianna Lombardi Department of Family Medicine, University of North Carolina at Chapel Hill, Chapel Hill, NC, USA

Cecil G. Sheps Center for Health Services Research, University of North Carolina at Chapel Hill, Chapel Hill, USA

Samantha L. Luu Peers for Progress, Department of Health Behavior, Gillings School of Global Public Health, University of North Carolina at Chapel Hill, Chapel Hill, NC, USA

Alexa Mieses Malchuk Department of Family Medicine, University of North Carolina at Chapel Hill, Chapel Hill, NC, USA

Jennifer Martini Department of Family Medicine, University of North Carolina at Chapel Hill School of Medicine, Chapel Hill, NC, USA

Mallory McClester Brown Department of Family Medicine, University of North Carolina at Chapel Hill, Chapel Hill, NC, USA

Morgan A. McEachern Department of Family Medicine, University of North Carolina at Chapel Hill, Chapel Hill, NC, USA

Eneida A. Mendonca Division of Biomedical Informatics, Department of Pediatrics, Cincinnati Children's Hospital and University of Cincinnati, Cincinnati, OH, USA

Carlton Moore Department of Medicine, University of North Carolina at Chapel Hill, Chapel Hill, NC, USA

Modjulie Moore Department of Family Medicine, University of North Carolina at Chapel Hill, Chapel Hill, NC, USA

Richard Moore Department of Family Medicine, University of North Carolina at Chapel Hill, School of Medicine, Chapel Hill, NC, USA

Nailah Adams Morancie Department of Family Medicine, University of North Carolina at Chapel Hill, Chapel Hill, NC, USA

Mary Mulcare Weill Cornell Medical College, New York, NY, USA

Linda Myerholtz Department of Family Medicine, University of North Carolina at Chapel Hill, Chapel Hill, NC, USA

Dana Neutze Department of Family Medicine, University of North Carolina at Chapel Hill, Chapel Hill, NC, USA

Jonathan Oberlander Department of Social Medicine, University of North Carolina at Chapel Hill, Chapel Hill, NC, USA

Department of Health Policy and Management, University of North Carolina at Chapel Hill, Chapel Hill, NC, USA

Cristy Page University of North Carolina at Chapel Hill School of Medicine, Chapel Hill, NC, USA

Zachary J. Pettigrew Pediatric Teaching Program, Cone Health, Greensboro, NC, USA

Debbie Phipps Department of Family Medicine, University of North Carolina at Chapel Hill, Chapel Hill, NC, USA

Deborah S. Porterfield Gillings School of Global Public Health, University of North Carolina at Chapel Hill, Chapel Hill, NC, USA

Amy N. Prentice Department of Family Medicine, University of North Carolina at Chapel Hill, Chapel Hill, NC, USA

Vinay Reddy Department of Family Medicine, University of North Carolina at Chapel Hill, Chapel Hill, NC, USA

Ashley Rietz Department of Family Medicine, University of North Carolina School of Medicine, Chapel Hill, NC, USA

Michelle Del Rio Indiana University School of Public Health, Bloomington, IN, USA

Caroline Collins Roberts, MD Department of Family Medicine, University of North Carolina at Chapel Hill, Chapel Hill, NC, USA

Kimberly A. Sanders University of North Carolina Eshelman School of Pharmacy, Chapel Hill, NC, USA

University of North Carolina Adams School of Dentistry, Chapel Hill, NC, USA

Samantha Schilling Department of Pediatrics, University of North Carolina at Chapel Hill, Chapel Hill, NC, USA

Christina Shenvi University of North Carolina at Chapel Hill School of Medicine, Chapel Hill, NC, USA

Kimberly A. Shoenbill Department of Family Medicine, Program on Health and Clinical Informatics, University of North Carolina at Chapel Hill, Chapel Hill, NC, USA

Lineberger Comprehensive Cancer Center, University of North Carolina Health Care System, Chapel Hill, NC, USA

Pam Silberman Department of Health Policy and Management, Gillings School of Global Public Health, University of North Carolina at Chapel Hill, Chapel Hill, NC, USA

Rachel Sandler Silva Department of Medicine, Hennepin Healthcare, University of Minnesota, Minneapolis, MN, USA

Kelly Lacy Smith School of Medicine, University of North Carolina at Chapel Hill, Chapel Hill, NC, USA

Nathaniel A. Sowa Department of Psychiatry, University of North Carolina at Chapel Hill, Chapel Hill, NC, USA

Jenny T. van der Steen Department of Public Health and Primary Care, Leiden University Medical Center, Leiden, the Netherlands

Radboudumc Alzheimer Center and Department of Primary and Community Care, Radboud University Medical Center, Nijmegen, the Netherlands

Liza Straub Department of Family Medicine, University of North Carolina at Chapel Hill, Chapel Hill, NC, USA

Patrick Y. Tang Peers for Progress, Department of Health Behavior, Gillings School of Global Public Health, University of North Carolina at Chapel Hill, Chapel Hill, NC, USA

Alexandra Targan Department of Family Medicine, University of Michigan, Ann Arbor, MI, USA

Maria Thekkekandam Department of Family Medicine at Chapel Hill, University of North Carolina, Chapel Hill, NC, USA

Margaret C. Wang Office of the Chief Quality Officer, Stanford Health Care, Palo Alto, CA, USA

Ashley A. Weiner Lineberger Comprehensive Cancer Center, University of North Carolina Health Care System, Chapel Hill, NC, USA

Department of Radiation Oncology, University of North Carolina at Chapel Hill, Chapel Hill, NC, USA

Brian Wiggs Department of Family Medicine, University of North Carolina at Chapel Hill, Chapel Hill, NC, USA

Ciara Zachary Department of Health Policy and Management, Gillings School of Global Public Health, University of North Carolina at Chapel Hill, Chapel Hill, NC, USA

Matthew Zeitler Department of Family Medicine, University of North Carolina at Chapel Hill, Chapel Hill, NC, USA

Adam Zolotor Department of Family Medicine, University of North Carolina at Chapel Hill, Chapel Hill, NC, USA

Part I

Individual Influences on Chronic Illness

Genetic Contributions and Personalized Medicine

J. Kevin Hicks

Role of Genetics in Chronic Disease

There are multiple factors that contribute to the development of chronic disease including lifestyle behaviors, environmental exposure, social determinants, and in certain instances genetics. Genomic alterations may increase the risk of having a chronic disorder, and genetic susceptibility can be potentiated by lifestyle choices or social and environmental factors. For example, mutations in the lipid homeostasis genes *LDLR*, *APOB*, or *PCSK9* can result in familial hypercholesterolemia, thus enhancing the probability of premature cardiovascular disease, although individuals may remain asymptomatic [1, 2]. Harboring mutations in these lipid homeostasis genes concomitantly with tobacco use or obesity exacerbates the risk for cardiovascular disease [3].

For certain chronic conditions, such as cystic fibrosis, genetic polymorphisms alone can directly result in disease. An autosomal recessive genetic disorder, cystic fibrosis is caused by mutations in the cystic fibrosis transmembrane conductance regulator (*CFTR*) gene [4]. Because of advances in management and treatment, cystic fibrosis has transitioned from a disease associated with substantial childhood mortality to a chronic condition with a life expectancy of over 40 years [4]. Other examples of inherited genomic variations that can enhance the risk for chronic disease include familial cardiomyopathy (e.g., mutations in heart muscle genes such as *TNNI3*, *TNNT2*, *MYH7*), inherited neuropathies (e.g., mutations in myelin genes such as *PMP22*, *EGR2*), Alzheimer's disease (e.g., mutations in genes associated with amyloid plaques such as *APOE ε4*), and cancer (e.g., mutations in genomic stability genes such as *BRCA1*, *BRCA2*, *MSH6*) [5–8].

In addition to contributing to the development of chronic disorders, genetic polymorphisms influence the response to pharmacological treatment. Patients with a single chronic disease are likely to take at least one maintenance medication, whereas those with multiple chronic conditions may be treated with 10 or more drugs [9, 10]. Within a population diagnosed with the same chronic disease and prescribed similar medications, the response to a particular drug or occurrence of an adverse drug reaction may vary greatly among individuals. Inter-individual differences in pharmacotherapy response have been attributed to genomic alterations encoding proteins affecting the pharmacokinetics (i.e., metabolism or transport) or pharmacodynamics (i.e., target) of a drug [11–13]. The *CFTR* gene, which encodes for a chloride channel that is a vital regulator of ion and fluid transport, is an example of how polymorphisms influence drug response [4]. Over 1900 *CFTR* mutations have been observed that can have deleterious effects such as disruption of biosynthesis or folding and trafficking of the CFTR protein, along with mutations that cause the ion gate to be in a mostly closed position [14]. Ivacaftor is a drug that increases the likelihood of the ion gate being in an open configuration. Thus, within a population of cystic fibrosis patients only those harboring mutations (e.g., *CFTR G551D*) that affect ion channel gating would benefit from taking ivacaftor [14]. Dependent on the drug and associated polymorphism, approximately 20–95% of observed variability in drug response can be attributed to inheritance [11, 12].

Adverse drug reactions and non-response to pharmacotherapy are major causes of morbidity and mortality. Serious or fatal adverse drug reactions are estimated to affect millions of patients each year and are thought to be a leading cause of death in the US [15, 16]. For individuals with a chronic condition requiring multiple medications, there is a greater probability for an adverse drug event. Understanding associations between genomic variation and drug effectiveness, and identifying polymorphisms predictive of adverse drug risk, has the potential to decrease morbidity and mortality caused by gene–drug interactions [17].

Pharmacogenetics is the study of how genetic variants influence drug response and was first described in the 1950s regarding observed inter-individual differences in drug

J. K. Hicks (✉)
Department of Individualized Cancer Management, Moffitt Cancer Center, Tampa, FL, USA
e-mail: james.hicks@moffitt.org; James.Hicks@moffit.org

metabolism [18–20]. Single nucleotide polymorphisms (SNPs) are the most commonly observed genetic variants that affect drug response. SNPs can cause loss of protein function or, if located in the promoter region, can influence gene expression [21–23]. Over 40 million SNPs were identified in the initial sequencing of the human genome and it is estimated that one SNP occurs in every 600 DNA base pairs [24, 25]. Other genetic variants that influence drug response include DNA base pair insertions or deletions (indels), short DNA sequence repeats, and copy number variation (i.e., gain or loss of a gene) [26, 27]. The term allele is used to describe the SNPs or other genetic variants harbored within a gene. Dependent on how genetic variants affect protein function, a phenotype can be assigned based on an individual's diplotype (i.e., summary of the inherited maternal and paternal allele). In the context of drug metabolizing enzymes, a predicted phenotype may be ultra-rapid, rapid, normal, intermediate, or poor metabolizer [28]. In most instances, phenotypes at the extremes of the drug metabolic continuum have the greatest potential to affect pharmacotherapy outcomes.

For many chronic conditions, there are numerous pharmacotherapies for treatment. Therapeutic options to treat major depressive disorder, for example, include tricyclic antidepressants, selective serotonin reuptake inhibitors, and serotonin norepinephrine reuptake inhibitors. Even when adhering to current guidelines and best practices, multiple treatment strategies exist [29, 30]. Each drug has its own unique side effect profile, and dependent on an individual's genetic profile, the risk for an adverse event may be greater for some drugs than others. Utilizing pharmacogenetic results in a similar manner to kidney or liver function tests, rational drug prescribing strategies can be established to allow for the selection of a drug with lower potential for an adverse event among the many drugs that would be a suitable treatment option. For certain gene–drug pairs the evidence demonstrating an association between polymorphisms and drug response is sufficiently strong to warrant clinical implementation [31–33]. This chapter provides an overview of genetics in clinical care across the continuum of chronic disease including screening, prevention strategies in genetically susceptible populations, and treatment strategies (Fig. 1.1).

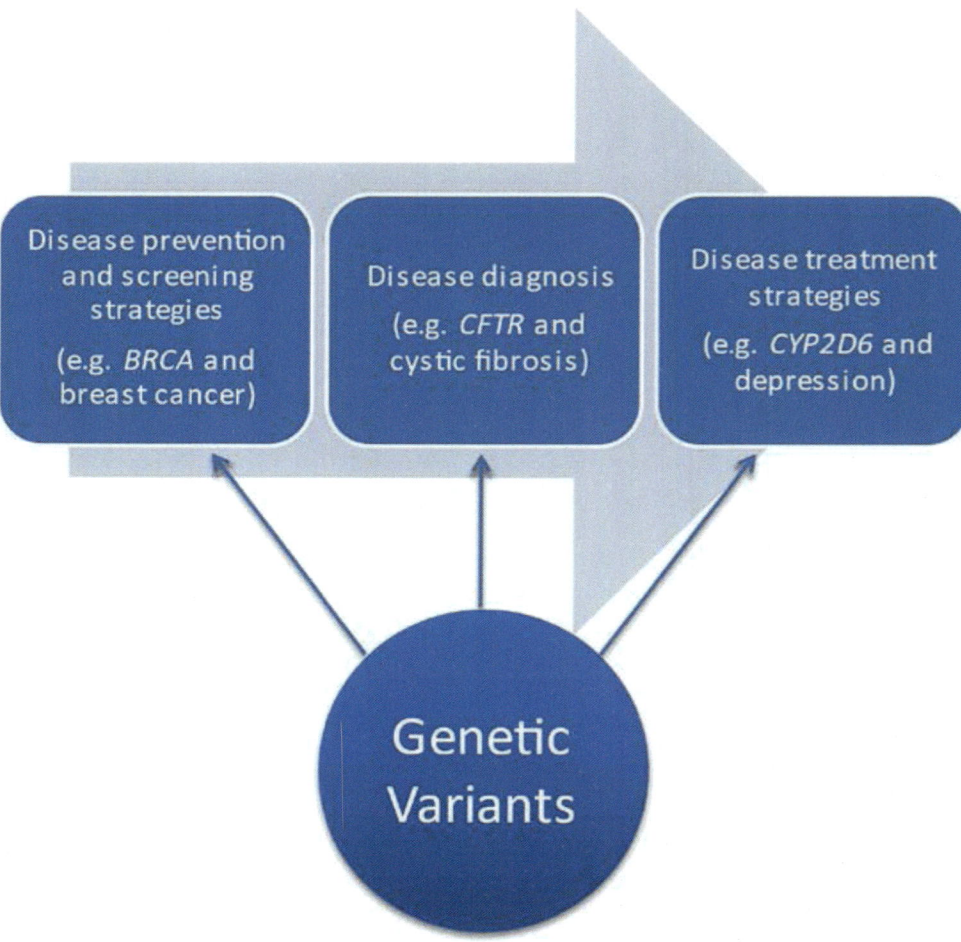

Fig. 1.1 Applications of genomic medicine in chronic disease

Gene–Drug Considerations for Chronic Disease

Substantial evidence supports linkages between genetic variation and chronic disease, and associations between genetic polymorphisms and response to pharmacotherapies. This section highlights several gene–drug pairs that are currently considered in clinical settings or have the potential for adoption in coming years.

Autoimmune Disorders

Multiple chronic autoimmune diseases, including rheumatoid arthritis, lupus, and inflammatory bowel diseases, can be pharmacologically managed with the thiopurine drug class. Azathioprine and mercaptopurine are relatively inexpensive drugs and are often prescribed before initiation of tumor necrosis factor-α inhibitors. Thiopurine methyltransferase (TPMT) degrades azathioprine and mercaptopurine to compounds with less pharmacological activity [34, 35]. In the absence of TPMT activity, thiopurines are converted at a greater rate than expected to thioguanine nucleotides, which at high concentrations can cause bone marrow toxicity. Those who inherit 1 non-functional *TPMT* allele (intermediate metabolizers) are at an increased risk of myelosuppression whereas those who inherit two non-functional *TPMT* alleles (poor metabolizers) are at very high risk of myelosuppression if prescribed standard doses of thiopurines due to high thioguanine nucleotide concentrations. For TPMT intermediate metabolizers, it is recommended to decrease the initial dose of azathioprine or mercaptopurine by 30–60% and then titrate the dose based on response [36, 37]. The azathioprine or mercaptopurine dose should be reduced by 90% and administered three times per week instead of daily for TPMT poor metabolizers [36, 37].

Cancer

Cancer susceptibility and drug response can be influenced by both germline variations and somatic mutations. Germline polymorphisms are inherited from maternal and paternal alleles, where somatic mutations are not inherited but rather acquired after conception. Inheritance of *BRCA1* or *BRCA2* variations increases the risk for certain types of cancer; however, those with *BRCA1/BRCA2* variations are more likely to respond to the poly(ADP-ribose) polymerase inhibitors such as olaparib [38–40]. Likewise, inheritance of *MSH6* polymorphisms increases the risk of Lynch syndrome (also known as hereditary nonpolyposis colorectal cancer) where immunotherapy may be a treatment option [41]. Treatment regimens for hematologic malignancies such as acute lymphocytic leukemia include mercaptopurine. Dosing strategies for TPMT intermediate and poor metabolizers are the same as the dosing strategies described for autoimmune diseases [36, 37]. Dihydropyrimidine dehydrogenase, encoded by the *DPYD* gene, is responsible for the elimination of the chemotherapeutic drug 5-fluorouracil [42]. In rare instances, an individual may inherit two non-functional *DPYD* alleles and if exposed to 5-fluorouracil can experience severe or even fatal toxicities [43, 44]. DPYD poor metabolizers should avoid 5-fluorouracil, whereas a 50% dose reduction should be considered for intermediate metabolizers [43–45].

Interrogating tumor biopsies for somatic mutations is becoming increasingly common, and for some cancers (e.g., advanced lung cancer) somatic testing is considered standard practice. For example, epidermal growth factor receptor (*EGFR*) mutations drive the selection of EGFR-tyrosine kinase inhibitors (TKI) that are used to treat lung cancer patients [46, 47]. *EGFR* exon 19 deletions can be targeted by EGFR-TKIs such as erlotinib, whereas EGFR^{T790M} mutations are resistant to first- and second-generation TKIs but susceptible to the third-generation EGFR-TKI osimertinib. The FLAURA trial showed that osimertinib has superior efficacy for certain EGFR mutations (e.g., EGFR^{L858R} and *EGFR* exon 19 deletions) and is now considered frontline therapy for metastatic lung cancer harboring those particular EGFR mutations [48]. Precision oncology is revolutionizing the treatment of cancer as many of the targeted therapies can be taken orally, have less severe side effects than the older chemotherapeutic agents, and may be more effective. Numerous targeted anti-cancer agents that have specific mutations listed in the Indications and Usage section of the package label are now entering the drug market (Table 1.1). As clinical trials enroll patients based on the presence of specific somatic mutations and independent of tumor histology, the number of approved anti-cancer agents targeting specific somatic mutations is predicted to grow [49].

Infectious Diseases

Although there is currently no cure for the human immunodeficiency virus (HIV), antiretroviral therapy has drastically increased survival, with studies suggesting that the life expectancy of HIV-infected individuals may be comparable to the general population [50–52]. Early initiation of antiretroviral therapy along with medication compliance is essential for viral suppression and improved outcomes. Antiviral agents, though, can induce serious and sometimes life-threatening side effects that disrupt therapy or compromise compliance. Abacavir is a nucleoside-analogue reverse-transcriptase inhibitor with potent antiviral activity and is a component of numerous combination therapies. Approximately 6% of individuals exposed to abacavir will experience a hypersensitivity reaction that in rare instances can be fatal [53, 54].

Table 1.1 Examples of anti-cancer agents that target specific somatic mutations

Drug	Genomic variant
Ado-Trastuzumab emtansine	*ERBB2* gene amplification
Afatinib	*EGFR* exon 19 deletion EGFR^{L858R}
Alectinib	*ALK* fusion
Alpelisib	*PIK3CA* mutations
Amivantamab	*EGFR* exon 20 insertion
Brigatinib	*ALK* fusion
Bosutinib	*BCR-ABL1* fusion
Capmatinib	*MET* exon 14 skipping
Ceritinib	*ALK* fusion
Cetuximab	*EGFR* gene amplification
Cobimetinib	BRAF^{V600E} BRAF^{V600K}
Crizotinib	*ALK* fusion, *ROS1* fusion
Dabrafenib	BRAF^{V600E}
Entrectinib	*NTRK* fusion, *ROS1* fusion
Erlotinib	*EGFR* exon 19 deletion EGFR^{L858R}
Fam-trastuzumab deruxtecan-nxki	*ERBB2* mutations
Gefitinib	*EGFR* exon 19 deletion EGFR^{L858R}
Imatinib	*BCR-ABL1* fusion
Lapatinib	*ERBB2* gene amplification
Larotrectinib	*NTRK* fusion
Lorlatinib	*ALK* fusion
Mobocertinib	*EGFR* exon 20 insertion
Nilotinib	*BCR-ABL1* fusion
Olaparib	*BRCA1* deleterious mutations *BRCA2* deleterious mutations
Osimertinib	*EGFR* mutations
Pertuzumab	*ERBB2* gene amplification
Pralsetinib	*RET* fusion
Selpercatinib	*RET* fusion
Sotorasib	KRAS^{G12C}
Tepotinib	*MET* exon 14 skipping
Trametinib	BRAF^{V600E} BRAF^{V600K}
Trastuzumab	*ERBB2* gene amplification
Vemurafenib	BRAF^{V600E}

Human leukocyte antigen B (HLA-B) is a member of the major histocompatibility complex and has a role in immune response including drug-induced immune reactions. Although the mechanism of action is poorly understood, it is hypothesized that HLAs recognize drugs as foreign (non-self) and present drug–peptide complexes to the immune system inducing a hypersensitivity reaction [55]. The *HLA-B*57:01* allele has been demonstrated to be predictive of abacavir-induced hypersensitivity reactions [56–58]. A prospective, randomized, double-blind study investigating the use of genomics to guide abacavir prescribing found that preemptive *HLA-B*57:01* screening significantly reduced the incidence of hypersensitivity reactions (3.4% genotyping group versus 7.8% control group, $p<0.001$) [59]. The Food and Drug Administration (FDA) placed a warning in the drug package insert stating that patients should be screened for *HLA-B*57:01* before being prescribed abacavir.

Atazanavir is a protease inhibitor that is concomitantly prescribed with other antiretrovirals as part of HIV treatment [60, 61]. A side effect of atazanavir is hyperbilirubinemia due to inhibition of uridine diphosphate glucuronosyltransferase (UGT) 1A1. UGT1A1 converts bilirubin into a water-soluble conjugated form that can be eliminated from the body. DNA sequence repeats in the *UGT1A1* promoter region, such as *UGT1A1*28* defined by an extra TA, causes a reduction in protein expression resulting in Gilbert's syndrome [23, 62]. Carriers of *UGT1A1*28* who are prescribed atazanavir have a higher treatment discontinuation rate due to hyperbilirubinemia that can cause discoloration of the skin and eyes [63, 64]. Incorporating preemptive genotyping of *HLA-B*57:01* and *UGT1A1* into HIV antiretroviral treatment algorithms could assist with identifying those at increased risk of hypersensitivity reactions or premature discontinuation and further guide drug prescribing strategies [54, 59, 65, 66].

Chronic hepatitis C infection is a major cause of liver disease including cirrhosis and hepatocellular carcinoma [67, 68]. Pegylated interferon-α concomitantly with ribavirin is an effective treatment as measured by sustained virological response—defined as absence of viremia 24 weeks after treatment—and is associated with decreased morbidity and mortality [69]. Approximately 30–45% of patients will not achieve a sustained virological response when treated with pegylated interferon-α/ribavirin [69–72]. Because therapy lasts up to 48 weeks and causes multiple adverse effects that can be severe, identifying those less likely to respond could assist in clinical decision making. A genome wide association study in 1,137 hepatitis C patients discovered that a SNP in *IFNL3* (also known as *IL28B*) was predictive of an unfavorable response to interferon-α based therapy [72]. Those with an unfavorable genotype had an approximately 30% chance for a sustained virological response with attainment of response doubling to 60% if a protease inhibitor was added to the pegylated interferon-α/ribavirin regimen [73]. Individuals with a favorable genotype are eligible for shortened therapy (24–28 weeks versus 48 weeks) [73]. *IFNL3* genotyping has been integrated into clinical practice; though newer more effective antiviral therapeutic regimens (e.g., ledipasvir/sofosbuvir) are lessening the clinical use of *IFNL3* for guiding hepatitis C treatment decisions.

Invasive fungal infections are more commonly observed in chronic diseases that involve immune defense mechanisms, such as HIV and cystic fibrosis [74]. Medications that treat autoimmune disorders or cancer can weaken the immune system and often require antifungal prophylaxis. Voriconazole is an antifungal agent that is considered a first line treatment for aspergillosis [75]. Voriconazole has a narrow therapeutic range (1–6 mcg/mL) with sub-therapeutic plasma concentrations associated with progressive fungal infections and poor outcomes [76, 77]. CYP2C19 metabolizes voriconazole to compounds with less anti-fungal activity. Approximately 25% of the population carries a SNP (c.-806C>T) in the *CYP2C19* gene promoter region, referred to as *CYP2C19*17*, that causes upregulation of gene expression and increased metabolic capacity [22, 78]. *CYP2C19*17* carriers metabolize voriconazole to a greater extent than normal metabolizers resulting in lower drug plasma concentrations and increased risk of progressive fungal infections [76, 79, 80]. *CYP2C19* genotyping in populations at risk of a fungal infection has the potential to identify those requiring higher initial voriconazole doses or those who may benefit from selection of an antifungal agent not metabolized by CYP2C19 [81, 82].

Psychiatric and Neurologic Conditions

Major depressive disorder is a leading cause of disease burden and may emerge as the most prevalent disease in developed countries [83, 84]. Depression may be considered a chronic disorder itself, or can be a comorbidity due to another chronic disease such as cancer, chronic obstructive pulmonary disease or congestive heart failure [85]. Approximately 30–50% of patients fail initial therapy due to intolerance or ineffectiveness, and it is estimated that antidepressant-induced adverse events result in over 25,000 emergency department visits per year in the US [86–88]. The majority of antidepressants are metabolized by polymorphic cytochrome P450 enzymes including CYP2D6 and CYP2C19. There is a substantial body of evidence demonstrating an association between *CYP2D6* or *CYP2C19* polymorphisms and pharmacokinetic parameters along with treatment outcomes for the selective serotonin reuptake inhibitors (SSRIs) and tricyclic antidepressants (TCAs) [89–91]. Initial clinical implementation studies showed that using pharmacogenomic testing to guide drug prescribing in patients with depression resulted in better response rates and was cost effective when compared to those who were not genotyped, although further studies are needed to support these findings [92–95]. Due to high initial pharmacotherapy failure rates and no single drug demonstrating unequivocal efficacy, pharmacogenomic testing has the potential to become part of routine care for those with depression to assist with drug prescribing strategies [96, 97].

CYP2D6 and *CYP2C19* gene-based dosing guidelines are available for the SSRIs and TCAs [89–91]. CYP2D6 ultra-rapid metabolizers are at risk of therapeutic failure due to low drug plasma concentrations, and it is recommended to prescribe an SSRI or TCA that is not metabolized by the CYP2D6 enzyme for those patients. CYP2D6 poor metabolizers have an increased risk of adverse drug effects due to elevated drug plasma concentrations. An initial 50% dose reduction of SSRIs and TCAs is recommended with titration to response. For the SSRI and TCA drugs metabolized by CYP2C19, similar recommendations exist for CYP2C19 ultra-rapid or poor metabolizers [89, 90]. There are currently limited gene-based guidelines for other antidepressants that are metabolized by CYP2D6 or CYP2C19, though guidelines are likely to be developed [98]. In addition to drug metabolizing enzymes, there is a growing body of literature suggesting that polymorphisms in serotonin receptors and transporters may influence antidepressant response [99, 100].

Drugs metabolized by CYP2C19 and CYP2D6 that treat chronic neurologic disorders include clobazam, cholinesterase inhibitors, and tetrabenazine. Clobazam is used to treat Lennox-Gastaut syndrome, which requires life-long therapeutic management of seizures. CYP2C19 poor metabolizers have a 3–5 times higher exposer to the metabolite n-desmethylclobazam, which is thought to be associated with an elevated risk of side effects [101]. Although the clinical utility of *CYP2C19* genotyping to dose clobazam is evolving, the FDA approved drug insert suggests that for adult CYP2C19 poor metabolizers the initial dose should be reduced by 50% and titrated carefully based on clinical response. Cholinesterase inhibitors (e.g., donepezil and galantamine) are used to treat Alzheimer's disease. Both donepezil and galantamine are metabolized by CYP2D6, but currently there are no strong correlations between *CYP2D6* genotype and drug response [102]. CYP2D6 poor metabolizers may have a greater exposure to galantamine than normal metabolizers per the drug package insert, and care should be taken during dose titration. Chorea associated with Huntington's disease can be treated with tetrabenazine. Limited evidence suggests that those who are CYP2D6 poor metabolizers may be more likely to experience tetrabenazine-induce side effects such as suicidality, particularly at higher doses [103]. The drug insert recommends *CYP2D6* genotyping before titrating to higher doses, and for those who are CYP2D6 poor metabolizers limiting the maximum single dose to 25 mg and maximum daily dose to 50 mg.

Carbamazepine can be utilized for the management of many chronic conditions including seizures, nerve pain such as trigeminal neuralgia or diabetic neuropathy, migraine prophylaxis, and other neurological disorders. Severe side effects such as Stevens-Johnson syndrome and toxic epidermal necrolysis can be caused by carbamazepine, and is fatal in up to 30% of individuals diagnosed with these cutaneous adverse events. A small study consisting of 44 patients with pathology proven Stevens-Johnson syndrome found that all patients were positive for the *HLA-B*15:02* allele [104]. Subsequent studies confirmed this finding and suggested that those who carry the *HLA-B*15:02* allele are approximately

100-fold more likely to develop carbamazepine-induced Stevens-Johnson syndrome/toxic epidermal necrolysis; though the occurrence of this side effect is low with a positive predictive value of about 8% [105]. A prospective study consisting of 4335 individuals found that *HLA-B*15:02* preemptive genotyping completely prevented Stevens-Johnson syndrome/toxic epidermal necrolysis in the study population by prescribing alternative medications to those positive for the *HLA-B*15:02* allele [106]. The FDA placed a warning in the drug package insert stating that particular patient populations should be screened for *HLA-B*15:02* before prescribing carbamazepine.

Chronic Pain

One in three individuals in the US is reported to suffer from chronic pain [107]. Genomic alterations in genes encoding proteins involved in pain perception (e.g., *COMT*) along with the metabolism (e.g., *CYP2D6*), transport (e.g., *ABCB1*), and targets (e.g., *OPRM1*) of pain treatment drugs can affect treatment response [108]. One investigation suggested that two-thirds of observed inter-individual variability to morphine response may be due to genetic variation [109]. Catechol-O-methyltransferase (COMT) is an important regulator of dopamine, epinephrine, and norepinephrine in the pain perception pathway [110]. Four SNPs in *COMT* have been proposed to influence pain perception, and dependent on how many SNPs an individual harbors, the sensitivity to pain can be predicted as low, average, or high [111–113]. At the time of this chapter being published, there was limited clinical data supporting the use of *COMT* genotypes to guide opioid therapy [114].

Chronic pain treatment will vary based on the type of pain (e.g., neuropathic pain, nociceptive pain) and severity. Tricyclic antidepressants, typically at low doses, can be used to treat neuropathic pain. CYP2D6 ultra-rapid metabolizers have an increased risk of drugs such as amitriptyline not being effective due to faster than expected metabolism that can lead to low or undetectable drug plasma concentrations [90, 91]. Dose adjustments may not be needed for CYP2D6 poor metabolizers, as the typically lower amitriptyline doses may not place a patient at risk of side effects due to high drug concentrations. If higher doses of tricyclics are used for treating neuropathic pain, gene-based dosing strategies can be considered. Nonsteroidal anti-inflammatory drugs (NSAIDs) may be used for chronic pain conditions such as arthritis. The NSAID celecoxib is metabolized by the polymorphic P450 drug metabolizing enzyme CYP2C9. Two *CYP2C9* variants that cause decreased enzyme function, *CYP2C*2* and *CYP2C9*3*, are associated with a longer elimination half-life of celecoxib [115]. The FDA package insert for celecoxib suggests a 50% dose reduction for known CYP2C9 poor metabolizers. The Clinical Pharmacogenetics Implementation Consortium published a guideline for adjusting NSAID therapy based on *CYP2C9* genotype [116].

Opioids may be prescribed for chronic pain. Codeine is a prodrug that is converted to the more active compound morphine by CYP2D6. Multiple deaths have been reported in children who were prescribed normal doses of codeine [117]. It was later recognized that these children were CYP2D6 ultra-rapid metabolizers and converted codeine to morphine to a greater extent than normal metabolizers, likely resulting in a morphine overdose. Other pain medications metabolized by CYP2D6 include tramadol, hydrocodone, and oxycodone. For CYP2D6 ultra-rapid metabolizers, a pain medication not metabolized by CYP2D6 should be considered [114, 118]. Because CYP2D6 converts these medications to more active compounds, those who are CYP2D6 poor metabolizers are less likely to benefit from tramadol, codeine, hydrocodone, and oxycodone [114, 118]. Opioids target the μ-opioid receptor, OPRM1. Polymorphisms in *OPRM1*, such as *OPRM1 A118G*, have been associated with the need for higher opioid doses [119, 120]. Research is ongoing to determine the potential for utilizing *OPRM1* genetic variants to predict opioid doses that may better treat pain. Currently there is limited clinical data supporting the use of *OPRM1* genotypes to guide opioid therapy [114].

Cardiovascular Disease

Cardiovascular disease is a leading cause of morbidity and mortality and accounts for approximately one in three deaths in the US [121]. Hypertension is a major risk factor for cardiovascular disease, with genetic polymorphisms influencing the response to anti-hypertensive agents. Results from the Veterans Affairs Cooperative Studies revealed that patients with Northern European ancestry responded better to angiotensin-converting enzyme inhibitors and β-blockers while patients with West African ancestry responded better to calcium-channel blockers and diuretics [122–124]. This observed difference is thought to be due to polymorphisms in genes affecting plasma renin activity [125]. Polymorphisms in *NEDD4L* are associated with sodium retention, hypertension, and greater blood pressure and lower response to thiazide diuretics [126–128]. Two variants in *ADRB1*, rs1801252 and rs1801253, are associated with a decreased response to β-blockers [129–131]. However, there are currently limited practical applications of hypertension pharmacogenomics with enough validity to be implemented in clinical practice. This may be due to the relatively low effect size of each individual variant, with combinatorial gene studies and polygenic risk scores needed to create a large enough effect size to achieve genetically guided antihypertension treatments.

Dyslipidemia is a modifiable risk factor for cardiovascular disease. Familial hypercholesterolemia (FH) is an inherited dyslipidemia characterized by high low density lipoprotein (LDL) concentrations [132]. Familial hypercholesterolemia is an autosomal dominant disorder with variants in *LDLR* accounting for 79% of FH cases followed by variants in *ApoB*, *PCSK9*, and *LDLRAP1* [3]. About 15% of cases are either polygenic or have an unknown genetic cause. Like other forms of dyslipidemia, statins are a mainstay of treatment. Patients treated with statins and carrying variants in *HMGCR* and *LDLR* have smaller reductions in LDL level than non-carriers [133]. The *SLCO1B1* variant rs4149056 has been shown to attenuate the LDL lowering effects of rosuvastatin, pravastatin, and simvastatin [134–136]. This *SLCO1B1* variant encodes for a reduced function hepatic uptake transporter. Additionally, this variant has been associated with increased myopathies for patients treated with simvastatin [137]. There are dosing guidelines for simvastatin and *SLCO1B1* [138, 139].

Antiplatelet therapy with aspirin, clopidogrel, prasugrel, or ticagrelor is indicated to prevent ischemic events following acute coronary syndrome (ACS) and percutaneous coronary intervention. Clopidogrel is metabolized in the liver by several cytochrome P450 enzymes including CYP2C19 to its active form which irreversibly inhibits platelet activation and aggregation. CYP2C19 poor metabolizers are at an increased risk of therapeutic failure due to non-activation of clopidogrel. A meta-analysis found patients who have the *CYP2C19*2* variant are at an increased risk of major adverse cardiovascular events and stent thrombosis compared to wild-type patients, hazard ratio 1.55 and 2.67 for heterozygotes and 1.76 and 3.97 for homozygotes respectfully. This effect is strongest in high-risk ACS patients. Dosing guidelines are available for clopidogrel and *CYP2C19* [140, 141].

Anticoagulation therapy is a standard of most atrial fibrillation treatment. Warfarin is the historical drug of choice and is metabolized mainly by CYP2C9. The *CYP2C9*2* and **3* variants are associated with lower warfarin dose requirement and an increased risk of bleeding in European ancestry [142, 143]. These variants are less prevalent in those of African ancestry; *CYP2C9*5*, **8*, and **11* are more commonly observed [144, 145]. VKORC1 is the rate-limiting enzyme of vitamin K and variants in the promoter region of *VKORC1* affect warfarin dosing requirements [146]. The FDA package labeling contains dosing recommendations for warfarin using a combination of *CYP2C9* and *VKORC1*. The Clinical Pharmacogenetics Implementation Consortium published a guideline for adjusting warfarin therapy based on *CYP2C9* and *VKORC1* genotype [145]. Two randomized controlled trials evaluated the clinical benefit of genetically guided warfarin dosing, the EU-PACT and COAG trials [147], and had conflicting results. The EU-PACT trial, which had a greater than 90% white population, reported better outcomes from the genetically guided warfarin dosing arm. The COAG trial, which had a more than 20% black study population, found no difference between a clinical dosing algorithm and genetically guided warfarin dosing. It should be noted that neither trial genotyped patients for *CYP2C9*5*, **6*, **8*, or **11*, which may improve dosing prediction particularly in African Americans [140].

Diabetes Mellitus

Diabetes mellitus is a major worldwide health problem. There are two major subgroups of diabetes: Type-1 (autoimmune) and Type-2 (non-autoimmune). Diabetes occurs when genetic predisposition collides with environmental and lifestyle factors [148]. Genetic associations with occurrence and treatment of diabetes is an area of intense research; however, few findings, especially related to genotype-guided treatment, have progressed to clinical practice. Type-1 diabetes is estimated to have 80% heritability [149]. Variants in multiple genes have been linked to autoimmune diabetes: *HLA*, *INS*, *CTLA4*, *PTPN22*, *PTPN2*, *IL2RA*, *IFIH1*, *CAPSLIL7R*, and *CLEC16A* [150]. Type-2 diabetes is estimated to have 26–73% heritability [151]. More than 100 loci are associated with non-autoimmune diabetes [111, 152, 153].

No genetic variants have been found to be associated with treatment response to insulin. Metformin, a first line agent to treat Type-2 diabetes, has been studied in-depth for genetic links to response. The pharmacokinetics of metformin are affected by variants in *SLC22A1* and *SLC47A1*; however, no consistent effect on clinical outcomes has been found [154–157]. Sulfonylureas are inactivated by CYP2C9. Patients with *CYP2C9* reduced function variants (**2* and **3*) are consistently observed to have greater glycemic response than those who do not carry these variants [157]. Two forms of Type-2 diabetes are caused by variations in single genes and are highly sensitive to sulfonylureas: maturity-onset diabetes of the young (*HNF1A*) and neonatal diabetes mellitus (*KCNJ11* or *ABCC8*) [158, 159].

Implementation of Personalized Medicine

Identifying those with genetic susceptibility to chronic conditions can promote prevention including education about lifestyle changes and individualized plans for disease screening [160, 161]. For those diagnosed with a chronic disorder, integrating pharmacogenomics into clinical practice can guide medication prescribing strategies by identifying gene–drug interactions predictive of poor response. Although it has been recognized for decades that genetic variants are associated with chronic disease development and pharmacotherapy outcomes, genomic medicine is only in the early stages of implementation in clinical practice. Changes in health care delivery is one of the factors contributing to the growing interest in genomic medicine implementation. Reimbursement for medical services is transitioning away from a volume incentive model to a value-based model that takes into account both costs and outcomes [162]. In value-based health care, utilizing genetic testing to identify at-risk patient populations that lead to preventative measures may translate into better care and lower costs. Furthermore, advances in technology have led to decreasing genotyping costs that make genomic medicine financially feasible. The adoption of electronic health records, incentivized by the 2009 American Recovery and Reinvestment Act, facilitates the curation of genomic information and dissemination of clinical decision support at the point of computerized drug order entry [163]. Besides family health history that be used as a tool to detect familial syndromes, pharmacogenomics has been integrated into routine clinical practice to a greater extent than other areas of genomic medicine. Lessons learned from pharmacogenomic implementation can be extrapolated to other areas of genomic medicine.

Barriers to Implementation

Pharmacogenomic data has potential for informing clinical care across the lifespan of a patient. It is not practical for clinicians to remember the genetic variants of their patients, the associated phenotype, and associated gene-based dosing recommendations. Electronic health records (EHRs) can be utilized to discretely curate important genomic information and provide clinical decision support associated with gene–drug interactions [164, 165]. Most EHR systems are not optimized to store and present genomic data in meaningful ways for clinicians. In many instances, genetic test results are scanned into the EHR as a PDF or entered as unstructured data and organized in a time-dependent manner. Locating a particular genetic result often requires a cumbersome search strategy. Ideally, genetic test results should be discretely summarized in an easily accessed section of the EHR and organized in a time-independent manner so results can be readily displayed.

The greatest barrier for integrating genomic results into the EHR may be the lack of machine-readable codes to discretely convey information. Logical Observation Identifiers Names and Codes (LOINC) or Systematized Nomenclature of Medicine terminology allows for discrete transmission of results between a reference laboratory and EHR software. There are currently few standardized LOINC or SNOMED genomic terms that enable discrete transmission of results [28]. Without discrete entry of results, datamining the EHR for pharmacogenomic data is difficult and prevents translation to clinical decision support tools [166]. There are multiple national groups that are working on optimization efforts

and development of best practices for integrating genomics into the EHR, including the Electronic Medical Records and Genomics (eMERGE) network, Implementing Genomics in Practice (IGNITE) network, and the Displaying and Integrating Genetic Information Through the EHR Action Collaborative [167–169]. Other potential barriers for implementation include paucity of third-party reimbursement for genomic testing or clinical services, knowledge deficiency regarding what to do clinically with test results, and integration of genetic testing and distribution of pharmacogenomic knowledge in a manner that complements existing clinical workflows [170].

Pharmacogenomic Implementation Tools

The Clinical Pharmacogenetics Implementation Consortium (CPIC), a collaboration between the Pharmacogenomics Knowledgebase and the Pharmacogenomics Research Network, publishes peer-reviewed gene-based dosing guidelines that can be found at www.cpicpgx.org [31]. Guidelines for over 40 gene–drug pairs have been published, with the number of unique gene–drug pair dosing guidelines growing

Table 1.2 CPIC gene–drug pair guidelines

Specialty	Gene	Drug
Cardiology	CYP2C19	Clopidogrel
	SLCO1B1	Simvastatin
	CYP2C9/ VKORC1	Warfarin
Infectious disease	CYP2C19	Voriconazole
	CYP2B6	Efavirenz
	IFNL3	Peginterferon
	MT-RNR1	Aminoglycosides
	UGT1A1	Atazanavir
	HLA-B	Abacavir
Oncology	G6PD	Rasburicase
	DPYD	Capecitabine, fluorouracil, tegafur
Pain	CYP2C9	NSAIDS
	CYP2D6	Opioids
Psychiatry	CYP2C19/ CYP2D6	Amitriptyline, clomipramine, doxepin, imipramine, trimipramine
	CYP2C19	Citalopram, escitalopram, sertraline,
	CYP2D6	Desipramine, fluvoxamine, nortriptyline, paroxetine
Other	CYP2C19	Proton pump inhibitors
	CFTR	Ivacaftor
	CYP2C9/ HLA-B	Phenytoin
	CYP3A5	Tacrolimus
	TPMT/ NUDT15	Azathioprine, mercaptopurine, thioguanine
	HLA-B	Allopurinol
	HLA-B	Carbamazepine

every year (Table 1.2). These guidelines do not inform clinicians if a test should be performed, but rather how to apply the results to patient care. Every CPIC guideline has available a comprehensive pharmacogenenetic translation table that links all possible diplotypes to a phenotype, priority notation (i.e., actionable or non-actionable result), and interpretation language [165]. Over 100 drugs have pharmacogenetic information in the FDA package insert, and for certain drugs specific gene-based prescribing recommendations are provided. Another resource for gene-based dosing recommendations is the Dutch Pharmacogenetics Working Group [171].

Although commercial gene–drug interaction software is expanding, most early pharmacogenomic adopters have created local solutions for EHR clinical decision support. The CPIC Informatics Working Group provides examples of EHR agnostic clinical decision support tools that complement each CPIC guideline [172]. The eMERGE and IGNITE networks recently created the Clinical Decision Support Knowledgebase (www.cdskb.org) that provides tools for developing and disseminating genomic decision support. These decision support resources provide clinical workflow templates, considerations for when interruptive alerts should be activated, and recommendations on preventing alert fatigue. As the number of clinically important gene–drug interactions increases, the utilization of interruptive alerts to notify clinicians of important information will become overwhelming. Indeed, many health care systems have significantly reduced the number of drug interaction and drug duplication pop-up notifications because of alert fatigue. Other long-term solutions besides interruptive alerts will be needed for presenting genomic information to clinicians, for example passively displaying pharmacogenomic data during computerized drug order entry [164]. Additional implementation tools include the IGNITE network (www.ignite-genomics.org) toolbox that contains resources for clinicians and educators along with the Pharmacogenomics Knowledgebase (www.pharmgkb.org).

Implementation Strategies

Strategies for implementing genomic medicine will depend on the needs and goals of individual health care systems. For earlier adopters of pharmacogenomics, common approaches have emerged that may apply to other health care settings [33, 164, 173]. First, multiple strategic partners should be engaged early in the implementation process, including executive leadership, pathology, health informatics, financial services, and end users such as patients, physicians, and pharmacists. It may be difficult to identify key stakeholders, but lack of support from any of these groups has the potential to derail the formation of a precision medicine service. A second consideration is the utilization of preexisting committees to guide the integration of personalized medicine into patient care. For example, most health care systems have a Pharmacy & Therapeutics committee that reviews and approves practices pertaining to drug utilization. A Pharmacy & Therapeutics committee may have the capacity and authority to approve decision support language for gene–drug interactions and approve alternative drugs or doses. Creating implementation cost models that utilize institution-specific data could help formulate meaningful business plans [78]. Furthermore, certain genotype tests (e.g., *HLA-B*57:01*, *HLA-B*15:02*, *TPMT*, *CYP2C19*) are reimbursed by third parties, dependent on the clinical scenario and necessity. An initial implementation strategy may include focusing on those gene–drug pairs where the testing is reimbursed [164].

Certain genomic variants are more likely to be observed in specific ancestries and ethnicities. The allele frequency for *HLA-B*15:02* is 0–0.02% for those of West African or Northern European descent, whereas the allele frequency among some Asian ethnicities is as high as 10–12% [174]. Patient populations should be taken into consideration when selecting gene–drug pairs for systematic implementation. Taking the approach of *HLA-B*15:02* genotyping for every patient prescribed carbamazepine would be of limited cost-effectiveness for health systems with more homogeneous populations consisting of those with West African and Northern European ancestry. A better implementation approach may be clinical decision support that reminds providers to assess ancestry and order an *HLA-B*15:02* genotype when appropriate. Implementation strategies may also consist of selecting a reference laboratory or testing platform. A genotype test should include variants representative of the patient population. For example, CYP2C9 metabolizes warfarin, with *CYP2C9* polymorphisms predictive of warfarin dose [175]. *CYP2C9* genotype tests may only interrogate a limited number of variants such as *CYP2C9*2* and *CYP2C9*3*. However, variants such as *CYP2C9*8* may be important predictors of warfarin dose for those of West African ancestry, and a warfarin pharmacogenomics clinic that serves patients of African descent and includes *CYP2C9* testing with important variants would be preferable [176].

Future of Personalized Medicine

Genomics is the first step in precision medicine, as additional data from proteomics, epigenomic, metabolomics, and other omics will need to be integrated into personalized medicine. The future of genomic medicine will need to focus on developing the guidelines and best practices for integrating specific gene–drug pairs with an emerging evidence base for clinical applicability to patient care. As more patients receive genotyping, additional gene-chronic disease and gene–drug associations will be discovered. One challenge of personalized medicine going forward will be translating the expanding clinically significant genomic information into patient care, while other barriers include understanding and managing the genetic variants that alone have mild to moderate penetrance but in combination predict severe phenotypes. The large-scale adoption and sustained implementation of personalized medicine will be informed by genomic medicine studies that demonstrate clinical utility and cost-effectiveness. Other future considerations will need to include ethical, legal, and social implications of available genomic information.

References

1. Sharifi M, Rakhit RD, Humphries SE, Nair D. Cardiovascular risk stratification in familial hypercholesterolaemia. Heart. 2016;102(13):1003–8.
2. Soutar AK, Naoumova RP. Mechanisms of disease: genetic causes of familial hypercholesterolemia. Nat Clin Pract Cardiovasc Med. 2007;4(4):214–25.
3. Wiegman A, Gidding SS, Watts GF, Chapman MJ, Ginsberg HN, Cuchel M, et al. Familial hypercholesterolaemia in children and adolescents: gaining decades of life by optimizing detection and treatment. Eur Heart J. 2015;36(36):2425–37.
4. Elborn JS. Cystic fibrosis. Lancet. 2016;388(10059):2519–31.
5. Cahill TJ, Ashrafian H, Watkins H. Genetic cardiomyopathies causing heart failure. Circ Res. 2013;113(6):660–75.
6. Li J. Inherited neuropathies. Semin Neurol. 2012;32(3):204–14.
7. Miki Y, Swensen J, Shattuck-Eidens D, Futreal PA, Harshman K, Tavtigian S, et al. A strong candidate for the breast and ovarian cancer susceptibility gene BRCA1. Science. 1994;266(5182):66–71.
8. Cuyvers E, Sleegers K. Genetic variations underlying Alzheimer's disease: evidence from genome-wide association studies and beyond. Lancet Neurol. 2016;15(8):857–68.
9. Coleman CI, Limone B, Sobieraj DM, Lee S, Roberts MS, Kaur R, et al. Dosing frequency and medication adherence in chronic disease. J Manag Care Pharm. 2012;18(7):527–39.
10. Loffler C, Drewelow E, Paschka SD, Frankenstein M, Eger J, Jatsch L, et al. Optimizing polypharmacy among elderly hospital patients with chronic diseases—study protocol of the cluster randomized controlled POLITE-RCT trial. Implement Sci. 2014;9:151.
11. Kalow W, Tang BK, Endrenyi L. Hypothesis: comparisons of inter- and intra-individual variations can substitute for twin studies in drug research. Pharmacogenetics. 1998;8(4):283–9.
12. Evans WE, McLeod HL. Pharmacogenomics—drug disposition, drug targets, and side effects. N Engl J Med. 2003;348(6):538–49.
13. Wang L, McLeod HL, Weinshilboum RM. Genomics and drug response. N Engl J Med. 2011;364(12):1144–53.
14. Clancy JP, Johnson SG, Yee SW, McDonagh EM, Caudle KE, Klein TE, et al. Clinical Pharmacogenetics Implementation Consortium (CPIC) guidelines for ivacaftor therapy in the context of CFTR genotype. Clin Pharmacol Ther. 2014;95(6):592–7.
15. Davies EC, Green CF, Mottram DR, Pirmohamed M. Adverse drug reactions in hospitals: a narrative review. Current Drug Safety. 2007;2(1):79–87.
16. Lazarou J, Pomeranz BH, Corey PN. Incidence of adverse drug reactions in hospitalized patients: a meta-analysis of prospective studies. JAMA. 1998;279(15):1200–5.
17. Finkelstein J, Friedman C, Hripcsak G, Cabrera M. Pharmacogenetic polymorphism as an independent risk factor for frequent hospitalizations in older adults with polypharmacy: a pilot study. Pharmgenomics Pers Med. 2016;9:107–16.
18. Kalow W. Familial incidence of low pseudocholinesterase level. Lancet. 1956;2:576.
19. Kalow W. Human pharmacogenomics: the development of a science. Hum Genomics. 2004;1(5):375–80.
20. Weinshilboum R. Inheritance and drug response. N Engl J Med. 2003;348(6):529–37.
21. Hicks JK, Swen JJ, Gaedigk A. Challenges in CYP2D6 phenotype assignment from genotype data: a critical assessment and call for standardization. Curr Drug Metab. 2014;15(2):218–32.
22. Sim SC, Risinger C, Dahl ML, Aklillu E, Christensen M, Bertilsson L, et al. A common novel CYP2C19 gene variant causes ultrarapid drug metabolism relevant for the drug response to proton pump inhibitors and antidepressants. Clin Pharmacol Ther. 2006;79(1):103–13.
23. Bosma PJ, Chowdhury JR, Bakker C, Gantla S, de Boer A, Oostra BA, et al. The genetic basis of the reduced expression of bilirubin UDP-glucuronosyltransferase 1 in Gilbert's syndrome. N Engl J Med. 1995;333(18):1171–5.
24. 1000 Genomes Project Consortium. A map of human genome variation from population-scale sequencing. Nature. 2010;467(7319):1061–73.
25. Altshuler DM, Gibbs RA, Peltonen L, Dermitzakis E, Schaffner SF, Yu F, et al. Integrating common and rare genetic variation in diverse human populations. Nature. 2010;467(7311):52–8.
26. He Y, Hoskins JM, McLeod HL. Copy number variants in pharmacogenetic genes. Trends Mol Med. 2011;17(5):244–51.
27. Gaedigk A. Complexities of CYP2D6 gene analysis and interpretation. Int Rev Psychiatry. 2013;25(5):534–53.
28. Caudle KE, Dunnenberger HM, Freimuth RR, Peterson JF, Burlison JD, Whirl-Carrillo M, et al. Standardizing terms for clinical pharmacogenetic test results: consensus terms from the Clinical Pharmacogenetics Implementation Consortium (CPIC). Genet Med. 2016;
29. Cleare A, Pariante CM, Young AH, Anderson IM, Christmas D, Cowen PJ, et al. Evidence-based guidelines for treating depressive disorders with antidepressants: a revision of the 2008 British Association for Psychopharmacology guidelines. J Psychopharmacol. 2015;29(5):459–525.
30. Qaseem A, Barry MJ, Kansagara D. Clinical Guidelines Committee of the American College of P. Nonpharmacologic versus pharmacologic treatment of adult patients with major depressive disorder: a clinical practice guideline from the american college of physicians. Ann Intern Med. 2016;164(5):350–9.
31. Relling MV, Klein TE. CPIC: clinical pharmacogenetics implementation consortium of the pharmacogenomics research network. Clin Pharmacol Ther. 2011;89(3):464–7.
32. Relling MV, Evans WE. Pharmacogenomics in the clinic. Nature. 2015;526(7573):343–50.
33. Dunnenberger HM, Crews KR, Hoffman JM, Caudle KE, Broeckel U, Howard SC, et al. Preemptive clinical pharmacogenetics implementation: current programs in five US medical centers. Annu Rev Pharmacol Toxicol. 2015;55:89–106.
34. Relling MV, Hancock ML, Rivera GK, Sandlund JT, Ribeiro RC, Krynetski EY, et al. Mercaptopurine therapy intolerance and heterozygosity at the thiopurine S-methyltransferase gene locus. J Natl Cancer Inst. 1999;91(23):2001–8.
35. McLeod HL, Siva C. The thiopurine S-methyltransferase gene locus—implications for clinical pharmacogenomics. Pharmacogenomics. 2002;3(1):89–98.
36. Relling MV, Gardner EE, Sandborn WJ, Schmiegelow K, Pui CH, Yee SW, et al. Clinical Pharmacogenetics Implementation Consortium guidelines for thiopurine methyltransfer-

ase genotype and thiopurine dosing. Clin Pharmacol Ther. 2011;89(3):387–91.
37. Relling MV, Schwab M, Whirl-Carrillo M, Suarez-Kurtz G, Pui CH, Stein CM, et al. Clinical Pharmacogenetics Implementation Consortium guideline for thiopurine dosing based on TPMT and NUDT15 genotypes: 2018 update. Clin Pharmacol Ther. 2019;105(5):1095–105.
38. Fong PC, Boss DS, Yap TA, Tutt A, Wu P, Mergui-Roelvink M, et al. Inhibition of poly(ADP-ribose) polymerase in tumors from BRCA mutation carriers. N Engl J Med. 2009;361(2):123–34.
39. de Bono J, Mateo J, Fizazi K, Saad F, Shore N, Sandhu S, et al. Olaparib for metastatic castration-resistant prostate cancer. N Engl J Med. 2020;382(22):2091–102.
40. Golan T, Hammel P, Reni M, Van Cutsem E, Macarulla T, Hall MJ, et al. Maintenance olaparib for germline BRCA-mutated metastatic pancreatic cancer. N Engl J Med. 2019;381(4):317–27.
41. Westdorp H, Fennemann FL, Weren RD, Bisseling TM, Ligtenberg MJ, Figdor CG, et al. Opportunities for immunotherapy in microsatellite instable colorectal cancer. Cancer Immunol Immunother. 2016;65(10):1249–59.
42. Thorn CF, Marsh S, Carrillo MW, McLeod HL, Klein TE, Altman RB. PharmGKB summary: fluoropyrimidine pathways. Pharmacogenet Genomics. 2011;21(4):237–42.
43. Caudle KE, Thorn CF, Klein TE, Swen JJ, McLeod HL, Diasio RB, et al. Clinical Pharmacogenetics Implementation Consortium guidelines for dihydropyrimidine dehydrogenase genotype and fluoropyrimidine dosing. Clin Pharmacol Ther. 2013;94(6):640–5.
44. Amstutz U, Henricks LM, Offer SM, Barbarino J, Schellens JHM, Swen JJ, et al. Clinical Pharmacogenetics Implementation Consortium (CPIC) guideline for dihydropyrimidine dehydrogenase genotype and fluoropyrimidine dosing: 2017 update. Clin Pharmacol Ther. 2018;103(2):210–6.
45. Henricks LM, Lunenburg C, de Man FM, Meulendijks D, Frederix GWJ, Kienhuis E, et al. DPYD genotype-guided dose individualisation of fluoropyrimidine therapy in patients with cancer: a prospective safety analysis. Lancet Oncol. 2018;19(11):1459–67.
46. Ke EE, Wu YL. EGFR as a pharmacological target in EGFR-mutant non-small-cell lung cancer: where do we stand now? Trends Pharmacol Sci. 2016;37(11):887–903.
47. Sharma SV, Bell DW, Settleman J, Haber DA. Epidermal growth factor receptor mutations in lung cancer. Nat Rev Cancer. 2007;7(3):169–81.
48. Soria JC, Ohe Y, Vansteenkiste J, Reungwetwattana T, Chewaskulyong B, Lee KH, et al. Osimertinib in untreated EGFR-mutated advanced non-small-cell lung cancer. N Engl J Med. 2018;378(2):113–25.
49. Redig AJ, Janne PA. Basket trials and the evolution of clinical trial design in an era of genomic medicine. J Clin Oncol. 2015;33(9):975–7.
50. Hunt PW. HIV and aging: emerging research issues. Curr Opin HIV AIDS. 2014;9(4):302–8.
51. Samji H, Cescon A, Hogg RS, Modur SP, Althoff KN, Buchacz K, et al. Closing the gap: increases in life expectancy among treated HIV-positive individuals in the United States and Canada. PLoS One. 2013;8(12):e81355.
52. Deeks SG, Lewin SR, Havlir DV. The end of AIDS: HIV infection as a chronic disease. Lancet. 2013;382(9903):1525–33.
53. Escaut L, Liotier JY, Albengres E, Cheminot N, Vittecoq D. Abacavir rechallenge has to be avoided in case of hypersensitivity reaction. AIDS. 1999;13(11):1419–20.
54. Martin MA, Klein TE, Dong BJ, Pirmohamed M, Haas DW, Kroetz DL, et al. Clinical pharmacogenetics implementation consortium guidelines for HLA-B genotype and abacavir dosing. Clin Pharmacol Ther. 2012;91(4):734–8.
55. Hershfield MS, Callaghan JT, Tassaneeyakul W, Mushiroda T, Thorn CF, Klein TE, et al. Clinical Pharmacogenetics Implementation Consortium guidelines for human leukocyte antigen-B genotype and allopurinol dosing. Clin Pharmacol Ther. 2013;93(2):153–8.
56. Martin AM, Nolan D, Gaudieri S, Almeida CA, Nolan R, James I, et al. Predisposition to abacavir hypersensitivity conferred by HLA-B*5701 and a haplotypic Hsp70-Hom variant. Proc Natl Acad Sci USA. 2004;101(12):4180–5.
57. Mallal S, Nolan D, Witt C, Masel G, Martin AM, Moore C, et al. Association between presence of HLA-B*5701, HLA-DR7, and HLA-DQ3 and hypersensitivity to HIV-1 reverse-transcriptase inhibitor abacavir. Lancet. 2002;359(9308):727–32.
58. Hetherington S, Hughes AR, Mosteller M, Shortino D, Baker KL, Spreen W, et al. Genetic variations in HLA-B region and hypersensitivity reactions to abacavir. Lancet. 2002;359(9312):1121–2.
59. Mallal S, Phillips E, Carosi G, Molina JM, Workman C, Tomazic J, et al. HLA-B*5701 screening for hypersensitivity to abacavir. N Engl J Med. 2008;358(6):568–79.
60. Lennox JL, Landovitz RJ, Ribaudo HJ, Ofotokun I, Na LH, Godfrey C, et al. Efficacy and tolerability of 3 nonnucleoside reverse transcriptase inhibitor-sparing antiretroviral regimens for treatment-naive volunteers infected with HIV-1: a randomized, controlled equivalence trial. Ann Intern Med. 2014;161(7):461–71.
61. Molina JM, Andrade-Villanueva J, Echevarria J, Chetchotisakd P, Corral J, David N, et al. Once-daily atazanavir/ritonavir versus twice-daily lopinavir/ritonavir, each in combination with tenofovir and emtricitabine, for management of antiretroviral-naive HIV-1-infected patients: 48 week efficacy and safety results of the CASTLE study. Lancet. 2008;372(9639):646–55.
62. Bosma P, Chowdhury JR, Jansen PH. Genetic inheritance of Gilbert's syndrome. Lancet. 1995;346(8970):314–5.
63. Lubomirov R, Colombo S, di Iulio J, Ledergerber B, Martinez R, Cavassini M, et al. Association of pharmacogenetic markers with premature discontinuation of first-line anti-HIV therapy: an observational cohort study. J Infect Dis. 2011;203(2):246–57.
64. Ribaudo HJ, Daar ES, Tierney C, Morse GD, Mollan K, Sax PE, et al. Impact of UGT1A1 Gilbert variant on discontinuation of ritonavir-boosted atazanavir in AIDS Clinical Trials Group Study A5202. J Infect Dis. 2013;207(3):420–5.
65. Vardhanabhuti S, Ribaudo HJ, Landovitz RJ, Ofotokun I, Lennox JL, Currier JS, et al. Screening for UGT1A1 genotype in study A5257 would have markedly reduced premature discontinuation of atazanavir for hyperbilirubinemia. Open Forum Infect Dis. 2015;2(3):ofv085.
66. Gammal RS, Court MH, Haidar CE, Iwuchukwu OF, Gaur AH, Alvarellos M, et al. Clinical Pharmacogenetics Implementation Consortium (CPIC) guideline for UGT1A1 and atazanavir prescribing. Clin Pharmacol Ther. 2016;99(4):363–9.
67. Bandiera S, Billie Bian C, Hoshida Y, Baumert TF, Zeisel MB. Chronic hepatitis C virus infection and pathogenesis of hepatocellular carcinoma. Curr Opin Virol. 2016;20:99–105.
68. Easterbrook PJ, Group WHOGD. Who to test and how to test for chronic hepatitis C infection—2016 WHO testing guidance for low- and middle-income countries. J Hepatol. 2016;65(1 Suppl):S46–66.
69. van der Meer AJ, Veldt BJ, Feld JJ, Wedemeyer H, Dufour JF, Lammert F, et al. Association between sustained virological response and all-cause mortality among patients with chronic hepatitis C and advanced hepatic fibrosis. JAMA. 2012;308(24):2584–93.
70. Manns MP, McHutchison JG, Gordon SC, Rustgi VK, Shiffman M, Reindollar R, et al. Peginterferon alfa-2b plus ribavirin compared with interferon alfa-2b plus ribavirin for initial treatment of chronic hepatitis C: a randomised trial. Lancet. 2001;358(9286):958–65.

71. Fried MW, Shiffman ML, Reddy KR, Smith C, Marinos G, Goncales FL Jr, et al. Peginterferon alfa-2a plus ribavirin for chronic hepatitis C virus infection. N Engl J Med. 2002;347(13):975–82.
72. Ge D, Fellay J, Thompson AJ, Simon JS, Shianna KV, Urban TJ, et al. Genetic variation in IL28B predicts hepatitis C treatment-induced viral clearance. Nature. 2009;461(7262):399–401.
73. Muir AJ, Gong L, Johnson SG, Lee MT, Williams MS, Klein TE, et al. Clinical Pharmacogenetics Implementation Consortium (CPIC) guidelines for IFNL3 (IL28B) genotype and PEG interferon-alpha-based regimens. Clin Pharmacol Ther. 2014;95(2):141–6.
74. Pilmis B, Puel A, Lortholary O, Lanternier F. New clinical phenotypes of fungal infections in special hosts. Clin Microbiol Infect. 2016;22(8):681–7.
75. Walsh TJ, Anaissie EJ, Denning DW, Herbrecht R, Kontoyiannis DP, Marr KA, et al. Treatment of aspergillosis: clinical practice guidelines of the Infectious Diseases Society of America. Clin Infect Dis. 2008;46(3):327–60.
76. Owusu Obeng A, Egelund EF, Alsultan A, Peloquin CA, Johnson JA. CYP2C19 polymorphisms and therapeutic drug monitoring of voriconazole: are we ready for clinical implementation of pharmacogenomics? Pharmacotherapy. 2014;34(7):703–18.
77. Miyakis S, van Hal SJ, Ray J, Marriott D. Voriconazole concentrations and outcome of invasive fungal infections. Clin Microbiol Infect. 2010;16(7):927–33.
78. Mason NT, Bell GC, Quilitz RE, Greene JN, McLeod HL. Budget impact analysis of CYP2C19-guided voriconazole prophylaxis in AML. J Antimicrob Chemother. 2015;70(11):3124–6.
79. Hicks JK, Gonzalez BE, Zembillas AS, Kusick K, Murthy S, Raja S, et al. Invasive Aspergillus infection requiring lobectomy in a CYP2C19 rapid metabolizer with subtherapeutic voriconazole concentrations. Pharmacogenomics. 2016;17(7):663–7.
80. Hicks JK, Crews KR, Flynn P, Haidar CE, Daniels CC, Yang W, et al. Voriconazole plasma concentrations in immunocompromised pediatric patients vary by CYP2C19 diplotypes. Pharmacogenomics. 2014;15(8):1065–78.
81. Moriyama B, Obeng AO, Barbarino J, Penzak SR, Henning SA, Scott SA, et al. Clinical Pharmacogenetics Implementation Consortium (CPIC) guidelines for CYP2C19 and voriconazole therapy. Clin Pharmacol Ther. 2017;102(1):45–51.
82. Hicks JK, Quilitz RE, Komrokji RS, Kubal TE, Lancet JE, Pasikhova Y, et al. Prospective CYP2C19-guided voriconazole prophylaxis in patients with neutropenic acute myeloid leukemia reduces the incidence of subtherapeutic antifungal plasma concentrations. Clin Pharmacol Ther. 2020;107(3):563–70.
83. Kessler RC, Berglund P, Demler O, Jin R, Koretz D, Merikangas KR, et al. The epidemiology of major depressive disorder: results from the National Comorbidity Survey Replication (NCS-R). JAMA. 2003;289(23):3095–105.
84. Mathers CD, Loncar D. Projections of global mortality and burden of disease from 2002 to 2030. PLoS Med. 2006;3(11):e442.
85. Kessler RC. The costs of depression. Psychiatr Clin North Am. 2012;35(1):1–14.
86. Barak Y, Swartz M, Baruch Y. Venlafaxine or a second SSRI: switching after treatment failure with an SSRI among depressed inpatients: a retrospective analysis. Prog Neuropsychopharmacol Biol Psychiatry. 2011;35(7):1744–7.
87. Hampton LM, Daubresse M, Chang HY, Alexander GC, Budnitz DS. Emergency department visits by adults for psychiatric medication adverse events. JAMA Psychiatry. 2014;71(9):1006–14.
88. Kennedy SH, Giacobbe P. Treatment resistant depression—advances in somatic therapies. Ann Clin Psychiatry. 2007;19(4):279–87.
89. Hicks JK, Bishop JR, Sangkuhl K, Muller DJ, Ji Y, Leckband SG, et al. Clinical Pharmacogenetics Implementation Consortium (CPIC) guideline for CYP2D6 and CYP2C19 genotypes and dosing of selective serotonin reuptake inhibitors. Clin Pharmacol Ther. 2015;98(2):127–34.
90. Hicks JK, Swen JJ, Thorn CF, Sangkuhl K, Kharasch ED, Ellingrod VL, et al. Clinical Pharmacogenetics Implementation Consortium guideline for CYP2D6 and CYP2C19 genotypes and dosing of tricyclic antidepressants. Clin Pharmacol Ther. 2013;93(5):402–8.
91. Hicks JK, Sangkuhl K, Swen JJ, Ellingrod VL, Muller DJ, Shimoda K, et al. Clinical pharmacogenetics implementation consortium guideline (CPIC) for CYP2D6 and CYP2C19 genotypes and dosing of tricyclic antidepressants: 2016 update. Clin Pharmacol Ther. 2017;102(1):37–44.
92. Altar CA, Carhart JM, Allen JD, Hall-Flavin DK, Dechairo BM, Winner JG. Clinical validity: Combinatorial pharmacogenomics predicts antidepressant responses and healthcare utilizations better than single gene phenotypes. Pharmacogenomics J. 2015;15(5):443–51.
93. Hall-Flavin DK, Winner JG, Allen JD, Carhart JM, Proctor B, Snyder KA, et al. Utility of integrated pharmacogenomic testing to support the treatment of major depressive disorder in a psychiatric outpatient setting. Pharmacogenet Genomics. 2013;23(10):535–48.
94. Winner JG, Carhart JM, Altar CA, Goldfarb S, Allen JD, Lavezzari G, et al. Combinatorial pharmacogenomic guidance for psychiatric medications reduces overall pharmacy costs in a 1 year prospective evaluation. Curr Med Res Opin. 2015;31(9):1633–43.
95. Oslin DW, Lynch KG, Shih MC, Ingram EP, Wray LO, Chapman SR, et al. Effect of pharmacogenomic testing for drug-gene interactions on medication selection and remission of symptoms in major depressive disorder: the PRIME care randomized clinical trial. JAMA. 2022;328(2):151–61.
96. Thompson C, Steven PH, Catriona H. Psychiatrist attitudes towards pharmacogenetic testing, direct-to-consumer genetic testing, and integrating genetic counseling into psychiatric patient care. Psychiatry Res. 2015;226(1):68–72.
97. Walden LM, Brandl EJ, Changasi A, Sturgess JE, Soibel A, Notario JF, et al. Physicians' opinions following pharmacogenetic testing for psychotropic medication. Psychiatry Res. 2015;229(3):913–8.
98. de Leon J, Armstrong SC, Cozza KL. Clinical guidelines for psychiatrists for the use of pharmacogenetic testing for CYP450 2D6 and CYP450 2C19. Psychosomatics. 2006;47(1):75–85.
99. Lohoff FW, Aquino TD, Narasimhan S, Multani PK, Etemad B, Rickels K. Serotonin receptor 2A (HTR2A) gene polymorphism predicts treatment response to venlafaxine XR in generalized anxiety disorder. Pharmacogenomics J. 2013;13(1):21–6.
100. Wilkie MJ, Smith G, Day RK, Matthews K, Smith D, Blackwood D, et al. Polymorphisms in the SLC6A4 and HTR2A genes influence treatment outcome following antidepressant therapy. Pharmacogenomics J. 2009;9(1):61–70.
101. de Leon J, Spina E, Diaz FJ. Clobazam therapeutic drug monitoring: a comprehensive review of the literature with proposals to improve future studies. Ther Drug Monit. 2013;35(1):30–47.
102. Miranda LF, Gomes KB, Silveira JN, Pianetti GA, Byrro RM, Peles PR, et al. Predictive factors of clinical response to cholinesterase inhibitors in mild and moderate Alzheimer's disease and mixed dementia: a one-year naturalistic study. J Alzheimers Dis. 2015;45(2):609–20.
103. Mehanna R, Hunter C, Davidson A, Jimenez-Shahed J, Jankovic J. Analysis of CYP2D6 genotype and response to tetrabenazine. Mov Disord. 2013;28(2):210–5.
104. Chung WH, Hung SI, Hong HS, Hsih MS, Yang LC, Ho HC, et al. Medical genetics: a marker for Stevens-Johnson syndrome. Nature. 2004;428(6982):486.

105. Yip VL, Marson AG, Jorgensen AL, Pirmohamed M, Alfirevic A. HLA genotype and carbamazepine-induced cutaneous adverse drug reactions: a systematic review. Clin Pharmacol Ther. 2012;92(6):757–65.
106. Chen P, Lin JJ, Lu CS, Ong CT, Hsieh PF, Yang CC, et al. Carbamazepine-induced toxic effects and HLA-B*1502 screening in Taiwan. N Engl J Med. 2011;364(12):1126–33.
107. Hardt J, Jacobsen C, Goldberg J, Nickel R, Buchwald D. Prevalence of chronic pain in a representative sample in the United States. Pain Med. 2008;9(7):803–12.
108. Sadhasivam S, Chidambaran V. Pharmacogenomics of opioids and perioperative pain management. Pharmacogenomics. 2012;13(15):1719–40.
109. Ross JR, Rutter D, Welsh K, Joel SP, Goller K, Wells AU, et al. Clinical response to morphine in cancer patients and genetic variation in candidate genes. Pharmacogenomics J. 2005;5(5):324–36.
110. Zubieta JK, Heitzeg MM, Smith YR, Bueller JA, Xu K, Xu Y, et al. COMT val158met genotype affects mu-opioid neurotransmitter responses to a pain stressor. Science. 2003;299(5610):1240–3.
111. Diatchenko L, Slade GD, Nackley AG, Bhalang K, Sigurdsson A, Belfer I, et al. Genetic basis for individual variations in pain perception and the development of a chronic pain condition. Hum Mol Genet. 2005;14(1):135–43.
112. Kim H, Neubert JK, San Miguel A, Xu K, Krishnaraju RK, Iadarola MJ, et al. Genetic influence on variability in human acute experimental pain sensitivity associated with gender, ethnicity and psychological temperament. Pain. 2004;109(3):488–96.
113. Rakvag TT, Ross JR, Sato H, Skorpen F, Kaasa S, Klepstad P. Genetic variation in the catechol-O-methyltransferase (COMT) gene and morphine requirements in cancer patients with pain. Mol Pain. 2008;4:64.
114. Crews KR, Monte AA, Huddart R, Caudle KE, Kharasch ED, Gaedigk A, et al. Clinical pharmacogenetics implementation consortium guideline for CYP2D6, OPRM1, and COMT genotypes and select opioid therapy. Clin Pharmacol Ther. 2021;110(4):888–96.
115. Kirchheiner J, Stormer E, Meisel C, Steinbach N, Roots I, Brockmoller J. Influence of CYP2C9 genetic polymorphisms on pharmacokinetics of celecoxib and its metabolites. Pharmacogenetics. 2003;13(8):473–80.
116. Theken KN, Lee CR, Gong L, Caudle KE, Formea CM, Gaedigk A, et al. Clinical Pharmacogenetics Implementation Consortium Guideline (CPIC) for CYP2C9 and nonsteroidal anti-inflammatory drugs. Clin Pharmacol Ther. 2020;108(2):191–200.
117. Kelly LE, Rieder M, van den Anker J, Malkin B, Ross C, Neely MN, et al. More codeine fatalities after tonsillectomy in North American children. Pediatrics. 2012;129(5):e1343–7.
118. Crews KR, Gaedigk A, Dunnenberger HM, Leeder JS, Klein TE, Caudle KE, et al. Clinical Pharmacogenetics Implementation Consortium guidelines for cytochrome P450 2D6 genotype and codeine therapy: 2014 update. Clin Pharmacol Ther. 2014;95(4):376–82.
119. Chou WY, Yang LC, Lu HF, Ko JY, Wang CH, Lin SH, et al. Association of mu-opioid receptor gene polymorphism (A118G) with variations in morphine consumption for analgesia after total knee arthroplasty. Acta Anaesthesiol Scand. 2006;50(7):787–92.
120. Janicki PK, Schuler G, Francis D, Bohr A, Gordin V, Jarzembowski T, et al. A genetic association study of the functional A118G polymorphism of the human mu-opioid receptor gene in patients with acute and chronic pain. Anesth Analg. 2006;103(4):1011–7.
121. Mensah GA, Brown DW. An overview of cardiovascular disease burden in the United States. Health Aff (Millwood). 2007;26(1):38–48.
122. Materson BJ, Reda DJ, Cushman WC, Massie BM, Freis ED, Kochar MS, et al. Single-drug therapy for hypertension in men. A comparison of six antihypertensive agents with placebo. The Department of Veterans Affairs Cooperative Study Group on Antihypertensive Agents. N Engl J Med. 1993;328(13):914–21.
123. Johnson JA, Gong Y, Bailey KR, Cooper-DeHoff RM, Chapman AB, Turner ST, et al. Hydrochlorothiazide and atenolol combination antihypertensive therapy: effects of drug initiation order. Clin Pharmacol Ther. 2009;86(5):533–9.
124. Mahmud A, Feely J. Choice of first antihypertensive: simple as ABCD? Am J Hypertens. 2007;20(8):923–7.
125. Schwartz GL, Bailey K, Chapman AB, Boerwinkle E, Turner ST. The role of plasma renin activity, age, and race in selecting effective initial drug therapy for hypertension. Am J Hypertens. 2013;26(8):957–64.
126. Dahlberg J, Nilsson LO, von Wowern F, Melander O. Polymorphism in NEDD4L is associated with increased salt sensitivity, reduced levels of P-renin and increased levels of Nt-proANP. PLoS One. 2007;2(5):e432.
127. Dahlberg J, Sjogren M, Hedblad B, Engstrom G, Melander O. Genetic variation in NEDD4L, an epithelial sodium channel regulator, is associated with cardiovascular disease and cardiovascular death. J Hypertens. 2014;32(2):294–9.
128. Luo F, Wang Y, Wang X, Sun K, Zhou X, Hui R. A functional variant of NEDD4L is associated with hypertension, antihypertensive response, and orthostatic hypotension. Hypertension. 2009;54(4):796–801.
129. Johnson JA, Zineh I, Puckett BJ, McGorray SP, Yarandi HN, Pauly DF. Beta 1-adrenergic receptor polymorphisms and antihypertensive response to metoprolol. Clin Pharmacol Ther. 2003;74(1):44–52.
130. Liu J, Liu ZQ, Yu BN, Xu FH, Mo W, Zhou G, et al. beta1-Adrenergic receptor polymorphisms influence the response to metoprolol monotherapy in patients with essential hypertension. Clin Pharmacol Ther. 2006;80(1):23–32.
131. Wu D, Li G, Deng M, Song W, Huang X, Guo X, et al. Associations between ADRB1 and CYP2D6 gene polymorphisms and the response to beta-blocker therapy in hypertension. J Int Med Res. 2015;43(3):424–34.
132. Sjouke B, Kusters DM, Kindt I, Besseling J, Defesche JC, Sijbrands EJ, et al. Homozygous autosomal dominant hypercholesterolaemia in the Netherlands: prevalence, genotype-phenotype relationship, and clinical outcome. Eur Heart J. 2015;36(9):560–5.
133. Poduri A, Khullar M, Bahl A, Sehrawat BS, Sharma Y, Talwar KK. Common variants of HMGCR, CETP, APOAI, ABCB1, CYP3A4, and CYP7A1 genes as predictors of lipid-lowering response to atorvastatin therapy. DNA Cell Biol. 2010;29(10):629–37.
134. Akao H, Polisecki E, Kajinami K, Trompet S, Robertson M, Ford I, et al. Genetic variation at the SLCO1B1 gene locus and low density lipoprotein cholesterol lowering response to pravastatin in the elderly. Atherosclerosis. 2012;220(2):413–7.
135. Thompson JF, Man M, Johnson KJ, Wood LS, Lira ME, Lloyd DB, et al. An association study of 43 SNPs in 16 candidate genes with atorvastatin response. Pharmacogenomics J. 2005;5(6):352–8.
136. Chasman DI, Giulianini F, MacFadyen J, Barratt BJ, Nyberg F, Ridker PM. Genetic determinants of statin-induced low-density lipoprotein cholesterol reduction: the Justification for the Use of Statins in Prevention: an Intervention Trial Evaluating Rosuvastatin (JUPITER) trial. Circ Cardiovasc Genet. 2012;5(2):257–64.
137. Group SC, Link E, Parish S, Armitage J, Bowman L, Heath S, et al. SLCO1B1 variants and statin-induced myopathy—a genomewide study. N Engl J Med. 2008;359(8):789–99.
138. Ramsey LB, Johnson SG, Caudle KE, Haidar CE, Voora D, Wilke RA, et al. The clinical pharmacogenetics implementation consor-

tium guideline for SLCO1B1 and simvastatin-induced myopathy: 2014 update. Clin Pharmacol Ther. 2014;96(4):423–8.
139. Cooper-DeHoff RM, Niemi M, Ramsey LB, Luzum JA, Tarkiainen EK, Straka RJ, et al. The Clinical Pharmacogenetics Implementation Consortium Guideline for SLCO1B1, ABCG2, and CYP2C9 genotypes and statin-associated musculoskeletal symptoms. Clin Pharmacol Ther. 2022;111(5):1007–21.
140. Scott SA, Sangkuhl K, Stein CM, Hulot JS, Mega JL, Roden DM, et al. Clinical Pharmacogenetics Implementation Consortium guidelines for CYP2C19 genotype and clopidogrel therapy: 2013 update. Clin Pharmacol Ther. 2013;94(3):317–23.
141. Lee CR, Luzum JA, Sangkuhl K, Gammal RS, Sabatine MS, Stein CM, et al. Clinical Pharmacogenetics Implementation Consortium Guideline for CYP2C19 genotype and clopidogrel therapy: 2022 update. Clin Pharmacol Ther. 2022;112:959–67.
142. Aithal GP, Day CP, Kesteven PJ, Daly AK. Association of polymorphisms in the cytochrome P450 CYP2C9 with warfarin dose requirement and risk of bleeding complications. Lancet. 1999;353(9154):717–9.
143. Limdi NA, McGwin G, Goldstein JA, Beasley TM, Arnett DK, Adler BK, et al. Influence of CYP2C9 and VKORC1 1173C/T genotype on the risk of hemorrhagic complications in African-American and European-American patients on warfarin. Clin Pharmacol Ther. 2008;83(2):312–21.
144. Limdi NA, Arnett DK, Goldstein JA, Beasley TM, McGwin G, Adler BK, et al. Influence of CYP2C9 and VKORC1 on warfarin dose, anticoagulation attainment and maintenance among European-Americans and African-Americans. Pharmacogenomics. 2008;9(5):511–26.
145. Johnson JA, Caudle KE, Gong L, Whirl-Carrillo M, Stein CM, Scott SA, et al. Clinical Pharmacogenetics Implementation Consortium (CPIC) guideline for pharmacogenetics-guided warfarin dosing: 2017 update. Clin Pharmacol Ther. 2017;102(3):397–404.
146. Rieder MJ, Reiner AP, Gage BF, Nickerson DA, Eby CS, McLeod HL, et al. Effect of VKORC1 haplotypes on transcriptional regulation and warfarin dose. N Engl J Med. 2005;352(22):2285–93.
147. Kimmel SE, French B, Kasner SE, Johnson JA, Anderson JL, Gage BF, et al. A pharmacogenetic versus a clinical algorithm for warfarin dosing. N Engl J Med. 2013;369(24):2283–93.
148. Stankov K, Benc D, Draskovic D. Genetic and epigenetic factors in etiology of diabetes mellitus type 1. Pediatrics. 2013;132(6):1112–22.
149. Noble JA, Erlich HA. Genetics of type 1 diabetes. Cold Spring Harb Perspect Med. 2012;2(1):a007732.
150. Morahan G. Insights into type 1 diabetes provided by genetic analyses. Curr Opin Endocrinol Diabetes Obes. 2012;19(4):263–70.
151. Medici F, Hawa M, Ianari A, Pyke DA, Leslie RD. Concordance rate for type II diabetes mellitus in monozygotic twins: actuarial analysis. Diabetologia. 1999;42(2):146–50.
152. Morris AP, Voight BF, Teslovich TM, Ferreira T, Segre AV, Steinthorsdottir V, et al. Large-scale association analysis provides insights into the genetic architecture and pathophysiology of type 2 diabetes. Nat Genet. 2012;44(9):981–90.
153. Altshuler D, Hirschhorn JN, Klannemark M, Lindgren CM, Vohl MC, Nemesh J, et al. The common PPARgamma Pro12Ala polymorphism is associated with decreased risk of type 2 diabetes. Nat Genet. 2000;26(1):76–80.
154. Becker ML, Visser LE, van Schaik RH, Hofman A, Uitterlinden AG, Stricker BH. Genetic variation in the organic cation transporter 1 is associated with metformin response in patients with diabetes mellitus. Pharmacogenomics J. 2009;9(4):242–7.
155. Graham GG, Punt J, Arora M, Day RO, Doogue MP, Duong JK, et al. Clinical pharmacokinetics of metformin. Clin Pharmacokinet. 2011;50(2):81–98.
156. Shu Y, Sheardown SA, Brown C, Owen RP, Zhang S, Castro RA, et al. Effect of genetic variation in the organic cation transporter 1 (OCT1) on metformin action. J Clin Invest. 2007;117(5):1422–31.
157. Zhou K, Donnelly LA, Kimber CH, Donnan PT, Doney AS, Leese G, et al. Reduced-function SLC22A1 polymorphisms encoding organic cation transporter 1 and glycemic response to metformin: a GoDARTS study. Diabetes. 2009;58(6):1434–9.
158. Gloyn AL, Pearson ER, Antcliff JF, Proks P, Bruining GJ, Slingerland AS, et al. Activating mutations in the gene encoding the ATP-sensitive potassium-channel subunit Kir6.2 and permanent neonatal diabetes. N Engl J Med. 2004;350(18):1838–49.
159. Pearson ER, Starkey BJ, Powell RJ, Gribble FM, Clark PM, Hattersley AT. Genetic cause of hyperglycaemia and response to treatment in diabetes. Lancet. 2003;362(9392):1275–81.
160. Wilson CJ, de la Haye K, Coveney J, Hughes DL, Hutchinson A, Miller C, et al. Protocol for a randomized controlled trial testing the impact of feedback on familial risk of chronic diseases on family-level intentions to participate in preventive lifestyle behaviors. BMC Public Health. 2016;16:965.
161. Vassy JL, Donelan K, Hivert MF, Green RC, Grant RW. Genetic susceptibility testing for chronic disease and intention for behavior change in healthy young adults. J Community Genet. 2013;4(2):263–71.
162. Teng K, DiPiero J, Meese T, Doerr M, Leonard M, Daly T, et al. Cleveland Clinic's Center for personalized healthcare: setting the stage for value-based care. Pharmacogenomics. 2014;15(5):587–91.
163. CMS. Centers for Medicare & Medicaid Services EHR Incentive Programs. https://www.cms.gov/Regulations-and-Guidance/Legislation/EHRIncentivePrograms/index.html?redirect=/ehrincentiveprograms.
164. Hicks JK, Stowe D, Willner MA, Wai M, Daly T, Gordon SM, et al. Implementation of clinical pharmacogenomics within a large health system: from electronic health record decision support to consultation services. Pharmacotherapy. 2016;36(8):940–8.
165. Hicks JK, Crews KR, Hoffman JM, Kornegay NM, Wilkinson MR, Lorier R, et al. A clinician-driven automated system for integration of pharmacogenetic interpretations into an electronic medical record. Clin Pharmacol Ther. 2012;92(5):563–6.
166. Bell GC, Crews KR, Wilkinson MR, Haidar CE, Hicks JK, Baker DK, et al. Development and use of active clinical decision support for preemptive pharmacogenomics. J Am Med Inform Assoc. 2014;21(e1):e93–9.
167. (AC) DaIGITtEACD. Establishing connectivity and pharmacogenomic clinical decision support rules to protect patients carrying HLA-B*57:01 and TPMT Variants; 2015. http://iom.nationalacademies.org/~/media/Files/Activity%20Files/Research/GenomicBasedResearch/Action%20Collaboratives/DIGITizE%20Abacavir%20and%20TPMT%20CDS%20Implementation%20Guide%20-%20Final%201_0.pdf?la=en.
168. Rasmussen-Torvik LJ, Stallings SC, Gordon AS, Almoguera B, Basford MA, Bielinski SJ, et al. Design and anticipated outcomes of the eMERGE-PGx project: a multicenter pilot for preemptive pharmacogenomics in electronic health record systems. Clin Pharmacol Ther. 2014;96(4):482–9.
169. Weitzel KW, Alexander M, Bernhardt BA, Calman N, Carey DJ, Cavallari LH, et al. The IGNITE network: a model for genomic medicine implementation and research. BMC Med Genomics. 2016;9(1):1.
170. Levy KD, Blake K, Fletcher-Hoppe C, Franciosi J, Goto D, Hicks JK, et al. Opportunities to implement a sustainable genomic medicine program: lessons learned from the IGNITE Network. Genet Med. 2019;21(3):743–7.
171. Swen JJ, Nijenhuis M, de Boer A, Grandia L, Maitland-van der Zee AH, Mulder H, et al. Pharmacogenetics: from bench to byte—an update of guidelines. Clin Pharmacol Ther. 2011;89(5):662–73.

172. Hoffman JM, Dunnenberger HM, Kevin Hicks J, Caudle KE, Whirl Carrillo M, Freimuth RR, et al. Developing knowledge resources to support precision medicine: principles from the Clinical Pharmacogenetics Implementation Consortium (CPIC). J Am Med Inform Assoc. 2016;23(4):796–801.
173. Dunnenberger HM, Biszewski M, Bell GC, Sereika A, May H, Johnson SG, et al. Implementation of a multidisciplinary pharmacogenomics clinic in a community health system. Am J Health Syst Pharm. 2016;73(23):1956–66.
174. Leckband SG, Kelsoe JR, Dunnenberger HM, George AL Jr, Tran E, Berger R, et al. Clinical Pharmacogenetics Implementation Consortium guidelines for HLA-B genotype and carbamazepine dosing. Clin Pharmacol Ther. 2013;94(3):324–8.
175. Johnson JA, Gong L, Whirl-Carrillo M, Gage BF, Scott SA, Stein CM, et al. Clinical Pharmacogenetics Implementation Consortium Guidelines for CYP2C9 and VKORC1 genotypes and warfarin dosing. Clin Pharmacol Ther. 2011;90(4):625–9.
176. Nagai R, Ohara M, Cavallari LH, Drozda K, Patel SR, Nutescu EA, et al. Factors influencing pharmacokinetics of warfarin in African-Americans: implications for pharmacogenetic dosing algorithms. Pharmacogenomics. 2015;16(3):217–25.

Obesity and Chronic Disease

Debbie Phipps and Margaret R. Helton

Prevalence and Impact

Obesity is a disease which is extraordinarily prevalent in the United States (US), with over 40% of American adults meeting the criteria for obesity [1]. The prevalence of severe obesity in adults is 9.2%. Among adults, the prevalence of both obesity and severe obesity was highest in Black American adults compared to other groups. Worldwide, obesity has nearly tripled since 1975 with over 1.9 billion adults overweight and 650 million of them considered obese [2]. Over 340 million children and adolescents were overweight or obese in 2016. Most of the world's population live in countries where overweight and obesity kills more people than being underweight. These trends are of great concern in terms of the future health of most populations and the burgeoning costs of this condition and the associated morbidities for health care systems.

It need not be this way, as obesity is preventable. Environmental and societal factors strongly influence the rising tide of this obesity epidemic, including increasing palatability, convenience, and accessibility of food, and decreased physical activity at work and during leisure time. The understanding of obesity as a disease state, rather than simply an association with other chronic diseases, is crucial to the discussion of risk factors as well as treatment. Risk factors for obesity include an obesogenic environment, genetic predisposition, psychological stress, medication-adverse events, hormonal shifts (e.g., pregnancy or perimenopause), and life events such as smoking cessation [3, 4].

D. Phipps · M. R. Helton (✉)
Department of Family Medicine, University of North Carolina at Chapel Hill, Chapel Hill, NC, USA
e-mail: dleech@email.unc.edu; debbie_Phipps@med.unc.edu; margaret_helton@med.unc.edu

Defining Obesity

People are considered overweight if their body mass index (BMI) is ≥ 25.0 kg/m^2 and obese if their BMI is ≥ 30.0 kg/m^2 (Table 2.1) [5]. These cutpoints were established in 1998 and remain widely accepted [6]. Evidence supports these ranges as there is a direct relationship between increasing BMI and a higher risk for fatal coronary heart disease in both men and women, starting at the upper end of normal weight (BMI 18.5–24.9 kg/m^2) [7]. BMI is calculated by weight (in kilograms) divided by height (in meters squared). One limitation of the BMI system is that it accounts poorly for the heterogeneity of individuals within each class and serves only as an estimation for adiposity, which is the condition of having too much fatty tissue in the body. Waist circumference and waist-to-hip ratio are used as indirect anthropometric measures to act as a proxy for visceral adipose tissue (VAT). VAT can be directly measured with magnetic resonance imaging (MRI) or computed tomography, but this imaging is currently too expensive to be utilized on a large scale. Increasing VAT raises the risk of metabolic and cardiac disease [8]. There are differences across genders and ethnic backgrounds which can limit the utility of these anthropometric measures.

The Edmonton Obesity Staging System (EOSS) accounts for physical and psychological co-morbidities as well as functionality when considering one's health status. It accounts better for individual risk related to excess

Table 2.1 Defining adult overweight and obesity. Centers for Disease Control and Prevention [5]

Weight status	BMI (kg/m^2)
Underweight	<18.5
Normal weight	18.5–24.9
Overweight	25–29.9
Class I obesity	30–34.9
Class II obesity	35–39.9
Class III obesity	>40

visceral fat than the BMI system, which is better suited to population-based data [9]. The EOSS exists in Stages 0–4, where physical, psychological, and functional limitations are classified as absent (Stage 0), mild (Stage 1), moderate (Stage 2), severe (Stage 3), or end-stage (Stage 4). EOSS stages 3–4 have been linked to increased post-operative mortality rate following bariatric surgery as compared to EOSS 0–2. Higher EOSS is linked to increased mortality risk, and polypharmacy and health care services use [10, 11].

Obesity as a Chronic Disease

It is a common experience among patients with obesity that early success with weight loss is difficult to maintain, which is discouraging to people who struggle with obesity, making obesity itself a chronic condition with a physiologic basis. The human body is designed to preserve energy and survive in conditions of food scarcity. Body weight is regulated by the hypothalamus with hormonal input from the pancreas, gastrointestinal tract, and adipose tissue [12]. The body responds to caloric restriction by reducing energy expenditure and levels of leptin and cholecystokinin, while increasing levels of ghrelin, which stimulates hunger, all of which promotes weight gain. Other factors in the physiology of energy include the hormones peptide YY, glucagon-like peptide 1, and the melanocortin peptides and their receptors. These hormones signal nutrition depletion and satiety and modulate energy intake and expenditure, and are the focus of research involving causes of as well as treatment for obesity [13].

The many compensatory responses to low-calorie diets are not temporary, and persist for a year after weight loss, even if weight is regained, indicating that the failure to maintain weight loss has a strong physiological basis and is not just due to the personal weaknesses of the individual [14].

Obesity and Comorbid Conditions

Obesity is a disease state. As BMI rises, the body is at risk for other diseases, including both fat mass disease (physical consequences) and sick fat disease (metabolic consequences). Co-morbidities of obesity include hypertension, osteoarthritis, stroke, varicose veins, intertrigo, gastroesophageal reflux disorder, fatty liver disease, heart failure, pulmonary embolism, asthma, obstructive sleep apnea/obesity hypoventilation syndrome, idiopathic intracranial hypertension, striae distensae (stretch marks), and depression. Most of these conditions result from abnormal physical forces of carrying extra weight, cardiovascular effects, pulmonary constriction, or psychosocial factors, including internalization of weight bias and stigma [15].

Adiposopathy, or "sick fat disease," relates to the abnormal endocrine and immune response to obesity. Metabolic consequences of obesity include hyperandrogenism, hirsutism, polycystic ovary syndrome, gestational diabetes mellitus, pre-eclampsia, erectile dysfunction, infertility, pelvic organ prolapse, and increased risk of multiple kinds of malignancy. Obesity increases the risk of cancer through mechanisms involving adiposopathic cytokines (tumor necrosis factor-alpha and interleukin-6) damaging cellular DNA, promoting gene mutations, promoting cell proliferation, and contributing to endothelial damage to allow for metastasis [15].

Obesity and COVID-19

COVID-19 infection can present with a range of symptoms, from mild or asymptomatic disease to severe symptoms requiring hospitalization and intensive care, and even leading to death. Risk factors for severe illness include obesity, hypertension, diabetes, chronic kidney disease, asthma, cancer, and heart disease. Obesity is noted to increase the risk of hospitalization, intensive care unit (ICU) admission, invasive mechanical ventilation, and death in those with COVID-19 [16, 17]. This association is strongest in young adults <50 years old [18]. BMI may not be the best indicator for measuring outcomes related to COVID-19 in patients with obesity; EOSS 0–1 patients actually had lower mortality related to COVID-19 than individuals with normal weight, whereas EOSS 2 and 4 patients had higher rates of intubation and death from COVID-19 [19].

There are several obesity-related physiologic and anatomic changes that may predispose to increased disease severity, including increase in adipose tissue leading to high expression of angiotensin converting enzyme 2 (ACE2), chronic activation of renin-angiotensin-aldosterone system, impaired immune response, impaired inflammatory response, and impaired pulmonary function [20]. There are also challenges with diagnosis and management, including imaging quality, airway management, and responsiveness to prone positioning, which impact care of patients with obesity and COVID-19.

Obesity exponentially increases the mortality risk from SARS-CoV-2. There is a direct link between inflammatory states seen in metabolic syndrome and the cytokine storm that has been connected to worse outcomes with COVID-19. Obesity itself is a state of chronic, sub-clinical inflammation which can alter response to infectious disease through multiple mechanisms. Indeed, obesity can reduce immune cell functionality [21].

ACE2 is used by the SARS-CoV-2 spike protein as a point of entry to the host cell, and ACE2 is highly expressed in adipose tissue, leading to the theory that adipose tissue is a point of entry for infection. ACE2 is downregulated upon engagement with the spike protein, leading to accumulation of angiotensin II in the lungs, another site of ACE2 receptors. Angiotensin II accumulation results in increased vascular permeability, worsening pulmonary edema, and in many cases acute respiratory distress syndrome [22].

Obesity is known to influence major cardiovascular risk factors, including hyperlipidemia, diabetes, and hypertension. These conditions are also linked to worse outcomes for COVID-19. Increased levels of circulating pro-inflammatory cytokines, including TNF-alpha, IL-6, and leptin, may impair the immune response [22, 23].

Health Disparities in Obesity

Obesity prevalence is highest in people from rural, economically disadvantaged, and racial and ethnic minority backgrounds [24]. Obesity is less prevalent among people with a college education [25]. Prevalence of obesity is higher among lesbian women than among heterosexual women, and this disparity begins in adolescence [26]. Obesity and the related co-morbidities of hypertension, coronary heart disease, and stroke are disproportionately more common among non-Hispanic Black and Hispanic/Latino populations compared to non-Hispanic Whites [27]. These racial disparities are present in pregnancy, where Black and Hispanic women are more likely to be overweight or obese than White women [24]. The rate of infant weight gain independently contributes to the racial and ethnic disparities in childhood obesity, where rapid weight gain in infancy is a strong risk factor for childhood obesity [28]. In infancy and early childhood, lower rates of breastfeeding, early introduction of solid foods, increased intake of sugar-sweetened beverages, and increased fast food consumption also significantly impact this disparity. Black and Hispanic children are more likely to be exposed to lower-quality diets, including fast food and sugar-sweetened beverages. In addition, lack of access to organized sports and playgrounds in neighborhoods with lower socioeconomic status leads to higher BMI in childhood [24].

A strong and consistent association exists between poor communities and increased density of fast food restaurants with limited access to healthy food, a phenomenon known as a "food desert." Compounding the problem is the fact that areas with increased poverty have lower "walkability" scores due to lower perceived safety and lack of sidewalks or parks, which increases physical inactivity. This occurs in both rural and urban settings. Rural Americans are more likely to have obesity and are also less likely to report regular physical activity and intake of fruits and green vegetables [29].

Parental, particularly maternal, mental health is also correlated to childhood overweight and obesity; positive mental health in mothers is associated with lower odds of overweight and obesity in children, even after adjusting for family food security, child physical activity, and child screen time [30]. There is a link between women who report food insecurity and obesity, but this relationship is complex as it is not found in men [31].

With regard to research, most genome studies have been performed on individuals of European descent, even though a disproportionate number of Black or Hispanic American people are affected by obesity. This lack of research limits the understanding of the genetics of obesity and precision medicine treatment options [32].

Treating Obesity

Given the challenges of achieving weight loss and the lifestyle changes in eating and physical activity patterns required to effectively maintain the weight loss, patients must feel motivated to do so and clinicians must have the skill set to counsel and support patients in this effort. Lifestyle Medicine is an emerging medical training process where clinicians can be certified in lifestyle interventions that help patients manage their chronic conditions, including obesity, using healthy eating, avoidance of harmful substance use, physical activity, restorative sleep, stress management, and social interactions (https://lifestylemedicine.org/). The US Preventive Services Task Force recommends referral of patients with obesity to intensive, multicomponent behavioral weight loss programs [33]. The American Heart Association advises that collaborative team efforts that include physicians and nutritionists working at both the individual and population health level are imperative to meet the massive public health and economic burdens from chronic disease including cardiovascular disease and obesity [34].

The effort is worth it as there is evidence of a dose–response relationship between weight loss in overweight and obese adults and reduction in cardiovascular disease risk factors (diabetes, hypertension, and hyperlipidemia) [7]. Weight loss can reduce the risk of type 2 diabetes in overweight and obese adults, with weight loss of 2.5–5.5 kg for two or more years lowering the risk by 30–60 percent. For those who already have type 2 diabetes, weight loss of 5–10% is associated with hemoglobin A1c reductions of 0.6–1.0 and reduced need for diabetes medications.

Approach to Patient

The medical assessment of a patient with obesity begins with asking permission to have the discussion about weight. How the discussion is initiated and the language used may influence the patient's reaction and participation in weight loss efforts [35]. Obesity societies suggest using "people first language" to reduce stigma in patients with obesity seeking care. This involves not labeling a person by their disease but recognizing the person first and then the medical condition. For example, rather than saying "the obese patient" use the term "the patient with obesity" [36].

Surveys of primary care physicians suggest that many clinicians understand the disease of obesity and have competency to prescribe anti-obesity medications, but more than half noted that they would spend more time counseling on weight loss if they were better reimbursed for their time [37]. There is evidence from the National Health and Nutrition Examination Survey that the simple act of being told by their physician that they met BMI criteria for overweight or obesity is associated with significant weight loss [38].

To tailor weight management recommendations, a complete patient history focused on weight should be obtained. This includes assessing weight highs and lows at different points in life to identify events that may have impacted weight, such as accelerated weight gain during smoking cessation, starting a new medication, or postpartum periods. Assessing family history of obesity can help determine possible genetic predispositions to weight gain [35]. The patient's lifestyle should be assessed, including nutrition and eating behaviors, physical activity, sleep, and stress. Previous use of anti-obesity medication or other treatments should be noted.

Nutrition and Dietary Treatments

To successfully lose weight, a caloric or energy deficit is required. It is generally accepted that the daily energy requirement is 1200–1500 kcal per day for women and 1500–1800 kcal per day for men, and an energy deficit of 500–750 kcal per day is required for weight loss [39]. Popular diets such as such as high-protein diets, lacto-ovo, vegetarian, or vegan diets, low-carbohydrate diets, low-fat diets, macronutrient diets, and the Mediterranean diet can all be effective, as long as this reduced dietary energy deficit is achieved [7].

Though all of these diets lead to short-term weight loss, most people are unable to maintain the weight loss over the long term [40]. This can be discouraging to patient and provider alike, but people who incorporate regular physical activity into their lifestyle have better success at maintaining their weight loss.

Physical Activity for Weight Loss

Scores of clinical trials have shown that aerobic physical activity is effective in helping overweight or obese people lose weight, with better outcomes with increasing intensity, duration, or frequency of the exercise [41]. Patients should progressively increase the volume and intensity of exercise until they reach the goal of ≥150 min per week of moderate exercise performed during 3–5 daily sessions per week [42–44]. Exercise should include resistance training to preserve fat-free muscle mass while losing fat.

Weight Loss Medications

Pharmacotherapy for weight loss in overweight and obese adults is effective but should be used only as an adjunct to lifestyle therapy and not alone [41]. There are seven US Food and Drug Administration (FDA)-approved weight loss medications (orlistat, phentermine, phentermine-topiramate, liraglutide, lorcaserin, naltrexone and bupropion, and semaglutide) and all are associated with more weight loss and weight loss maintenance and a decreased incidence of progression to type 2 diabetes compared with placebo at up to 48 months of follow-up [45]. Six of these medications are approved for long-term weight management while phentermine is only approved for short-term use.

Weight loss medications work through a variety of physiologic mechanisms, are consistently associated with weight loss among obese individuals, and cause several side effects (Table 2.2). A large review of 28 randomized clinical trials involving 29,018 patients of whom 74% were women (median baseline body weight, 100.5 kg; median baseline body mass index, 36.1) showed that the percentage of patients who successfully lost at least 5% of their weight was 63% for liraglutide, 49% for lorcaserin, 55% for naltrexone-bupropion, 44% for orlistat, and 75% for phentermine-topiramate, with 23% of those taking placebo also losing this percentage of weight [46]. Semaglutide is the newest medication approved by the FDA for chronic weight management in adults with obesity or overweight with at least one weight-related condition (e.g., high blood pressure, type 2 diabetes, or high cholesterol), for use in addition to a reduced-calorie diet and increased physical activity. It is the first newly approved drug for chronic weight management in adults since 2014.

Although pharmacological therapies are associated with weight loss and improvements in weight-related chronic diseases, they are not "magic pills" and should only be used as a complement to lifestyle changes in diet and exercise. Weight loss medications often have significant side effects, and most have not been studied regarding clinically relevant long-term outcomes such as heart disease and stroke. Weight loss medications can be prohibitively expensive for patients and are often not covered by health insurance, limiting their widespread use [47, 48]. Many clinicians still believe that patients with obesity should have the willpower to make the

Table 2.2 Physiologic mechanisms and side effects of FDA-approved weight loss medications

Medication	Mechanism	Therapeutic effect in randomized clinical trials	Side effects
Liraglutide	GLP-1 receptor agonist. Acts on GLP-1 receptors in the brain to increase postprandial satiety and fullness, reducing hunger. Injected SQ once daily. Treats diabetes and is effective in weight loss	Additional 6% reduction in weight when added to lifestyle changes. Improvements in CV risk markers such as waist circumference, hemoglobin A1c, systolic blood pressure, triglycerides, and high-sensitivity C-reactive protein [64, 65]	Nausea, hypoglycemia (in diabetics), diarrhea, constipation, vomiting, headache, decreased appetite, dyspepsia, fatigue, dizziness, abdominal pain, and increased lipase. Associated with gastrointestinal disorders, increased heart rate, pancreatitis, acute gallbladder disease, and in animal studies, thyroid tumor
Lorcaserin	Agonist of 5-hydroxytryptamine 2C receptor to suppress appetite. 5-HT2c receptors are located on the pro-opiomelanocortin neurons in the arcuate nucleus and are part of the anorexigenic pathway	Weight loss of 5.8% with improvement in blood pressure and lipid levels [66, 67]	Headaches, dizziness, nausea, fatigue, constipation, dry mouth, hypoglycemia (in diabetics). Rare cognitive impairment. Is a serotonergic agonist so can interact with other serotonin medications to cause serotonin syndrome or neuroleptic malignant syndrome. Avoid use with SSRIs, SNRIs, tricyclic antidepressants, bupropion, triptans, MAOIs, lithium, dextromethorphan, and dopamine agonists [41]
Naltrexone/Bupropion (sustained-release combination)	Naltrexone (opioid receptor antagonist) and bupropion (weak inhibitor of neuronal reuptake of dopamine and norepinephrine). Together they reduce food intake via activation of the anorexigenic pathway, dampening reward pathways, reducing compulsive feeding behavior and the pleasure of feeding	Weight loss of 3–8% with improved cardiovascular risk markers, such as hemoglobin A1c, waist circumference, HDL cholesterol, and triglycerides [68, 69]	Nausea, vomiting, constipation, headache, dizziness, dry mouth. Avoid in patients who are regularly taking opioids or who are experiencing opiate withdrawal
Orlistat	Intestinal lipase inhibitor that reduces fat absorption by approximately 30%	Weight loss, reduction in the risk of diabetes and improvements in blood pressure, lipid profile, waist circumference [41, 70–72]	Fecal leakage and a decrease in the absorption of fat-soluble vitamins, which can be addressed by taking a daily multivitamin containing vitamins A, D, E, K, and beta-carotene
Phentermine	Norepinephrine-releasing agent that suppresses appetite, is approved only for short-term use (≤ 3 months)	Additional 3.6 kg of weight loss compared to placebo [73]	Palpitations, tachycardia, increased blood pressure, overstimulation, restlessness, dizziness, insomnia, euphoria, dysphoria, tremor, headache, rare psychotic episodes, dry mouth, unpleasant taste, diarrhea, constipation, gastrointestinal disturbances, impotence, changes in libido, urticaria. Pulmonary hypertension and valvular heart disease when taken with fenfluramine
Phentermine/Topiramate extended release	Phentermine (see mechanism above) is approved for long-term use when combined with topiramate, an anticonvulsant that has weight loss side effects	Weight loss of ~10%, and reduction in waist circumference, blood pressure, lipid profiles, and fasting serum glucose [41, 74–77]	Paresthesia, dry mouth, constipation, unpleasant taste, insomnia, and dizziness
Semaglutide	GLP-1 agonist that targets areas of the brain that regulate appetite and food intake. Once weekly SQ injection with dose increased gradually over 16 to 20 weeks to reduce gastrointestinal side effects	15% reduction (15.3 kg) in weight at 68 weeks; reduction in CV risk factors and increase in physical functioning [78]	Nausea and diarrhea which were typically transient and mild-to-moderate in severity and subsided with time

Abbreviations: GLP-1 Glucagon-like peptide-1, *SQ* Subcutaneously, *CV* Cardiovascular, *SSRIs* Selective serotonin reuptake inhibitors, *SNRIs* Serotonin-norepinephrine reuptake inhibitors, *MAOIs* Monoamine oxidase inhibitors

changes in diet and exercise necessary to lose weight and are reluctant to prescribe medications. Many primary care physicians are not familiar enough with the medications to prescribe them, including the necessary discussion on the risks and benefits of these drugs. Many physicians recall the problems of the weight loss regimen of Fen-Phen, the combination of fenfluramine and phentermine, which was popular in the 1990s until the fenfluramine component was associated with heart valvular regurgitation and pulmonary hypertension, leading to withdrawal of the combination from the market in 1997 amid many lawsuits [49].

Given the global epidemic of obesity, physicians will serve their patients better if they are comfortable and familiar with weight loss medications. The American Board of Obesity Medicine (ABOM) allows US and Canadian physicians who are board-certified in a specialty recognized by the American Board of Medical Specialties to become experts in obesity medicine. Candidates must complete a minimum of 60 Continuing Medical Education credits on the topic of obesity, at least 30 of which must meet ABOM special designations, within the 36 months prior to applying to sit for the certification exam, which is offered annually (https://www.abom.org/). With more physicians comfortable in prescribing medications, and if health insurance companies realize the long-term cost savings and improved outcomes of weight reduction and thereby cover the costs of weight loss pharmacotherapy, these medications are likely to be used more widely in the coming years.

Metabolic Surgery

Many people with severe obesity have tried repeatedly to lose weight and even when successful often see the weight re-accumulate, much to their discouragement. Those with obesity-related chronic diseases are increasingly turning to metabolic surgery to help them achieve and sustain meaningful weight loss. The term metabolic surgery is now preferred rather than bariatric surgery, given the metabolic effects of these surgical procedures beyond weight loss [50]. Approximately 256,000 metabolic surgeries were performed in the US in 2019, an increase of 32% over 5 years [51]. The field is rapidly evolving with updated guidelines to identify who are the best candidates for these procedures, what type of procedures should be offered, and how patients should be managed before and after surgery [50]. People with a BMI $\geq$40 kg/m^2 or a BMI $\geq$35 kg/m^2 plus one or more obesity-related chronic diseases are generally eligible for metabolic surgery.

Sleeve gastrectomy is the most common metabolic surgery and consists of the resection of most of the stomach, creating a long, narrow, tubular stomach [52]. A variation of this is creating an anastomosis of the sleeve to a duodenal-ileal bypass, which is likely to become more common either as the original surgery or a revision to previous sleeve surgery. Roux-en-Y gastric bypass involves the creation of a small stomach and joining it with the resected end of the jejunum so that food bypasses the stomach and upper small intestine, which both restricts the size of the stomach and causes malabsorption. Another option known as laparoscopic adjustable gastric banding is now less common due to a higher rate of complications and less successful weight loss [53].

Metabolic surgery is more successful in initial and sustained weight loss than lifestyle interventions or medications [7]. Weight loss at 3 years after a metabolic surgical procedure is typically 20–35% of the person's original weight. The mechanism of the weight loss is far more complex than simply altering the size of the stomach and involves neuroendocrine changes likely involving improved β-cell function, improved insulin sensitivity, and alterations in gut physiology, bile acid metabolism, and gut microbiota [54]. These changes are especially effective in the treatment and even remission of diabetes, including a decreased risk of microvascular and macrovascular complications [55–57]. In addition to the anatomic changes of the surgery, hormones including glucagon-like peptide-1, peptide YY, insulin, leptin, ghrelin, C-reactive protein, interleukin-6, tumor necrosis factor–alpha, and adiponectin are affected, with the cumulative resultant effect of enhanced insulin secretion, reduced insulin resistance, earlier satiety, and delayed gastric emptying [54, 58]. People who have had metabolic surgery are consistently found to have improvement in fasting glucose and insulin levels, with a favorable impact on obesity-related comorbid chronic conditions [7]. This includes a reduction in the development of hypertension, obstructive sleep apnea, dyslipidemia, ischemic heart disease, heart failure, and breast, colon, and endometrial cancers [59, 60]. The reduction in endometrial and breast cancer is due to their association with estrogen, which is produced in part by fat cells, so the reduction in body fat mass lowers the risk [61]. Among people with obesity, those who have had metabolic surgery live longer than those without, though mortality remains higher in both groups compared to the non-obese population [62]. Metabolic surgery is cost-effective over a lifetime due to decreased medication costs, improvement in chronic diseases related to obesity, and indirect costs due to increased productivity [63].

Future Directions

Obesity is a complex chronic disease that is influenced by a broad range of metabolic, genetic, emotional, social, and economic factors. Humans are designed to survive in conditions of food scarcity and those very factors work against modern humans who desire to lose weight amid an abundance of food in an era when physical activity is no longer a part of daily life for most people. The understanding of the endocrine factors that influence the metabolic caloric balance in humans is rapidly evolving and the number of identified modulators of appetite already includes leptin, ghrelin, peptide YY, insulin, cholecystokinin, and glucagon-like peptide 1, with more to be identified. This provides the opportunity to develop effective treatments to counteract the compensatory mechanisms that work against sustained weight loss. Further research to substantiate the benefits of weight loss may reinforce and prioritize weight loss as a strategy for managing and treating the chronic illnesses that are so prevalent in modern society.

Medications may prove effective but may not replace the need for lifestyle modifications. More study may elucidate which eating patterns are healthiest, and how counseling or education can best motivate and support patients in living in a healthier manner. This includes studying whether remote care including telemedicine, text messaging, the internet, apps, or other media is effective in delivering lifestyle interventions.

As the population ages, it will be important to examine the benefits as well as the negative health consequences of weight loss in older adults. Studies on the effects of childhood obesity are needed, as well as strategies to mitigate negative long-term consequences. A better understanding of both the causes and treatments of obesity among economically disadvantaged populations can improve health outcomes across people who are often systematically ignored.

Research into the long-term outcomes of metabolic surgery is necessary to understand the benefits as well as the risks of these surgical procedures, and to establish who are the best candidates for good long-term results.

Ongoing research that establishes the health care costs and resource utilization attributed to obesity-related chronic diseases is critically needed to encourage payors to cover the costs of programs that support treatments for obesity, which may involve long-term support to maintain a healthy lifestyle. Obesity is a modern epidemic with high prevalence and significant impact and should be a research priority in the effort to improve the health of the population and lower health care costs.

References

1. Hales CM, Carroll MD, Fryar CD, Ogden CL. Prevalence of obesity and severe obesity among adults: United States, 2017–2018. NCHS Data Brief, no 360. Hyattsville, MD: National Center for Health Statistics. 2020.
2. World Health Organization. Obesity and overweight [Internet]. [cited 2022 Sep 10]. https://www.who.int/news-room/fact-sheets/detail/obesity-and-overweight
3. Heymsfield SB, Wadden TA. Mechanisms, pathophysiology, and management of obesity. N Engl J Med. 2017;376(3):254–66.
4. Kushner RF, Ryan DH. Assessment and lifestyle management of patients with obesity: clinical recommendations from systematic reviews. JAMA. 2014;312(9):943–52.
5. CDC. Defining adult overweight and obesity [Internet]. Centers for Disease Control and Prevention; 2022 [cited 2022 Sep 5]. https://www.cdc.gov/obesity/basics/adult-defining.html
6. Clinical guidelines on the identification, evaluation, and treatment of overweight and obesity in adults—the evidence report. National Institutes of Health. Obes Res. 1998;6(Suppl 2):51S–209S.
7. Obesity Expert Panel, National Heart, Lung, and Blood Institute. Guidelines (2013) for managing overweight and obesity in adults. Obesity (Silver Spring). 2014;22(Suppl 2):S40.
8. Ruiz-Castell M, Samouda H, Bocquet V, Fagherazzi G, Stranges S, Huiart L. Estimated visceral adiposity is associated with risk of cardiometabolic conditions in a population based study. Sci Rep. 2021;11(1):9121.
9. Sharma AM, Kushner RF. A proposed clinical staging system for obesity. Int J Obes. 2009;33(3):289–95.
10. Padwal RS, Pajewski NM, Allison DB, Sharma AM. Using the Edmonton obesity staging system to predict mortality in a population-representative cohort of people with overweight and obesity. CMAJ. 2011;183(14):E1059–66.
11. Atlantis E, Sahebolamri M, Cheema BS, Williams K. Usefulness of the Edmonton obesity staging system for stratifying the presence and severity of weight-related health problems in clinical and community settings: a rapid review of observational studies. Obes Rev. 2020;21(11):e13120.
12. Schwartz MW, Woods SC, Porte D, Seeley RJ, Baskin DG. Central nervous system control of food intake. Nature. 2000;404(6778):661–71.
13. van der Klaauw AA, Farooqi IS. The hunger genes: pathways to obesity. Cell. 2015;161(1):119–32.
14. Sumithran P, Prendergast LA, Delbridge E, Purcell K, Shulkes A, Kriketos A, et al. Long-term persistence of hormonal adaptations to weight loss. N Engl J Med. 2011;365(17):1597–604.
15. Bays HE, McCarthy W, Christensen S, Seger J, Wells S, Long J, Shah NN, Primack C. Obesity algorithm slides, presented by the Obesity Medicine Association. www.obesityalgorithm.org; 2018–2019 [cited 2022 Sep 5]. https://obesitymedicine.org/obesity-algorithm-powerpoint/
16. Huang Y, Lu Y, Huang YM, Wang M, Ling W, Sui Y, et al. Obesity in patients with COVID-19: a systematic review and meta-analysis. Metabolism. 2020;113:154378.
17. Yang J, Hu J, Zhu C. Obesity aggravates COVID-19: a systematic review and meta-analysis. J Med Virol. 2021;93(1):257–61.
18. Hendren NS, de Lemos JA, Ayers C, Das SR, Rao A, Carter S, et al. Association of body mass index and age with morbidity and mortality in patients hospitalized with COVID-19. Circulation. 2021;143(2):135–44.
19. Rodríguez-Flores M, Goicoechea-Turcott EW, Mancillas-Adame L, Garibay-Nieto N, López-Cervantes M, Rojas-Russell ME, et al. The utility of the Edmonton obesity staging system for the prediction of COVID-19 outcomes: a multi-Centre study. Int J Obes. 2022;46(3):661–8.
20. Yu W, Rohli KE, Yang S, Jia P. Impact of obesity on COVID-19 patients. J Diabetes Complications [Internet]. 2021;35(3) https://www.proquest.com/docview/2486124588/abstract/7B59B2C2AF894005PQ/1
21. Petrakis D, Margină D, Tsarouhas K, Tekos F, Stan M, Nikitovic D, et al. Obesity—a risk factor for increased COVID-19 prevalence, severity and lethality. Mol Med Rep. 2020 Jul;22(1):9–19.
22. Albashir AAD. The potential impacts of obesity on COVID-19. Clin Med (Lond). 2020;20(4):e109–13.
23. Sanchis-Gomar F, Lavie CJ, Mehra MR, Henry BM, Lippi G. Obesity and outcomes in COVID-19: when an epidemic and pandemic collide. Mayo Clin Proc. 2020;95(7):1445–53.
24. Byrd AS, Toth AT, Stanford FC. Racial disparities in obesity treatment. Curr Obes Rep. 2018;7(2):130–8.
25. Ogden CL, Fakhouri TH, Carroll MD, Hales CM, Fryar CD, Li X, et al. Prevalence of obesity among adults, by household income and education - United States, 2011-2014. MMWR Morb Mortal Wkly Rep. 2017;66(50):1369–73.
26. Simenson AJ, Corey S, Markovic N, Kinsky S. Disparities in chronic health outcomes and health Behaviors between lesbian and heterosexual adult women in Pittsburgh: a longitudinal study. J Womens Health (Larchmt). 2020;29(8):1059–67.

27. Cuevas AG, Chen R, Slopen N, Thurber KA, Wilson N, Economos C, et al. Assessing the role of health behaviors, socioeconomic status, and cumulative stress for racial/ethnic disparities in obesity. Obesity (Silver Spring). 2020;28(1):161–70.
28. Wang G, Johnson S, Gong Y, Polk S, Divall S, Radovick S, et al. Weight gain in infancy and overweight or obesity in childhood across the gestational spectrum: a prospective birth cohort study. Sci Rep. 2016;6:29867.
29. Cohen SA, Greaney ML, Sabik NJ. Assessment of dietary patterns, physical activity and obesity from a national survey: rural-urban health disparities in older adults. PLoS One. 2018;13(12):e0208268.
30. Foster BA, Weinstein K, Mojica CM, Davis MM. Parental mental health associated with child overweight and obesity, examined within rural and urban settings, stratified by income. J Rural Health. 2020;36(1):27–37.
31. Hernandez DC, Reesor LM, Murillo R. Food insecurity and adult overweight/obesity: gender and race/ethnic disparities. Appetite. 2017;117:373–8.
32. Young KL, Graff M, Fernandez-Rhodes L, North KE. Genetics of obesity in diverse populations. Curr Diab Rep. 2018;18(12):145.
33. US Preventive Services Task Force. Behavioral weight loss interventions to prevent obesity-related morbidity and mortality in adults: US preventive services task force recommendation statement. JAMA. 2018;320(11):1163–71.
34. Aspry KE, Van Horn L, Carson JAS, Wylie-Rosett J, Kushner RF, Lichtenstein AH, et al. Medical nutrition education, training, and competencies to advance guideline-based diet Counseling by physicians: a science advisory from the American Heart Association. Circulation. 2018;137(23):e821–41.
35. Kushner RF. Clinical assessment and management of adult obesity. Circulation. 2012;126(24):2870–7.
36. Palad CJ, Stanford FC. Use of people-first language with regard to obesity. Am J Clin Nutr. 2018;108(1):201–3.
37. Foster GD, Wadden TA, Makris AP, Davidson D, Sanderson RS, Allison DB, et al. Primary care physicians' attitudes about obesity and its treatment. Obes Res. 2003;11(10):1168–77.
38. Pool AC, Kraschnewski JL, Cover LA, Lehman EB, Stuckey HL, Hwang KO, et al. The impact of physician weight discussion on weight loss in US adults. Obes Res Clin Pract. 2014;8(2):e131–9.
39. Joint FAO/WHO/UNU Expert Consultation. Energy and protein requirements. Geneva: World Health Organization; 1985; [Internet] https://apps.who.int/iris/bitstream/handle/10665/39527/WHO_TRS_724_(chp1-chp6).pdf?sequence=1
40. Anderson JW, Konz EC, Frederich RC, Wood CL. Long-term weight-loss maintenance: a meta-analysis of US studies. Am J Clin Nutr. 2001;74(5):579–84.
41. Garvey WT, Mechanick JI, Brett EM, Garber AJ, Hurley DL, Jastreboff AM, et al. American Association of Clinical Endocrinologists and American College of Endocrinology Comprehensive Clinical practice guidelines for medical care of patients with obesity. Endocr Pract. 2016;22(Suppl 3):1–203.
42. Piercy KL, Troiano RP, Ballard RM, Carlson SA, Fulton JE, Galuska DA, et al. The physical activity guidelines for Americans. JAMA. 2018;320(19):2020–8.
43. Jensen MD, Ryan DH, Apovian CM, Ard JD, Comuzzie AG, Donato KA, et al. 2013 AHA/ACC/TOS guideline for the management of overweight and obesity in adults: a report of the American College of Cardiology/American Heart Association Task Force on practice Guidelines and The Obesity Society. Circulation. 2014;129(25 Suppl 2):S102–38.
44. Donnelly JE, Blair SN, Jakicic JM, Manore MM, Rankin JW, Smith BK, et al. American College of Sports Medicine Position Stand. Appropriate physical activity intervention strategies for weight loss and prevention of weight regain for adults. Med Sci Sports Exerc. 2009;41(2):459–71.
45. LeBlanc ES, Patnode CD, Webber EM, Redmond N, Rushkin M, O'Connor EA. Behavioral and pharmacotherapy weight loss interventions to prevent obesity-related morbidity and mortality in adults: updated evidence report and systematic review for the US preventive services task force. JAMA. 2018;320(11):1172–91.
46. Khera R, Murad MH, Chandar AK, Dulai PS, Wang Z, Prokop LJ, et al. Association of Pharmacological Treatments for obesity with weight loss and adverse events: a systematic review and meta-analysis. JAMA. 2016;315(22):2424–34.
47. Bessesen DH, Van Gaal LF. Progress and challenges in anti-obesity pharmacotherapy. Lancet Diabetes Endocrinol. 2018;6(3):237–48.
48. Finkelstein EA, Kruger E. Meta- and cost-effectiveness analysis of commercial weight loss strategies. Obesity (Silver Spring). 2014;22(9):1942–51.
49. Cunningham JW, Wiviott SD. Modern obesity pharmacotherapy: weighing cardiovascular risk and benefit. Clin Cardiol. 2014;37(11):693–9.
50. Mechanick JI, Apovian C, Brethauer S, Garvey WT, Joffe AM, Kim J, et al. Clinical practice guidelines for the perioperative nutrition, metabolic, and nonsurgical support of patients undergoing bariatric procedures—2019 update: cosponsored by American Association of Clinical Endocrinologists/American College of Endocrinology, the Obesity Society, American Society for Metabolic & Bariatric Surgery, Obesity Medicine Association, and American Society of Anesthesiologists—executive summary. Endocr Pract. 2019;25(12):1346–59.
51. American Society for Metabolic and Bariatric Surgery. Estimate of bariatric surgery numbers, 2011-2020 [internet]. American Society for Metabolic and Bariatric Surgery; 2022 [cited 2022 Sep 10]. https://asmbs.org/resources/estimate-of-bariatric-surgery-numbers
52. Banerjee ES, Schroeder R. Metabolic surgery for adult obesity: common questions and answers. Am Fam Physician. 2022;105(6):9.
53. Coblijn UK, Verveld CJ, van Wagensveld BA, Lagarde SM. Laparoscopic Roux-en-Y gastric bypass or laparoscopic sleeve gastrectomy as revisional procedure after adjustable gastric band—a systematic review. Obes Surg. 2013;23(11):1899–914.
54. Cho YM. A gut feeling to cure diabetes: potential mechanisms of diabetes remission after bariatric surgery. Diabetes Metab J. 2014;38(6):406–15.
55. Mingrone G, Panunzi S, De Gaetano A, Guidone C, Iaconelli A, Capristo E, et al. Metabolic surgery versus conventional medical therapy in patients with type 2 diabetes: 10-year follow-up of an open-label, single-Centre, randomised controlled trial. Lancet. 2021;397(10271):293–304.
56. Sjöström L, Peltonen M, Jacobson P, Ahlin S, Andersson-Assarsson J, Anveden Å, et al. Association of bariatric surgery with long-term remission of type 2 diabetes and with microvascular and macrovascular complications. JAMA. 2014;311(22):2297–304.
57. Billeter AT, Eichel S, Scheurlen KM, Probst P, Kopf S, Müller-Stich BP. Meta-analysis of metabolic surgery versus medical treatment for macrovascular complications and mortality in patients with type 2 diabetes. Surg Obes Relat Dis. 2019;15(7):1197–210.
58. Khosravi-Largani M, Nojomi M, Aghili R, Otaghvar HA, Tanha K, Seyedi SHS, et al. Evaluation of all types of metabolic bariatric surgery and its consequences: a systematic review and meta-analysis. Obes Surg. 2019;29(2):651–90.
59. Wiggins T, Guidozzi N, Welbourn R, Ahmed AR, Markar SR. Association of bariatric surgery with all-cause mortality and incidence of obesity-related disease at a population level: a systematic review and meta-analysis. PLoS Med. 2020;17(7):e1003206.

60. Schauer DP, Feigelson HS, Koebnick C, Caan B, Weinmann S, Leonard AC, et al. Bariatric surgery and the risk of cancer in a large multisite cohort. Ann Surg. 2019;269(1):95–101.
61. Persson I. Estrogens in the causation of breast, endometrial and ovarian cancers—evidence and hypotheses from epidemiological findings. J Steroid Biochem Mol Biol. 2000;74(5):357–64.
62. Carlsson LMS, Sjöholm K, Jacobson P, Andersson-Assarsson JC, Svensson PA, Taube M, et al. Life expectancy after bariatric surgery in the Swedish obese subjects study. N Engl J Med. 2020;383(16):1535–43.
63. Xia Q, Campbell JA, Ahmad H, Si L, de Graaff B, Palmer AJ. Bariatric surgery is a cost-saving treatment for obesity-a comprehensive meta-analysis and updated systematic review of health economic evaluations of bariatric surgery. Obes Rev. 2020;21(1):e12932.
64. Pi-Sunyer X, Astrup A, Fujioka K, Greenway F, Halpern A, Krempf M, et al. A randomized, controlled trial of 3.0 mg of liraglutide in weight management. N Engl J Med. 2015;373(1):11–22.
65. Wadden TA, Hollander P, Klein S, Niswender K, Woo V, Hale PM, et al. Weight maintenance and additional weight loss with liraglutide after low-calorie-diet-induced weight loss: the SCALE maintenance randomized study. Int J Obes. 2013;37(11):1443–51.
66. Fidler MC, Sanchez M, Raether B, Weissman NJ, Smith SR, Shanahan WR, et al. A one-year randomized trial of lorcaserin for weight loss in obese and overweight adults: the BLOSSOM trial. J Clin Endocrinol Metab. 2011;96(10):3067–77.
67. Smith SR, Weissman NJ, Anderson CM, Sanchez M, Chuang E, Stubbe S, et al. Multicenter, placebo-controlled trial of lorcaserin for weight management. N Engl J Med. 2010;363(3):245–56.
68. Greenway FL, Fujioka K, Plodkowski RA, Mudaliar S, Guttadauria M, Erickson J, et al. Effect of naltrexone plus bupropion on weight loss in overweight and obese adults (COR-I): a multicentre, randomised, double-blind, placebo-controlled, phase 3 trial. Lancet. 2010;376(9741):595–605.
69. Hollander P, Gupta AK, Plodkowski R, Greenway F, Bays H, Burns C, et al. Effects of naltrexone sustained-release/bupropion sustained-release combination therapy on body weight and glycemic parameters in overweight and obese patients with type 2 diabetes. Diabetes Care. 2013;36(12):4022–9.
70. Torgerson JS, Hauptman J, Boldrin MN, Sjöström L. XENical in the prevention of diabetes in obese subjects (XENDOS) study: a randomized study of orlistat as an adjunct to lifestyle changes for the prevention of type 2 diabetes in obese patients. Diabetes Care. 2004;27(1):155–61.
71. Davidson MH, Hauptman J, DiGirolamo M, Foreyt JP, Halsted CH, Heber D, et al. Weight control and risk factor reduction in obese subjects treated for 2 years with orlistat: a randomized controlled trial. JAMA. 1999;281(3):235–42.
72. O'Meara S, Riemsma R, Shirran L, Mather L, ter Riet G. A systematic review of the clinical effectiveness of orlistat used for the management of obesity. Obes Rev. 2004;5(1):51–68.
73. Li Z, Maglione M, Tu W, Mojica W, Arterburn D, Shugarman LR, et al. Meta-analysis: pharmacologic treatment of obesity. Ann Intern Med. 2005;142(7):532–46.
74. Allison DB, Gadde KM, Garvey WT, Peterson CA, Schwiers ML, Najarian T, et al. Controlled-release phentermine/topiramate in severely obese adults: a randomized controlled trial (EQUIP). Obesity (Silver Spring). 2012;20(2):330–42.
75. Gadde KM, Allison DB, Ryan DH, Peterson CA, Troupin B, Schwiers ML, et al. Effects of low-dose, controlled-release, phentermine plus topiramate combination on weight and associated comorbidities in overweight and obese adults (CONQUER): a randomised, placebo-controlled, phase 3 trial. Lancet. 2011;377(9774):1341–52.
76. Garvey WT, Ryan DH, Bohannon NJV, Kushner RF, Rueger M, Dvorak RV, et al. Weight-loss therapy in type 2 diabetes: effects of phentermine and topiramate extended release. Diabetes Care. 2014;37(12):3309–16.
77. Garvey WT, Ryan DH, Look M, Gadde KM, Allison DB, Peterson CA, et al. Two-year sustained weight loss and metabolic benefits with controlled-release phentermine/topiramate in obese and overweight adults (SEQUEL): a randomized, placebo-controlled, phase 3 extension study. Am J Clin Nutr. 2012;95(2):297–308.
78. Wilding JPH, Batterham RL, Calanna S, Davies M, Van Gaal LF, Lingvay I, et al. Once-weekly Semaglutide in adults with overweight or obesity. N Engl J Med. 2021;384(11):989–1002.

Promoting Physical Activity

Nailah Adams Morancie, Catherine Ellis, Alyssa Heinrich, and Justin Lee

Relationship of Reduced Physical Activity and Chronic Disease

Infectious diseases have accounted for the majority of deaths for most of human history, but since the middle of the twentieth century chronic diseases have been the leading cause of death in the US [1, 2]. One cause of the increase in deaths from chronic disease is a decrease in physical activity, which is a major risk factor contributing to deaths and disease burden, even more so than obesity. Increasing physical activity in the general population would reduce all-cause mortality risk by mitigating the impact of cardiovascular disease, diabetes, and cancer [3].

The 2018 National Health Interview Survey showed 74% of US adults participate in leisure-time physical activity [4, 5]. Persons aged 65 years and older are the most sedentary age group, with only 78% participating in sufficient amounts of physical activity. As life expectancy continues to rise, those aged 60 years and older are the fastest growing population in the Western Hemisphere [6, 7]. This makes understanding the link between active aging, physical activity, and chronic disease prevention and treatment increasingly important [3].

Aging and Exercise

Physical performance comprises neuromuscular endurance, strength, capacity, and power, all of which decline after the age of 60 [7]. Sarcopenia, the gradual loss of muscle due to aging, results from reduced regenerative capacity and perfusion with increased oxidative stress, mitochondrial dysfunction, and chronic inflammation [8]. The physiologic changes that result in sarcopenia position it as a mediator between chronic diseases and frailty [9, 10]. Older, less active individuals have a low ratio of appendicular (arms and legs) lean mass to body mass index (ALM_{BMI}) and this is associated with a 50% increased risk of mortality [11]. ALM_{BMI} is measured using dual-energy Xray absorptiometry (DEXA) to calculate the sum of lean mass in the arms and legs only [12]. Physical activity and structured exercise can reverse the effects of sarcopenia and age-related decline in function and cognition.

VO_{2max} is the calculation used to estimate aerobic capacity and can be estimated by the following calculation: [(maximum heart rate ÷ resting heart rate) × 15.3]. Aerobic endurance training improves aerobic capacity (VO_{2max}), which helps to reduce frailty in older adults [8]. Aerobic exercise improves muscle insulin sensitivity and prevents decline in mitochondrial respiratory capacity, leading to increased muscle endurance. Resistance exercise induces remarkable gains in strength and power in older adults, showing increases in muscle mass of 16–23% after four months of resistance training [8, 13]. These improvements provide health benefits and increase quality of life.

Frailty

Frailty is an age-related condition caused by neurally modulated multisystem decline in physiologic reserve and function [14]. The Clinical Frailty Scale is a widely used tool to evaluate categories including comorbidity, function, cognition, and other domains to develop a frailty score associated with health outcomes ranging from very fit (score of 1) to terminally ill (score of 9) [15]. Frailty is associated with disability, falls, hospital admissions, premature death, and lower quality of life among community-dwelling older adults [16–18]. Pharmacologic and non-pharmacologic interventions, proteins to reduce cell damage, and exercise are being investigated as possible strategies to reduce frailty in aging adults. Adequate aerobic and resistance training prevent or reduce frailty through increased muscle mass, strength, and endurance, which improves physical function [8].

N. A. Morancie (✉) · A. Heinrich · J. Lee
Department of Family Medicine, University of North Carolina at Chapel Hill, Chapel Hill, NC, USA
e-mail: nailah_adams@med.unc.edu; justin_lee@med.unc.edu

C. Ellis
Departments of Family Medicine and Orthopedics, University of North Carolina at Chapel Hill, Chapel Hill, NC, USA

Obesity and Chronic Disease

Obesity is defined by the World Health Organization as a weight-for-height ratio, known as body mass index (BMI), of 30 kg/m^2 or higher [18]. Other methods of obesity classification include the Edmonton Obesity Staging System, which ranges from Stage 0 to Stage 4 and classifies obesity based on a person's metabolic profile, psychologic health, and physical function [19]. Body fat percentage and waist circumference have also been studied as definitions of obesity [20]. Normal weight obesity, defined in persons with BMIs within normal limits but high body fat percentages, significantly increase the risk of cardiovascular disease, metabolic syndrome, and mortality [19]. However, the measurer-dependent discrepancies in estimating body fat percentage and the need for advanced imaging such as computed tomography or DEXA scans for accurate measurements limit the use of this measure in directing clinical outcomes. Globally, the BMI remains the most widely used definition of obesity [20].

The prevalence of obesity in US adults is high, with 42% of adults considered obese and 9% severely obese. Adults aged 40–59 years, women, and non-Hispanic Black adults have higher rates of severe obesity than other age groups, men, and other ethnicities and races respectively [21]. The association of obesity with comorbid chronic diseases is well established. Abnormal fat deposition around vasculature disrupts adipokine and cytokine-mediated vasoregulation, which, combined with inappropriate immune response, altered bioavailability of nitric oxide, and increased production of reactive oxygen species and other inflammatory factors, leads to the endothelial dysfunction that is the cause of the deleterious sequelae of obesity [22, 23]. Adults with obesity have an increased risk of coronary artery disease, stroke, hypertension, diabetes, insulin resistance, end stage renal disease, dyslipidemia, gall bladder disease, asthma, sleep apnea, arthritis, and many cancers compared with adults of normal weight [24–26]. Even persons who meet the BMI criteria but have normal metabolic profiles, known as metabolically healthy obesity, are at increased risk of hypertension, cardiovascular disease, and earlier mortality [27, 28].

Furthermore, the fat increases and muscle mass decreases that can occur with aging, known as 'sarcopenic obesity,' can lead to metabolic and functional impairment [20, 21]. Eighty percent of patients with non-alcoholic fatty liver disease are obese, particularly those with high amounts of visceral adipose tissue, which exacerbates the chronic inflammation and free fatty acid deposition into the venous system [22]. Every 5 kg/m^2 increase in BMI above 25 kg/m^2 increases the risk of rheumatoid arthritis by 13%, deaths due to vascular complications and diabetes by 41% and 210% respectively, and overall mortality by 29%, with the top three causes of death in patients with obesity being heart disease, cancer, and diabetes [23, 24]. Obesity increases the risk of depression and anxiety, cancer, and cancer-related deaths [25–27]. People with a BMI of 40–59 kg/m^2 live up to 13.7 years less than those with normal BMI [28].

The financial ramifications of this are staggering, with the direct costs related to the care of these diseases totaling $149 billion dollars annually, with the cost predicted to increase to $957 billion by 2030 [29, 30]. Indirect costs related to loss of productivity and employee absenteeism range from 3 to 6 billion dollars [31]. The burdens of obesity are many, and the factors that contribute to this issue are complex. However, physical activity and exercise, along with a healthy diet, are effective means by which some of these burdens may be lessened. Balancing net energy intake from calories consumed each day with total energy expenditure used for exercise plays a part in maintenance of appropriate weight. Intentional weight loss may reduce insulin levels, insulin-like growth factor 1, cholesterol, glucose, and pro-inflammatory adipokines and cytokines, thereby reducing the risk of chronic diseases including cancer [32].

Primary Prevention of Chronic Disease

Exercise can affect longevity, with a dose–response relationship between exercise and mortality [33]. The American Heart Association recommends that adults engage in at least 150–300 min of *moderate* exercise per week or 75–150 min of *vigorous* exercise per week, both of which confer significant health benefits [34].

Energy expenditure is commonly measured in metabolic equivalency of task units, or METs. One MET is equivalent to the rate of energy expenditure of an individual at rest. Moderate-intensity exercise is classified as 3.0–5.9 METs, which is to say that the relative energy expenditure of moderate activities such as brisk walking and doubles tennis is 3–5.9 times more energy than a resting state. Vigorous physical activities, such as jogging, running, or carrying heavy loads, confer a MET of 6 or above. A common measurement for activity is the *MET minute*s, which is the MET multiplied by the time in minutes spent at that level of energy expenditure. Even individuals who engage in limited physical activity (defined as 0–1999 MET minutes/month) have survival benefits, with those engaging in five times the recommended amount of moderate to vigorous physical activity (>20,000 MET minutes/month) having the greatest benefit, with as much as a 45% risk reduction of all-cause mortality [35].

Cardiovascular disease is the leading cause of death in both men and women in the US [2]. Exercise can prevent coronary artery disease and stroke by increasing cardioprotective cholesterol, improving endothelial function, normalizing blood pressure, and reducing glucose [36, 37]. Men engaged in fitness lower their risk of stroke and subsequent mortality by 68% when compared to low-fitness counterparts [36, 38].

Physical activity is associated with lower risk of breast and colon cancer, likely due to a reduction of circulating sex hormone levels, increase in insulin-like growth factor receptor binding protein, and decrease in prostaglandin levels [38,

39]. Physical activity in the US population at the level recommended in the physical activity guidelines would prevent 46,000 cancer cases annually [40].

As of 2020, one in five US adults experience mental illness, and there is evidence that exercise intervention can reduce or prevent symptoms of anxiety and depression [41]. In patients with depression, regular exercise is effective in prevention and symptom reduction [42, 43]. In the short term, exercise can directly reduce acute anxiety states, while longer-term regular exercise can reduce anxiety traits in individuals both with and without anxiety disorders [44]. In school-aged children and adolescents, regular exercise reduces the risk of depression and improves academic performance, executive function, and memory, especially in certain conditions such as attention deficit and hyperactivity disorders [45]. Exercise also improves sleep quality and efficiency, which can help support equilibrium in anxious or depressive states [46, 47]. Exercise is also associated with decreased risk of cognitive decline and dementia [48–50]. Physical activity is a low-risk intervention, and is beneficial for the primary prevention of many conditions and can be modified to suit an individual's limitations. A summary of the health benefits associated with physical activity can be found in Table 3.1 [51].

Table 3.1 Health Benefits Associated with Regular Physical Activity (Adapted from *Physical Activity Guidelines for Americans 2nd edition*, 2018) [51]

Children and adolescents
• Improved bone health (ages 3 through 17 years)
• Improved weight status (aged 3 through 17 years)
• Improved cardiovascular and muscular fitness (ages 6 through 17 years)
• Improved cardiometabolic health (ages 6 through 17 years)
• Improved cognition (ages 6 through 13 years)
• Reduced risk of depression (ages 6 through 13 years)
Adults
• Lower risk of all-cause mortality
• Lower risk of cardiovascular disease mortality
• Lower risk of cardiovascular disease (including heart disease and stroke)
• Lower risk of hypertension
• Lower risk of type 2 diabetes
• Lower risk of adverse blood lipid profile
• Lower risk of cancers of the bladder, breast, colon, endometrium, esophagus, kidney, lung, and stomach
• Improved cognition
• Reduced risk of dementia (including Alzheimer's disease)
• Improved quality of life
• Reduced anxiety and depression
• Improved sleep
• Slowed or reduced weight gain
• Weight loss, particularly when combined with reduced calorie intake
• Prevention of weight regain after initial weight loss
• Improved bone health
• Improved physical function
• Lower risk of falls and fall-related injuries (older adults)

Note: The Advisory Committee rated the evidence of health benefits of physical activity as strong, moderate, limited, or grade not assignable. Only outcomes with strong or moderate evidence of effect are included in this table

Secondary Prevention of Chronic Disease

Diabetes Mellitus

Patients with poorly controlled diabetes have a three to four times higher risk of stroke and heart disease [52]. Exercise improves glycemic control and cardiovascular health [53]. A structured aerobic exercise program that includes resistance training, walking, cycling, or jogging reduces hemoglobin A1c values by 0.6%, which is significant given that a 1% decrease in hemoglobin A1c is associated with a 20% reduction in major cardiovascular events and a 37% reduction in microvascular complications [54]. The combination of both aerobic and resistance exercises is superior to either type of exercise alone in improving hemoglobin A1c due to increased insulin sensitivity, reduced ectopic fat, better lipid values, and lowered blood pressure [55]. Still, only 39% of adults with diabetes are physically active [56].

The American College of Sports Medicine and the American Diabetes Association recommend that patients with diabetes perform 30 min of moderate- to vigorous-intensity aerobic exercise at least five days a week or a total of 150 min per week [54, 57]. This activity should occur at least three days per week with no more than two days in a row without exercise. The US Preventive Services Task Force does not recommend pre-exercise program stress testing in asymptomatic individuals with a low coronary artery disease (CAD) risk (<10% risk of a cardiac event over 10 years). However, ECG stress testing may be indicated in patients with diabetes for more than 10 years or with signs of end-organ disease. Patients with certain complications of diabetes require special consideration [54]. For example, those with diabetic peripheral neuropathy are at increased risk of falls and benefit from balance exercises and activities with less fall risk, such as stationary bike and swimming. Patients with proliferative retinopathy from their diabetes are at risk of vitreous hemorrhage and retinal detachment with exercise and should avoid heavy lifting and vigorous exercise and focus instead on low-impact activities such as biking, walking in a pool, slow hiking, and elliptical machines.

Cardiovascular Diseases

Regular physical activity is an effective tool for secondary prevention of cardiovascular diseases [58–61]. Patients with coronary artery disease (CAD) have an increased risk of sudden cardiac death and/or acute myocardial infarction with vigorous exercise and therefore should undergo stress testing and assessment of left ventricular function prior to starting an exercise routine [62]. Clinicians and patients should then engage in shared decision-making regarding results, considering risks versus benefits of exercise. The recommended amount of physical activity is three to four 40-min sessions of moderate to vigorous aerobic activity per week, which improves both survival and quality of life in people with CAD. [58, 59, 61, 63, 64]

Hypertension is the most common modifiable cardiovascular condition among the general population, affecting 160 million US adults [64, 65]. Physical activity is effective as secondary prevention for hypertension and reduces the incidence of stroke and all-cause and cardiovascular mortality [66–68]. Both systolic blood pressure (SBP) and diastolic blood pressure (DBP) remain lower for up to 24 hours after aerobic exercise [69].

For those with stage 1 hypertension (SBP 140–159 mmHg or DBP 90–99 mmHg), there are no restrictions to initiating exercise, provided blood pressure is monitored every few months. Stage 1 patients with sustained hypertension following exercise should have an echocardiogram. Patients with stage 2 hypertension (SBP >160 mmHg or DBP >100 mmHg) should avoid high static sports (weightlifting, wrestling, etc.) until blood pressure is controlled [64].

Chronic Obstructive Pulmonary Disease

Chronic obstructive pulmonary disease (COPD) causes airflow obstruction, prolonged expiratory phase, air trapping, and inflammation [70]. COPD is the third leading cause of death in the US, accounting for more than 3 million deaths in 2019 [71]. Patients with COPD have fatigue, shortness of breath, poor functional status and quality of life, and poor exercise tolerance [72]. All of this improves with exercise, not by improving lung function, but by maximizing the function of other body systems. Gains in muscle strength and endurance allow a patient to work harder with delayed fatigue and decreased ventilation demand, which allows for more time for expiration of air [73, 74]. Psychological factors, such as increased tolerance to dyspnea, are positively affected with exercise [75]. This may be due to the antidepressant effects of exercise, social interaction, and distraction when participating in pulmonary rehabilitation programs with other people having the same condition or education of patients regarding their disease.

Although the benefit of exercise is clearly established in patients with COPD, there are risks. Musculoskeletal injury is a concern as most patients with COPD are debilitated and may need supervision [72]. Exercise-induced bronchospasm is not uncommon, and patients need to have their bronchodilators on hand. Patients with COPD are at increased risk for cardiovascular death and may need stress testing before starting an exercise program [76, 77].

Pulmonary rehabilitation is an interdisciplinary intervention that can be started at any stage of disease. Endurance and resistance exercise for the upper and lower extremities is central to any pulmonary rehabilitation program and improves function [72]. High-intensity workouts are preferred, targeting 60% of VO_{2max}, but even low-intensity exercise produces benefit. Health benefits are seen after just six weeks of exercise with longer programs likely sustaining benefit [78–80].

Osteoporosis

Osteoporosis is characterized by low bone mass and microarchitecture deterioration of bone tissue leading to bone fragility and increase in fracture risk. Over 200 million people are currently diagnosed with osteoporosis, and the incidence rate increases with age [81]. Between 30% and 50% of women and 15–20% of men will suffer an osteoporotic fracture in their lifetime, often as the presenting symptom of the disease [82].

Though there are pharmaceutical treatments for osteoporosis, physical activity is still the first recommendation in the prevention of osteoporosis and fragility fractures. Resistance training and weight-bearing exercises are likely to help build and preserve bone mass. Exercise enhances muscular strength and coordination, which reduces the risk of falling, the major risk factor for fragility fractures and the most common cause of mortality and morbidity from osteoporosis. A physically active lifestyle is associated with a 50% decrease of hip fractures, presumably related to a decrease in fall risk [83–85]. Exercises such as tai chi focus on posture and weight bearing using low-velocity movements of the body, which increases muscular strength and improves balance, postural stability, and flexibility, reducing the risk of falls in older adults by 50%. Starting physical activity at a young age likely contributes to higher peak bone mass later in life, and short-term gains in bone density can be measured in children and adolescents [86, 87].

In women, multi-component exercise programs with jogging, walking, or stair climbing and resistance training improve the bone density at both the lumbar spine and the femoral neck. Programs that focus solely on resistance training or weight-bearing exercise result in changes to only the lumbar spine and femoral neck, respectively [88–91]. Walking and endurance training alone have little to no effect on femoral neck or lumbar spine bone density. High-impact jumping programs without other exercises are also ineffective [92–96].

Studies on the effects of exercise on bones in men are limited but show that high-intensity progressive resistance training combined with moderate-impact to high-impact weight-bearing exercises performed at least three times a week can improve femoral neck bone density [82, 97]

Exercise programs that involve weight-bearing activities that are variable in nature and applied rapidly, such as skipping, dancing, jumping, and hopping, and are performed three to five times a week for up to 45 min per session are most effective in increasing bone strength [98–100]. In older adults where high-impact exercises may be contraindicated, low- to moderate-impact weight-bearing exercise in combination with progressive resistance and/or agility training is safe and effective [95, 97, 101]. In frail elderly patients who are prone to fall, regular low-impact aerobics, dance exercises, or resistance training on machines may be a safe option. In younger subjects, nonlinear high-impact and high-loading activities at least twice weekly are beneficial and safe [102–104].

Osteoarthritis

Osteoarthritis (OA) is a chronic degenerative joint disorder and the most frequent cause of disability among adults in the US [105]. It affects more than 50 million adults and is the fourth most common cause of hospitalization. In 2020, almost 1.8 million knee and hip replacements were performed at a cost of over $60 billion [106]. The risk of OA by age 85 is one in two and increases to two in three for those who are obese [6, 106, 107]. Other risk factors are family history, female sex, past trauma, muscular weakness, and advancing age.

OA often asymmetrically affects the hands, knees, hips, and spine. Although any joint can be affected, knees followed by hips are the most affected joints [108]. The disease process involves the whole joint, including cartilage, bone, ligament, and muscle, with joint pain the predominant symptom. OA is defined radiographically by joint space narrowing, bony osteophytes, bone contour deformity, and/or sclerosis, and clinically by descriptions that consider age, stiffness, warmth, crepitus, tenderness, and bony enlargement [109]. These symptoms lead to physical and psychological disabilities and impaired quality of life.

Despite evidence that exercise is beneficial, most people with OA do not achieve recommended levels of physical activity. This leads to muscle weakness which worsens joint biomechanics, making joints less stable and subject to pathologic shear, which causes microtrauma and cartilage degeneration, subchondral bone sclerosis, and malalignment [110]. Exercise and muscle strengthening is the cornerstone of nonsurgical management of OA and reduces pain while increasing physical function, so patients can pursue social, domestic, occupational, and recreational activities [111–113]. Land-based exercises reduce pain and improve physical function in those with knee OA [108]. There is less evidence regarding hip OA.

Any weight loss in beneficial, with weight loss of greater than 5% per week leading to significant improvement in disability and reductions in the load placed on the knee in individuals with knee osteoarthritis [114]. Incorporating strength training during weight loss helps prevent muscle wasting and increase lean mass while dieting to achieve weight loss [115].

Exercise therapy should be individualized with patient age, mobility, comorbidities, and preferences considered. Aquatic therapy or seated exercises may be better tolerated by patients who are deconditioned or obese. Exercise may be effectively delivered via individual treatments or supervised groups, or can be performed unsupervised [116]. Some supervision may lead to improvement in movement and walking pain in the long term. General exercise programs are safe and well tolerated for most people with lower limb OA but are often limited by discomfort at the affected joint, which may require modification to the exercise regimen. Adequate footwear, proper warm-up and cooldown, correct exercise technique, proper clothing, and gradual increases in exercise dose are recommended [117].

Promoting Physical Activity

There are innumerable benefits of physical activity for a host of chronic diseases. Most practitioners are at least partially aware of these benefits and the crucial role that exercise can play in a comprehensive treatment plan, yet many consistently fail to incorporate activity recommendations into the plan of care. Only a third of patients report that their physician has advised them to be physically active [118]. Many clinicians are uncertain as to how to write an appropriate exercise prescription or do not know what counseling strategies are effective. Only 6% of medical schools include exercise guidelines in their core curriculum [119, 120]. System factors include lack of time during visits, an emphasis on acute issues rather than preventive medicine, and lack of financial reimbursement for exercise counseling. Although these barriers exist, physicians can influence patients' physical activity. Patients provided with physician advice and written materials had about a 1 kcal/kg/day increase in physical activity six months after the initial encounter. In an 80 kg man, this would translate into almost a 600 kcal/week increase in physical activity, indicating that effective counseling on physical activity is a worthwhile use of time in a physician–patient encounter. Several successful models are highlighted below [121].

Exercise as a Vital Sign

Exercise is Medicine is a campaign that began as a collaboration between the American College of Sports Medicine, the American Medical Association, and the US Surgeon General. Part of this campaign is the concept of "Exercise as a Vital Sign," which encouraged providers to prescribe exercise to patients [122, 123]. In addition to the usual vital signs, patients were asked "On average, how many days per week do you engage in moderate to vigorous physical activity (like brisk walking)?" and "On average, how many minutes do you engage in physical activity at this level?" The answers were multiplied to obtain the total number of minutes of physical activity per week and recorded in the patient's medical record. These initiated discussions of physical activity highlight the importance of exercise, are associated with modest weight loss in overweight patients, and improve glucose control in people with diabetes. By recording physical activity in an electronic medical record, clinicians can track values over time and patient progression toward exercise goals. From a public health standpoint, aggregating physical activity data may be a tool for analysis of health discrepancies by geographical area.

The Exercise Prescription

Providing a written prescription for exercise may be effective in motivating patients to be more active. One effective and simple prescription is known as the FITT model and includes specific recommendations regarding **F**requency (number of days per week), **I**ntensity (moderate or vigorous), **T**ype (modality of activity, often dependent on the resources available to the patient, limitations of the chronic medical conditions, and their personal interests), and **T**ime (length of the session or the number of repetitions) [123]. As patients advance it is important to increase duration or frequency before increasing intensity. Exercise prescriptions should include a recommendation for two days/week of strength training. All sessions should include a dynamic warm-up, the main cardiorespiratory phase, and then a cooldown period [122].

Defining Physical Activity and Exercise

Physical activity is defined as bodily movement that is produced by the contraction of skeletal muscle and that substantially increases energy expenditure. Exercise is defined as a type of physical activity that is planned, structured, and repetitive bodily movement done to improve or maintain one or more components of physical fitness. Exercise occurs outside the expected or unexpected activities of the day [124].

Exercise can generally be divided into four subtypes [125]:

1. Aerobic/endurance: any activity requiring the body's large muscle groups to move in a rhythmic pattern for sustained periods of time. Examples include walking, hiking, jogging, cycling, and swimming.
2. Balance/neuromotor training: combination of activities to improve lower body strength and reduce the chances of falling. Examples include single leg stance, tandem walking, yoga, and tai chi.
3. Resistance/strength training: exercises that require muscles to work or hold against an applied force or weight. Examples include weight machines, handheld weights, push-ups, use of resistance bands, and heavy lifting (groceries, furniture, etc.).
4. Flexibility training: exercises designed to maintain or extend range of motion of joints. Examples include static stretching (holding a stretch for period of time), dynamic stretching (gradual transition from one body position to another), ballistic stretching (momentum of moving body part to produce the stretch), and proprioceptive neuromuscular facilitation (isometric contraction of muscle-tendon unit immediately followed by static stretching of same body part, i.e., contract-relax) [57].

Recommendations for Adults

The 2018 Department of Health and Human Services Physical Activity Guidelines recommend that all adults strive to be more active and sit less, and conclude that some physical activity is better than none [51]. To achieve substantial health benefits, adults should perform 150–300 min of moderate-intensity aerobic exercise per week or 75–150 min of vigorous-intensity aerobic exercise per week spread across three separate days [51, 57]. Additional health benefits can be achieved by increasing weekly physical activity above 300 min of moderate-intensity exercise or 150 min of vigorous-intensity exercise. The talk test is a practical, valid, and reliable test that can be used to determine if an exercise is of moderate to vigorous intensity. If a person can talk but not sing during aerobic activity, this is considered moderate intensity. If a person cannot say more than a few words without pausing to breathe, this is considered vigorous intensity [126]. Table 3.2 lists examples of activities classified as moderate or vigorous intensity [43].

Table 3.2 Examples of different aerobic physical activities and intensities, based on absolute intensity (adapted from *Physical Activity Guidelines for Americans 2nd edition*, 2018)

Moderate-intensity activities
• Walking briskly (2.5 miles per hour or faster)
• Recreational swimming
• Bicycling slower than 10 miles per hour on level terrain
• Tennis (doubles)
• Active forms of yoga (e.g.,, vinyasa or power yoga)
• Ballroom or line dancing
• General yard work and home repair work
• Exercise classes like water aerobics

Vigorous-intensity activities
• Jogging or running
• Swimming laps
• Tennis (singles)
• Vigorous dancing
• Bicycling faster than 10 miles per hour
• Jumping rope
• Heavy yard work (digging or shoveling, with heart rate increases)
• Hiking uphill or with a heavy backpack
• High-intensity interval training
• Exercises class like vigorous aerobic or kickboxing

Muscle strengthening exercises should be performed for all major muscle groups at least two days per week with at least one set of eight to 12 repetitions. The American College of Sports Medicine recommends flexibility exercises involving most major muscle groups at least two days per week as well as neuromotor/balance training at least two days per week [57].

Recommendations for Older Adults

Physical activity guidelines for older adults are the same as for their younger adult counterparts [51]. For those older adults who cannot do 150 min of moderate-intensity aerobic activity per week because of chronic conditions, it is recommended they determine their level of activity relative to their fitness level and be as physically active as their health allows. Older adults should incorporate balance training into their physical activity regimen along with aerobic and resistance training exercise.

Recommendations for Obese Patients

Though the benefits of exercise outweigh the risks in obese patients, there are some points to consider when recommending an exercise prescription to these patients. Gradual increase in duration and intensity level should be recommended [127]. This prevents stress fractures and other overuse injuries and allows for confidence building with each successfully completed level. Avoiding high-impact activities minimizes joint forces and lowers the risk for early osteoarthritis. Obese patients have lowered proprioception sense and joint awareness predisposing them to falls, acute ligament sprains, and muscle tears. Thermoregulation is diminished, so education regarding heat exhaustion and heat stroke is crucial and appropriate hydration strategies should be advised for before, during, and after exercise. Although the risk is low for a cardiac event during low-intensity exercise, a patient's risk factors for cardiovascular disease should be evaluated prior to initiating an exercise regimen [127, 128].

Current recommendations for exercise in adults suggest 150 min or greater of moderate-intensity exercise per week or 75 min per week of vigorous exercise [127, 129]. While any level of exercise improves health, a high-intensity regimen is required to produce significant weight loss. Patients should aim for gradual lessening of daily caloric intake with increasing levels of physical activity [127, 128, 130]. For able-bodied patients, 150–200 min of walking per week can prevent weight gain and improve cardiovascular fitness, but a minimum of 60 min of moderate-intensity exercise per day is often needed to achieve weight loss. Aerobic activity results in improved endurance, weight loss, and a decrease in abdominal and visceral fat. Resistance training demonstrates improved muscle mass and strength. Each of these exercise types is important for obese patients and should be included in exercise prescriptions [127, 128].

Recommendations for Children

Sedentary behavior in childhood is associated with poorer cardiometabolic health and weight status/adiposity (Fig. 3.1) [51]. Preschool-aged children (3–5 years of age) should be physically active for at least 3 h a day to support growth and development [51]. School-aged children and adolescents (6–17 years of age) should aim to do at least 60 min per day of moderate-to-vigorous physical activity. A variety of activities constitute physical activities in young people (Table 3.3). Much of this time should be devoted to moderate or vigorous

Fig. 3.1 Relationship of moderate-to-vigorous physical activity to all-cause mortality

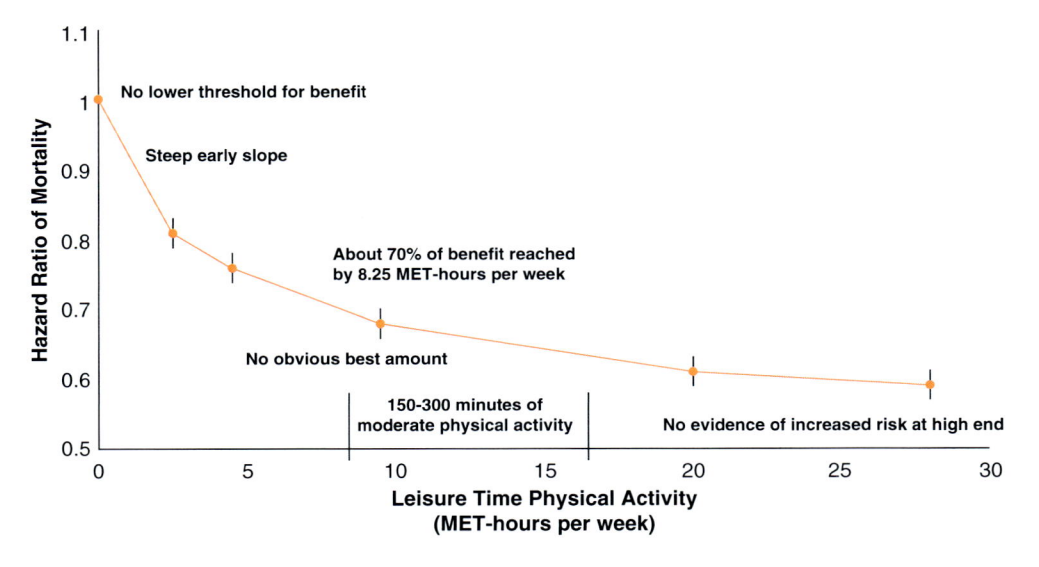

Source: Adapted from data found in Moore SC, Patel AV, Matthews CE. Leisure time physical activity of moderate to vigorous intensity and mortality: a large pooled cohort analysis. PLoS Med. 2012;9(11):e1001335. doi:10.1371/journal.pmed.1001335.

Table 3.3 Examples of aerobic, muscle-, and bone-strengthening physical activities for children and adolescents (adapted from *Physical Activity Guidelines for Americans 2nd edition*, 2018)

Type of physical activity	Preschool-aged children	School-aged children	Adolescents
Moderate-intensity aerobic	• Games such as tag or follow the leader • Playing on a playground • Tricycle or bicycle riding • Walking, running, skipping, jumping, dancing • Swimming • Playing games that require catching • Gymnastics or tumbling	• Brisk walking • Bicycle riding • Active recreation, such as hiking, riding a scooter without a motor, swimming • Playing games that require catching and throwing, such as baseball and softball	• Brisk walking • Bicycle riding • Active recreation, such as kayaking, hiking, swimming • Playing games that require catching and throwing, such as baseball and softball • House and yard work, such as sweeping or pushing a lawn mower • Some video games that include continuous movement
Vigorous-intensity aerobic	• Games such as tag or follow the leader • Playing on a playground • Tricycle or bicycle riding • Walking, running, skipping, jumping, dancing • Swimming • Playing games that require catching, throwing, and kicking • Gymnastics or tumbling	• Running • Bicycle riding • Active games involving running and chasing, such as tag or flag football • Jumping rope • Cross-country skiing. • Sports such as soccer, basketball, swimming, tennis • Martial arts • Vigorous dancing	• Running • Bicycle riding • Active games involving running and chasing, such as flag football • Jumping rope • Cross-country skiing • Sports such as soccer, basketball, swimming, tennis • Martial arts • Vigorous dancing
Muscle strengthening	• Games such as tug of war • Climbing on playground equipment • Gymnastics	• Games such as tug of war • Resistance exercises using body weight or resistance bands • Rope or tree climbing • Climbing on playground equipment • Some forms of yoga	• Games such as tug of war • Resistance exercises using body weight, resistance bands, weight machines, hand-held weights • Some forms of yoga
Bone strengthening	• Hopping, skipping, jumping • Jumping rope • Running • Gymnastics	• Hopping, skipping, jumping • Jumping rope • Running • Sports that involve jumping or rapid change in direction	• Jumping rope • Running • Sports that involve jumping or rapid change in direction

aerobic exercise, which includes muscle- and bone-strengthening exercises, at least three days per week. Adults should encourage and provide age-appropriate and enjoyable activities to inspire youth to be physically active.

Community and Clinic Initiatives

The cost of an individual gym or fitness program membership can be a barrier for many people. Some communities, health care systems, or corporations sponsor and encourage physical activity through free programs in local parks. Shopping mall walking programs positively impact individuals and communities [131, 132]. Physical education classes are often cut as part of cost-saving measures in school systems, which can be detrimental to the health of the students. The rise in childhood obesity and the well-documented individual and public health issues secondary to obesity should underscore why physical education and activity must remain a cornerstone of our school systems [133].

Future Trends

Primary care has an integral role in improving the lives of the population. The transition to value-based care payment models, where doctors are paid for keeping people well rather than for performing procedures, will appropriately incentivize care approaches that improve health and prevent disease [134, 135]. Physical activity is foundational in the health of individuals and populations, including in the prevention and management of chronic diseases.

References

1. Remington PL, et al. Fifty years of progress in chronic disease epidemiology and control. MMWR Suppl. 2011;60(4):70–7.
2. Murphy SL, et al. Mortality in the United States, 2020. NCHS Data Brief. 2021;427:1–8.
3. Bauman A, et al. Updating the evidence for physical activity: summative reviews of the epidemiological evidence, prevalence,

and interventions to promote "active aging". Gerontologist. 2016;56(Suppl 2):S268–80.
4. CDC, National Health Interview Survey. https://www.cdc.gov/nchs/nhis/index.htm
5. Whitfield GP, et al. Trends in aerobic physical activity participation across multiple domains among US adults, National Health and nutrition examination survey 2007/2008 to 2017/2018. J Phys Act Health. 2021;18(S1):S64–s73.
6. Murphy L, et al. Lifetime risk of symptomatic knee osteoarthritis. Arthritis Rheum. 2008;59(9):1207–13.
7. Mendonca GV, et al. Impact of aging on endurance and neuromuscular physical performance: the role of vascular senescence. Sports Med. 2017;47(4):583–98.
8. Angulo J, El Assar M, Rodriguez-Manas L. Frailty and sarcopenia as the basis for the phenotypic manifestation of chronic diseases in older adults. Mol Asp Med. 2016;50:1–32.
9. Singer JP, Lederer DJ, Baldwin MR. Frailty in pulmonary and critical care medicine. Ann Am Thorac Soc. 2016;13(8):1394–404.
10. Sinclair AJ, Rodriguez-Manas L. Diabetes and frailty: two converging conditions? Can J Diabetes. 2016;40(1):77–83.
11. Dodds RM, Sayer AA. Sarcopenia, frailty and mortality: the evidence is growing. Age Ageing. 2016;45(5):570–1.
12. Cawthon PM. Assessment of lean mass and physical performance in sarcopenia. J Clin Densitom. 2015;18(4):467–71.
13. Carter A, et al. Racial and ethnic health care disparities among women in the veterans affairs healthcare system: a systematic review. Womens Health Issues. 2016;26(4):401–9.
14. Xue QL. The frailty syndrome: definition and natural history. Clin Geriatr Med. 2011;27(1):1–15.
15. Sternberg SA, et al. The identification of frailty: a systematic literature review. J Am Geriatr Soc. 2011;59(11):2129–38.
16. Pamoukdjian F, et al. Measurement of gait speed in older adults to identify complications associated with frailty: a systematic review. J Geriatr Oncol. 2015;6(6):484–96.
17. Fried LP, et al. Frailty in older adults: evidence for a phenotype. J Gerontol A Biol Sci Med Sci. 2001;56(3):M146–56.
18. Rizzoli R, et al. Quality of life in sarcopenia and frailty. Calcif Tissue Int. 2013;93(2):101–20.
19. Oliveros E, et al. The concept of normal weight obesity. Prog Cardiovasc Dis. 2014;56(4):426–33.
20. Roubenoff R. Sarcopenic obesity: does muscle loss cause fat gain? Lessons from rheumatoid arthritis and osteoarthritis. Ann N Y Acad Sci. 2000;904:553–7.
21. Lim KI, et al. The association between the ratio of visceral fat to thigh muscle area and metabolic syndrome: the Korean Sarcopenic Obesity Study (KSOS). Clin Endocrinol. 2010;73(5):588–94.
22. Milic S, Lulic D, Stimac D. Non-alcoholic fatty liver disease and obesity: biochemical, metabolic and clinical presentations. World J Gastroenterol. 2014;20(28):9330–7.
23. Prospective Studies, C, et al. Body-mass index and cause-specific mortality in 900 000 adults: collaborative analyses of 57 prospective studies. Lancet. 2009;373(9669):1083–96.
24. Feng J, et al. Body mass index and risk of rheumatoid arthritis: a meta-analysis of observational Studies. Medicine (Baltimore). 2016;95(8):e2859.
25. Luppino FS, et al. Overweight, obesity, and depression: a systematic review and meta-analysis of longitudinal studies. Arch Gen Psychiatry. 2010;67(3):220–9.
26. Bhaskaran K, et al. Body-mass index and risk of 22 specific cancers: a population-based cohort study of 5.24 million UK adults. Lancet. 2014;384(9945):755–65.
27. Calle EE, et al. Overweight, obesity, and mortality from cancer in a prospectively studied cohort of U.S. adults. N Engl J Med. 2003;348(17):1625–38.
28. Kitahara CM, et al. Association between class III obesity (BMI of 40-59 kg/m2) and mortality: a pooled analysis of 20 prospective studies. PLoS Med. 2014;11(7):e1001673.
29. Kim DD, Basu A. Estimating the medical care costs of obesity in the United States: systematic review, meta-analysis, and empirical analysis. Value Health. 2016;19(5):602–13.
30. Finkelstein EA, et al. Annual medical spending attributable to obesity: payer-and service-specific estimates. Health Aff (Millwood). 2009;28(5):w822–31.
31. Trogdon JG, et al. Indirect costs of obesity: a review of the current literature. Obes Rev. 2008;9(5):489–500.
32. Gallagher EJ, LeRoith D. Obesity and diabetes: the increased risk of cancer and cancer-related mortality. Physiol Rev. 2015;95(3):727–48.
33. Ekelund U, et al. Does physical activity attenuate, or even eliminate, the detrimental association of sitting time with mortality? A harmonised meta-analysis of data from more than 1 million men and women. Lancet. 2016;388(10051):1302–10.
34. American Heart Association. American Heart Association recommendations for physical activity in adults and kids. [cited 2021 12 Dec]. https://www.heart.org/en/healthy-living/fitness/fitness-basics/aha-recs-for-physical-activity-in-adults.
35. Loprinzi PD. Dose-response association of moderate-to-vigorous physical activity with cardiovascular biomarkers and all-cause mortality: considerations by individual sports, exercise and recreational physical activities. Prev Med. 2015;81:73–7.
36. Prior PL, Suskin N. Exercise for stroke prevention. Stroke Vasc Neurol. 2018;3(2):59–68.
37. Hambrecht R, et al. Effect of exercise on coronary endothelial function in patients with coronary artery disease. N Engl J Med. 2000;342(7):454–60.
38. Bernstein L. Exercise and breast cancer prevention. Curr Oncol Rep. 2009;11(6):490–6.
39. Trojian TH, Mody K, Chain P. Exercise and colon cancer: primary and secondary prevention. Curr Sports Med Rep. 2007;6(2):120–4.
40. Minihan AK, et al. Proportion of cancer cases attributable to physical inactivity by US state, 2013-2016. Med Sci Sports Exerc. 2022;54(3):417–23.
41. Schuch FB, Stubbs B. The role of exercise in preventing and treating depression. Curr Sports Med Rep. 2019;18(8):299–304.
42. Mead GE, et al. Exercise for depression. Cochrane Database Syst Rev. 2009;3:Cd004366.
43. Martinsen EW. Physical activity in the prevention and treatment of anxiety and depression. Nord J Psychiatry. 2008;62(Suppl 47):25–9.
44. Saeed SA, Cunningham K, Bloch RM. Depression and anxiety disorders: benefits of exercise, yoga, and meditation. Am Fam Physician. 2019;99(10):620–7.
45. Neudecker C, et al. Exercise interventions in children and adolescents with ADHD: a systematic review. J Atten Disord. 2019;23(4):307–24.
46. Fullagar HH, et al. Sleep and athletic performance: the effects of sleep loss on exercise performance, and physiological and cognitive responses to exercise. Sports Med. 2015;45(2):161–86.
47. Kelley GA, Kelley KS. Exercise and sleep: a systematic review of previous meta-analyses. J Evid Based Med. 2017;10(1):26–36.
48. De la Rosa A, et al. Physical exercise in the prevention and treatment of Alzheimer's disease. J Sport Health Sci. 2020;9(5):394–404.
49. Alty J, Farrow M, Lawler K. Exercise and dementia prevention. Pract Neurol. 2020;20(3):234–40.
50. Cass SP. Alzheimer's disease and exercise: a literature review. Curr Sports Med Rep. 2017;16(1):19–22.
51. U.S. Department of Health and Human Services. Physical activity guidelines for Americans. 2nd ed. Washington, DC: U.S. Department of Health and Human Services; 2018. https://

health.gov/sites/default/files/2019-09/Physical_Activity_Guidelines_2nd_edition.pdf
52. Sigal RJ, et al. Effects of aerobic training, resistance training, or both on glycemic control in type 2 diabetes: a randomized trial. Ann Intern Med. 2007;147(6):357–69.
53. Dunstan DW, et al. High-intensity resistance training improves glycemic control in older patients with type 2 diabetes. Diabetes Care. 2002;25(10):1729–36.
54. Colberg SR, et al. Physical activity/exercise and diabetes: a position statement of the American Diabetes Association. Diabetes Care. 2016;39(11):2065–79.
55. Lee S, et al. Effects of exercise modality on insulin resistance and ectopic fat in adolescents with overweight and obesity: a randomized clinical trial. J Pediatr. 2019;206:91–98 e1.
56. Zhao G, et al. Compliance with physical activity recommendations in US adults with diabetes. Diabet Med. 2008;25(2):221–7.
57. Garber CE, et al. American College of Sports Medicine position stand. Quantity and quality of exercise for developing and maintaining cardiorespiratory, musculoskeletal, and neuromotor fitness in apparently healthy adults: guidance for prescribing exercise. Med Sci Sports Exerc. 2011;43(7):1334–59.
58. Ahmed HM, et al. Effects of physical activity on cardiovascular disease. Am J Cardiol. 2012;109(2):288–95.
59. Darden D, Richardson C, Jackson EA. Physical activity and exercise for secondary prevention among patients with cardiovascular disease. Curr Cardiovasc Risk Rep. 2013;7(6)
60. Eckel RH, et al. 2013 AHA/ACC guideline on lifestyle management to reduce cardiovascular risk: a report of the American College of Cardiology/American Heart Association Task Force on Practice Guidelines. J Am Coll Cardiol. 2014;63(25 Pt B):2960–84.
61. Smith SC Jr, et al. AHA/ACC guidelines for secondary prevention for patients with coronary and other atherosclerotic vascular disease: 2006 update: endorsed by the National Heart, Lung, and Blood Institute. Circulation. 2006;113(19):2363–72.
62. Thompson PD, et al. Eligibility and disqualification recommendations for competitive athletes with cardiovascular abnormalities: task force 8: coronary artery disease: a scientific statement from the American Heart Association and American College of Cardiology. J Am Coll Cardiol. 2015;66(21):2406–11.
63. Black DW, et al. Depression in veterans of the first Gulf War and comparable military controls. Ann Clin Psychiatry. 2004;16(2):53–61.
64. Black HR, et al. Eligibility and disqualification recommendations for competitive athletes with cardiovascular abnormalities: task force 6: hypertension: a scientific statement from the American Heart Association and the American College of Cardiology. Circulation. 2015;132(22):e298–302.
65. Writing Group Members, et al. Executive summary: heart disease and stroke statistics—2016 update: a report from the American Heart Association. Circulation. 2016;133(4):447–54.
66. Church TS, et al. Usefulness of cardiorespiratory fitness as a predictor of all-cause and cardiovascular disease mortality in men with systemic hypertension. Am J Cardiol. 2001;88(6):651–6.
67. Lee CD, Folsom AR, Blair SN. Physical activity and stroke risk: a meta-analysis. Stroke. 2003;34(10):2475–81.
68. Whelton SP, et al. Effect of aerobic exercise on blood pressure: a meta-analysis of randomized, controlled trials. Ann Intern Med. 2002;136(7):493–503.
69. Pescatello LS, et al. Short-term effect of dynamic exercise on arterial blood pressure. Circulation. 1991;83(5):1557–61.
70. Bellinger CR, Peters SP. Outpatient chronic obstructive pulmonary disease management: going for the GOLD. J Allergy Clin Immunol Pract. 2015;3(4):471–8; quiz 479–80.
71. CDC. COPD death rates in the United States. [cited 2022]. https://www.cdc.gov/copd/data.htm
72. Casaburi R, ZuWallack R. Pulmonary rehabilitation for management of chronic obstructive pulmonary disease. N Engl J Med. 2009;360(13):1329–35.
73. Spruit MA, et al. COPD and exercise: does it make a difference? Breathe (Sheff). 2016;12(2):e38–49.
74. Fiorentino G, Esquinas AM, Annunziata A. Exercise and chronic obstructive pulmonary disease (COPD). Adv Exp Med Biol. 2020;1228:355–68.
75. Haas F, Salazar-Schicci J, Axen K. Desensitization to dyspnea in chronic obstructive pulmonary disease. In: Casaburi R, Petty TL, editors. Principles and practice of pulmonary rehabilitation. Philadelphia: W. Saunders; 1993. p. 241–51.
76. Huiart L, Ernst P, Suissa S. Cardiovascular morbidity and mortality in COPD. Chest. 2005;128(4):2640–6.
77. van Eeden SF, Sin DD. Chronic obstructive pulmonary disease: a chronic systemic inflammatory disease. Respiration. 2008;75(2):224–38.
78. Nici L, et al. American Thoracic Society/European Respiratory Society statement on pulmonary rehabilitation. Am J Respir Crit Care Med. 2006;173(12):1390–413.
79. Wolf SL, et al. Reducing frailty and falls in older persons: an investigation of Tai Chi and computerized balance training. Atlanta FICSIT Group. Frailty and injuries: cooperative studies of intervention techniques. J Am Geriatr Soc. 1996;44(5):489–97.
80. Ries AL, et al. Pulmonary rehabilitation: joint ACCP/AACVPR evidence-based clinical practice guidelines. Chest. 2007;131(5 Suppl):4S–42S.
81. Wright NC, et al. The recent prevalence of osteoporosis and low bone mass in the United States based on bone mineral density at the femoral neck or lumbar spine. J Bone Miner Res. 2014;29(11):2520–6.
82. Office of the Surgeon General, Reports of the Surgeon General. In Bone health and osteoporosis: a report of the surgeon general, Office of the Surgeon General (US): Rockville (MD); 2004.
83. Gregg EW, Pereira MA, Caspersen CJ. Physical activity, falls, and fractures among older adults: a review of the epidemiologic evidence. J Am Geriatr Soc. 2000;48(8):883–93.
84. Karlsson MK, Nordqvist A, Karlsson C. Physical activity, muscle function, falls and fractures. Food Nutr Res. 2008:52.
85. Moayyeri A. The association between physical activity and osteoporotic fractures: a review of the evidence and implications for future research. Ann Epidemiol. 2008;18(11):827–35.
86. Nikander R, et al. Targeted exercise against osteoporosis: a systematic review and meta-analysis for optimising bone strength throughout life. BMC Med. 2010;8:47.
87. Hind K, Burrows M. Weight-bearing exercise and bone mineral accrual in children and adolescents: a review of controlled trials. Bone. 2007;40(1):14–27.
88. Kelley GA, Kelley KS. Efficacy of resistance exercise on lumbar spine and femoral neck bone mineral density in premenopausal women: a meta-analysis of individual patient data. J Womens Health (Larchmt). 2004;13(3):293–300.
89. Kelley GA, Kelley KS, Tran ZV. Resistance training and bone mineral density in women: a meta-analysis of controlled trials. Am J Phys Med Rehabil. 2001;80(1):65–77.
90. Wallace BA, Cumming RG. Systematic review of randomized trials of the effect of exercise on bone mass in pre- and postmenopausal women. Calcif Tissue Int. 2000;67(1):10–8.
91. Kelley GA, Kelley KS. Exercise and bone mineral density at the femoral neck in postmenopausal women: a meta-analysis of controlled clinical trials with individual patient data. Am J Obstet Gynecol. 2006;194(3):760–7.
92. Martyn-St James M, Carroll S. Meta-analysis of walking for preservation of bone mineral density in postmenopausal women. Bone. 2008;43(3):521–31.

93. Palombaro KM. Effects of walking-only interventions on bone mineral density at various skeletal sites: a meta-analysis. J Geriatr Phys Ther. 2005;28(3):102–7.
94. Wolff I, et al. The effect of exercise training programs on bone mass: a meta-analysis of published controlled trials in pre- and postmenopausal women. Osteoporos Int. 1999;9(1):1–12.
95. Martyn-St James M, Carroll S. A meta-analysis of impact exercise on postmenopausal bone loss: the case for mixed loading exercise programmes. Br J Sports Med. 2009;43(12):898–908.
96. Howe TE, et al. Exercise for preventing and treating osteoporosis in postmenopausal women. Cochrane Database Syst Rev. 2011;7:Cd000333.
97. Kukuljan S, et al. Effects of a multi-component exercise program and calcium-vitamin-D3-fortified milk on bone mineral density in older men: a randomised controlled trial. Osteoporos Int. 2009;20(7):1241–51.
98. Bailey CA, Brooke-Wavell K. Optimum frequency of exercise for bone health: randomised controlled trial of a high-impact unilateral intervention. Bone. 2010;46(4):1043–9.
99. Vainionpaa A, et al. Effect of impact exercise and its intensity on bone geometry at weight-bearing tibia and femur. Bone. 2007;40(3):604–11.
100. Vainionpää A, et al. Intensity of exercise is associated with bone density change in premenopausal women. Osteoporos Int. 2006;17(3):455–63.
101. Karinkanta S, et al. A multi-component exercise regimen to prevent functional decline and bone fragility in home-dwelling elderly women: randomized, controlled trial. Osteoporos Int. 2007;18(4):453–62.
102. Feskanich D, Willett W, Colditz G. Walking and leisure-time activity and risk of hip fracture in postmenopausal women. JAMA. 2002;288(18):2300–6.
103. Michaelsson K, et al. Leisure physical activity and the risk of fracture in men. PLoS Med. 2007;4(6):e199.
104. Cussler EC, et al. Exercise frequency and calcium intake predict 4-year bone changes in postmenopausal women. Osteoporos Int. 2005;16(12):2129–41.
105. CDC. Osteoarthritis. https://www.cdc.gov/arthritis/basics/osteoarthritis.htm.
106. Singh JA, et al. Rates of total joint replacement in the United States: future projections to 2020-2040 using the National Inpatient Sample. J Rheumatol. 2019;46(9):1134–40.
107. Bennell KL, Hinman RS. A review of the clinical evidence for exercise in osteoarthritis of the hip and knee. J Sci Med Sport. 2011;14(1):4–9.
108. Murphy L, Helmick CG. The impact of osteoarthritis in the United States: a population-health perspective: a population-based review of the fourth most common cause of hospitalization in U.S. adults. Orthop Nurs. 2012;31(2):85–91.
109. Prevalence of doctor-diagnosed arthritis and arthritis-attributable activity limitation—United States, 2010–2012. MMWR Morb Mortal Wkly Rep, 2013. 62(44): p. 869–873.
110. Farr JN, et al. Physical activity levels in patients with early knee osteoarthritis measured by accelerometry. Arthritis Rheum. 2008;59(9):1229–36.
111. Messier SP, et al. Exercise and dietary weight loss in overweight and obese older adults with knee osteoarthritis: the arthritis, diet, and activity promotion trial. Arthritis Rheum. 2004;50(5):1501–10.
112. O'Reilly SC, et al. Quadriceps weakness in knee osteoarthritis: the effect on pain and disability. Ann Rheum Dis. 1998;57(10):588–94.
113. Christensen R, et al. Effect of weight reduction in obese patients diagnosed with knee osteoarthritis: a systematic review and meta-analysis. Ann Rheum Dis. 2007;66(4):433–9.
114. Fransen M, McConnell S. Exercise for osteoarthritis of the knee. Cochrane Database Syst Rev. 2008;4:CD004376.
115. Fransen M, et al. Exercise for osteoarthritis of the knee: a Cochrane systematic review. Br J Sports Med. 2015;49(24):1554–7.
116. McCarthy CJ, et al. Supplementing a home exercise programme with a class-based exercise programme is more effective than home exercise alone in the treatment of knee osteoarthritis. Rheumatology (Oxford). 2004;43(7):880–6.
117. Mazieres B, et al. Adherence to, and results of, physical therapy programs in patients with hip or knee osteoarthritis. Development of French clinical practice guidelines. Joint Bone Spine. 2008;75(5):589–96.
118. Butts JF, et al. Implementing a physical activity consultation clinic during a global pandemic. Curr Sports Med Rep. 2021;20(8):389–94.
119. Joy EL, et al. Physical activity counselling in sports medicine: a call to action. Br J Sports Med. 2013;47(1):49–53.
120. Cardinal BJ, et al. If exercise is medicine, where is exercise in medicine? Review of U.S. medical education curricula for physical activity-related content. J Phys Act Health. 2015;12(9):1336–43.
121. Shuval K, et al. Physical activity counseling in primary care: insights from public health and behavioral economics. CA Cancer J Clin. 2017;67(3):233–44.
122. ACSM. Exercise is medicine ACSM's Rx for health. https://www.exerciseismedicine.org/eim-in-action/health-care/health-care-providers/.
123. Thompson PD, et al. ACSM's new preparticipation health screening recommendations from ACSM's guidelines for exercise testing and prescription, ninth edition. Curr Sports Med Rep. 2013;12(4):215–7.
124. Dasso NA. How is exercise different from physical activity? A concept analysis. Nurs Forum. 2019;54(1):45–52.
125. American College of Sports Medicine, et al. American College of Sports Medicine position stand. Exercise and physical activity for older adults. Med Sci Sports Exerc. 2009;41(7):1510–30.
126. Reed JL, Pipe AL. The talk test: a useful tool for prescribing and monitoring exercise intensity. Curr Opin Cardiol. 2014;29(5):475–80.
127. Donnelly JE, et al. American College of Sports Medicine Position Stand. Appropriate physical activity intervention strategies for weight loss and prevention of weight regain for adults. Med Sci Sports Exerc. 2009;41(2):459–71.
128. Mathus-Vliegen EM, O. Obesity management task force of the European Association for the study of, prevalence, pathophysiology, health consequences and treatment options of obesity in the elderly: a guideline. Obes Facts. 2012;5(3):460–83.
129. CDC, Overweight & obesity. https://www.cdc.gov/obesity/ Last accessed 14 Apr 23.
130. Davidson LE, et al. Effects of exercise modality on insulin resistance and functional limitation in older adults: a randomized controlled trial. Arch Intern Med. 2009;169(2):122–31.
131. Pollard TM, Guell C, Morris S. Communal therapeutic mobility in group walking: a meta-ethnography. Soc Sci Med. 2020;262:113,241.
132. Farren L, et al. Mall walking program environments, features, and participants: a scoping review. Prev Chronic Dis. 2015;12:E129.
133. Advocate, T.P.H. What's wrong with physical education. 2019 [cited 2022 6 Jan 2022]. https://pha.berkeley.edu/2019/12/01/whats-wrong-with-physical-education/.
134. Phillips RL Jr, McCauley LA, Koller CF. Implementing high-quality primary care: a report from the National Academies of Sciences, Engineering, and Medicine. JAMA. 2021;325(24):2437–8.
135. HealthCare.Gov. Wellness programs. https://www.healthcare.gov/glossary/wellness-programs/.

Tobacco Use and Dependence

Kimberly A. Shoenbill, M. Justin Byron, Ashley A. Weiner, and Adam O. Goldstein

Introduction

Tobacco use in the United States (US) has fallen over the last half-century but remains the leading preventable causes of death and disability [1]. From a peak of over 40% in 1965, cigarette smoking has declined to 12.5% among adults in 2020 [2]. When other tobacco products such as chewing tobacco, cigars, and e-cigarettes are included, 19% of adults in the US (47 million people) currently use a tobacco product [2]. Globally, smoking caused nearly 8 million deaths and 200 million disability-adjusted life years in 2019 [3].

Up to one out of three cardiovascular deaths and four out of ten cancer deaths are due to tobacco use [4, 5]. Sites of tobacco-related cancers include the lung, bladder, cervix, gastrointestinal tract, liver, pancreas, stomach, esophagus, larynx, oropharynx, and blood (myeloid leukemia) [1]. In addition, for every person who dies from tobacco-related disease, 30 more people suffer debilitating chronic illnesses, including diabetes, decreased immune function, rheumatoid arthritis, hip fractures, vascular disease, chronic obstructive pulmonary disease (COPD), blindness, cataracts, strokes, and pneumonia. [6] Exposure to secondhand smoke (SHS) increases risk of premature death and disease for people who have never smoked, and negatively impacts fetal development as well as the health of infants and children [7, 8]. In the US, tobacco use costs $600 billion (in 2018 dollars), including $240 billion in direct medical care, lost productivity from smoking-related illnesses and health conditions, lost productivity from early death related to smoking, and $7 billion in lost productivity due to death from secondhand tobacco exposure [6, 9–11].

Large disparities in tobacco use exist by region, state, age, race and ethnicity, social economic status, occupation, mental health, gender, and sexual orientation. In medical practice, smoking by people with one or more chronic diseases, including mental health and substance use, remains significantly higher than those with no comorbidities [12]. One of the largest factors in tobacco use is educational attainment, with tobacco use ranging from 40% among people with a high-school degree or equivalent to 8.6% among those with a graduate degree [2]. Income follows a similar trend, with smoking rates ranging from 25% among people with an annual household income of under $35,000 to 14% among people with an income of over $100,000 [2]. Mental health is also an important predictor, with tobacco use more common among people with generalized anxiety (30% use), major depression (36% use), and bipolar or psychotic disorders. People who identify as lesbian, gay, or bisexual also have a higher prevalence of tobacco use (25%) [2]. Cigarillo use, one of the most popular of all cigar types, is disproportionately higher among young adults and African American adults [13].

Since the 1964 US Surgeon General's report on smoking and health, a comprehensive tobacco control strategy has sought to decrease the initiation and prevalence of smoking through public health policy initiatives such as clean air statutes, media campaigns, taxes on cigarettes, and comprehensive state programs, including quitlines, websites, and apps. Despite advocacy for health care system change that supports treatment, evidence-based interventions remain under-prescribed by providers and under-utilized by patients [1, 14, 15].

Tobacco Use and Chronic Disease

Tobacco Use as a Chronic Disease

The US Public Health Service's Guidelines on Treating Tobacco Use and Dependence includes 10 key recommendations (Table 4.1). The first recommendation emphasizes that tobacco use and addiction are *chronic diseases* that often require repeated intervention and multiple attempts to quit and that effective treatments exist that can significantly increase rates of long-term abstinence [16]. Only a minority of people who use tobacco are able to achieve long-term abstinence in an initial attempt; rather, the experience of most patients involves multiple quit attempts, with periods of abstinence followed by periods of relapse, hence the ongoing, chronic nature of tobacco addiction. Like managing hypertension or diabetes, clinicians who acknowledge tobacco use as a chronic disease should include brief interventions in every patient encounter, give patients realistic expectations about achieving success, use behavioral therapy, encourage use of various approved pharmacotherapy agents and monitor compliance, refer patients to treatment specialists, and view relapse without judgment.

While over two-thirds of smokers want to quit smoking, and over one half try to quit each year, less than 10% who try on their own are successful in any given year, which is lower than successful abstention from heroin or alcohol [17, 18]. Tobacco cessation doubles with strong advice from the clinician to quit and achieves successful quit rates of 20–30% of patients when behavioral counseling is combined with pharmacotherapy [19].

Tobacco dependence is a chronic illness that involves changes in brain chemistry from the effects of nicotine and other compounds involved in the upregulation of nicotine receptors. When people stop using tobacco, physiologic changes in the brain cause urges and withdrawal symptoms. Like other chronic illnesses, tobacco dependence merits effective treatment and should be covered by health insurance [20].

Patients who smoke often feel isolated and tend to under-report or deny their tobacco use if they anticipate judgment from their doctor. Patients are more likely to successfully quit if their clinicians offer empathy and an acknowledgment of the difficulty of stopping tobacco use while providing resources for cessation [21].

Impact on Other Chronic Diseases

Tobacco use, especially smoking, damages nearly every organ in the body and has a significant impact on chronic diseases [6] (Fig. 4.1). From 2005 to 2013, adults with asthma, diabetes, heart disease, hypertension, and substance abuse did not reduce their rate of smoking as much as that of adults without chronic conditions, and those with substance use disorder or mental health problems continue to smoke at higher rates than the general population [12]. Almost half of cigarettes are consumed by those with serious mental illness, and smoking rates for individuals with schizophrenia and bipolar disorder are increasing. The stress of trying to stop a highly addictive behavior like smoking while living with a chronic disease can feel overwhelming to patients, who may struggle to give up the one thing that comforts them. Patients may also dislike the weight gain associated with stopping smoking. Still, most people are willing to contemplate stopping and understand that doing so will decrease the adverse outcomes of their chronic disease [22, 23].

Types of Tobacco Products

Tobacco use disorder involves tobacco use on a regular basis for which abstinence produces withdrawal symptoms, meeting criteria for addiction (Table 4.2). Tobacco products,

Table 4.1 US Public Health Service's ten guidelines on treating tobacco use and dependence [16]

Tobacco dependence is a chronic disease that often requires repeated intervention and multiple attempts to quit.
It is essential that clinicians and health care delivery systems consistently identify and document tobacco use status and treat every tobacco user seen in a health care setting.
Tobacco dependence treatments are effective across a broad range of populations. Clinicians should encourage every patient willing to make a quit attempt to use recommended counseling treatments and medications.
Brief tobacco dependence treatment is effective. Clinicians should offer every patient who uses tobacco at least brief treatments.
Individual, group, and telephone counseling are effective, and their effectiveness increases with treatment intensity. Practical counseling (problem-solving/skills training) and social support are especially effective.
Nicotine replacement (provided in gum, inhaler, lozenge, nasal spray, or patch) and two non-nicotine medications (bupropion SR and varenicline) are effective for tobacco dependence and their use should be encouraged, except when medically contraindicated or with specific populations for which there is insufficient evidence of effectiveness.
Counseling and medication are effective when used by themselves, and more so when used in combination.
Telephone quitline counseling is effective with diverse populations and has broad reach.
If a tobacco user is currently unwilling to make a quit attempt, clinicians should use motivational treatments to increase future quit attempts
Tobacco dependence treatments are both clinically effective and highly cost-effective. Providing coverage for these treatments increases quit rates. Insurers and purchasers should cover these services.

Cancers

- Oropharynx
- Larynx
- Esophagus
- Trachea, bronchus, and lung
- Acute myeloid leukemia
- Stomach
- Liver
- Pancreas
- Kidney and ureter
- Cervix
- Bladder
- Colorectal

Chronic Diseases

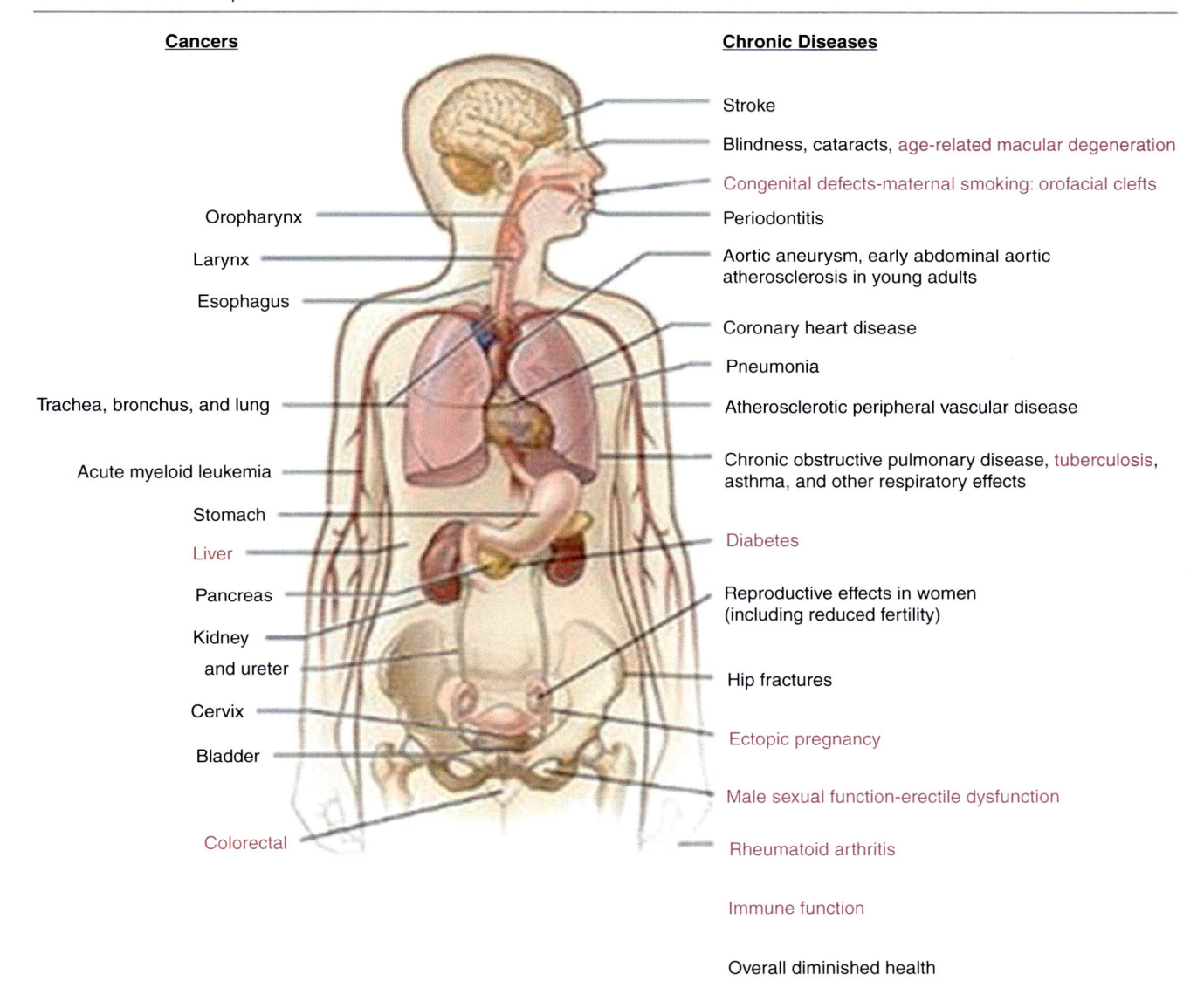

- Stroke
- Blindness, cataracts, age-related macular degeneration
- Congenital defects-maternal smoking: orofacial clefts
- Periodontitis
- Aortic aneurysm, early abdominal aortic atherosclerosis in young adults
- Coronary heart disease
- Pneumonia
- Atherosclerotic peripheral vascular disease
- Chronic obstructive pulmonary disease, tuberculosis, asthma, and other respiratory effects
- Diabetes
- Reproductive effects in women (including reduced fertility)
- Hip fractures
- Ectopic pregnancy
- Male sexual function-erectile dysfunction
- Rheumatoid arthritis
- Immune function
- Overall diminished health

Fig. 4.1 The health consequences causally linked to smoking. Notations in red were newly added to the 2014 Surgeon General's Report. Reprinted from public domain: http://www.cdc.gov/tobacco/data_statistics/fact_sheets/health_effects/effects_cig_smoking/

defined and regulated by the US Food and Drug Authority (FDA), include smoked, smokeless, and heated/vaporized. About one in five tobacco users use more than one product, which is referred to as poly-tobacco use and is especially prevalent in young adults (ages 18–24 years). Most poly-tobacco users use two products ("dual-use"), the most common of which are cigarette and e-cigarette use, followed by cigarettes and another combustible product (e.g., cigars), followed by cigarettes and smokeless tobacco [2]. It is important to ask about all tobacco product use.

Smoked (Combustibles)

All combustible tobacco products are carcinogenic and promote multiple respiratory and cardiac diseases. *Cigarettes* contain tobacco wrapped in a paper, usually with a filter to reduce the harshness (but not the toxicity) of the inhaled smoke. Cigarettes are a highly effective and efficient drug delivery system, delivering a bolus of nicotine to the brain within 10 seconds of inhalation [25]. A pack includes 20 cigarettes and can be sold as single packs or in cartons of 10 packs. Sale of single cigarettes ("loosies") is illegal, but common in some places. Previous attempts by tobacco companies to brand cigarettes as safer included "light" and "low tar" designations. These misleading labels are now prohibited, but still identifiable by color labels, for example, light products are often in gold packaging. Terms such as "natural" and "organic" have also been used to convey a less harmful product [26]. Congress banned all characterizing flavors in US cigarettes in 2009, with the notable exception of menthol, even though it may be the most harmful flavor.

Table 4.2 Tobacco use disorder definitions [24]

DSM-5 condition	ICD 10 codes	Description
Tobacco use disorder and dependence	305.1 (Z72.0)—Mild: 2–3 symptoms 305.1 (F17.200)—Moderate: 4–5 symptoms 305.1 (F17.200)—Severe: 6 or more symptoms	A problematic pattern of tobacco use leading to clinically significant impairment or distress, characterized by at least two of the following: loss of control (inability to stop using); persistent desire/unsuccessful efforts to stop using; craving (a strong desire to use the substance); failure to fulfill major role obligations due to use; a great deal of time is spent obtaining, using, and recovering from the use of substances; continued use of substances despite having social or interpersonal problems caused or made worse by the use; important activities are reduced or given up because of the use; substance use in situations where it is physically hazardous; continued use of substances despite having physical or psychological caused or made worse by the use; tolerance; or withdrawal.
Nicotine dependence	Z72.0 (F17.200)	Chronic, relapsing disease defined as a compulsive craving to use tobacco, despite social consequences, loss of control over tobacco intake, and emergence of withdrawal symptoms when quitting.
Nicotine dependence with withdrawal	292.0 (F17.213)	Daily use for at least several weeks, with abrupt cessation or reduction in tobacco use, followed by significant distress or impairment within 24 h characterized by four or more of the following: irritability, frustration, or anger; anxiety; difficulty concentrating; increased appetite; restlessness; depressed mood; or insomnia.

Abbreviations: DSM-5 Diagnostic and Statistical Manual of Mental Disorders, Fifth Edition, *ICD-10* International Classification of Disease

Menthol masks the harsh taste and feel of inhaled smoke and allows for deeper inhalation, with the ability to deliver higher levels of nicotine in fewer cigarettes. In 2020, 37% of all cigarettes sold in the US were mentholated [27]. Use of menthol makes it easier to start smoking and more difficult to stop [28]. Young people smoke menthol cigarettes at higher rates than adults and almost 75% of African Americans who smoke use menthol cigarettes [29]. The FDA announced in 2022 plans to ban menthol in cigarettes, a move that could dramatically decrease cigarette consumption if combined with increased support for cessation [30].

Cigars and cigarillos use tobacco leaf as the wrapper and range in size from cigarette-size (little cigars) to an intermediary size (cigarillos), to large cigars. Someone who smokes 20 cigarettes a day (one pack) and who switches to cigarillos will typically use about three cigarillos per day, stubbing them out and relighting them frequently to maintain nicotine levels. Because there are no minimum pack sizes, cigarillos can be sold individually or in small packages at inexpensive prices (e.g., 3 for $0.99). Currently no federal flavor limitations exist for cigar products, allowing a wide array of flavors, such as apple, grape, and cherry, which are popular with youth and young adults. The FDA may ban flavors in cigar products [30].

Pipe smoking involves use of different blends of tobacco stuffed into the pipe bowl, lit, and inhaled through the pipe stem. While it has the lowest prevalence among combustible tobacco products, it still delivers nicotine and carcinogens throughout the lungs and most organ systems.

Hookah or water pipe, originally from the Middle East, has become more popular in the US, particularly among youth and young adults, often in group settings [31]. Hookah use among college students is high, with over 20% of college students using hookah in any given year [32]. In a hookah, burned tobacco passes through a water pipe which filters out some chemicals, but the inhaled smoke still contains high levels of toxins that come from the burning of the charcoal, tobacco, and flavoring; hence, it is not a safe alternative to smoking cigarettes [31].

Smokeless (Non-combustibles)

Smokeless tobacco is placed in the mouth, where nicotine and other chemicals are absorbed through the oral mucosa. Smokeless tobacco includes chew, dip, snuff, and snus, and newer products like nicotine pouches. Smokeless tobacco (especially Swedish snus), while harmful, is substantially less harmful than cigarette use [33]. Chew and dip (also sometimes called moist snuff) [34] usually require expectoration of the liquid that pools in the lower jaw, hence the name spit tobacco. Nasal snuff may be sniffed up the nose. Snus, based on a Scandinavian product, contains tobacco in a small teabag-like pouch that does not require spitting. Nicotine pouch products also use a small pouch, but rather than containing ground tobacco leaves use a white powder that is a mix of nicotine, flavoring, sweeteners, and binding agents. Smokeless tobaccos contain a number of carcinogens and cause oral cancer, esophageal cancer, and pancreatic cancer [34]. Smokeless tobacco use can also lead to leukoplakia, gum disease, tooth decay, and tooth loss. Use of smokeless tobacco increases the risk of death from heart disease and stroke and use during pregnancy increases the risk of pre-term delivery and stillbirth and affects fetal brain development [35].

E-Cigarettes (Vapes) and Heated Tobacco Products

E-cigarettes (also called vape pens) deliver nicotine by using a battery to heat a solution of nicotine, flavoring, and carrier chemicals (propylene glycol and/or glycerin) to create an aerosol that is inhaled or "vaped." The small, discrete size of e-cigarettes, the variety of flavors available, and social media marketing make e-cigarettes popular among youth.

Heated tobacco products (also called "heat-not-burn" tobacco products, for example, Philip Morris's IQOS brand) use a battery-powered device to heat a heavily modified type of tobacco cigarette. These products are increasingly popular internationally and are recently available in the US.

While people who use e-cigarettes and heated tobacco products are not exposed to the carbon monoxide, tars, or carcinogens of smoked tobacco, these products are not harmless and research is underway to determine their carcinogenicity and toxicity. The FDA has started the process of regulating e-cigarettes.

Second- and Thirdhand Smoke Exposure

While those who use combustible tobacco products receive the most concentrated exposure to toxic chemicals, the effects can be experienced by others. Secondhand smoke (SHS) is a combination of smoke that comes directly from burning cigarettes, cigars, or pipes, called "side-stream smoke," and smoke that is exhaled by the person smoking, or "main-stream" smoke. Side-stream smoke comprises 85% of SHS. SHS can remain in the air for hours which increases the time others are vulnerable [7]. Nonsmokers who are exposed to SHS increase their risk of developing heart disease by 25–30%, yet providers rarely ask nonsmokers about SHS exposure [6].

Thirdhand smoke (THS) refers to the residual nicotine and carcinogens found in tobacco smoke adhering to surfaces long after a cigarette has been finished. [36] These lingering toxins are found in hair, skin, clothes, carpets, furniture, walls, insulation, and vehicles. The molecules react with oxidants in the air and other compounds in the environment to generate secondary contaminants that can be more toxic to humans than the original contaminants [37]. These toxic effects have been shown in cells, animal models, and children, including in neonates. While more research is needed to understand long-term effects of these exposures, it is prudent to decrease such exposure [38].

Individuals exposed to SHS and THS can suffer the same adverse health effects as those who smoke voluntarily [7]. Adults exposed to tobacco smoke in the environment have increased adverse effects on their cardiovascular system and can develop lung cancer. In the US, SHS annually causes about 3,400 lung cancer deaths and 42,000 heart disease deaths in people who do not smoke. Children who are exposed to smoke have elevated risk for sudden infant death syndrome (SIDS), acute respiratory infections, ear infections, and asthma [7]. In the US, this translates to hundreds of thousands of lower respiratory tract infections in children younger than 18 months. Approximately 14% of US children live in a household with at least one person who smokes, which increases their vulnerability to tobacco smoke and the resulting consequences [39].

African Americans, children, people with incomes below the poverty level, and those who rent their homes are more likely to be exposed to SHS than other populations. Especially vulnerable are people living in multi-unit housing like apartments and condominiums. Even if they adopt smoke-free policies for their own living units, they can be exposed to smoke from nearby units and shared areas. Tobacco-free policies in workplaces and public places, including public housing, have contributed to reducing exposure to SHS and THS for many people in the US, but such policies vary widely by state and locality [40].

Children are at the greatest risk of exposure to THS, as they more frequently touch surfaces on which the toxic particles reside. They also can be exposed over long periods of time, from in utero until leaving home as young adults. Exposure to nicotine and tobacco-specific nitrosamines is of particular concern [41]. Thirdhand smoke is not easily removed and can take months to years to dissipate [42]. Although the risks of exposure are not fully known, human and in vitro animal studies link THS to DNA damage, altered fibroblast migration involved in wound healing, and impaired respiratory development [43–45].

Public health experts advocate that all clinicians ask adults and children if they are or have been exposed to smoke from tobacco products in their usual environment [46]. Secondhand smoke exposure is an ICD 10 code (Z77.22) that can be used to indicate a diagnosis for reimbursement purposes [47].

Benefits of Cessation in Patient Populations

Asymptomatic Patients and Disease Prevention

People who stop using tobacco decrease the risk for cancer, lung disease, and cardiovascular disease and add years to life expectancy [48] (Fig. 4.2). They report increased sense of taste and smell, overall well-being and sense of accomplishment, a new-found freedom, and increased self-efficacy for making other behavior changes. The 2020 report of the US Surgeon General summarizes the health benefits of smoking cessation on multiple health systems and diseases (Table 4.3) [1]. The benefits of stopping tobacco use on individual chronic conditions are discussed below [22, 23].

Cardiovascular Disease

For patients at risk for or with current cardiovascular disease (CVD), stopping smoking can be the single best intervention for improving cardiovascular health and has greater cost-effectiveness than treatment for hypertension and hyperlipidemia [49]. Benefits begin immediately, including decrease in

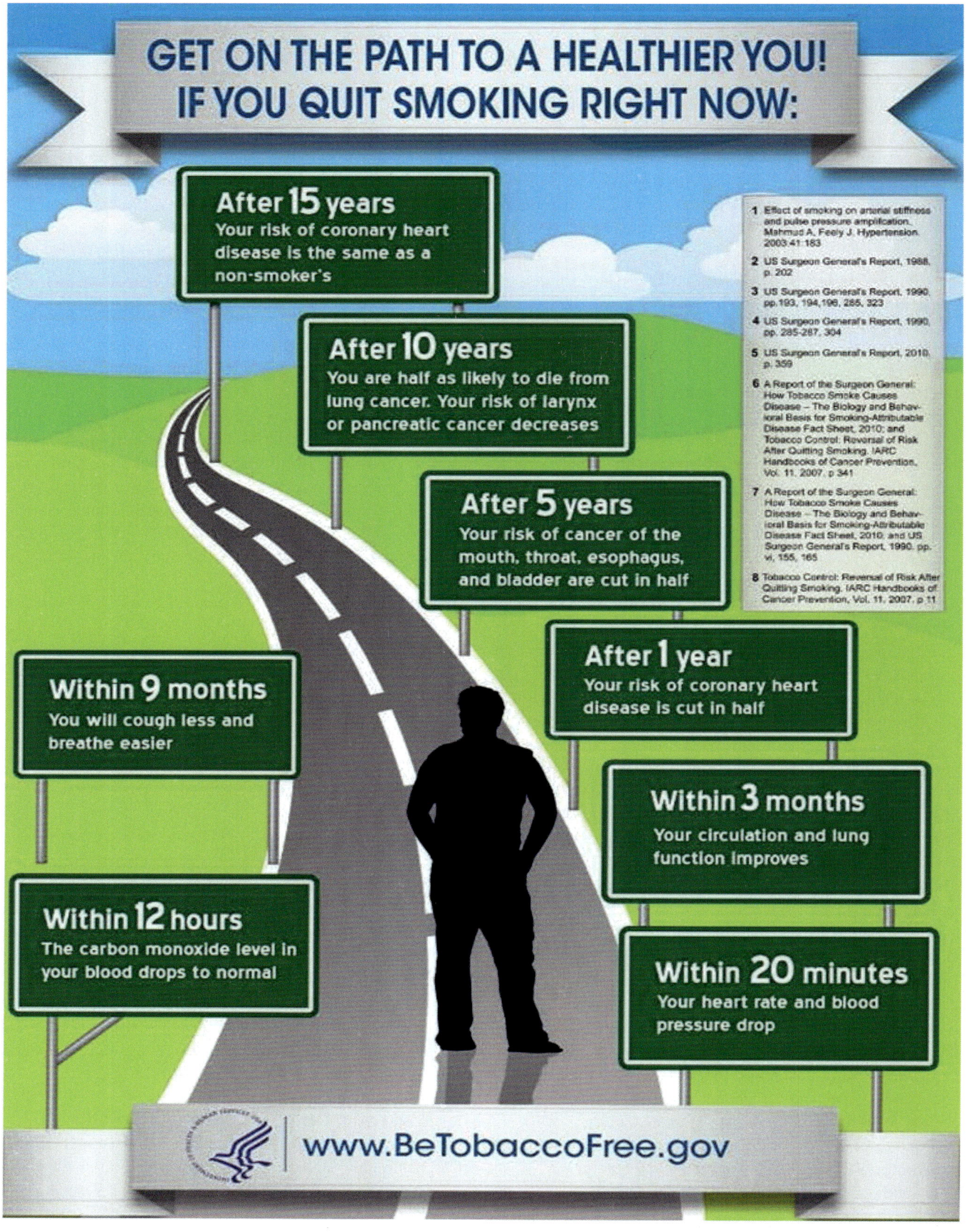

Fig. 4.2 Positive outcomes from stopping tobacco use. Reprinted from public domain: www.BeTobaccoFree.gov

Table 4.3 Smoking cessation: a report of the surgeon general—2020, key findings [1]

Smoking cessation is beneficial at any age, improves health status, and enhances quality of life.
Smoking cessation reduces the risk of premature death and can add as much as a decade to life expectancy.
Smoking places a substantial financial burden on people who smoke, health care systems, and society. Smoking cessation reduces this burden, including smoking-attributable health care expenditures.
Smoking cessation reduces risk for many adverse health effects, including reproductive health outcomes, cardiovascular diseases, chronic obstructive pulmonary disease (COPD), and cancer. Quitting smoking is beneficial to those with heart disease and COPD.
More than three out of five US adults who have ever smoked cigarettes have quit. Although most people who smoke cigarettes make a quit attempt each year, less than one-third use cessation medications approved by the FDA or behavioral counseling to support quit attempts.
Disparities exist in the prevalence of smoking across the US population, with higher prevalence in some subgroups. Smoking cessation attempts, support, and treatment also vary across the population, with lower prevalence in some subgroups. These disparities are defined by educational attainment, poverty, age, health insurance status, race/ethnicity, and geography.
Smoking cessation medications approved by the FDA and behavioral counseling are cost-effective strategies and increase the likelihood of successfully quitting smoking, particularly when used in combination. Using combinations of nicotine replacement therapies can further increase the likelihood of quitting.
Insurance coverage for smoking cessation treatment that is comprehensive, barrier free, and widely promoted increases the use of these treatment services, leads to higher rates of successful quitting, and is cost-effective.
E-cigarettes, a continually changing and heterogeneous group of products, are used in a variety of ways. There is presently inadequate evidence to conclude that e-cigarettes increase smoking cessation.
Smoking cessation can be increased by raising the price of cigarettes, adopting comprehensive smokefree policies, implementing mass media campaigns, requiring pictorial health warnings, and maintaining comprehensive statewide tobacco control programs.

Abbreviations: US United States, *FDA* US Food & Drug Administration

sudden cardiac death, and within a few years the risk for acute myocardial infarction is decreased (Fig. 4.2) [50]. Cessation also decreases the risk of stroke [51]. All FDA-approved tobacco use treatment medications can be effectively used with patients who have CVD. While misconceptions about use of nicotine replacement therapy (NRT) persist, no clinical evidence links NRT and CVD, even if patients smoke while using NRT [52]. Intensive behavioral therapy can significantly increase quit rates in patients with CVD [53].

Diabetes

Long-term effects of stopping smoking for people with diabetes include improved blood lipid levels and rates of inhaled insulin absorption that approach those of people who do not smoke [54, 55]. Varenicline is well tolerated in people with diabetes and can help achieve continuous abstinence rates of 18%, which is double that of placebo, with an average weight gain in those who stopped smoking similar to study participants who did not have diabetes (around 2 kg) [56].

Chronic Obstructive Pulmonary Disease

In early chronic obstructive pulmonary disease (COPD), people who stop smoking can reduce disease progression [57]. Even in advanced COPD, decreasing lung function can be slowed, and risk of death decreases compared to continued smoking [58, 59]. Interventions that include pharmacotherapy, educational materials, and behavioral strategies demonstrate significant abstinence rates and effectiveness in patients, regardless of perceived readiness or motivation [60].

Asthma

Smoking cessation improves asthma control, with significant reductions in chest tightness and nighttime symptoms, improved lung function, decreased sputum neutrophil count, and reduced inhaled steroid use [61]. People with asthma can quit, but they may experience slower declines in nicotine withdrawal symptoms and cravings compared to people without asthma [62]. Promising treatment approaches include peer interventions with adolescents, mobile applications, and tailoring for specific needs of asthma patients [63].

Cancer

With increasing survival following cancer diagnosis, the need for addressing continued tobacco use in cancer care is critical. Surgery, radiation, and chemotherapy treatments are more effective when patients stop using tobacco, and patients who are tobacco free have lower rates of cancer recurrence and higher quality-of-life measures [6, 64]. Effective interventions include pharmacotherapy and intensive behavioral strategies [65–68].

HIV/AIDS

While effective treatments for people living with human immunodeficiency virus (HIV) have extended life expectancy, those who smoke have twice the decreased life expectancy as HIV itself [69]. People with HIV smoke at higher rates (42%) and are less likely to quit than the general population [70]. Those who stop smoking in the course of HIV treatment can gain up to 5.7 years of life by decreasing risks of pneumonia, thrush, and hairy leukoplakia, as well as cancer, cardiovascular disease, and respiratory disease [69]. Pilot studies on treatment that include adherence-focused interventions, such as peer counseling, prepaid cell phones, or texting, have demonstrated effectiveness [71–73].

Mental Health and Substance Use

Having a mental health or substance use problem is associated with significantly higher rates of tobacco use compared to the general population [74]. Such conditions often occur in environments that normalize smoking, with concomitant less access to tobacco use treatment [75]. People with mental health disorders who stop smoking experience decreased depression, anxiety, and stress, with improved mood and quality of life compared to those who continue to smoke [76]. Studies also show increased abstinence from illicit drug and alcohol use in those who stop smoking [75, 77]. Effective treatment includes intensive pharmacotherapy and behavioral interventions, often over a long period of time. Peer counseling and integrated treatment models are also effective.

Inpatients

The inpatient setting, which is invariably smoke-free, is an ideal environment for patients to receive tobacco cessation counseling [78]. The Joint Commission has implemented inpatient tobacco treatment measures (TTMs) which involve identifying patients who have used tobacco within 30 days, offering nicotine replacement therapy and counseling while inpatient, and providing nicotine replacement therapy and referral for outpatient tobacco cessation counseling at discharge. Standardized pathways in an electronic medical record can improve inpatient ordering of nicotine replacement therapy, tobacco cessation counseling, and care coordination of tobacco cessation treatments [79]. Evidence-based inpatient tobacco treatment programs are successful, easy to access, offer appropriate smoking cessation medications, and save the inpatient team time [80]. Patients who receive bedside cessation counseling as an inpatient followed by 6 months of outpatient counseling after hospital discharge have abstinence rates of 78% at 4 weeks and 59% at 6 months [81]. In contrast, patients who only receive counseling while in the hospital have low (less than 20%) success rates of smoking cessation at 3 or 6 months [82]. Patients on inpatient psychiatry services randomized to receive group counseling, free nicotine patches at time of hospital discharge, free post-discharge counseling (quitline, text- or web-based), and post-discharge automatic interactive calls and/or texts are more likely to use smoking cessation treatments than a control group (74.6 vs 40.5%) and to achieve abstinence from tobacco use (8.9 vs 3.5%) [83]. Patients with admission for cardiovascular diagnoses have higher smoking cessation rates than patients admitted with respiratory or neurologic diagnoses after enrollment in an inpatient smoking cessation program, suggesting that some diagnoses provide better teachable moments than others [84]. One pharmacist-led smoking cessation program during hospital stays did not improve smoking cessation rates, which may be due to the "Hawthorne effect," in which participants in the control group of a study modify their behaviors due to an awareness of being observed [85]. Still, hospitalizations may serve as an entry point to tobacco cessation education and counseling, and further studies may determine what strategies have the most impact.

The Chronic Care Model and Tobacco Dependence

Effective chronic care management requires understanding of the chronic nature of tobacco dependence and utilization of effective evidence-based treatments. The Chronic Care Model (CCM) improves health outcomes through system changes that include patient-centered and evidence-based care, team care, planned interventions, self-management, community resources, decision support, patient registries, and information technology [86].

A Comprehensive Approach

Effective approaches such as the 5As model for tobacco use (described below) should be utilized at every health care visit [87]. Effective use of information technology to support this model includes integrating the 5As into electronic health records (EHRs). Most EHRs include *Ask* in vital signs. If *Assess* and *Advise* are also in the vital signs, counseling rates for smoking cessation increase [88]. The American Academy of Family Physicians recommends an abbreviated version known as *Ask and Act* [89].

Physicians and other health care providers must view tobacco use as a long-term condition and routinely assess motivation and interest in medications and referral to specialized or community resources, utilizing shared decision making. Clinicians should address patient concerns such as failure, boredom, addiction, weight gain, and loss of a social circle, and understand the barriers to the use of medications, such as cost, availability, or misinformation.

Team Approach

While providers are in the best position to relate tobacco use to health outcomes, the involvement of clinic staff and other health care professionals increases delivery and success rates of treatment [89–91]. Team-based care demonstrates the importance of addressing tobacco use and increases efficiency by introducing the topic before the physician sees the patient. Supportive, non-judgmental comments such as "We are happy that you are trying to quit, and our team looks forward to seeing you again soon."

Family and Social Support

Social networks and families can support a person's cessation efforts and increase the intention and success rate of smoking cessation [92–94]. Having family or friends who are quitting tobacco increases the probability that patients will also quit [95]. Interactions with former smokers or peer-support groups increase successful quit attempts in patients with less social support, such as those experiencing homelessness or historically marginalized populations [96, 97]. Since smoking behavior is often similar in family and friends, it is important to determine who in the patient's social network is willing and able to support the patient [98, 99]. Partners often undertake behavior changes together, including smoking cessation [100]. Optimizing support for the patient's quit attempt often means working with family members on cessation including discussing how a tobacco-free environment improves everyone's health and saves money [101]. Children who live in tobacco-free homes are less likely to initiate use.

Social connections can also negatively influence a person's attempt to quit. Family or friends may not believe that tobacco use is a chronic disease and may not be empathetic or supportive of patients who struggle with continued use despite health complications [102]. If others in the family smoke, the patient may change the status quo in the home which may result in conflict or family stress regarding continued smoking in a family member [103, 104]. Clinicians can try to motivate family members to consider cessation or supportive behaviors such as not smoking in the home [105].

Public Health Interventions

Tobacco's massive cost to society for health care and lost productivity is a public health concern. Public health initiatives can counter efforts that promote smoking. The tobacco industry spends billions of dollars in advertising and promotion or nearly $22 million per day in the US [106]. In addition to direct advertising and coupons, marketing dollars are paid directly to retailers or wholesalers to reduce the price of cigarettes and fund promotions such as two for one pricing. Much of the advertising is historically targeted to younger populations, women, racial and ethnic communities. Community-based coalitions across the US can advocate for federal, state, and local policy initiatives, including youth empowerment efforts, taxes, or minimum prices to raise the cost of tobacco products, strong clean air regulations, preventing youth access to tobacco products, smoke-free homes and cars, banning flavored tobacco products, promoting strong warnings on tobacco products, and supporting comprehensive state funding for tobacco-free initiatives.

Emotional Support

When individuals understand that tobacco use is a chronic disease, they may feel less of a sense of failure if they struggle to quit. Understanding the relapsing nature of the addiction, while knowing that support and effective treatment exist, can increase self-efficacy. Misperceptions can be barriers to successful management of this chronic condition. One misperception is that the responsibility for change rests entirely on the individual who uses tobacco, viewing tobacco use as "just a bad habit" or "just a mind thing." This view reinforces judgment and shame. In fact, the highly addictive nature of tobacco products, which deliver nicotine to the brain in less than 10 seconds, makes tobacco use an automatic, ingrained repetitive behavior. Effective abstinence requires continued practice to relearn new behaviors while dealing with the difficult symptoms of withdrawal. Willpower alone rarely succeeds, especially with patients who deal with multiple chronic diseases, financial insecurity, or other life stress.

Another misperception is the association of smoking with stress relief. Nicotine triggers the release of dopamine, leading to a temporary feeling of well-being and enhanced cognitive performance. However, this is a "cruel illusion." [107] While the immediate hit of nicotine causes feelings of well-being, it also puts stress on the heart by increasing heart rate and blood pressure and, after a few hours, adds the stress of withdrawal that can only be relieved by smoking again. It is important that both patient and provider understand this phenomenon as they work to find effective strategies to improve health.

The 5As Model for Tobacco Cessation

Effective systems addressing tobacco dependence follow a strong theoretical intervention, such as the 5As model for tobacco use: Ask, Advise, Assess, Assist, and Arrange, which should be addressed at every health care visit (Fig. 4.3). [21, 87, 108, 109]

Ask

Team-based care starts with *Ask*, meaning a nurse or medical assistant inquiries about tobacco use while taking vital signs. Asking about smoking behaviors in a non-judgmental manner acknowledges the chronic nature of tobacco dependence and that tobacco cessation is not a linear accomplishment for most patients [110]. A straight forward "Have you ever used tobacco products?" with a positive response followed by "Do you currently smoke or use any other tobacco products, including e-cigarettes?" has a very different feel than the

Fig. 4.3 The Five A's for treating tobacco use (Reprinted from public domain)

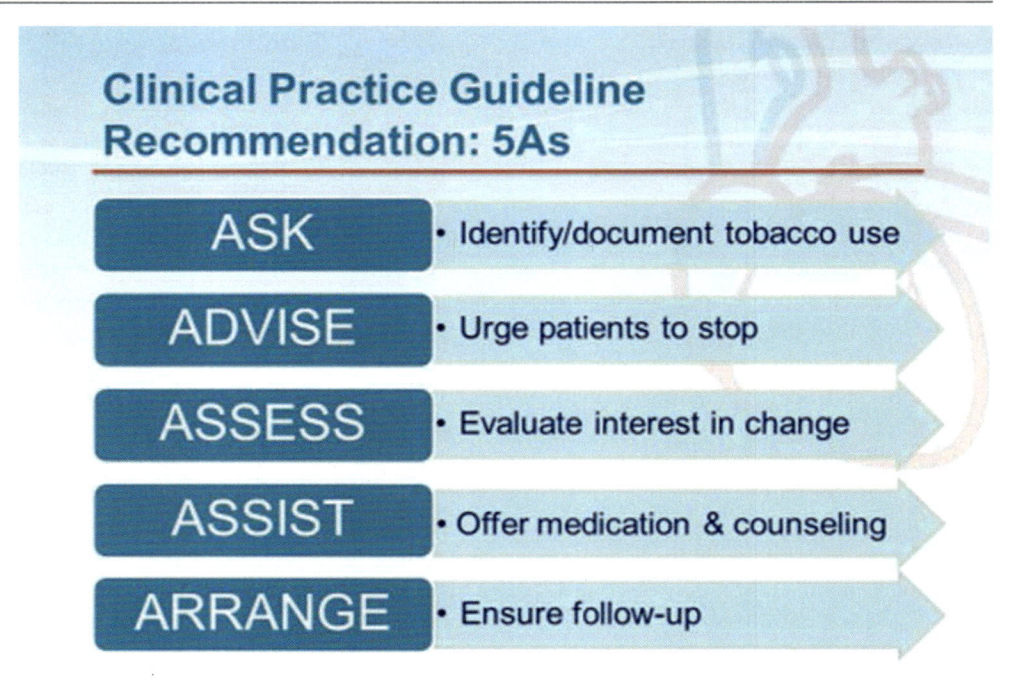

Clinical Practice Guideline Recommendation: 5As

- ASK • Identify/document tobacco use
- ADVISE • Urge patients to stop
- ASSESS • Evaluate interest in change
- ASSIST • Offer medication & counseling
- ARRANGE • Ensure follow-up

accusatory tone of "Are you (still) a smoker?" or "You don't smoke, do you?" Asking the patient if they are exposed to secondhand smoke allows for conversations on ways to reduce that exposure. Patients may be embarrassed or reluctant to be truthful regarding tobacco use. The term "smoker" reinforces judgment and stigmatization, labeling a person by the disease or addiction. Alternative language such as "a person who smokes" labels the behavior instead of the person, allowing clinicians to see patients who use tobacco as people who are caught in a cycle of addiction that has both individual and societal determinants. This reframing can increase empathy toward the patient who is being asked to change daily routines that revolve around smoking, while fighting off cravings and irritability.

Advise

Many patients report that their doctor told them to quit smoking but did not offer any help or information about how to quit. Patients do not like being preached to or having fingers wagged or hearing about all the bad things that will happen if they continue to smoke. Instead, they benefit from specific information related to individual circumstances, for example, "Stopping all tobacco use is one of the best things you can do for your health. You will notice significant reductions in your asthma symptoms, without having to rely on higher doses of medications. I understand how difficult this change can be. We have effective medications and resources for supporting you in becoming tobacco-free." In this brief message, the clinician voices belief in positive outcomes of stopping tobacco use, demonstrates empathy, and offers resources to the patient. Positive messaging or "gain-framed" statements, such as the benefits that will accrue after stopping tobacco use for 1 day, 1 month, or 1 year, may be positive moderators of treatment [111].

Assess

Assessment has typically been framed as a yes/no question such as "Are you ready to quit?" with an affirmative answer required for further assistance. This is insufficient. Seventy percent of people who smoke say they want to stop, but may not say they are ready to quit because of perceived stress, lack of success in previous efforts, or not knowing how. An open-ended prompt, such as "I'd like to hear your thoughts about cutting down or stopping smoking" or "Tell me about your smoking and your interest in making any changes," is better and allows patients to state their concerns and give clinicians clues about how to best approach efforts to become tobacco free. The clinician can listen for patient fears and perceived difficulties, then address those with empathy, education, and resources.

If the patient is not interested in quitting, **motivational interviewing** using empathetic open-ended questions is an evidenced-based strategy to help patients consider treatment [112, 113]. Effective motivational interviewing creates teachable moments when a patient may be more receptive to considering a behavior change due to a health scare (e.g., chronic disease diagnosis, hospitalization, or cancer diagnosis related to complications from smoking) or due to renewed interest in health optimization (e.g., annual physical exam) [114–118]. Teachable moments occur in the inpatient, outpatient, and emergency department setting but are often lost opportunities to increase patient motivation and commitment to change [119, 120].

The OARS framework can guide motivational interviewing:

- **O**pen-ended questions to invite further dialogue with the patient, such as "What has worked when you have tried to stop smoking in the past?"
- **A**ffirming to identify positive attributes in the patient, such as "That is great that you were able to cut down by 5 cigarettes."
- **R**eflective or active listening to communicate back to patient that their message was heard and they have your attention, such as "I hear that it has been difficult for you to quit tobacco and that you have tried many different approaches to quitting."
- **S**ummarizing the conversation to gather important points within the current session and/or link salient information from prior sessions, transition to a new topic, or signal the end of a session, such as "It sounds like you're saying that despite many previous attempts to quit on your own that were not fully successful, you are ready to try medications and counseling."

Asking the patient open-ended questions such as "Help me understand why you are not ready to quit given what you know about the health effects of tobacco use" or "What would it take to get you interested in quitting?" often elicits information that motivates change. Follow-up questions might help overcome resistance, such as "If we could relieve your cravings, would you consider quitting?" or "Knowing that it is not easy, how can I best help you do so?" Physician-delivered motivational interviewing is associated with a 3.5-fold increased rate of quitting tobacco compared to usual care or limited brief advice [121].

Motivational interviewing can elicit both strengths and challenges to quitting. Strengths can be found even in statements such as "I've tried a hundred times and failed," which can be countered with the statement "You've had a lot of practice and it sounds like you can be quite persistent." The patient may reference a past situation that prevented abstinence such as "I quit for a few months but then my husband lost his job" and the clinician can reply "You were able to quit, and a very stressful situation set you back." Finding strengths can be useful in suggesting strategies to deal with the challenge of changing tobacco habits. Some patients end up stopping smoking even when they do not indicate a readiness to quit. When provided treatment, patients who said they were not ready to quit had higher rates of six-month abstinence than those stating they were planning to quit [122, 123].

Assist

Evidence-based treatment includes a combination of pharmacotherapy and behavioral counseling. The strength of the addiction to nicotine and other substances means that changing behavior immediately and without intervention ("cold turkey") will be extremely difficult for most people [19].

Cutting-Down-to-Quit (Nicotine Fading)

The traditional advice is that a person using tobacco should set a quit date and abruptly quit on that date [124]. An alternative approach is to gradually reduce the amount of tobacco used (e.g., cutting down from 10 cigarettes per day to 1 cigarette per day over the course of a few weeks) as both abrupt and gradual cessation approaches are similarly effective [125]. Clinicians should support the approach that the patient believes will work best for them.

Behavioral Counseling

Even brief behavioral interventions for tobacco dependence treatment can promote abstinence [126]. Given the chronic nature of tobacco dependence, repeated, longitudinal interventions and multiple quit attempts may be necessary for long-term cessation. Comprehensive treatment strategies benefit most people who use tobacco, and intensive counseling increases patient satisfaction even in those patients who are not ready to quit smoking [127–129]. Individual, group, and telephone counseling can all be effective strategies. There is a dose-response between counseling and effectiveness suggesting that increasing the duration or frequency of counseling will improve outcomes. While even 3 minutes of counseling can have impact, 10 or more minutes is ideal, with increasing effectiveness with four or more sessions. Counseling via different strategies (i.e., problem-solving skills vs social support), by different personnel (both clinicians and non-clinicians) and inclusion of nicotine replacement therapies and/or non-nicotine pharmacologic management compliment tobacco cessation counseling and increase abstinence rates.

Pharmacotherapy

Physical and psychological tobacco use dependence is most effectively managed with medications that alleviate nicotine withdrawal symptoms and reduce the strength and frequency of urges to use tobacco. Medications can double initial quit rates but sustained abstinence requires behavioral interventions that address the routines, stressors, and psychological factors that reinforce tobacco use.

The Food and Drug Administration (FDA) has approved varenicline, bupropion, and various types of nicotine replacement therapy (NRT) for tobacco cessation treatment (Table 4.4). The two most effective pharmacotherapy approaches are single-use varenicline or combination NRT,

Table 4.4 FDA-approved tobacco cessation medications; table adapted from Duke-UNC Tobacco Treatment Specialist Training Program Manual

Medication (and doses)	Contraindications	Potential Side Effects (Mitigation)	Mechanism of Action	Dosing
Nicotine patch (7 mg, 14 mg, 21 mg)	Systemic allergic reaction (hives) to adhesive; Latex allergy; Pregnant women may consider use if behavioral treatments fail	Local skin irritation (helps to rotate patch site); vivid dreams/sleep disturbance (helps to remove patch at night and have short-acting nicotine medication available upon awakening if withdrawal symptoms)	Sustained nicotine receptor agonist	7 mg if 14 mg not tolerated or while decreasing dose[a]; 14 mg for ≤10 cigarettes/day for 12 weeks[b]; 21 mg for 11–20 cigarettes/day for 12 weeks[b]
Nicotine gum (2 mg, 4 mg)	Dental work/problems preventing gum use	Headache, hiccups, jaw pain (chew until tingling sensation felt then park in cheek and stop chewing); mouth, esophageal, and gastric irritation; nausea/vomiting; palpitations	Immediate release nicotine receptor agonist	If first cigarette is: >30 min after waking, use 2 mg; ≤30 min after waking, use 4 mg
Nicotine lozenge or mini lozenge (2 mg, 4 mg)	Pregnant women may consider use if behavioral treatments fail	Headache, hiccups, jaw pain (chew until tingling sensation felt then park in cheek and stop chewing); mouth, esophageal, and gastric irritation; nausea/vomiting; palpitations	Immediate release nicotine receptor agonist. Mini lozenge has faster absorption than original lozenge.	If first cigarette is: >30 min after waking, use 2 mg; ≤30 min after waking, use 4 mg
Nicotine nasal spray 10 mg/mL	Pregnant women may consider use if behavioral treatments fail	Cough, headache, nasal irritation, rhinitis, throat irritation	Immediate release nicotine receptor agonist	1 spray in each nostril 1–2 times/hour up to 10 sprays per hour
Nicotine inhaler 10 mg/cartridge	Pregnant women may consider use if behavioral treatments fail	Cough, mouth irritation, throat irritation	Immediate release nicotine receptor agonist	Puff into mouth 6–16 cartridges/day as needed
Varenicline; Chantix (0.5 mg, 1 mg)	Not recommended for women who are pregnant or breast feeding	Abnormal dreams, headache, insomnia, nasopharyngitis, nausea/vomiting, xerostomia	Sustained nicotine receptor agonist and antagonist (so prevents immediate, larger nicotine stimulation nicotine inhaled from cigarettes)	Day 1–3: 0.5 mg once daily; Day 4–7: 0.5 mg twice daily; Day 8 and onward: 1 mg twice daily
Bupropion SR; Zyban (150 mg)	Not recommended for those with risk of seizure (seizure history, alcohol dependence, stroke, head injury, MAO inhibitors, anorexia or bulimia) or for women who are pregnant or breast feeding	Constipation, diaphoresis, dizziness, headache, insomnia, nausea/vomiting, weight loss, xerostomia	Blocks re-uptake of dopamine and norepinephrine	150 mg SR once daily for 3 days then increase to 150 mg twice daily

[a] Some patients prefer step-down dosing of patch
[b] Minimum recommended dosing for nicotine replacement is 12 weeks. Some patients may require longer dosing indefinitely

such as a long-acting patch plus short-acting gum or lozenge. Varenicline is a nicotine agonist and is proven safe, even in people with mental health diagnoses [130]. Patients do not need to quit smoking before starting varenicline. Combination NRT allows for self-dosing of nicotine to reduce withdrawal symptoms, which is the most common cause for relapse or inability to stop use. Step-down dosing of the patch strength over weeks to months is a common approach, with use of NRT gum or lozenge dosing as needed for cravings. Informing patients of medication cost and potential side effects improves compliance with therapy.

The amount of nicotine delivered per cigarette has increased in the past decades, which makes quitting more difficult and NRT less effective. E-cigarette use practices make this clear, as patients liberally self-dose. Nicotine withdrawal symptoms include agitation, anhedonia, anxiety, depression, foggy thoughts, irritability, cravings for tobacco, and restlessness. Over medicating with nicotine can also cause symptoms such as nausea, dizziness, light-headedness, and insomnia. Effective management of withdrawal symptoms allows the energy and focus necessary to develop the behavioral changes that will support long-term abstinence, such as strategies to manage triggers and cues, cognitive therapy to reframe feelings of weakness or lack of willpower, and nutritional and physical activity to reduce resultant weight gain.

Arrange

As with any chronic illness, long-term follow-up improves outcomes. Immediate follow-up to new quit attempts helps patients adhere to medications and manage side effects and improves cessation outcomes [131]. Patients may be referred to a quitline or a tobacco treatment specialist or other behavioral health provider. Quitlines are free, live, evidence-based, and are available in every US state by calling 1-800-QUIT NOW (1-800-784-8669). Automated text-messaging interventions are effective, but smartphone apps remain unproven.

Referrals to quitlines can be integrated into EHRs or faxed. Hospitals, clinics, and other organizations may employ certified tobacco treatment specialists who undergo evidence-based training, including didactic sessions on the biomedical and psychosocial aspects of tobacco dependence, counseling techniques, and 240 hours of documented tobacco cessation counseling with patients, prior to becoming certified [132]. They skillfully provide short- and long-term follow-up with patients including counseling, coaching, and medication management.

Long-term follow-up focuses on relapse prevention, reinforces the positives of a tobacco-free life, and anticipates challenges or cause for return to tobacco use. Inquiring as to progress in cessation takes only a few moments at follow-up visits. This individual care along with community resources increases the success rate of tobacco cessation.

Telehealth

The COVID-19 pandemic increased virtual care delivery including tobacco cessation treatment. Telehealth for smoking cessation is efficient and effective [133–137]. It has potential as an effective tool for tobacco cessation but disparities in access to telehealth tools (i.e., computers, cell phones, tablets, and/or broadband) exacerbate inequities in care delivery [138–140]. In the US, the Federal Communication Commission is investing billions of dollars to improve broadband connectivity to rural and lower-income regions [139, 141, 142]. Greater access will help overcome barriers to virtual tobacco treatment [143]. Ongoing research and implementation evaluations regarding best practices have the potential to improve effective access to tobacco use treatment, ensuring equitable access for all populations [143, 144].

Population Health and the Health Care System

Tobacco use is so detrimental to the health of individuals that efforts to promote cessation should be prominent in the health care system. Addressing tobacco use may be a consideration in recognition as a Patient-Centered Medical Home (PCMH). Tobacco use treatment should be streamlined into patient visits, including integration of protocols into EHRs which can assist with patient and cohort identification, care documentation, patient follow-up, guideline adherence, and benchmarking. EHR registries can identify patients with a disease of interest and facilitate population health tracking and interventions for these patients [145]. Dashboards use demographic data from registries and associated interventions to track process, financial, quality, and clinical outcome measures. Dashboards that present data in an accessible and comprehensible way to clinicians improve care processes and outcomes [146]. Visualization dashboards present data to clinicians in graphic formats that are easy to read and time efficient, thereby reducing clinician errors and cognitive load and improving evidence-based guideline adherence [147].

The Centers for Disease Control and Prevention (CDC) recommends use of tobacco registries and treatment tracking in all patients who smoke though it is not yet clear which types of digital support are used and which are most effective [148]. Tobacco registries standardize tobacco use treatment leading to increased referrals to quitlines, tobacco use counseling, and medication prescriptions [149]. EHRs can send Best Practice Advisories to clinicians during an encounter, reminding them to *Ask, Advise, Assess, Assist,* and *Arrange,* while providing decision support, pharmacotherapy guidance, and behavioral treatment referrals which can include access to community resources [145]. These digital supports provide population-level interventions to standardize outreach and tracking of patients who use tobacco, send targeted messages to patients (via patient portals or mailings), and provide billing prompts for rendered services [149].

Federal population-based tobacco use treatment efforts include the National Cancer Institute's smokefree.gov initiative, which offers free evidence-based support to the public [150]. These digital supports augment traditional quitlines and individual counseling sessions with websites, text-messaging programs, and mobile applications that can target the general population or specific populations such as military veterans, women, adolescents, Spanish-speakers, and older adults. With over 7 million users a year, the benefits of multiple intervention modalities are apparent [150].

Quality Improvement

Quality improvement (QI) efforts can dramatically increase tobacco use treatment [101, 151]. QI processes such as Lean continuous improvement to systematically evaluate workflows and processes can improve care delivery [152, 153]. QI studies may use Plan-Do-Study-Act (PDSA) cycles to iteratively evaluate, implement, and test patient care improvement efforts. Systematic methods to improve workflows and patient care processes in tobacco use can improve site-specific tobacco treatment and inform similar work at other institutions resulting in shared knowledge and continuous process improvements across institutions [154–156].

Insurance Changes

The 2010 Affordable Care Act requires insurance companies to cover evidence-based services that have a rating of "A" or "B" from the US Preventive Services Task Force (USPSTF), an independent panel of clinicians and scientists commissioned by the Agency for Healthcare Research and Quality, including tobacco use counseling and medication. Treatment is covered up to four sessions twice a year with 12 weeks of pharmacotherapy coverage. While these provisions are a start, they do not acknowledge the long-term nature of behavioral change, especially in people who are trying to address mental health or other substance use at same time, or for whom smoking is a coping strategy for grief, stress, discomfort, and loneliness.

Future Directions

Social Media, mHealth, and eHealth

Mobile health interventions, such texting, may increase quitting success. There are numerous smartphone cessation apps but their quality varies and evidence is still lacking on their efficacy or effectiveness [157]. Online and text-based interventions are common with peer recruiting through social media showing some promise with one online social network (Share2Quit) quadrupling peer recruitment [158]. Given the ubiquity of social media and digital devices, more options for tobacco cessation support are likely to develop.

New Pharmacotherapies

There are several novel pharmacotherapies in clinical trials [159]. Nicotine vaccines and galenic formulations of varenicline may be effective in producing antibody levels that reduce side effects. Efforts should also continue to address misperceptions about the currently available medications, including the low risk of these agents compared to the enormous health risks of continued smoking.

E-Cigarettes for Quitting Cigarettes

Electronic cigarettes have grown in popularity, and some people who smoke use them to try to quit cigarette smoking even those that are not an approved cessation product. While likely less harmful than cigarettes, e-cigarettes are not harmless and the long-term health effects remain unknown [160]. E-cigarettes may be more effective than nicotine replacement therapy in randomized clinical trials, but evidence is conflicting, especially in the long term (more than 1 year) [161, 162]. Observational studies of consumer e-cigarette use have not found them to be associated with smoking cessation [163]. Rather than using e-cigarettes to completely quit smoking, many smokers use e-cigarettes as a supplement, for example, vaping in places where they can't smoke [164]. About half of e-cigarette users still smoke cigarettes with the associated ongoing health risks [165]. E-cigarette users should be encouraged to fully quit cigarettes and only use e-cigarettes or, better yet, use an approved cessation product.

Behavioral Therapies

Mindfulness, as both primary and adjunct therapy for becoming tobacco free, can reduce craving and manage stress, which may improve smoking abstinence and relapse prevention [166–168]. This approach may be especially helpful when combined with other established treatments.

Genetics

Research on the human genome has opened a new dimension for understanding tobacco use and dependence. An association between the nicotinic receptor alpha 5 (CHRNA5) and increased risk of addiction-associated phenotypes may explain why some people smoke more heavily than others. The potential for using genetic data includes individualized treatment as well as the ability to target prevention efforts [169–171].

Adolescents and Young Adults

Tobacco use and habituation usually start in adolescence or young adulthood [172, 173]. In 2020, 24% of high-school students and 7% of middle-school students reported use of a tobacco product in the previous 30 days. Primary treatment for tobacco use in adolescents focuses on behavioral interventions with little research showing efficacy of pharmacotherapy in youth [174]. Characteristics of effective behavioral cessation programs include voluntary and fun sessions, motivational interviewing focused on intrinsic and extrinsic motivations to quit, frequent counseling sessions (10 sessions have been efficacious), using social and community support for cessation, extrinsic rewards for quitting, and education on handling stress, social situations, and peer pressure [175]. The National Cancer Institute's Smokefree Teen website provides online resources for teens including text messaging, apps, and access to counselors with age-appropriate cessation support [176]. Several resources are also available for parents and caregivers to support adolescents in cessation efforts [177, 178]. The Truth Initiative has a texting program for youth and young adult vaping called "This is Quitting" that has been shown effective. [179]

Prenatal Treatment

Behavioral treatment is also emphasized during pregnancy, given the concerns of medication use. A 2021 USPSTF guideline recommends (grade A recommendation) that clinicians ask and advise cessation for pregnant people who smoke and provide behavioral counseling to assist in cessation [131]. This guideline also states there is insufficient evidence (grade I recommendation) to adequately determine the risks and benefits of cessation medication use in pregnancy.

Education to Health Care Team Members

Team-based care is a growing concept in our health care system. All health care providers in practice or training, including physicians, nurses, dentists, physical and occupational therapists, and advanced practice practitioners, should be well-versed in the harms of tobacco use and taught the skills to address this leading cause of preventable disease and death.

References

1. U.S. Department of Health and Human Services. Smoking cessation: a report of the surgeon general; 2020. https://www.hhs.gov/surgeongeneral/reports-and-publications/tobacco/2020-cessation-sgr-factsheet-key-findings/index.html. Accessed 01 Jul 2020
2. Cornelius ME, Loretan CG, Wang TW, Jamal A, Homa DM. Tobacco product use among adults—United States, 2020. MMWR Morb Mortal Wkly Rep. 2022;71:397–405. https://doi.org/10.15585/mmwr.mm7111a1external.
3. Reitsma MB, Kendrick PJ, Ababneh E, et al. Spatial, temporal, and demographic patterns in prevalence of smoking tobacco use and attributable disease burden in 204 countries and territories, 1990–2019: a systematic analysis from the global burden of disease study 2019. Lancet. 2021;397(10292):2337–60. https://doi.org/10.1016/s0140-6736(21)01169-7.
4. Jacobs EJ, Newton CC, Carter BD, et al. What proportion of cancer deaths in the contemporary United States is attributable to cigarette smoking? Ann Epidemiol. 2015;25(3):179–82. e1. https://doi.org/10.1016/j.annepidem.2014.11.008.
5. Islami F, Goding Sauer A, Miller KD, et al. Proportion and number of cancer cases and deaths attributable to potentially modifiable risk factors in the United States. CA Cancer J Clin. 2018;68(1):31–54. https://doi.org/10.3322/caac.21440.
6. The health consequences of smoking—50 years of progress: a report of the surgeon general; 2014.
7. The health consequences of involuntary exposure to tobacco smoke: a report of the surgeon general; 2006.
8. Meernik C, Goldstein AO. A critical review of smoking, cessation, relapse and emerging research in pregnancy and post-partum. Br Med Bull Jun 2015;114(1):135–146. doi:https://doi.org/10.1093/bmb/ldv016.
9. Xu X, Shrestha SS, Trivers KF, Neff L, Armour BS, King BA. U.S. healthcare spending attributable to cigarette smoking in 2014. Prev Med. 2021:106529. https://doi.org/10.1016/j.ypmed.2021.106529.
10. Shrestha SS, Ghimire R, Wang X, Trivers KF, Homa DM, Armour BS. Cost of cigarette smoking attributable productivity losses, U.S., 2018. Am J Prev Med. 2022; https://doi.org/10.1016/j.amepre.2022.04.032.
11. Max W, Sung HY, Shi Y. Deaths from secondhand smoke exposure in the United States: economic implications. Am J Public Health. 2012;102(11):2173–80. https://doi.org/10.2105/AJPH.2012.300805.
12. Stanton CA, Keith DR, Gaalema DE, et al. Trends in tobacco use among US adults with chronic health conditions: National Survey on drug use and health 2005-2013. Prev Med. 2016;92:160–8. https://doi.org/10.1016/j.ypmed.2016.04.008.
13. Kong AY, Queen TL, Golden SD, Ribisl KM. Neighborhood disparities in the availability, advertising, promotion, and youth appeal of little cigars and cigarillos, United States, 2015. Nicotine Tob Res. 2020;22(12):2170–7. https://doi.org/10.1093/ntr/ntaa005.
14. Edwards SA, Bondy SJ, Callaghan RC, Mann RE. Prevalence of unassisted quit attempts in population-based studies: a systematic review of the literature. Addict Behav. 2014;39(3):512–9. https://doi.org/10.1016/j.addbeh.2013.10.036.
15. Danesh D, Paskett ED, Ferketich AK. Disparities in receipt of advice to quit smoking from health care providers: 2010 National Health Interview Survey. Prev Chronic Dis. 2014;11:E131. https://doi.org/10.5888/pcd11.140053.
16. Fiore M, Jaen CR, Baker T, et al. Treating tobacco use and dependence: 2008 update. Rockville, MD: US Department of Health and Human Services; 2008.
17. Creamer MR, Wang TW, Babb S, et al. Tobacco product use and cessation indicators among adults-United States, 2018. MMWR. 2019;68(45):1013–9.
18. Heyman GM. Do addicts have free will? An empirical approach to a vexing question. Addict Behav Rep Jun 2017;5:85–93. doi:https://doi.org/10.1016/j.abrep.2017.02.001.
19. Lemmens VOA, Knut IK, Brug J. Effectiveness of smoking cessation interventions among adults: a systematic review of reviews. Eur J Cancer Prevention. 2008;17(6):535–44. https://doi.org/10.1097/CEJ.0b013e3282f75e48.
20. Steinberg MB, Schmelzer AC, Richardson DL, Foulds J. The case for treating tobacco dependence as a chronic disease. Ann Intern Med. 2008;148(7):554–6.
21. Halladay JR, Vu M, Ripley-Moffitt C, Gupta SK, O'Meara C, Goldstein AO. Patient perspectives on tobacco use treatment in primary care. Prev Chronic Dis. 2015;12:E14. https://doi.org/10.5888/pcd12.140408.
22. Gritz ER, Vidrine DJ, Fingeret MC. Smoking cessation: a critical component of medical management in chronic disease populations. Am J Prev Med. 2007;33(6):S414–22.
23. Rojewski AM, Baldassarri S, Cooperman NA, et al. Exploring issues of comorbid conditions in people who smoke. Nicotine Tob Res. 2016;18(8):1684–96. https://doi.org/10.1093/ntr/ntw016.
24. Reis RK, Miller SC. The ASAM principles of addiction medicine. Wolters Kluwer Health; 2014.
25. Berridge MS, Apana SM, Nagano KK, Berridge CE, Leisure GP, Boswell MV. Smoking produces rapid rise of [11C]nicotine in human brain. Psychopharmacology. 2010;209(4):383–94. https://doi.org/10.1007/s00213-010-1809-8.
26. Byron MJ, Baig SA, Moracco KE, Brewer NT. Adolescents' and adults' perceptions of 'natural', 'organic' and 'additive-free' cigarettes, and the required disclaimers. Tob Control. 2016;25(5):517. https://doi.org/10.1136/tobaccocontrol-2015-052560.
27. Commission USFT. U.S. Federal Trade Commission (FTC), Cigarette Report for 2020, 2021. 2021.
28. Levy DT, Blackman K, Tauras J, et al. Quit attempts and quit rates among menthol and nonmenthol smokers in the United States. Am J Public Health. 2011;101(7):1241–7. https://doi.org/10.2105/ajph.2011.300178.

29. Keeler C, Max W, Yerger V, Yao T, Ong MK, Sung HY. The association of menthol cigarette use with quit attempts, successful cessation, and intention to quit across racial/ethnic groups in the United States. Nicotine Tob Res. 2016; https://doi.org/10.1093/ntr/ntw215.
30. FDA proposes rules prohibiting menthol cigarettes and Flavored cigars to prevent youth initiation, significantly reduce tobacco-related disease and death. FDA; 04/28/2022. https://www.fda.gov/news-events/press-announcements/fda-proposes-rules-prohibiting-menthol-cigarettes-and-flavored-cigars-prevent-youth-initiation
31. Office on Smoking and Health NCfCDPaHP. Hookahs. U.S. Department of Health & Human Services; 2022. https://www.cdc.gov/tobacco/data_statistics/fact_sheets/tobacco_industry/hookahs/index.htm. Accessed 29 Aug 2022.
32. General USPHSOotS, Prevention NCfCD, Smoking HPOo. Preventing tobacco use among youth and young adults: a report of the surgeon general. US Government Printing Office; 2012.
33. Biener L, Nyman AL, Stepanov I, Hatsukami D. Public education about the relative harms of tobacco products: an intervention for tobacco control professionals. Tob Control. 2014;23(5):385. https://doi.org/10.1136/tobaccocontrol-2012-050814.
34. Organization WH. IARC Monographs on the evaluation of carcinogenic risks to humans. Volume 89: smokeless tobacco and some tobacco-specific N-nitrosamines; 2007.
35. Prevention UCfDCa. Smokeless tobacco: health effects. Office on Smoking and Health, US Center for Disease Control and Prevention. Updated August 13, 2020. https://www.cdc.gov/tobacco/data_statistics/fact_sheets/smokeless/health_effects/index.htm. Accessed 9 Sep 2022.
36. Burton A. Does the smoke ever really clear? Thirdhand smoke exposure raises new concerns. Environ Health Perspect. 2011;119(2):A70–4.
37. Protano C, Vitali M. The new danger of thirdhand smoke: why passive smoking does not stop at secondhand smoke. Environ Health Perspect. 2011;119(10):A422. https://doi.org/10.1289/ehp.1103956.
38. Diez-Izquierdo A, Cassanello-Penarroya P, Lidon-Moyano C, Matilla-Santander N, Balaguer A, Martinez-Sanchez JM. Update on thirdhand smoke: a comprehensive systematic review. Environ Res. 2018;167:341–71. https://doi.org/10.1016/j.envres.2018.07.020.
39. U.S. Department of Health and Human Services. America's health rankings analysis of National Survey of Children's Health. (MCHB) MaCHB; 2021. https://www.americashealthrankings.org. Accessed 15 Sep 2022
40. CDC. Vital signs: nonsmokers' exposure to secondhand smoke—United States, 1999–2008. MMWR Morb Mortal Wkly Rep. 2010;59(35):1141–6.
41. Northrup TF, Matt GE, Hovell MF, Khan AM, Stotts AL. Thirdhand smoke in the homes of medically fragile children: assessing the impact of indoor Smoking levels and Smoking bans. Nicotine Tob Res. 2016;18(5):1290–8. https://doi.org/10.1093/ntr/ntv174.
42. Bahl V, Jacob P 3rd, Havel C, Schick SF, Talbot P. Thirdhand cigarette smoke: factors affecting exposure and remediation. PLoS One. 2014;9(10):e108258. https://doi.org/10.1371/journal.pone.0108258.
43. Hang B, Sarker AH, Havel C, et al. Thirdhand smoke causes DNA damage in human cells. Mutagenesis. 2013;28(4):381–91. https://doi.org/10.1093/mutage/get013.
44. Rehan VK, Sakurai R, Torday JS. Thirdhand smoke: a new dimension to the effects of cigarette smoke on the developing lung. Am J Physiol Lung Cell Mol Physiol. 2011;301(1):L1–8. https://doi.org/10.1152/ajplung.00393.2010.
45. Díez-Izquierdo A, Cassanello-Peñarroya P, Lidón-Moyano C, Matilla-Santander N, Balaguer A, Martínez-Sánchez JM. Update on thirdhand smoke: a comprehensive systematic review. Environ Res. 2018;167:341–71. https://doi.org/10.1016/j.envres.2018.07.020.
46. Klein JD, Chamberlin ME, Kress EA, et al. Asking the right questions about secondhand smoke. Nicotine Tob Res. 2021;23(1):57–62. https://doi.org/10.1093/ntr/ntz125.
47. ICD10.Data.com. ICD10-CM Codes. https://www.icd10data.com/ICD10CM/Codes/Z00-Z99/Z77-Z99/Z77-/Z77.22. Accessed 29 Aug 2022.
48. Jha P, Ramasundarahettige C, Landsman V, et al. 21st-century hazards of smoking and benefits of cessation in the United States. N Engl J Med. 2013;368(4):341–50. https://doi.org/10.1056/NEJMsa1211128.
49. Bullen C. Impact of tobacco smoking and smoking cessation on cardiovascular risk and disease. Expert Rev Cardiovasc Ther. 2008;6(6):883–95. https://doi.org/10.1586/14779072.6.6.883.
50. Burns DM. Epidemiology of smoking-induced cardiovascular disease. Prog Cardiovasc Dis. 2003;46(1):11–29.
51. Robbins AS, Manson JE, Lee IM, Satterfield S, Hennekens CH. Cigarette smoking and stroke in a cohort of U.S. male physicians. Ann Intern Med. 1994;120(6):458–62.
52. McRobbie H, Hajek P. Nicotine replacement therapy in patients with cardiovascular disease: guidelines for health professionals. Addiction. 2001;96(11):1547–51. https://doi.org/10.1080/09652140120080688.
53. Barth J, Critchley J, Bengel J. Efficacy of psychosocial interventions for smoking cessation in patients with coronary heart disease: a systematic review and meta-analysis. Ann Behav Med. 2006;32(1):10–20. https://doi.org/10.1207/s15324796abm3201_2.
54. Mikhailidis DP, Papadakis JA, Ganotakis ES. Smoking, diabetes and hyperlipidaemia. J R Soc Health. 1998;118(2):91–3.
55. Becker RH, Sha S, Frick AD, Fountaine RJ. The effect of smoking cessation and subsequent resumption on absorption of inhaled insulin. Diabetes Care. 2006;29(2):277–82.
56. Tonstad S, Lawrence D. Varenicline in smokers with diabetes: a pooled analysis of 15 randomized, placebo-controlled studies of varenicline. J Diabetes Investig. 2016; https://doi.org/10.1111/jdi.12543.
57. Anthonisen NR. Lessons from the lung health study. Proc Am Thorac Soc. 2004;1(2):143–5. https://doi.org/10.1513/pats.2306033.
58. Burnes D. Chronic obstructive pulmonary disease In: Tobacco: science, policy and public health. Oxford University Press; 2004.
59. Godtfredsen NS, Lam TH, Hansel TT, et al. COPD-related morbidity and mortality after smoking cessation: status of the evidence. Eur Respir J. 2008;32(4):844–53. https://doi.org/10.1183/09031936.00160007.
60. Hilberink SR, Jacobs JE, Bottema BJ, de Vries H, Grol RP. Smoking cessation in patients with COPD in daily general practice (SMOCC): six months' results. Prev Med. 2005;41(5–6):822–7. https://doi.org/10.1016/j.ypmed.2005.08.003.
61. Lazarus SC, Chinchilli VM, Rollings NJ, et al. Smoking affects response to inhaled corticosteroids or leukotriene receptor antagonists in asthma. Am J Respir Crit Care Med. 2007;175(8):783–90. https://doi.org/10.1164/rccm.200511-1746OC.
62. McLeish AC, Farris SG, Johnson AL, Bernstein JA, Zvolensky MJ. Evaluation of smokers with and without asthma in terms of smoking cessation outcome, nicotine withdrawal symptoms, and craving: findings from a self-guided quit attempt. Addict Behav. 2016;63:149–54. https://doi.org/10.1016/j.addbeh.2016.07.021.
63. Perret JL, Bonevski B, McDonald CF, Abramson MJ. Smoking cessation strategies for patients with asthma: improving patient outcomes. J Asthma Allergy. 2016;9:117–28. https://doi.org/10.2147/jaa.s85615.
64. Balduyck B, Sardari Nia P, Cogen A, et al. The effect of smoking cessation on quality of life after lung cancer surgery. Eur J Cardio-

65. Nayan S, Gupta MK, Strychowsky JE, Sommer DD. Smoking cessation interventions and cessation rates in the oncology population: an updated systematic review and meta-analysis. Otolaryngol Head Neck Surg. 2013;149(2):200–11. https://doi.org/10.1177/0194599813490886.
66. Sheeran P, Jones K, Avishai A, et al. What works in smoking cessation interventions for cancer survivors? A meta-analysis. Health Psychol. 2019;38(10):855–65. https://doi.org/10.1037/hea0000757.
67. Goldstein AO, Shoenbill KA, Jolly TA. Intensive smoking cessation counseling for patients with cancer. JAMA. 2020;324(14):1401–3. https://doi.org/10.1001/jama.2020.13102.
68. Park ER, Perez GK, Regan S, et al. Effect of sustained smoking cessation counseling and provision of medication vs shorter-term counseling and medication advice on smoking abstinence in patients recently diagnosed with cancer: a randomized clinical trial. JAMA. 2020;324(14):1406–18. https://doi.org/10.1001/jama.2020.14581.
69. Reddy KP, Parker RA, Losina E, et al. Impact of cigarette smoking and smoking cessation on life expectancy among people with HIV: a US-based modeling study. J Infect Dis. 2016;2016 https://doi.org/10.1093/infdis/jiw430.
70. Mdodo R, Frazier EL, Dube SR, et al. Cigarette smoking prevalence among adults with HIV compared with the general adult population in the United States: cross-sectional surveys. Ann Intern Med. 2015;162(5):335–44. https://doi.org/10.7326/m14-0954.
71. Tseng TY, Krebs P, Schoenthaler A, et al. Combining text messaging and telephone counseling to increase varenicline adherence and smoking abstinence among cigarette smokers living with HIV: a randomized controlled study. AIDS Behav. 2016; https://doi.org/10.1007/s10461-016-1538-z.
72. Wewers ME, Neidig JL, Kihm KE. The feasibility of a nurse-managed, peer-led tobacco cessation intervention among HIV-positive smokers. J Assoc Nurses AIDS Care. 2000;11(6):37–44. https://doi.org/10.1016/s1055-3290(06)60353-1.
73. Vidrine DJ, Arduino RC, Lazev AB, Gritz ER. A randomized trial of a proactive cellular telephone intervention for smokers living with HIV/AIDS. AIDS (London, England). 2006;20(2):253–60. https://doi.org/10.1097/01.aids.0000198094.23691.58.
74. Gfroerer JDS, King BA, Garrett BE, Babb S, McAfee T. Vital signs: currrent cigarette smoking among adults aged ≥18 years with mental illness, United States 2009–2011. MMWR Morb Mortal Wkly Rep. 2013;62:81–7.
75. Schroeder SA, Morris CD. Confronting a neglected epidemic: tobacco cessation for persons with mental illnesses and substance abuse problems. Annu Rev Public Health. 2010;31:297–314. 1p following 314. https://doi.org/10.1146/annurev.publhealth.012809.103701.
76. Taylor G, McNeill A, Girling A, Farley A, Lindson-Hawley N, Aveyard P. Change in mental health after smoking cessation: systematic review and meta-analysis. BMJ. 2014;348:g1151. https://doi.org/10.1136/bmj.g1151.
77. Tsoh JY, Chi FW, Mertens JR, Weisner CM. Stopping smoking during first year of substance use treatment predicted 9-year alcohol and drug treatment outcomes. Drug Alcohol Depend. 2011;114(2–3):110–8. https://doi.org/10.1016/j.drugalcdep.2010.09.008.
78. Kopsaftis Z, van Agteren J, Carson K, O'Loughlin T, Smith B. Smoking cessation in the hospital setting: a systematic review and meta-analysis. Eur Respir J. 2017;50(suppl 61):PA1271. https://doi.org/10.1183/1393003.congress-2017.PA1271.
79. Iannello J, Levitt MP, Poetter D, et al. Improving inpatient tobacco treatment measures: outcomes through standardized treatment, care coordination, and electronic health record optimization. J Healthc Qual. 2021;43(1):48–58. https://doi.org/10.1097/JHQ.0000000000000251.
80. Trout S, Ripley-Moffitt C, Meernik C, Greyber J, Goldstein AO. Provider satisfaction with an inpatient tobacco treatment program: results from an inpatient provider survey. Int J General Med. 2017;10:363–9. https://doi.org/10.2147/IJGM.S136965.
81. Park HY, Choe YR, Oh IJ, et al. Efficacy of an inpatient smoking cessation program at a single regional cancer center: a prospective observational study. Medicine (Baltimore). 2021;100(6):e24745. https://doi.org/10.1097/MD.0000000000024745.
82. Matuszewski PE, Joseph K, O'Hara NN, DiClemente C, O'Toole RV. Prospective randomized trial on smoking cessation in orthopaedic trauma patients: results from the let's STOP (smoking in trauma orthopaedic patients) now trial. J Orthop Trauma. 2021;35(7):345–51. https://doi.org/10.1097/BOT.0000000000002028.
83. Brown RA, Minami H, Hecht J, et al. Sustained care Smoking cessation intervention for individuals hospitalized for psychiatric disorders: the helping HAND 3 randomized clinical trial. JAMA Psychiatry. 2021;78(8):839–47. https://doi.org/10.1001/jamapsychiatry.2021.0707.
84. See JJH, See KC. Impact of admission diagnosis on the Smoking cessation rate: a brief report from a multi-Centre inpatient smoking cessation programme in Singapore. J Prev Med Public Health. 2020;53(5):381–6. https://doi.org/10.3961/jpmph.20.134.
85. Thomas D, Abramson MJ, Bonevski B, et al. Integrating smoking cessation into routine care in hospitals—a randomized controlled trial. Addiction. 2016;111(4):714–23. https://doi.org/10.1111/add.13239.
86. Coleman K, Austin BT, Brach C, Wagner EH. Evidence on the chronic care model in the new millennium. Health Aff (Millwood). 2009;28(1):75–85. https://doi.org/10.1377/hlthaff.28.1.75.
87. Wagner EH, Bennett SM, Austin BT, Greene SM, Schaefer JK, Vonkorff M. Finding common ground: patient-centeredness and evidence-based chronic illness care. J Altern Complement Med. 2005;11(supplement 1):s-7–s-15.
88. McCullough A, Fisher M, Goldstein AO, Kramer KD, Ripley-Moffitt C. Smoking as a vital sign: prompts to ask and assess increase cessation counseling. J Am Board Fam Med. 2009;22(6):625–32. https://doi.org/10.3122/jabfm.2009.06.080211.
89. Theobald M, Botelho RJ, Saccocio SC, Houston TP, McAfee T, Mullins S, Weida TJ. Treating tobacco dependence practice manual, a systems-change approach. Am Acad Fam Phys; 2017.
90. Whittet MN, Capesius TR, Zook HG, Keller PA. The role of health systems in reducing tobacco dependence. Am J Accountable Care. 2019;7(2):4–11.
91. Lindson N, Pritchard G, Hong B, Fanshawe TR, Pipe A, Papadakis S. Strategies to improve smoking cessation rates in primary care. Cochrane Database Syst Rev. 2021;9(9):Cd011556. https://doi.org/10.1002/14651858.CD011556.pub2.
92. Soulakova JN, Tang CY, Leonardo SA, Taliaferro LA. Motivational benefits of social support and behavioural interventions for smoking cessation. J Smok Cessat. 2018;13(4):216–26. https://doi.org/10.1017/jsc.2017.26.
93. Cohen S, Lichtenstein E. Partner behaviors that support quitting smoking. J Consult Clin Psychol. 1990;58(3):304–9. https://doi.org/10.1037//0022-006x.58.3.304.
94. Derrick JL, Leonard KE, Homish GG. Perceived partner responsiveness predicts decreases in smoking during the first nine years of marriage. Nicotine Tob Res. 2013;15(9):1528–36. https://doi.org/10.1093/ntr/ntt011.
95. Christakis NFJ. The collective dynamics of smoking in a large social network. New Engl J Med. 2008;358(21):2248–58.
96. Ford P, Clifford A, Gussy K, Gartner C. A systematic review of peer-support programs for smoking cessation in disadvantaged groups. Int J Environ Res Public Health. 2013;10(11):5507–22. https://doi.org/10.3390/ijerph10115507.

97. Goldade K, Des Jarlais D, Everson-Rose SA, et al. Knowing quitters predicts smoking cessation in a homeless population. Am J Health Behav. 2013;37(4):517–24. https://doi.org/10.5993/ajhb.37.4.9.
98. Ruge J, Ulbricht S, Schumann A, Rumpf HJ, John U, Meyer C. Intention to quit smoking: is the partner's smoking status associated with the smoker's intention to quit? Int J Behav Med. 2008;15(4):328–35. https://doi.org/10.1080/10705500802365607.
99. vanDellen MR, Boyd SM, Ranby KW, MacKillop J, Lipkus IM. Willingness to provide support for a quit attempt: a study of partners of smokers. J Health Psychol. 2016;21(9):1840–9. https://doi.org/10.1177/1359105314567209.
100. Falba TA, Sindelar JL. Spousal concordance in health behavior change. Health Serv Res. 2008;43(1 Pt 1):96–116. https://doi.org/10.1111/j.1475-6773.2007.00754.x.
101. Ruebush E, Mitra S, Meyer C, Sisler L, Goldstein AO. Using a family systems approach to treat tobacco use among Cancer patients. Int J Environ Res Public Health. 2020;17(6) https://doi.org/10.3390/ijerph17062050.
102. Lobchuk MM, McClement SE, McPherson CJ, Cheang M. Impact of patient smoking behavior on empathic helping by family caregivers in lung cancer. Oncol Nurs Forum. 2012;39(2):E112–21.
103. Bottorff JL, Robinson CA, Sullivan KM, Smith ML. Continued family smoking after lung cancer diagnosis: the patient's perspective. Oncol Nurs Forum. 2009;36(3):E126–32. https://doi.org/10.1188/09.ONF.E126-E132.
104. Robinson CA, Bottorff JL, Smith ML, Sullivan KM. "Just because you've got lung cancer doesn't mean I will": lung cancer, smoking, and family dynamics. J Fam Nurs. 2010;16(3):282–301. https://doi.org/10.1177/1074840710370747.
105. Bottorff JL, Robinson CA, Sarbit G, Graham R, Kelly MT, Torchalla I. A motivational, gender-sensitive smoking cessation resource for family members of patients with lung cancer. Oncol Nurs Forum. 2015;42(4):363–70. https://doi.org/10.1188/15.Onf.42-04ap.
106. Federal Trade Commission Cigarette Report for 2019 (Federal Trade Commission); 2021, pp. 1–35.
107. Cleveland Clinic. Stress, stress Management, and Smoking. Cleveland Clinic. http://my.clevelandclinic.org/health/healthy_living/hic_Stress_Management_and_Emotional_Health/hic_Stress_Stress_Management_and_Smoking. Accessed 6 Jan 2017.
108. Wagner EH, Austin BT, Von Korff M. Organizing care for patients with chronic illness. Milbank Q. 1996:511–44.
109. Gould GS. Patient-centred tobacco management. Drug Alcohol Rev. 2014;33(1):93–8. https://doi.org/10.1111/dar.12082.
110. Bernstein SL, Toll BA. Ask about smoking, not quitting: a chronic disease approach to assessing and treating tobacco use. Addict Sci Clin Pract. 2019;14(1):29. https://doi.org/10.1186/s13722-019-0159-z.
111. Toll BA, Rojewski AM, Duncan LR, et al. "Quitting smoking will benefit your health": the evolution of clinician messaging to encourage tobacco cessation. Clin Cancer Res. 2014;20(2):301–9. https://doi.org/10.1158/1078-0432.ccr-13-2261.
112. Apodaca TR, Longabaugh R. Mechanisms of change in motivational interviewing: a review and preliminary evaluation of the evidence. Addiction. 2009;104(5):705–15. https://doi.org/10.1111/j.1360-0443.2009.02527.x.
113. Heckman CJ, Egleston BL, Hofmann MT. Efficacy of motivational interviewing for smoking cessation: a systematic review and meta-analysis. Tob Control. 2010;19(5):410–6. https://doi.org/10.1136/tc.2009.033175.
114. Cohen DJ, Clark EC, Lawson PJ, Casucci BA, Flocke SA. Identifying teachable moments for health behavior counseling in primary care. Patient Educ Couns. 2011;85(2):e8–15. https://doi.org/10.1016/j.pec.2010.11.009.
115. Dresler C, Warren GW, Arenberg D, et al. "Teachable moment" interventions in lung cancer: why action matters. J Thorac Oncol. 2018;13(5):603–5. https://doi.org/10.1016/j.jtho.2018.02.020.
116. Lawson PJ, Flocke SA. Teachable moments for health behavior change: a concept analysis. Patient Educ Couns. 2009;76(1):25–30. https://doi.org/10.1016/j.pec.2008.11.002.
117. Puleo GE, Borger T, Bowling WR, Burris JL. The state of the science on cancer diagnosis as a "Teachable Moment" for smoking cessation: a scoping review. Nicotine Tob Res. 2021; https://doi.org/10.1093/ntr/ntab139.
118. Xiang X. Chronic disease diagnosis as a teachable moment for health behavior changes among middle-aged and older adults. J Aging Health. 2016;28(6):995–1015. https://doi.org/10.1177/0898264315614573.
119. Buchbinder M, Wilbur R, Zuskov D, McLean S, Sleath B. Teachable moments and missed opportunities for smoking cessation counseling in a hospital emergency department: a mixed-methods study of patient-provider communication. BMC Health Serv Res. 2014;14:651. https://doi.org/10.1186/s12913-014-0651-9.
120. Gritz ER, Fingeret MC, Vidrine DJ, Lazev AB, Mehta NV, Reece GP. Successes and failures of the teachable moment: smoking cessation in cancer patients. Cancer. 2006;106(1):17–27. https://doi.org/10.1002/cncr.21598.
121. Lindson-Hawley N, Thompson TP, Begh R. Motivational interviewing for smoking cessation. Cochrane Database Syst Rev. 2015;(3):CD006936. https://doi.org/10.1002/14651858.CD006936.pub3.
122. Ellerbeck EF, Mahnken JD, Cupertino AP, et al. Effect of varying levels of disease management on smoking cessation: a randomized trial. Ann Intern Med. 2009;150(7):437–46.
123. Pisinger C, Vestbo J, Borch-Johnsen K, Jorgensen T. It is possible to help smokers in early motivational stages to quit. The Inter99 study. Prev Med. 2005;40(3):278–84. https://doi.org/10.1016/j.ypmed.2004.06.011.
124. Tan J, Zhao L, Chen H. A meta-analysis of the effectiveness of gradual versus abrupt smoking cessation. Tob Induc Dis. 2019;17:09. https://doi.org/10.18332/tid/100557.
125. Lindson N, Klemperer E, Hong B, Ordóñez-Mena JM, Aveyard P. Smoking reduction interventions for smoking cessation. Cochrane Database Syst Rev. 2019;(9) https://doi.org/10.1002/14651858.CD013183.pub2.
126. Lancaster T, Stead L. Physician advice for smoking cessation. Cochrane Database Syst Rev. 2004;(4):CD000165. https://doi.org/10.1002/14651858.CD000165.pub2.
127. Alterman AI, Gariti P, Mulvaney F. Short- and long-term smoking cessation for three levels of intensity of behavioral treatment. Psychol Addict Behav. 2001;15(3):261–4.
128. Hilleman DE, Mohiuddin SM, Packard KA. Comparison of conservative and aggressive smoking cessation treatment strategies following coronary artery bypass graft surgery. Chest. 2004;125(2):435–8. https://doi.org/10.1378/chest.125.2.435.
129. Barzilai DA, Goodwin MA, Zyzanski SJ, Stange KC. Does health habit counseling affect patient satisfaction? Prev Med. 2001;33(6):595–9. https://doi.org/10.1006/pmed.2001.0931.
130. Anthenelli RM, Benowitz NL, West R, et al. Neuropsychiatric safety and efficacy of varenicline, bupropion, and nicotine patch in smokers with and without psychiatric disorders (EAGLES): a double-blind, randomised, placebo-controlled clinical trial. Lancet. 2016;387(10037):2507–20. https://doi.org/10.1016/s0140-6736(16)30272-0.
131. USPSTF, Krist AH, Davidson KW, et al. Interventions for tobacco smoking cessation in adults, including pregnant persons: US preventive services task force recommendation statement. JAMA. 2021;325(3):265–79. https://doi.org/10.1001/jama.2020.25019.

132. National Association for Alcoholism and Drug Abuse Counselors (NAADAC). National certificate in tobacco treatment practice. https://www.naadac.org/NCTTP. Accessed 10 Dec 2021.
133. American Academy of Family Physicians (AAFP). Tobacco cessation telehealth guide; 2020. https://www.aafp.org/dam/AAFP/documents/patient_care/tobacco/tobacco-cessation-telehealth-guide.pdf. Accessed 02 May 2021.
134. American Lung Association. Tobacco cessation, telehealth and a pandemic: a changing landscape; 2020. https://www.lung.org/getmedia/83628722-434c-432b-84f4-754b25ea0cce/tobacco-cessation-and-telehealth_final.pdf. Accessed 05 Feb 2021.
135. Kotsen C, Dilip D, Carter-Harris L, et al. Rapid scaling up of telehealth treatment for tobacco-dependent cancer patients during the COVID-19 outbreak in New York City. Telemed J E Health. 2020;27(1):20–9. https://doi.org/10.1089/tmj.2020.0194.
136. Mujcic A, Blankers M, Bommele J, et al. The effectiveness of distance-based interventions for smoking cessation and alcohol moderation among cancer survivors: a meta-analysis. Psychooncology. 2020;29(1):49–60. https://doi.org/10.1002/pon.5261.
137. Shoenbill KA, Newcomer E, Valcourt-Hall C, Baca-Atlas M, Smith CA, Goldstein AO. An analysis of inpatient tobacco use treatment transition to telehealth. Nicotine Tob Res. 2021; https://doi.org/10.1093/ntr/ntab233.
138. Cantor JH, McBain RK, Pera MF, Bravata DM, Whaley CM. Who is (and is not) receiving telemedicine care during the COVID-19 pandemic. Am J Prev Med. 2021;61(3):434–8. https://doi.org/10.1016/j.amepre.2021.01.030.
139. Hirko KA, Kerver JM, Ford S, et al. Telehealth in response to the COVID-19 pandemic: implications for rural health disparities. J Am Med Inform Assoc. 2020;27(11):1816–8. https://doi.org/10.1093/jamia/ocaa156.
140. Arlington Research. Telehealth take-up: the risks and opportunities; Healthcare Report 2021. November 30, 2021. https://media.kasperskycontenthub.com/wp-content/uploads/sites/43/2021/11/22125239/Kaspersky_Healthcare-report-2021_eng.pdf.
141. Federal Communications Commission. COVID-19 Telehealth Program. Federal Communications Commission. https://www.fcc.gov/covid-19-telehealth-program. Accessed 05 Apr 2021.
142. HHS invests $8 million to address gaps in rural telehealth through the telehealth broadband pilot program. 01/11/2021, 2021. Accessed 15 Jan 2021. https://www.hhs.gov/about/news/2021/01/11/hhs-invests-8-million-to-address-gaps-in-rural-telehealth-through-telehealth-broadband-pilot.html
143. Slater JS, Nelson CL, Parks MJ, Ebbert JO. Connecting low-income smokers to tobacco treatment services. Addict Behav. 2016;52:108–14. https://doi.org/10.1016/j.addbeh.2015.10.013.
144. Darrat I, Tam S, Boulis M, Williams AM. Socioeconomic disparities in patient use of telehealth during the coronavirus disease 2019 surge. JAMA Otolaryngol Head Neck Surg. 2021;147(3):287–95. https://doi.org/10.1001/jamaoto.2020.5161.
145. Neutze D, Ripley-Moffitt C, Gwynne M, Goldstein AO. The implementation of a tobacco use registry in an academic family practice. J Am Board Fam Med. 2015;28(2):214–21. https://doi.org/10.3122/jabfm.2015.02.140117.
146. Dowding D, Randell R, Gardner P, et al. Dashboards for improving patient care: review of the literature. Int J Med Inform 2015;84(2):87–100. doi:https://doi.org/10.1016/j.ijmedinf.2014.10.001.
147. Khairat SS, Dukkipati A, Lauria HA, Bice T, Travers D, Carson SS. The impact of visualization dashboards on quality of care and clinician satisfaction: integrative literature review. JMIR Hum Factors. 2018;5(2):e22. https://doi.org/10.2196/humanfactors.9328.
148. Centers for Disease Control and Prevention. Best practices for comprehensive tobacco control programs—2014; 2014.
149. Ripley-Moffitt C, Neutze D, Gwynne M, Goldstein AO. Patient care outcomes of a tobacco use registry in an academic family practice. J Am Board Fam Med. 2015;28(2):205–13. https://doi.org/10.3122/jabfm.2015.02.140121.
150. Prutzman YM, Wiseman KP, Grady MA, et al. Using digital technologies to reach tobacco users who want to quit: evidence from the National Cancer Institute's Smokefree.gov initiative. Am J Prev Med. 2021;60(3 Suppl 2):S172–84. https://doi.org/10.1016/j.amepre.2020.08.008.
151. Kowitt SD, Goldstein AO, Cykert S. A heart healthy intervention improved tobacco screening rates and cessation support in primary care practices. J Prev Dent. 2022;43(3):375–86. https://doi.org/10.1007/s10935-022-00672-5.
152. Meyer C, Mitra S, Ruebush E, Sisler L, Wang K, Goldstein AO. A lean quality improvement initiative to enhance tobacco use treatment in a cancer hospital. Int J Environ Res Public Health. 2020;17(6) https://doi.org/10.3390/ijerph17062165.
153. Sisler L, Omofoye O, Paci K, Hadar E, Goldstein AO, Ripley-Moffitt C. Using lean quality improvement tools to increase delivery of evidence-based tobacco use treatment in hospitalized neurosurgical patients. Jt Comm J Qual Patient Saf. 2017;43(12):633–41. https://doi.org/10.1016/j.jcjq.2017.06.012.
154. Croyle RT, Morgan GD, Fiore MC. Addressing a core gap in cancer care—the NCI moonshot program to help oncology patients stop smoking. N Engl J Med. 2019;380(6):512–5. https://doi.org/10.1056/NEJMp1813913.
155. Ugalde A, White V, Rankin NM, et al. How can hospitals change practice to better implement smoking cessation interventions? A systematic review. CA Cancer J Clin. 2021; https://doi.org/10.3322/caac.21709.
156. Wiseman KP, Hauser L, Clark C, et al. An evaluation of the process and quality improvement measures of the University of Virginia Cancer Center Tobacco Treatment Program. Int J Environ Res Public Health. 2020;17(13) https://doi.org/10.3390/ijerph17134707.
157. Whittaker R, McRobbie H, Bullen C, Rodgers A, Gu Y, Dobson R. Mobile phone text messaging and app-based interventions for smoking cessation. Cochrane Database Syst Rev. 2019;10:CD006611. https://doi.org/10.1002/14651858.CD006611.pub5.
158. Sadasivam RS, Cutrona SL, Luger TM, et al. Share2Quit: online social Network peer marketing of tobacco cessation systems. Nicotine Tob Res. 2016; https://doi.org/10.1093/ntr/ntw187.
159. Beard E, Shahab L, Cummings DM, Michie S, West R. New pharmacological agents to aid Smoking cessation and tobacco harm reduction: what has been investigated, and what is in the pipeline? CNS Drugs. 2016;30(10):951–83. https://doi.org/10.1007/s40263-016-0362-3.
160. National Academies of Sciences E, Medicine. Public health consequences of E-cigarettes. The National Academies Press; 2018. p. 774.
161. Hartmann-Boyce J, McRobbie H, Butler AR, et al. Electronic cigarettes for smoking cessation. Cochrane Database Syst Rev. 2021;(9) https://doi.org/10.1002/14651858.CD010216.pub6.
162. Ibrahim S, Habiballah M, Sayed IE. Efficacy of electronic cigarettes for smoking cessation: a systematic review and meta-analysis. Am J Health Promot. 2021;35(3):442–55. https://doi.org/10.1177/0890117120980289.
163. Wang RJ, Bhadriraju S, Glantz SA. E-cigarette use and adult cigarette smoking cessation: a meta-analysis. Am J Public Health. 2021;111(2):230–46. https://doi.org/10.2105/ajph.2020.305999.
164. Harlow AF, Cho J, Tackett AP, et al. Motivations for E-cigarette use and associations with vaping frequency and smoking abstinence among adults who smoke cigarettes in the United States. Drug Alcohol Depend. 2022;238:109583. https://doi.org/10.1016/j.drugalcdep.2022.109583.

165. Mirbolouk M, Charkhchi P, Kianoush S, et al. Prevalence and distribution of E-cigarette use among U.S. adults: behavioral risk factor surveillance system, 2016. Ann Intern Med. 2018;169(7):429–38. https://doi.org/10.7326/m17-3440.
166. de Souza IC, de Barros VV, Gomide HP, et al. Mindfulness-based interventions for the treatment of smoking: a systematic literature review. J Altern Complement Med. 2015;21(3):129–40. https://doi.org/10.1089/acm.2013.0471.
167. Davis JM, Manley AR, Goldberg SB, Smith SS, Jorenby DE. Randomized trial comparing mindfulness training for smokers to a matched control. J Subst Abus Treat. 2014;47(3):213–21. https://doi.org/10.1016/j.jsat.2014.04.005.
168. Elwafi HM, Witkiewitz K, Mallik S, Thornhill TA, Brewer JA. Mindfulness training for smoking cessation: moderation of the relationship between craving and cigarette use. Drug Alcohol Depend. 2013;130(1–3):222–9. https://doi.org/10.1016/j.drugalcdep.2012.11.015.
169. Wen L, Jiang K, Yuan W, Cui W, Li MD. Contribution of variants in CHRNA5/A3/B4 gene cluster on chromosome 15 to tobacco smoking: from genetic association to mechanism. Mol Neurobiol. 2016;53(1):472–84. https://doi.org/10.1007/s12035-014-8997-x.
170. Bierut LJ, Johnson EO, Saccone NL. A glimpse into the future—personalized medicine for smoking cessation. Neuropharmacology Jan 2014;76(Pt B):592-599. doi:https://doi.org/10.1016/j.neuropharm.2013.09.009.
171. O'Loughlin J, Sylvestre MP, Labbe A, et al. Genetic variants and early cigarette smoking and nicotine dependence phenotypes in adolescents. PLoS One. 2014;9(12):e115716. https://doi.org/10.1371/journal.pone.0115716.
172. Office on Smoking and Health NCfCDPaHP. Youth and Tobacco Use. 09/09/2022.
173. Barrington-Trimis JL, Braymiller JL, Unger JB, et al. Trends in the age of cigarette smoking initiation among young adults in the US from 2002 to 2018. JAMA Netw Open. 2020;3(10):e2019022. https://doi.org/10.1001/jamanetworkopen.2020.19022.
174. Stanton A, Grimshaw G. Tobacco cessation interventions for young people. Cochrane Database Syst Rev. 2013;(8):CD003289. https://doi.org/10.1002/14651858.CD003289.pub5.
175. American Lung Association. N-O-T: Not On Tobacco—proven teen smoking and vaping cessation program. https://www.lung.org/quit-smoking/helping-teens-quit/not-on-tobacco. Accessed 11 Sep 2022.
176. U.S. Department Health and Human Services. Smokefree Teen. Accessed 09 Sep 2022. https://teen.smokefree.gov.
177. Mayo Foundation for Medical Education and Research. Mayo Clinic: teen smoking: how to help your teen quit. https://www.mayoclinic.org/healthy-lifestyle/tween-and-teen-health/in-depth/teen-smoking/art-20046474. Accessed 09 Sep 2022.
178. MD Anderson Cancer Network. How to help your teen quit vaping. https://www.mdanderson.org/publications/focused-on-health/how-to-help-your-teen-quit-vaping.h13-1593780.html. Accessed 09 Sep 2022.
179. Graham AL, Amato MS, Cha S, Jacobs MA, Bottcher MM, Papandonatos GD. Effectiveness of a vaping cessation text message program among young adult e-cigarette users: a randomized clinical trial. JAMA Intern Med. 2021;181(7):923–30. https://doi.org/10.1001/jamainternmed.2021.1793.

Chronic Disease Self-Management

Liza Straub and Maria Thekkekandam

Introduction

Approximately half of all US adults have at least one chronic health condition and over 25% live with two or more chronic diseases [1]. The most recent data (from 2016) demonstrate that the total costs of chronic diseases in the US, including economic productivity loss, totaled 3.7 trillion dollars [2]. Redesigning and implementing health care delivery systems in ways that support patient self-management improve outcomes and reduce costs [3]. The concept of *self-management* encompasses the reality that patients dictate their own chronic disease outcomes by their day-to-day decisions. In this chapter, we share specific and practical examples of self-management that can be celebrated and promoted by health systems.

Historical Developments

Health care systems were developed primarily to manage acute episodic care. The changing epidemiology of health care has forced a shift in focus to providing quality long-term chronic disease care. This shift has posed many challenges. One development in this changing environment is the patient-centered medical home (PCMH), which emphasizes comprehensive team-based care that is patient-centered [4]. The pillars of the PCMH are providing quality health care at lower cost, improved patient and staff satisfaction, and better health outcomes. To achieve these goals, patients must be empowered in the self-management of their chronic diseases.

Another major change to the landscape of chronic disease management is the growth of telemedicine/virtual care. Prior to 2020, some practices in the US were already providing telemedicine visits; however, reimbursement was still a barrier. The COVID-19 pandemic forced the Centers for Medicare and Medicaid Services (CMS) to quickly expand their reimbursement for telehealth visits. This expansion of virtual care has required patients to rely more on their own self-management and highlighted the importance of supporting and empowering patients.

Principles of Self-Management

Limitations of Physician-Directed Care

Western medicine developed to care for acute conditions by physicians specializing in separate body systems. In the 1960s, during a time of social restructuring such as the US civil rights movement and the Vietnam War protests, people began to push for holistic care over the course of a lifespan. Consistent with these ideals, Family Medicine emerged as a new specialty [5]. Continuity of care is a foundational tenet of the discipline and includes treating chronic conditions longitudinally [6]. This poses challenges for the physician, as good outcomes require high levels of patient involvement in their own care. Prescriptions from the physician may not simply be a medication or procedure but may include lifestyle changes, routine symptom monitoring (e.g., symptoms of hyperglycemia in a patient with diabetes), and attending recommended visits (e.g., for an annual diabetic eye exam with an ophthalmologist). The reality is that regular follow-through lies in the hands of the patient and can be impeded by competing physiological factors based on a patient's comorbid health conditions and personal psychosocial factors, such as mental illness or poverty. Physicians may be discouraged when patients do not or cannot follow advice that would likely lead to improved outcomes [7]. *Self-management* is a concept describing how the significant and constant patient influence on health outcomes can be supported to counteract barriers and work toward improving outcomes.

L. Straub (✉) · M. Thekkekandam
Department of Family Medicine, University of North Carolina at Chapel Hill, Chapel Hill, NC, USA
e-mail: Liza_Straub@med.unc.edu; Maria_Thekkekandam@med.unc.edu

Fig. 5.1 The Chronic Care Model

The Chronic Care Model

```
         Community                          Health systems
   Resources and policies             Organization of Health Care
          Self-
       Management            Delivery      Decision     Clinical
         Support             System        Support    Information
                             Design                     Systems
```

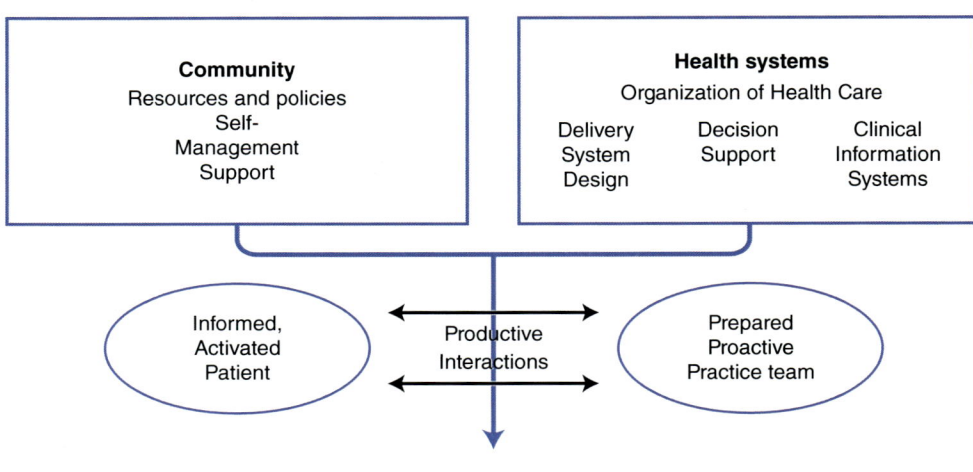

Informed, Activated Patient ↔ Productive Interactions ↔ Prepared Proactive Practice team

Improved outcomes

Chronic Care Model

The Chronic Care Model (CCM) was developed by Ed Wagner, MD, MPH, at the MacColl Institute for Healthcare Innovation in the mid-1990s, to assist health care organizations in supporting high-quality chronic disease management (Fig. 5.1). The CCM was based on evidence showing the most improved chronic disease patient outcomes were tied to interventions that increased providers' expertise, educated and supported patients, improved care delivery (utilizing planning and team-based care), or used registry-based information systems [8]. Combining these interventions leads to even more improved patient outcomes [9]. The CCM does this, incorporating six critical areas of focus (Table 5.1) [10].

Limitations of the CCM include the costs of changing practices in this way, applying the model across multiple chronic diseases (as many of the studies focused on a single condition), and the practicality of a given health care organization applying this framework to its own specific practice conditions. While these topics require further research, the overall findings suggest the CCM improves health care outcomes [9].

Table 5.1 Six fundamental areas that form a system that encourages high-quality chronic disease management [10]

Area	Description
Self-Management Support	Encourage and support patients to be active participants in their care.
Delivery System Design	Ensure the care reaches the patient by communicating information in a way patients can understand, having case management available for complex patients, and planning regular follow-up by a team member.
Decision Support	Utilize shared decision-making by engaging in discussion with patients that provides evidence-based recommendations and elicits patient preferences.
Clinical Information Systems	Use patient and population data to identify at-risk groups and care gaps for proactive care, create reminders for providers and patients, enable communication between team members and patients for care coordination, and assess team performance.
Organization of Health Care	Foster a culture of high-quality care
Community	Help meet patient care needs by connecting them with available community resources and advocating for improved patient care policies.

Empowerment

Empowerment is the feeling that one can influence change and is critical to the successful practice of self-management. Empowerment is a main pillar of high-quality care in diabetes, a chronic condition that is often challenging to treat successfully [11]. Helping patients feel empowered encourages them to participate in their own health care. Empowerment means patients are confident they have a working understanding of a given medical diagnosis and relevant treatment options with the power to choose the direction of their care and management. The process to develop this requires resources that help with decisions and implement treatment. When challenges arise, patients should know where to find help.

Patients must have a foundational understanding of their medical diagnosis and treatment options prior to making any decisions regarding their own care. If a patient with hepatitis C facing administrative challenges to obtaining treatment does not first understand what hepatitis C is or its implications on her health, she cannot be expected to care about solving the challenges and obtaining the needed medication. Clinicians have limitations on their time and patients have limitations on their medical knowledge that can hamper this understanding. Patients often do not know where to begin or what questions to ask. An asymmetry of knowledge and the relationship hierarchy that is inherent in the doctor-patient relationship can limit the ability to overcome this knowledge gap [12]. Implementation of delivery system design tools in the CCM can bridge this gap by having team members provide education on a given health topic pertinent to the patient. Team members include diabetic educators, pharmacists who review medication dosing and side effects, and asthma educators. Patient handouts, community presentations on a given health topic, and peer support groups can be helpful. One study found knowledge of osteoporosis and vitamin D intake improved after implementing patient education interventions such as a handout of calcium-rich foods, though further methods were needed to increase dietary intake [13].

Once patients feel confident that they are informed on a particular disease and treatment options, they should be reminded that they can choose their treatment path. Patients frequently feel they are a secondary member of their health care team, when in fact their participation is of primary importance. If a patient does not feel invested in the treatment, they are less likely to adhere to it [14]. Further discussions with the physician and utilizing decision aid tools may enhance the sense of empowerment. One such tool is bedsider.org, a website that facilitates decision-making regarding contraceptives [15]. Another is the Mayo Clinic's Statin Choice Decision Aid, which allows patients to visualize risk in terms of colored dots, with yellow dots showing the number of people with identical risk factors to the patient who will have a heart attack out of 100 people, once the patient has entered their own data such as age, gender, race, total and LDL cholesterol, smoking status, presence of diabetes, and blood pressure [16]. In a study of patient choice of diabetic medications, using a decision aid improved patient involvement in treatment decisions [17].

Challenges to treatment may arise, including psychological factors regarding the diagnosis (anger, frustration), comorbidities (depression, intellectual disability), or the involvement of multiple family members in the decision-making (e.g., children of people with cognitive impairment). In these cases, it is still important for the patient or their decision-maker(s) to feel supported and empowered. This may involve additional appointments, adequately treating concomitant diagnoses, and spending the time to bring in other members of the patient's team, such as family or a designated health care power of attorney.

Shared Decision-Making

Shared decision-making (SDM) is the process by which providers and patients together make decisions regarding the patient's health, considering both high-quality evidenced-based recommendations and patient values. This is the central tenet of the *Decision Support* part of the CCM and can be utilized as a general communication style between providers and patients, as it places priority on patient engagement in the conversation to promote a patient making value-congruent choices [18]. The Agency for Healthcare Research and Quality (AHRQ) has created a useful acronym for this approach, called the **SHARE** approach (**S**eek your patient's participation, **H**elp them explore/compare treatment options, **A**ssess their values/preferences, **R**each a decision, and **E**valuate this decision) [19].

While SDM can be of benefit in nearly every discussion between physicians and patients, some classic applications include:

- Screening for conditions where the balance of benefits and harms is equivocal, such as prostate cancer screening with a Prostate Specific Antigen blood test. This is now a grade C recommendation from the US Preventive Services Task Force for men aged 55–69 years [20]. Prior to ordering the test, a physician should go through the SDM process with a patient.
- Discussing treatment for any medical condition, as every option has the potential for side effects. SDM should be employed to assess the patient's understanding and comfort with both the possible side effects and the consequences of the condition remaining untreated.
- Discussing challenging situations such as end of life care.

One challenge to SDM is providing recommendations without being overly prescriptive. Conversely, one must avoid providing the treatments or screenings a patient wants without any evidence-based guidance [21]. Instead, SDM works toward a collaborative approach where the medical recommendations and the patient preferences contribute equally to a final decision.

Reasons to perform SDM include that ethically, it places value on autonomy. Furthermore, patients want to participate in decision-making [22]. SDM improves outcomes and reduces health care costs, due to more patient engagement in a decision, better follow-through with a plan, and less missed appointments or unfulfilled orders caused by a provider simply ordering something that was not agreed upon [23–26]. Limitations to SDM include competing requirements on a physician's time and low health literacy on the part of the patient.

Health Literacy

Health literacy (HL) describes a patient's level of understanding of basic health information. One study of college students showed that only 49% self-reported adequate health literacy [27]. According to a national survey of HL in 2003, which is one of the more recent surveys of its kind, only 12%

of US adults reported no difficulty with HL [28]. No matter how well-intentioned a clinician may be in informing and empowering a patient, this effort can be thwarted by providing information that is too advanced for the patient to understand. Understanding the HL level of one's audience is crucial to providing information in the most appropriate and user-friendly manner so that it can be utilized by patients to improve their self-management capability. Following are practices that can improve HL:

- Patients should have access to health information tools such as handouts that are concise and easy to read.
- Clinicians should utilize the Teach-Back method, where they invite patients to display their understanding of discussions with the provider.
- Patients can be encouraged to use the *Ask Me Three* method that empowers them to participate in their care discussion by asking specific questions of their provider ("What is my main problem? What do I need to do? Why is it important I do this?") [29].
- Clinicians should include decision aids in health management discussions with patients, as they provide easy-to-understand depictions of benefits and harms, often using graphics to help conceptualize the comparisons involved in each decision.

Practicalities of Self-Management

Managing Chronic Disease at Home

Patients carry out most of their chronic disease management outside of the medical office, in their daily decisions regarding lifestyle choices and medication compliance. Managing chronic disease successfully can be challenging for patients, as it is influenced by many competing community and personal psychosocial factors, from financial constraints to interpersonal or psychological stressors. The following are examples of tools that can simplify these processes for patients, from the day-to-day monitoring of their health to simplifying medication use instructions, thus allowing them to achieve their self-management goals.

One of the most prevalent chronic conditions is type 2 diabetes mellitus. In 2016 there were 26.6 million individuals in the US living with type 2 diabetes, at a total cost of 530 million dollars [2]. Diabetes is a chronic condition that demands a significant amount of self-management from those living with it, including blood glucose monitoring, dietary maintenance, medication administration, and, when applicable, insulin titration. While routine blood glucose monitoring is not necessary for non-insulin-treated type 2 diabetes [30], it is required for the safe management of insulin-dependent diabetes. Continuous blood glucose monitors are new devices that streamline self-management. They continuously measure blood glucose levels and transmit those readings to the patient's smart device, allowing timely action when indicated while avoiding multiple finger sticks. A systematic review is currently underway to determine the benefits of continuous glucose monitoring compared to flash glucose monitoring in the primary care setting [31]. A newer treatment for type 2 diabetes is a glucagon-like peptide 1 (GLP-1) agonist, such as semaglutide, dulaglutide, and exenatide. These medications empower patients with their own home self-management, lower A1c, and help with weight loss [32]. The GLP-1 agonists are once or twice weekly injections, which increase adherence compared to daily injections [33]. Other conveniently dosed treatments, such as once weekly basal insulin injections, are in development [34].

Another chronic condition that requires daily, as well as episodic flare-up, management is asthma. The asthma action plan is a tool that assists both pediatric and adult patients in the self-management of their asthma. This tool classifies the patient's symptoms into green, yellow, and red zones and has provider-prescribed, patient-specific actions for each zone. Asthma action plans increase the number of days spent in the desired green zone and decrease emergency department visits and hospitalizations [35]. Complimentary self-management education that includes self-monitoring of symptoms, a written asthma action plan, and regular review of asthma control decreases asthma morbidity in both adults and children [36]. Given their efficacy, asthma action plans are recommended for all patients with asthma by the Global Initiative for Asthma (GINA) 2021 Report, *Global Strategy for Asthma Management and Prevention* [37]. A sample asthma action plan template from GINA is shown in Fig. 5.2 [38].

Technological Advancements

Technological advancements through the emerging field of consumer health informatics provide helpful tools that assist patients with self-management. Online patient portals that make personal health records available via electronic platforms are a prime example of patients at the forefront of their own health and self-management. Patients now have access to their medication lists, blood work results, imaging reports, health prevention "gaps," clinic visit notes/documentation by their provider, growth charts, weight and blood pressure flow sheets, immunization records, and more. Additionally, patients can schedule appointments, ask questions, and

ASTHMA ACTION PLAN

Name: _____
Phone: _____

Action plan updated: M _____ / D _____ / Y _____

Bring this action plan to your doctor/nurse at each visit.

Doctor's Contact Details: _____
Nurse/Educator Details: _____

In an emergency call: _____
OR CALL AN AMBULANCE IMMEDIATELY.

YOUR EMERGENCY CONTACT PERSON

Name: _____
Phone: _____
Relationship: _____

IF YOUR ASTHMA IS WELL CONTROLLED
You need your reliever inhaler less than 3 times per week, you do not wake up with asthma and, and your asthma does not limit your activities (including exercise) (If used, peak flow over _____L/min)

Your controller medication is: _____ (name) _____ (strength)

Take: _____ puffs/tablet _____ times EVERY DAY

☐ Use a spacer with your controller inhaler

Your reliever/rescue medication is: _____ (name) _____ (strength)

Take _____ puffs if needed to relieve asthma symptoms like wheezing, coughing, shortness of breath

☐ Use a spacer with your reliever inhaler

Other medications: _____ (name) _____ (strength) _____ (how often)

_____ (name) _____ (strength) _____ (how often)

Before exercise take: _____ (name) _____ (strength) _____ (how many puffs/tablets)

IF YOUR ASTHMA IS GETTING WORSE
You need your reliever more often than usual, you wake up with asthma, or you cannot do your normal activities (including exercise) because of your asthma (If used, peak flow between _____ and _____ L/min)

Take your reliever/rescue medication: _____ (name) _____ (strength) _____ (how often)

☐ Use a spacer with your controller inhaler

Take your controller medication: _____ (name) _____ (strength)

Take: _____ puffs/tablet _____ times EVERY DAY

☐ Use a spacer with your reliever inhaler   ☐ Contact your doctor

Other medications: _____ (name) _____ (strength) _____ (how often)

IF YOUR ASTHMA SYMPTOMS ARE SEVERE
You need your reliever again more often than every 3-4 hours, your breathing is difficult, or you often wake up with asthma
(if used, Peak Flow under _____L/min)

Take your reliever/rescue medication: _____ (name) _____ (strength) _____ (how often)

Take prednisone/prednisolone: _____ (name) _____ (strength)

Take: _____ tablet _____ times every day

CONTACT A DOCTOR TODAY OR GO TO THE EMERGENCY DEPARTMENT

Additional comments: _____

Fig. 5.2 Asthma Action Plan template from the Global Initiative for Asthma Implementation Toolbox [38]

request medication refills through their patient portal. Patients with diabetes who use their patient portals have improved glycemic control, although it is not clear whether the improved control is a direct result of using the patient portal or if confounding factors exist [39]. Such technology helps connect patients seamlessly to various aspects of their health care, allowing them to be more active and informed participants.

Electronic health tools can also be used for medication monitoring, allowing patients and caregivers to directly input symptom improvement, side effects, or other clinical outcomes. For instance, some patient portals allow patients to input their home blood pressure measurements into a flow sheet that is sent to their provider for review and medication adjustment. Patients generally find these tools to be a useful way to improve communication with their provider, and they improve health-related outcomes in frequent users [40].

Mobile/text messaging is used to promote health improvement and behavior change. Mobile messaging is an effective intervention for self-management of diabetes, weight loss, physical activity, smoking cessation, and medication adherence for antiretroviral therapy [41]. More studies are needed to determine cost-effectiveness of this strategy of promoting self-management as well as to inform the most effective mobile messaging intervention characteristics.

Numerous health mobile applications, known as apps, are available to consumers to assist in self-management efforts, usually for free or at low cost. These include weight loss apps (Noom, Weight Watchers, NutriSystem), physical activity apps (Map My Run, Fitness Buddy, MyFitnessPal, Nike Training Club), mental health apps (Moodkit, Talkspace, Calm, Headspace), and women's health apps (Ovia, Flo), to list just a few. While the use of apps has yet to show statistically significant improved health outcomes [42], they show great promise and evidence of their effectiveness in improving health outcomes is likely to grow.

Tobacco cessation counseling through telephone services, or quitlines, offers patients convenient and often free support for their self-management of tobacco cessation. Participating in multiple quitline counseling sessions improves long-term cessation for patients who smoke [43]. For example, QuitlineNC offers residents of North Carolina free, evidence-based tobacco treatment services. Printable resources are available on their website to keep in the office setting to encourage patients to call [44].

Suicide hotlines offer free and timely counseling and information through phone calls, virtual support, and text messaging. Their effectiveness has not been well studied given the ethical concerns surrounding randomized controlled trials for patients having mental health crises, though they may be helpful for young people [45]. Adolescents do engage with hotline services, suggesting that they are a good mental health self-management option.

Chat-based hotlines are a similar virtual support option that provide real-time communication between patients and trained professionals by utilizing mainstream chat applications such as WhatsApp and Facebook Messenger. Chat-based hotlines are an effective means of providing crisis and emotional support [46], with many patients preferring instant messenger applications over other modalities such as email, text messaging, phone calls, and in-person counseling. Positive and statistically significant mental health outcomes are noted regarding depression, anxiety, well-being, and suicidality. Chat-based hotlines have potential for providing additional support outside clinic walls in a medium that is mainstream and preferred by many consumers.

Peer Support

Peer support is an effective and cost-effective way to improve health outcomes [47]. Social support decreases morbidity and mortality, increases self-efficacy, and reduces use of emergency services [48]. Peer support is an effective means of reaching groups who would otherwise have little contact with the health care system [49]. The American Academy of Family Physicians Foundation developed *Peers for Progress*, an international collaborative learning network made up of peer support researchers, experts, and advocates. They have developed a toolkit that assists with developing a peer support program to help patients with their chronic disease self-management [50].

Group visits are another way that peer support promotes improved health outcomes in chronic disease management. For example, the University of North Carolina Family Medicine Center utilizes group visits for weight management and medication management of opioid use disorder. Additionally, they offer a longitudinal *Living Healthy* course, which supports patients with any chronic disease by helping them to develop action plans and thus take control of their own health. The program focuses on topics such as exercise, nutrition, stress management, and important questions to ask your provider [51].

Case Management/Population Health Services

Self-management needs ongoing support from the health care team; however, providing adequate support can be difficult for providers to fit into a busy clinic schedule, where the standard appointment time for primary care visits may not extend beyond 20 minutes regardless of the complexity of the patient's medical conditions. Care managers thus emerge as vital members of the clinical team, to help bridge care from the office to the community. Care managers provide additional support and services to patients such as motivational interviewing, locating and disseminating resources, coordinating care, and addressing social barriers. Their services are a crucial component to providing patients with adequate support for their own self-management outside the clinic walls.

One example of a successful program is *Chronic Care Management (CCM)* at the University of North Carolina Family Medicine center in Chapel Hill. This program helps patients with chronic conditions in their own self-management via periodic check-ins that involve coaching through motivational interviewing; reminding patients of health maintenance items due; connecting patients to community resources; helping to secure appointments; helping to obtain durable medical equipment; case management; and coordination of care. The care managers in the CCM program serve as a conduit between the patient and the provider outside the clinic visit, which means fewer office visits, as patients can self-manage more at home. The CCM program reduces emergency department utilization and inpatient admissions for patients receiving its services [52]. Programs like this are increasingly important as payment models move from fee-for-service to value-based reimbursement.

Another successful model of care management is Community Care of North Carolina (CCNC), a partnership between North Carolina Medicaid and community primary care physicians in North Carolina that was developed with the goal of providing cost-effective, high-quality care for Medicaid recipients. This program improves the quality of care while reducing costs and utilization of health care resources by maintaining a focus on population health, care coordination, and quality improvement efforts [53]. Their Population Health Outreach and Care Coordination team comprises certified health coaches who work with patients on wellness coaching and disease management coaching, thus placing emphasis for patients on individual goal setting and taking control of their own health [54]. In July 2021, approximately 1.6 million Medicaid beneficiaries in North Carolina transitioned to a Medicaid Managed Care health plan. CCNC entered into agreements with the managed care health plans with the goal of providing a uniform approach to care management and quality improvement across all plans.

Future Directions

The COVID-19 pandemic sparked rapid change in health care delivery with the expansion of reimbursement for virtual visits. Telehealth is a safe and effective option for supporting patients in their self-management [55]. With ongoing technological advancements that support patients in managing their chronic conditions at home, health care delivery will likely continue to shift toward more virtual care, allowing providers to support patients safely and effectively in their self-management. The report *Implementing High-Quality Primary Care* from the National Academies of Sciences, Engineering, and Medicine (NASEM) recommends that the Centers for Medicare & Medicaid Services make permanent the expansion of reimbursement for virtual (not in person) and telehealth visits [56].

Current fee-for-service payment models do not support the wrap-around services of a patient-centered medical home. Care managers, health coaches, online patient portals (and the time spent by health care staff and providers managing the requests through the portals), and many other services are beneficial and necessary to support self-management by patients. The NASEM report presents multiple objectives that will support self-management by patients, including *Pay for primary care teams to care for people, not doctors to deliver services* [56]. Other recommendations include designing information technology that supports the continuous contact and relationships needed to promote patient self-management, interprofessional care teams, and research for continuous improvement. During the transition to alternative payment models, payors reimbursing with fee-for-service for primary care should shift toward value-based care by using a hybrid (fee-for-service and capitated) payment model that prospectively pays for team-based care, including care managers, and encourages investment in online patient portals.

Payment reform in our health care system must support the move toward increased patient self-management, given the many examples of benefits of the various methods described above, from implementing the Chronic Care Model to utilizing new and emerging technologies to promote patient engagement. New reimbursement systems and research to establish best practices will fulfill the promising potential of putting the patient at the center of their health care, a vantage point from which they can best understand their own health and most effectively foster positive change.

References

1. Boersma P, Black LI, Ward BW. Prevalence of multiple chronic conditions among US adults, 2018. Prev Chronic Dis. 2020;17:E106.
2. Waters H, Graf M. THE costs of chronic disease in the U.S [Internet]. Milken Institute; 2018 Aug [cited 2021 Nov 28]. https://milkeninstitute.org/sites/default/files/reports-pdf/ChronicDiseases-HighRes-FINAL_2.pdf
3. Reynolds R, Dennis S, Hasan I, Slewa J, Chen W, Tian D, et al. A systematic review of chronic disease management interventions in primary care. BMC Fam Pract. 2018;19(1):11.
4. Health Care Accreditation, Health Plan Accreditation Organization—NCQA—NCQA [Internet]. [cited 2021 Nov 29]. https://www.ncqa.org/
5. Gutierrez C, Scheid P. The history of family medicine and its impact in US health care delivery [Internet]. Primary Care Symposium; 2002 [cited 2021 Nov 28]. https://www.aafpfoundation.org/content/dam/foundation/documents/who-we-are/cfhm/FMImpactGutierrezScheid.pdf

6. Britt E, Hudson SM, Blampied NM. Motivational interviewing in health settings: a review. Patient Educ Couns. 2004;53(2):147–55.
7. Lorig KR, Holman H. Self-management education: history, definition, outcomes, and mechanisms. Ann Behav Med. 2003;26(1):1–7.
8. Renders CM, Valk GD, Griffin S, Wagner EH, Eijk JT, Assendelft WJ. Interventions to improve the management of diabetes mellitus in primary care, outpatient and community settings. Cochrane Database Syst Rev. 2001;(1):CD001481.
9. Coleman K, Austin BT, Brach C, Wagner EH. Evidence on the chronic care model in the new millennium. Health Aff (Millwood). 2009;28(1):75–85.
10. Changes to Improve Chronic Care | IHI—Institute for Healthcare Improvement [Internet]. [cited 2021 Nov 28]. http://www.ihi.org/resources/Pages/Changes/ChangestoImproveChronicCare.aspx.
11. Lambrinou E, Hansen TB, Beulens JW. Lifestyle factors, self-management and patient empowerment in diabetes care. Eur J Prev Cardiol. 2019;26(2_suppl):55–63.
12. Ariss SM. Asymmetrical knowledge claims in general practice consultations with frequently attending patients: limitations and opportunities for patient participation. Soc Sci Med. 2009;69(6):908–19.
13. Bohaty K, Rocole H, Wehling K, Waltman N. Testing the effectiveness of an educational intervention to increase dietary intake of calcium and vitamin D in young adult women. J Am Acad Nurse Pract. 2008;20(2):93–9.
14. Graffigna G, Barello S. Spotlight on the Patient Health Engagement model (PHE model): a psychosocial theory to understand people's meaningful engagement in their own health care. Patient Prefer Adherence. 2018;12:1261–71.
15. Bedsider Birth Control Support Network [Internet]. [cited 2021 Nov 28]. https://www.bedsider.org/
16. Statin Choice Decision AID—Site [Internet]. [cited 2021 Nov 28]. https://statindecisionaid.mayoclinic.org/
17. Mullan RJ, Montori VM, Shah ND, Christianson TJH, Bryant SC, Guyatt GH, et al. The diabetes mellitus medication choice decision aid: a randomized trial. Arch Intern Med. 2009;169(17):1560–8.
18. Stacey D, Légaré F, Lewis K, Barry MJ, Bennett CL, Eden KB, et al. Decision aids for people facing health treatment or screening decisions. Cochrane Database Syst Rev. 2017;4:CD001431.
19. The SHARE Approach | Agency for Healthcare Research and Quality [Internet]. [cited 2021 Nov 28]. https://www.ahrq.gov/health-literacy/professional-training/shared-decision/index.html
20. Recommendation: Prostate Cancer: Screening | United States Preventive Services Taskforce [Internet]. [cited 2021 Nov 28]. https://www.uspreventiveservicestaskforce.org/uspstf/recommendation/prostate-cancer-screening
21. Grad R, Légaré F, Bell NR, Dickinson JA, Singh H, Moore AE, et al. Shared decision making in preventive health care: What it is; what it is not. Can Fam Physician. 2017;63(9):682–4.
22. Chewning B, Bylund CL, Shah B, Arora NK, Gueguen JA, Makoul G. Patient preferences for shared decisions: a systematic review. Patient Educ Couns. 2012;86(1):9–18.
23. Charles C, Gafni A, Whelan T. Shared decision-making in the medical encounter: what does it mean? (or it takes at least two to tango). Soc Sci Med. 1997;44(5):681–92.
24. Sheridan SL, Harris RP, Woolf SH, Shared Decision-Making Workgroup of the U.S. Preventive Services Task Force. Shared decision making about screening and chemoprevention. a suggested approach from the U.S. Preventive Services Task Force. Am J Prev Med. 2004;26(1):56–66.
25. Makoul G, Clayman ML. An integrative model of shared decision making in medical encounters. Patient Educ Couns. 2006;60(3):301–12.
26. Berwick DM, Nolan TW, Whittington J. The triple aim: Care, health, and cost. Health Aff (Millwood). 2008;27(3):759–69.
27. Patil U, Kostareva U, Hadley M, Manganello JA, Okan O, Dadaczynski K, et al. Health literacy, digital health literacy, and covid-19 pandemic attitudes and behaviors in U.S. college students: implications for interventions. Int J Environ Res Public Health. 2021;18(6)
28. Liang L, Brach C. Health literacy universal precautions are still a distant dream: analysis of U.S. data on health literate practices. Health Lit Res Pract. 2017;1(4):e216–30.
29. Ask Me 3: Good Questions for Your Good Health | IHI—Institute for Healthcare Improvement [Internet]. [cited 2021 Nov 29]. http://www.ihi.org/resources/Pages/Tools/Ask-Me-3-Good-Questions-for-Your-Good-Health.aspx
30. Young LA, Buse JB, Weaver MA, Vu MB, Mitchell CM, Blakeney T, et al. Glucose self-monitoring in non-insulin-treated patients with type 2 diabetes in primary care settings: a randomized trial. JAMA Intern Med. 2017;177(7):920–9.
31. Kieu A, Govender RD, Östlundh L, King J. Benefits of the addition of continuous or flash glucose monitoring versus standard practice using self-monitored blood glucose and haemoglobin A1c in the primary care of diabetes mellitus: a systematic review protocol. BMJ Open. 2021;11(8):e050027.
32. Nauck MA, Quast DR, Wefers J, Meier JJ. GLP-1 receptor agonists in the treatment of type 2 diabetes—state-of-the-art. Mol Metab. 2021;46:101102.
33. Weiss T, Carr RD, Pal S, Yang L, Sawhney B, Boggs R, et al. Real-world adherence and discontinuation of glucagon-like peptide-1 receptor agonists therapy in type 2 diabetes mellitus patients in the United States. Patient Prefer Adherence. 2020;14:2337–45.
34. Rosenstock J, Bajaj HS, Janež A, Silver R, Begtrup K, Hansen MV, et al. Once-weekly insulin for Type 2 diabetes without previous insulin treatment. N Engl J Med. 2020;383(22):2107–16.
35. Farag H, Abd El-Wahab EW, El-Nimr NA, Saad El-Din HA. Asthma action plan for proactive bronchial asthma self-management in adults: a randomized controlled trial. Int Health. 2018;10(6):502–16.
36. Pinnock H, Parke HL, Panagioti M, Daines L, Pearce G, Epiphaniou E, et al. Systematic meta-review of supported self-management for asthma: a healthcare perspective. BMC Med. 2017;15(1):64.
37. 2021 GINA Main Report—Global Initiative for Asthma—GINA [Internet]. [cited 2021 Nov 28]. https://ginasthma.org/gina-reports/
38. GINA Implementation ToolBox. [cited 2021 Nov 28]. https://ginasthma.org/wp-content/uploads/2019/01/GINA-Implementation-Toolbox-2019.pdf
39. Alturkistani A, Qavi A, Anyanwu PE, Greenfield G, Greaves F, Costelloe C. Patient portal functionalities and patient outcomes among patients with diabetes: systematic review. J Med Internet Res. 2020;22(9):e18976.
40. Lancaster K, Abuzour A, Khaira M, Mathers A, Chan A, Bui V, et al. The use and effects of electronic health tools for patient self-monitoring and reporting of outcomes following medication use: systematic review. J Med Internet Res. 2018;20(12):e294.
41. Hall AK, Cole-Lewis H, Bernhardt JM. Mobile text messaging for health: a systematic review of reviews. Annu Rev Public Health. 2015;(36):393–415.
42. Iribarren SJ, Akande TO, Kamp KJ, Barry D, Kader YG, Suelzer E. Effectiveness of mobile apps to promote health and manage disease: systematic review and meta-analysis of randomized controlled trials. JMIR Mhealth Uhealth. 2021;9(1):e21563.
43. Stead LF, Perera R, Lancaster T. A systematic review of interventions for smokers who contact quitlines. Tob Control. 2007;16(Suppl 1):i3–8.
44. QuitlineNC.com [Internet]. [cited 2021 Nov 28]. https://www.quitlinenc.com/
45. Mathieu SL, Uddin R, Brady M, Batchelor S, Ross V, Spence SH, et al. Systematic review: the state of research into youth helplines. J Am Acad Child Adolesc Psychiatry. 2021;60(10):1190–233.
46. Brody C, Star A, Tran J. Chat-based hotlines for health promotion: a systematic review. Mhealth. 2020;6:36.

47. Fisher EB, Ballesteros J, Bhushan N, Coufal MM, Kowitt SD, McDonough AM, et al. Key features of peer support in chronic disease prevention and management. Health Aff (Millwood). 2015;34(9):1523–30.
48. The Science Behind Peer Support [Internet]. [cited 2021 Nov 29]. http://peersforprogress.org/learn-about-peer-support/science-behind-peer-support/.
49. Sokol R, Fisher E. Peer support for the hardly reached: a systematic review. Am J Public Health. 2016;106(7):e1–8.
50. Advocating and planning for a behavioral health peer support program. [cited 2021 Nov 29]. http://peersforprogress.org/wp-content/uploads/2014/03/20140313_advocating_and_planning_for_a_behavioral_health_peer_support_program.pdf
51. Living Healthy—Department of Family Medicine [Internet]. [cited 2021 Nov 29]. https://www.med.unc.edu/fammed/service-to-the-community/health-education/living-healthy-classes/
52. Daaleman TP, Hay S, Prentice A, Gwynne MD. Embedding care management in the medical home: a case study. J Prim Care Community Health. 2014;5(2):97–100.
53. Steiner BD, Denham AC, Ashkin E, Newton WP, Wroth T, Dobson LA. Community care of North Carolina: improving care through community health networks. Ann Fam Med. 2008;6(4):361–7.
54. Population Health Outreach & Care Coordination | Community Care of North Carolina [Internet]. [cited 2021 Nov 28]. https://www.communitycarenc.org/what-we-do/care-management/population-health-outreach-and-care-coordination
55. Hanlon P, Daines L, Campbell C, McKinstry B, Weller D, Pinnock H. Telehealth interventions to support self-management of long-term conditions: a systematic metareview of diabetes, heart failure, asthma, chronic obstructive pulmonary disease, and cancer. J Med Internet Res. 2017;19(5):e172.
56. National Academies of Sciences, Engineering, and Medicine, Health and Medicine Division, Board on Health Care Services, Committee on Implementing High-Quality Primary Care. In: Robinson SK, Meisnere M, Phillips RL, McCauley L, editors. Implementing high-quality primary care: rebuilding the foundation of health care. Washington (DC): National Academies Press (US); 2021.

Alcohol and Drug Use Disorders

Michael H. Baca-Atlas, Stefani N. Baca-Atlas, and Kelly Bossenbroek Fedoriw

Introduction

Alcohol and drug use exist on a spectrum ranging from occasional use without consequences to a devastating chronic illness. Given the prevalence and impact, diagnosing and treating alcohol and substance use disorders is an essential skill in primary care and successful treatments are available. An estimated 20 million Americans aged 12 years and older have at least one substance use disorder and 37 million have used an illicit substance (other than marijuana) in the past 12 months [1]. Marijuana is the most used illicit substance with 48 million people using it in 2019 followed by 10 million people misusing prescription pain relievers. Thirty-four percent of adults aged 18–25 years report binge drinking in the past month, defined by the Substance Abuse and Mental Health Services Administration (SAMHSA) as consuming five or more drinks for men or four or more drinks for women on the same occasion, and 18% of people aged 12–20 years report underage drinking in the past month. Approximately two thirds of adults report increased alcohol consumption during the COVID-19 pandemic [2]. The pandemic also saw a dramatic increase in overdose deaths to an estimated 100,306 during the 12-month period ending in April 2021; an increase of 28.5% from the 78,056 deaths during the same period the year prior [3].

Estimates of the financial cost to society of alcohol and substance use disorders range from 400 to 600 billion dollars annually [4, 5]. However, treatment substantially reduces cost, overdoses, and deaths from substance use disorders.

M. H. Baca-Atlas (✉) · K. B. Fedoriw
Department of Family Medicine, University of North Carolina at Chapel Hill, Chapel Hill, NC, USA
e-mail: michael_baca-atlas@med.unc.edu; kelly_fedoriw@med.unc.edu

S. N. Baca-Atlas
University of North Carolina at Chapel Hill School of Social Work, Chapel Hill, NC, USA
e-mail: sbaca-atlas@unc.edu

Studies show a return on investment between four and seven times for substance use treatment not including the benefits of recovery to individual patients and families [5, 6]. A history of systemic inequities and racism has contributed to poorer outcomes regarding substance use, treatment, and consequences among minoritized groups compared to non-Latine[1] White Americans [7–10].

Substance Use Disorders and Chronic Conditions

A substance use disorder (SUD) is defined as "recurrent use of alcohol and/or drugs causing clinically significant impairment, including health problems, disability, and failure to meet major responsibilities at work, school, or home" [1]. The *Diagnostic and Statistical Manual of Mental Disorders (DSM-5)*, the standard classification of mental disorders in the US, documents specific symptoms and criteria for making the diagnosis [11]. Not every person who uses alcohol or illicit substances develops negative consequences or a use disorder. Approximately 16% of nicotine users, 15% of cocaine users, 11% of alcohol users, and 6% of cannabis users develop use disorders within a decade after first use [12]. Some groups are at higher risk for drug use including young adults (aged 18–25 years, 24% rate of illicit drug use) compared to adolescents and older adults; males (14%) compared to females (9%); Native American/Indigenous people (18%) and those identifying with two or more races (17%) compared to African American/Black people (13%), White people (12%), Native Hawaiians or Pacific Islanders (10%), Latines (10%), and people of Asian descent (4.5%) [13].

---

[1] *Latine(s)* (Lah-tEENn-eh) is a pan-ethnic, gender-inclusive form of the word *Latino(s)*. Rather than *Latinx*, which is not congruent with Spanish orthography, *Latine* replaces the gendered *o/a* with an *e*, already in use in some Spanish words (e.g., *estudiante*.). It is best practice to ask patients about their preferences regarding these terms.

Additional experiences that increase risk for developing a SUD include a history of childhood trauma, personal or family history of addiction, and/or pre-existing psychiatric disorders [14–16].

Substance use is intertwined with other aspects of health. Substance use disorders may exist on their own, exacerbate chronic conditions, or cause other chronic illnesses. Consider worsening diabetes or hypertension from alcohol use, chronic obstructive pulmonary disease arising from cigarette smoking, and methamphetamine-associated cardiomyopathy. Patients with SUD experience a high prevalence of chronic pain, and each condition can increase vulnerability to the other [17]. These relationships can be challenging for providers to assess and treat. In addition, negative consequences can occur with just one exposure (cocaine induced myocardial infarction) or with cumulative effects of repeated use (hyperemesis syndrome from chronic marijuana use) [18, 19].

Approximately half of patients with a substance use disorder also have a co-occurring mental illness [20]. Patients with co-occurring diagnoses have worse outcomes than patients with only a mental illness or SUD including greater functional impairment and increased disability [21]. Treating the underlying mental illness is essential to treating the SUD. Differentiating between substance-induced mental disorders and mental illness without comorbid substance use is often challenging and relies on an accurate history and a period of abstinence. For example, if depressive symptoms were present prior to the initiation of substance use and do not resolve when the substance has not been used for at least a month, the patient likely has a co-occurring diagnosis of depression. Over 70% of patients in treatment for a SUD also use cigarettes and have worse outcomes than patients who do not smoke. Addressing tobacco use in the SUD population is essential as it is associated with increased mortality [22].

Screening Approaches and Diagnostic Criteria

Screening for unhealthy alcohol and drug use is part of obtaining a comprehensive medical history and has implications for the diagnosis and management of numerous medical and psychiatric conditions. The U.S. Preventive Services Task Force (USPSTF) and several professional medical organizations support screening for alcohol and other drug use in primary care clinics among adults aged 18 years and older and pregnant/postpartum women [23, 24]. The USPSTF concluded that current evidence is insufficient to access the benefits and harms of screening for unhealthy alcohol and drug use in adolescents, although the American Academy of Pediatrics and Bright Futures Initiative support screening [23–25]. Although there is no direct evidence of the benefits or harms of screening for drug use, several screening instruments with acceptable sensitivity and specificity are available. An unintended consequence of screening, particularly in pregnant/postpartum women, is provider bias in testing and subsequent referrals to child welfare system when screening is positive, placing disproportionate burden on marginalized women and their families [26].

Screening tools must be brief and validated for primary care populations and are not intended to diagnose substance use disorders. Patients with positive screening results may need further diagnostic assessments to diagnose an alcohol or drug use disorder. Evidence to guide the optimal interval for screening in adults is limited [23, 24]. Alcohol screening ranks among the highest-performing preventive services, based on cost-effectiveness and health impact, comparable to other recommended preventive services such as screening for hypertension, immunizations (influenza, pneumococcal), and colorectal cancer [27]. However, screening for alcohol use occurs at a much lower rate than other preventive health services with even lower rates of screening in African American patients compared to White patients [28].

Brief screening instruments can detect unhealthy alcohol use in primary care with satisfactory sensitivity and specificity (Table 6.1). One- to three-item tools, such as the Alcohol Use Disorders Identification Test-Concise (AUDIT-C) and Single Alcohol Screening Questionnaire (SASQ), accurately assess unhealthy alcohol use in adults 18 years or older [29]. AUDIT-C is indicated for pregnant women, college students, veterans, and people who are arrested/incarcerated [30–32]. The CAGE questionnaire, a well-known tool for alcohol screening, detects more severe use rather than the full spectrum of unhealthy alcohol use [33]. The CAGE questionnaire generally performs equally well among Black, Latine, and White racial/ethnic participants [34, 35]. However, this screening test may not be effective for White or pregnant women, college students, and people who do not drink as heavily [36]. Screening tools for prescription misuse include brief one-item measures such as the Single-Item Screening Questions (SISQ) and Tobacco, Alcohol, Prescription Medications, and other Substances (TAPS) [37, 38]. Because SISQ/SASQ have low specificity for identifying an alcohol or drug use disorder, positive responses should be followed by an additional screening tool such as the AUDIT-C, Drug Abuse Screening Test (DAST-10), or an interview [37, 39].

The diagnosis of a substance use disorder is based on 11 criteria from the *DSM-5* (Table 6.2). Critiques of the lack of cultural validity of the DSM criteria for SUD are well documented [40]. The terms abuse and dependence were eliminated and combined into one disorder with the release of the *DSM-5* in 2013 [41]. Criteria are the same whether diagnosing an alcohol or drug use disorder and occur over a 12-month

Table 6.1 Screening instruments for alcohol and drug use disorders (Source: [29, 30, 31, 32, 37, 38, 39, 142])

Tool	Full name	Number of items	Population
AUDIT	Alcohol Use Disorders Identification Test	10	Adults
AUDIT-C	Alcohol Use Disorders Identification Test–Concise	3	Adults, Older Adults, Pregnancy
CAGE	Cut, Annoyed, Guilty, Eye Opener (EtOH)	4	Adults
CRAFFT	Car, Relax, Alone, Forget, Friends, Trouble (EtOH)	6	Adolescents
DAST-10	Drug Abuse Screening Test	10	Adults, Pregnancy
SISQ	Single Item Screening Question (drug use)	1	Adults
SASQ	Single Alcohol Screening Question	1	Adults, Adolescents
TAPS-1	Tobacco, Alcohol, Prescription medication, and other Substance use; followed by TAPS-2 if {+}	4	Adults

Abbreviations: EtOH Alcohol
http://lib.adai.washington.edu/instruments/
https://www.drugabuse.gov/nidamed-medical-health-professionals/screening-tools-resources/chart-screening-tools

Table 6.2 DSM-5 criteria for substance use disorder (Source: [11])

Using larger amounts or over longer period than intended
Persistent desire or unsuccessful efforts to cut down/control use
Great deal of time spent obtaining, using, recovering from use
Craving
Recurrent use resulting in a failure to fulfill major role obligations at work, school, or home
Continued use despite persistent or recurrent social or interpersonal problems caused or exacerbated by substance
Important activities given up or reduced because of use
Recurrent use in situations in which it is physically hazardous
Continued use despite knowledge of having a persistent or recurrent physical or psychological problem caused or exacerbated by use
Tolerance
Withdrawal

period leading to clinically significant impairment or distress. An individual must meet two criteria to receive the diagnosis, and severity is based on the number of criteria met. A minimum of two to three criteria is required for the diagnosis of mild SUD, while four to five is moderate, and six or more is severe. The diagnosis is substance specific, so an individual may have co-occurring disorders (e.g., mild cannabis use disorder, moderate benzodiazepine use disorder, and severe alcohol use disorder simultaneously).

The diagnosis of SUD is based primarily on patient interview rather than a single test result. Although some laboratory results such as urine toxicology can provide collateral information, toxicology alone cannot diagnose SUD. Several diagnostic instruments have demonstrated reliability and validity [42]. However, these tools were predominantly developed for research and are too time consuming to be adopted in a busy primary care setting [43].

A common area for confusion in clinical practice exists among individuals prescribed opioids for chronic pain who develop tolerance and withdrawal over time. If individuals are prescribed a substance such as an opioid under appropriate medical supervision, tolerance and withdrawal in the absence of other criteria do not indicate an opioid use disorder [41].

Treatment of Substance Use Disorders

Substance use disorder is conceptualized as a chronic disease [44]. SUD treatment approaches are generally successful at reducing disease symptoms and improving health and functioning [43]. Interventions are not meant to "cure" SUD, rather induce remission and prevention of return to use. Similar to other chronic diseases, effective treatment is heavily dependent on adherence to a medical regimen and failure to follow advice is as common as it is in other chronic diseases including asthma, diabetes, and hypertension [45]. Treatment may consist of a combination of psychosocial therapy, pharmacotherapy, and recovery support provided in a variety of care settings.

After diagnosing a SUD, providers should partner with the patient to determine the appropriate treatment setting (e.g., inpatient vs. outpatient). A patient-centered approach incorporating patients' unique needs and preferences is associated with improved patient engagement in effective SUD treatment services [46]. A biopsychosocial-spiritual assessment of the patient is important, and motivational interviewing can engage patients who are precontemplative or contemplative about treatment. Behavioral strategies are important particularly during early treatment as alcohol and drug use impair brain functioning around decision making. Patient-centered care considers patients' preferences, needs, culture (e.g., race/ethnicity, gender, sexuality, age, spirituality, ability status, language skills/literacy, socioeconomic status, immigration status) and history (e.g., treatment history, trauma history, history of incarceration, comorbid physical, and mental health problems) [47]. Attention to culturally relevant interventions based on the patient population improves engagement and retention among marginalized groups [48, 49].

Typically, SUD treatment programs exist independently from general medical care and are limited to special settings, particularly when SUD is severe or complex. Specialty treatment settings are often organized by the intensity and resources of the care setting, which range from outpatient to medically managed inpatient care. The American Society of Addiction Medicine (ASAM) criteria is the most widely used classification system for placement, continued stay, transfer, or discharge of patients with addiction and co-occurring conditions (Fig. 6.1) [50]. The ASAM criteria utilizes six dimensions to determine an individual's risk, needs, and strengths to match the patient to the appropriate level of care. The six dimensions include: (1) acute intoxication and/or withdrawal potential; (2) biomedical conditions and complications; (3) emotional/behavioral/cognitive conditions and complications; (4) readiness to change; (5) relapse/continued use/continued problem potential, and (6) recovery environment.

A traditional path through the treatment system begins with short-term, medically managed detoxification, followed by one or more months of intensive residential treatment, followed by continuing care in an outpatient treatment program, with or without additional recovery supportive housing [4]. Despite this recognized pathway for treatment, evidence supporting residential treatment over outpatient treatment is unclear [51]. Residential treatment may be beneficial for individuals with few social supports (e.g., homelessness or a social network limited to people with SUD), or for individuals with limited success in outpatient programs. The Ecological Systems Model, applied to substance use disorders, highlights the interconnected relationships between individuals and their recovery environments (Fig. 6.2).

Barriers to Treatment

The 2019 National Survey on Drug Use and Health estimated that 22 million people aged 12 years and older needed substance use treatment in the previous year and only 1.4 million received it [1]. A significant barrier to substance use treatment is lack of access. Of the 813,000 people surveyed who perceived a need for substance use treatment and did not receive it, 24% did not know where to go for treatment, 21% were not able to afford the cost of treatment, and 40% were not ready for cessation. As of 2020, 31% of all counties in the US have no substance use treatment facilities at any level of care and only 6% offer all six levels of care (from outpatient to intensively managed inpatient) [52]. The dearth of services is more acute in rural areas with fewer referrals made, fewer services available, and higher treatment costs to patients [5, 53]. Black, Indigenous, and People of Color (BIPOC) face traditional barriers to treatment in addition to lack of evidence-based cross-cultural treatment, more burdensome and/or stigmatizing treatment, and multiple forms of racism [54].

One goal of inpatient SUD treatment is to address barriers individuals' experience in their community. Patients with frequent inpatient admissions face major barriers reflected in their use of the hospital as temporary housing, lack of planning for long-term treatment while inpatient, and unsuccessful follow up after hospitalization, which could be addressed with supportive housing, transportation, and support for patients after discharge [55]. Healthcare providers can reduce the risk of patients' SUD relapse with long-term treatment

ASAM CONTINUUM OF CARE

▶ ADULT

- .5 Early Intervention
- 1 Outpatient Services
- 2.1 Intensive Outpatient Services
- 2.5 Partial Hospitalization Services
- 3.1 Clinically Managed Low-Intensity Residential Services
- 3.3 Clinically Managed Population-Specific High-Intensity Residential Services
- 3.5 Clinically Managed High-Intensity Residential Services
- 3.7 Medically Monitored Intensive Inpatient Services
- 4 Medically Managed Intensive Inpatient Services

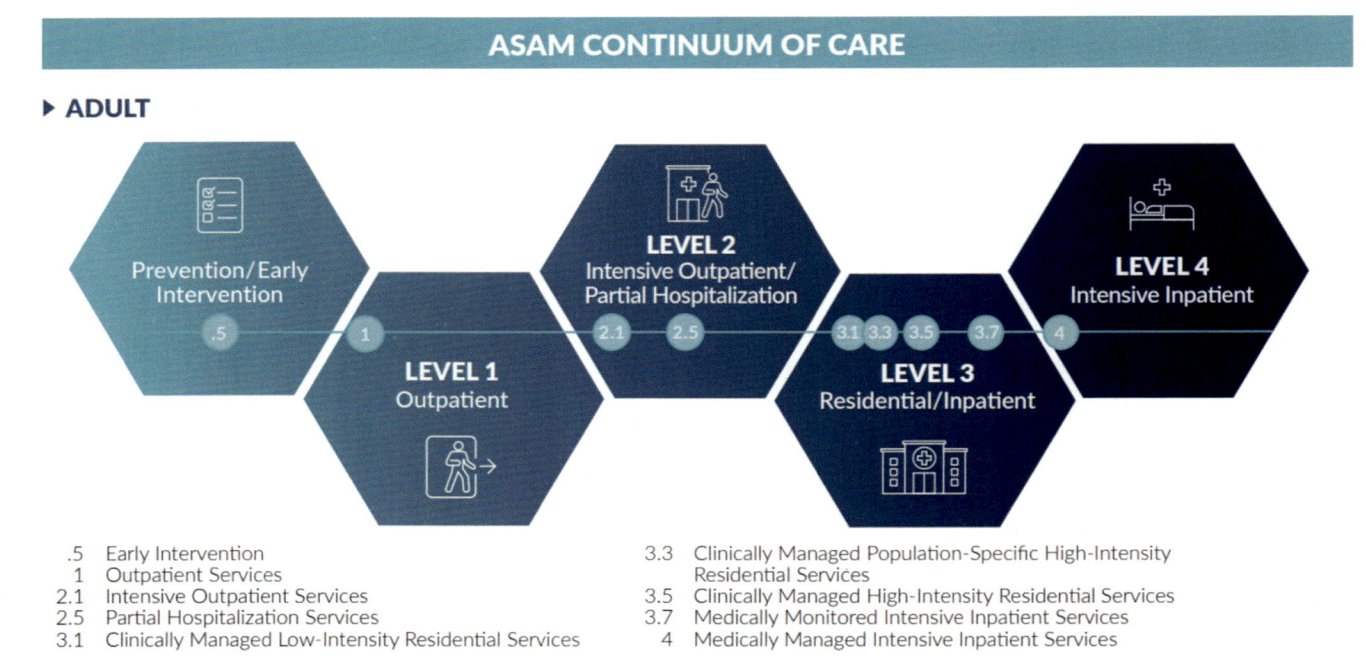

Fig. 6.1 American Society of Addiction Medicine (ASAM) levels of care for adults (Source: [146])

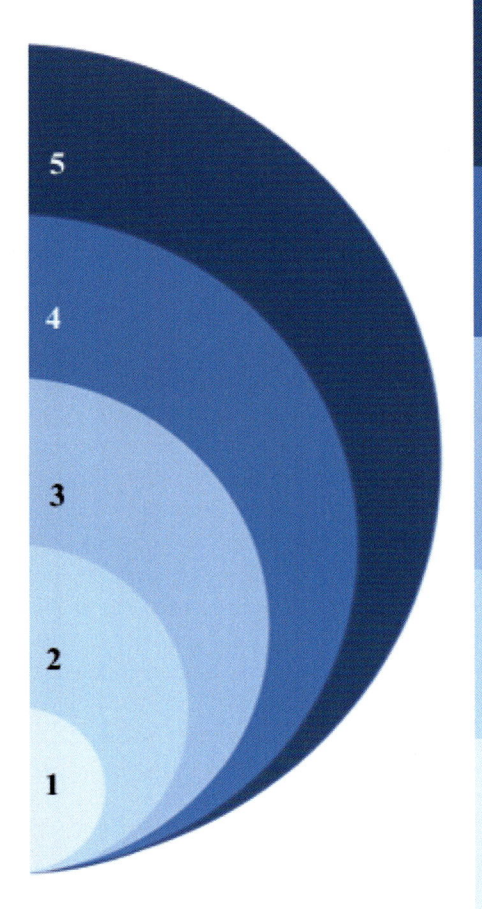

Domain 5: Macrosystem/Society. Goal: Support harm reduction strategies at state and federal level. Examples: Increase mental health and substance use treatment access and parity. Promote just naloxone laws. Decriminalize cannabis. Update buprenorphine practice guidelines.

Domain 4: Exosystem/Community. Goal: Create a local context that supports harm reduction. Change attitudes to support access to addiction treatment and harm reduction services. Fund syringe exchange programs. Equip local social workers and teachers with naloxone. Include naloxone administration in First Aid training.

Domain 3: Provider. Goal: Support patients in their recovery and promote population health with an eye on at risk populations. Prescribe pharmacotherapy. Provide patient-centered care. Celebrate positive gains. Collaborate with harm reduction agencies. Educate colleagues about benefits of harm reduction strategies. Engage in continuing education. Provide culturally relevant care.

Domain 2: Microsystem/Family[1]. Goal: Support family, help family support individual and other domains. Examples: Attend support groups. Foster communication, model healthy behavior. Obtain and learn to administer naloxone. Learn triggers, create contingency plans. Lobby for safe injection sites.

Domain 1: Individual. Goal: Reduce harm to individuals and others. Examples: Obtain treatment with pharmacotherapy. Obtain and adhere to PrEP, use safe sex practices. Obtain vaccinations (Hep A/B/COVID-19). Obtain and learn to administer naloxone. Know needle exchange and testing center locations.

Time: Allow time for establishing services, relapse, building relationships

Fig. 6.2 The Ecological Systems Model describes the interconnected and bi-directional relationship between individuals and their environments. The individual is in the center, nested within all the domains [147]
Abbreviations: PrEP Pre-exposure prophylaxis, *Hep* Hepatitis

Notes: (1) *Family* is conceptualized as the group of people who the individual perceives as family. In some cases, the birth family may be a protective factor, and in other situations the birth family may serve as a barrier to care

plans including close follow up and support after hospitalization. Other barriers include patients' perception of a lack of privacy during treatment [53].

Despite a recent reduction in the societal stigma of mental health problems, the stigma of SUD persists and is another barrier to treatment. Healthcare providers' stigmatizing attitudes toward people with SUD is associated with poor quality treatment and low patient engagement in care [56]. Stigmatizing attitudes from primary care providers is associated with a lower likelihood of supporting practice and policies of treating opioid use disorder with medication [57]. Use of non-stigmatizing, person-first language can improve quality of care for patients and should be used in all healthcare settings (Table 6.3) [58].

Harm Reduction

Harm reduction, an approach commonly utilized in substance use treatment settings, refers to policies and programs aimed at reducing the negative consequences of substance use rather than eliminating use altogether [59]. Specific examples include medications for opioid use disorder (e.g., methadone, buprenorphine), syringe exchange programs, safe injection facilities, naloxone distribution, and overdose prevention programs [60]. Harm reduction programs are occasionally met with resistance despite applications to patients across the behavioral health spectrum, including those with HIV/AIDS, eating disorders, intimate partner violence, and obesity. Harm reduction can be a universal precaution with a set of principles applied to all individuals in healthcare settings regardless of the presence of negative health behaviors (Table 6.4). Some opponents promote abstinence-only interventions based on the concern that harm reduction encourages ongoing use and is detrimental at the community level. However, existing literature provides compelling evidence for the feasibility, effectiveness, and cost-effectiveness of harm reduction interventions for substance use [60–64]. For example, individuals who utilize syringe service programs are five times more likely to enter treatment and three times more likely to stop using substances compared to those who do not use these programs [65].

Pharmacotherapy

Effective treatment for alcohol and drug use disorders includes the use of pharmacotherapy. Medications have a degree of efficacy in reducing return to use similar to treatment effectiveness of antidepressants for major depression and statins for prevention of coronary events. Despite the availability of efficacious medications approved by the US Food and Drug Administration (FDA), access to treatment remains limited, particularly in rural settings [66].

Three medications for the treatment of opioid use disorder (methadone, buprenorphine, and naltrexone) and three for alcohol use disorder (acamprosate, disulfiram, and naltrexone) are approved by the FDA (Tables 6.5 and 6.6). As of 2021, FDA-approved medications are not available for treatment of stimulant, sedative, or cannabis use disorders, although some medications have modest evidence in small studies, such as topiramate for cocaine use disorder, N-acetylcysteine for cannabis use disorder, and extended-release naltrexone and bupropion for methamphetamine use disorder [67–70].

The evidence base is strongest for medications for treatment of opioid use disorder (OUD) with methadone and buprenorphine; however, clinical trials have primarily been conducted with treatment-seeking individuals, overlooking Black, Indigenous, and People of Color (BIPOC) [24].

Table 6.3 Non-stigmatizing, clinically accurate language for SUD (Source: [58])

Avoid	Prefer
Abuse	Use (or specify low-risk or unhealthy use)
Addicted baby	Baby experiencing substance withdrawal
Addict, abuser, alcoholic, junkie	Person with substance use disorder or addiction
Drunk, strung out	Intoxicated
Detoxification	Withdrawal, withdrawal management
Medication assisted treatment	Opioid agonist treatment, medication treatment, treatment
Relapse	Return to use, recurrence of symptoms/disorder
Dirty vs. clean urine	Positive or negative, detected or not detected

Table 6.4 Harm reduction principles (Source: [143])

Principle	Approaches
Humanism	Avoid making moral judgments and holding grudges against patients; Accept patients' choices.
Pragmatism	Do not assume abstinence is the goal; Providers may experience moral ambiguity since they may support individuals with behaviors that may cause negative health outcomes.
Individualism	Assess strengths and needs on an individual basis; Tailor messaging and interventions to specific needs of each patient while maximizing treatment options.
Autonomy	Highlight provider-patient partnership; Engage in patient-centered care and shared decision making.
Incrementalism	Celebrate any positive gains; Recognize that all patients at times have negative courses or periods of stagnation.
Accountability without termination	Avoid penalizing backward movement and assist patients with understanding the effect of behaviors and choices on their health.

Table 6.5 Medications for opioid use disorder (Source: [144])

	Methadone (PO)	Buprenorphine (SL)	Naltrexone (IM)
Mechanism of Action	Full Agonist—Opioid Receptor	Partial Agonist—Opioid Receptor	Antagonist—Opioid Receptor
Dosing	80 mg–120 mg	4–32 mg	380 mg IM injection
Advantages	• Provided in highly structured setting (OTP), diversion unlikely • May be effective for those who have not benefitted from other treatment medications • Used in pregnancy	• Improved safety due to partial agonism • Available in primary care setting • Available in several formulations (SC injection, implant, buccal) • Used in pregnancy	• No addictive potential or diversion risk • No withdrawal upon cessation • Available in primary care settings • Option for individuals wanting to avoid opioids

Abbreviations: *PO* Oral, *SL* Sublingual, *IM* Intramuscular, *OTP* Opioid treatment program, *SC* Subcutaneous

Table 6.6 Medications for alcohol use disorder (Source: [84, 85, 145])

Medication	Mechanism of action	Dosing regimen
Acamprosate	Thought to modulate hyperactive glutamatergic NMDA receptors	Oral: 666 mg 3 times/day
Disulfiram	Inhibits ALDH2, causing accumulation of acetaldehyde during alcohol consumption, resulting in unpleasant effects such as nausea, dizziness, and flushing	Oral: 250–500 mg daily
Naltrexone	Opioid antagonist blocking the effects of ethanol-induced endogenous opioid release	Oral: 50–100 mg daily IM injection: 380 mg/month
Topiramate[a]	Normalizes GABA neuronal activity and suppresses ethanol-induced dopamine release	Oral: 200–300 mg/day
Gabapentin[a]	Calcium channel GABAergic modulator, benefits alcohol-induced insomnia and negative affect	Oral: 900–1800 mg/day

Abbreviations: ALDH2 Aldehyde dehydrogenase 2, *IM* Intramuscular, *GABA* Gamma-aminobutyric acid, *NMDA* N-Methyl-D-aspartic acid
[a]Non-FDA approved

Methadone, utilized in the US for more than 50 years, reduces opioid use, overdose, and HIV/Hep C acquisition. Methadone improves treatment retention, lowers rates of cellulitis, and is associated with a reduction in criminal behavior [71, 72]. In the US, methadone must be administered in an opioid treatment program and observed daily dosing is initially combined with integrated counseling. Daily dosing can be logistically challenging for patients who are employed or those with limited transportation. These issues in addition to stigma are often cited as reasons methadone is less appealing for treatment [73]. This burdensome treatment is disproportionately less available for BIPOC [74]. In contrast, buprenorphine can be prescribed in a provider's office and taken at home with similar effectiveness compared to methadone. Recognizing the evidence supporting methadone and buprenorphine treatment, the World Health Organization includes both on its list of essential medications [75]. Methadone and buprenorphine are recommended as first line treatment for OUD in pregnancy with buprenorphine reducing the severity of neonatal opioid withdrawal syndrome [76]. Each medication has its advantages and disadvantages and having more than one option for patients maximizes patient-centered treatment and engagement.

Naltrexone, an opioid antagonist, is available in a once daily oral formulation or in an extended release monthly intramuscular injection. Oral naltrexone is not widely used for treatment of OUD because of high rates of medication non-adherence and difficulty remaining abstinent for the necessary time before treatment initiation [77]. Extended-release naltrexone is as effective as buprenorphine at increasing treatment retention and preventing relapse but may be associated with a higher risk of overdose [78–80]. Naloxone, a rapid-acting opioid antagonist that reverses the effects of an opioid overdose, is a lifesaving medication for individuals with OUD rather than a form of treatment like methadone or buprenorphine. Naloxone distribution is a key component of harm reduction and should be readily accessible to patients and their caregivers along with training on proper use. People who inject drugs, BIPOC individuals, and those experiencing homelessness are less likely to have received naloxone compared to their White counterparts [81].

Medications for alcohol use disorder can increase abstinence, decrease heavy drinking, and improve protracted withdrawal symptoms. Despite the availability, safety, ease of prescribing, and demonstrated efficacy, medications are underutilized with only 1.6% of eligible patients using this treatment [82]. Naltrexone and acamprosate are more effective than disulfiram, which provides no benefit unless dispensed as directly observed treatment [83]. Topiramate and gabapentin are not FDA approved for alcohol use disorder, but randomized controlled trials support their use to reduce heavy drinking and increase abstinence [84, 85]. Treatment regimens often combine these medications to take advantage of varied mechanisms of action and effects in the brain to promote recovery.

Individuals with moderate or severe alcohol use disorder should be offered either oral naltrexone or acamprosate in combination with behavioral therapies [86, 87]. Oral naltrexone plus brief behavioral support by clinicians yields comparable results to state-of-the-art outpatient addiction therapy, suggesting that increasing treatment availability in primary care settings would significantly enhance access to effective care [88, 89]. Behavioral support includes reviewing medication adherence and side effects, assessing current alcohol use and consequences, and validating abstinence or efforts to reduce consumption.

Psychosocial Interventions

The USPSTF recommends evidence-based psychosocial interventions, such as cognitive behavioral therapy, motivational interviewing, contingency management, and mindfulness, as part of a comprehensive treatment plan, noting that most research in this field is conducted with treatment-seeking individuals [90]. This suggests BIPOC perspectives are missing since those individuals are less likely than White counterparts to have access to treatment with fewer opportunities to engage in health research [91]. Thus, interventions should be suggested with caution and additional research specific to minoritized groups is needed.

Cognitive behavioral therapy (CBT) is a common behavioral intervention to address SUD and aims to increase coping skills and improve self-efficacy [92]. The goals of CBT are to identify and avoid triggers and learn strategies to face triggers or high-risk situations [93]. CBT is appropriate for individuals with alcohol, cannabis, opioid, stimulant, and tobacco use disorders [94–96]. Between 42 and 75% of people with mental health disorders have a substance use disorder [5]. CBT may promote positive effects among individuals with a co-occurring mental health disorder. Although CBT performs better than treatment as usual or no intervention, CBT does not show superior efficacy compared to other evidence-based modalities such as motivational interviewing, contingency management, or mindfulness [90, 92]. Contingency management is based on principles of positive reinforcement in return for pre-specified goals (e.g., treatment attendance, days abstinent), and can complement CBT and be effective in treating alcohol, cannabis, opioids, nicotine, and stimulant use disorders including cocaine and methamphetamine, and polysubstance use [95, 97–99].

Mindfulness is a practice that promotes non-judgmental, moment-by-moment awareness and acceptance of the mind and body and can reduce the frequency and severity of substance misuse, cravings, and stress [100]. Mindfulness alters cognitive regulation and neurocognitive mechanisms of addiction [101].

Motivational interviewing is a behavior change intervention that promotes a therapeutic alliance that is non-judgmental and assesses patient readiness, motivations for and barriers to engaging in behavior change, and adherence to treatment [102–105]. Motivational interviewing may not be as effective as CBT in treating methamphetamine use disorder nor with African American patients, who may prefer health education [94, 106]. Motivational enhancement therapy is a brief intervention focused on helping the individual create a plan for change and consists of a four-session intervention with treatment efficacy similar to CBT and 12-step programs [93].

Peer-Based Recovery

Treatment led by peers is just as efficacious as that led by professionals [107]. Peer-based recovery is the practice of laypersons providing support to patients with shared experiences to those of the peer [108]. Peer support specialists are typically employed by an institution from whom they receive non-clinical training that prepares them for patient-centered relationships that are not transactional in nature [109].

Alcoholics Anonymous (AA) and Narcotics Anonymous (NA) are well-known community-based mutual support groups that include shared experiences but are distinct from peer support professionals [110]. Characterized by 12-step facilitation, these programs are efficacious and increase the rates of continuous abstinence at 12 months, reduce the number of drinks per drinking day, and reduce alcohol-related consequences compared to other behavioral interventions [111]. Benefits of AA include being widely available and free with support available and accessible during times of crisis. These programs have a strong religious component and an abstinence policy that may serve as a deterrent for some individuals [112]. Pressures from group members to discontinue medications for treatment of SUD, particularly opioid use disorder, can be harmful because premature and/or rapid discontinuation is associated with higher healthcare expenditures, return to use, and elevated risk of mortality [113–115]. AA and the 12-step program are beneficial for individuals who find the mission a good fit for their needs and recovery goals and may be a helpful resource for lesbian, gay, and bisexual patients, particularly for women who are older with income less than $40,000 and with greater alcohol use disorder severity [116]. Patient-centered care requires discussing potential stigma and/or supplying information about alternatives to AA/NA and the 12-step program so patients may make choices that reflect their needs and interests [117]. Alternatives to the 12-step approach for people with low religiosity include Women for Sobriety, LifeRing, and SMART Recovery [118].

Monitoring Treatment Effectiveness

Monitoring response to treatment is an expected and routine part of medical care for chronic conditions including substance use disorders. Unlike illnesses such as hypertension and diabetes, substance use treatment does not have a standard of care to which treatment effectiveness can be compared. Recovery from a substance use disorder is defined as "a process of change through which individuals improve their health and wellness, live a self-directed life, and strive to reach their full potential" [119]. The process of recovery may involve periods of abstinence and return to use, and a treated patient is neither "cured" if abstinent nor a "treatment failure" if there is return to use. Documenting patient progress includes assessing diagnoses, drug use and related programs, and urine testing [120].

Recovery Management Checkups (RMC), a long-term clinical approach to following-up with patients with substance use disorder, is cost-effective in terms of its ability to increase abstinence and decrease substance use-related problems and involves check-ups every 3 months for 4 years [121, 122]. At each check-up, individuals are asked about past 90-day substance use, substance use-related problems, withdrawal symptoms, and if the person feels the need to intensify treatment services. Individuals who report no substance use submit a toxicology specimen and discrepancies are addressed with a reminder that any substance use serves as an opportunity for enhanced care. The ongoing management for SUD in the RMC model, similar to chronic disease surveillance for other common conditions, involves symptom management, treatment adherence, laboratory testing, and modifying individualized treatment as needed.

Integrating Treatment into Primary Care

Integration of SUD treatment into the primary care setting starts with screening but does not end there. Full integration requires pharmacotherapy and other treatments which are within the scope of primary care. Treatment of alcohol and opioid use disorders within primary care reduces hospitalizations and emergency department utilization [123]. Patients who receive at least 3 months of buprenorphine as treatment for OUD from their primary care provider (PCP) rather than a psychiatrist also have improvements in nationally recommended preventive primary care screenings [124].

Primary care offices are already structured to care for chronic illnesses using a team-based approach and comprehensive care. The optimal system for delivery of OUD treatment is unclear, though a coordinated, multidisciplinary approach appears to be the most successful in retaining patients and supporting prescribers [125]. This approach may include utilizing non-physician/advanced practice provider team members to help manage/schedule appointments, obtain urine toxicology screens, review clinic expectations, and provide behavioral counseling and between-visit support.

An early intervention model often used to integrate SUD treatment is screening, brief intervention, and referral to treatment for patients using risky substances (SBIRT) [126]. Brief interventions include using motivational interviewing to raise awareness about risky use and empower the patient toward behavioral change. SBIRT services can be offered by various primary care team members and are often covered by Medicaid, although some states have training requirements [127].

Treatment for opioid and alcohol use disorders often requires more than a brief intervention, and referral to a higher level of care is sometimes indicated. Building relationships with local addiction medicine specialists and opioid treatment programs can facilitate referrals in both directions. Often patients are stabilized at a higher level of support (e.g., daily visits at an opioid treatment program, psychiatric management of mental health disorders, inpatient detoxification) and then return to a primary care practice for ongoing management.

Local and national supports are available for PCPs working to integrate SUD treatment into their practice. SAMHSA offers opportunities for further education including the Providers Clinical Support System which offers free discussion forums, ask an expert, and one-to-one mentoring (https://pcssnow.org/mentoring/). In recent years, several hub and spoke models of support have spread across the country [127]. These systems foster relationships between experts (hub) and primary care clinics (spokes) to support and enable PCPs to expand their scope of practice.

Telehealth for Substance Use Disorder

Telehealth, also known as virtual care, describes the care patients receive from healthcare providers via or as a result of electronic communication (e.g., virtual visits, patient-provider chats, remote monitoring, physician-to-physician communication) [128]. Telehealth promotes engagement and adherence, increases access to care, and prevents return to use [129]. Mobile or wireless devices provide mobile health (mHealth), which may support craving management and coping skills and reduce substance use among adults and adolescents [130–132]. Efforts to limit exposure to COVID-19 required rapid advancement of telehealth and, as of 2021, federal policy and some state policies support the use of telemedicine for substance use treatment including utilizing an emergency exception to the Ryan Haight Online Pharmacy Consumer Protection Act of 2008 to allow providers to prescribe controlled substances via telemedicine without first conducting an in-person examination [133]. The proliferation of cell phones and other mobile devices makes electronic and wireless device-based interventions accessible to most patients [134]. Telehealth has the potential to increase access to services among rural-dwelling individuals and remove obstacles related to availability of services [135]. Still, not all patients have access to necessary resources (e.g., the Internet, minutes on a cell phone) or skills to navigate technology, which may compound existing inequities in substance use treatment [136].

Future Directions

Integration of SUD treatment into primary care settings has increased due to passage of several important policies and increased emphasis on addiction education in medical training. Passage of the Comprehensive Addiction Recovery Act (CARA) in 2016 expanded prescribing privileges for buprenorphine to nurse practitioners and physician assistants, previously limited to physicians [137]. In 2021, the Practice Guidelines for the Administration of Buprenorphine for Treating Opioid Use Disorder addressed barriers to prescribing buprenorphine by exempting practitioners from the certification requirements related to training and counseling to increase the availability of OUD treatment [138]. In 2022, the Mainstreaming Addiction Treatment Act removed the waiver requirement to prescribe buprenorphine for opioid use disorder expanding access to buprenorphine for the treatment of opioid use disorder [139]. Policies expanding access to treatment are critical as only about 10% of people with a SUD receive any type of specialty treatment and even less receive pharmacotherapy [82, 140]. Medical students receive only 2–10 h of education about addiction, leaving clinicians inadequately prepared to treat substance use disorders and co-occurring clinical conditions [141]. Medical schools and other medical training programs should expand addiction education. Addiction medicine fellowships accredited by the Accreditation Council on Graduate Medical Education (ACGME) are growing in the US with graduates eligible for certification through the American Board of Preventive Medicine. The SUD treatment ecosystem in the US must address the need for an expanded workforce and provide low barrier access to person-centered, high-quality, and evidence-based treatment to overcome the addiction epidemic.

References

1. Substance Abuse and Mental Health Services Administration, National Survey of Substance Abuse Treatment Services (N-SSATS): 2020. Data on substance abuse treatment facilities. Rockville, MD: Substance Abuse and Mental Health Services Administration; 2021.
2. Grossman ER, Benjamin-Neelon SE, Sonnenschein S. Alcohol consumption during the COVID-19 pandemic: a cross-sectional survey of US adults. Int J Environ Res Public Health. 2020;17(24):9189. Published 2020 Dec 9. https://doi.org/10.3390/ijerph17249189.
3. Ahmad FB, Rossen LM, Sutton P. Provisional drug overdose death counts. National Center for health. Statistics. 2021; (CDC)
4. U.S. Department of Health and Human Services (HHS), Office of the Surgeon General. Facing addiction in America: the surgeon general's report on alcohol, drugs, and health. Washington, DC: HHS; 2016.
5. NIDA. Is drug addiction treatment worth its cost?; 2020, June 3. https://www.drugabuse.gov/publications/principles-drug-addiction-treatment-research-based-guide-third-edition/frequently-asked-questions/drug-addiction-treatment-worth-its-cost. Accessed 16 Dec 2021.
6. Miller T, Hendrie D. Substance abuse prevention dollars and cents: a cost-benefit analysis, DHHS Pub. No. (SMA) 07-4298. Center for Substance Abuse Prevention, Substance Abuse and Mental Health Services Administration: Rockville, MD; 2008.
7. Jordan A, Mathis M, Haeny A, Funaro M, Paltin D, Ransome Y. An evaluation of opioid use in black communities: a rapid review of the literature. Harv Rev Psychiatry. 2021;29(2):108–30. https://doi.org/10.1097/HRP.0000000000000285.
8. Lopez-Vergara HI, Yang M, Weiss NH, Stamates AL, Spillane NS, Feldstein Ewing SW. The cultural equivalence of measurement in substance use research. Exp Clin Psychopharmacol. 2021;29(5):456–65. https://doi.org/10.1037/pha0000512.
9. Netherland J, Hansen H. White opioids: pharmaceutical race and the war on drugs that wasn't. BioSocieties. 2017;12(2):217–38. https://doi.org/10.1057/biosoc.2015.46.
10. Pinedo M. A current re-examination of racial/ethnic disparities in the use of substance abuse treatment: do disparities persist? Drug Alcohol Depend. 2019;202:162–7. https://doi.org/10.1016/j.drugalcdep.2019.05.017.
11. Diagnostic and statistical manual of mental disorders: DSM-5. 5th ed., American Psychiatric Association; 2013.
12. Lopez-Quintero C, Pérez de los Cobos J, Hasin DS, Okuda M, Wang S, Grant BF, Blanco C. Probability and predictors of transition from first use to dependence on nicotine, alcohol, cannabis, and cocaine: results of the National Epidemiologic Survey on Alcohol and Related Conditions (NESARC). Drug Alcohol Depend. 2011;115(1–2):120–30. https://doi.org/10.1016/j.drugalcdep.2010.11.004. Epub 2010 Dec 8.
13. Center for Behavioral Health Statistics and Quality. Results from the 2017 National Survey on drug use and health: detailed tables. Substance Abuse and Mental Health Services Administration; 2018. Accessed 24 Dec 2021.
14. Harrington M, Robinson J, Bolton SL, Sareen J, Bolton J. A longitudinal study of risk factors for incident drug use in adults: findings from a representative sample of the US population. Can J Psychiatr. 2011;56(11):686–95. https://doi.org/10.1177/070674371105601107.
15. LeTendre ML, Reed MB. The effect of adverse childhood experience on clinical diagnosis of a substance use disorder: results of a nationally representative study. Subst Use Misuse. 2017;52(6):689–97. https://doi.org/10.1080/10826084.2016.1253746. December 24, 2021, 4:51 PM.
16. Schmaling KB, Blume AW, Skewes MC. Negative life events and incident alcohol use disorders among ethnic minorities. J Ethn Subst Abus. 2020;19(2):327–42. https://doi.org/10.1080/15332640.2018.1548322.
17. Sheu R, Lussier D, Rosenblum A, et al. Prevalence and characteristics of chronic pain in patients admitted to an outpatient drug and alcohol treatment program. Pain Med. 2008;9(7):911–7.
18. Galli JA, Sawaya RA, Friedenberg FK. Cannabinoid hyperemesis syndrome. Curr Drug Abuse Rev. 2011;4(4):241–9. https://doi.org/10.2174/1874473711104040241.
19. Rezkalla SH, Kloner RA. Cocaine-induced acute myocardial infarction. Clin Med Res. 2007;5(3):172–6. https://doi.org/10.3121/cmr.2007.759.
20. NIDA. Part 1: the connection between substance use disorders and mental illness. National Institute on Drug Abuse website; 2021. https://www.drugabuse.gov/publications/research-reports/common-comorbidities-substance-use-disorders/part-1-connection-between-substance-use-disorders-mental-illness. Accessed 6 Nov 2021.
21. Iqbal MN, Levin CJ, Levin FR. Treatment for substance use disorder with co-occurring mental illness. Focus (American Psychiatric Publishing). 2019;17(2):88–97. https://doi.org/10.1176/appi.focus.20180042.
22. McHugh RK, Votaw VR, Fulciniti F, et al. Perceived barriers to smoking cessation among adults with substance use disorders. J Subst Abus Treat. 2017;74:48–53. https://doi.org/10.1016/j.jsat.2016.12.008.
23. O'Connor EA, Perdue LA, Senger CA, et al. Screening and behavioral counseling interventions to reduce unhealthy alcohol use in adolescents and adults: updated evidence report and systematic review for the US preventive services task force. JAMA. 2018;320(18):1910–28. https://doi.org/10.1001/jama.2018.12086.
24. Patnode CD, Perdue LA, Rushkin M, et al. Screening for unhealthy drug use: updated evidence report and systematic review for the

US preventive services task force. JAMA. 2020;323(22):2310–28. https://doi.org/10.1001/jama.2019.21381.
25. Hagan JF, Shaw JS, Duncan P, editors. Bright futures: guidelines for health supervision of infants, children, and adolescents. 4th ed. Elk Grove Village, IL: American Academy of Pediatrics; 2017.
26. Price HR, Collier AC, Wright TE. Screening pregnant women and their neonates for illicit drug use: consideration of the integrated technical, medical, ethical, legal, and social issues. Front Pharmacol. 2018;9. https://www.frontiersin.org/article/10.3389/fphar.2018.00961. Accessed 20 Jan 2022.
27. Solberg LI, Maciosek MV, Edwards NM. Primary care intervention to reduce alcohol misuse ranking its health impact and cost effectiveness. Am J Prev Med. 2008;34(2):143–52. https://doi.org/10.1016/j.amepre.2007.09.035.
28. Denny CH, Hungerford DW, McKnight-Eily LR, et al. Self-reported prevalence of alcohol screening among U.S. adults. Am J Prev Med. 2016;50:380–3.
29. Smith PC, Schmidt SM, Allensworth-Davies D, Saitz R. Primary care validation of a single-question alcohol screening test. J Gen Intern Med. 2009;24(7):783–8.
30. Burns E, Gray R, Smith LA. Brief screening questionnaires to identify problem drinking during pregnancy: a systematic review. Addiction. 2010;105(4):601–14. https://doi.org/10.1111/j.1360-0443.2009.02842.x.
31. Campbell CE, Maisto SA. Validity of the AUDIT-C screen for at-risk drinking among students utilizing university primary care. J Am Coll Heal. 2018;66(8):774–82. https://doi.org/10.1080/07448481.2018.1453514.
32. Crawford EF, Fulton JJ, Swinkels CM, Beckham JC, Calhoun PS. Diagnostic efficiency of the AUDIT-C in U.S. veterans with military service since September 11, 2001. Drug Alcohol Depend. 2013;132(1):101–6. https://doi.org/10.1016/j.drugalcdep.2013.01.012.
33. Samet JH, O'Connor PG. Alcohol abusers in primary care: readiness to change behavior. Am J Med. 1998;105(4):302–6.
34. Frank D, DeBenedetti AF, Volk RJ, Williams EC, Kivlahan DR, Bradley KA. Effectiveness of the AUDIT-C as a screening test for alcohol misuse in three race/ethnic groups. J Gen Intern Med. 2008;23(6):781–7. https://doi.org/10.1007/s11606-008-0594-0.
35. Saitz R, Lepore MF, Sullivan LM, Amaro H, Samet JH. Alcohol abuse and dependence in Latinos living in the United States: validation of the CAGE (4M) questions. Arch Intern Med. 1999;159(7):718–24. https://doi.org/10.1001/archinte.159.7.718.
36. Xuan B, Li P, Yang L, Li M, Zhou J. Similarities and differences in diagnostic scales. In: Zhang X, Shi J, Tao R, eds. Substance and non-substance addiction. Advances in experimental medicine and biology. Springer; 2017:133–168. doi:https://doi.org/10.1007/978-981-10-5562-1_8.
37. McNeely J, Cleland CM, Strauss SM, Palamar JJ, Rotrosen J, Saitz R. Validation of self-administered single-item screening questions (SISQs) for unhealthy alcohol and drug use in primary care patients. J Gen Intern Med. 2015;30(12):1757–64. https://doi.org/10.1007/s11606-015-3391-6.
38. McNeely J, Wu L, Subramanian G, et al. Performance of the tobacco, alcohol, prescription medication, and other substance use (TAPS) tool for substance use screening in primary care patients. Ann Intern Med. 2016;165(10):690–9.
39. Yudko E, Lozhkina O, Fouts A. A comprehensive review of the psychometric properties of the drug abuse screening test. J Subst Abus Treat. 2007;32(2):189–98. https://doi.org/10.1016/j.jsat.2006.08.002.
40. Gonzalez Suitt K, Castro Y, Caetano R, Field CA. Predictive utility of alcohol use disorder symptoms across race/ethnicity. J Subst Abus Treat. 2015;56:61–7. https://doi.org/10.1016/j.jsat.2015.03.001.
41. Hasin DS, O'Brien CP, Auriacombe M, et al. DSM-5 criteria for substance use disorders: recommendations and rationale. Am J Psychiatry. 2013;170(8):834–51. https://doi.org/10.1176/appi.ajp.2013.12060782.
42. Forman RF, Svikis D, Montoya ID, Blaine J. Selection of a substance use disorder diagnostic instrument by the National Drug Abuse Treatment Clinical Trials Network. J Subst Abus Treat. 2004;27(1):1–8.
43. Samet S, Waxman R, Hatzenbuehler M, Hasin DS. Assessing addiction: concepts and instruments. Addict Sci Clin Pract. 2007;4(1):19–31.
44. ASAM's 2019 definition of addiction. https://www.asam.org/docs/default-source/qualityscience/asam's-2019-definition-of-addiction-(1).pdf?sfvrsn=b8b64fc2_2. Published 15 Sep 2019. Accessed 15 Jan 2022.
45. McLellan AT, Lewis DC, O'Brien CP, Kleber HD. Drug dependence, a chronic medical illness: implications for treatment, insurance, and outcomes evaluation. JAMA. 2000;284(13):1689–95.
46. Park SE, Mosley JE, Grogan CM, et al. Patient-centered care's relationship with substance use disorder treatment utilization. J Subst Abus Treat. 2020;118:108125.
47. VA DOD Clinical Practice Guideline for The Management of Substance Use Disorders. healthquality.va.gov. https://www.healthquality.va.gov/guidelines/MH/sud/VADoDSUDCPG.pdf. Published August 2021. Accessed January 15, 2022.
48. Guerrero EG. Enhancing access and retention in substance abuse treatment: the role of Medicaid payment acceptance and cultural competence. Drug Alcohol Depend. 2013;132(3):555–61. https://doi.org/10.1016/j.drugalcdep.2013.04.005.
49. Williams DR, Lawrence JA, Davis BA, Vu C. Understanding how discrimination can affect health. Health Serv Res. 2019;54(S2):1374–88. https://doi.org/10.1111/1475-6773.13222.
50. Mee-Lee D. Understanding the new ASAM criteria. NCADD Webinar. April 23, 2015. Available online: https://www.naadac.org/understanding-the-new-asam-criteria. Accessed 15 Jan 2022.
51. Reif S, George P, Braude L, Dougherty RH, Daniels AS, Ghose SS, Delphin-Rittmon ME. Residential treatment for individuals with substance use disorders: assessing the evidence. Psychiatr Serv. 2014;65(3):301–12. https://doi.org/10.1176/appi.ps.201300242.
52. GAO-21-58, substance use disorder: Reliable data needed for substance abuse and prevention and treatment block grant program. https://www.gao.gov/assets/gao-21-58.pdf. Accessed 15 Jan 2022.
53. Browne T, Priester MA, Clone S, Iachini A, DeHart D, Hock R. Barriers and facilitators to substance use treatment in the rural south: a qualitative study. J Rural Health. 2016;32(1):92–101.
54. Amaro H, Sanchez M, Bautista T, Cox R. Social vulnerabilities for substance use: stressors, socially toxic environments, and discrimination and racism. Neuropharmacology. 2021;188:108518. https://doi.org/10.1016/j.neuropharm.2021.108518.
55. Raven MC, Carrier ER, Lee J, Billings JC, Marr M, Gourevitch MN. Substance use treatment barriers for patients with frequent hospital admissions. J Subst Abus Treat. 2010;38(1):22–30.
56. van Boekel LC, Brouwers EP, van Weeghel J, Garretsen HF. Stigmatiserende van pati''enten met een verslaving en de gevolgen voor de hulpverlening: een; 2015.
57. Stone EM, Kennedy-Hendricks A, Barry CL, Bachhuber MA, McGinty EE. The role of stigma in U.S. primary care physicians' treatment of opioid use disorder. Drug Alcohol Depend. 2021;221:108627.
58. Saitz R, Miller SC, Fiellin DA, Rosenthal RN. Recommended use of terminology in addiction medicine. J Addict Med. 2021;15(1):3–7. https://doi.org/10.1097/ADM.0000000000000673.
59. Des Jarlais DC. Harm reduction—a framework for incorporating science into drug policy. Am J Public Health. 1995;85:10–2.
60. Ritter A, Cameron J. A review of the efficacy and effectiveness of harm reduction strategies for alcohol, tobacco and

61. illicit drugs. Drug Alcohol Rev. 2006;25(6):611–24. https://doi.org/10.1080/09595230600944529.
62. Anderson KO, Green CR, Payne R. Racial and ethnic disparities in pain: causes and consequences of unequal care. J Pain. 2009;10(12):1187–204. https://doi.org/10.1016/j.jpain.2009.10.002.
63. Burton R, Henn C, Lavoie D, O'Connor R, Perkins C, Sweeney K, Greaves F, Ferguson B, Beynon C, Belloni A, et al. A rapid evidence review of the effectiveness and cost-effectiveness of alcohol control policies: an English perspective. Lancet. 2017;389:1558–80.
64. Cook C, Bridge J, Stimson GV. The diffusion of harm reduction in Europe and beyond. Monographs. 2010:37–56.
65. Kerr T, Small W, Buchner C, Zhang R, Li K, Montaner J, Wood E. Syringe sharing and HIV incidence among injection drug users and increased access to sterile syringes. Am J Public Health. 2010;100:1449–53.
66. Des Jarlais DC, Nugent A, Solberg A, Feelemyer J, Mermin J, Holtzman D. Syringe service programs for persons who inject drugs in urban, suburban, and rural areas—United States, 2013. MMWR Morb Mortal Wkly Rep. 2015;64(48):1337–41. https://doi.org/10.15585/mmwr.mm6448a3.
67. Ghertner R. U.S. trends in the supply of providers with a waiver to prescribe buprenorphine for opioid use disorder in 2016 and 2018. Drug Alcohol Depend. 2019;204:107527. https://doi.org/10.1016/j.drugalcdep.2019.06.029.
68. Baldaçara L, Cogo-Moreira H, Parreira BL, et al. Efficacy of topiramate in the treatment of crack cocaine dependence: a double-blind, randomized, placebo-controlled trial. J Clin Psychiatry. 2016;77(3):398–406.
69. Singh M, Keer D, Klimas J, Wood E, Werb D. Topiramate for cocaine dependence: a systematic review and meta-analysis of randomized controlled trials. Addiction. 2016;111(8):1337–46.
70. Gray KM, Carpenter MJ, Baker NL, DeSantis SM, Kryway E, Hartwell KJ, McRae-Clark AL, Kathleen T. Brady a double-blind randomized controlled trial of N-acetylcysteine in cannabis-dependent adolescents. Am J Psychiatr. 2012;169(8):805–12.
71. Trivedi MH, Walker R, Ling W, et al. Bupropion and naltrexone in methamphetamine use disorder. N Engl J Med. 2021;384(2):140–53. https://doi.org/10.1056/NEJMoa2020214.
72. Fullerton CA, Kim M, Thomas CP, Lyman DR, Montejano LB, Dougherty RH, Delphin-Rittmon ME. Medication-assisted treatment with methadone: assessing the evidence. Psychiatr Serv. 2014;65(2):146–57.
73. Schwartz RP, Jaffe JH, O'Grady KE, Kinlock TW, Gordon MS, Kelly SM, et al. Interim methadone treatment: impact on arrests. Drug Alcohol Depend. 2009;103(3):148–54.
74. Yarborough BJ, Stumbo SP, McCarty D, Mertens J, Weisner C, Green CA. Methadone, buprenorphine and preferences for opioid agonist treatment: a qualitative analysis. Drug Alcohol Depend. 2016;160:112–8.
75. Andraka-Christou B. Addressing racial and ethnic disparities in the use of medications for opioid use disorder. Health Aff. 2021;40(6):920–7. https://doi.org/10.1377/hlthaff.2020.02261.
76. Executive summary: The selection and use of essential medicines 2021: Report of the 23rd WHO expert committee on the selection and use of essential medicines. World Health Organization. https://www.who.int/publications/i/item/WHO-MHP-HPS-EML-2021.01. Accessed 15 Jan 2022.
77. Jones HE, Kaltenbach K, Heil SH, et al. Neonatal abstinence syndrome after methadone or buprenorphine exposure. N Engl J Med. 2010;363(24):2320–31. https://doi.org/10.1056/NEJMoa1005359.
78. Sullivan MA, Garawi F, Bisaga A, Comer SD, Carpenter K, Raby WN, Nunes EV. Management of relapse in naltrexone maintenance for heroin dependence. Drug Alcohol Depend. 2007;91(2–3):289–92.
79. Lee JD, Nunes EV Jr, Novo P, et al. Comparative effectiveness of extended-release naltrexone versus buprenorphine-naloxone for opioid relapse prevention (X:BOT): a multicentre, open-label, randomised controlled trial. Lancet. 2018;391(10118):309–18. https://doi.org/10.1016/S0140-6736(17)32812-X.
80. Tanum L, Solli KK, Latif Z, et al. Effectiveness of injectable extended-release naltrexone vs daily buprenorphine-naloxone for opioid dependence: a randomized clinical noninferiority trial. JAMA Psychiatry. 2017;74(12):1197–205. https://doi.org/10.1001/jamapsychiatry.2017.3206.
81. Ajazi EM, Dasgupta N, Marshall SW, et al. Revisiting the X:BOT naltrexone clinical trial using a comprehensive survival analysis. J Addict Med. 2022;16(4):440–6. https://doi.org/10.1097/ADM.0000000000000931.
82. Kinnard EN, Bluthenthal RN, Kral AH, Wenger LD, Lambdin BH. The naloxone delivery cascade: identifying disparities in access to naloxone among people who inject drugs in Los Angeles and San Francisco, CA. Drug Alcohol Depend. 2021;225:108759. https://doi.org/10.1016/j.drugalcdep.2021.108759.
83. Han B, Jones CM, Einstein EB, Powell PA, Compton WM. Use of medications for alcohol use disorder in the US: results from the 2019 National Survey on Drug Use and Health [published online ahead of print, 2021 Jun 16]. JAMA Psychiatry. 2021;78(8):922–4. https://doi.org/10.1001/jamapsychiatry.2021.1271.
84. Garbutt JC, West SL, Carey TS, et al. Pharmacological treatment of alcohol dependence: a review of the evidence. JAMA. 1999;281(14):1318–25.
85. Johnson BA, Ait-Daoud N. Topiramate in the new generation of drugs: efficacy in the treatment of alcoholic patients. Curr Pharm Des. 2010;16(19):2103–12.
86. Mason BJ, Quello S, Shadan F. Gabapentin for the treatment of alcohol use disorder. Expert Opin Investig Drugs. 2018;27(1):113–24. https://doi.org/10.1080/13543784.2018.1417383.
87. National Collaborating Centre for Mental Health, National Institute for Health & Clinical Excellence. Alcohol-use disorders: the NICE guidelines on diagnosis, assessment and management of harmful drinking and alcohol dependence. The British Psychological Society and The Royal College of Psychiatrists; 2011. https://www.nice.org.uk/guidance/CG115/chapter/1-Guidance#interventions-for-alcohol-misuse. Accessed 14 Sep 2021.
88. Reus VI, Fochtmann LJ, Bukstein O, et al. The American Psychiatric Association practice guideline for the pharmacological treatment of patients with alcohol use disorder. Am J Psychiatry. 2018;175(1):86–90. https://doi.org/10.1176/appi.ajp.2017.1750101.
89. Anton RF, et al. Combined pharmacotherapies and behavioral interventions for alcohol dependence: the COMBINE study: a randomized controlled trial. JAMA. 2006;295(17):2003–17.
90. O'Malley SS, et al. Initial and maintenance naltrexone treatment for alcohol dependence using primary care vs specialty care: a nested sequence of 3 randomized trials. Arch Intern Med. 2003;163(14):1695–704.
91. Ray LA, Meredith LR, Kiluk BD, Walthers J, Carroll KM, Magill M. Combined pharmacotherapy and cognitive Behavioral therapy for adults with alcohol or other drug use disorders: a systematic review and meta-analysis. JAMA Netw Open. 2020;3(6):e208279. https://doi.org/10.1001/jamanetworkopen.2020.8279.
92. Skewes MC, Hallum-Montes R, Gardner SA, Blume AW, Ricker A, FireMoon P. Partnering with native communities to develop a culturally grounded intervention for substance use disorder. Am J Community Psychol. 2019;64(1–2):72–82. https://doi.org/10.1002/ajcp.12354.
93. Magill M, Tonigan JS, Kiluk B, Ray L, Walthers J, Carroll K. The search for mechanisms of cognitive Behavioral therapy for

alcohol or other drug use disorders: a systematic review. Behav Res Ther. 2020;131(August):103648. https://doi.org/10.1016/j.brat.2020.103648.
93. Glasner S, Drazdowski TK. Evidence-based Behavioral treatments for substance use disorders. In: Danovitch I, Mooney L, editors. The assessment and treatment of addiction: best practices and new frontiers. Elsevier Health Sciences; 2018.
94. Cohen JY, Huguet G, Cohen J, Vera L, Dardennes R. Cognitive-behavioural therapies and motivational interviewing for methamphetamine use disorders: a systematic review. J Addict Med Ther. Published online. 2017;6:1030.
95. Gates PJ, Sabioni P, Copeland J, Le Foll B, Gowing L. Psychosocial interventions for cannabis use disorder. Cochrane Database Syst Rev. 2016;(5):CD005336. https://doi.org/10.1002/14651858CD005336.pub4.
96. Magill M, Ray L, Kiluk B, et al. A meta-analysis of cognitive-behavioral therapy for alcohol or other drug use disorders: treatment efficacy by contrast condition. J Consult Clin Psychol. 2019;87(12):1093–105. https://doi.org/10.1037/ccp0000447.
97. McKay JR, Lynch KG, Coviello D, et al. Randomized trial of continuing care enhancements for cocaine-dependent patients following initial engagement. J Consult Clin Psychol. 2010;78(1):111–20. https://doi.org/10.1037/a0018139.
98. Ainscough TS, McNeill A, Strang J, Calder R, Brose LS. Contingency management interventions for non-prescribed drug use during treatment for opiate addiction: a systematic review and meta-analysis. Drug Alcohol Depend. 2017;178:318–39. https://doi.org/10.1016/j.drugalcdep.2017.05.028.
99. Davis DR, Kurti AN, Skelly JM, Redner R, White TJ, Higgins ST. A review of the literature on contingency management in the treatment of substance use disorders, 2009–2014. Prev Med. 2016;92:36–46. https://doi.org/10.1016/j.ypmed.2016.08.008.
100. Li W, Howard MO, Garland EL, McGovern P, Lazar M. Mindfulness treatment for substance misuse: a systematic review and meta-analysis. J Subst Abus Treat. 2017;75:62–96. https://doi.org/10.1016/j.jsat.2017.01.008.
101. Garland E, Froeliger B, Howard M. Mindfulness training targets neurocognitive mechanisms of addiction at the attention-appraisal-emotion interface. Front Psych. 2014;4:173. https://doi.org/10.3389/fpsyt.2013.00173.
102. Kelly TM, Daley DC, Douaihy AB. Treatment of substance abusing patients with comorbid psychiatric disorders. Addict Behav. 2012;37(1):11–24. https://doi.org/10.1016/j.addbeh.2011.09.010.
103. DiClemente CO, Velasquez MM. Motivational interviewing and the stages of change. In: Miller WR, Rollnick S, editors. Motivational interviewing: preparing people for change. 2nd ed. The Guilford Press; 2002. p. 201–16.
104. SAMHSA TIP 35: enhancing motivational interviewing for change in substance use disorder treatment. Substance Abuse and Mental Health Services Administration, U.S. Department of Health and Human Services; 2019. Accessed 18 Dec 2021. https://store.samhsa.gov/sites/default/files/d7/priv/tip35_final_508_compliant_-_02252020_0.pdf.
105. Lundahl B, Burke BL. The effectiveness and applicability of motivational interviewing: a practice-friendly review of four meta-analyses. J Clin Psychol. 2009;65(11):1232–45. https://doi.org/10.1002/jclp.20638.
106. Grobe JE, Goggin K, Harris KJ, Richter KP, Resnicow K, Catley D. Race moderates the effects of motivational interviewing on smoking cessation induction. Patient Educ Couns. 2020;103(2):350–8. https://doi.org/10.1016/j.pec.2019.08.023.
107. Beaulieu M, Tremblay J, Baudry C, Pearson J, Bertrand K. A systematic review and meta-analysis of the efficacy of the long-term treatment and support of substance use disorders. Soc Sci Med. 2021;285(September):114289. https://doi.org/10.1016/j.socscimed.2021.114289.
108. White W. Peer-based addiction recovery support: history, theory, practice, and scientific evaluation. Chicago, IL: Great Lakes Addiction Technology Transfer Center and Philadelphia Department of Behavioral Health and Mental Retardation Services; 2009.
109. Bassuk EL, Hanson J, Greene RN, Richard M, Laudet A. Peer-delivered recovery support Services For Addictions In the United States: a systematic review. J Subst Abus Treat. 2016;63:1–9. https://doi.org/10.1016/j.jsat.2016.01.003.
110. Jack HE, Oller D, Kelly J, Magidson JF, Wakeman SE. Addressing substance use disorder in primary care: the role, integration, and impact of recovery coaches. Subst Abus. 2018;39(3):307–14. https://doi.org/10.1080/08897077.2017.1389802.
111. Kelly JF, Humphreys K, Ferri M. Alcoholics anonymous and other 12-step programs for alcohol use disorder. Cochrane Database Syst Rev. 2020;2020(3):CD012880. https://doi.org/10.1002/14651858.CD012880.pub2.
112. Zemore SE, Kaskutas LA, Mericle A, Hemberg J. Comparison of 12-step groups to mutual help alternatives for AUD in a large, national study: differences in membership characteristics and group participation, cohesion, and satisfaction. J Subst Abus Treat. 2017;73:16–26. https://doi.org/10.1016/j.jsat.2016.10.004.
113. Agbese E, Leslie DL, Manhapra A, Rosenheck R. Early discontinuation of buprenorphine therapy for opioid use disorder among privately insured adults. PS. 2020;71(8):779–88. https://doi.org/10.1176/appi.ps.201900309.
114. Binswanger IA, Glanz JM, Faul M, et al. The association between opioid discontinuation and heroin use: a nested case-control study. Drug Alcohol Depend. 2020;217:108248. https://doi.org/10.1016/j.drugalcdep.2020.108248.
115. Stein BD, Sherry TB, O'Neill B, Taylor EA, Sorbero M. Rapid discontinuation of chronic, high-dose opioid treatment for pain: prevalence and associated factors. J Gen Intern Med. 2021; https://doi.org/10.1007/s11606-021-07119-3.
116. McGeough BL, Karriker-Jaffe KJ, Zemore SE. Rates and predictors of alcoholics anonymous attendance across sexual orientations. J Subst Abus Treat. 2021;129:108400. https://doi.org/10.1016/j.jsat.2021.108400.
117. Andraka-Christou B, Totaram R, Randall-Kosich O. Stigmatization of medications for opioid use disorder in 12-step support groups and participant responses. Subst Abus. 2021:1–10. https://doi.org/10.1080/08897077.2021.1944957.
118. Zemore SE, Lui C, Mericle A, Hemberg J, Kaskutas LA. A longitudinal study of the comparative efficacy of women for sobriety, LifeRing, SMART recovery, and 12-step groups for those with AUD. J Subst Abus Treat. 2018;88:18–26. https://doi.org/10.1016/j.jsat.2018.02.004.
119. SAMHSA.gov. SAMHSA's working definition of recovery: ten guiding principles of recovery. 2012. PEP12-RECDEF. https://store.samhsa.gov/sites/default/files/d7/priv/pep12-recdef.pdf. Accessed 21 Dec 2021.
120. Carroll KM, Rounsaville BJ. On beyond urine: clinically useful assessment instruments in the treatment of drug dependence. Behav Res Ther. 2002;40(11):1329–44.
121. McCollister KE, French MT, Freitas DM, Dennis ML, Scott CK, Funk RR. Cost-effectiveness analysis of recovery management Checkups (RMC) for adults with chronic substance use disorders: evidence from a 4-year randomized trial. Addiction. 2013;108(12):2166–74.
122. Scott CK, Dennis ML. Recovery management check-ups: an early re-intervention model. 2003. http://www.williamwhitepapers.com/pr/Recovery%20Management%20Checkup%20Manual%20Scott%20%26%20Dennis%202003.pdf. Accessed 21 Nov 2021.
123. Wakeman S, Rigotti N, Chang Y, Herman G, Erwin A, Regan S, et al. Effect of integrating substance use disorder treatment into

123. primary care on inpatient and emergency department utilization. J Gen Intern Med. 2019;34(6):871–7.
124. Haddad M, Zelenev A, Altice F. Buprenorphine maintenance treatment retention improves nationally recommended preventive primary care screenings when integrated into urban federally qualified health centers. J Urban Health. 2015;92(1):193–213.
125. Lagisetty P, Klasa K, Bush C, Heisler M, Chopra V, Bohnert A. Primary care models for treating opioid use disorders: what actually works? A systematic review. PLoS One. 2017;12(10):e0186315.
126. Babor T, McRee B, Kassebaum P, Grimaldi P, Ahmed K, Bray J. Screening, brief intervention, and referral to treatment (SBIRT). Subst Abus. 2007;28(3):7–30. https://doi.org/10.1300/J465v28n03_03.
127. Townley C, Dorr H. Integrating substance use disorder treatment and primary care. National Academy for State Health Policy; 2017.
128. Tuckson RV, Edmunds M, Hodgkins ML. Telehealth. N Engl J Med. 2017;377(16):1585–92. https://doi.org/10.1056/NEJMsr1503323.
129. Tofighi B, Abrantes A, Stein MD. The role of technology-based interventions for substance use disorders in primary care: a review of the literature. Med Clin North Am. 2018;102(4):715–31. https://doi.org/10.1016/j.mcna.2018.02.011.
130. Carreiro S, Newcomb M, Leach R, Ostrowski S, Boudreaux ED, Amante D. Current reporting of usability and impact of MHealth interventions for substance use disorder: a systematic review. Drug Alcohol Depend. 2020;215(October):108201. https://doi.org/10.1016/j.drugalcdep.2020.108201.
131. Gonzales R, Ang A, Murphy DA, Glik DC, Douglas Anglin M. Substance use recovery outcomes among a cohort of youth participating in a mobile based texting aftercare pilot program. J Subst Abus Treat. 2014;47(1):20–6. https://doi.org/10.1016/j.jsat.2014.01.010.
132. Ondersma SJ, Ellis JD, Resko SM, Grekin E. Technology-delivered interventions for substance use among adolescents. Pediatr Clin N Am. 2019;66(6):1203–15. https://doi.org/10.1016/j.pcl.2019.08.009.
133. McDonnell A, MacNeill C, Chapman B, Gilbertson N, Reinhardt M, Carreiro S. Leveraging digital tools to support recovery from substance use disorder during the COVID-19 pandemic response. J Subst Abus Treat. 2021;124:108226. https://doi.org/10.1016/j.jsat.2020.108226.
134. Lin L(A), Casteel D, Shigekawa E, Weyrich MS, Roby DH, McMenamin SB. Telemedicine-delivered treatment interventions for substance use disorders: a systematic review. J Subst Abus Treat. 2019;101(June):38–49. https://doi.org/10.1016/j.jsat.2019.03.007.
135. Lister JJ, Weaver A, Ellis JD, Himle JA, Ledgerwood DM. A systematic review of rural-specific barriers to medication treatment for opioid use disorder in the United States. Am J Drug Alcohol Abuse. 2020;46(3):273–88. https://doi.org/10.1080/00952990.2019.1694536.
136. Rodriguez JA, Betancourt JR, Sequist TD, Ganguli I. Differences in the use of telephone and video telemedicine visits during the COVID-19 pandemic. Am J Manag Care. 2021;27(1):21–6. https://doi.org/10.37765/ajmc.2021.88573.
137. Text—S.524—114th Congress (2015–2016): comprehensive addiction and recovery act of 2016. Congress.gov, Library of Congress; 22 July 2016, https://www.congress.gov/bill/114th-congress/senate-bill/524/text.
138. Practice guidelines for the administration of buprenorphine for treating opioid use disorder, 21 U.S.C. 823(g)(2)(H)(i)(II). (2021). https://www.govinfo.gov/content/pkg/FR-2021-04-28/pdf/2021-08961.pdf.
139. https://www.pewtrusts.org/en/research-and-analysis/articles/2022/12/30/president-signs-bipartisan-measure-toimprove-addiction-treatment.
140. Center for Behavioral Health Statistics and Quality. Results from the 2015 National Survey on drug use and health: detailed tables. Rockville, MD: Substance Abuse and Mental Health Services Administration; 2016.
141. Lipari RN, Hedden SL, Hughes A. Substance use and mental health estimates from the 2013 National Survey on drug use and health: overview of findings. 2014 Sep 4. In: The CBHSQ Report. Rockville, MD: Substance Abuse and Mental Health Services Administration (US); 2013. https://www.ncbi.nlm.nih.gov/books/NBK385055/.
142. Knight JR, Sherritt L, Shrier LA, Harris SK, Chang G. Validity of the CRAFFT substance abuse screening test among adolescent clinic patients. Arch Pediatr Adolesc Med. 2002;156(6):607–14. https://doi.org/10.1001/archpedi.156.6.607.
143. Hawk M, Coulter RWS, Egan JE, et al. Harm reduction principles for healthcare settings. Harm Reduct J. 2017;14:70. https://doi.org/10.1186/s12954-017-0196-4.
144. Schuckit MA. Treatment of opioid-use disorders. N Engl J Med. 2016;375(4):357–68. https://doi.org/10.1056/NEJMra1604339.
145. Agency for Healthcare Research and Quality. Pharmacotherapy for adults with alcohol-use disorders in outpatient settings; executive summary; 2014. http://effectivehealthcare.ahrq.gov/index.cfm/search-for-guides-reviews-and-reports/?pageaction=displayproduct&productid=1907 Accessed 18 Jan 2017.
146. About the ASAM criteria [Internet]. American Society of Addiction Medicine. [cited 2022 Mar 7]. https://www.asam.org/asam-criteria/about-the-asam-criteria
147. Bronfenbrenner U. The ecology of human development: experiments by nature and design. Harvard University Press; 1979.

Part II
Family, Social, and Community Support

Family and Other Caregivers

Alexandra Targan and Caroline Collins Roberts

Introduction

An informal caregiver is a friend or relative who provides unpaid assistance to a person with a chronic or disabling condition [1]. Caregivers are needed for individuals who have a chronic condition, trauma, or illness which limits their ability to carry out basic self-care tasks such as bathing, toileting, dressing, and eating, known as *activities of daily living* (ADLs), or chores, meal preparation, household cleaning, and money management, known as *instrumental activities of daily living* (IADLs).

Demographics of Caregivers

In 2020, more than 1 in 5 Americans identify themselves as caregivers, having provided care to an adult or child with special needs at some time in the past 12 months, which is a 3% increase since 2015. This increase is due to the aging baby boomer population, shortages in the health or long-term formal care systems, increasing state and federal efforts to facilitate home- and community-based services, and an increased rate of self-identification as caregivers by Americans. As people age and live longer, the US population's collective health status is more complex with more chronic medical conditions, calling upon unpaid caregiving to provide the backbone of in-home, community, and long-term care to the many recipients of that care [2].

The Olmstead Decision by the US Supreme Court (July 1999) guaranteed the right of individuals to receive care in the community, as opposed to an institution, whenever possible, leading to the increased availability and utilization of community-based services. Two out of three (66%) older adults with disabilities who receive long-term care at home get their caregiving needs met exclusively from an informal caregiver, while another quarter (26%) receive some combination of informal care and paid help; only 9% receive paid caregiving help exclusively [3]. Among the older adult population who require assistance for tasks due to multiple functional limitations, 80% live in private homes in the community, not in institutions [4].

Most adults who identify as caregivers are caring for a relative, with 50% of adult care recipients being a parent or parent-in-law, 12% being a spouse or partner, 8% being a grandparent or grandparent-in-law, and 6% being an adult child. The remaining group of caregivers (around 10%) provide care to a neighbor or a friend. Older caregivers tend to take care of similar-aged recipients, with 74% of caregivers aged 75 years and older also caring for a recipient aged 75 years or older. Caregivers in the US are a diverse population, spanning all genders, ages, races and cultures, socioeconomic statuses, educational levels, family makeup, gender identities, and sexual orientations. The average age of caregivers is 49 years old, with a median age of 51. Three in five caregivers are women and two in five are men. Sixty-one percent of caregivers report being non-Hispanic white, 17% are Hispanic or Latino, 14% African American or black, and 5% Asian American and Pacific Islander [2].

The needs of care recipients are increasingly complex as care recipients age and technology improves, resulting in a greater number of comorbid conditions in individuals. The three most common conditions requiring caregiving, in order of frequency, are (1) physical conditions, (2) memory problems and dementia, and (3) emotional or mental health issues [2].

The informal caregiver is essential in sustaining healthcare delivery in community-based long-term care (LTC) settings, such as Program for All-Inclusive Care (PACE), which provides comprehensive medical and social services to older adults still living in the community, most of whom are dually

A. Targan
Department of Family Medicine, University of Michigan,
Ann Arbor, MI, USA
e-mail: ltargan@med.umich.edu; alexandra_targan@med.unc.edu

C. C. Roberts (✉)
Department of Family Medicine, University of North Carolina at Chapel Hill, Chapel Hill, NC, USA
e-mail: caroline_roberts@med.unc.edu

eligible for both Medicare and Medicaid. Improving direct support for family caregivers improves health outcomes and the quality of care the recipient receives and keeps the recipient out of more costly nursing home care.

In 2017, about 41 million family caregivers in the US provided an estimated 34 billion hours of care to an adult with limitations in daily activities [5]. The estimated economic value of their unpaid contributions was approximately $470 billion, more than all out-of-pocket spending on US health care in 2017 ($366 billion) [6].

The Effects of Caregiving

Positive Effects of Caregiving

Though caregiving is often conceptualized as a burden on those providing care, newer research has found benefits of being a caregiver. For example, after a landmark study reported higher mortality rates for spouse caregivers, five subsequent population-based studies showed reduced mortality and extended longevity for caregivers compared to non-caregiving counterparts [7, 8]. This could be explained by overall better health of caregivers compared to non-caregivers that enables them to provide care for another person, or by the great deal of meaning derived from caregiving. Several studies that emphasize negative effects of caregiving do not distinguish the stress of having an ill family member from actually providing care for that person. In contrast, studies on population-based samples using rigorous methods to control for confounding and that distinguish stress from caregiver status often show better health outcomes for caregivers [8]. Additionally, because caregiving can be both psychologically challenging and provide gratification and a sense of purpose simultaneously, measurements of both positive and negative factors should be obtained when assessing the effects of caregiving [8, 9].

Health Consequences of Caregiving

Risk Factors for Caregiver Burden

Caregiver burden is an individual's perception of overload during the caregiving process in one or more of four realms: physical, psychological, social, and financial [10]. Risk factors can be categorized into the types of assistance caregivers are tasked to provide (ADL and IADL related, health management, and health system logistics), caregiver characteristics, and care recipient characteristics. Caregivers are significantly more likely to experience increased burden if they are required to assist with more ADLs (specifically, incontinence and mobility) and IADLs, health management tasks, and health system logistics, all of which have equal potential to increase the risk for caregiver burden. Specific caregiver characteristics associated with increased burden include female sex, being an adult child, self-reported fair or poor health, the need to use respite care, and anxiety symptoms [11, 12]. If the caregiver is retired or has a pension, they are less likely to experience a significant burden [12]. For healthcare recipients, characteristics associated with increased caregiver burden include age over 80 years, aggressive tendencies (especially violence), and dementia, regardless of whether the dementia causes substantial disability [11, 12].

Certain factors place caregivers at risk for psychological health consequences, such as depression, anxiety, and reduced overall well-being. Some of the factors that affect psychological outcomes are the relationship of the caregiver to the recipient, with parents and spouses of care recipients having higher psychological burden. In addition, caregiving intensity, chronicity of disease, living as co-residents, the quality of relationships between caregiver and care receiver, and the caregiver's age and ethnicity (specifically being white and Asian American) are associated with lower levels of life satisfaction and more perceived psychological symptoms. Family caregivers with perceived choices in caregiving reported better psychological well-being than those who felt they did not have a choice [13].

Physical Consequences
Several physical effects of caregiving have been noted. Higher mean levels of inflammatory markers such as interleukin-6 (IL-6) and D-dimer among caregivers for patients with Alzheimer's dementia are reported which could increase the risk of cardiovascular disease in the caregiver, though age may be a confounder [14]. Caregiving strain is significantly associated with higher estimated stroke risk with greatest effects for men, particularly African American men providing caregiving to their wives [15]. Other physical effects of caregiving include higher rates of insomnia and depression, lower likelihood of engaging in preventive care, and subjective sense of worsening health [7, 8, 16, 17]. However, these physical effects are not often distinguished between caregivers and people with an ill family member regardless or if they are providing the care themselves. While increased mortality for caregiving spouses is reported, other population-based studies show significantly lower mortality among caregivers [7, 8]. Most caregivers (55%) do not see their caregiving role as a detriment to their own health [2].

Psychological Consequences
Caregiving is often cited as a chronic stress experience. Caregiving creates longitudinal strain due to unpredictable and uncontrollable situations, requires high level of vigilance, and creates secondary stress in social domains such as work and family relationships [18]. Informal caregivers are more likely to report symptoms of depression and other indi-

cators of psychological distress than non-caregivers [8]. Those who perceive a higher strain of caregiving report a worse quality of life, more problems with emotional distress, worse physical functioning, and fewer social contacts than non-caregivers [19]. Four in 10 caregivers rate their caregiving situation to be highly stressful with one in four reporting moderate emotional stress, with an emotional stress score of 3 out of 5. One in five caregivers strongly agree or agree with the statement "I Feel Alone," which is associated with feelings of stress and strain [2].

Younger caregivers (less than 65 years old) have a higher propensity toward adverse mental health outcomes, leading to increased rates of binge drinking, heavy drinking, and cigarette smoking [20].

Financial Consequences

About half (45%) of caregivers experience negative financial impact from caregiving [2]. These include (in descending order of frequency) interruption of long-term financial saving, addition of debt, exhaustion of personal short-term savings, delay or inability to pay bills, borrowing money from family or friends, and taking on more work or delaying retirement [2]. Younger caregivers and younger recipients suffer greater financial impact than their older counterparts [2].

In 2015–2016 in the US, an estimated 3.2 million caregivers for people with dementia averaged 1278 h of caregiving per year, totaling more than 4.1 billion hours of care, with an estimated economic value of $41.5 billion [21]. The annual cost of the provision of informal care for patients with dementia was estimated at over $18,000 per patient, due mostly to caregivers' lost earnings [22]. For cardiovascular disease patients, the costs of informal caregiving were estimated to be $61 billion in 2015 and are projected to increase to $128 billion in 2035, with over half of that cost attributed to informal caregiving for patients with stroke [23, 24].

Specific Conditions and Caregiving

There are many shared experiences among informal caregivers, from psychological and physical impacts to financial implication. Some patient conditions can present specific challenges and familiarity with these issues can be helpful in providing caregiver support.

Chronically Ill Children

Caregivers for chronically ill children are at increased risk from physical, psychological, and financial stress related to caregiving. The primary caregivers for chronically ill children are usually parents or legal guardians, but caregiver tasks may fall to the entire extended family [25]. Increased weight of the child and the increased illness acuity of the child (more severe limitations and behavioral issues) are associated with worsening caregiver well-being [26, 27]. Medical advances have improved survival rates in children who are chronically ill and allowed more advanced care at home of young family members with increasingly complex medical conditions [25, 28]. Day-to-day responsibilities are often the most challenging for caregivers, and interventions aimed at reducing these demands are most effective at reducing caregiver burden [27].

Children with multiple interacting primary and co-morbid diagnoses and functional limitations are particularly stressful for caregivers [24]. These children require medical assistive devices, such as feeding tubes and ventilators, and ongoing acute, rehabilitation, and community health services [25]. Both the children and the caregivers prefer care in the home, which is associated with reduced stress and improved well-being [29, 25]. Effective care in the home includes structured programs which provide coordinated, comprehensive, and family-centered care including respite services, peer support, financial aid, and medical home technologies. Caregivers are better able to cope with caregiving duties when provided breaks in daily demands via respite care and assistive technology. They also benefit from efforts that limit the financial impact on the family and flexible work opportunities. Caregivers have improved mental and physical well-being when provided easy service access by telehealth, case workers, and peer support [25]. Caregivers of children with life-limiting conditions or life-threatening illnesses have higher rates of poor sleep and low back pain, which can improve with peer support, respite care, and professional support for the children's medical needs [26]. Parents caring for children with cancer find that the most difficult part of their caregiving responsibilities is the provision of emotional support to the afflicted child and to other children in the family [30].

Caring for children on the Autism Spectrum Disorder (ASD) poses special challenges, compounded by the stigma associated with the condition. Caregivers' well-being is affected by the children's experience with public stigma (social rejection and loneliness), courtesy stigma (experienced by caregivers), and affiliate stigma (caregiver self-stigmatization based on public stereotypes of both the children and their caregiver), all of which leads to negative thinking and diminished mental health, quality of life, and caregiver well-being. Financial burden compounds these negative effects and leads to social isolation of the caregiver. Public education that reduces stigma toward children with autism, such as Sesame Street's *See Amazing in All Children*, is beneficial to caregivers [31].

Protective factors that reduce the burden of providing care to children with disabilities include support, positive family dynamics, higher socioeconomic status, and access to respite care. Caregiver burden is also less for children who do not suffer from behavioral and sleep difficulties or diminished cognitive and motor skills. Finding positive meaning in the face of adversity, family collaboration in problem solving, positive reappraisal, and adaptive humor styles (self-enhancing and affiliative) are protective strategies to reduce stress [32].

Dementia

Caring for people with dementia can be distressful, especially in the presence of behavioral problems and limited social support to the caregiver. Dementia can require many hours of care depending on severity, averaging 80 hours per week [17]. Physicians and other members of the healthcare team should assess the level of caregiver distress and provide supportive resources, especially since family caregivers play a crucial role in the optimal care of these patients [33]. The accompanying experience for the family starts at diagnosis, at which time the caregivers may feel relief to hear what they already suspected, understand the gravitas of the diagnosis, grieve, process the patient's reaction, and eventually accept the diagnosis and commit to care [34]. Respite care has mixed results to both patient and caregiver, depending on type (daytime, temporary admission, or community-based), with some decrease in caregiver burden and in behavioral/psychological symptoms but also accelerated time to nursing home admission [35]. When the patient does eventually transition to a long-term care facility, caregivers typical feel grief and loneliness, coupled with feelings of relief and the reassurance that their relative or friend will be well cared for and safe [36].

Behavioral and psychological symptoms of dementia are the primary factors associated with caregiver burden and the most frequent reason for institutionalization [37, 38]. Conceptualizing these distressing actions or conduct as an expression of an unmet need rather than a problem behavior is vital to caregiver success in addressing the patient's needs and improving both their and their loved one's care experience [39]. Caregiver education should focus on recognizing and addressing the underlying cause of the behavioral symptoms.

Caregivers for patients with dementia report poorer sleep quality than controls, independent of caregiver age [17]. However, caregivers' subjective sense of poor sleep due to increased nighttime awakenings is not associated with poorer global sleep quality (sleep onset latency, duration, sleep medication use, sleep efficiency, sleep disturbances, and daytime dysfunction sleep efficiency).

The COVID-19 pandemic has elucidated the vital contribution that family caregivers provide in preventing dementia progression for their loved ones given the rapid decline in many people with dementia that occurred in the caregiver's absence [40].

As with other conditions, the caregiver's experience depends on the level of support as well as their own mental health, perceptions, knowledge of the disease, and coping strategies. Caregivers of people with dementia benefit from resources provided by the Alzheimer's Association, among other organizations. Respite care and individual psychosocial interventions are moderately effective in reducing caregiver stress, with group interventions having a modest, though still positive, effect [41]. Specific individual psychosocial interventions include anger management, behavioral activation, and managing disruptive patient behaviors [33]. Though group interventions are less effective than individual interventions, they are often more readily available. The acceptance or rejection of supportive services for caregivers of people with dementia differs by type of service; whereas physical health, mental health, and social/legal/financial resources are readily accepted, support groups are of less interest but become more so as the ability to conduct activities of daily living by the person with dementia declines [42].

Mental Health Disorders

Caring for people with mental health disorders puts caregivers at increased risk of psychological burden [13]. The level of caregiver distress is directly related to the severity of the patient's mental illness, level of functioning, tasks associated with caregiving, and the caregiver's personality traits (such as neuroticism), perceived support, time spent in caregiving, subjective burden, and perceived experience [43]. Caregivers of patients with emotional or mental health issues do not, on average, provide more assistance with activities of daily living (ADLs), but when they do so, they find it especially difficult. It is common for caregivers of patients with mental health disorders to provide more instrumental activities of daily living (IADLs) and caregivers report more difficulty with care coordination and finding affordable care services [2].

Given the influence of the caregiver's personality and subjective experiences on well-being, individualized interventions that support strategies to cope with stress, similar to those used in supporting caregivers of patients with dementia, may be effective [43]. Caregivers of those with mental and emotional health problems rely on technological services to help with caregiving, including using the internet for searches for services, aides, facilities or other help, purchasing medicines and groceries online, watching videos to learn care tasks, creating an online or shared calendar to organize caregiving schedules, using a ride-share service, or connecting with other caregivers [2].

Physical Disabilities

Caring for an adult with a long-term physical disability is common, with 6 out of 10 caregivers reporting this as a reason for providing care. The challenges of caring for a person with long-term disability are associated with psychological burden in the caregiver [2].

Stroke is the leading cause of neurological disability in adults worldwide [44]. Stroke survivors have unique needs and face many limitations, including behavioral, physical, communication, and memory impairments. Strokes are usually unexpected, leaving caregivers unprepared to seek support or adjust to isolation from their social networks, which is made more challenging by the older age of both the stroke survivor and the caregiver. These factors contribute to psychological problems, such as anxiety, and an overall decline in physical health for the caregiver. Caregivers of stroke survivors need education on medication administration, physical care, diet, and safety with transfers. Interventions aimed at individualized educational, social, health, and emotional support needs before hospital discharge improve the quality of life for the caregiver and the quality of care provided [45]. It is not uncommon for caregivers of those with a stroke to describe their role as a "full time job," which results in caregivers restructuring their lives, including their relationships. Specifically, relationships between stroke survivors and the caregiver can be affected, including a lack of intimacy between spouses and frustration between children and parents. This changing relationship dynamic can lead to a sense of loss and emotional challenges for caregivers but can also positively impact communication in the caregiving dyad [46].

There are many novel strategies to support caregivers of people with long-term physical disabilities secondary to neurological disorders, such as amyotrophic lateral sclerosis (ALS) or Parkinson's disease. These include using paid caregivers instead of informal caregivers, psychological support for partners, psychoeducational programs, and assistive home technologies, though none of these have shown widespread success and are not yet incorporated into common care practices [47]. These caregivers find respite care helpful and are likely to use technology for assistance and caregiver support services but have a harder time finding affordable care services [2].

Environmental strategies reduce caregiver burden for those caring for people with disabilities, including modifying the home and physical objects, simplifying task performance, and introducing assistive devices. Home occupational and physical therapists play an important role in preparing caregivers to use assistive devices in the home. Training caregivers to use assistive devices increases safety, reduces caregiver responsibilities, expands ability to manage care, and maximizes functional performance [48]. An excellent resource on assistive devices is available through The Family Caregiver Alliance's website www.caregiver.org (https://www.caregiver.org/resource/assistive-technology/) [49].

Caregiving During the COVID-19 Pandemic

The COVID-19 pandemic has heightened several shortcomings of healthcare systems worldwide, including the US and Canada's heavy dependence on informal caregivers [40, 50–53]. In long-term care, isolation from family caregivers due to visitor restrictions highlighted caregivers' essential role in preventing negative patient outcomes such as social isolation, decreased quality of life, and disease progression for people living with dementia [50]. In care transitions, such as when a hospitalized patient with COVID-19 returns home, family caregivers depend on reliable guidance from community health workers, social workers, nurses, and primary care physicians in light of ever-changing recommendations during an evolving pandemic [51]. Parents of children both with and without chronic illnesses have demonstrated increased caregiver burden, anxiety, and depression during the COVID-19 pandemic compared to non-parent counterparts [52, 53].

End-of-Life Care

As with caregivers for all conditions, the support available and health of the caregiver affect their experience in caregiving. Caregivers of patients with terminal illnesses who are themselves in poor health report a higher caregiver burden, and caregivers who develop effective coping strategies such as self-confidence and reframing have a better caregiving experience [54]. Not surprisingly, caregiver burden increases as the care recipient's activities of daily living decline and care tasks increase [54, 55]. A caregiver's experience, whether burdensome or beneficial, can impact their perception of the care recipient's end-of-life care [56].

To support family caregivers of patients with end-stage cancer, a CARES model has been proposed, which includes: **C**onsidering caregivers as part of the unit of care; **A**ssessing the caregiver's situation, perceptions, and needs; **R**eferring to appropriate services and resources including palliative care teams, respite care, hospice, social work, psychology, and community resources; **E**ducating about practical aspects of caregiving; and **S**upporting caregivers through bereavement [57].

Caregivers of people dying of cancer can experience "preloss grief," which is severe in 15% of caregivers and associated with depressive symptoms, high caregiver burden, low preparedness for death, inadequate communication about dying, and too much prognostic information, the latter suggesting there is a balance to be struck in the provision of information [58].

Evaluating and Supporting Caregivers

Caregivers as Invisible Patients

Informal caregiving is associated with financial burden, feelings of isolation, decreased emotional and psychological well-being, and physical diminishment. Acting as a caregiver also has positive benefits including personal fulfillment and satisfaction from helping to relieve another's suffering. Family caregivers receive little support and assistance, despite situations which cause mental toil and include physically taxing tasks, supervising patient behavior, and accessing and negotiating healthcare services [1]. Physicians and other members of the healthcare team, including nurses, social workers, and care managers, play a crucial role in assessing caregivers as patients themselves to identify and relieve the negative consequences of caregiving. If caregivers are not supported and sustained, the ability to provide care for patients at home or in the community is negatively impacted. The Family Caregiver Alliance's National Consensus Development Conference for Caregiver Assessment states "A key concern is that the continued reliance on family caregivers, without better recognition of their own support needs, could negatively affect the ability of family caregivers to provide care in the future and result in even greater emotional, physical and financial strain" [1].

To assist with physician assessment, the National Consensus Development Conference for Caregiver Assessment developed a set of guiding principles and practice guidelines which are incorporated into the Guided Care model as key components for chronic care delivery. It approaches issues from the caregiver's perspective and culture, focuses on what assistance the caregiver may need and the outcomes the family member wants for support, and seeks to maintain the caregiver's own health and well-being [1]. Physicians can identify caregivers during primary care or other health visits in which the caregiver accompanies the care recipient. Physicians may refer a caregiver for a formal assessment if the individual self-identifies as a caregiver or as someone providing assistance to a friend or family member. Other opportunities to refer individuals for a formal caregiver assessment include transitions of care (home health appointments or upon hospital discharge), or times where there is a change in functional status of the care recipient [59]. While it is recommended that caregivers be referred for formal assessment if their care recipient has a condition associated with higher levels of burden, such as dementia,

Table 7.1 Key principles of caregiver assessment [1]

Principle 1	Public and private programs should recognize key dimensions of family caregiving, focusing on both the care recipient and caregiver as a unit and part of the care team with services being consumer directed and family focused.
Principle 2	The form, content, and process for caregiver assessment should be tailored based upon the caregiving context, service setting, and program.
Principle 3	The purpose of the caregiver assessment should be clear to both assessor and caregiver. The aims are to: 1. Identify the primary caregiver/informal caregivers 2. Improve caregiver understanding of their role and needed abilities 3. Understand the caregiving situation (service needs, unresolved problems, and potential risks) 4. Identify services available for the caregiver and provide appropriate and timely referral for services. 5. Determine the care recipient's eligibility for services that also help the caregiver.
Principle 4	Assessment findings should be used in care planning and service interventions to guide informed decisions and link caregivers with community services.
Principle 5	Available information technology should be used to share assessment findings and make it easier for the caregiver to access help.

cancer, or stroke, others benefit as well and referral for assessment should be considered for all caregivers, regardless of the condition of the patient. Assessments should occur upon initial identification of a caregiver and as the care recipient's or caregiver's condition changes [59]. The caregiver assessment guidelines established by the National Consensus Development Conference rely on five key principles, laid out in Table 7.1.

Validated tools exist to meet the goals of the Caregiver Assessment guidelines, such as an online toolkit from the Family Caregiver Alliance that helps practitioners assess the needs of family caregivers (Caregivers Count Too!; https://www.caregiver.org/resource/caregivers-count-too-toolkit/) [49]. Several additional well-validated tools exist which specifically address caregiver burden, including the Caregiver Burden Inventory and the Adapted Zarit Interview [59].

Interventions

Two categories of intervention improve caregiver burden: psychosocial and environmental [48]. Psychosocial interventions address the "interior life" of those providing care and reduce emotional and subjective burden. Interventions include psychoeducation, counseling, and skill building in stress reduction and coping techniques [60]. Positive effects of psychosocial interventions are overall positive feelings in caregivers and delayed patient admissions to nursing homes, though this does not occur consistently, and the reduction in caregiver stress or emotional distress can be minimal to moderate. Environmental interventions focus on the ecological models that caregivers need to improve the situation of the individual helped [60]. Environmental strategies include modifying physical objects and the home environment, simplifying task performance, and training in using assistive devices [48].

Social workers are critical in connecting caregivers with local support services. *The National Family Caregiver Support Program (NFCSP)* provides grants to states and territories to fund programs that assist caregivers such as individual counseling, support groups, accessing existing services, and respite care. Caregivers for people with dementia can find resources through professional organizations such as the Alzheimer's Association, local county Departments of Aging, and various books [61, 62]. Education of health professionals such as nurses and social workers to better understand their role in supporting caregivers and the resources available is beneficial to patients and caregivers alike [16].

Public Policy and Caregiving

Increased understanding of public policies and financial reimbursement strategies can improve caregivers' ability to provide optimal care and reduce their own burnout and stress. Public policies related to caregiver support span many arenas, from financial reimbursement to workplace rights and securities, to the provision of information and support. The 2020 AARP Report *Caregiving in the USA* reports that two thirds of caregivers would find an income tax credit helpful, two thirds would find a program to pay caregivers helpful, and more than half feel that a partially paid leave of absence from work would be helpful, especially for those who work more than 30 hours a week [2].

Several policies exist which define caregivers, their scope of responsibilities, and how best to support them. Some of the best-known policies and programs are described in Table 7.2.

Caregivers were first recognized by a federally funded program in 2000 when NFCSP was implemented via the Older Americans Act. NFCSP provides grants to states and territories to support caregivers with information and assistance on available services, individual counseling, organization of support groups, and caregiver training, respite care, and supplemental services [68]. Medicaid is the largest provider of caregiving services and defines a caregiver as family members, friends, or neighbors who provide unpaid assistance to a person with a chronic illness or disabling condition. Caregivers benefit from Medicaid's standard set of benefits, known as Community Alternatives Program for Disabled Adults, which includes home health services, respite services, meal preparation and delivery, and specialized medical supplies. Enrollees can also use Medicaid funding to pay an

Table 7.2 Policies and programs for caregivers

Program/policy	Year of implementation	Description
National Family Caregiver Support Program (NFCSP) [63]	2000	• Allocates resources to provide support services to family caregivers • Administered by state and local agencies on aging
Lifespan Respite Care Act [64]	2006	• Awards $2.5 million annually in grants to states to develop, operate, or supplement services that give respite to caregivers
Program of All-Inclusive Care of the Elderly (PACE) [65]	1990	• Delivers medical and supportive services to individuals 55+ years old with chronic care needs, certified by their state to need nursing home care and able to live safely in the community • Provides adult day care, medical care, home health and personal care, prescription drugs, social services, medical specialties, respite care • Provided by Medicaid and Medicare (for dually eligible individuals)
RAISE Family Caregivers Act [66]	2018	• Tasked US Department of Health and Human Services with establishing a national family caregiving agenda and improving coordination across government programs that assist caregivers and care recipients
Caregiver Advise, Record, Enable (CARE) Act [67]	2014	• Supports better communication between healthcare professionals and family caregivers in providing complex care at home • Requires that hospitals identify a family caregiver upon and during admission to a hospital, records the caregiver's name and contact information in the health record, and provides notice about discharge timing, consultation, and discusses caregiver role in discharge plan • Individual state specific adaptation of CARE Act law • As of Dec 2020, 40 states and territories have enacted CARE Act law
Family and Medical Leave Act (FMLA) [64]	1993	• Allows employees of public employers and those with private employees with at least 50 employees to take unpaid leave for a minimum of 12 weeks for family and personal medical reasons without risking job loss.

(continued)

Table 7.2 (continued)

Program/policy	Year of implementation	Description
National Alliance for Caregiving [63]	1996	• Conducts Family Caregiving in the US national survey in conjunction with AARP
Home and Community Based Service (HCBS) [64]	2012	• Provides for the coverage of some respite care • Offered via Medicaid and US Department of Veterans Affairs
Community Alternatives Program for Disabled Adults (CAP) [64]	2005	• Allows states to establish self-directed care programs that permit family members to be hired as paid caregivers

informal caregiver. The challenge in these programs and policies is the fact that they are state regulated, meaning there is inconsistency across the states including variation in the definitions of caregivers and "serious medical condition," and the presence or absence of waivers. Medicaid expansion improves access to care, health, and finances in the general population and is associated with overall improved mental well-being in caregivers [69]. Another limitation of current policies is that the focus is usually on the disease or disability of the person receiving care rather than the characteristics and circumstances of the caregiver, limiting support for younger, older, minority, and rural caregivers [70].

Policies addressing workplace issues can support caregivers who continue to work. The Family and Medical Leave Act (FMLA) provides support to many caregivers in the US, yet the scope is limited by FMLA's definition of caregivers as those supporting a "child, spouse, or parent with a serious health condition," while ignoring other relationships (in-laws, grandparents, and friendships) for whom care may be provided [70]. Social disparities may also be exacerbated by FMLA policies, as working women, Latinos, low-wage workers, and less-educated employees are less likely to have access to FMLA or paid sick leave and family leave [71]. Like Medicaid, FMLA is regulated on a state level, allowing for inconsistencies in definitions of caregivers and eligible medical conditions [70]. Since the COVID-19 pandemic, many employers allow flexible scheduling and telecommuting, both of which can be helpful to caregivers.

Cultural Aspects of Caregiving

Acting as a caregiver affects health and well-being and is often underrecognized. These challenges can be exacerbated for caregivers and patients who belong to underrepresented and minority groups, highlighting the importance of being cognizant of the cultural aspects of caregiving and closing racial and other health disparities. As the demographics of the growing population of older adults in the US diversifies, knowledge of cultural influences on caregiving is essential.

According to the 2020 report *Caregiving in the US*, white and Asian American caregivers more often report that caregiving has a negative effect on their health as compared to Latinx caregivers [2]. Asian American caregivers report higher levels of emotional stress than African American or Latinx caregivers. Latinx caregivers report absence of a reliable source for help or information, more than African American or Asian American caregivers, suggesting that Latinx caregivers may rely less on health professionals. African American caregivers experience increased negative impact on financial status due to caregiving responsibilities, compared to other racial groups, though this disparity is limited to those with incomes over $50,000 and is eliminated in households with lower incomes. Latinx and African American caregivers provide more hours of care and higher intensity care than other groups, while reporting more positive psychological outcomes, such as having a greater sense of purpose and being less emotionally stressed [2]. These positive perceptions persist even in high-burden caregiving situations (such as dementia) or when corrected for lower income, education, and socioeconomic status [72].

A common experience of immigrant caregivers is generational reciprocity, in which first-generation immigrants have the same filial values, expectations, and obligations as their country of origin, while second- or later-generation caregivers born in the US are challenged by their acculturation into American society. First-generation caregivers who are grounded in the cultural values and norms of their native country experience lower burden, although they may face challenges given limited English language abilities or limited knowledge of available services. Social disparities also exist for first-generation caregivers as they are more likely to work in an unsupportive workplace culture with supervisors who may be less accommodating, causing the caregiver to leave their work position. Challenges for the older first-generation immigrant care recipient include lack of a retirement pension or other financial resources [73, 74]. Black and Latinx caregivers of foreign-born care recipients report a higher caregiver burden but better psychological well-being and self-rated health overall. For all caregivers of foreign-born care recipients, a healthy relationship with the care recipient is associated with less burden and better caregiver emotional and self-rated health [74].

Chronically ill people who identify as lesbian, gay, bisexual, transgender, or queer (LGBTQ+) are more likely to rely on close friends (commonly referred to as their chosen family) as caregivers rather than their biological family. Without written protections in place, the chosen family may not be legally recognized, and their role could be contested by a biological family member [75]. The US Supreme Court's landmark decision in Obergefill v. Hodges has advanced LGBTQ+ rights by allowing same-sex couples the federally recognized right to legally marry, though many patients and caregivers who identify as LGBTQ+ face legal and financial hurdles. LGBTQ+ caregivers can feel isolated, experience discrimination in the workplace, and experience financial strain [2].

LGBTQ+ patients and their caregivers experiencing chronic disease, such as cancer, benefit from inclusive and effective provider communication, clarifying the patient's choice of family, and the consideration of spiritual needs [76]. Collecting Sexual Orientation and Gender Identity (SOGI) information is key in providing holistic care and doing so in a safe and comfortable space results in greater comfort level, higher overall healthcare satisfaction rates, improved patient-caregiver-provider alignment, improved well-being, and enhanced quality of care for the LGBTQ+ patients and their caregivers. Organizations like LGBT HealthLink, National Center for Lesbian Rights, Transgender Law Center, Lambda Legal, and the National LGBT Cancer Network have raised awareness of best practices for the provision of care for the LGBTQ+ community.

Future Directions

Electronic and digital resources assist caregivers and are widely used [2]. These technologies connect caregivers to transportation resources, health records, improved methods of family coordination and communication, medication management, remote monitoring, and telehealth [2, 59, 77, 78]. Ongoing studies are assessing the utility of free smartphone applications and other technologies such as wearable devices in assisting caregivers, some of which have proven effective at reducing caregiver stress [79, 80, 81]. These technological advances can benefit patients, caregivers, and providers.

References

1. Family Caregiver Alliance. Caregiver assessment: principles, guidelines and strategies for change. Report from a national consensus development conference. Vol. 1. San Francisco, CA: Family Caregiver Alliance [Internet]; 2006. http://www.caregiver.org/caregiver/jsp/content/pdfs/v1_consensus.pdf [cited 2021 Nov 16]. https://www.caregiver.org/uploads/legacy/pdfs/v1_consensus.pdf
2. AARP, National Alliance for Caregiving. Caregiving in the U.S. 2020. Washington, DC: AARP; 2020.
3. Doty P. The evolving balance of formal and informal, institutional and non-institutional long-term care for older Americans: a thirty-year perspective. Public Policy Aging Report. 2010;20(1):3–9.
4. Congressional Budget Office. Rising demand for long-term services and supports for elderly people; 2013.
5. Reinhard SC, Feinberg LF, Houser A, Choula R, Evans M. Valuing the invaluable: 2019 update: charting a path forward. Washington, DC: AARP; 2019.
6. Centers for Medicare and Medicaid Services. NHE Fact Sheet [Internet]. National Health Expenditure Fact Sheet. 2021 [cited 2022 Jan 10]. https://www.cms.gov/research-statistics-data-and-systems/statistics-trends-and-reports/nationalhealthexpenddata/nhe-fact-sheet
7. Schulz R, Beach SR. Caregiving as a risk factor for mortality: the caregiver health effects study. JAMA. 1999;282(23):2215–9.
8. Roth DL, Fredman L, Haley WE. Informal caregiving and its impact on health: a reappraisal from population-based studies. Gerontologist. 2015;55(2):309–19.
9. Beach SR, Schulz R, Yee JL, Jackson S. Negative and positive health effects of caring for a disabled spouse: longitudinal findings from the caregiver health effects study. Psychol Aging. 2000;15(2):259–71.
10. Chou KR. Caregiver burden: a concept analysis. J Pediatr Nurs. 2000;15(6):398–407.
11. Riffin C, Van Ness PH, Wolff JL, Fried T. Multifactorial examination of caregiver burden in a national sample of family and unpaid caregivers. J Am Geriatr Soc. 2019;67(2):277–83.
12. Rodríguez-González A-M, Rodríguez-Míguez E, Claveria A. Determinants of caregiving burden among informal caregivers of adult care recipients with chronic illness. J Clin Nurs. 2021;30(9-10):1335–46.
13. Li L, Lee Y. Caregiving choice and caregiver-receiver relation: effects on psychological well-being of family caregivers in Canada. Can J Aging. 2020;39(4):634–46.
14. von Känel R, Dimsdale JE, Mills PJ, Ancoli-Israel S, Patterson TL, Mausbach BT, et al. Effect of Alzheimer caregiving stress and age on frailty markers interleukin-6, C-reactive protein, and D-dimer. J Gerontol A Biol Sci Med Sci. 2006;61(9):963–9.
15. Haley WE, Roth DL, Howard G, Safford MM. Caregiving strain and estimated risk for stroke and coronary heart disease among spouse caregivers: differential effects by race and sex. Stroke. 2010;41(2):331–6.
16. Kelly K, Reinhard SC, Brooks-Danso A. Professional partners supporting family caregivers. Am J Nurs. 2008;108(9 Suppl):6–12.
17. Simpson C, Carter P. Dementia behavioural and psychiatric symptoms: effect on caregiver's sleep. J Clin Nurs. 2013;22(21-22):3042–52.
18. Schulz R, Sherwood PR. Physical and mental health effects of family caregiving. Am J Nurs 2008;108(9 Suppl):23–7; quiz 27.
19. Roth DL, Perkins M, Wadley VG, Temple EM, Haley WE. Family caregiving and emotional strain: associations with quality of life in a large national sample of middle-aged and older adults. Qual Life Res. 2009;18(6):679–88.
20. Grenard DL, Valencia EJ, Brown JA, Winer RL, Littman AJ. Impact of caregiving during emerging adulthood on frequent mental distress, smoking, and drinking behaviors: United States, 2015-2017. Am J Public Health. 2020;110(12):1853–60.
21. Rabarison KM, Bouldin ED, Bish CL, McGuire LC, Taylor CA, Greenlund KJ. The economic value of informal caregiving for persons with dementia: results from 38 states, the District of Columbia, and Puerto Rico, 2015 and 2016 BRFSS. Am J Public Health. 2018;108(10):1370–7.
22. Moore MJ, Zhu CW, Clipp EC. Informal costs of dementia care: estimates from the National Longitudinal Caregiver Study. J Gerontol B Psychol Sci Soc Sci. 2001;56(4):S219–28.
23. Dunbar SB, Khavjou OA, Bakas T, Hunt G, Kirch RA, Leib AR, et al. Projected costs of informal caregiving for cardiovascular disease: 2015 to 2035: a policy statement from the American Heart Association. Circulation. 2018;137(19):e558–77.
24. Joo H, Dunet DO, Fang J, Wang G. Cost of informal caregiving associated with stroke among the elderly in the United States. Neurology. 2014;83(20):1831–7.

25. Edelstein H, Schippke J, Sheffe S, Kingsnorth S. Children with medical complexity: a scoping review of interventions to support caregiver stress. Child Care Health Dev. 2017;43(3):323–33.
26. Hartley J, Bluebond-Langner M, Candy B, Downie J, Henderson EM. The physical health of caregivers of children with life-limiting conditions: a systematic review. Pediatrics. 2021;148(2)
27. Raina P, O'Donnell M, Rosenbaum P, Brehaut J, Walter SD, Russell D, et al. The health and well-being of caregivers of children with cerebral palsy. Pediatrics. 2005;115(6):e626–36.
28. Wightman A. Caregiver burden in pediatric dialysis. Pediatr Nephrol. 2020;35(9):1575–83.
29. Cohen E, Patel H. Responding to the rising number of children living with complex chronic conditions. Can Med Assoc J. 2014;186(16):1199–200.
30. Svavarsdottir EK. Caring for a child with cancer: a longitudinal perspective. J Adv Nurs. 2005;50(2):153–61.
31. Papadopoulos C, Lodder A, Constantinou G, Randhawa G. Systematic review of the relationship between autism stigma and informal caregiver mental health. J Autism Dev Disord. 2019;49(4):1665–85.
32. Fritz HL. Coping with caregiving: humor styles and health outcomes among parents of children with disabilities. Res Dev Disabil. 2020;104:103700.
33. Haley WE. The family caregiver's role in Alzheimer's disease. Neurology. 1997;48(5 Suppl 6):S25–9.
34. Champlin BE. The informal caregiver's lived experience of being present with a patient who receives a diagnosis of dementia: a phenomenological inquiry. Dementia. 2020;19(2):375–96.
35. Vandepitte S, Van Den Noortgate N, Putman K, Verhaeghe S, Verdonck C, Annemans L. Effectiveness of respite care in supporting informal caregivers of persons with dementia: a systematic review. Int J Geriatr Psychiatry. 2016;31(12):1277–88.
36. Crawford K, Digby R, Bloomer M, Tan H, Williams A. Transitioning from caregiver to visitor in a long-term care facility: the experience of caregivers of people with dementia. Aging Ment Health. 2015;19(8):739–46.
37. Chiao CY, Wu HS, Hsiao CY. Caregiver burden for informal caregivers of patients with dementia: a systematic review. Int Nurs Rev. 2015;62(3):340–50.
38. Afram B, Stephan A, Verbeek H, Bleijlevens MHC, Suhonen R, Sutcliffe C, et al. Reasons for institutionalization of people with dementia: informal caregiver reports from 8 European countries. J Am Med Dir Assoc. 2014;15(2):108–16.
39. Song J-A, Park M, Park J, Cheon HJ, Lee M. Patient and caregiver interplay in behavioral and psychological symptoms of dementia: family caregiver's experience. Clin Nurs Res. 2018;27(1):12–34.
40. Borges-Machado F, Barros D, Ribeiro Ó, Carvalho J. The effects of COVID-19 home confinement in dementia care: physical and cognitive decline, severe neuropsychiatric symptoms and increased caregiving burden. Am J Alzheimers Dis Other Dement. 2020;35:1533317520976720.
41. Knight BG, Lutzky SM, Macofsky-Urban F. A meta-analytic review of interventions for caregiver distress: recommendations for future research. Gerontologist. 1993;33(2):240–8.
42. Zwingmann I, Dreier-Wolfgramm A, Esser A, Wucherer D, Thyrian JR, Eichler T, et al. Why do family dementia caregivers reject caregiver support services? Analyzing types of rejection and associated health-impairments in a cluster-randomized controlled intervention trial. BMC Health Serv Res. 2020;20(1):121.
43. Hegde A, Chakrabarti S, Grover S. Caregiver distress in schizophrenia and mood disorders: the role of illness-related stressors and caregiver-related factors. Nord J Psychiatry. 2019;73(1):64–72.
44. Katan M, Luft A. Global burden of stroke. Semin Neurol. 2018;38(2):208–11.
45. Camak DJ. Addressing the burden of stroke caregivers: a literature review. J Clin Nurs. 2015;24(17–18):2376–82.
46. Kokorelias KM, Lu FKT, Santos JR, Xu Y, Leung R, Cameron JI. Caregiving is a full-time job "impacting stroke caregivers" health and well-being: a qualitative meta-synthesis. Health Soc Care Community. 2020;28(2):325–40.
47. Schischlevskij P, Cordts I, Günther R, Stolte B, Zeller D, Schröter C, et al. Informal caregiving in amyotrophic lateral sclerosis (ALS): a high caregiver burden and drastic consequences on caregivers' lives. Brain Sci. 2021;11(6)
48. Chen T-Y(A), Mann WC, Tomita M, Nochajski S. Caregiver involvement in the use of assistive devices by frail older persons. The. Occup Ther J Res. 2000 Jul;20(3):179–99.
49. National Center on Caregiving. Family caregiver alliance [Internet]. Family caregiver alliance. [cited 2021 Nov 16]. http://www.caregiver.org
50. Hindmarch W, McGhan G, Flemons K, McCaughey D. COVID-19 and long-term care: the essential role of family caregivers. Can Geriatr J. 2021;24(3):195–9.
51. Naylor MD, Hirschman KB, McCauley K. Meeting the transitional care needs of older adults with COVID-19. J Aging Soc Policy. 2020;32(4-5):387–95.
52. Russell BS, Hutchison M, Tambling R, Tomkunas AJ, Horton AL. Initial challenges of caregiving during COVID-19: caregiver burden, mental health, and the parent-child relationship. Child Psychiatry Hum Dev. 2020;51(5):671–82.
53. Dhiman S, Sahu PK, Reed WR, Ganesh GS, Goyal RK, Jain S. Impact of COVID-19 outbreak on mental health and perceived strain among caregivers tending children with special needs. Res Dev Disabil. 2020;107:103790.
54. Joanna Briggs Institute. Caregiver burden of terminally-ill adults in the home setting. Nurs Health Sci. 2012;14(4):435–7.
55. Riffin C, Van Ness PH, Wolff JL, Fried T. Family and other unpaid caregivers and older adults with and without dementia and disability. J Am Geriatr Soc. 2017;65(8):1821–8.
56. Luth EA, Pristavec T. Do caregiver experiences shape end-of-life care perceptions? Burden, benefits, and care quality assessment. J Pain Symptom Manag. 2020;59(1):77–85.
57. Alam S, Hannon B, Zimmermann C. Palliative care for family caregivers. J Clin Oncol. 2020;38(9):926–36.
58. Nielsen MK, Neergaard MA, Jensen AB, Vedsted P, Bro F, Guldin M-B. Preloss grief in family caregivers during end-of-life cancer care: a nationwide population-based cohort study. Psychooncology. 2017;26(12):2048–56.
59. Swartz K, Collins LG. Caregiver Care. Am Fam Physician. 2011;99(11):699–706.
60. Gitlin LN, Corcoran MA. Managing dementia at home. Top Geriatr Rehabil. 1996;12(2):28–39.
61. Sloane P, editor. Alzheimer's medical advisor: a caregiver's guide to common medical and behavioral signs and symptoms in persons with dementia. Illustrated. Sunrise River Press; 2017.
62. Mace NL, Rabins PV. The 36-hour day: a family guide to caring for people who have Alzheimer disease and other dementias (a Johns Hopkins press health book). 7th ed. Johns Hopkins University Press; 2021.
63. Historical overview. Am J Nurs. 2008;108(9):22.
64. Lipson DJ. The policy and political environment of family caregiving. Family caregiving in the new normal. Elsevier; 2015. p. 137–51.
65. National PACE Association. The history of PACE [internet]. National PACE Association; 2022. [cited 2022 Jan 12]. https://www.npaonline.org/policy-advocacy/value-pace
66. AARP. RAISE act promises Federal Help for family caregivers. American Association of Retired Persons (AARP): Politics & Society Advocacy; 2021.
67. Reinhard SC, Young H, Choula RB, Ryan E. The CARE Act implementation: progress and promise [Internet]. AARP Public Policy Institute; 2019. [cited 2022 Jan 12]. Available from:

https://www.aarp.org/content/dam/aarp/ppi/2019/03/the-care-act-implementation-progress-and-promise.pdf
68. U.S. Department of Health and Human Services, Administration for Community Living. National Family Caregiver Support Program | ACL Administration for Community Living [Internet]. https://acl.gov/programs/support-caregivers/national-family-caregiver-support-program. 2021 [cited 2021 Nov 17]. https://acl.gov/programs/support-caregivers/national-family-caregiver-support-program
69. Torres ME, Capistrant BD, Karpman H. The effect of Medicaid expansion on caregiver's quality of life. Soc Work Public Health. 2020;35(6):473–82.
70. Raj M, Singer PM. Redefining caregiving as an imperative for supporting caregivers: challenges and opportunities. J Gen Intern Med. 2021;36:3844–6.
71. Chen M-L. The growing costs and burden of family caregiving of older adults: a review of paid sick leave and family leave policies. Gerontologist. 2016;56(3):391–6.
72. Liu C, Badana ANS, Burgdorf J, Fabius CD, Roth DL, Haley WE. Systematic review and meta-analysis of racial and ethnic differences in dementia caregivers' well-being. Gerontologist. 2021;61(5):e228–43.
73. Lahaie C, Earle A, Heymann J. An uneven burden. Res Aging. 2013;35(3):243–74.
74. Moon HE, Haley WE, Rote SM, Sears JS. Caregiver well-being and burden: variations by race/ethnicity and care recipient nativity status. Innov. Aging. 2020;4(6):igaa045.
75. Metlife Mature Market Institute®2. The lesbian and gay aging issues ne. Out and aging: the metlife study of lesbian and gay baby boomers. J GLBT Fam Stud. 2010;6(1):40–57.
76. Cloyes KG, Hull W, Davis A. Palliative and end-of-life care for lesbian, gay, bisexual, and transgender (LGBT) cancer patients and their caregivers. Semin Oncol Nurs. 2018;34(1):60–71.
77. Yellowlees P, Nesbitt T, Cole S. Telemedicine: the use of information technology to support rural caregiving. In: Talley RC, Chwalisz K, Buckwalter KC, editors. Rural caregiving in the United States. New York, NY, Springer New York; 2011. p. 161–77.
78. Catalyzing technology to support family caregiving.
79. Lucero RJ, Jaime-Lara R, Cortes YI, Kearney J, Granja M, Suero-Tejeda N, et al. Hispanic dementia family caregiver's knowledge, experience, and awareness of self-management: foundations for health information technology interventions. Hisp Health Care Int. 2018;17(2):49–58.
80. Ferré-Grau C, Raigal-Aran L, Lorca-Cabrera J, Ferré-Bergadá M, Lleixà-Fortuño M, Lluch-Canut MT, et al. A multi-centre, randomized, 3-month study to evaluate the efficacy of a smartphone app to increase caregiver's positive mental health. BMC Public Health. 2019;19(1):888.
81. Hu C, Kung S, Rummans TA, Clark MM, Lapid MI. Reducing caregiver stress with internet-based interventions: a systematic review of open-label and randomized controlled trials. J Am Med Inform Assoc. 2015;22(e1):e194–209.

Domestic Violence, Abuse, and Neglect

Samantha Schilling and Adam Zolotor

Introduction

The Centers for Disease Control and Prevention defines intimate partner violence (IPV) as "physical violence, sexual violence, stalking, and psychological aggression (including coercive tactics) by a current or former intimate partner (i.e., spouse, boyfriend/girlfriend, dating partner, or ongoing sexual partner)" [1]. Specifically, physical violence is defined as the intentional use of physical force with the potential for causing death, disability, injury, or harm and includes scratching, pushing, shoving, throwing, grabbing, biting, choking, shaking, hair-pulling, slapping, punching, hitting, burning, use of a weapon (gun, knife, or other object), and use of restraints or one's body, size, or strength against another person. Sexual violence is defined as a sexual act that is committed or attempted by another person without freely given consent of the victim or against someone who is unable to consent or refuse. Stalking is a pattern of repeated, unwanted attention and contact that causes fear or concern for one's own safety or the safety of someone else (e.g., family member, close friend), and psychological aggression is the use of verbal and non-verbal communication with the intent to harm another person mentally or emotionally, and/or exert control over another person [1].

Over the course of a lifetime, more than one in three women and more than one in four men in the US experience rape, physical violence, and/or stalking by an intimate partner [2]. Approximately one third of homicides of women are committed by intimate partners [3]. Because victims of IPV tend to have high rates of physical and mental health morbidity, they are frequent users of the health care system. IPV is thus a condition that physicians and other providers can expect to encounter frequently in their care settings.

The Child Abuse Prevention and Treatment Act was enacted in 1974, which defines child maltreatment as "any recent act or failure to act on the part of a parent or caretaker, which results in death, serious physical or emotional harm, sexual abuse or exploitation, or an act or failure to act which presents an imminent risk of serious harm" [4]. While federal legislation sets minimum standards for states, each state provides its own definitions of maltreatment within civil and criminal statutes. Each year in the US, Child Protective Service (CPS) agencies receive more than three million reports of suspected child maltreatment and investigate more than two million of these reports; more than 650,000 children are substantiated by child welfare as maltreatment victims [5]. Most maltreated children are victims of neglect (78.5%), 17.6% are victims of physical abuse, and 9.1% are victims of sexual abuse. More than 1500 child deaths are attributed annually to child abuse or neglect.

A substantial body of research indicates that child maltreatment and IPV are public health problems with lifelong health consequences for survivors [6]. A landmark project, the Adverse Childhood Experience study, demonstrated a gradient risk among adults for both health risk behaviors and chronic diseases based on the number of childhood adversities and trauma experienced. For example, those with greater adversity had 4–12 times greater risk, compared to those with less adversity, for alcoholism, drug abuse, and suicide attempt. Similarly, those with greater adversity had higher rates of cancer, heart disease, lung disease, and liver disease compared to those with less adversity [7]. Not all childhood adversities are traumatic events. For example, living with a household member with mental illness may be stressful but not-traumatic. The Centers for Disease Control and Prevention defines trauma as "an event or series of events that causes a moderate or severe stress reaction … characterized by a sense of horror, helplessness, serious injury, or threat of serious injury or death" [8]. People who experience or witness traumatic events may have stress reactions. Most stress reactions resolve in a short period of time, but some people develop post-traumatic stress disorder. Many victims or child maltreatment and IPV will have post-traumatic stress reactions and post-traumatic stress disorder.

At the other end of the life course is elder mistreatment. An expert panel convened by the National Academy of Sciences defines elder maltreatment broadly as the intentional actions that cause harm or create a serious risk of harm (whether or not harm is intended), to a vulnerable elder by a caregiver or other person who stands in a trusted relationship to the elder, or failure by a caregiver to satisfy the elder's basic needs or to protect the elder from harm [9]. Multiple types of elder maltreatment exist, including physical abuse, psychological abuse, sexual assault, neglect, and financial exploitation. Estimates of elder abuse vary between 2% and 10%. In a probability sample of elderly people living in Boston, the overall abuse rate was 3.2% [10]. The extent of elder abuse is sufficiently large that physicians who care for elderly adults are likely to encounter it routinely.

Physicians and other care providers play a key role is identifying and treating maltreatment and family violence, as well as understanding physical and mental health problems in their patients in the context of challenging life events, such as chronic illness. This chapter will first provide general guidelines for clinicians who may encounter IPV, child maltreatment, and elder mistreatment. The next section will outline evaluation approaches for patients who may present for medical care, and will be followed by management strategies. The chapter will close with future trends in this important area.

General Guidelines

Because maltreatment and family violence are widely prevalent, all health care providers will encounter patients who have experienced this trauma. Furthermore, although there are subspecialists with expertise in the evaluation and management of child maltreatment and family violence, the vast majority of identification and treatment occurs by primary care clinicians. The identification of abuse can be difficult for many reasons; abuse is rarely witnessed, disclosure by the perpetrator is uncommon, and victims are often non-verbal, too severely injured, or too frightened to disclose. Furthermore, injuries may be non-specific in the case of physical abuse or absent in the case of sexual abuse.

Intimate Partner Violence (IPV)

Assessing for IPV in the clinical setting can be universal or selective, based on presentation or risk factors. The United States Preventive Services Task Force (USPSTF) recommends screening all women of childbearing age and referring those who screen positive for intervention services [11]. This recommendation is based on evidence that IPV can be accurately detected using currently available screening instruments, that effective interventions can mitigate the adverse health outcomes of IPV, and that screening causes minimal harm [11].

Physicians and other providers should be aware of the clusters of symptoms that are common in victims of IPV. When patients present with signs and symptoms suggestive of IPV (e.g., frequent somatic complaints, unexplained injuries, injuries to the face or trunk, frequent mental health complaints), clinicians should inquire about IPV, not only because intervention may be beneficial, but also because knowledge of IPV may inform the treatment plan or help the clinician understand barriers to treatment. A physician perception of poor adherence to medical recommendations may in fact be associated with the abuse a patient is experiencing, since impeding access to health care may be part of the control that abusers exert in their partners' lives [12]. Physicians who diagnose IPV, and therefore begin to understand the barriers that their abused patients face, may be able to develop more effective therapeutic relationships. Identifying IPV also provides an important opportunity for providing the patient with empathic support; educating them regarding the dynamics of IPV and the future risks it poses to the patient and their children.

Several questionnaires for assessing for IPV have been validated in a variety of settings and are practical in primary care, such as HITS, Woman Abuse Screening Tool (WAST), the Ongoing Violence Assessment Tool (OVAT), and the Partner Violence Screen [13]. Whether a clinician uses a structured instrument or simply asks questions informally in the context of a patient interview, several principles are important to follow. Physicians should ensure a private setting, without friends or family members present. They should assure patients of confidentiality, but notify them of any reporting requirements. It is often helpful to preface questions about IPV with normalizing statements, for example, "Because violence is a common problem, I routinely ask my patients about it," or "Many people with [condition] have worse symptoms if they have been physically, emotionally, or sexually abused in the past."

Child Abuse

Existing instruments designed to screen for social determinants of health often inquire about parental concern for child abuse [14]. Asking a caregiver about abuse is important and underscores the centrality of these problems to child health. A negative response, however, should not preclude an evaluation for abuse if other concerns are identified. Indeed, the best available screen for child abuse at this time remains a high index of suspicion and a thorough physical examination.

Although the maltreatment of children has been recognized for decades, there are ongoing challenges in identifying and ensuring the health and safety of abused and neglected children. There is abundant evidence that physicians often miss opportunities for early intervention of injuries that are concerning for physical abuse [15–17]. Sentinel injuries are minor injuries such as bruises or intraoral injuries that are noted before more severe injuries lead to a diagnosis of child abuse. Such injuries are often identified by physicians, but are incorrectly attributed to accidental trauma or not reported to CPS for investigation despite physician suspicion for abuse [15, 16, 18].

There is considerable variability in the diagnostic evaluation for physical abuse. All children younger than two years of age in whom physical abuse is suspected, for example, require a skeletal survey, the standard tool for detecting occult fractures [19]. However, race and socioeconomic status appear to influence a physician's decision to obtain skeletal surveys when children younger than two years present with skeletal trauma or traumatic brain injury, leading to both the over-reporting and under-reporting of abuse in different populations [20–22].

Variability has also been observed in performing recommended testing for sexually transmitted infections (STIs) and pregnancy, and administering recommended prophylaxis and emergency contraception when adolescents present to pediatric emergency departments following acute sexual abuse [23]. Studies have also shown that many physicians have not been properly trained in anogenital examination of children [24, 25].

Although neglect is by far the most widespread form of child maltreatment and results in significant morbidity and mortality, the focus of public and professional attention is largely on physical and sexual abuse. A greater and ongoing challenge is that neglect is difficult to define. For instance, although a health care provider might view repeated non-adherence to medications as neglect, this may not meet a state's CPS statute for neglect unless harm has resulted from this inaction. Neglect can involve failure to supervise a child resulting in harm or increasing risk of harm. Neglect can also involve failure to provide food, housing, education, medical care, or an emotionally supportive environment. In some states, child neglect statues exclude failure to provide when that failure is due to poverty or inadequate resources. In other states, these statutes are not related to intent, but only to the needs of the child.

Toxic Stress, Child Maltreatment, and IPV

The lifetime consequences of early trauma are substantial and enduring. Researchers have found that most causes of morbidity and mortality, including obesity, heart disease, alcoholism, and drug use, are directly associated with child maltreatment and childhood exposure to IPV [7, 26, 27]. Children need an environment in which a responsive, attentive caregiver meets their basic needs, including nurturance, love, and protection for normal growth and development. In this fundamental caregiver–child relationship, the child also depends on the caregiver to mediate and buffer life's stressors [27]. When stressors are overwhelming, or when caregivers are unable to help children buffer them, significant adversities can challenge the normal development of healthy coping mechanisms, learning, emotional health, and physical health [26, 27].

Stress that is unbuffered and overwhelming leads to potentially maladaptive neuroendocrine changes that impede a child's capacity to protect themselves from threats that are experienced and perceived in their world. When a child faces profound and chronic adversity such as abuse, neglect, and household IPV, significant biologic changes can occur. Excessive activation of the physiologic stress response system can lead to changes to: hypothalamic–pituitary–adrenal gland axis activation; epigenetic gene translation; altered immune response; and impaired neurodevelopment involving brain structures responsible for cognition, rational thought, emotional regulation, activity level, attention, impulse control, and executive function [27]. These biological processes manifest in specific behavioral, learning, and health problems which are seen in many children who have been maltreated or exposed to IPV. Adverse childhood experiences are closely link conceptually and empirically with toxic stress [28].

In the health care setting, physicians and other providers may address some of the changes in bodily function associated with trauma's influence on the brain. Sleep problems may include difficulty initiating or maintaining sleep, or experiencing nightmares. Children who have experienced trauma may demonstrate rapid eating, lack of satiety, food hoarding, or loss of appetite. Toileting problems include constipation, encopresis, enuresis, and regression of toileting skills [29]. Neuroendocrine changes can impact the immune and inflammatory response. In addition, an increased risk of infection and rates of asthma and allergy, and an increased risk of metabolic syndrome can all be linked to trauma [30, 31].

There has been increasing interest in screening for adverse childhood experiences since screening identifies a large percentage of children who experience one or more adversities [32]. What remains less clear is the right type of intervention to ameliorate the impact of these adversities. Some experts have, for example, advocated for focusing on prevention rather than screening for adversities that have already occurred. Another approach is to screen for unmet social care needs or social determinants of health, such as transportation challenges, food or housing insecurity, or barriers to medical care [33]. Increasingly, health care systems, providers, and insurers seek to find ways to help people get services to address these unmet needs as a path to improved outcomes and lower costs. Social determinants of health are a concept closely aligned with adverse childhood experiences, and typically include experiences of violence. It is important that screening for adverse events or social determinants be undertaken only when there are evidence-informed interventions available to the family [34, 35].

Elder Mistreatment

There are no validated instruments for the screening or evaluation of elder mistreatment. Clues about potential mistreatment frequently come from ancillary staff members or home care nurses who observe the abuser–victim dyad away from the health care provider [36]. A general sense that something is concerning in the patient's environment such as an abrasive interaction between the elder and the caregiver, poor hygiene, frequently missed medical appointments, or failure to adhere with a clearly designated treatment strategy can all be important indicators.

There are no diagnostic signs or symptoms of elder abuse and clinicians need to consider elder mistreatment in the differential of many clinical presentations they encounter. Significant injuries and severe neglect are obvious, but many prevalent chronic diseases that afflict the elderly also have clinical manifestations of abuse and vice versa. For instance, fractures may result from osteoporosis or physical abuse. Malnutrition may be the result of progressive malignancy or the withholding of nourishment. Most often, chronic disease and elder abuse co-occur making the identification of elder mistreatment one of the most difficult clinical challenges in geriatric medicine.

Patient Evaluation

Suspected IPV

When IPV is detected in the clinical setting, clinicians should respond in a way that builds trust and sets the stage for an ongoing therapeutic relationship. Key components of an initial interaction should include validation of the patient's concerns, education regarding the dynamics and consequences of IPV, safety assessment, and referral to local resources. A growing body of evidence suggests that a variety of counseling and advocacy interventions are effective at reducing violence and mitigating its negative health effects [37]. IPV is usually a chronic problem that will not be mitigated in one or two visits, but rather addressed overtime [38].

An initial response to a disclosure of IPV should include listening to the patient empathically and non-judgmentally, expressing concern for their health and safety, and affirming a commitment to help them address the problem. Victims of abuse may believe that the abuse is their fault. Health care providers can help counter this belief, reassuring patients that although partner violence is common, it is unacceptable and not the fault of the victim. Clinicians should also convey respect for IPV victims' choices regarding how to respond to the violence. Victims of IPV may have a clearer understanding than their health care providers about what courses of action may result in increased danger. If patients need to move slowly, frequent office visits can be helpful by providing ongoing support and addressing medical problems.

Suspected Child Abuse

Child abuse and neglect result from a complex interaction of child, parent, and environmental factors (Fig. 8.1). Most often multiple factors coexist and are interrelated and increase the child's vulnerability to maltreatment [39]. Even if there is no single factor that overwhelms the caregiver, a combination of several stressors may precipitate an abusive crisis [40].

Individual characteristics that predispose a child to maltreatment include those that make a child more difficult to care for, or may be at odds with parental expectations. Adolescents are more likely than younger children to suffer physical abuse and neglect, however infants and toddlers are particularly vulnerable to severe and fatal maltreatment because of their smaller size and developmental phase [41]. Girls may be at higher risk for sexual abuse, although this may be in part because boys are more likely to delay disclosure of sexual abuse [42]. Children with physical or developmental disabilities, special health care needs, or chronic illnesses may also be at increased risk [43]. Physical aggression, resistance to parental direction, and antisocial behaviors also more commonly characterize maltreated children [44].

Parent characteristics associated with child maltreatment include young age, being a single parent, and low educational achievement [45]. Factors that decrease a parent's ability to cope with stress and increase the potential for maltreatment include low self-esteem, poor impulse control, substance abuse, and mental illness [46]. In addition, parents who were themselves victims of child maltreatment are more likely to have children who are abused or neglected [47]. Parents who maltreat their children are more likely to have unrealistic developmental expectations for child behavior, and to have a negative perception of normal behavior. In addition, parents with punitive parenting styles are more likely to maltreat their children [47].

Poverty and unemployment are also associated with maltreatment [48]. When low-income working parents have

Fig. 8.1 Factors that place a child at risk for maltreatment

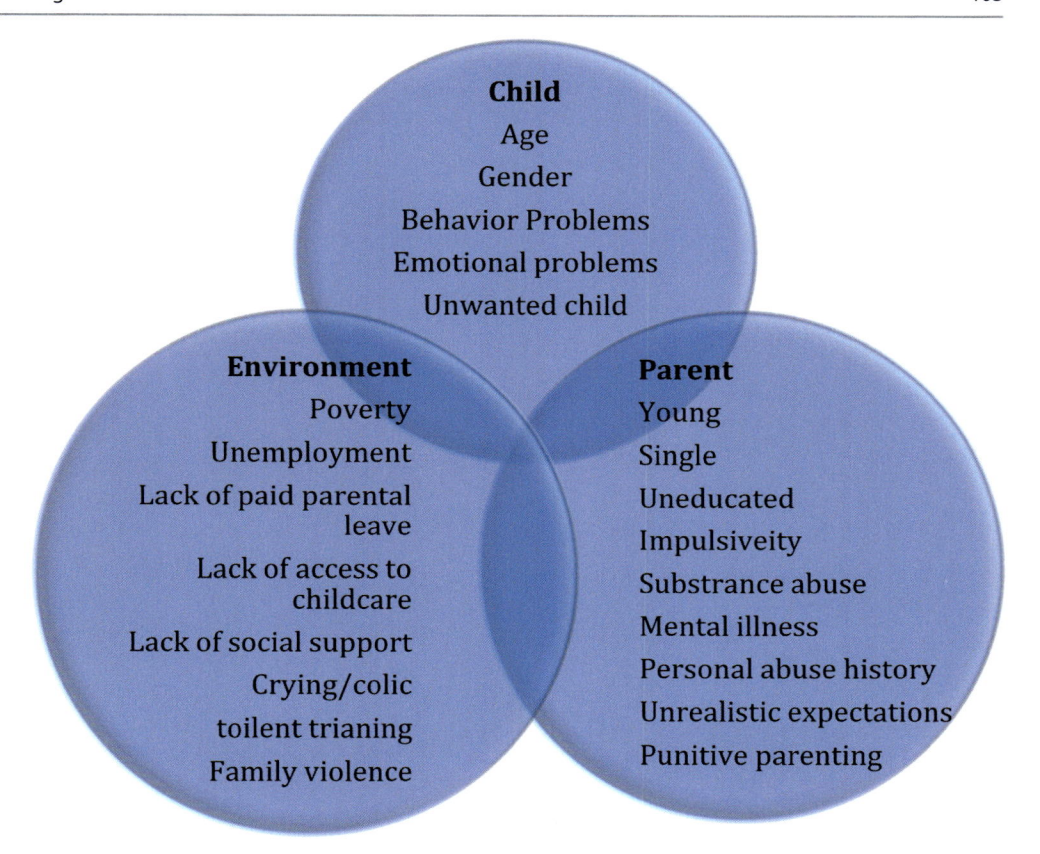

Child
Age
Gender
Behavior Problems
Emotional problems
Unwanted child

Environment
Poverty
Unemployment
Lack of paid parental leave
Lack of access to childcare
Lack of social support
Crying/colic
toilent trianing
Family violence

Parent
Young
Single
Uneducated
Impulsiveity
Substrance abuse
Mental illness
Personal abuse history
Unrealistic expectations
Punitive parenting

challenges accessing affordable and safe childcare, substandard childcare can present an elevated risk for child abuse [49]. The absence of a robust family social support system places the child at increased risk for maltreatment [48]. Young children who live in households with unrelated adults are at exceptionally high risk for abuse [50]. Children living in homes with IPV are at increased risk of being physically abused, in addition to suffering the negative emotional, behavioral, and cognitive consequences from exposure to this family violence [51–53].

High-stress situations can increase the potential for child abuse. Circumstances that occur during the course of normal child development, including colic, nighttime awakenings, and toilet training, are potential triggers for maltreatment [39]. In particular, crying is a common trigger for abusive head trauma [54]. Infant crying generally peaks between two and four months, and the incidence of abusive head trauma parallels this crying trajectory [55]. Accidents surrounding toilet training are another potential trigger. Immersion burns may be inflicted in response to encopresis or enuresis when a caregiver believes that children should be able to control these bodily functions [56]. The average age of children who have been intentionally burned is 32 months, by which time abusive parents may have expected their children to have mastered bodily functions [39].

Physical Abuse

Almost no injury is pathognomonic for abuse or accident without careful consideration of the history, a thorough physical examination, and targeted radiographic or laboratory analysis. When an accidental history is offered by the caregiver, the clinician must consider if the accidental mechanism is a plausible explanation for the identified injury/injuries, and whether the mechanism is consistent with the child's developmental abilities. When abuse is suspected as the cause of an injury, the clinician may conduct tests to screen for other injuries, and to identify potential medical etiologies in the differential diagnosis of abuse. The extent of diagnostic testing depends on several factors, including the severity of the injury, the type of injury, and the age and developmental level of the child. Table 8.1 summarizes tests that may be used during a medical assessment for suspected physical abuse.

Skin Injuries

Bruises are universal in active children. Bruises are also the most common injury resulting from physical abuse, the most easily recognized sign of physical abuse, and the most common direct sign of physical abuse to be missed. For these reasons, it is critical that children's skin be fully examined during medical encounters. Patterned bruises, such as slap marks or

Table 8.1 Laboratory and radiologic testing for the evaluation of suspected physical abuse

Injury	Laboratory Testing	Radiologic Testing
Bruises	CBC PT, INR, PTT VWF antigen, VWF activity Factor VIII level, factor IX level	Skeletal survey for non-ambulatory infants with bruises Skeletal survey for children <2 years with suspicious bruising CT head/MRI head for infants <6 months or infants with suspicious bruising
Fractures	Calcium, phosphorous, ALKP Consider 25OHD, PTH Consider DNA analysis for osteogenesis imperfecta	Skeletal survey CT head/MRI head for infants <6 months
Abdominal injury	AST, ALT	CT abdomen with contrast Skeletal survey in children <2 years
Head injury	CBC PT/INR/aPTT Factor VIII level, factor IX level Fibrinogen, d-dimer Review newborn screen Consider urine organic acids	CT head MRI head and spine Skeletal survey in children <2 years

CBC complete blood count, *PT* prothrombin time, *INR* international normalized ratio, *PTT* Partial thromboplastin time, *VWF* von willebrand factor, *ALKP* alkaline phosphatase, *25OHD* 25-hydroxy vitamin D, *PTH* parathyroid hormone, *DNA* Deoxyribonucleic acid, *AST* aspartate aminotransferase, *ALT* alanine transaminase, *CT* computed tomography, *MRI* magnetic resonance imagine

marks caused by a looped cord, are highly suggestive of abuse. Bruises in healthy children tend to be distributed over bony prominences; bruises isolated to the torso, ears, cheek, or neck should raise concern [57]. Bruises in non-ambulatory infants are unusual and are highly concerning for physical abuse [58]. Many diseases are associated with bruises, including coagulopathies and vasculitis, and children who present with suspicious bruises may require screening for these hematologic disorders [59]. Bite marks are characterized by ecchymoses, abrasions, or lacerations that are found in an elliptical or ovoid pattern [60]. Bite marks can be inflicted by an adult, another child, an animal, or the patient.

Approximately 6–20% of children hospitalized with burns are victims of abuse [61]. Abusive scalds due to neglect outnumber those due to intentional injury by a factor of 9:1 [62]. Inflicted burns can be the result of contact with hot objects such as irons, radiators, stoves, or cigarettes, and from immersion injuries. Although both inflicted and accidental contact burns may be patterned, inflicted contact burns are characteristically deep and leave a clear imprint of the hot instrument. In contrast to accidental scald injuries, inflicted scald burns have clear demarcation, uniformity of burn depth, and a characteristic pattern [63]. Dermatologic and infectious diseases can mimic abusive burns, including toxin-mediated staphylococcal and streptococcal infections, impetigo, phytophotodermatitis, and chemical burns of the buttocks from laxatives [64].

Fractures

Unexplained fractures, fractures in non-ambulatory infants, and the presence of multiple fractures raise suspicion for physical abuse [65]. Certain fracture types also have a higher specificity for abuse, such as rib fractures and classic metaphyseal lesions. Skeletal survey is the standard tool for detecting occult fractures in possible victims of child abuse [19]. Repeating skeletal surveys 2–3 weeks after an initial presentation of suspected abuse improves diagnostic sensitivity and specificity for identifying skeletal trauma in abused infants [66, 67]. Expert consensus guidelines recommend obtaining a skeletal survey in the setting of a fracture: (1) if a fracture is attributed to abuse, IPV, or being hit with a toy; (2) when there is no history of trauma; and (3) in children younger than 12 months regardless of the fracture type or reported history, with rare exceptions [68]. Vitamin and mineral deficiencies, and genetic diseases may be considered in the differential diagnosis of unexplained fractures when appropriate [69].

Abdominal Injuries

Abdominal injury is the second leading cause of mortality from physical abuse [70]. Compared with children who sustain accidental abdominal trauma, victims of abuse tend to be younger, more likely to have hollow viscera injury, more likely to have delayed presentations to medical care, and have a higher mortality rate [71, 72]. Symptomatic children can present with signs of hemorrhage or peritonitis, but many children will not display overt findings. Therefore liver enzymes are important to obtain in all children who present with serious trauma, even if they do not display acute abdominal symptoms [73]. Contrast-enhancing computed tomography (CT) is warranted if these screening laboratory tests indicate possible abdominal trauma and in all cases of symptomatic injury.

Head Injuries

Abusive head trauma is the leading cause of mortality and morbidity from physical abuse [74]. Multiple mechanisms contribute to the cerebral, spinal, and cranial injuries that result from inflicted head injury, including both shaking and blunt impact [74]. For symptomatic children, CT of the head will identify abnormalities that require immediate surgical intervention and is preferred over MRI for identifying acute hemorrhage and skull fractures and scalp swelling from blunt injury. MRI is the optimal modality for assessing intracranial injury, including cerebral hypoxia and ischemia, and is used for all children with abnormal CT scans and asymptomatic infants with non-cranial abusive injuries [75].

An examination using indirect ophthalmoscopy is indicated in the evaluation of abusive head trauma because severe retinal hemorrhages are highly associated with abuse [76]. Conditions that may be confused with abusive head trauma include accidental/birth trauma, and metabolic, genetic, or hematologic diseases with associated vascular or coagulation defects [77]. Many of these can be ruled out through careful medical, developmental, and family history, and thorough physical examination.

Suspected Neglect

Neglect occurs when a child's basic needs are not adequately met. Physical neglect, the most common form of neglect, includes failure to provide food, clothing, stable housing, supervision, or protection. Educational neglect occurs when a child's educational needs have not been met, often by failure to enroll a child in school or by chronic truancy. Emotional neglect refers to exposing a child to conditions that could result in psychological harm such are ignoring a child's need for stimulation, isolating a child, threatening a child, or verbally ridiculing a child. Medical neglect refers to lack of appropriate medical or mental health care or treatment. The general examination, including careful measurement of growth parameters, may reveal evidence of neglect, including malnutrition, extensive dental caries, or neglected wound care.

Sexual Abuse

Sexual abuse is rarely discovered because it is witnessed or due to a physical exam finding or STI diagnosis. In the vast majority of cases, suspicion for sexual abuse arises from the child's disclosure. In fact, the child's disclosure is the most important evidence in making a diagnosis of sexual abuse and therefore must be carefully documented in the medical record. Many communities have child advocacy centers where children can be referred when concerns of sexual abuse arise. Depending on the community services available, the physician should be prepared to conduct a basic medical interview with a verbal child when there is a concern regarding sexual abuse. Any disclosure should be recorded word for word in the medical record [78]. If the sexual abuse occurred in the distant past and the asymptomatic child is going to be referred to a specialty center for medical evaluation, examination might be deferred. However, if the abuse is recent and the child is reporting genital or anal pain or bleeding, examination should be performed to rule out injury.

Most sexually abused children have normal anogenital examinations [79]. The sexual abuse of children may not result in injury and when injury does occur the anogenital tissue often heals quickly and completely [80]. A normal examination of the genitalia and anus does not rule out sexual abuse [81].

Sexually abused adolescents should be tested for chlamydia, gonorrhea, trichomonas, and pregnancy [82, 83]. In addition, the CDC suggests hepatitis B testing in unimmunized victims and consideration of human immunodeficiency virus (HIV) and syphilis testing in populations in which there is a high incidence of infection, or when the victim requests these tests [84]. STIs in pre-pubertal children evaluated for abuse are rare and thus a targeted approach is recommended [85]. Factors that may prompt testing include vaginal or anal penetration, abuse by a stranger, abuse by a perpetrator infected or at risk of infection with an STI, having a household contact with an STI, or signs or symptoms of an STI. Positive results should be confirmed using additional tests in populations with a low prevalence of the infection or when a false-positive test could have an adverse outcome. If diagnosed with an STI, the child should be treated promptly. Children who have had recent sexual contact should be immediately referred to a specialized clinic or emergency department capable of forensic evidence collection [86]. Most states recommend that forensic evidence be collected in less than 72 or 96 hours since the assault.

Suspected Elder Mistreatment

Spouses and adult children are the most common perpetrators of elder abuse [87]. Living with another adult is a major risk factor for elder abuse, perhaps due to increased opportunities for contact and conflict in a shared living arrangement [10, 87]. An exception to this pattern is financial abuse, for which victims are more likely to live alone [88]. Several studies have reported higher rates of physical abuse in patients with dementia [89, 90]. A likely mechanism is the high rate of disruptive and aggressive behaviors of patients, which are a major cause of stress and distress to caregivers. Social isolation has been identified as a risk factor for elder abuse [91]. There are certain perpetrator-specific risk factors as well, including mental illness and alcohol misuse [89, 92]. Finally, elder abusers tend to be heavily financially dependent on the person they are mistreating [93].

Once the possibility of elder abuse has been raised, a comprehensive assessment is necessary. If there are no cognitive limitations, the patient should be interviewed alone and asked directly about the etiology of any concerning findings [94]. Often patients are initially unwilling to speak openly about being an elder abuse victim due to embarrassment, shame, or fear of retribution from the perpetrator who is frequently a caregiver [94]. Interview of the suspected abuser is a potentially hazardous undertaking and not necessary [94]. Elder abusers who are presented with an empathetic, non-judgmental ear to describe their stresses and actions will sometimes describe their situations at great length and in great detail. However, all forms of domestic abuse share a pattern wherein abusers gain and control access to their victims. An elder abuser confronted with allegations of mistreatment may move to sequester a victim in such a way that a fragile, isolated adult loses access to critically needed medical, and social services [94].

Management Strategies

Mandated Reporting

In every state, health care providers are mandated by law to identify and report all cases of suspected child abuse and neglect. Yet, much of the abuse that is recognized by physicians does not get reported to CPS for investigation [16]. In part this is because clinicians may incorrectly believe that making a report requires certainty in their diagnosis of child abuse, rather than having a *reasonable suspicion* for maltreatment as the law requires. In addition, many clinicians believe that reporting to CPS is not an effective intervention and distrust the ability of the child welfare system to protect children [17]. In all states, the law provides immunity for good faith reporting. However, failing to report may result in malpractice suits, criminal offenses, licensing penalties, and continued abuse to the child. Mandated reporters must become familiar with their state-specific reporting procedures and laws. Most states, for example, have specific language about threat of harm or substantial risk to health or welfare in physical abuse statutes. Failure to educate is included in neglect statutes in about half of states, while medical neglect is defined in ten states [95].

Prenatal exposure to some drugs may cause a neonatal abstinence syndrome or neurodevelopmental consequences. Evidence of substance exposure at birth or prenatal exposure to illegal substances is considered child abuse in about half of states. Parenting after birth can be profoundly impacted by substance use, leading to risk for abuse, neglect, and exposure to production and distribution of illegal substances. Sixteen percent of child abuse reports include alcohol abuse as an additional risk factor and 29% include drug abuse as an additional risk factor [5]. In addition, alcohol or drug abuse is one of the reasons for child removal from the home in 39% of cases [96]. Most states have specific laws regarding maltreatment reporting and additional penalties for parent substance use and related exposures, but the laws vary by state [97].

Health care provider cooperation with CPS investigations is critical to effective decision making by investigators. Health Insurance Portability and Accountability Act rules allow disclosure of protected health information to CPS without authorization by a legal guardian when the clinician has made a mandatory report, but state laws differ regarding the release of health information during and after investigations are complete [98]. More than half of states specify circumstances of the child witnessing IPV that constitutes maltreatment. These statutes often include language around witnessing that includes a child within sight or sound of the IPV, and/or IPV that is escalating or involves a weapon [99]. Clinicians should know their specific state's reporting requirements before screening and inform the caregiver accordingly. In most states cases of elder abuse must be reported to adult protective services. Websites such as www.endabuse.org, http://www.childwelfare.gov, or http://www.eldercare.gov/Eldercare.NET/Public/Index.aspx provide information on state-specific laws about mandated reporting and available resources.

Trauma-Informed Care

About half of adults report one or more adverse child experiences, experiences that can contribute to a variety of acute and chronic health conditions. Because of the important role of adversity in health and well-being, there has been steady advocacy, research, change in reimbursement, and practice to support trauma-informed care. Trauma-informed care is defined by the National Traumatic Stress Network as "medical care in which all parties involved assess, recognize, and respond to the traumatic effects of stress on children, caregivers, and healthcare providers" [100]. The American Academy of Pediatrics has published recent guidance for practitioners in delivering trauma-informed care. Understanding the role stress plays in emotional and behavioral symptoms, evidence-based screening for such symptoms using validated tools to screen for depression and anxiety, treatment for disorders when diagnosed, and avoiding re-traumatization by the use of non-threatening language and exam procedures are all important components of trauma-informed care [100]. The training required for a truly trauma-informed practice can be a barrier to providing this care.

Many experts encourage screening for adverse childhood experiences as a part of trauma-informed care with the rationale that adversities are common and are linked to a variety of acute and chronic health conditions. However, adverse childhood experiences screening tools are quite varied, not validated, and may screen for events that occurred in the past and do not need to be addressed in the present. There is also a lack of tools to address these events, such as neighborhood violence [35]. The state of California reimburses practices for adverse childhood experience screening and recently passed legislation to require commercial insurers to reimburse for adverse childhood experience screening [101]. Other states may follow this example. Screening for recent or ongoing trauma as well as unmet social needs such as food and housing insecurity represents an alternative approach to adverse childhood experience screening that can be incorporated in trauma-informed care [35].

Approaching Intimate Partner Violence

Clinicians should educate patients on the dynamics of partner violence and potential effects on victims and their children, helping them understand that once violent dynamics are established in a relationship, the violence generally continues and escalates over time. Health care providers can convey concern to patients regarding the negative physical and mental effects that IPV may have on patients and their children. Although addressing IPV is usually a long-term process, health care providers should be alert to crisis situations that indicate imminent danger (e.g., escalating violence, use of or threat with a weapon, drug or alcohol use). Assessing for these risk factors provides an opportunity to educate patients about what situations indicate increased risk.

Health care providers should refer victims of IPV to local resources that can provide advocacy and support. Physicians and others should be familiar with organizations in their communities that provide assistance to victims of IPV, including organizations' capacity to accommodate specific populations such as immigrants, specific ethnic or cultural groups, teens, lesbian, gay, bisexual or transgender clients, or persons with disabilities. Resources can also include community-based advocacy groups, shelters, law enforcement agencies, or social workers. The National DV Hotline (800-799-SAFE) can serve as an information source. If immediate concerns for safety exist, the health care providers can offer to contact these resources for the patient directly from the office. A follow-up visit should be scheduled, and IPV should be readdressed at future visits.

Approach to Child Maltreatment

The treatment of child maltreatment is complex and challenging. Many of the approaches developed by child welfare agencies, health care providers, therapists, and others have not been rigorously tested, and many families suffer from chronic dysfunction and a multitude of challenges that require broad approaches to management.

Abuse-Focused Cognitive Behavioral Therapy (AF-CBT) and Parent–Child Interaction Therapy (PCIT) are considered "best-practice" interventions for the treatment of physical abuse [102]. Both are dyadic interventions designed to alter specific maladaptive patterns of interaction in parent–child relationships. AF-CBT represents an approach to working with abused children and their offending caregivers based on learning theory and behavioral principles that target child, parent, and family characteristics related to the maltreatment [103]. The approach is designed to promote the expression of appropriate/prosocial behavior and to discourage the use of coercive, aggressive, or violent behavior. PCIT is a highly specified, step-by-step, live-coached behavioral parent training model. Immediate prompts are provided to a parent by a therapist while the parent interacts with their child. Over the course of 14–20 weeks, parents are coached to develop specific positive relationship skills, which then results in child compliance to parent commands [104, 105].

Table 8.2 Trauma resources

Resource	Website
AAP Healthy Foster Care America	www.aap.org/fostercare
AAP Cope with Trauma Guide	www.aap.org/traumaguide
AAP Medical Home for Children and Adolescents Exposed to Violence	www.aap.org/medhomecev
National Child Traumatic Stress Network	http://nctsn.org
SAMHSA National Center for Trauma-Informed Care	www.samhsa.gov/nctic/trama.asp

When abused children develop post-traumatic stress disorder symptoms, Trauma-Focused Cognitive Behavioral Therapy (TF-CBT) is effective [106]. TF-CBT has been most widely used for children who have been sexually abused or have witnessed IPV and involves structured individual and parent trauma-focused models with skills-based components followed by more trauma-specific components with gradual exposure integrated into each component [106].

Clinicians should become familiar with programs in their geographic area of practice, which provide evidence-based interventions for children who have experienced abuse or IPV exposure. Additional information on trauma-informed care resources is listed in Table 8.2.

Enhanced Health Care Needs of Maltreated Children

Maltreated children, particularly those in foster care, exhibit high rates of acute and chronic physical, developmental, and mental health conditions [107–110]. In fact, nearly 80% of children in foster care have significant physical, mental, and developmental health care needs [111]. Exposures such as insufficient prenatal care, prematurity, or in-utero toxins as well as chronic abuse/neglect have direct and indirect effects on the health and well-being of this population.

The interplay of chronic or prolonged stress, physiologic response to that toxic stress, and behavioral adaptations to this stress impact the health of children over the life course. Maltreated children may require more frequent preventive health visits due to multiple environmental and social issues that can adversely impact their health. Furthermore, this medically vulnerable population requires intensive, integrated behavioral and medical care.

Approach to Elder Mistreatment

There are no evidence-based interventions regarding treatment for elder abuse and clinicians should view elder abuse as multifactorial rather than as a homogeneous condition. However, clinicians can offer interventions that may mitigate the impact of the abuse. Table 8.3 lists potential interventions to be considered in the treatment of elder maltreatment. Resources for clinicians and families who are dealing with elder mistreatment can be found at Area Agencies on Aging (http://www.n4a.org).

Prevention of Family Violence

More focus is needed on the prevention of family violence, child maltreatment, and elder mistreatment. Within the social–ecological context, prevention of family violence can be targeted to the individual level, the family/relationship level, the community level, and the societal/policy level. For instance, on the individual level, addressing known risk factors for family violence within an individual at risk of perpetrating abuse such as depression or substance addiction, may be an effective prevention strategy. Parent education programs, parenting programs that focus on strengthening parent–child relationship and positive parenting skills, and intensive home visiting are among the most evaluated programs for family/relationship level interventions [112–115]. Intensive home visiting has a substantial evidence base in the prevention of child maltreatment. Despite this demonstrated track record, it remains poorly disseminated, engagement and retention in this type of program is limited, and outcomes are hard to reproduce.

Community-based programs that seek to change social norms around parenting and family dynamics have also been shown to be successful [116]. These programs are often implemented in combination with some level of individual or family level intervention. Finally, at the societal level, there are untapped opportunities for prevention. Large societal factors influencing family violence include the health, economic, educational, and social policies that help to maintain economic and social inequalities between groups in society. For example, policies addressing Medicaid expansion, paid family leave, earned income tax credit, and lack of waitlists to access subsidized child care have each independently been associated with decreases in child maltreatment [117–119].

Future Directions

Child abuse, family violence, and elder mistreatment are tied to substantial burdens of suffering and associated costs to communities (e.g., health care, criminal justice, mental illness, substance use). These conditions and maladaptations should ultimately be viewed as problems of the individuals involved, as well as the family, the community, and the greater social environment. For health care providers, there is ample opportunity to: (1) identify families at risk, (2) provide resources and referral, (3) treat the sequelae, and (4) advocate for the most constructive programs and policies to reduce the burden of suffering.

The most important frontiers in research will be the development, adoption, and sustained implementation of programs—prevention and intervention—for families across the life course who are at risk and victimized by violence. The most effective types of intervention for child maltreatment, for example, is intensive home visiting [115, 120], however, these programs are available to relatively few families who may benefit, and recruitment and retention rates are low. In addition, although these approaches require significant resources per person, they can be adapted and scaled across a broader range of settings, such as primary care, early care and education, schools, and long-term care. Finally, research is needed on how to most effectively engage and retain families in effective prevention and treatment programs.

The COVID-19 pandemic created and amplified multiple risk areas for family violence, including unemployment, social isolation, disruptions of childcare, and stress associated with loss, illness, and death. These stressors contributed to a remarkable increase in substance use, with more than one in ten adults reporting they started or increased the use of alcohol or drugs to cope with the pandemic [121]. Rates of depres-

Table 8.3 Interventions to consider for elder abuse

Abuse Trigger to Target	Potential Interventions
Alleviating caregiver stress	Respite services Adult daycare Caregiver education program Recruitment of other family, informal, or paid caregivers to share burden of care Social integration of caregiver to reduce isolation
Treating specific caregiver deficiency	Treatment for caregiver depression or mental illness Referral to alcohol or drug misuse rehabilitation program
Aggressive symptoms in patient with dementia	Geriatric medical assessment of causes of underlying behavior and treatment of aggressive symptoms
Long-standing spousal violence	Marital counseling Support groups Shelters Orders of protection Victim advocacy
Financial exploitation by family member	Guardianship proceedings Power of attorney Adult Protective Services
Financial exploitation by paid caregiver	Legal services Law enforcement Adult Protective Services

sion also increased with 32.8% of US adults experiencing elevated depressive symptoms in 2021 compared to 8.5% pre-pandemic [122]. In spite of these increased risks, there was not a significant rise in child maltreatment related to COVID-19 [123–125]. The sharp decrease in reports of maltreatment to child protective services at the beginning of the pandemic was initially thought to be attributed not to an actual decrease in maltreatment, but to surveillance bias because children were at home, with limited access to mandated reporters (e.g., teachers, daycare providers). However, large increases in reporting were not observed with the return to in-person school and multiple studies indicate that abuse-related hospitalizations did not increase during the COVID-19 pandemic [123–125]. Although this paradox is not fully understood, it may provide insight into family violence prevention, indicating that federal financial assistance to at-risk families was protective or contributed to increased parental presence at home, leading to stronger parent–child relationships. At this time, there has been limited research that has examined the impact of the pandemic on IPV or elder mistreatment.

References

1. Breiding MJ, Basile KC, Smith SG, Black MC, Mahendra R. Intimate partner violence surveillance: uniform definitions and recommended data elements, version 2.0. National Center for Injury Prevention and Control, Centers for Disease Control and Prevention: Atlanta, GA; 2015.
2. Black MBK, Breiding M. The National Intimate Partner and Sexual Violence Survey (NISVS): 2010 summary report. Atlanta, GA: National Center for Injury Prevention and Control, Centers for Diseases Control and Prevention; 2010.
3. U.S. Department of Justice BoJS, editor. Homicide trends in the United States, 1980–2008. 2011.
4. The Child Abuse Prevention and Treatment Act (CAPTA) Reauthorization Act of 2010, Pub. L. No. P.L. 111-320(12/20/2010, 2010).
5. US Department of Health & Human Services. Child maltreatment 2019. 2021.
6. Middlebrooks JS, Audage NC. The effects of childhood stress on health across the lifespan; 2008.
7. Felitti VJ, Anda RF, Nordenberg D, Williamson DF, Spitz AM, Edwards V, et al. Relationship of childhood abuse and household dysfunction to many of the leading causes of death in adults: the Adverse Childhood Experiences (ACE) Study. Am J Prev Med. 1998;14(4):245–58.
8. https://www.cdc.gov/masstrauma/factsheets/professionals/coping_professional.pdf.
9. Sciences NAo. Elder abuse: abuse, neglect, and exploitation in an aging America. In: Bonnie R WR, editor. Washington DC: National Academy Press; 2002.
10. Pillemer K, Finkelhor D. The prevalence of elder abuse: a random sample survey. The Gerontologist. 1988;28(1):51–7.
11. Moyer VA. Screening for intimate partner violence and abuse of elderly and vulnerable adults: US Preventive Services Task Force recommendation statement. Ann Intern Med. 2013;158(6):478–86.
12. Plichta SB. Intimate partner violence and physical health consequences policy and practice implications. J Interpers Violence. 2004;19(11):1296–323.
13. Rabin RF, Jennings JM, Campbell JC, Bair-Merritt MH. Intimate partner violence screening tools: a systematic review. Am J Prev Med. 2009;36(5):439–45.e4.
14. Pai N, Kandasamy S, Uleryk E, Maguire JL. Social risk screening for pediatric inpatients. Clin Pediatr. 2015:0009922815623498.
15. Jenny C, Hymel KP, Ritzen A, Reinert SE, Hay TC. Analysis of missed cases of abusive head trauma. JAMA. 1999;281(7):621–6.
16. Sheets LK, Leach ME, Koszewski IJ, Lessmeier AM, Nugent M, Simpson P. Sentinel injuries in infants evaluated for child physical abuse. Pediatrics. 2013;131(4):701–7.
17. Jones R, Flaherty EG, Binns HJ, Price LL, Slora E, Abney D, et al. Clinicians' description of factors influencing their reporting of suspected child abuse: report of the Child Abuse Reporting Experience Study Research Group. Pediatrics. 2008;122(2):259–66.
18. King WK, Kiesel EL, Simon HK. Child abuse fatalities: are we missing opportunities for intervention? Pediatr Emerg Care. 2006;22(4):211–4.
19. Christian CW, Crawford-Jakubiak JE, Flaherty EG, Leventhal JM, Lukefahr JL, Sege RD, et al. The evaluation of suspected child physical abuse. Pediatrics. 2015;135(5):e1337–e54.
20. Lane WG, Rubin DM, Monteith R, Christian CW. Racial differences in the evaluation of pediatric fractures for physical abuse. JAMA. 2002;288(13):1603–9.
21. Lane WG, Dubowitz H. What factors affect the identification and reporting of child abuse-related fractures? Clin Orthop Relat Res. 2007;461:219–25.
22. Wood JN, Hall M, Schilling S, Keren R, Mitra N, Rubin DM. Disparities in the evaluation and diagnosis of abuse among infants with traumatic brain injury. Pediatrics. 2010;126(3):408–14.
23. Schilling S, Samuels-Kalow M, Gerber JS, Scribano PV, French B, Wood JN. Testing and treatment after adolescent sexual assault in pediatric emergency departments. Pediatrics. 2015;136(6):e1495–503.
24. Lentsch KA, Johnson CF. Do physicians have adequate knowledge of child sexual abuse? The results of two surveys of practicing physicians, 1986 and 1996. Child Maltreat. 2000;5(1):72–8.
25. Starling SP, Heisler KW, Paulson JF, Youmans E. Child abuse training and knowledge: a national survey of emergency medicine, family medicine, and pediatric residents and program directors. Pediatrics. 2009;123(4):e595–602.
26. Garner AS, Shonkoff JP, Siegel BS, Dobbins MI, Earls MF, McGuinn L, et al. Early childhood adversity, toxic stress, and the role of the pediatrician: translating developmental science into lifelong health. Pediatrics. 2012;129(1):e224–e31.
27. Shonkoff JP, Garner AS, Committee on Psychosocial Aspects of Child and Family Health; Committee on Early Childhood, Adoption, and Dependent Care; Section on Developmental and Behavioral Pediatrics. The lifelong effects of early childhood adversity and toxic stress. Pediatrics. 2012;129(1):e232–e46.
28. Shonkoff JP, Garner AS, Siegel BS, Dobbins MI, Earls MF, McGuinn L, et al. The lifelong effects of early childhood adversity and toxic stress. Pediatrics. 2012;129(1):e232–e46.
29. Forkey H, Szilagyi M. Foster care and healing from complex childhood trauma. Pediatr Clin N Am. 2014;61(5):1059–72.
30. Johnson SB, Riley AW, Granger DA, Riis J. The science of early life toxic stress for pediatric practice and advocacy. Pediatrics. 2013;131(2):319–27.
31. Dantzer R, O'Connor JC, Freund GG, Johnson RW, Kelley KW. From inflammation to sickness and depression: when the immune system subjugates the brain. Nat Rev Neurosci. 2008;9(1):46–56.
32. Petruccelli K, Davis J, Berman T. Adverse childhood experiences and associated health outcomes: a systematic review and meta-analysis. Child Abuse Negl. 2019;97:104127.
33. DeCamp M, DeSalvo K, Dzeng E. Ethics and spheres of influence in addressing social determinants of health. J Gen Intern Med. 2020;35(9):2743–5.

34. Berkowitz SA, Kangovi S. Health care's social movement should not leave science behind. Milbank Quarterly Opinion. September 3, 2020. https://doi.org/10.1599/mqop.2020.0826.
35. Dubowitz HFD, Zolotor A, Kleven J, Davis N. Addressing adverse childhood experiences in primary care: challenges and considerations. Pediatrics. 2022;149:e2021052641.
36. Lachs MS. Elder abuse. In: Halter JB, Ouslander JG, Stephanie S, High KP, Asthana S, Supiano MA, Ritchie C, editors. Hazzard's geriatic medicine and gerontology. 7th ed. McGraw-Hill Education; 2016.
37. Nelson HD, Bougatsos C, Blazina I. Screening women for intimate partner violence: a systematic review to update the US Preventive Services Task Force recommendation. Ann Intern Med. 2012;156(11):796–808.
38. Rivas C, Ramsay J, Sadowski L, Davidson LL, Dunne D, Eldridge S, et al. Advocacy interventions to reduce or eliminate violence and promote the physical and psychosocial well-being of women who experience intimate partner abuse. The Cochrane Library; 2015.
39. Flaherty EG, Stirling J. The pediatrician's role in child maltreatment prevention. Pediatrics. 2010;126(4):833–41.
40. Brown J, Cohen P, Johnson JG, Salzinger S. A longitudinal analysis of risk factors for child maltreatment: findings of a 17-year prospective study of officially recorded and self-reported child abuse and neglect. Child Abuse Negl. 1998;22(11):1065–78.
41. Finkelhor D, Ormrod R, Turner H, Hamby SL. The victimization of children and youth: a comprehensive, national survey. Child Maltreat. 2005;10(1):5–25.
42. O'Leary PJ, Barber J. Gender differences in silencing following childhood sexual abuse. J Child Sex Abus. 2008;17(2):133–43.
43. Hibbard RA, Desch LW, American Academy of Pediatrics Committee on Child A, Neglect, American Academy of Pediatrics Council on Children with D. Maltreatment of children with disabilities. Pediatrics. 2007;119(5):1018–25.
44. Kolko DJ. Characteristics of child victims of physical violence research findings and clinical implications. J Interpers Violence. 1992;7(2):244–76.
45. Sidebotham P, Heron J. Child maltreatment in the "children of the nineties": a cohort study of risk factors. Child Abuse Negl. 2006;30(5):497–522.
46. Kelleher K, Chaffin M, Hollenberg J, Fischer E. Alcohol and drug disorders among physically abusive and neglectful parents in a community-based sample. Am J Public Health. 1994;84(10):1586–90.
47. Oates RK, Davis AA, Ryan MG. Predictive factors for child abuse. J Paediatr Child Health. 1980;16(4):239–43.
48. Kotch JB, Browne DC, Dufort V, Winsor J, Catellier D. Predicting child maltreatment in the first 4 years of life from characteristics assessed in the neonatal period. Child Abuse Negl. 1999;23(4):305–19.
49. Fortson B, Klevens J, Merrick M, Gilbert L, Alexander S. Preventing child abuse and neglect: a technical package for policy, norm, and programmatic activities. National Center for Injury Prevention and Control; 2016.
50. Schnitzer PG, Ewigman BG. Child deaths resulting from inflicted injuries: household risk factors and perpetrator characteristics. Pediatrics. 2005;116(5):e687–e93.
51. Christian CW, Scribano P, Seidl T, Pinto-Martin JA. Pediatric injury resulting from family violence. Pediatrics. 1997;99(2):e8.
52. Holt S, Buckley H, Whelan S. The impact of exposure to domestic violence on children and young people: a review of the literature. Child Abuse Negl. 2008;32(8):797–810.
53. Zolotor AJ, Theodore AD, Coyne-Beasley T, Runyan DK. Intimate partner violence and child maltreatment: overlapping risk. Brief Treat Crisis Interv. 2007;7(4):305.
54. Brewster AL, Nelson JP, Hymel KP, Colby DR, Lucas DR, McCanne TR, et al. Victim, perpetrator, family, and incident characteristics of 32 infant maltreatment deaths in the United States air Force. Child Abuse Negl. 1998;22(2):91–101.
55. Barr RG, Trent RB, Cross J. Age-related incidence curve of hospitalized shaken baby syndrome cases: convergent evidence for crying as a trigger to shaking. Child Abuse Negl. 2006;30(1):7–16.
56. Daria S, Sugar NF, Feldman KW, Boos SC, Benton SA, Ornstein A. Into hot water head first: distribution of intentional and unintentional immersion burns. Pediatr Emerg Care. 2004;20(5):302–10.
57. Pierce MC, Kaczor K, Aldridge S, O'Flynn J, Lorenz DJ. Bruising characteristics discriminating physical child abuse from accidental trauma. Pediatrics. 2010;125(1):67–74.
58. Sugar NF, Taylor JA, Feldman KW. Bruises in infants and toddlers: those who don't cruise rarely bruise. Arch Pediatr Adolesc Med. 1999;153(4):399–403.
59. Anderst JD, Carpenter SL, Abshire TC, Hord J, Crouch G, Hale G, et al. Evaluation for bleeding disorders in suspected child abuse. Pediatrics. 2013;131(4):e1314–e22.
60. Kellogg N. Oral and dental aspects of child abuse and neglect. Pediatrics. 2005;116(6):1565–8.
61. Peck MD, Priolo-Kapel D. Child abuse by burning: a review of the literature and an algorithm for medical investigations. J Trauma Acute Care Surg. 2002;53(5):1013–22.
62. Chester DL, Jose RM, Aldlyami E, King H, Moiemen NS. Non-accidental burns in children—are we neglecting neglect? Burns. 2006;32(2):222–8.
63. Purdue GF, Hunt JL, Prescott PR. Child abuse by burning-an index of suspicion. J Trauma Acute Care Surg. 1988;28(2):221–4.
64. Leventhal JM, Griffin D, Duncan KO, Starling S, Christian CW, Kutz T. Laxative-induced dermatitis of the buttocks incorrectly suspected to be abusive burns. Pediatrics. 2001;107(1):178–9.
65. Leventhal JM, Thomas SA, Rosenfield NS, Markowitz RI. Fractures in young children: distinguishing child abuse from unintentional injuries. Am J Dis Child. 1993;147(1):87–92.
66. Kleinman PK, Nimkin K, Spevak MR, Rayder SM, Madansky DL, Shelton YA, et al. Follow-up skeletal surveys in suspected child abuse. AJR Am J Roentgenol. 1996;167(4):893–6.
67. Zimmerman S, Makoroff K, Care M, Thomas A, Shapiro R. Utility of follow-up skeletal surveys in suspected child physical abuse evaluations. Child Abuse Negl. 2005;29(10):1075–83.
68. Wood JN, Fakeye O, Feudtner C, Mondestin V, Localio R, Rubin DM. Development of guidelines for skeletal survey in young children with fractures. Pediatrics. 2014;134(1):45–53.
69. Flaherty EG, Perez-Rossello JM, Levine MA, Hennrikus WL, Christian CW, Crawford-Jakubiak JE, et al. Evaluating children with fractures for child physical abuse. Pediatrics. 2014;133(2):e477–e89.
70. Barnes PM, Norton CM, Dunstan FD, Kemp AM, Yates DW, Sibert JR. Abdominal injury due to child abuse. Lancet. 2005;366(9481):234–5.
71. Wood J, Rubin DM, Nance ML, Christian CW. Distinguishing inflicted versus accidental abdominal injuries in young children. J Trauma Acute Care Surg. 2005;59(5):1203–8.
72. Maguire SA, Upadhyaya M, Evans A, Mann MK, Haroon M, Tempest V, et al. A systematic review of abusive visceral injuries in childhood—their range and recognition. Child Abuse Negl. 2013;37(7):430–45.
73. Lindberg DM, Shapiro RA, Blood EA, Steiner RD, Berger RP. Utility of hepatic transaminases in children with concern for abuse. Pediatrics. 2013;131(2):268–75.
74. Christian CW, Block R. Abusive head trauma in infants and children. Pediatrics. 2009;123(5):1409–11.
75. Boos M. Abusive head trauma part II: radiological aspects. Eur J Pediatr. 2012;171:617–23.

76. Vinchon M, de Foort-Dhellemmes S, Desurmont M, Delestret I. Confessed abuse versus witnessed accidents in infants: comparison of clinical, radiological, and ophthalmological data in corroborated cases. Childs Nerv Syst. 2010;26(5):637–45.
77. Sirotnak A. Medical disorders that mimic abusive head trauma. Abusive head trauma in infants and children. St Louis, MO: GW Medical Publishing; 2006. p. 191–214.
78. Jenny C, Crawford-Jakubiak JE, Christian CW, Flaherty EG, Leventhal JM, Lukefahr JL, et al. The evaluation of children in the primary care setting when sexual abuse is suspected. Pediatrics. 2013;132(2):e558–e67.
79. Heger A, Ticson L, Velasquez O, Bernier R. Children referred for possible sexual abuse: medical findings in 2384 children. Child Abuse Negl. 2002;26(6):645–59.
80. McCann J, Miyamoto S, Boyle C, Rogers K. Healing of non-hymenal genital injuries in prepubertal and adolescent girls: a descriptive study. Pediatrics. 2007;120(5):1000–11.
81. Kellogg ND, Menard SW, Santos A. Genital anatomy in pregnant adolescents: "normal" does not mean "nothing happened.". Pediatrics. 2004;113(1):e67–e9.
82. Kaufman M. Care of the adolescent sexual assault victim. Pediatrics. 2008;122(2):462–70.
83. Sexually transmitted infections. In: Pediatrics AAo, editor. Red book: 2003 report of the Committee of Infectious Diseases 29th ed. Elk Grove Village, IL: American Academy of Pediatrics; 2012. p. 157–67.
84. Workowski KA, Berman SM. Centers for Disease Control and Prevention sexually transmitted disease treatment guidelines. Clin Infect Dis. 2011;53(suppl 3):S59–63.
85. Adams JA, Kellogg ND, Farst KJ, Harper NS, Palusci VJ, Frasier LD, et al. Updated guidelines for the medical assessment and care of children who may have been sexually abused. J Pediatr Adolesc Gynecol. 2016;29(2):81–7.
86. Kairys S, Alexander R, Block R, Everett V, Hymel K, Johnson C, et al. Guidelines for the evaluation of sexual abuse of children: subject review. Pediatrics. 1999;103(1):186–91.
87. Lachs MS, Williams C, O'Brien S, Hurst L, Horwitz R. Risk factors for reported elder abuse and neglect: a nine-year observational cohort study. The Gerontologist. 1997;37(4):469–74.
88. Choi NG, Kulick DB, Mayer J. Financial exploitation of elders: analysis of risk factors based on county adult protective services data. J Elder Abuse Negl. 1999;10(3–4):39–62.
89. Paveza GJ, Cohen D, Eisdorfer C, Freels S, Semla T, Ashford JW, et al. Severe family violence and Alzheimer's disease: prevalence and risk factors. The Gerontologist. 1992;32(4):493–7.
90. Dyer CB, Pavlik VN, Murphy KP, Hyman DJ. The high prevalence of depression and dementia in elder abuse or neglect. J Am Geriatr Soc. 2000;48(2):205–8.
91. Lachs MS, Berkman L, Fulmer T, Horwitz RI. A prospective community-based pilot study of risk factors for the investigation of elder mistreatment. J Am Geriatr Soc. 1994;42(2):169–73.
92. Campbell Reay A, Browne K. Risk factor characteristics in carers who physically abuse or neglect their elderly dependants. Aging Ment Health. 2001;5(1):56–62.
93. Greenberg JR, McKibben M, Raymond JA. Dependent adult children and elder abuse. J Elder Abuse Negl. 1990;2(1–2):73–86.
94. Lachs MS, Pillemer K. Elder abuse. Lancet. 2004;364(9441):1263–72.
95. Child Welfare Information Gateway. Definitions of child abuse and neglect. Washington, DC: U.S. Department of Health and Human Services, Children's Bureau; 2019.
96. https://ncsacw.samhsa.gov/research/child-welfare-and-treatment-statistics.aspx [Internet].
97. Child Welfare Information Gateway. Parental substance use as child abuse. Washington, DC: U.S. Department of Health and Human Services, Children's Bureau; 2020.
98. Jenny C, Christian CW, Crawford J, Flaherty E, Hibbard R, Kaplan R, et al. Policy statement-child abuse, confidentiality, and the health insurance portability and accountability act. Pediatrics. 2010;125(1):197–201.
99. Child Welfare Information Gateway. Child witnesses to domestic violence. U.S. Department of Health and Human Services, Administration for Children and Families, Children's Bureau; 2021.
100. Forkey H, Szilagyi M, Kelly ET, Duffee J, Springer SH, Fortin K, et al. Trauma-informed care. Pediatrics. 2021;148:2.
101. Health care coverage: adverse childhood experiences screenings, Legislative Counsel of California; 2021.
102. Chaffin M, Friedrich B. Evidence-based treatments in child abuse and neglect. Child Youth Serv Rev. 2004;26(11):1097–113.
103. Kolko D, Swenson CC. Assessing and treating physically abused children and their families: a cognitive-behavioral approach. Sage Publications; 2002.
104. Timmer SG, Urquiza AJ, Zebell NM, McGrath JM. Parent-child interaction therapy: application to maltreating parent-child dyads. Child Abuse Negl. 2005;29(7):825–42.
105. Chaffin M, Silovsky JF, Funderburk B, Valle LA, Brestan EV, Balachova T, et al. Parent-child interaction therapy with physically abusive parents: efficacy for reducing future abuse reports. J Consult Clin Psychol. 2004;72(3):500.
106. Cohen JA, Mannarino AP, Deblinger E. Treating trauma and traumatic grief in children and adolescents. Guilford Press; 2006.
107. Justin RG. Medical needs of foster children. Am Fam Physician. 2003;67(3):474, 6-, 6.
108. Hansen RL, Mawjee FL, Barton K, Metcalf MB, Joye NR. Comparing the health status of low-income children in and out of foster care. Child Welfare. 2004;83(4):367.
109. Kools S, Paul SM, Jones R, Monasterio E, Norbeck J. Health profiles of adolescents in foster care. J Pediatr Nurs. 2013;28(3):213–22.
110. Jee SH, Barth RP, Szilagyi MA, Szilagyi PG, Aida M, Davis MM. Factors associated with chronic conditions among children in foster care. J Health Care Poor Underserved. 2006;17(2):328–41.
111. Brown KE. Foster care: state practices for assessing health needs facilitating service delivery, and monitoring children's: Care: DIANE Publishing; 2009.
112. Zolotor AJ, Runyan DK, Shanahan M, Durrance CP, Nocera M, Sullivan K, et al. Effectiveness of a statewide abusive head trauma prevention program in North Carolina. JAMA Pediatr. 2015;169(12):1126–31.
113. Schilling S, French B, Berkowitz SJ, Dougherty SL, Scribano PV, Wood JN. Child adult relationship enhancement in primary care: a randomized trial of a parent training for child behavior problems. Acad Pediatr. 2016;
114. Dubowitz H, Lane WG, Semiatin JN, Magder LS. The seek model of pediatric primary care: can child maltreatment be prevented in a low-risk population? Acad Pediatr. 2012;12(4):259–68.
115. Selph SS, Bougatsos C, Blazina I, Nelson HD. Behavioral interventions and counseling to prevent child abuse and neglect: a systematic review to update the US Preventive Services Task Force recommendation. Ann Intern Med. 2013;158(3):179–90.
116. Sanders MR, Ralph A, Sofronoff K, Gardiner P, Thompson R, Dwyer S, et al. Every family: a population approach to reducing behavioral and emotional problems in children making the transition to school. J Prim Prev. 2008;29(3):197–222.
117. Brown EC, Garrison MM, Bao H, Qu P, Jenny C, Rowhani-Rahbar A. Assessment of rates of child maltreatment in states with Medicaid expansion vs states without Medicaid expansion. JAMA Netw Open. 2019;2(6):e195529.
118. Klevens J, Luo F, Xu L, Peterson C, Latzman NE. Paid family leave's effect on hospital admissions for pediatric abusive head trauma. Inj Prev. 2016;22(6):442–5.

119. Klevens J, Barnett SBL, Florence C, Moore D. Exploring policies for the reduction of child physical abuse and neglect. Child Abuse Negl. 2015;40:1–11.
120. MacMillan HL, Wathen CN, Barlow J, Fergusson DM, Leventhal JM, Taussig HN. Interventions to prevent child maltreatment and associated impairment. Lancet. 2009;373(9659):250–66.
121. Substance use issues are worsening alongside access to care. https://www.kff.org/policy-watch/substance-use-issues-are-worsening-alongside-access-to-care/. Accessed 20 Jan 2022.
122. Ettman CK, Cohen GH, Abdalla SM, Sampson L, Trinquart L, Castrucci BC, et al. Persistent depressive symptoms during COVID-19: a national, population-representative, longitudinal study of US adults. Lancet Regional Health-Americas. 2022;5:100091.
123. Swedo E, Idaikkadar N, Leemis R, Dias T, Radhakrishnan L, Stein Z, et al. Trends in US emergency department visits related to suspected or confirmed child abuse and neglect among children and adolescents aged< 18 years before and during the COVID-19 pandemic—United States, January 2019–September 2020. Morb Mortal Wkly Rep. 2020;69(49):1841.
124. Maassel NL, Asnes AG, Leventhal JM, Solomon DG. Hospital admissions for abusive head trauma at children's hospitals during COVID-19. Pediatrics. 2021;148:e2021050361.
125. Kaiser SV, Kornblith AE, Richardson T, Pantell MS, Fleegler EW, Fritz CQ, et al. Emergency visits and hospitalizations for child abuse during the COVID-19 pandemic. Pediatrics. 2021;147(4):e2020038489.

Peer Support

Edwin B. Fisher, Patrick Y. Tang, Muchieh Coufal, Yuexing Liu, Samantha L. Luu, Megan Evans, and Weiping Jia

Introduction

Peer support (PS) provided by "community health workers" (CHWs), "lay health advisors," "*promotores*," "patient navigators," "peer supporters," and individuals with a number of other designations has been shown to play influential roles in health and the delivery of health care [1]. Although medical care and self-management programs may help individuals understand what to do to stay healthy, people often find themselves disconnected from resources and left on their own to manage a complex set of health behaviors. In response, PS links people living with a chronic disease or condition with others who share knowledge and experience that health care providers often do not have [2]. This approach offers emotional, social, and practical assistance to promote complex behaviors and activities that are critical for managing conditions and staying healthy [3–7]. It can also complement health care by enhancing self-care, providing motivation and coping skills to individuals who have the stressors of chronic disease, and linking them to their health care providers [8–11]. The contributions and complementarity of PS were summarized in a paper "Teaching How, Not What" [12]. Adults with diabetes pointed out that clinicians teach what to do whereas the peer supporter "taught me a lot about how to control my diabetes, how to eat healthy, and how to do my exercise" (p. 213S).

The average person may spend about 6 h each year in a health care environment (e.g., outpatient clinic), which leaves 8760 h a year for individuals to manage their health conditions. The importance of 8760 is recognized, for example, by the distinction between education and ongoing support for sustaining diabetes self-management in the *National Standards for Diabetes Self-Management Education and Support* developed by the American Diabetes Association, the Association of Diabetes Care & Education Specialists, and the American Dietetic Association [13]. PS interventions have been shown to be an effective disease management strategy to enhance linkages to care and attend to the dynamic and evolving conditions of "real world" environments and circumstances that influence health behavior [14–22].

Peer support has been broadly applied across demographics, health conditions, stages of disease, and care settings to enhance a variety of health outcomes. Employing multiple modalities (e.g., face-to-face, group-based, telephone-based, digital health), peer support may be adapted to the unique needs of its organizational home and can utilize a population focus. Peer support can occur organically in group medical visits and patient-education classes as patients take advantage of opportunities to share their experiences. Organized peer support, with trained volunteers or certified CHWs or Peer Support Specialists, can provide individual counseling, support daily self-management of chronic diseases, connect patients with social services, and provide a basic level of care coordination.

Peers for Progress [23–26] (peersforprogress.org) has facilitated research on and dissemination of peer support in health care and prevention since 2007. Peer support has been recognized as the provision of assistance and emotional support in chronic care and chronic disease management, in addition to connecting individuals to appropriate care and

E. B. Fisher (✉) · P. Y. Tang · S. L. Luu
Peers for Progress, Department of Health Behavior, Gillings School of Global Public Health, University of North Carolina at Chapel Hill, Chapel Hill, NC, USA
e-mail: edfisher@unc.edu; fishere@email.unc.edu; ptang@unc.edu; samantha@downtownchapelhill.com

M. Coufal
Peers for Progress, Department of Health Behavior, Gillings School of Global Public Health, University of North Carolina-Chapel Hill, Chapel Hill, NC, USA

Asian Center for Health Education, Plano, TX, USA
e-mail: mcoufal@acheusa.org

Y. Liu · W. Jia
Shanghai Jiaotong University Affiliated Sixth People's Hospital and Shanghai Diabetes Institute, Shanghai, China
e-mail: wpjia@sjtu.edu.cn

M. Evans
Department of Psychiatry, Yale University, New Haven, CT, USA
e-mail: megan.evans@yale.edu

resources in their community. Although using peers to teach time-limited health courses [27], or to promote health screening or immunization [28], is important, Peers for Progress has emphasized peer support more broadly focused to support and encourage the ongoing behaviors and patterns that are central to healthy living through 8760 h a year, 24/7 for the rest of one's life. This chapter is grounded in this orientation and provides an overview to PS.

The first two sections of the chapter, "Understanding Peer Support" and "Foundations of Peer Support," discuss key definitional issues around PS and then historical and intellectual foundations of the field. Next, the section "Evidence Base of PS" is presented with a particular focus on diabetes mellitus. The subsequent section identifies "Implementation and Dissemination Approaches" through which PS may contribute to improved population and public health. The next section "Peer Support Applications in Primary Care" highlights integration strategies including the Chronic Care Model (CCM). The next section identifies "Organizational and Fiscal Considerations." Sections on "Peer Support and Health Information Technologies" and the "Peer Support Workforce" precede then with a final section on "Future Directions."

Understanding Peer Support

There is ongoing discussion in the peer support field regarding the requirement of supporters to have the lived experience of those they assist in addition to other features, such as volunteer versus reimbursement for the services rendered. In light of this conversation and recognizing the challenge of developing a model that could be adopted across different nations with varied cultures and health systems, Peers for Progress initiated a consultation organized through the World Health Organization in 2007 [29]. Representatives from over 20 countries pointed out that key aspects of PS could be generalizable across differences in settings, although PS programs would have to be tailored to individual health systems, cultures, and patient populations. Accordingly, Peers for Progress has pursued a strategy of defining PS not by specific implementation protocols or details but according to "key functions of support" [30, 31]. This follows a strategy of "standardization by function, not content" [32, 33].

Initial work [24, 25, 31] identified four key functions of peer support: (1) assistance in daily management; (2) social and emotional support to encourage management behaviors and coping with negative emotions; (3) linkage to clinical care and community resources; and (4) ongoing support because chronic disease is for the rest of one's life [31]. With tailoring according to needs and strengths of a specific setting or health challenge, these functions have become a template for planning and evaluating PS programs [30]. The hardiness of this approach was demonstrated by its application in programs in Cameroon, South Africa, Thailand, and Uganda and the benefits they achieved across clinical, self-management, and quality-of-life indicators [30].

A fifth function, "being there," emerged through a study of telephone peer support for US military veterans, police, and other high risk groups [34] who identified the value of voicemails not only as ways to arrange contacts, but as an important mode of connection in and of themselves. As one client put it most powerfully, "I have listened to every one of the voicemails you left for me. You are the only one who continued to reach out. Because of you there is one less dead Marine" [35]. Being there or the value of presence [36] overlaps with social and emotional support, but emphasizes that, even without transactions or a substantive focus of support, just being there for people is of great value.

A sixth key PS function, advocacy, emerges from scoping and realist reviews of peer support for those with schizophrenia [37, 38]. Peers and those they help can strategize about how to influence or transform the mental health care system. Peers can also promote self-advocacy such as with health care providers for their own care needs and preferences. Advocacy overlaps with other functions, including linkage to clinical care and community resources, but includes a dimension of what resources *should* be in place, not just which ones are available.

There is a continuum of peer support from natural helpers embedded in their communities to certified paraprofessionals [39]. At the informal end of the continuum, "*natural helping*" includes those who meet qualifications "set by a community" and "have a reputation in their community for good judgment, sound advice, a caring ear, and being discreet" [39]. Often, they may be volunteers. At the other end of the continuum, paraprofessional community health workers can extend the reach of health care and social services delivery systems. Pros and cons surround the points along the continuum, the natural help of volunteers from one's neighborhood, the greater training and reliable availability of a CHW working through an organized program, the risk of professionalism compromising peerness, loyalty potentially split among those served versus employers [39, 40]. Consequently, programs should select peer support models that best fit their objectives and the population served.

Foundations of Peer Support

In the late eighteenth century, the Bicêtre Hospital in Paris employed former patients recovering from mental health problems as hospital staff who were praised for being "gentle, honest, and humane," "averse from active cruelty," and "disposed to kindness" [41]. A century later, peer-facilitated recovery emerged through Alcoholics Anonymous and has been adopted by other peer groups [42]. A group of consumers in the 1950s calling themselves *We Are Not Alone* developed a clubhouse approach to provide mutual support after they left a state hospital. This program was adapted in building an intentional therapeutic community comprising both people with serious mental illness and staff who worked in the facility [43]. Community mental health professionals advocated for lay counselors to help mentally ill patients in the late 1960s [44], a philosophy that was adopted by mental health consumers in the 1970s as state mental hospitals in the United States were being shuttered.

Research on the social influences that underlie peer support date back to Harry Harlow's classic study showing that, although a wire surrogate mother was the source of food, young monkeys spent more time on a warmer, more inviting terry-cloth surrogate. Counter to thinking that affectional bonds are based on association with food and other necessities, Harlow argued that "contact comfort" and the relationships that provide it are of value in and of themselves, not derivative of other needs [45]. A large body of subsequent research reinforces the idea that social support has direct and independent effects on health. For example, among healthy volunteers exposed to rhinoviruses and quarantined in a laboratory setting for 1 week, variety of social ties predicted symptom response [46]. In women with ovarian cancer, high levels of reported social support were associated with lower levels of factors associated with invasive and metastatic growth [47]. These demonstrations of fundamental roles of social connections are reflected in major epidemiological reviews [48, 49], showing the effects on mortality of social isolation to be comparable to cigarette smoking. More recently, the widespread isolation that has accompanied the worldwide COVID pandemic led to numerous reports of profound effects on psychology and emotions [50], bringing to everyday experience just how undermining social isolation can be [51].

The value of social support and the direct influence on important biological processes have important implications for PS programs. In addition to benefits through enhanced health behaviors, PS may directly influence disease processes. Thus, in addition to training supporters in skills for promoting self-management and behavior change, it may often be of value to encourage their simple availability and emotional support of those they help [52]. These aspects of "being there" may be of substantial value in health as well as quality of life.

Evidence Base of Peer Support

Multiple reviews have examined the evidence base of PS interventions for people with chronic conditions, most of which report moderate effect sizes in a variety of outcome domains. One review [53] focused on PS through community health worker interventions as a bridge between community members—especially hard-to-reach populations—and health care systems, and found "moderate" evidence for impacts on knowledge, health behaviors, utilization, and cost/cost effectiveness. Another review of PS for underserved groups in the United States [1] reported enhanced uptake in preventive services, such as mammography and cervical cancer screening. A 2014 review [54] identified the contributions of community health workers to basic health needs in low-income countries (e.g., reducing childhood undernutrition), to primary care and health promotion in middle-income countries, and to disease management in the United States and other countries with developed economies.

A comprehensive review conducted by Peers for Progress [55] included PS interventions from around the world, addressing a wide variety of prevention and health objectives entailing sustained behavior change (in contrast to relatively isolated acts such as cancer screening). Sixty-five papers (United States—34 papers, Canada—7, Bangladesh, England, Pakistan, and Scotland—4 each) included 12 from low-income, low-middle, and high-middle-income countries. They addressed a variety of health conditions including drug, alcohol, and tobacco addiction (3 papers), cardiovascular disease (10), diabetes (9), HIV/AIDS (6), other chronic diseases (12), maternal and child health (17), and mental health (8) [55]. Among 43 reporting RCT or other controlled designs and utilizing objective or standardized outcome measures, 31 (72.1%) reported significant between-condition effects favoring PS [55]. Additionally, across 19 reviews of peer support included in this systematic review, a median of 64.5% of studies reviewed reported significant effects of PS [55].

Thirty papers in the review focused on diabetes, among which 17 (56.7%) reported significant, between-group differences favoring PS. Among the 24 diabetes studies utilizing controlled designs and either objective and/or standardized outcome measures, 16 (66.7%) reported significant between-condition effects favoring PS. Among the 23 reporting changes in HbA1c among those receiving PS, the average reduction of HbA1c was 0.76 points ($p < 0.001$), for example, a reduction of 8.76% to 8%.

A recent review of reviews [56] on PS interventions for people with one or more chronic conditions found that, of the 31 studies included in the analysis, most reviews reported positive but non-significant effects on measured outcomes. Of the 51 outcome domains identified, quality of life and self-efficacy were the most common. Focusing on type 2 diabetes, another recent review and meta-analysis [57] found that PS integrated with diabetes self-management education significantly improves glycemic control.

PS interventions with smaller group sizes, shorter duration, and high frequency of contacts were associated with lower HbA1c levels.

Implementation and Dissemination Approaches

Engaging the Hardly Reached

PS can be effective in redressing the avoidable, costly, distressing, and ineffective care for those who are often not reached by clinical services. A systematic review of PS for those too often "hardly reached" found that 94% reported significant changes favoring peer support [58]. For example, peer asthma coaches were able to engage 89.7% of mothers of Medicaid-covered children who were hospitalized for asthma. The coaches sustained that engagement, averaging 21.1 contacts per parent over a two-year intervention, and reducing rehospitalization by 52% [8]. In a PS intervention for diabetes management among ethnic minority patients of safety net clinics in San Francisco [59], the impact of PS over usual care alone was *greatest* among those initially reporting low medication adherence and self-management [60]. Among US military veterans with diabetes [61], dyadic support led to improvements in blood glucose that were greatest among those with initially low levels of diabetes support or health literacy [62]. In Pakistan, PS for post-partum depression was most effective relative to controls among women with household debt and/or relatively low levels of economic empowerment [63].

Reaching Populations

Many studies of PS have focused on selected samples, shedding little light on the challenge of reaching populations. A collaboration of Alivio Medical Center, an Federally Qualified Health Center (FQHC) in Chicago, the National Council of La Raza, Peers for Progress, and the former TransforMed^{SM} sought to reach the entire population of an estimated 3500–4000 Latino adults with type 2 diabetes whom Alivio serves. The initiative, *Compañeros en Salud*, reached 88% of 471 patients considered as "High Need" (i.e., high HbA1c, distress or depression symptoms, viewed by their primary care providers as especially likely to benefit) [25]. Participants initially received biweekly phone calls, reduced to monthly, and then quarterly as progress warranted. *Compañeros* also engaged 82% of 3316 assigned to regular care that included group classes and activities and quarterly contacts via phone or during regular clinical appointments. Across all 3787 Alivio patients with diabetes, HbA1c declined from 8.22% to 8.14% ($p < 0.05$) over 2 years. Among patients in the High Need group, HbA1c declined from 9.43% to 9.16% ($p < 0.01$) and the proportion with moderate to good HbA1c control ($\leq 8\%$) increased from 19% to 26% [25]. Although modest in comparison to larger changes in smaller samples, these outcomes indicate PS may benefit populations of those with diabetes and other health problems.

Addressing Social Determinants of Health

Social determinants of health (SDOH) are the "conditions in the environments where people are born, live, learn, work, play, worship, and age that affect a wide range of health, functioning, and quality-of-life outcomes and risks" [64]. They can be grouped into five domains: economic stability, education access and quality, health care assess and quality, neighborhood and built environment, and social and community context. PS can help individuals solve their most immediate problems and access social services that can help them overcome barriers related to SDOH [65]. One systematic review [66] found that CHW programs have reduced inequities relating to place of residence, gender, education, and socio-economic position. Beyond individual-level interventions, PS can also address upstream factors at the community and policy levels through community mobilization and advocacy [67, 68]. Data from the 2014 National Community Health Worker Advocacy Survey [69] showed a significant, positive association between CHW advocacy and change in community conditions.

Academic-community partnerships are increasingly exploring ways to train, empower, and support CHWs in advocating for community changes and address SDOH. In the Acción para la Salud program, CHWs in Arizona conducted community advocacy to raise awareness about SDOH, identify neighborhood solutions, and create community opportunities [70]. Another program in Louisiana empowered community members to advocate for changes in community conditions through a CHW training curriculum focused on SDOH, leadership, and advocacy [71].

Reaching Out for Behavioral Health

Chronic disease is often accompanied by psychosocial and mental health problems including depression and anxiety disorders [72]. A broad range of factors influence psychological and physical health, from the epigenetic effects of early maternal care to the social and economic contexts of family and social relationships, and larger organizational, economic, and cultural factors [72]. Those disadvantaged across these determinants are likely to experience both physical and psychological problems and a disproportionate utilization of emergency and hospital services [72]. The importance of social contact and emotional support in general [73] as well as in psychopathology suggests that simple, frequent, affirming, and pleasant PS may be especially helpful to those with emotional distress [74]. Indeed, PS has been found to reduce distress and associated hospitalizations among adults with diabetes in Hong Kong [75]. "Lady Health Workers" in Pakistan implemented a cognitive-behavioral, problem-solving intervention that greatly reduced post-partum depression [76], while PS achieved reductions in the prevalence of depression and other common mental disorders and days out of work in India [77].

Schizophrenia is associated with challenges in daily living along with medication and symptom management. As such, peer support would appear to be an especially apt strategy, but research addressing it is sparse. A systematic review examining the effectiveness of peer support interventions on hospital admission, relapse, functioning, quality of life, death, and cost to society for people with schizophrenia identified only 13 studies for inclusion and only 2 of these specified measured outcomes [78]. Furthermore, many peer support interventions that reach people with schizophrenia are intended for a broader audience of people with a variety of serious mental illnesses. In a scoping review, only half of the 20 identified peer interventions focused exclusively on people with schizophrenia or related psychoses, while the remainder were delivered to mixed-diagnosis groups [38]. Careful attention to the unique needs of people with schizophrenia and tailoring program components to meet these needs may be warranted [38].

Notable exceptions to the general lack of evidence with schizophrenia provide promising findings of the utility of PS. For example, peer-led mutual support groups for people with schizophrenia and their families in China resulted in consistently greater improvements over 3 years in overall functioning and a reduction in duration and number of hospitalizations compared to standard care [79–82]. In this intervention, the peer supporters were family members of people with schizophrenia, highlighting the importance of cultural tailoring. Results from the systematic scoping review of the literature referenced above [38] showed that seven of nine studies measuring at least one key outcome (acute care utilization, patient functioning, positive or negative symptoms) found significant effects favoring peer-delivered intervention. Given the difficulty of addressing negative symptoms such as apathy and withdrawal, it is noteworthy that three of four studies measuring negative symptoms reported a reduction [38].

Cultural Considerations: Adaptable Standardization in China

Peers for Progress has carried out extensive collaboration with the Chinese Diabetes Society and other colleagues in China since 2011 [25]. Updating these activities, over 500 program managers, clinicians, and diabetes educators have been trained to develop and implement programs. Notably, training has included ongoing consultation by conference call to facilitate coping with problems in developing and implementing PS programs. The impact is reflected in over 35 programs being developed, the expansion of the section on patient education and management of the Chinese Diabetes Society [25], and a demonstration project of the Beijing Diabetes Prevention and Treatment Association that engaged 50 hospitals and community health centers (CHCs) and over 5000 individuals with diabetes [83].

One demonstration project in community health centers in Anhui province trained adults with diabetes to co-lead monthly informational and educational meetings with staff of community health centers [84]. In addition to informal support through neighborhood activities, peer leaders also led discussion groups that provided greater opportunity for participants to talk about self-management plans, obstacles encountered, and successes. The project achieved significant benefits relative to controls for knowledge, self-efficacy, blood pressure control, and both fasting and 2-h postprandial blood glucose [84].

The Shanghai Sixth People's Hospital (S6PH) has developed the Shanghai Integration Model (SIM) that improves patterns of care and clinical outcomes through integration of primary, specialty, and hospital care for diabetes. The project has been led by Professor Weiping Jia, who, at the time the project was developed, provided leadership as President of the S6PH and of the Chinese Diabetes Society. Under the umbrella of the SIM, peer support programs were developed in nine health centers with peer supporters leading group- and neighborhood-based activities, including those focused on diabetes management such as healthy diet, exercise, and regular clinical care, but also activities intended to create a sense of solidarity and community among those with diabetes [85]. Biometric and quality-of-life indicators showed improvement through the first 12 months of the program, especially among those with greater risk [85]. Further, these benefits were sustained after the intensive phase of program implementation and through 18 months from the start of the program [86].

Peer Support Applications in Primary Care

The Affordable Care Act and health care reform in the United States emphasize primary care and greater engagement of preventive services, effective chronic disease management, and timely access to appropriate care [87]. Within that framework, the Chronic Care Model (CCM) has been an important organizing framework that incorporates several elements: (1) organization of health care; (2) delivery system design; (3) decision support; (4) clinical information systems; (5) self-management support; and (6) community resources [88, 89]. Peer support (PS) can enhance CCM, especially through personalized care planning [90], providing self-management support, and accessing community resources [25]. For example, a study of primary care practices that demonstrated team-based primary care found that many incorporated health coaching that was often provided by medical assistants and lay people [91].

Although the evidence for PS is robust, the implementation and application in clinical care is evolving. The Baylor Health Care System used the CCM to integrate CHWs into primary care teams to address health inequities in five community clinics serving low-income Latino adults with diabetes [92, 93]. As part of system redesign, CHWs were recruited from medical assistants and were trained in general peer support skills and diabetes-specific information as part of clinical teams. Although they were part of those clinical teams, they reported to an offsite nurse manager who coordinated their work. CHWs and primary care providers indicated a number of ways in which the CHWs addressed key functions of PS, including self-management support and providing social and emotional support [92, 93].

In Appalachia, collaborators from Marshall University, several foundations, 11 Federally Qualified Health Centers, and 3 rural hospitals in southern Ohio, eastern Kentucky, and West Virginia established a model centered on a Chronic Care Management Team consisting of a nurse practitioner or physician's assistant, a nurse, and a community health worker (CHW) [94]. The team receives referrals from clinicians, insurers, or community programs and coordinates care with PCPs as it develops and executes care plans. A key component is the CHW who makes weekly home visits to review progress, identify challenges, and address barriers to care, such as assisting a woman with diabetes in securing a new refrigerator for her insulin. Reflecting the Peers for Progress key function of ongoing support, those receiving the CHW support strenuously objected to plans for its termination when their clinical statuses stabilized, so that the CHW support is now ongoing. Evaluation includes enrollment of 729 over 2.5 years from the 14 collaborating clinical sites. Among the 456 with diabetes, 282 (61.8%) reduced their HbA1c, reducing an average of 2.4 points, from a baseline mean of 10.3 to follow-up of 7.9%.

Additional applications of PS with the Chronic Care Model are noted in Table 9.1. In addition to self-management

Table 9.1 Examples of peer support in chronic care

Clinical condition (citation)	Interventions
Chronic kidney disease prevention in ethnic/racial minority and low SES groups [95]	PS as part of multidisciplinary team. Improved blood pressure control, knowledge, self-management behaviors (e.g., appointment keeping), and appropriate utilization of health services.
Macular degeneration [96, 97]	Chronic care coaches monitored treatment, including telephone reminders, patient information, self-management support, including patients' weekly self-administration of the Amsler test for monitoring vision problems, and action plan for dealing with symptoms, estimating severity, and reacting to deterioration.
African Americans with hypertension [154]	Patients with well-controlled hypertension provided self-management support for reducing blood pressure, CVD risks through three bimonthly phone calls over 6 months, alternating with staff visits. Calls addressed healthy diet, exercise, medication adherence, and smoking cessation.
Latino adults with diabetes in Federally Qualified Health Center [98]	Variety of activities for assistance in daily management (setting individual behavioral goals, developing strategies to overcome barriers, and feedback and support)
Practice redesign for pediatric asthma [155]	CHWs for outreach, encouraging engagement in care and follow-up. Program elements include quarterly visits, medication management, and attention to trigger exposures.
Smoking cessation initiated during hospital stays [156]	Quit-line counselors provided follow-up and communicated with primary care providers to integrate telephone counseling into ongoing care.

support and skills, PS included outreach and engagement in prevention and care, and interaction as part of the care team, such as the smoking cessation quit-line counselors communicating with PCPs to facilitate integration with ongoing care.

CCM applications often address individuals' needs for social and emotional support in general and management of chronic conditions. The study of prevention of kidney disease in Table 9.1 noted the contributions of peer support to providing social support [95]. Along these lines, a number of interventions included peer group meetings or support sessions that provide social support [96–98]. The study of team-based care also identified emotional support as among the contributions of medical assistants and lay people such as in conducting group visits [91].

An important dimension of clinical care teams can be recruiting staff and lay people from communities that they serve and establishing partnerships with community organizations. This can result in valuable ties among staff and lay people from communities, other members of the clinical team, community resources, and can be a base for advocacy around structural problems and social determinants of health [91]. In addition to helping individuals identify and gain access to care, peer support also provides a kind of advocacy to enhance the relationships between individuals and their care providers.

Organizational and Fiscal Considerations

There are organizational and fiscal challenges with incorporating PS in clinical environments [99]. The initial structure of PS in outpatient settings may begin with clinicians and team members identifying patients who may be suited to providing PS. Care must be taken, though, to avoid focusing on "model patients" who may provide "mastery" models rather than the "coping" models that are most effective in promoting new behaviors [100] and with whom others can identify. Peer supporters may be organized through clinical teams and/or as extensions of care managers [99]. Another approach is to introduce them through group patient-education programs [101] or through group medical visits. Peers have utilized skills learned in training for the Chronic Disease Self-Management Program [102] to provide a number of other services. PS programs can be based in community settings but with close ties to clinical providers [103]. For example, Columbia University and New York Presbyterian Health System developed a program that funded community-based organizations to offer PS services that were then coordinated with clinical care at the university health center [104].

Key considerations for organizing PS in primary care include communication and collaboration among organizational units, acceptance among clinical professionals, and supervision and quality control. Communication was highlighted in a study of community health workers and chronic care management [105]. In a study that expanded collaborative care for depression, CHWs noted problems with availability of and coordination with clinical resources ([106], p. S1-49). These challenges of integrating community outreach with clinical and other resources are especially a problem in mental health care. An assessment of services to address the diverse needs of those with mental health problems in North Carolina found a wide variety of types of available services, but sporadic availability and, most important, lack of systems for coordination of care [107].

Numerous informal reports and published studies have noted concerns and even opposition to PS among some clinicians, often centering around the potential for misinformation or harm, and alienation of patients from clinical care [108]. In a survey of pediatric providers' views on services for pediatric obesity, 100% indicated that it was very important (83.3%) or important to address obesity. Only 24%, however, thought they should be the ones to provide behavioral management interventions, opting instead for those to be implemented by a health educator or health coach [109]. The importance of clinical supervision and back up was illustrated in a study among Lady Health Workers in Pakistan. In response to low trust in their ability to address diarrhea and pneumonia and concern over their inability to provide medications [110], supportive mentorship including feedback cards was developed with supervisors. These were effective in raising trust and willingness to contact Lady Health Workers and also increased community members' perceptions of their skills in education and screening as well as providing appropriate medications [111].

The successful adoption of peer supporters in care teams can be tied to their incorporation as part of the routine system, not as an "add on." This is evidenced in the SUCCEED trial in which CHWs were paired with Advanced Practice Clinicians in a study of survivors of stroke and transient ischemic attacks [112]. The protocol was comprehensive in a combination of clinic and home visits, inclusion of psychosocial indicators, and flexibility in response to participants' needs. The intervention group surpassed controls in improvements in self-reported salt intake and C-reactive protein, but not with systolic blood pressure [113], attributable perhaps to mediocre participation. Among those offered the intervention, 89.6% had some participation but only 14.5% accepted the "full dose."

The way that peer support is organized may have major impacts on its pattern of benefits. A Peers for Progress report [114] included important observations from two projects in Mingo County, Georgia. One was community-based in a social service agency while the other was based in a health system. The former reached more people but with more modest average improvements in glucose control, while the clinic-based program reached fewer people but with greater average impacts. Clearly, what is the "right" approach will depend on the objectives and strategies of the program and its role within the organizations or communities that host it.

Financing PS Services. Financial models are critical to the adoption and sustained implementation of PS in clinical care. A conference led by Peers for Progress [114] identified both broad evidence for cost effectiveness of PS and several models for its financing. Among these, the Affordable Care Act (ACA) includes several provisions for financial support of PS, generally referred to as provided by CHWs. Among these provisions, the Health Home or Chronic Health Home [115] is a financing mechanism for a variety of supportive services for patients with chronic conditions. Many of the services outlined in the regulations could readily be carried out by peer supporters. The organization of such services is left for states to propose, creating the opportunity for a variety of organizational strategies in clinical as well as community settings.

The project in Appalachia described earlier and centered on Care Management Teams that include CHWs [94] has worked closely with insurers and managed care organizations (MCOs) to develop plans for financial sustainability of the program. As of 2020, two insurers had agreed with two Federally Qualified Health Centers (FQHCs) for an equitable payment model to support the program. Continued collaboration with payers, MCOs, and the FQHCs and hospitals is oriented toward preparing for value-based care as it emerges.

Other approaches to financing PS [99] include value-based reimbursement, in which clinical providers and health care systems would be able to support PS through enhanced quality incentives and by reducing avoidable health care costs. The Centennial Care initiative, for example, utilized capitated payment in New Mexico and stratified Medicaid beneficiaries into Level I (individuals with good to excellent health), Level II (those with long-term chronic disease or high cost conditions), and Level III (those with very complex health needs such as multiple chronic conditions, high hospitalization rates, high prescription drug use rates, and high emergency department usage) [116]. PS services are matched to each level and address health literacy challenges, such as navigating the health care system or understanding the importance of medication adherence, and non-clinical support such as assistance with transportation or obtaining food stamps. The highest-need individuals receive intensive individualized patient support services [116].

In the initiative, per member per month costs ranged from $321 for those receiving the intensive intervention to $5.75 for Levels I and II individuals receiving less intense, community-based services [116]. The long-term savings have been significant with an estimated ROI for a 3-year program of 1.5:1. This favorable financial analysis may be tied to PS services that mitigate the progression of beneficiaries to complex, high cost, and high utilizers. A 2018 simulation study that considered the savings of integrating CHWs in PCMHs to enhance attention to social determinants of health supports this assumption [117]. The simulation estimated that integration of CHWs would result in 7.1% annual savings relative to 1.7% for PCMH alone [117].

Peer Support and Health Information Technologies

Health information technologies (e.g., computer, mobile, web-based) have been studied for their potential to enhance, extend, and scale up peer support. These platforms create environments for the exchange of organic and/or structured peer support, provide patient education, encourage self-management behaviors, and collect and analyze patient data to deliver personalized messages and guide clinical decision-making [118]. Digital health technologies are able to respond in real-time, delivering support that is contextual, accessible, and convenient. Some people prefer digital modalities because they allow for the exchange of rich, thoughtful information and unique avenues of self-expression [119]. Additionally, digital health can facilitate PS across geographic distances, enabling those with rare diseases to find others with the same condition and improving access to support and affordability of care. A recent scoping review of web-based PS for people with chronic conditions found evidence for decreasing emotional distress and social isolation and increasing self-efficacy and health service navigation [120].

In both urban and more remote areas of Australia, Telephone Linked Care [121] provided messages and reminders that were personalized according to individual self-management and clinical measures, all monitored through data entered in patients' smartphones. Mean HbA1c values declined from 8.8% to 8.0% and were accompanied by improvements on quality-of-life indicators that exceeded those in a usual care control condition. Medication costs were lower as well: AUD $1542 versus AUD $1821 on average. A more recent version of this program using a smartphone, *My Diabetes Coach*, includes *Laura*, a "conversational agent" guiding users through modules addressing key components of diabetes management (e.g., healthy eating, medication). Individualized algorithms for projecting and guiding progress are also tailored according to recommendations of participants' PCPs. An effectiveness-implementation study [122] found good engagement and acceptability with users averaging 243 min of interaction over 12 months. Relative to controls, the intervention led to a significant improvement in health-related quality of life. Changes in HbA1c between the two groups were not significant, which was attributed to most participants beginning the study with HbA1c levels already meeting guidelines at less than 7%. Conversational agents such as Laura appear to have great potential to increase access and engage a wide range of users across a variety of health services, for example, screening, self-management, and home health care [123].

Online communities (e.g., forums, social media) are frequently consumer-driven networks whose purpose is to facilitate the exchange of peer support while providing linkages to health care professionals [124]. These online communities can be responsive to the needs of their members, leading to high levels of satisfaction. One review concluded that computer-mediated environments enhance an individual's ability to interact with peers while increasing the convenience of obtaining personalized support [125].

Technological developments in mobile phone applications (e.g., text messaging, mobile apps) can offer interactive features, monitoring tools, and personalized feedback that can enhance the quality of peer support interactions [126]. In collaboration with Vanguard Medical Group, a primary care practice in New Jersey, and WellDoc, a digital health company, Peers for Progress pilot tested a lay health coaching intervention enhanced with a diabetes self-management app (BlueStar™) [127]. Health coaches provided telephone-based diabetes self-management support and encouraged the routine use of BlueStar for day-to-day self-management tasks. Patient-generated data in BlueStar were shared with the health coaches and the care coordinators to guide highly personalized care. Patients that participated in the intervention made behavior changes and experienced a significant drop in HbA1c [128]. The most important observation from the study, however, may be the apparent complementarity of the high and low tech. The correlation between contacts with coaches and entries into the web app was 0.613, indicating complementarity rather than one substituting for the other. Additionally, participants' comments indicated complementarity, such as one participant who noted "it's okay because there [web app] you put numbers and whatever you are day-to-day. The coaching is different. … It's someone that you're listening to." Similarly, one of the coaches suggested the app "would be more of the day-to-day, and the role of the coaching would be … discuss things that maybe aren't so day-to-day" ([128] p. 7).

The complementarity of information technologies and PS has implications for comprehensive approaches to care. Offering both peer support and digital health increases patient choice depending on the support they need or prefer. Digital health can address the routine tasks and monitoring needed for chronic disease self-management, leaving peer supporters to provide highly individualized support for more complex problems. Digital platforms can extend peer support to more people and integrate the efficiencies of high tech with the humanizing force of personal contact [129]. Researchers are particularly interested in integrating digital health technologies for peer supporters that have the capacity to generate actionable data, prompt timely, context-sensitive outreach, and guide decision-making [130]. Such high tech/soft touch programs would be able to reach entire populations while maximizing the efforts of peer supporters and clinical staff.

Combining PS and digital health could provide tiered approaches to populations with a chronic disease. With diabetes, for example, patients who are well controlled may only be offered digital supports. Those with clinical or psychosocial indicators of mild concern might be offered the digital resources along with minimal PS to encourage adoption. Moderate concern might lead to more intensive peer support and encouragement of use of digital resources. Greater concern might then be met with intensive peer support focusing on self-management and other problems and using digital as ancillary resources [29].

Peer Support Workforce

Calls-to-action [131] and policy recommendations [132, 133] have repeatedly emphasized the importance of CHWs and peer supporters in chronic disease care. The World Health Organization's Global Health Workforce Alliance emphasized the essential role of CHWs in health care and the need for stronger integration at local and national levels [134]. In the United States, key agencies such as the Centers for Disease Control and Prevention [135] and the Health Resources and Services Administration [136] have encouraged the adoption of CHW interventions to address some of the country's most pressing public health concerns. The Affordable Care Act includes numerous provisions for supporting services of CHWs [137]. This near universal support of CHWs among public health authorities is a clear signal of a robust evidence base.

Selecting, training, supporting, compensating, and retaining the peer workforce is an enormous challenge. According to the US Bureau of Labor Statistics, there were roughly 61,000 people working as CHWs in 2021 [138]. Mental Health America estimates that there are over 24,000 mental health peer specialists in the United States [139]. For comparison, there were 715,600 social workers in the United States in 2020 [140]. These estimates of the US peer support workforce focus on the paraprofessional end of the PS continuum, and exclude the thousands of volunteers and part-time workers who contribute to chronic care. Using the world's estimated 387 million people with diabetes [141] as an example, if one CHW can serve 10 people, then 39 million will be required. If formal systems increase caseloads to 100 per CHW, nearly 4 million would still be needed.

The numbers of peer workers needed worldwide may appear overwhelming. But there are clear models for scaling up. In Thailand, Village Health Volunteers have been part of the public health system since 1978 [142, 143]: a system that spends US $296 per capita on health care (in 2019), relative to US $10,921 in the United States [144, 145]. In Pakistan, about 100,000 "Lady Health Workers" support maternal and child services through the primary care system that reaches an estimated 80% of Pakistan's rural population [76].

Formal training programs, including degree-granting programs through post-secondary education in the United States, are gaining popularity as an approach to increasing the peer support workforce. As with other professionals and recognized members of the health care team, the credentialing of CHWs will enhance the recognition and legitimacy not only of individuals credentialed, but of the field itself and the services it entails. However, areas of uncertainty remain about the importance of maintaining the "peerness" of those providing PS and the capacity of under-resourced organizations to manage the certification and maintenance of PS volunteers and/or staff [146]. Furthermore, for individuals that volunteer or work part-time, gaining and maintaining credentials may pose a barrier to entry and limit PS to the more "professionalized" end of the PS continuum.

In response, Peers for Progress and its collaborators have proposed model guidelines for the option of accrediting PS *programs* as a complement to individual credentialing [146]. Programs should be able to document the quality of their training, supervision, and services and then gain financial support for those services, without individuals working in the programs having to secure state certification or licensing. Additionally, credentialing of programs can promote high-quality implementation, deployment, and integration of PS that credentialing of individuals, alone, cannot provide. In mental health, the Council on Accreditation of Peer Recovery Support Services [147] provides program accreditation on a national level. Similarly, American Diabetes Association Education Recognition Program [148] credentials diabetes education programs based on the National Standards for Diabetes Self-Management Education and Support [13]. These types of structures are needed to ensure that organizations have the flexibility to engage a range of peer supporters and the ability to deploy them effectively.

Future Directions

Many peer support interventions and activities grew out of broader, community health promotion initiatives designed to recruit not only peers but a variety of community and social forces to promote healthy behaviors (e.g., [149, 150]). For example, the *Neighborhood Asthma Coalition* for asthma among children in predominantly African American neighborhoods of St. Louis [151] included as one program element *CASS workers* ("Change Asthma with Social Support," the name developed by neighborhood advisory groups). Amid other program features, contacts with CASS workers were predictive of reductions in the need for acute care health services [151].

The importance of community organization as the context for peer support is reflected in the growth of the PS program for diabetes management in Shanghai, described earlier. In its initial phase, implemented through nine community health centers (CHCs), the program showed benefits in biometric and quality-of-life indicators including through 18 months from program initiation [86]. Analyses, however, showed appreciable variation in outcomes linked to individual CHCs' level of implementation of the program [85]. This led to recognition that not all CHCs are able to host such a program effectively and, as a result, identification of other organizations that could be engaged in the program.

A second phase of the program in Shanghai is now implemented in 12 additional communities [152]. To broaden the community base for the program, sub-district or community level health staff are responsible for coordination and facilitation. This includes CHCs but also with Residential Committees, Community Self-Management Groups, and other community organizations. Residential Committees are government linked and responsible for guiding varied activities and implementation of government policies within their neighborhoods. Community Self-Management Groups, of which Shanghai includes about 6000, are composed of volunteers sharing a particular interest, such as hypertension control, diet, or diabetes. To provide content that any community group could implement, a first level of protocols includes just simple messages and materials that can be distributed without any special training. A second level includes group activities emphasizing diabetes management, and a third includes individual and family support requiring more extensive training and skills of peer supporters.

In the United States, peer support at the University of North Carolina at Chapel Hill (UNC-CH) began with a community organization approach to initiate and promote varied peer support activities addressing mental health challenges on campus [153]. At the time of initial challenges of COVID in March 2020, Peers for Progress staff began encouraging varied informal peer support groups and other activities. A presentation to the provost's regular meeting of deans and other campus leaders led to a meeting with representatives from several schools and other units to discuss how such activities could be broadened. Over the following 2 years, the *Carolina Peer Support Collaborative* (CPSC), named by its members, has grown to include representatives from over 50 schools, departments, offices, student and staff organizations, and other groups on campus.

Informal groups or "Pods" have formed among students identified by specific programs or majors, as well as pods defined by self-identification, such as an Asian, Asian-

American, and Pacific Islander pod for staff, students, and faculty; an early career faculty pod; or a pod for graduate students who are mothers. Peers for Progress staff have continued to consult widely across campus to encourage development of peer support activities as well as greater attention to existing peer support activities such as in sororities, fraternities, and other student organizations or in existing counseling and student services such as for "first gen" and BIPOC students. Under this umbrella, two student peer support programs have emerged. One, *Peer to Peer*, was developed and continues to be led by students (uncpeer2peer.com) and provides telephone support. A website provides access to the program and includes descriptions of peer responders with whom students can request linkage. A second program called *LSN* (listen, support, navigate) was developed with campus stakeholders utilizing a "Heels Care Network" website (care. unc.edu) that integrates information about mental health and well-being. As trained peer support volunteers, LSNers staff an online chat resource that is available at scheduled times suited to students' activity patterns throughout the week.

The overlap of peer support and community approaches to health promotion illustrates just one portion of the broad range of potential approaches to establishing and sustaining PS programs. The field has moved beyond providing evidence of efficacy to emerging research that is focusing on application, adoption, and sustained implementation. As shown here, knowledge is growing about how to define PS to support "bending the curve" of health care. We now need to address how to tailor PS to different problems, populations, and settings; what organizational and management structures it requires; and how to pay for it [114]. The fundamental importance of social connections in human behavior and health and the bulk of evidence on PS make clear that its contributions can be substantial.

Acknowledgments Hannah Barker and Caroline Carpenter provided broad, skillful, and invaluable contributions to the development of the peer support activities at the University of North Carolina at Chapel Hill described in this chapter. Preparation of this chapter has been supported by the Michigan-UNC Peer Support Research Core of the Michigan Center for Diabetes Translational Research (P30DK092926 from the National Institute of Diabetes and Digestive and Kidney Diseases, PI: William Herman) and by funding from the Merck Foundation, Sanofi China, Novo Nordisk, and the Shanghai Municipal Government and the Shanghai Health Bureau.

References

1. Gibbons MC, Tyus NC. Systematic review of U.S.-based randomized controlled trials using community health workers. Prog Community Health Partnersh. 2007;1(4):371–81.
2. Solomon P. Peer support/peer provided services: underlying processes, benefits, and critical ingredients. Psychiatr Rehabil J. 2004;27:392–401.
3. Davidson L, Chinman M, Kloos B, Weingarten R, Stayner D, Tebes JK. Peer support among individuals with severe mental illness: a review of the evidence. Clin Psychol Sci Pract. 1999;6(2):165–87.
4. Parry M, Watt-Watson J. Peer support intervention trials for individuals with heart disease: a systematic review. Eur J Cardiovasc Nurs. 2010;9(1):57–67.
5. Brownson CA, Heisler M. The role of peer support in diabetes care and self-management. Patient. 2009;2(1):5–17.
6. Dunn J, Steginga SK, Rosoman N, Millichap D. A review of peer support in the context of cancer. J Psychosoc Oncol. 2003;21(2):55–67.
7. Fisher EB, Brownson CA, O'Toole ML, Shetty G, Anwuri VV, Glasgow RE. Ecologic approaches to self-management: the case of diabetes. Am J Public Health. 2005;95(9):1523–35.
8. Fisher EB, Strunk RC, Highstein GR, Kelley-Sykes R, Tarr KL, Trinkaus K, et al. A randomized controlled evaluation of the effect of community health workers on hospitalization for asthma: the asthma coach. Arch Pediatr Adolesc Med. 2009;163(3):225–32.
9. Krieger J. Home visits for asthma: we cannot afford to wait any longer. Arch Pediatr Adolesc Med. 2009;163(3):279.
10. Whitley EM, Everhart RM, Wright RA. Measuring return on investment of outreach by community health workers. J Health Care Poor Underserved. 2006;17(1 Suppl):6–15.
11. Woolf SH. A closer look at the economic argument for disease prevention. JAMA. 2009;301(5):536–8.
12. Davis KL, O'Toole ML, Brownson CA, Llanos P, Fisher EB. Teaching how, not what: the contributions of community health workers to diabetes self-management. Diabetes Educ. 2007;33(Suppl 6):208S–15S.
13. Davis J, Fischl AH, Beck J, Browning L, Carter A, Condon JE, et al. 2022 National Standards for diabetes self-management education and support. Diabetes Care. 2022;45(2):484–94.
14. Norris SL, Chowdhury FM, Van Let K, Horsley T, Brownstein JN, Zhang X, et al. Effectiveness of community health workers in the care of persons with diabetes. Diabet Med. 2006;23:544–56.
15. Swider SM. Outcome effectiveness of community health workers: an integrative literature review. Public Health Nurs. 2002;19:11–20.
16. Andrews JO, Felton G, Wewers ME, Heath J. Use of community health workers in research with ethnic minority women. J Nurs Scholarsh. 2004;36(4):358–65.
17. Colella TJF, King KM. Peer support. An under-recognized resource in cardiac recovery. Eur J Cardiovasc Nurs. 2004;3(3):211–7.
18. Haines A, Sanders D, Lehmann U, Rowe AK, Lawn JE, Jan S, et al. Achieving child survival goals: potential contribution of community health workers. Lancet. 2007;369(9579):2121–31.
19. Brownstein JN, Chowdhury FM, Norris SL, Horsley T, Jack L. Effectiveness of community health workers in the care of people with hypertension. Am J Prev Med. 2007;32(5):435–47.
20. Hoey LM, Ieropoli SC, White VM, Jefford M. Systematic review of peer-support programs for people with cancer. Patient Educ Couns. 2008;70(3):315–37.
21. Cherrington A, Ayala GX, Amick H, Allison J, Corbie-Smith G, Scarinci I. Implementing the community health worker model within diabetes management: challenges and lessons learned from programs across the United States. Diabetes Educ. 2008;34(5):824–33.
22. Postma J, Karr C, Kieckhefer G. Community health workers and environmental interventions for children with asthma: a systematic review. J Asthma. 2009;46(6):564–76.
23. Boothroyd RI, Fisher EB. Peers for progress: promoting peer support for health around the world. Fam Pract. 2010;27(Suppl 1):i62–8.
24. Fisher EB, Ayala GX, Ibarra L, Cherrington AL, Elder JP, Tang TS, et al. Contributions of peer support to health, health care,

and prevention: papers from peers for Progress. Ann Fam Med. 2015;13(Suppl 1):S2–8.
25. Fisher EB, Ballesteros J, Bhushan N, Coufal MM, Kowitt SD, McDonough AM, et al. Key features of peer support in chronic disease prevention and management. Health Aff (Millwood). 2015;34(9):1523–30.
26. Fisher EB, Bhushan N, Coufal MM, Kowitt S, Parada H, Sokol RL, et al. Peer support in prevention, chronic disease management, and well being. In: Fisher EB, Cameron LD, Christensen AJ, Ehlert U, Guo Y, Oldenburg B, et al., editors. Principles and concepts of behavioral medicine: a global handbook. New York: Springer; 2018.
27. Lorig K, Ritter PL, Plant K. A disease-specific self-help program compared with a generalized chronic disease self-help program for arthritis patients. Arthritis Rheum. 2005;53(6):950–7.
28. Earp JA, Eng E, O'Malley MS, Altpeter M, Rauscher G, Mayne L, et al. Increasing use of mammography among older, rural African American women: results from a community trial. Am J Public Health. 2002;92(4):646–54.
29. World Health Organization. Peer support programmes in diabetes: report of a WHO consultation. Geneva: World Health Organization; 2008.
30. Fisher EB, Boothroyd RI, Coufal MM, Baumann LC, Mbanya JC, Rotheram-Borus MJ, et al. Peer support for self-management of diabetes improved outcomes in international settings. Health Aff (Millwood). 2012;31(1):130–9.
31. Fisher EB, Earp JA, Maman S, Zolotor A. Cross-cultural and international adaptation of peer support for diabetes management. Fam Pract. 2010;27(Suppl 1):i6–i16.
32. Hawe P, Shiell A, Riley T. Complex interventions: how "out of control" can a randomised controlled trial be? BMJ. 2004;328(7455):1561–3.
33. Aro A, Smith J, Dekker J. Contextual evidence in clinical medicine and health promotion. The European Journal of Public Health. 2008;18(6):548.
34. Evans M, Tang PY, Bhushan N, Fisher EB, Dreyer Valovcin D, Castellano C. Standardization and adaptability for dissemination of telephone peer support for high-risk groups: general evaluation and lessons learned. Transl Behav Med. 2020;10(3):506–15.
35. Fisher EB, Tang PY, Evans M, Bhushan N, Graham MA, Dreyer D, et al. The fundamental value of presence in peer and mutual support: observations from telephone support for high risk groups. The global journal of community psychology. Practice. 2020;11(2)
36. Castellano C. Reciprocal peer support (RPS): a decade of not so random acts of kindness. Int J Emerg Ment Health. 2012;14(2):105–10.
37. Evans MS. Peer-delivered services and support reaching people with schizophrenia: considerations for research and practice. In: Hill UoNCaC, editor. Doctoral Dissertation; 2022.
38. Evans BA, Barker H, Peddireddy S, Zhang A, Luu S, Qian Y, et al. Peer-delivered services and peer support reaching people with schizophrenia: a scoping review. Int J Ment Health. 2021; https://doi.org/10.1080/00207411.2021.1975441.
39. Eng E, Parker E, Harlan C. Lay health advisor intervention strategies: a continuum from natural helping to paraprofessional helping. Health Educ Behav. 1997;24(4):413–7.
40. Tang PY, Fisher EB. The peer workforce in chronic care: lessons and observations from peers for progress. N C Med J. 2021;82(5):357–61.
41. Davidson L, Bellamy C, Guy K, Miller R. Peer support among persons with severe mental illnesses: a review of evidence and experience. World Psychiatry. 2012;11(2):123–8.
42. Clay S, Schell B, Corrigan PW, Ralph RO, editors. On our own, together: peer programs for people with mental illness. Nashville, TN: Vanderbilt University Press; 2005.
43. Campbell J. The historical and philosophical development of peer-run support programs. In: Clay S, Schell B, Corrigan PW, Ralph RO, editors. On our own, together: peer programs for people with mental illness. Nashville, TN: Vanderbilt University Press; 2005.
44. Carkhuff RR, Truax CB. Lay mental health counseling. The effects of lay group counseling. J Consult Psychol. 1965;29(5):26–31.
45. Harlow HF. The nature of love. Am Psychol. 1958;13:673–85.
46. Cohen S, Doyle WJ, Skoner DP, Rabin BS, Gwaltney JM. Social ties and susceptibility to the common cold. J Am Med Assoc. 1997;277(24):1940–4.
47. Lutgendorf SK, Lamkin DM, Jennings NB, Arevalo JM, Penedo F, DeGeest K, et al. Biobehavioral influences on matrix metalloproteinase expression in ovarian carcinoma. Clin Cancer Res. 2008;14(21):6839–46.
48. House JS, Landis KR, Umberson D. Social relationships and health. Science. 1988;241:540–4.
49. Holt-Lunstad J, Smith TB, Baker M, Harris T, Stephenson D. Loneliness and social isolation as risk factors for mortality: a meta-analytic review. Perspect Psychol Sci. 2015;10(2):227–37.
50. Collaborators C-MD. Global prevalence and burden of depressive and anxiety disorders in 204 countries and territories in 2020 due to the COVID-19 pandemic. Lancet. 2021;398(10312):1700–12.
51. Fisher EB, Barreiro-Rosado JA, Carpenter C, Evans MS, Luu SL, Rams AR, et al. Social isolation and loneliness: ubiquity, complexity, importance. In: Revenson TA, Abraido-Lanza AF, editors. Handbook of health psychology, vol. 3. Washington, D.C.: American Psychological Association; 2023.
52. Green L, Fisher EB. Economic substitutability: some implications for health behavior. In: Bickel WK, Vuchinich RE, editors. Reframing health behavior change with behavioral economics. Mahwah, NJ: Lawrence Erlbaum Associates; 2000. p. 115–44.
53. Viswanathan M, Kraschnewski JL, Nishikawa B, Morgan LC, Honeycutt AA, Thieda P, et al. Outcomes and costs of community health worker interventions: a systematic review. Med Care. 2010;48(9):792–808.
54. Perry HB, Zulliger R, Rogers MM. Community health workers in low-, middle-, and high-income countries: an overview of their history, recent evolution, and current effectiveness. Annu Rev Public Health. 2014;35:399–421.
55. Fisher EB, Boothroyd RI, Elstad EA, Hays L, Henes A, Maslow GR, et al. Peer support of complex health Behaviors in prevention and disease management with special reference to diabetes: systematic reviews. Clin Diabetes Endocrinol. 2017;3(4)
56. Thompson DM, Booth L, Moore D, Mathers J. Peer support for people with chronic conditions: a systematic review of reviews. BMC Health Serv Res. 2022;22(1):427.
57. Azmiardi A, Murti B, Febrinasari RP, Tamtomo DG. The effect of peer support in diabetes self-management education on glycemic control in patients with type 2 diabetes: a systematic review and meta-analysis. Epidemiol Health. 2021;43:e2021090.
58. Sokol R, Fisher E. Peer support for the hardly reached: a systematic review. Am J Public Health. 2016;106(7):1308.
59. Thom DH, Ghorob A, Hessler D, De Vore D, Chen E, Bodenheimer TA. Impact of peer health coaching on glycemic control in low-income patients with diabetes: a randomized controlled trial. Ann Fam Med. 2013;11(2):137–44.
60. Moskowitz D, Thom DH, Hessler D, Ghorob A, Bodenheimer T. Peer coaching to improve diabetes self-management: which patients benefit most? J Gen Intern Med. 2013;28(7):938–42.
61. Heisler M, Vijan S, Makki F, Piette JD. Diabetes control with reciprocal peer support versus nurse care management: a randomized trial. Ann Intern Med. 2010;153(8):507–15.
62. Piette JD, Resnicow K, Choi H, Heisler M. A diabetes peer support intervention that improved glycemic control: mediators and moderators of intervention effectiveness. Chronic Illn. 2013;9(4):258–67.
63. Rahman A, Sikander S, Malik A, Ahmed I, Tomenson B, Creed F. Effective treatment of perinatal depression for women in debt

and lacking financial empowerment in a low-income country. Br J Psychiatry. 2012;201(6):451–7.
64. Office of Disease Prevention and Health Promotion. Social Determinants of Health: Office of the Assistant Secretary for Health, Office of the Secretary, U.S. Department of Health and Human Services. https://health.gov/healthypeople/priority-areas/social-determinants-health.
65. Schechter SB, Lakhaney D, Peretz PJ, Matiz LA. Community health worker intervention to address social determinants of health for children hospitalized with asthma. Hosp Pediatr. 2021;11(12):1370–6.
66. McCollum R, Gomez W, Theobald S, Taegtmeyer M. How equitable are community health worker programmes and which programme features influence equity of community health worker services? A systematic review. BMC Public Health. 2016;16:419.
67. Perez LM, Martinez J. Community health workers: social justice and policy advocates for community health and well-being. Am J Public Health. 2008;98(1):11–4.
68. Heisler M, Tang PY, Fisher EB. Working conference on peer support and social determinants of health. Ann Arbor, MI: Michigan-UNC Peer Support Research Core, Michigan Center for Diabetes Translational Research; 2019.
69. Sabo S, Flores M, Wennerstrom A, Bell ML, Verdugo L, Carvajal S, et al. Community health workers promote civic engagement and organizational capacity to impact policy. J Community Health. 2017;42(6):1197–203.
70. Ingram M, Schachter KA, Sabo SJ, Reinschmidt KM, Gomez S, De Zapien JG, et al. A community health worker intervention to address the social determinants of health through policy change. J Prim Prev. 2014;35(2):119–23.
71. Wennerstrom A, Silver J, Pollock M, Gustat J. Action to improve social determinants of health: outcomes of leadership and advocacy training for community residents. Health Promot Pract. 2022;23(1):137–46.
72. Fisher EB, Chan JCN, Kowitt S, Nan H, Sartorius N, Oldenburg B. Conceptual perspectives on the co-occurrence of mental and physical disease: diabetes and depression as a model. In: Sartorius N, Maj M, Holt R, editors. Comorbidity of mental and physical disorders. Basel: Karger; 2015.
73. Harlow HF, Harlow M. Learning to love. Am Sci. 1966;54:244–72.
74. Pfeiffer PN, Heisler M, Piette JD, Rogers MA, Valenstein M. Efficacy of peer support interventions for depression: a meta-analysis. Gen Hosp Psychiatry. 2011;33(1):29–36.
75. Chan JC, Sui Y, Oldenburg B, Zhang Y, Chung HH, Goggins W, et al. Effects of telephone-based peer support in patients with type 2 diabetes mellitus receiving integrated care: a randomized clinical trial. JAMA Intern Med. 2014;174(6):972–81.
76. Rahman A, Malik A, Sikander S, Roberts C, Creed F. Cognitive behaviour therapy-based intervention by community health workers for mothers with depression and their infants in rural Pakistan: a cluster-randomised controlled trial. Lancet. 2008;372(9642):902–9.
77. Patel V, Weiss HA, Chowdhary N, Naik S, Pednekar S, Chatterjee S, et al. Lay health worker led intervention for depressive and anxiety disorders in India: impact on clinical and disability outcomes over 12 months. Br J Psychiatry. 2011;199(6):459–66.
78. Chien WT, Clifton AV, Zhao S, Lui S. Peer support for people with schizophrenia or other serious mental illness. Cochrane Database Syst Rev. 2019;4
79. Chien W-T, Norman I. The effectiveness and active ingredients of mutual support groups for family caregivers of people with psychotic disorders: a literature review. Int J Nurs Stud. 2009;46(12):1604–23.
80. Chien W-T, Thompson DR, Norman I. Evaluation of a peer-led mutual support group for Chinese families of people with schizophrenia. Am J Community Psychol. 2008;42(1–2, 122):–34.
81. Chien WT. Effectiveness of psychoeducation and mutual support group program for family caregivers of Chinese people with schizophrenia. Open Nurs J. 2008;2:28.
82. Chien WT, Thompson DR. An RCT with three-year follow-up of peer support groups for Chinese families of persons with schizophrenia. Psychiatr Serv. 2013;64(10):997–1005.
83. Wang Q. Diabetics help each other treat disease. China Daily; 2012 November 15, 2012.
84. Zhong X, Wang Z, Fisher EB, Tanasugarn C. Peer support for diabetes management in primary care and community settings in Anhui Province, China. Ann Fam Med. 2015;13(Suppl 1):S50–8.
85. Liu Y, Wu X, Cai C, Tang PY, Coufal MM, Qian Y, et al. Peer support in Shanghai's commitment to diabetes and chronic disease self-management: program development, program expansion, and policy. Transl Behav Med. 2020;10(1):13–24.
86. Liu Y, Cai C, Wu X, Tang PY, Coufal MM, Qian Y, et al. Eighteen month follow up of peer support for diabetes management in shanghai integration model. New Orleans: American Diabetes Association; 2022.
87. Peers for Progress. Opportunities for peer support in the affordable care act; 2014.
88. Wagner EH, Austin BT, Davis C, Hindmarsh M, Schaefer J, Bonomi A. Improving chronic illness care: translating evidence into action. Health Aff (Millwood). 2001;20:54–78.
89. Wagner EH, Austin BT, Von Korff M. Organizing care for patients with chronic illness. Milbank Q. 1996;74:511–44.
90. Bolton RE, Bokhour BG, Hogan TP, Luger TM, Ruben M, Fix GM. Integrating personalized care planning into primary care: a multiple-case study of early adopting patient-centered medical homes. J Gen Intern Med. 2020;35(2):428–36.
91. Wagner EH, Flinter M, Hsu C, Cromp D, Austin BT, Etz R, et al. Effective team-based primary care: observations from innovative practices. BMC Fam Pract. 2017;18(1):13.
92. Collinsworth AW, Vulimiri M, Snead C, Walton J. Community health workers in primary care practice: redesigning health care delivery systems to extend and improve diabetes care in underserved populations. Health Promot Pract. 2014;15(2 Suppl):51S–61S.
93. Collinsworth AW, Vulimiri M, Schmidt KL, Snead CA. Effectiveness of a community health worker-led diabetes self-management education program and implications for CHW involvement in care coordination strategies. Diabetes Educ. 2013;39(6):792–9.
94. Crespo R, Christiansen M, Tieman K, Wittberg R. An emerging model for community health worker-based chronic care management for patients with high health care costs in rural Appalachia. Prev Chronic Dis. 2020;17:E13.
95. Greer R, Boulware LE. Reducing CKD risks among vulnerable populations in primary care. Adv Chronic Kidney Dis. 2015;22(1):74–80.
96. Frei A, Woitzek K, Wang M, Held U, Rosemann T. The chronic care for age-related macular degeneration study (CHARMED): study protocol for a randomized controlled trial. Trials. 2011;12:221.
97. Markun S, Dishy A, Neuner-Jehle S, Rosemann T, Frei A. The Chronic Care for Wet Age Related Macular Degeneration (CHARMED) study: a randomized controlled trial. PLoS One. 2015;10(11):e0143085.
98. Liebman J, Heffernan D, Sarvela P. Establishing diabetes self-management in a community health center serving low-income Latinos. Diabetes Educ. 2007;33(Suppl 6):132S–8S.
99. Daaleman TP, Fisher EB. Enriching patient-Centered medical homes through peer support. Ann Fam Med. 2015;13(Suppl 1):S73–8.
100. Meichenbaum DH. Examination of model characteristics in avoidance behavior. J Pers Soc Psychol. 1971;17:298–307.
101. Thanh DTN, Deoisres W, Keeratiyutawong P, Baumann LC. Effectiveness of a diabetes self-management support inter-

102. Lorig KR, Ritter P, Stewart AL, Sobel DS, William Brown B, Bandura A, et al. Chronic disease self-management program: 2-year health status and health care utilization outcomes. Med Care. 2001;39:1217–23.
103. Ingram M, Torres E, Redondo F, Bradford G, Wang C, O'Toole ML. The impact of promotoras on social support and glycemic control among members of a farmworker community on the US-Mexico border. Diabetes Educ. 2007;33(Suppl 6):172S–8S.
104. Findley S, Rosenthal M, Bryant-Stephens T, Damitz M, Lara M, Mansfield C, et al. Community-based care coordination: practical applications for childhood asthma. Health Promot Pract. 2011;12(6 Suppl 1):52S–62S.
105. Polletta VL, LeBron AMW, Sifuentes MR, Mitchell-Bennett LA, Ayala C, Reininger BM. Facilitators and barriers of a chronic care management intervention addressing diabetes among Mexican-origin adults. Health Educ Behavior. 2021;48(6):831–41.
106. Wennerstrom A, Vannoy SD 3rd, Allen CE, Meyers D, O'Toole E, Wells KB, et al. Community-based participatory development of a community health worker mental health outreach role to extend collaborative care in post-Katrina New Orleans. Ethn Dis. 2011;21(3 Suppl 1):S1-45–51.
107. Rusch ALF, Fisher EB. Comprehensive mental health care in North Carolina: key functions and availability. Chapel Hill, North Carolina: Peers for Progress and Gillings School of Global Public Health, University of North Carolina-Chapel Hill; 2017.
108. Brodar K, Carlisle V, Tang YP, Fisher EB. Program managers' report of implementation challenges and strategies for peer support programs in cancer. Annual meeting of the Society of Behavioral Medicine, April; New Orleans; 2018.
109. Rhee KE, Kessl S, Lindback S, Littman M, El-Kareh RE. Provider views on childhood obesity management in primary care settings: a mixed methods analysis. BMC Health Serv Res. 2018;18(1):55.
110. Aftab W, Shipton L, Rabbani F, Sangrasi K, Perveen S, Zahidie A, et al. Exploring health care seeking knowledge, perceptions and practices for childhood diarrhea and pneumonia and their context in a rural Pakistani community. BMC Health Serv Res. 2018;18(1):44.
111. Rabbani F, Khan HA, Piryani S, Pradhan NA, Shaukat N, Feroz AS, et al. Changing perceptions of rural frontline workers and caregivers about management of childhood diarrhea and pneumonia despite several inequities: the Nigraan plus trial in Pakistan. J Multidiscip Healthc. 2021;14:3343–55.
112. Towfighi A, Cheng EM, Ayala-Rivera M, McCreath H, Sanossian N, Dutta T, et al. Randomized controlled trial of a coordinated care intervention to improve risk factor control after stroke or transient ischemic attack in the safety net: Secondary stroke prevention by Uniting Community and Chronic care model teams Early to End Disparities (SUCCEED). BMC Neurol. 2017;17(1):24.
113. Towfighi A, Cheng EM, Ayala-Rivera M, Barry F, McCreath H, Ganz DA, et al. Effect of a coordinated community and chronic care model team intervention vs usual care on systolic blood pressure in patients with stroke or transient ischemic attack: the SUCCEED randomized clinical trial. JAMA Netw Open. 2021;4(2):e2036227.
114. Peers for Progress. Economic analysis in peer support: breadth of approaches and implications for peer support programs. American Academy of Family Physicians Foundation; 2014. http://peersforprogress.org/wp-content/uploads/2015/04/150417-economic-analysis-in-peer-support.pdf
115. Medicaid.Gov. Health Homes. https://www.medicaid.gov/medicaid/ltss/health-homes/index.html.
116. Kaufman A, Alfero C, Moffett M, Page-Reeves J, Nkouaga C. "Upstream" community health workers: a white paper on developing economic evaluation of an innovative payment model; 2014.
117. Moffett ML, Kaufman A, Bazemore A. Community health workers bring cost savings to patient-centered medical homes. J Community Health. 2018;43(1):1–3.
118. Greenwood DA, Gee PM, Fatkin KJ, Peeples M. A systematic review of reviews evaluating technology-enabled diabetes self-management education and support. J Diabetes Sci Technol. 2017;11(5):1015–27.
119. Wright K. Social networks, interpersonal social support, and health outcomes: a health communication perspective. Frontiers. Communication. 2016:1.
120. Hossain SN, Jaglal SB, Shepherd J, Perrier L, Tomasone JR, Sweet SN, et al. Web-based peer support interventions for adults living with chronic conditions: scoping review. JMIR Rehabil Assist Technol. 2021;8(2):e14321.
121. Williams ED, Bird D, Forbes AW, Russell A, Ash S, Friedman R, et al. Randomised controlled trial of an automated, interactive telephone intervention (TLC diabetes) to improve type 2 diabetes management: baseline findings and six-month outcomes. BMC Public Health. 2012;12:602.
122. Gong E, Baptista S, Russell A, Scuffham P, Riddell M, Speight J, et al. My diabetes coach, a mobile app-based interactive conversational agent to support type 2 diabetes self-management: randomized effectiveness-implementation trial. J Med Internet Res. 2020;22(11):e20322.
123. Dingler T, Kwasnicka D, Wei J, Gong E, Oldenburg B. The use and promise of conversational agents in digital health. Yearb Med Inform. 2021;30(1):191–9.
124. Cotter AP, Durant N, Agne AA, Cherrington AL. Internet interventions to support lifestyle modification for diabetes management: a systematic review of the evidence. J Diabetes Complicat. 2014;28(2):243–51.
125. Lewinski AA, Fisher EB. Social interaction in type 2 diabetes computer-mediated environments: how inherent features of the channels influence peer-to-peer interaction. Chronic Illn. 2016;12(2):116–44.
126. Quinn CC, Shardell MD, Terrin ML, Barr EA, Ballew SH, Gruber-Baldini AL. Cluster-randomized trial of a mobile phone personalized behavioral intervention for blood glucose control. Diabetes Care. 2011;34(9):1934–42.
127. Kowitt SD, Tang PY, Peeples M, Duni J, Peskin S, Fisher EB. Combining the high tech with the soft touch: population health management using eHealth and peer support. Popul Health Manag. 2016;20:3–5.
128. Tang PY, Duni J, Peeples MM, Kowitt SD, Bhushan N, Sokol RL, et al. Complementarity of digital health and peer support: "this is what's coming". Front Clin Diabetes Healthcare. 2021;2 https://doi.org/10.3389/fcdhc.2021.646963.
129. Lauckner HM, Hutchinson SL. Peer support for people with chronic conditions in rural areas: a scoping review. Rural Remote Health. 2016;16(1):3601.
130. Aikens JE, Zivin K, Trivedi R, Piette JD. Diabetes self-management support using mHealth and enhanced informal caregiving. J Diabetes Complicat. 2014;28(2):171–6.
131. Center for Health Law and Policy Innovation at Harvard Law School, National Council of La Raza (NCLR), Peers for Progress, Society of Behavioral Medicine. Call to action: integrating peer support in prevention and health care under the affordable care act; 2015.
132. Purington K. Using peers to support physical and mental health integration for adults with serious mental illness. National Academy for State Health Policy; 2016.
133. Mental Health America. Position statement 37: peer support services; 2013.
134. Global Health Workforce Alliance. Global experience of community health workers for delivery of health related millennium development goals: a systematic review, country case studies, and

recommendations for integration into National Health Systems. Geneva: World Health Organization; 2010.
135. CDC. Addressing chronic disease through community health workers: a policy and systems-level approach; 2011.
136. Health Resources and Services Administration. Community health workers evidence-based models toolbox. HRSA Office of Rural Health Policy: US Department of Health and Human Services; 2011.
137. Islam N, Nadkarni SK, Zahn D, Skillman M, Kwon SC, Trinh-Shevrin C. Integrating community health workers within Patient Protection and Affordable Care Act implementation. J Public Health Manag Pract. 2015;21(1):42–50.
138. Bureau of Labor Statistics. Occupational employment and wages, May 2021, 21-1094 Community Health Worker; 2022.
139. Mental Health America. What is a Peer?; 2017. http://www.mentalhealthamerica.net/conditions/what-peer.
140. Bureau of Labor Statistics. Occupational outlook handbook, social workers; 2022.
141. International Diabetes Federation. IDF Diabetes Atlas. Brussels, Belgium: International Diabetes Federation; 2019.
142. Bhutta Z, Lassi Z, Pariyo G, Huicho L. Global experience of community health workers for delivery of health related millennium development goals: a systematic review, country case studies, and recommendations for integration into national health systems. Geneva: Global Health Workforce Alliance; 2010.
143. Kowitt SD, Emmerling D, Fisher EB, Tanasugarn C. Community health workers as agents of health promotion: Analyzing Thailand's village health volunteer program. J Community Health. 2015;40(4):780–8.
144. World Health Organization. Global Health Expenditure Database; 2022.
145. World Bank. Health expenditure per capita (current US$). http://data.worldbank.org/indicator/SH.XPD.PCAP.
146. Center for Health Law and Policy Innovation at Harvard Law School, National Council of La Raza (NCLR), Peers for Progress. Recommended model guidelines for credentialing community health worker programs and community health workers; 2015.
147. Council on Accreditation of Peer Recovery Support Services. Council on Accreditation of Peer Recovery Support Services Washington, D.C.; 2022. https://caprss.org/.
148. American Diabetes Association. Education Recognition Program; 2022. https://professional.diabetes.org/diabetes-education.
149. Linnan L, Fisher EB, Hood S. The power and potential of peer support in workplace interventions. Am J Health Promot. 2013;28(1):TAHP2–10.
150. Fisher EB Jr, Auslander W, Sussman L, Owens N, Jackson-Thompson J. Community organization and health promotion in minority neighborhoods. Ethn Dis. 1992;2(3):252–72.
151. Fisher EB, Strunk RC, Sussman LK, Sykes RK, Walker MS. Community organization to reduce the need for acute care for asthma among African American children in low-income neighborhoods: the neighborhood asthma coalition. Pediatrics. 2004;114:116–23.
152. Evans M, Liu Y, Wu X, Cai C, Tang PT, Coufal MM, et al. Community organization guides standardization, adaptability, and innovation: lessons from peer support in the Shanghai integration model. Under Review.
153. Fisher E, Luu S, Tang P, Barker H, Carpenter C, editors. Leveraging peer support for student, staff, and faculty mental health at the University of North Carolina at Chapel Hill. San Diego: American College Health Association; 2022.
154. Turner BJ, Hollenbeak CS, Liang Y, Pandit K, Joseph S, Weiner MG. A randomized trial of peer coach and office staff support to reduce coronary heart disease risk in African-Americans with uncontrolled hypertension. J Gen Intern Med. 2012;27(10):1258–64.
155. Fifield J, McQuillan J, Martin-Peele M, Nazarov V, Apter AJ, Babor T, et al. Improving pediatric asthma control among minority children participating in Medicaid: providing practice redesign support to deliver a chronic care model. J Asthma. 2010;47(7):718–27.
156. Katz D, Vander Weg M, Fu S, Prochazka A, Grant K, Buchanan L, et al. A before-after implementation trial of smoking cessation guidelines in hospitalized veterans. Implement Sci. 2009;4:58.

Government Agencies and Community Organizations

Sherry Shackelford Hay and Marni Gwyther Holder

Introduction

The number of Americans living with chronic disease, which is both preventable and associated with high costs of care, continues to increase. The Centers for Disease Control and Prevention reported that in 2018, 51.8% of civilian, non-institutionalized US adults—129 million people—had at least one chronic health condition, and 27.2% (68 million) had multiple chronic conditions (MCC), defined as two or more chronic conditions [1]. Approximately 90% of US health care spending now goes to caring for individuals living with chronic conditions, and the cost of care increases proportionally with the number of chronic conditions, with 12% of Americans with five or more chronic conditions accounting for 41% of costs [2].

Beyond genetics, individual behavior, and the contributions of clinical care, there is growing attention to the impact of social determinants of health (SDOH) on individual health and chronic disease outcomes. Moreover, social determinants of health are the conditions in the environments where people are born, live, learn, work, play, worship, and age [3]. These factors include but are not limited to economic opportunity; neighborhood safety and the built environment; access to quality health care, education, and food; and social and community context. The distribution of SDOH-related resources in communities, impacted by power and policy, has a profound impact on health, as evidenced by large variations in life expectancy at the level of a zip code or census tract in which an individual resides [4]. There is growing recognition of racism as a powerful structural and social determinant of health that impacts the distribution of power, resources, and opportunities, contributing to health inequity in communities of color, including inequities in chronic disease [5].

The Chronic Care Model identifies partnerships with community resources, the mobilization of these resources, as well as advocating for policy change, as key domains in providing high-quality chronic disease care [6]. The National Academy of Sciences 2021 Report *Implementing High-Quality Primary Care: Rebuilding the Foundation of Health Care* defines high-quality primary care as "the provision of whole-person, integrated, accessible, and equitable health care by interprofessional teams who are accountable for addressing the majority of an individual's health and wellness needs across settings and through sustained relationships with patients, families, and communities" [7]. In the current age of value-based care, there are new opportunities and challenges in bridging the gap between health care and public health to address the upstream factors impacting health outcomes. As such, health care providers caring for those with chronic disease need to have a thorough understanding of how governmental agencies and non-governmental community-based organizations can help to meet patient and population health objectives.

This chapter offers a brief introduction to US government agencies and non-governmental organizations that may interface with chronic illness care, impact health care disparities, and promote health equity. Two sections provide an inventory of specific federal and state agencies and community-based organizations and resources. An approach for primary care practice engagement with community organizations is described in the subsequent section, and the chapter closes with some examples of successful cross-sector community partnerships.

Government Agencies

For many years in the US, the focus of public health, biomedical research, and health care delivery stakeholders was on treating acute, largely infectious diseases, rather than on chronic disease and health promotion. The shift to an emphasis on chronic disease and health promotion was the result of

S. S. Hay · M. G. Holder (✉)
Department of Family Medicine, University of North Carolina at Chapel Hill, Chapel Hill, NC, USA
e-mail: marni_holder@med.unc.edu

several influences converging over time: a decline in the infectious disease death rate due to vaccinations and effective antimicrobial therapies, an aging population, increased health care expenditures, a decline in the birthrate, and emerging evidence that behavioral risk factors play a role in disease onset [8].

US Department of Health and Human Services (HHS)

The US Department of Health and Human Services (HHS) was officially established on May 4, 1980, when the then Department of Health, Education, and Welfare (HEW) created in 1953 under President Eisenhower was reorganized under the Department of Education Organization Act of 1979 to create a separate Department of Education [9]. The mission of HHS is "to enhance the health and well-being of all Americans, by providing for effective health and human services and by fostering sound, sustained advances in the sciences underlying medicine, public health, and social services" [10]. HHS, as required by law, develops a strategic plan every four years [11]. The 2022–2026 draft strategic plan has five objectives: (1) protect and sustain equitable access to high-quality and affordable health care; (2) safeguard and improve national and global health conditions and outcomes; (3) strengthen social well-being, equity, and economic resilience; (4) restore trust and accelerate advancements in science and research for all; and (5) advance strategic management to build trust, transparency, and accountability [12].

HHS's top leadership position, the Secretary, is nominated by the President and then voted on by Congress. There are 11 operating divisions, eight of which comprise the US Public Health Service and three additional human services agencies, that together administer a wide variety of health and human services and that fund and conduct biomedical and health services research. The 11 HHS operating divisions include: Administration for Children and Families (ACF), Administration for Community Living (ACL), Agency for Healthcare Research and Quality (AHRQ), Agency for Toxic Substances and Disease Registry (ATSDR), Centers for Disease Control and Prevention (CDC), The Centers for Medicare & Medicaid Services (CMS), Food and Drug Administration (FDA), Health Resources and Services Administration (HRSA), Indian Health Service (IHS), National Institutes of Health (NIH) and Substance Abuse and Mental Health Services Administration (SAMHSA) [13]. HHS is responsible for almost a quarter of all federal outlays and administers more grant dollars than all other federal agencies combined [14].

Centers for Medicare and Medicaid Services (CMS)

The Centers for Medicare and Medicaid Services (CMS) is the federal agency that is responsible for administering Medicare, Medicaid, the Children's Health Insurance Program (CHIP), and the Affordable Care Act's Health Insurance Marketplace [15]. Individuals must apply for and meet certain eligibility guidelines to qualify for benefits or financial support for Medicare, Medicaid, CHIP, and the Health Insurance Marketplace. As the major public payer for health services, CMS plays a major role in paying for chronic illness-related care, shaping US health care reimbursement policy, and testing new models of care.

Medicare is a health insurance program available to individuals who are 65 or older, who are under 65 with certain disabilities or people of any age with end-stage renal disease [16]. There are three parts to the Medicare benefit: hospital insurance (Part A), medical insurance (Part B), and a drug benefit (Part D). Part A covers inpatient costs, skilled nursing, hospice, and some home health costs, while Part B will cover outpatient physician costs, some occupational and physical therapy, and some home health that Part A does not cover. Part D, established in 2006, covers prescription drugs and is provided by private companies [16].

Medicaid provides health insurance coverage to low-income adults, children, pregnant women, and people with disabilities. Medicaid is administered by the states, according to federal requirements and the program is funded jointly by the states and the federal government [17]. While there are defined, mandatory Medicaid services that all states are required to cover, states determine financial eligibility limits and optional benefits as approved by their legislature and outlined in their state Medicaid plans [18]. The Children's Health Insurance Plan (CHIP) created in 1997, extended health care coverage to millions of children from low-income families who earned too much to qualify for Medicaid. All 50 states and the District of Columbia now have CHIP plans, with most extending coverage to at least 200% of the federal poverty level [19].

To highlight three CMS programs of importance to chronic illness care in the community, Medicaid services benefits for children up to age 21 called *Early, Periodic, Screening, Diagnosis, and Treatment (EPSDT)*, were enacted into law in 1967 in response to high rejection rates for new military draftees who had untreated childhood illness [20]. The goal of EPSDT is the early identification and treatment of conditions that could impede a child's growth and development and the service package includes coverage for comprehensive health and developmental assessments, vision, hearing, and dental services [21].

Home and community-based services (HCBS) provide important options for Medicaid beneficiaries with limitations in activities of daily living to receive services in their own home or community settings rather than in facilities such as assisted living facilities and nursing homes. These programs serve a variety of Medicaid recipients with special needs, such as intellectual, developmental, or physical disabilities, and/or mental illness. HCBS first became available in 1983 when Congress added section 1915(c) to the Social Security Act giving states authority to request a waiver of Medicaid rules governing institutional care [22].

Lead agencies and other service providers are responsible for HCBS care. A lead agency, such as a county's department of human and social services, acts as the primary care coordinator for a defined area. Service providers contract with the lead agency in their area to provide services [23]. HCBS includes both health services and human services and programs may offer a combination of both types of services and do not necessarily offer all services from either category [23]. Table 10.1 lists an inventory of health services and human services that are often provided through HCBS.

HCBS programs provide many benefits to both individuals and communities; however, states may limit the number of people who can receive the waiver benefits, creating significant waitlists for services once enrollment caps are reached. There are several additional challenges with administering this type of program, which are listed in Table 10.2.

A third program, the *Program for All-Inclusive Care for the Elderly, or PACE*, is a voluntary option under Medicare and state Medicaid plans that helps older adults age 55 or older, who would otherwise qualify for nursing home care, to stay in the community for as long as it is safely possible to do so, receiving health care in community-based settings. PACE organizations serve defined service areas and are fully at risk for the total cost of medically necessary care to those they serve. Most services are provided at a PACE Center by an interdisciplinary care team (IDT) and as payers of care PACE organizations contract with many health care services providers, including hospitals, nursing homes, physicians, allied health, and hospice care. PACE organizations are required to meet state and federal safety requirements and are reimbursed via per member per month capitation for the total care of their participants [24].

The Patient Protection and Affordable Care Act (ACA) of 2010 aimed to reduce the number of uninsured Americans and improve access to care. It created the Health Insurance Marketplace exchanges where consumers could purchase health care coverage from private insurers with substantial subsidies, and it additionally provided federal funding to states electing to expand Medicaid to adults up to 138% of the federal poverty level. Among other payment and delivery system reforms impacting those with chronic conditions, the ACA protected those with pre-existing conditions from discrimination by insurance plans and eliminated cost sharing for evidence-based preventive services. Looking at the year following implementation of coverage expansions (January 1, 2014), a study demonstrated that among adults with chronic health conditions aged 18–64, health insurance rates increased 4.9% (more in states that implemented Medicaid expansions), not having to forego a physician visit increased by 2.4%, and having a check-up increased by 2.7% [25]. A subsequent study looking at the first five years of ACA implementation for the same population found coverage increases for those with vs. without chronic conditions of 6.9% vs. 5.4% [26].

Centers for Disease Control and Prevention (CDC)

The Centers for Disease Control and Prevention (CDC) was established in 1946 as the communicable disease center that arose from the work of the Malaria Control in War Areas

Table 10.1 Health and human services provided through home and community-based services (adapted from reference [23])

Health Services	Human Services

• Home health care, such as:
  – Skilled nursing care
  – Therapies: occupational, speech, and physical
  – Dietary management by registered dietician
  – Pharmacy
• Durable medical equipment
• Case management
• Personal care
• Caregiver and client training
• Health promotion and disease prevention
• Hospice care (palliative care for patients likely to die from their medical conditions)
	• Senior centers
	• Adult daycares
	• Congregate meal sites
	• Home-delivered meal programs
	• Personal care (dressing, bathing, toileting, eating, transferring to or from a bed or chair, etc.)
	• Transportation and access
	• Home repairs and modifications
	• Home safety assessments
	• Homemaker and chore services
	• Information and referral services
	• Financial services
	• Legal services, such as help preparing a will
	• Telephone reassurance

Table 10.2 Benefits and challenges of home and community-based services (adapted from reference [23])

Benefits	Challenges
• Cost-effectiveness: usually less than half the cost of residential care • Culturally responsive: spiritual and cultural activities and support available • Familiarity: patient enjoys the comfort of their own home or small residential facility in the community • Can provide counseling or clergy to assist with bereavement • Some waivers permit family members to be paid caregivers	• Access to providers • Availability of qualified caregivers • Caregiver burnout • Lack of 24/7 medical professional availability • Non-family caregivers may have limited access in remote locations, especially during winter • Potential cultural bias or barriers in the acuity assessment process • Skilled nursing care includes only medical services performed by a registered nurse. Other daily tasks fall primarily to family members • Those needing care do not always want family members to act as their caregivers due to potential for abuse or financial manipulation • Tribes need to complete processes that are often long and complex, such as creating an elder abuse code or establishing a memorandum of understanding with the state, to create an HCBS program

(MCWA). The mission of CDC is to serve as the national focus for developing and applying disease prevention and control, environmental health, and health promotion and health education activities designed to improve the health of the people of the US [27].

The National Center for Chronic Disease Prevention and Health Promotion (NCCDPHP) is a division of the CDC that supports a variety of activities that improve the nation's health by preventing chronic diseases and their risk factors as depicted in Fig. 10.1. Program activities include one or more major functions: supporting states' implementation of public health programs; public health surveillance; translation research; health communication; and, developing tools and resources for stakeholders at the national, state, and community levels [28]. The center works with partners to strengthen health for states, tribes, localities, and territories through four primary strategies: (1) tracking chronic diseases and risk factors through surveys and research, (2) improving environments to make it easier for people to make healthy choices, (3) strengthening health care systems to deliver prevention services that keep people well and diagnose diseases early, and (4) connecting clinical services to community programs that help people prevent and manage their chronic diseases and conditions [28].

The NCCDPHP connects clinical services to community programs and strives to increase the use of evidence-based, community-delivered interventions that help individuals prevent and/or manage their chronic diseases. Examples include the Diabetes Self-Management Education (DSME), the Diabetes Prevention Program (DPP) and the tobacco cessation services like Quit Lines. It promotes use of community-based health workers such as community pharmacists, community health workers and patient navigators to help people manage their health [29].

The NCCDPHP also supports programs focused on reducing health care disparities and increasing health equity in chronic disease outcomes. One program is Racial and Ethnic Approaches to Community Health (REACH), discussed later in this chapter, supports community coalitions that design, implement, and evaluate community-driven strategies to eliminate health disparities among African Americans, American Indians, Hispanic/Latinos, Asian Americans, Alaskan Natives, and Pacific Islanders [30].

Administration for Community Living

The Administration for Community Living (ACL) aims to maximize the independence, well-being, and health of older adults, people with disabilities across the lifespan, and their families and caregivers. With the ACL, the Administration on Aging (AOA) is charged with implementing provisions of the Older Americans Act of 1965 (OAA). The Act empowers the federal government to distribute funds to states for supportive services for individuals over the age of 60, funds which are distributed through a network of aging services organizations, including state units on aging (SUA), aging and disabilities resource center (ADRC), regional areas on

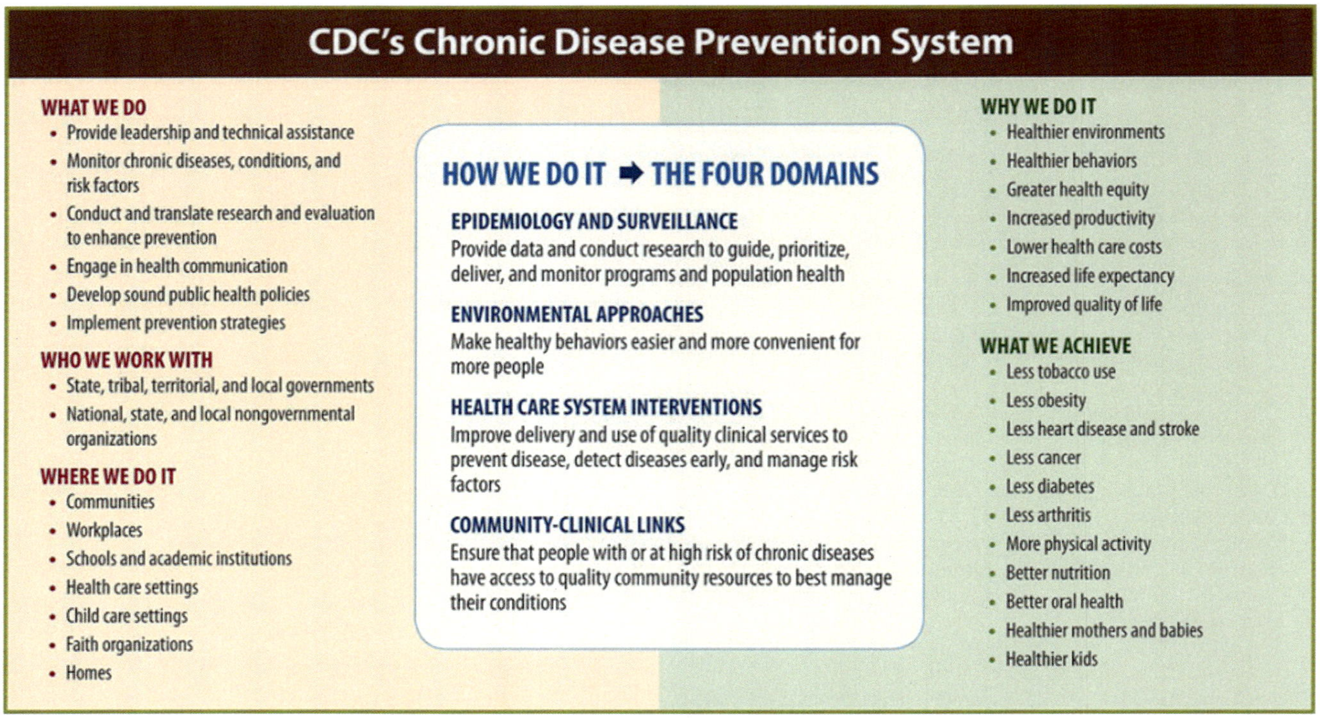

CDC's Chronic Disease Prevention System

WHAT WE DO
- Provide leadership and technical assistance
- Monitor chronic diseases, conditions, and risk factors
- Conduct and translate research and evaluation to enhance prevention
- Engage in health communication
- Develop sound public health policies
- Implement prevention strategies

WHO WE WORK WITH
- State, tribal, territorial, and local governments
- National, state, and local nongovernmental organizations

WHERE WE DO IT
- Communities
- Workplaces
- Schools and academic institutions
- Health care settings
- Child care settings
- Faith organizations
- Homes

HOW WE DO IT ➡ THE FOUR DOMAINS

EPIDEMIOLOGY AND SURVEILLANCE
Provide data and conduct research to guide, prioritize, deliver, and monitor programs and population health

ENVIRONMENTAL APPROACHES
Make healthy behaviors easier and more convenient for more people

HEALTH CARE SYSTEM INTERVENTIONS
Improve delivery and use of quality clinical services to prevent disease, detect diseases early, and manage risk factors

COMMUNITY-CLINICAL LINKS
Ensure that people with or at high risk of chronic diseases have access to quality community resources to best manage their conditions

WHY WE DO IT
- Healthier environments
- Healthier behaviors
- Greater health equity
- Increased productivity
- Lower health care costs
- Increased life expectancy
- Improved quality of life

WHAT WE ACHIEVE
- Less tobacco use
- Less obesity
- Less heart disease and stroke
- Less cancer
- Less diabetes
- Less arthritis
- More physical activity
- Better nutrition
- Better oral health
- Healthier mothers and babies
- Healthier kids

Fig. 10.1 CDC's chronic disease prevention system

aging (AAA), senior centers, and supportive services providers. The AOA funds services and programs designed to help older adults live independently in their homes and communities [31]. There are several divisions within the AOA:

Office of Supportive and Caregiver Services provides home and community-based services to millions of older persons through the programs funded under the AOA. Services provided include transportation, adult day care, caregiver supports and health promotion programs [31].

Office of Nutrition and Health Promotion Programs manages health, prevention, and wellness programs for older adults, including behavioral health, chronic disease self-management education programs, diabetes self-management, disease prevention and health promotion services, falls prevention programs, HIV/AIDS education, nutrition services, and oral health promotion [31].

Office of Elder Justice and Adult Protective Services manages programs specific to elder abuse prevention, legal assistance development, and pension counseling. It also leads the development and implementation of comprehensive Adult Protective Services systems that provide a coordinated response to adult victims of abuse and to prevent abuse [31]. This unit also develops standards to improve delivery and effectiveness of these types of services and provides support for the Elder Justice Coordinating Council.

Office for American Indian, Alaska Natives, and Native Hawaiian Programs administers programs for the provision of nutrition and supportive services for Native Americans (American Indians, Alaska Natives, and Native Hawaiians), as well as caregiver support services. Eligible [31] tribal organizations are eligible for grants that support home and community-based services for their elders, including nutrition services and support for family and informal caregivers.

Office of Long-Term Care Ombudsman Programs began as a demonstration program in 1972 and now operates in all states, the District of Columbia, Puerto Rico, and Guam [31]. Each state has an Office of the State Long-Term Care Ombudsman, headed by a full-time state ombudsman. As part of statewide programs, thousands of local ombudsman staff and volunteers assist residents in long-term care and their families by providing a voice for this vulnerable population.

Administration for Children and Families (ACF)

The Administration for Children and Families (ACF) was established in 1991 and aims to promote the economic and social well-being of families and children through funding, training, and technical support [32]. ACF programs have several aims: (1) to empower families and individuals to increase their economic independence and productivity; (2) to encourage strong communities that have a positive impact on quality of life and the development of children; (3) to create partnerships with service providers in order identify and implement solutions that transcend traditional program boundaries; (4) to improve access to services through planning, reform and integration; and (5) to address the needs, strengths, and capacities of vulnerable populations, such as people with developmental disabilities, refugees, and migrants [33].

The ACF funds states, territories, local and tribal organizations to provide family assistance, child support enforcement, childcare, child welfare, and other programs (e.g., low-income energy assistance, refugee resettlement) to support children and families. Many programs are supervised by state divisions of social services, with assistance programs administered via local departments of social services or other local providers. For example, Head Start is an ACF childcare service that collaborates with childcare centers and in-home childcare in local communities to provide free learning and development services to children and pregnant women from low-income families [34]. Candidates for these services apply to a Head Start or Early Head Start program in their community, where the local program determines eligibility.

There are resources for adults within family households, such as family violence prevention, adoption, and Temporary Assistance for Needy Families (TANF). TANF is designed to help low-income families achieve self-sufficiency. TANF can provide monthly cash assistance payments to low-income families with children, as well as a wide range of services that align with TANF's four broad purposes: childcare assistance, reducing reliance on government benefits by promoting job preparation, work and marriage; preventing and reducing the incidence of out-of-wedlock pregnancies, and encouraging the formation of two-parent families [35].

Health Resources and Services Administration (HRSA)

The mission of the Health Resources and Services Administration (HRSA) is to improve health outcomes and achieving health equity through access to quality services, a skilled health workforce and innovative, high-value programs [36]. HRSA's programs provide health care to people who are geographically isolated, socioeconomically or medically vulnerable, which includes people living with HIV/AIDS, pregnant women, mothers, and their families and those in need of high-quality primary health care [36]. HRSA also supports the training of health professionals, the distribution of providers to workforce shortage areas and improvements in health care delivery.

There are now six bureaus in HRSA. *The Bureau of Health Workforce* administers programs to strengthen the health care workforce and to connect skilled professionals to rural, urban, and tribal underserved communities nationwide [37]. The *Bureau of Primary Health Care* oversees the Health Center Program, a national network of health centers that provide comprehensive primary health care services to more than 27 million people annually. Services are provided on a sliding fee scale and regardless of the ability to pay. Special populations of focus in the health center program include people experiencing homelessness, those living in public housing, and migrant and seasonal farmworkers.

The Healthcare Systems Bureau focuses on protecting the public health and improving the health of individuals, supporting the following services: solid organ, bone marrow, and cord blood transplantation; poison control center services; countermeasure and vaccine injury compensation; Hansen's Disease direct patient care, provider education, and research; the Medical Claims Review Panel; and the 340B Drug Pricing Program [37]. *The HIV/AIDS Bureau* is responsible for the Ryan White HIV/AIDS Program, which provides a comprehensive system of care for people living with HIV [37]. The Program works with cities, states, and local community-based organizations to support HIV treatment services. The Maternal and Child Health Bureau's (MCHG) programs serves and estimated 55 million women, children, and families each year. MCHB provides Title V block grants to states to help focus on six focus areas; maternal/women's, child, adolescent/young adult, perinatal/infant, children with special health care needs, and a cross cutting life course [38]. Finally, the Provider Relief Bureau was created in response to the COVID-19 pandemic to reimburse providers for health care-related expenses and lost revenue attributable to the coronavirus pandemic.

Substance Abuse and Mental Health Services Administration (SAMHSA)

The Substance Abuse and Mental Health Services Administration (SAMHSA) is the federal agency that leads public health efforts to promote the behavioral health of the nation. SAMHSA's mission is to reduce the impact of substance abuse and mental illness on America's communities [39]. SAMHSA's 2019–2023 Strategic Plan has identified the following five agency priorities: (1) combatting the opioid crisis through the expansion of prevention, treatment, and recovery services; (2) addressing serious mental illness and serious emotional disturbances; (3) advancing prevention, treatment, and recovery support services for substance use; (4) improving data collection, analysis, dissemination, and program and policy evaluation, and (5) strengthening health practitioner and training and education. The work of the agency is guided by the following core principles: (1) supporting the adoption of evidence-based practice; (2) increasing access to the full continuum of services for mental health and substance use disorder; (3) engaging in outreach to clinicians, grantees, patients, and the American public; (4) collecting, analyzing, and disseminating data to inform policies, programs, and practices; and (5) recognizing that the availability of mental and substance abuse disorder services is integral to everyone's health [40].

US Department of Agriculture (USDA)

The Food and Nutrition Service (FNS) is an agency of the US Department of Agriculture (USDA's) Food, Nutrition, and Consumer Services. The mission of FNS is to increase food security and reduce hunger by providing children and low-income people access to food, a healthful diet and nutrition education in a way that supports American agriculture and inspires public confidence. FNS administers 15 federal nutrition assistance programs, including the WIC, Supplemental Nutrition Assistance Program (SNAP), and child nutrition programs described below. Most programs are administered at the state and local levels [41].

Supplemental Nutrition Assistance Program (SNAP)

SNAP is the largest program in the federal hunger safety net and offers nutrition assistance to millions of eligible, low-income individuals and families [42]. FNS works with state agencies, nutrition educators, and neighborhood and faith-based organizations to ensure that those eligible for nutrition assistance can make informed decisions about applying for the program and can access benefits. To receive SNAP benefits, households must meet certain tests, including resource and income tests [43]. FNS also works with state partners and the retail community to improve program administration and ensure program integrity. In 2021, for the first time in 45 years, the UDSA re-evaluated its *Thrifty Food Plan* used to calculate SNAP benefits. As a result, the average SNAP benefit will increase, and the plan's benefits have been adjusted to meet current cost realities and dietary guidance [44].

Special Supplemental Nutrition Program for Women, Infants, and Children (WIC)

The Special Supplemental Nutrition Program for Women, Infants, and Children (WIC) provides federal funding to states for supplemental foods, health care referrals, and nutrition education for low-income pregnant, breastfeeding, and non-breastfeeding postpartum women, and to infants and children up to age 5 who are at nutritional risk [45]. The program is administered through the Food and Nutrition Service (FNS) of the US Department of Agriculture and is not an entitlement program, but a federal grant program which Congress authorizes a specific amount of funds each year for the program. WIC is organized through 90 WIC state agencies, by 1900 local agencies in 10,000 clinical sites with approximately 47,000 authorized retailers [46].

Child Nutrition Programs

FNS also administers several programs that provide healthy food to children, including the National School Lunch Program, School Breakfast Program, Child and Adult Care Food Program, Summer Food Service Program, Fresh Fruit and Vegetable Program, and Special Milk Program [47]. These programs are administered by state agencies and targets hunger and obesity by reimbursing organizations such as schools, childcare centers, and after-school programs for providing healthy meals to children [47].

State and Local Health Agencies

The organization and governance models of state public health agencies are variable and can either be an independent agency or a unit of a larger agency [48]. Local health departments are units led by local governments, which make most of the programmatic and fiscal decisions. In a mixed model, some local health departments are led by state government and some are led by local government; no one arrangement predominates. A central model subsumes all local health departments as units of state government.

Services offered by local public health departments (LHD) vary widely according to structure, size and staffing and are adapted to local needs of diverse populations. A study of LHD services found the following most common activities: adult and childhood immunization; communicable disease surveillance, tuberculosis screening and treatment; community outreach and education (e.g., nutrition education, chronic disease prevention); Women, Infant, Child (WIC) nutrition program; tobacco control; environmental health services; food, school/daycare, and septic monitoring/regulation and safety. Personal health services tend to focus on prevention/wellness spectrum, including commonly STD screening and treatment and maternal/child health care [49]. Many LHDs are shifting away from personal health services toward population-based health services [50].

State health and social service agencies often assume programmatic and fiscal responsibility for a variety of federal initiatives, many of which were described earlier [48]. These agencies often provide technical assistance to a variety of partners in different areas, most commonly on quality improvement, performance, and accreditation [48]. For example, nearly all state health agencies provide training to local health agencies on disease prevention and tobacco control. Most state health agencies engage in activities to promote access to health care, health disparities and minority health initiatives, and rural health, and report providing financial incentives to primary care providers.

There are several services related to population-based primary prevention, screening, and treatment of diseases and conditions that are provided by state agencies. Most of these services are tied to tobacco, HIV, and sexually transmitted disease counseling [48]. State health agencies provide variety of functions related to surveillance, data collection, and laboratory functions, primarily in the areas of bioterror agent testing, foodborne illness testing, and influenza typing [48].

Non-government Organizations

A plethora of non-governmental organizations intersect with chronically ill patients and their caregivers. Several associations focus on a specific chronic disease, some provide social and legal support, while others are based in faith communities.

American Heart Association (AHA)

The American Heart Association (AHA) was founded in 1924 by six cardiologists and is the nations' oldest voluntary organization fighting heart disease and stroke [51]. The organization funds research, advocates for stronger public health policies, and provides tools and information for professionals and consumers. The AHA provides public health education as the nation's leader in CPR education training and promotes the importance of healthy lifestyle choices. For clinicians, the AHA provides evidence-based treatment guidelines to help them care for their patients, and advocates for policy changes to improve cardiovascular health. The AHA has a large grant portfolio and has funded more than $3.8 billion in heart disease and stroke research, more than any organization outside the federal government [51].

American Cancer Society (ACS)

The American Cancer Society (ACS) is a nationwide, community-based voluntary health organization dedicated to eliminating cancer [52]. The ACS is engaged in many areas that are focused on cancer: (1) encouraging prevention; (2) providing support for cancer patients and caregivers; (3) funding and conduct lifesaving research to better understand, prevent, and find cures for cancer; (4) working with policymakers and lawmakers to promote cancer care; and (5) promoting access to cancer care for millions of underinsured and uninsured Americans, and supporting multicultural communities to help reduce the risk of cancer. The ACS has a local presence in over 5000 communities and regional and local offices are organized to engage communities in their work, delivering potentially lifesaving programs and services and raising money at the local level [53].

American Diabetes Association (ADA)

The American Diabetes Association (ADA) is an organization comprised of volunteers, health professionals, and staff that leads the fight against the deadly consequences of diabetes and advocates for those affected by diabetes [54]. The ADA funds research to prevent, cure, and manage diabetes, provides services to hundreds of communities, and disseminates health information. In addition to 76 offices across the US, there are online resources that support the clinical practice and patient education [54].

Alzheimer's Association

The mission of the Alzheimer's Association is to lead the way to end Alzheimer's and all other dementia by accelerating global research, driving risk reduction and early detection, and maximizing quality care and support. The Association advocates for the needs of those impacted by Alzheimer's disease and other dementias and is the largest non-profit funder of Alzheimer's research. The Association has partnered with government and professional organizations to develop clinical care guidelines for patients with dementia and to support clinician training. The Association operates a national helpline and online forum, and Alzheimer's Association chapters in every state work to connect individuals with Alzheimer's and other dementias and their caregivers to community resources, convene support groups and offer education programs [55].

Legal Aid

Legal Services Corporation (LSC) is an independent non-profit established by Congress in 1974 to provide financial support for civil legal aid to low-income Americans [56]. LSC promotes provides funding to 134 independent non-profit legal aid programs in every state, the District of Columbia, and US territories, and serves thousands of low-income individuals, children, families, seniors, and veterans in every congressional district [56]. LSC is a grant-making organization and awards grants through a competitive process and currently funds 134 independent legal aid organizations.

LSC grantees handle the basic civil legal needs of the poor, addressing matters involving safety, subsistence, and family stability [56]. Most legal aid practices are focused on family law, including domestic violence, and child support and custody, and on housing matters, including evictions and foreclosures. LSC ensures grantee compliance with statutory and regulatory requirements and with sound financial management practices, LSC conducts regular on-site fiscal and programmatic compliance reviews and investigations. LSC also assesses the quality of legal services its grantees deliver and provides training and technical assistance to them.

Legal aid services are provided through a variety of public law firms and/or community legal clinics. In addition to legal aid services in the community, medical-legal aid partnerships are available in many states. The mission of the partnerships is to improve the health and well-being of people in communities by leading health, public health and legal sectors in an integrated, upstream approach to combating health-harming social conditions [57]. The partnership embeds lawyers and/or paralegals in health care settings who work as an extension of the care team to: (1) train health care teams in identifying health-harming social conditions; (2) assist patients in addressing the identified social issues which ranging from triage and consultations to legal representation; (3) transform clinic practice and institutional policies to better respond to patients' health-harming social conditions; and (4) prevent health-harming social conditions broadly by detecting patterns and improving policies and regulations that have an impact on population health [58].

National Alliance on Mental Illness (NAMI)

Founded in 1979, the mission of the National Alliance on Mental Illness (NAMI) is providing advocacy, education, support, and public awareness so that individuals and families affected by mental illness can build better lives. NAMI seeks to raise public awareness of and shape sound public policy on mental illness. It operates a national helpline to provide free information and support. More than 600 affiliates in 48 states work in local communities to provide support and mental health education to those with mental illness and their loved ones [59].

United Way

The United Way is a worldwide non-profit organization focused on creating community-based and community-led solutions that strengthen the cornerstones for a good quality of life: education, financial stability, and health [60]. It is a coalition of public and not-for-profit partners who identify and resolve issues facing communities and has 1200 local offices located throughout the US. Much of United Way's work is in triaging individuals to local community resources, particularly in the areas of education, financial stability, and health. In the area of health, the United Way promotes healthy eating and physical activity, expanding access to quality health care and integrating health for all people [60].

Faith-Based Organizations

Faith-based organizations can have a tremendous impact on the health and wellness of the faith communities they serve. Faith communities are natural venues for health education, screening outreach, chronic disease management support, and emotional and instrumental support in addressing individuals' social determinants of health. There are many positive examples of collaboration between the public health, primary care and faith sectors to address wellness and chronic disease, often with vulnerable populations at high risk of poor health outcomes. For example, a recent literature review on faith community nursing programs found that these programs can impact behavioral outcomes by reinforcing and clarifying information from primary care providers, emphasizing the importance of chronic illness management, emphasizing medication adherence and safety, and contributing to early screening and diagnosis of chronic disease. The strongest evidence for improved chronic illness outcomes is with hypertension, with promising work in the realm of diabetes and hospital discharge transitions [61]. Organizations such as YMCAs across the nation have been focused on expanding their impact on chronic disease, partnering with the CDC, public health departments and chronic disease expert groups (e.g., American Diabetes Association) to deliver effective chronic disease prevention and control programs focused on diabetes prevention, hypertension monitoring, falls prevention, cancer survivorship, and childhood obesity [62].

Engaging with Community Organizations

Both the Chronic Care and Patient-Centered Medical Home models have identified partnerships with community resources as a key domain in providing high-quality chronic disease care and addressing the social determinants of health [63]. There is a continuum of engagement that health care providers may have with governmental and non-governmental community organizations, ranging from basic awareness, to collaboration with community organizations through individual referral mechanisms, to active participation in formal cross-sector partnerships seeking to address the social determinants of health.

Primary Care Practice Connection to Community-Based Organizations

The American Academy of Family Physicians' *EveryONE Project: Addressing Health Equity in Every Community* outline key steps that primary care practices can take to create a culture of health equity and work with community organizations to address the social determinants of health. To understand the communities in which their patients live, practices can explore existing sources of community health data, such as the Robert Wood Johnson Foundation's County Health Rankings and Road Maps [64] or local community health assessments. These data can be supplemented by practice-level data on patient demographics, health literacy, and common conditions that can help a practice to prioritize collaboration goals and identify community partners. Practices can then implement a team-based process for *asking* about social determinants of health through implementation of a standardized screening tool, *identifying* resources in the community to address these needs, and *acting* to help connect individuals to these resources. This workflow can then be monitored for process improvements using data from the practice electronic health record and patient feedback [65].

With a thorough understanding of patient needs, several strategies can be adopted by primary care practice to strengthen linkage to community organizations on behalf of those they serve:

- Create a community resource directory: Map out existing community assets from existing resource lists (e.g., United Way 211 directory) or available community health assessments from hospital or public health partners [66]. Add resources to the directory based on the identified needs of the clinic population [66] and organize based on type of assistance or services needed, such as chronic disease, financial, or transportation. The Resource Directory can be made available in print and electronic format and produced in languages appropriate to the populations served.
- Provide a dedicated community resource space: Designate a space in a clinical practice as a community resource area for patients [66]. This area could be as simple as providing wall space for posters or brochures on community services with contact information for respective agencies, to providing a telephone and/or computer kiosk for use by individuals in connecting to community services or online chronic disease education information, to offering space for group activities [66].
- Co-locate staff from community agencies in the practice: Provide dedicated practice space to house staff from local community organizations [66]. For example, the space could house a rotation of community staff from a range of services [66] such as legal aid staff through a medical-legal partnership, Medicaid assistance services provided by a local department of social services worker, or nutrition services provided by a health department registered dietician. Seek to integrate these community resource members as part of the practice team by incorporating these individuals in staff meetings.
- Hire practice team members dedicated to enhancing community linkages: Care management services are increasingly provided in clinical settings by social workers or nurses as part of a team care approach. These services usually include comprehensive care planning, assistance in identifying and accessing community resources, and coordinating care across the community. Often the work of the care managers is supported by registry functionality in the practice electronic health record.
- Hire peer support staff: Peer support is an evidence-based approach to delivering cost-effective care for people liv-

ing with chronic disease that is individualized to a person's needs and includes offering emotional support, home visiting, and personal care services [67]. Peer support staff are often members of the community being served, sharing factors such as ethnicity, language, socioeconomic status, and lived experience with those they serve [68]. These individuals can be volunteers or paid members of a care team and may be designated as community health workers, lay health advisors, health coaches, patient navigators, and doulas [67].

- Commit to participation in a community partnership or coalition: Health care practices can seek to create formal community partnerships or lend their expertise to extant community coalitions to address community health priorities. Recognizing the growing importance of coalitions in addressing pressing health issues, a multi-agency task force updated and republished Principles of Community Engagement in 2011 [69]. Useful to any stakeholder undertaking collaborative work, the document describes both a continuum of community engagement (see Table 10.3) and nine principles for implementing successful partnerships (summarized in Table 10.4). See further discussion of formal cross-sector partnerships in the next section.

Cross-sector Community Partnership Models to Address Health Equity and Social Determinants of Health

There is increasing national recognition that sustained cross-sector collaboration between the health sector, public health agencies, and community-based organizations is necessary to effectively advancing health equity by addressing the social and environmental "upstream" determinants of health that impact overall health and well-being. Recognizing the funding silos inherent in health and social service funding streams, much of this work has been grant-funded, including significant investments by both government and philanthropic sectors. Several examples of grant-funded collaborations follow.

Racial and Ethnic Approaches to Community Health (REACH): The CDC began funding the Racial and Ethnic Approaches to Community Health (REACH) program in 1999. Funds are provided to states, tribes, universities, and community-based organizations that work collaboratively to reduce racial/ethnic disparities in groups with high incidence of chronic disease. More than 180 communities have received funding and technical assistance to develop local, culturally tailored programs to impact chronic disease disparities in conditions such as diabetes, asthma, cardiovascular disease, cancer, and obesity through prevention-focused interventions and clinic-community collaboration [71]. Looking at the impacts from the last completed round of five-year collaboratives (2014–2018), REACH-funded communities provided 2.9 million people with better access to fruit and vegetables, 322,000 benefitted from smoke and tobacco-free environments, 1.4 million people had more opportunities to be physically active, and 830,000 accessed local chronic disease programs linked to clinics [72]. An evaluation of the impact of the REACH coalitions published in 2010 demonstrated significant changes in community policies impacting health and significant reductions in disparities for minorities in REACH communities compared to national benchmarks [73].

Table 10.3 Principles of community engagement (adapted from *Principles of Community Engagement*, 2nd edition, 2011 available at https://www.atsdr.cdc.gov/communityengagement/pdf/PCE_Report_508_FINAL.pdf)

Increasing Level of Community Involvement, Impact, Trust, and Communication Flow →				
Outreach	**Consult**	**Involve**	**Collaborate**	**Shared Leadership**
Some Community Involvement	More Community Involvement	Better Community Involvement	Community Involvement	Strong Bidirectional Relationship
Communication flows from one to the other, to inform	Communication flows to the community and then back, answer seeking	Communication flows both ways, participatory form of communication	Communication flow is bidirectional	Final decision making is at community level.
Provides community with information.	Gets information or feedback from the community.	Involves more participation with community on issues.	Forms partnerships with community on each aspect of project from development to solution.	Entities have formed strong partnership structures.
Entities coexist.	Entities share information.	Entities cooperate with each other.	Entities form bidirectional communication channels.	Outcomes: Broader health outcomes affecting broader community. Strong bidirectional trust built.
Outcomes: Optimally, establishes communication channels and channels for outreach.	Outcomes: Develops connections.	Outcomes: Visibility of partnership established with increased cooperation.	Outcomes: Partnership building, trust building.	

Reference: Modified by the authors from the International Association for Public Participation.

Table 10.4 Principles of community engagement [70]

Principle	Key Elements
Set goals	• Clarify the purposes/goals of the engagement effort • Specify populations and/or communities
Study community	• Economic conditions • Political structures • Norms and values • Demographic trends • History • Experience with engagement efforts • Perceptions of those initiating the engagement activities
Build trust	• Establish relationships • Work with the formal and informal leadership • Seek commitment from community organizations and leaders • Create processes for mobilizing the community
Encourage self-determination	• Community self-determination is the responsibility and right of all people • No external entity should assume that it can bestow on a community the power to act in its own self-interest
Establish partnerships	• Equitable partnerships are necessary for success
Respect diversity	• Utilize multiple engagement strategies • Explicitly recognize cultural influences
Identify community assets and develop capacity	• View community structures as resources for change and action • Provide experts and resources to assist with analysis, decision-making, and action • Provide support to develop leadership training, meeting facilitation, skill building
Release control to the community	• Include as many elements of a community as possible • Adapt to meet changing needs and growth
Make a long-term commitment	• Recognize different stages of development and provide ongoing technical assistance

Community-Centered Health Home (CCHH): Community-Centered Health Home (CCHH) is a model developed by the Prevention Institute [74] in 2011. Based on the work of John Hatch and Jack Geiger, pioneers of the community health center movement, as well as current primary care medical home concepts, the model outlines steps that community health centers and other health care organizations can take to support community prevention. Clinicians are typically trained to collect data, diagnose a problem, and develop a treatment plan for individual patients. CCHH has parallel activities, which are termed inquiry, analysis, and action [74]. The inquiry step is collecting data on prevalence of disease and other social and economic factors in the community. The analysis step involves setting priorities and strategies with community partners while the action step involves both implementing coordinated strategies and making policy change for better health in the community [74].

This process is fueled by innovative leadership, diverse staff, and staff education in the clinic. Leadership creates a culture of innovation and continual quality improvement while providing staff with the tools and resources it needs to understand and work with patients to improve the adverse impacts of social determinants on health [74]. The diversity of staff speaks to the need of having the right mix of skills within clinic to meet the needs of the community. Strategies for identifying and convening partners outside of the clinic walls is also key. The Prevention Institute has created an interactive tool, The Collaboration Multiplier, which can be used to identify and engage with community partners [75].

A case study of the model is St. John's Well Child and Family Center in California. Clinicians at St. John's noticed a growing number of patients coming to the clinic with lead poisoning, cockroaches in the ears, and rodent bites [74]. The staff identified a potential association of these findings with area housing and a patient survey was conducted which included questions about housing [74]. This data provided the foundation for a partnership between the clinic and housing and human rights organizations to develop a strategic plan to improve local housing conditions. An evaluation of this intervention showed both improved housing and health outcomes [74].

Culture of Health Initiative: The Robert Wood Johnson Foundation (RWJF) launched its Culture of Health initiative in 2013, an effort "to enable all in our diverse society to lead healthier lives now and for generation to come" [76]. RWJF and the RAND Corporation developed a four-part Action Framework to "set a national agenda to improve health, equity and well-being" [77]. The four areas of the Action Framework are: (1) making health a shared value, (2) fostering cross-sector collaboration, (3) creating healthier, more equitable communities, and (4) strengthening integration of health services and systems. Regarding fostering cross-sector collaboration, the Foundation is tracking the number and quality of cross-sector partnerships, including local health department collaborations with non-health sector community partners and school and workplace-based efforts to support a culture of health; total financial investment in cross-sector collaboration by the corporate sector and through federal allocations; and changes in public policies that support collaboration with focus on community relations and policing, climate adaption and mitigation, and health in all policies approaches [78]. Per a progress report that summarized learning from cross-sector collaborative projects across the nation, key factors in effective collaborations include shared goals, stable collaboration focused on well-defined problems and tactics, and federal and state policies that enhance or deter collaboration [79]. A more recent progress report finds that cross-sector work fosters the development of all the other action areas [80].

BUILD Health Challenge: Since 2015, a consortium of philanthropies has supported the BUILD Health Challenge (BUILD stand for **B**old **U**pstream **I**ntegrated **L**ocal **D**ata-Driven), which funds collaborative partnerships between hospitals/health systems, public health agencies and community-based organizations, the latter serving as lead agencies for the supported projects [81]. To date, 55 projects in 24 states have been funded to create sustainable, systems-level change to advance health equity, and each coalition receives technical assistance as part of a learning community [81]. One example case study from the first cohort is the San Pablo Area Revitalization Collaborative (SPARC). SPARC worked with a historically African American Community in three neighborhoods/census tracts in West Oakland, California that experienced high crime rates, limited amenities, gentrification, and high rates of diabetes and hypertension. Working with partnership residents and non-profit developers, 30% of the neighborhood will have deeded affordable housing by 2025, with the City of Oakland prioritizing the SPARC corridor for affordable housing development. SPARC also resulted in an $11 million investment in a new grocery store, the first in more than a decade [82].

The Emerging Role of Payers in Clinical/Community Partnerships

As value-based care continues to accelerate, payers are now helping to support linkages between clinical care and community organizations that can impact the social determinants of health and chronic illness outcomes. These investments will be key to expanding and sustaining collaboration and to building the capacity of community-based organizations to improve population health. Several examples of payer demonstrations and incentives include:

Accountable Health Communities demonstration: Launched in 2017, the Accountable Health Communities is a five-year demonstration testing whether systemically identifying and addressing health-related social needs of Medicare and Medicaid beneficiaries through screening, referral, and navigation will reduce health care costs and utilization. Twenty-nine "bridge" organizations are participating in the model funded to serve as hubs for SDOH screening, with high-cost, high-needs beneficiaries offered navigation assistance. Moreover, eleven bridge organizations are assigned to the Assistance Track, providing health-related social needs screening to all and navigation to eligible beneficiaries, while the other eighteen are in the Alignment Track, providing screening and navigation combined with engagement with key stakeholders in continuous quality improvement to align community resources. Community partner agency capacity is not funded through this initiative. Early evaluation findings demonstrate that 15% of Medicare beneficiaries screen eligible for navigation services, having at least one of five health-related social needs and two emergency department visits in the 12 months prior to screening. Further, Medicare FFS beneficiaries receiving navigation from Assistance Track organizations have demonstrated 9% decline in ED visits compared to those in a control group, but no Medicare savings or impacts on other outcomes have been realized in the first year [83].

Accountable Care Organizations (ACOs): ACOs focus on providing comprehensive care to groups of beneficiaries, for which they receive shared savings if they meet spending and quality benchmarks. As these organizations seek to decrease costs associated with high-risk, high-health care utilizer beneficiaries, an increasing number of ACOs are focusing on the social determinants of health. Moreover, a recent qualitative survey of ACOs (107 respondents) showed that 84% considered SDOH in assessing the needs of high-risk identified individuals, and the top five socioeconomic needs identified by the ACOs were transportation (85%), food insecurity (82%), housing stability (79%), social isolation (77%), and access to healthy food (65%). Three-quarters of respondents reported collaboration with community-based organizations to address SDOH [84].

Medicare Advantage Plan(s) social determinants of health benefits: For plan year 2020, CMS finalized new supplemental benefit provisions for Medicare Advantage Health Plans, encouraging plans to support access to healthy foods, transportation to medical appointments, home maintenance related to chronic disease, and health and wellness education. The plans receive rebates from CMS for holding spending below benchmarks and can use these rebates on supplemental benefits or reduced premiums. Thus, plans have available funding to support community partnership and SDOH interventions [85]. More than 1000 Advantage Plans will soon participate in the CMS Innovation Center's Medicare Advantage Value-Based Insurance Design (VBID) Model in 2022, which tests the effect of customized benefits that are designed to better manage their chronic conditions and meet a wide range of social needs, from food insecurity to social isolation [86].

Medicaid Section 1115 waivers and managed care plans: States are working to encourage collaboration with community-based organizations on behalf of their Medicaid populations. Section 1115 waivers allow states to conduct demonstration projects that can add non-clinical benefits to the Medicaid program. Some state Medicaid managed care plans are allowing non-medical offerings aimed at reducing costs and improving the health of beneficiaries [85]. For example, a Section 1115 waivers program in North Carolina is funding Healthy Opportunities Pilots in three regions of the state beginning in 2022. An investment of $650 million will test and evaluate whether paying for non-medical services related to housing, food, transportation, and interpersonal safety will reduce costs and improve health. If successful, these services can then be added to the state's Medicaid managed care plan [87].

Future Directions

Providing chronic illness care has been historically challenging for many reasons: the chasm between health care services and community-level resources, the profound impact to which social determinants adversely impact health, and the increased number of Americans who are aging and living with multiple chronic conditions. New value-based health care delivery models are a promising catalyst for building partnerships with government agencies and community service partners who can provide complementary expertise and resources in caring for people living with chronic disease. Such collaborative work is hard and requires time, resources, and expertise. Although difficult, this important work must be done in partnership to identify shared goals and connect resources, so that equitable health care solutions can be available to everyone in our communities.

References

1. Boersma P, Black LI, Ward BW. Prevalence of multiple chronic conditions among US adults, 2018. Prev Chronic Dis. 2020;17:200130. https://doi.org/10.5888/pcd17.200130.
2. Buttorff C, Ruder T, Bauman M. Multiple chronic conditions in the United States. Santa Monica, CA: Rand Corporation; 2017.
3. Healthy People 2030, U.S. Department of Health and Human Services, Office of Disease Prevention and Health Promotion. https://health.gov/healthypeople/objectives-and-data/social-determinants-health. Accessed 14 Nov 2021.
4. Tejada-Vera B, Bastian B, Arias E, Escobedo LA., Salant B, Life Expectancy estimates by U.S. Census Tract, 2010–2015. National Center for Health Statistics 2020.
5. Paradies Y, Ben J, Denson N, et al. Racism as a determinant of health: a systematic review and meta-analysis. PLoS One. 2015;10(9):e0138511. Published 2015 Sep 23. https://doi.org/10.1371/journal.pone.0138511.
6. Wagner EH. Chronic disease management: what will it take to improve care for chronic illness? Eff Clin Pract. 1998;1(1):2–4.
7. National Academies of Sciences, Engineering, and Medicine. Implementing high-quality primary care: rebuilding the foundation of health care. Washington, DC: The National Academies Press; 2021. https://doi.org/10.17226/25983.
8. McLeroy K, Crump C. Health promotion and disease prevention: a historical perspective. Preventive Healthcare and Health Promotion for Older Adults; Spring 1994, pp. 9–17.
9. Department of Health and Human Services. https://www.hhs.gov/about/historical-highlights/index.html. Accessed 14 Nov 2021.
10. Department of Health and Human Services. https://www.hhs.gov/about/strategic-plan/introduction/index.html#mission. Accessed 14 Nov 2021.
11. Department of Health and Human Services, https://www.hhs.gov/about/strategic-plan/introduction/index.html?language=es#overview (accessed 11/14/2021).
12. Department of Health and Human Services. https://www.hhs.gov/about/draft-strategic-plan/index.html. Accessed 14 Nov 2021.
13. Department of Health and Human Services. http://www.hhs.gov/about/agencies/orgchart/index.html
14. Department of Health and Human Services. https://www.hhs.gov/about/strategic-plan/introduction/index.html?language=es#overview. Accessed 14 Nov 2021.
15. Centers for Medicare and Medicaid. https://www.cms.gov/About-CMS/About-CMS.html
16. Centers for Medicare and Medicaid. https://www.cms.gov/Medicare/Medicare-General-Information/MedicareGenInfo/index.html
17. Centers for Medicare and Medicaid. https://www.medicaid.gov/medicaid/index.html
18. Centers for Medicare and Medicaid. https://www.medicaid.gov/medicaid/benefits/list-of-benefits/index.html
19. https://www.medicaid.gov/about-us/program-history/index.html. Accessed 14 Nov 2021.
20. Early and periodic screening, diagnostic, and treatment services, Kaiser Commission on Medicaid facts; October 2005, pg. 34–35. Wwwl.kff.org/kcmu.
21. Centers for Medicare and Medicaid, https://www.medicaid.gov/medicaid/benefits/epsdt/index.html
22. Centers for Medicare and Medicaid. https://www.medicaid.gov/medicaid/hcbs/authorities/index.html
23. Centers for Medicare and Medicaid. https://www.cms.gov/Outreach-and-Education/American-Indian-Alaska-Native/AIAN/LTSS-TA-Center/info/hcbs.html
24. Centers for Medicare and Medicaid. https://www.medicaid.gov/medicaid/ltss/pace/pace-benefits/index.html
25. Torres H, Poorman E, Tadepalli U, Schoettler C, Fung CH, Mushero N, Campbell L, Basu G, McCormick D. Coverage and access for Americans with chronic disease under the affordable care act: a quasi-experimental study. Ann Intern Med. 2017;166(7):472–9. https://doi.org/10.7326/M16-1256. Epub 2017 Jan 24.
26. Rebecca M, Samuel C. Coverage for adults with chronic disease under the first 5 years of the affordable care act. Medical Care. 2020;58(10):861–6. https://doi.org/10.1097/MLR.0000000000001370.
27. Center for Disease Control and Prevention. https://www.cdc.gov/about/organization/cio-orgcharts/pdfs/CDCfs-508.pdf.
28. National Center for Chronic Disease Prevention and Health Promotion. https://www.cdc.gov/chronicdisease/resources/publications/aag/nccdphp.htm
29. https://www.cdc.gov/chronicdisease/center/nccdphp/how.htm
30. https://www.cdc.gov/nccdphp/dnpao/state-local-programs/reach/index.htm
31. Department of Health and Human Services, Administration for Community Living. https://aoa.acl.gov/
32. Administration for Children and Families. http://www.acf.hhs.gov/
33. Administration for Children and Families. https://www.acf.hhs.gov/about/what-we-do
34. Administration for Children and Families. https://eclkc.ohs.acf.hhs.gov/hslc/hs/directories/apply/howdoiapplyfo.htm
35. Administration for Children and Families. https://www.acf.hhs.gov/ofa/programs/tanf/about.
36. Health Resources and Services Administration. https://www.hrsa.gov/about/index.html
37. Health Resources and Services Administration. https://www.hrsa.gov/about/organization/bureaus/index.html
38. Health Resources and Services Administration. https://www.hrsa.gov/about/organization/bureaus/mchb/index.html
39. SAMSHA. http://www.samhsa.gov/about-us
40. https://www.samhsa.gov/sites/default/files/samhsa_strategic_plan_fy19-fy23_final-508.pdf

41. US Department of Agriculture, Food, and Nutrition Services. https://www.fns.usda.gov.
42. US Department of Agriculture, Food, and Nutrition Services. https://www.fns.usda.gov/snap/supplemental-nutrition-assistance-program-snap
43. US Department of Agriculture, Food, and Nutrition Services https://www.fns.usda.gov/snap/eligibility
44. https://www.fns.usda.gov/news-item/usda-0179.21
45. US Department of Agriculture, Food, and Nutrition Services. https://www.fns.usda.gov/wic/women-infants-and-children-wic
46. https://www.fns.usda.gov/wic/about-wic-glance
47. US Department of Agriculture, Food, and Nutrition Services. https://www.fns.usda.gov/school-meals/child-nutrition-programs
48. Association of State and Territorial Health Officials. Astho Profile of State Public Health, Volume 3, 2014. http://www.astho.org/Profile/Volume-Three/
49. Shah GH, Luo H, Sotnikov S. Public health services most commonly provided by local health departments in the United States. Front Public Health Serv. Syst Res. 2014;3(1) https://doi.org/10.13023/FPHSSR.0301.02.
50. Gebbie K, Rosenstock L, Hernandez LM, editors. Institute of Medicine (US) Committee on Educating Public Health Professionals for the 21st Century. Washington, DC: National Academies Press (US); 2003.
51. American Heart Association. http://www.heart.org/HEARTORG/General/About-Us%2D%2D-American-Heart-Association_UCM_305422_SubHomePage.jsp
52. American Cancer Society. https://www.cancer.org/about-us/what-we-do.html
53. American Cancer Society. https://www.cancer.org/about-us/who-we-are/fact-sheet.html
54. American Diabetes Association. http://www.diabetes.org/about-us/?loc=util-header_aboutus
55. Alzheimer's Association. https://www.alz.org/about/our-impact
56. Legal Services Corporation. http://www.lsc.gov/
57. National Center for Medical-Legal Partnerships. http://medical-legalpartnership.org/
58. National Center for Medical-Legal Partnerships. http://medical-legalpartnership.org/mlp-response/
59. https://www.nami.org/About-NAMI/Who-We-Are
60. United Way. http://www.unitedway.org/about
61. Warren G. The impact of faith community nursing programs for chronic disease screening and management in vulnerable populations: a comprehensive review of the literature. Int J Faith Community Nurs. 2021;6(1):8. https://digitalcommons.wku.edu/ijfcn/vol6/iss1/8
62. https://www.ymca.org/what-we-do/social-responsibility/advocate/preventing-disease.
63. 2016–2017 Improving Chronic Illness Care, Group Health Research Institute. http://www.improvingchroniccare.org/index.php?p=The_Community&s=19
64. University of Wisconsin Population Health Institute, County Health Rankings & Roadmaps. https://www.countyhealthrankings.org/. Accessed 14 Nov 2021.
65. https://www.aafp.org/dam/AAFP/documents/patient_care/everyone_project/team-based-approach.pdf
66. American Academy of Pediatrics, Bright Futures, Implementation Community Resources Implementation Tip Sheet; April 2015.
67. Peers for Progress. Global evidence for peer support: humanizing health care. Report from an international conference hosted by peers for Progress and the National Council of La Raza. Leawood, KS: American Academy of Family Physicians Foundation; 2014.
68. Gibbons MC, Tyus NC. Systematic review of U.S.-based randomized controlled trials using community health workers. Prog Community Health Partnersh. 2007;1(4):371–81.
69. https://www.atsdr.cdc.gov/communityengagement/pdf/PCE_Report_508_FINAL.pdf.
70. Principles of community engagement: Edition 2. Clinical and Translational Science Awards Consortium Community Engagement Key Function Committee Task Force on Principles of Community Engagement, 2011; Table of principles summarized by Plumb, J, Weinstein, LD, Brawer, R and Scott, K. (2012). Community-based partnerships for improving chronic disease management. Department of Family and Community Medicine Faculty papers. Paper 29: http://jdc.jefferson/fnfp/29. Complete set of community engagement principles available at https://www.atsdr.cdc.gov/communityengagement/pdf/PCE-report_508_final.pdf
71. https://www.cdc.gov/nccdphp/dnpao/state-local-programs/reach/20th-anniversary/index.html
72. https://www.cdc.gov/nccdphp/dnpao/state-local-programs/reach/program_impact/index.htm
73. Giles WH. The US perspective: lessons learned from the racial and ethnic approaches to community health (REACH) program. J R Soc Med. 2010;103(7):273–6. https://doi.org/10.1258/jrsm.2010.100029.
74. Community-Centered Health Homes: Bridging the Gap between health services and prevention, executive summary. https://www.preventioninstitute.org/sites/default/files/publications/Executive%20Summary.Final.pdf
75. The Prevention Institute. https://www.preventioninstitute.org/tools/collaboration-multiplier
76. https://www.evidenceforaction.org/about-us/what-culture-health/
77. https://www.rwjf.org/en/how-we-work/building-a-culture-of-health.html
78. Robert Wood Johnson Foundation. From vision to action: a framework and measures to mobilize a culture of health; 2015.
79. Grob G. Building a culture of health progress report, year one. Princeton, NJ: Robert Wood Johnson Foundation; 2018.
80. Rog DJ, Abbruzzi E. Culture of health progress report, phase 2 findings and conclusions (draft report). Rockville MD: Westat; 2020.
81. https://buildhealthchallenge.org/about/
82. https://buildhealthchallenge.org/resources/case-study-san-pablo-area-revitalization-collaborative/
83. https://innovation.cms.gov/data-and-reports/2020/ahc-first-eval-rpt-fg
84. An initial assessment of initiatives to improve care for high-need, high-cost individuals in accountable care organizations, Health Affairs Blog; 2019. doi: https://doi.org/10.1377/hblog20190411.143015
85. Healthify. Funding community-based efforts to address social determinants of health. https://www.helathify.us/funding-community-based-efforts-to-address-sdoh
86. https://www.cms.gov/newsroom/press-releases/cms-releases-2022-premiums-and-cost-sharing-information-medicare-advantage-and-prescription-drug
87. https://www.ncdhhs.gov/about/department-initiatives/healthy-opportunities/healthy-opportunities-pilots

Part III

Providing Chronic Illness Care

Screening and Secondary Prevention

Erik Butler and Katrina Donahue

Introduction

Screening and secondary prevention are important components of chronic illness care. Screening is a systematic approach to detect disease in asymptomatic individuals through laboratory and imaging tests, physical and/or other observational examinations, and specific procedures [1]. The goal of secondary prevention is to identify disease in the earliest stages or before signs and symptoms develop, in order to recommend preventive strategies or provide treatment that can mitigate disease morbidity, improve quality of life, and decrease disease mortality [2]. For example, measured blood pressure is routinely recorded at primary care visits in patients with and without a diagnosis or symptoms of hypertension. The detection of high blood pressure in an asymptomatic patient should ideally lead to discussion and interventions that might include lifestyle changes and/or medication to decrease cardiovascular risk. Clinicians and other healthcare team members should be familiar with the benefits and risks of screening, factors that influence effective screening, and individual considerations when screening for disease.

Principles That Inform Screening

Sensitivity and Specificity

High sensitivity and specificity are preferred characteristics of an effective screening test. Sensitivity is the ability of a screening test to detect all people who have a specific condition or disease. In brief, "true positives" represent the proportion of people who screen positive that actually have the underlying disease [3]. Specificity is the ability of screening test to correctly identify all patients who do not have the disease. These "true negatives" are the proportion of people who screen negative that do not have the disease [3]. Sensitivity and specificity are often the only parameters of the screening test that are considered and clinicians should not rely on a screening test's sensitivity and specificity to estimate the probability of disease in individual patients [4]. The positive and negative predictive values (PPV, NPV) of a screening test provide additional information.

Positive and Negative Predictive Value

Positive and negative predictive values (PPV, NPV) inform *how likely* a screening test accurately identifies whether an individual patient does or does not have the target condition, based on a positive or negative result [3]. As a result, the PPV depicts the ability of a test to readily identify all those who have the disease and test positive for that disease. While NPV is the ability of a test to accurately rule out a disease when the screening result is negative. Figure 11.1 expresses the relationship between sensitivity, specificity, PPV, and NPV.

The Effect of Disease Prevalence

The disease prevalence in populations that are being screened affects both positive and negative predictive values of the screening test. Prevalence is defined as the proportion of a population who have a disease or condition at a specific time [5]. The higher the prevalence of a disease in a population, the more likely a positive test means that the individual has the disease and the higher the PPV. Figure 11.2 expresses the relationship between disease prevalence and predictive value.

Clinicians should be aware of the effect that disease prevalence has on positive and negative predictive value when screening for disease. As the prevalence of disease increases, so does the positive predictive value of the screening test and the likelihood of a positive test. Negative predictive value however declines with increasing disease prevalence [6]. Ideally screening is best implemented in the asymptomatic

E. Butler (✉) · K. Donahue
Department of Family Medicine, University of North Carolina at Chapel Hill, Chapel Hill, NC, USA
e-mail: erik_butler@med.unc.edu; katrina_donahue@med.unc.edu

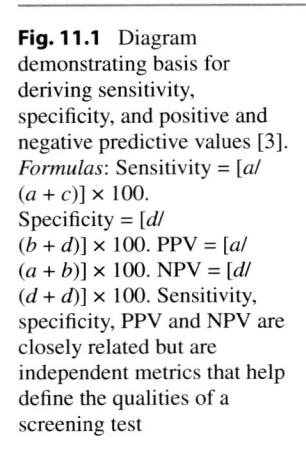

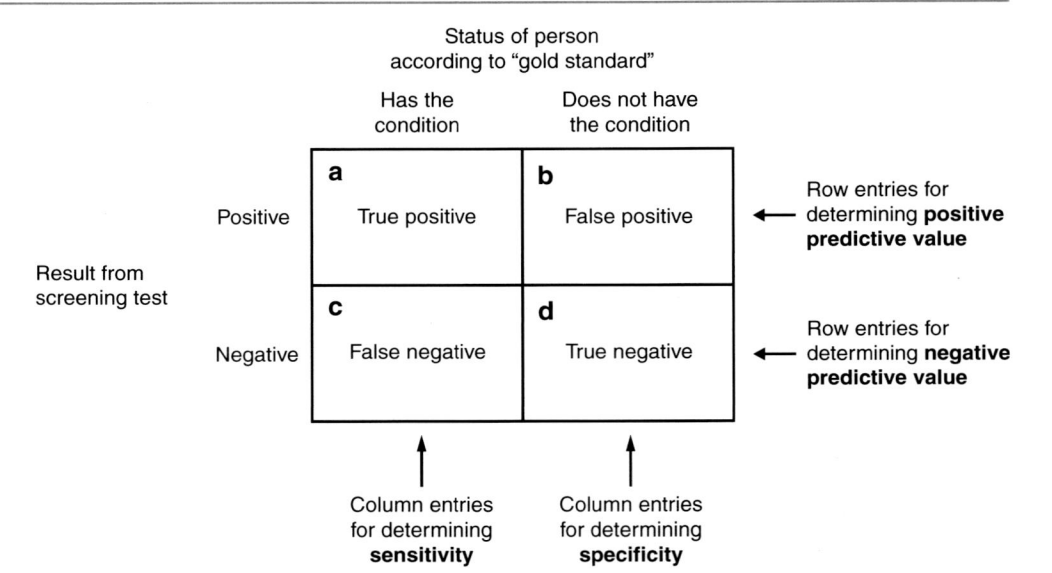

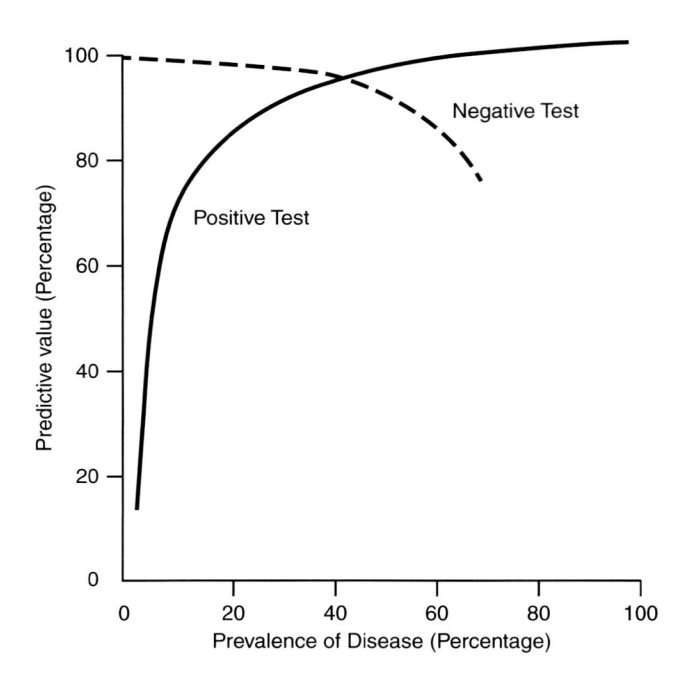

Fig. 11.1 Diagram demonstrating basis for deriving sensitivity, specificity, and positive and negative predictive values [3]. *Formulas*: Sensitivity = [$a/(a + c)$] × 100. Specificity = [$d/(b + d)$] × 100. PPV = [$a/(a + b)$] × 100. NPV = [$d/(d + d)$] × 100. Sensitivity, specificity, PPV and NPV are closely related but are independent metrics that help define the qualities of a screening test

Fig. 11.2 Relationship between disease prevalence and predictive value in a test with 95% sensitivity and 85% specificity [6]

period of a condition that has a relatively high prevalence and carries significant morbidity and mortality if undetected and untreated [7].

Levels of Screening

Clinicians and their healthcare teams can help patients navigate the extensive array of screening tests that are available. It can be overwhelming for both clinical teams and patients who have multiple, and frequently changing, screening recommendations, including mammography for breast cancer, Pap smear and HPV testing for cervical cancer, low-dose CT scan for lung cancer, PSA for prostate cancer, lipid levels for heart disease, and hepatitis C antibody for chronic hepatitis C. Screening recommendations can be organized into population-based screening, individual screening, and opportunistic screening.

Population-Based Screening

Population-based screening initiatives have been developed from evidence that supports screening in reducing morbidity and mortality from the target disease. This approach emphasizes that regardless of family history or risk factors, patients in a defined age group should be screened for a specific disease or condition, such as colorectal cancer (CRC) screening for all adults aged 50–75 years [8]. Population-based screening allows for clinicians, multidisciplinary care teams, health systems and insurers to work together to maximize screening rates and subsequently reduce disease burden in individuals and populations [9]. For example, health systems, health insurers and clinics promote fecal occult blood testing (FBT) using mailed fecal immunochemical test (FIT) kits as a strategy to increase colorectal screening rates [9]. Other directed approaches, including patient navigation, to colon cancer screening and FBT outreach improved CRC screening rates by almost 20% [10].

Individual Screening

Individualized screening focuses on identifying individuals for screening based on family history and/or additional risk factors (e.g., age, race, sex, family history, and/or lifestyle habits), as well as patient preference and health status in situations with insufficient evidence for population-level screening. Prostate cancer screening, for example, has insufficient evidence that all men of a specific age should be screened for prostate cancer using a prostate specific antigen (PSA) test [11]. A significant number of men with an elevated PSA (i.e.,

>4.0) at screening will have a false positive result, or have a prostate cancer that will not progress to become clinically symptomatic [12]. When considering individual screening, healthcare providers should take into account patient goals, risk factors, overall health, life expectancy and patient understanding of the risks and benefits of screening [11].

Opportunistic Screening

Opportunistic screening is initiated when a patient seeks healthcare office for a symptom or condition unrelated to screening, and are offered a testing to screen for a specific condition [13]. Routine blood pressure measurement to screen for hypertension is a common example. Offering chlamydia and gonorrhea screening in all sexually active females 24 years or younger is another example since these infections are frequently asymptomatic and can lead to pelvic inflammatory disease, ectopic pregnancy, infertility, and chronic pelvic pain [14].

Benefits and Risks of Screening

Clinical decision making regarding screening is challenging, given the availability and increasing number of screening tests, and due to conflicting screening recommendations from various public and private organizations [15]. In addition, longitudinal studies of common cancer screening tests have identified misperceptions about screening that lead to overdiagnosis and overtreatment [16–18] and often occur because of overestimation of potential benefits and under appreciation of potential harms of screening [15, 19]. Concomitantly, there is underutilization of screening in underrepresented populations, when compared to individuals with better access to care [15]. As a result, healthcare teams and systems need to improve outreach and engagement to provide high-value and cost-effective screening targeted to populations where screening benefits outweigh harms [15].

Overdiagnosis and Overtreatment

Screening can sometimes detect indolent, pre-clinical disease, resulting in overdiagnosis, which is the diagnosis of a medical condition that would never have caused symptoms or death if it had gone undetected and followed its natural course [20]. Screening can also increase the risk of overdiagnosis which may result in fear, anxiety, and potential harm patients [12, 13]. Overdiagnosis also leads to overtreatment, which is the treatment or intervention of a pre-clinical disease or condition that would have resolved on its own or never caused symptoms [21]. Figure 11.3 illustrates these concepts.

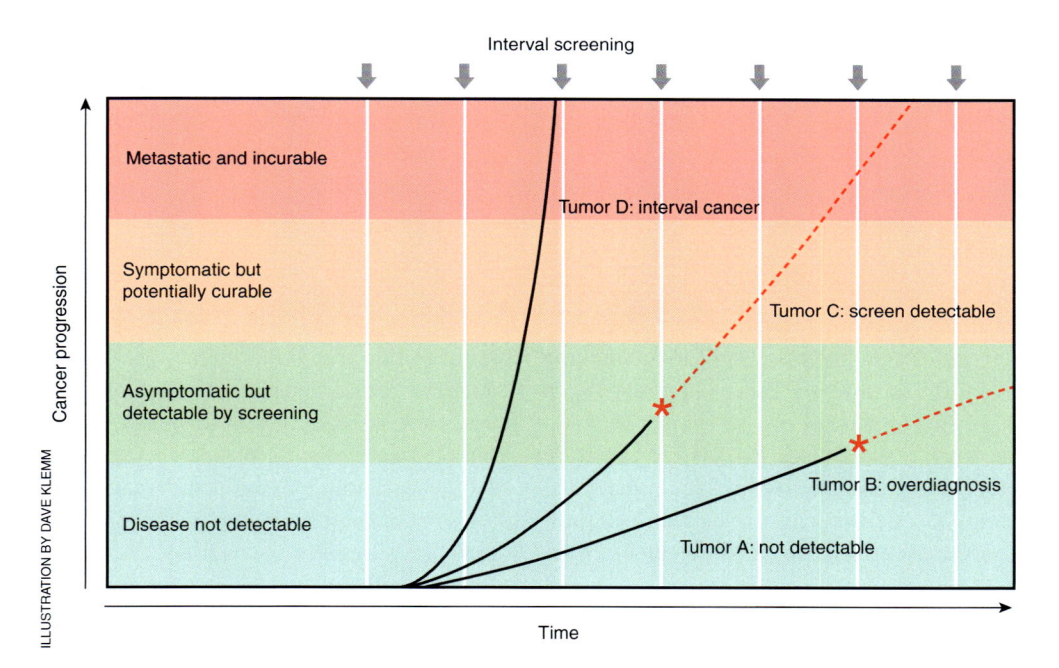

Fig. 11.3 Overdiagnosis in cancer screening. In this hypothetical example, the probability of detecting disease is related to the growth rate of each tumor. *Tumor A* remains microscopic and undetectable with the current screening test. *Tumor B* eventually becomes detectable by screening (asterisk), but its growth rate is so slow that it will not cause symptoms during the life of the individual; its detection will result in overdiagnosis. *Tumor C* (the only cancer with potential to benefit from screening in this example) is capable of metastasizing, but it grows slowly enough that it can be detected by screening (asterisk); for some, this early detection will result in survival. *Tumor D* grows very quickly and therefore is usually not detected by screening. This will present in the interval between screening examinations and has a poor prognosis. Red dashed lines represent the natural history of these tumors in the absence of detection by screening [22]

Implementing Effective Screening

The goal of screening is to reduce mortality by the early detection and early treatment of a condition [23]. Screening is important for individual health and has public health relevance, particularly with effective screening programs that can reduce the burden of illness in populations [24]. A screening program may be considered if adequate and consistent evidence supports, with at least moderate certainty, that the benefits of screening outweigh potential harms [23, 24]. Many conditions are not amenable to screening due to failure of this criterion. For example, although selective screening may be considered in high-risk patients, pancreatic cancer is not amenable to mass screening in the general population because of very low disease prevalence, increased risk of harms due to limited accuracy of available screening tests, invasive diagnostic tests, and generally poor outcomes of treatment [25].

Screening often occurs in primary care settings and can be incorporated into clinical practice. There are several components that promote effective screening in primary care: assessment of patient health risk factors, guidelines, or protocols for preventive services, a reminder system for past and currently due preventive services, a team-based approach to perform counseling and screening, and a follow-up system for test results and future preventive services [26]. Preventive services should be offered during most outpatient visits, such as annual exams and acute care visits. Electronic health record reminder systems, such a "Best Practice Alert" (BPA) can facilitate the initiation and receipt of preventive services by tracking prior and currently due health screenings [25, 27].

In community-based settings, there have been effective screening programs in locations such as barbershops [28], strategies that utilize lay health advisors [29], and leveraging relationships in faith-based settings [30]. For example, faith-based organizations have hosted programs, including screening for high blood pressure, diabetes, weight loss, smoking cessation, and cancer screening. These initiatives can increase knowledge and trust, improve screening behavior and readiness to change [30]. Lay Health Advisors can serve as a trusted member of the community to discuss fears and encourage screening [29]. Barbers can also be seen as important health advocates to overcome barriers to screening in the community [28].

Engagement in screening requires a complex interaction of the patient with the healthcare system. This has been referred to as the five A's of access: affordability, availability, accessibility, accommodation, and acceptability [31, 32]. Affordability relates to a person's ability and willingness to pay for services. Availability includes the personnel and technology to meet the person's needs. Accessibility encompasses geography and how easily a person can reach health care. Accommodation relates to healthcare meeting the constraints and preferences of the person, which include clinic hours that expand past work hours. Finally, engagement includes acceptability, where the person is comfortable with the provider, which can include immutable characteristics (e.g., age, racial/ethnic gender considerations to foster relationship) as well as the diagnosis [32].

Both clinical and community-based screening programs provide opportunities to promote health equity and mitigate health disparities. In addition to the earlier examples of faith base organizations and lay health advisors [28–30], decision aids, physician reminders and tailored office materials for cancer screening, smoking cessation and weight loss have been effective strategies [33]. However, there are multiple challenges and barriers to effective screening programs. Individuals may be reluctant to engage in screening programs for reason such as fear, medical mistrust, poor clinician communication, socioeconomic challenges such as access to care and insurance, fewer years of education, cultural norms, and individual perceptions of risk [22, 34, 35]. For example, African American patients may be less likely to be screened for colorectal cancer (CRC), and have a higher incidence of, and mortality from, CRC than white patients due to mistrust of the medical community [36, 37].

Evidence gaps in screening recommendations also contribute to health disparities in breast cancer screening in African American women, prostate cancer screening in African American men, and illicit drugs use in children and adolescents [38, 39]. Most of the breast cancer screening trials were based in Europe and the UK and enrolled predominantly white women [40]. There is little evidence whether tailoring screening approaches based on race/ethnicity or family history reduces prostate cancer mortality risk in higher-risk men [32, 41]. More research is needed to examine the screening for unhealthy drug use in adolescents, prevention of marijuana use, potential harms of intervention use as well as examine health and social outcomes [38]. There are inequities across the screening-to-treatment continuum, including access, quality of screening and quality of treatment [42]. If screening is to reduce health disparities and promote health equity, physicians and other providers will need to be mindful of factors that influence screening among diverse populations and implement evidence-based interventions to improve screening rates among different sub-populations.

Evidence Base of Screening

There are several information sources and groups that provide evidence-based recommendations for screening, including the National Institute for Health and Care Excellence in the UK (NICE), the Cochrane Library, and the US

Preventative Service Task Force (USPSTF). NICE aims to improve outcomes for people using the UK's National Health System by providing health and social care practitioners with evidence-based guidance and advice, as well as developing quality standards for public health and social services within the UK and internationally [43]. It has provided guidance on screening programs and improving quality of care both in the UK and around the world [44]. The Cochrane Library is an international network of researchers that provide systematic reviews of the clinical literature and is a well-known source of evidence-based guidance for healthcare professionals, patients and policymakers [45].

The US Preventive Services Task Force (USPSTF) was created in 1984 and works to improve the health of people nationwide by making evidence-based recommendations on clinical preventive services [46]. They are comprised of an independent volunteer group of national experts in prevention and evidence-based medicine. The USPSTF assigns an evidence grade to summarize the benefits versus harms of a screening program or other preventive service, based on the consistency, quality, and quantity of published evidence [47].

The grades range from A for a recommended service with high certainty that the net benefit is substantial, to D for moderate or high certainty that the service has no net benefit or that the harms outweigh the benefits, or I indicate that evidence is insufficient to assess the balance of benefits and harm (Table 11.1).

Clinicians can also utilize a point-of-care mobile decision tool by downloading the USPSTF electronic preventive services selector app at https://www.uspreventiveservicestaskforce.org/apps/.

Below are examples of screening using the USPSTF rating system.

Screening with Strong Evidence (A, B): Lung Cancer

Lung cancer is the leading cause of cancer death with a generally poor prognosis [48]. Major risk factors are smoking and older age, as well as environmental exposures, prior radiation, other noncancerous lung disease and family his-

Table 11.1 US Preventive Services Task Force (USPSTF) Grading Criteria for strength of recommendation

Grade	Definition	Suggestion for Practice
A	The USPSTF recommends the service. There is high certainty that the net benefit is substantial.	Offer or provide this service.
B	The USPSTF recommends the service. There is high certainty that the net benefit is substantial.	Offer or provide this service.
C	The USPSTF recommends selectively offering or providing this service to individual patients based on professional judgment and patient preferences. There is at least moderate certainty that the net benefit is small.	Offer or provide this service for selected patients depending on individual circumstances.
D	The USPSTF recommends against the service. There is moderate or high certainty that the service has no net benefit or that the harms outweigh the benefits.	Discourage the use of this service.
I Statement	The USPSTF concludes that the current evidence is insufficient to assess the balance of benefits and harms of the service. Evidence is lacking, of poor quality, or conflicting, and the balance of benefits and harms cannot be determined.	Read the clinical considerations section of USPSTF Recommendation Statement. If the service is offered, patients should understand the uncertainty about the balance of benefits and harms.

Source: Grade Definitions and Suggestions for Practice ("Grade Definitions After 2012"). Current as of June 2018. US Preventive Services Task Force; Rockville, MD. https://www.uspreventiveservicestaskforce.org/Page/Name/grade-definitions#grade-definitions-after-july-2012

tory [49]. The incidence of lung cancer and death rates are highest among African American men [48]. The USPSTF recommends annual screening for lung cancer with low-dose computed tomography (LDCT) in adults aged 50–80 years who have a 20 pack-year smoking history and currently smoke or who have quit within the past 15 years [50].

Potential Benefits

There are an estimated 235,000 new cases of lung cancer in 2021 [51]. LDCT has good sensitivity to detect early-stage lung cancer and adequate evidence that annual screening of high-risk persons can reduce lung cancer mortality [52, 53]. The USPSTF concludes with moderate certainty based on available evidence from clinical trials and cohort studies that annual screening with LDCT is of moderate benefit for persons at high risk based on age, total cumulative exposure to tobacco smoke and years quit since smoking [50].

Potential Harms

Patient age, smoking exposure, and functional status and comorbidities are considerations for discontinuing screening due to harms risks [54]. The USPSTF recommends discontinuing screening over the age of 80, if a person has not smoked for over 15 years, or if a patient is unwilling or unable to have lung surgery [50].

Implementation

The uptake of lung cancer screening is low [55]. Shared decision making is important in patients at high risk and who are more likely to benefit [56]. The discussion should include the risk of false positive findings that lead to subsequent work up, and the anxiety of living with a finding that may be cancer. Patient age, tobacco use-pack year and current smoking status can inform screening eligibility [50]. LDCT should ideally be at a center with expertise in lung cancer screening. Smoking cessation should be provided to current smokers.

Screening with Shared Decision Making (B, C): Breast Cancer and Mammography

Breast cancer is now the most diagnosed cancer globally accounting for 12% of all new cancers annually [57]. In the US approximately one in eight women who reach 80 years of age will develop invasive breast cancer in her lifetime, and it is the second leading cause of cancer death among women [58]. The US Preventative Task Force recommends bi-annual screening with mammography for all women aged 50–74 years (B recommendation). The decision to begin screening before age 50 should be individualized and take into consideration risk factors as well as potential benefits and harms (C recommendation) [59].

Potential Benefits

There is evidence that women who participate in mammography screening have a significantly lower risk of dying from breast cancer compared to women who do not have regular mammograms [60]. However, most of the benefit of screening is in women ages 50–74, with the greatest benefit at ages 60–69 years. Results of meta-analysis of clinical trials showed that for every 10,000 women screened by repeat mammography over ten years, 3 deaths will be avoided in women aged 40–49 years, 8 in women aged 50–59 years, 21 in the 60- to 69-year age group, and 13 in the 70- to 74-year age group [40]. In addition, women aged 40–49 years who have a first-degree relative with breast cancer are at a similar risk of breast cancer, and share comparable benefits and harms to biannual screening as women aged 50–59 [61, 62].

Potential Harms

Breast cancer screening with mammography at any age carries a risk of false positive results, overdiagnosis, and patient harm, including patient distress and overtreatment [59]. The risk of false positive results is more likely in younger women and those who undergo annual screening [40]. For example, if 1000 40-year-old women get a mammogram every year for ten consecutive years approximately 60% will be called back at least once for additional imaging [63]. In addition, all women undergoing regular mammography are at risk of being diagnosed and treated for breast cancer that would not have become clinically apparent or a threat to their health. It is estimated that 11–22% of cases may result in overdiagnosis [40].

Implementation

Age is the most important risk factor for breast cancer. Other factors include family history, genetics, personal history of breast cancer, race/ethnicity, being overweight, pregnancy history, breastfeeding history, drinking alcohol, dense breasts, lack of exercise, and smoking [64]. Presently there is not consensus among medical organizations regarding screening for breast cancer before age 50 for average-risk women. The American Cancer Society recommends annual screening mammography at age 45 until age 55, then every two years after age 55 [65]. The American College of Obstetricians and Gynecologists recommends offering annual screening beginning at age 40 years but emphasizes an individualized approach and shared decision making [66]. The American College of Radiology recommends annual screening mammograms starting at age 40 for average-risk women [67].

Clinicians should recognize the conflicting recommendations regarding breast cancer screening and be mindful that the benefits of screening appear to increase with age; the greatest benefit realized in women in their 60s. The benefit of screening average-risk women in their 40s is small and appear to gradually increase as they advance through their 40s. In each case, the decision to screen before age 50 should be individualized based on personal values as to the benefits and harms.

Screening with Risk of Harm (D): Asymptomatic Carotid Artery Stenosis

Asymptomatic carotid artery stenosis is a risk factor for stroke and one of the leading causes of death in the US, though the prevalence is low [68]. Additional risk factors for carotid artery stenosis include older age, male sex, smoking, and comorbidities, including hypertension, hyperlipidemia, diabetes mellitus, and heart disease [69]. The US Preventive Services Task Force recommends against screening for asymptomatic carotid artery stenosis in the general population [70].

Potential Harms
Several factors contribute to potential harms for screening for asymptomatic carotid artery stenosis. There are minimal predictive modalities that can reliably determine who is at high risk for asymptomatic carotid artery stenosis, or who is at increased risk for stroke when disease is present [71]. There is adequate evidence that duplex ultrasound can detect carotid artery stenosis but ultrasounds yield many false positive results [71]. Additionally, traditional auscultation of the neck for bruits is not reliable with poor accuracy [72]. False positive screening leads to follow-up testing and surgical recommendations that includes serious risks, including stroke, heart attacks, or death.

Implementation
Reducing the risk of stroke and associated cardiovascular diseases ideally focuses on preventive health services that are of higher value. This includes controlling high blood pressure, cholesterol, not smoking, maintaining a healthy weight, being physically active and eating a healthy diet [73].

Secondary Prevention

In addition to screening for disease, secondary prevention can involve a medical intervention or treatment of established disease to prevent its progression or its recurrence [74]. An example of secondary prevention is the use of statins and aspirin to prevent future cardiovascular disease (CVD) events, such as stroke or myocardial infarction in patients with known CVD [75]. CVD is the leading cause of death worldwide with ischemic heart disease and stroke accounting for 16% and 11% of all deaths respectively [76]. Given CVD global significance, secondary prevention plays an important role at reducing its morbidity and mortality [77]. Clinicians and associated healthcare teams should be knowledgeable about secondary prevention guidelines for CVD, and skilled in strategies to implement them, which include low-dose aspirin therapy, high potency statin therapy, education on smoking cessation, diet, physical activity, and blood pressure control [77].

Social Determinants of Health

Social Determinants of Health (SDoHs) are defined as "conditions in the environments in which people are born, live, learn, work, play, worship, and age that affect a wide range of health, functioning, and quality-of-life outcomes and risks" [78]. Access to food, transportation, safe housing, as well as exposure to violence and unemployment are proven to have a strong impact on health and well-being [79]. Despite wide-spread recognition on the importance of SDoHs, consensus screening guidelines for SDoHs have been slow to evolve due to insufficient evidence assessing the effect of interventions, and concern about the ethics of screening without available evidence-based interventions [80].

The USPTF recognizes the critical need for addressing SDoHs and included screening recommendations for intimate partner violence, elder abuse and abuse of vulnerable adults as well as screening for drugs, tobacco and alcohol in children and adolescence [80]. Identifying health-related socials needs is the first step in connecting individuals with community resources. Healthcare systems, medical practices and community health centers are increasingly developing tools and systems for screening for social needs [81, 82]. In addition, the Center for Medicare and Medicaid Services and the American Academy of Family Physicians offer brief screening tools for SDoHs that can help identify social needs in clinical practice [83, 84]. When screening for SDoHs, resources should be available to address these needs.

Future Directions

Future directions in screening will need to focus on health disparities and gaps in medically vulnerable and underserved populations in order to understand the individual and larger social factors that are at play. In response, healthcare systems and front-line clinicians will need to develop approaches that can effectively screen for social determinants of health and use that information to improve the social needs of patients and communities. The quality and quantity of evidence associated with screening tests is ever changing and clinicians and healthcare providers will need to keep a current understanding of screening tests and maintain the communication skills that promote informed patient discussions regarding benefits and harms, recognize individual considerations, and use shared decision making. Impactful screening practices will incorporate an appreciation and responsiveness to patient preferences by gauging personal and cultural beliefs and recognize the structural elements in health care that contribute to health disparities.

References

1. Whitby LG. Screening for disease: definitions and criteria. Lancet. 1974;2(7884):819–22.
2. WHO/Europe | Publications – Screening programmes: a short guide. Increase effectiveness, maximize benefits and minimize harm [Internet]. 2020 [cited 2022 Jan 30]. https://www.euro.who.int/en/publications/abstracts/screening-programmes-a-short-guide.-increase-effectiveness,-maximize-benefits-and-minimize-harm-2020.
3. Trevethan R. Sensitivity, specificity, and predictive values: foundations, pliabilities, and pitfalls in research and practice. Front Public Health. 2017;5:307.
4. Akobeng AK. Understanding diagnostic tests 1: sensitivity, specificity and predictive values. Acta Paediatr. 2007;96(3):338–41.
5. Prevalence | epidemiology | Britannica [Internet]. [cited 2021 Sep 7]. https://www.britannica.com/science/prevalence.
6. Mausner JS, Kramer S. Epidemiology: an introductory text. Philadelphia: Saunders; 1985.
7. Wilson JM, Jungner YG. Principles and practice of mass screening for disease. Bol Oficina Sanit Panam. 1968;65(4):281–393.
8. US Preventive Services Task Force, Bibbins-Domingo K, Grossman DC, Curry SJ, Davidson KW, Epling JW, et al. Screening for colorectal cancer: US Preventive Services Task Force recommendation statement. JAMA. 2016;315(23):2564–75.
9. Verma M, Sarfaty M, Brooks D, Wender RC. Population-based programs for increasing colorectal cancer screening in the United States. CA Cancer J Clin. 2015;65(6):497–510.
10. Dougherty MK, Brenner AT, Crockett SD, Gupta S, Wheeler SB, Coker-Schwimmer M, et al. Evaluation of interventions intended to increase colorectal cancer screening rates in the United States: a systematic review and meta-analysis. JAMA Intern Med. 2018;178(12):1645–58.
11. US Preventive Services Task Force, Grossman DC, Curry SJ, Owens DK, Bibbins-Domingo K, Caughey AB, et al. Screening for prostate cancer: US preventive services task force recommendation statement. JAMA. 2018;319(18):1901–13.
12. Kilpeläinen TP, Tammela TLJ, Roobol M, Hugosson J, Ciatto S, Nelen V, et al. False-positive screening results in the European randomized study of screening for prostate cancer. Eur J Cancer. 2011;47(18):2698–705.
13. Benefits and risks of screening tests – InformedHealth.org – NCBI Bookshelf [Internet]. 2019 [cited 2022 Jan 31]. https://www.ncbi.nlm.nih.gov/books/NBK279418/.
14. US Preventive Services Task Force, Davidson KW, Barry MJ, Mangione CM, Cabana M, Caughey AB, et al. Screening for chlamydia and gonorrhea: US Preventive Services Task Force recommendation statement. JAMA. 2021;326(10):949–56.
15. Kaysin A, Gourlay ML. Screening for chronic disease. In: Daaleman TP, Helton MR, editors. Chronic illness care. Cham: Springer International Publishing; 2018. p. 163–73.
16. Kapp JM, Yankaskas BC, LeFevre ML. Are mammography recommendations in women younger than 40 related to increased risk? Breast Cancer Res Treat. 2010;119(2):485–90.
17. Harris RP, Wilt TJ, Qaseem A, High Value Care Task Force of the American College of Physicians. A value framework for cancer screening: advice for high-value care from the American College of Physicians. Ann Intern Med. 2015;162(10):712–7.
18. Jørgensen KJ, Gøtzsche PC, Kalager M, Zahl P-H. Breast cancer screening in Denmark. Ann Intern Med. 2017;167(7):524.
19. Hoffmann TC, Del Mar C. Patients' expectations of the benefits and harms of treatments, screening, and tests: a systematic review. JAMA Intern Med. 2015;175(2):274–86.
20. Welch HG, Black WC. Overdiagnosis in cancer. J Natl Cancer Inst. 2010;102(9):605–13.
21. Gupta P, Gupta M, Koul N. Overdiagnosis and overtreatment; how to deal with too much medicine. J Family Med Prim Care. 2020;9(8):3815–9.
22. Gates TJ. Screening for cancer: concepts and controversies. Am Fam Physician. 2014;90(9):625–31.
23. Screening Programmes: a short guide. [cited 2021 Sep 13]. https://apps.who.int/iris/bitstream/handle/10665/330829/9789289054782-eng.pdf.
24. Procedure Manual Section 2. Topic selection, prioritization, and updating | United States Preventive Services Taskforce [Internet]. [cited 2021 Sep 13]. https://www.uspreventiveservicestaskforce.org/uspstf/about-uspstf/methods-and-processes/procedure-manual/procedure-manual-section-2-topic-selection-prioritization-and-updating.
25. US Preventive Services Task Force, Owens DK, Davidson KW, Krist AH, Barry MJ, Cabana M, et al. Screening for pancreatic cancer: US Preventive Services Task Force reaffirmation recommendation statement. JAMA. 2019;322(5):438–44.
26. Hensrud DD. Clinical preventive medicine in primary care: background and practice: 2. Delivering primary preventive services. Mayo Clin Proc. 2000;75(3):255–64.
27. Sawaya GF, Guirguis-Blake J, LeFevre M, Harris R, Petitti D, U.S. Preventive Services Task Force. Update on the methods of the U.S. Preventive Services Task Force: estimating certainty and magnitude of net benefit. Ann Intern Med. 2007;147(12):871–5.
28. Osorio M, Ravenell JE, Sevick MA, Ararso Y, Young T, Wall SP, et al. Community-based hemoglobin A1C testing in barbershops to identify black men with undiagnosed diabetes. JAMA Intern Med. 2020;180(4):596–7.
29. Earp JA, Flax VL. What lay health advisors do: an evaluation of advisors' activities. Cancer Pract. 1999;7(1):16–21.
30. DeHaven MJ, Hunter IB, Wilder L, Walton JW, Berry J. Health programs in faith-based organizations: are they effective? Am J Public Health. 2004;94(6):1030–6.
31. Penchansky R, Thomas JW. The concept of access: definition and relationship to consumer satisfaction. Med Care. 1981;19(2):127–40.
32. McLaughlin CG, Wyszewianski L. Access to care: remembering old lessons. Health Serv Res. 2002;37(6):1441–3.
33. Nelson HD, Cantor A, Wagner J, Jungbauer R, Quiñones A, Fu R, et al. Achieving health equity in preventive services. Rockville, MD: Agency for Healthcare Research and Quality (US); 2019.
34. Steele CB, Rim SH, Joseph DA, King JB, Seeff LC, Centers for Disease Control and Prevention (CDC). Colorectal cancer incidence and screening – United States, 2008 and 2010. MMWR Suppl. 2013;62(3):53–60.
35. Adams LB, Richmond J, Corbie-Smith G, Powell W. Medical mistrust and colorectal cancer screening among African Americans. J Commun Health. 2017;42(5):1044–61.
36. Bromley EG, May FP, Federer L, Spiegel BMR, van Oijen MGH. Explaining persistent under-use of colonoscopic cancer

37. Katz ML, James AS, Pignone MP, Hudson MA, Jackson E, Oates V, et al. Colorectal cancer screening among African American church members: a qualitative and quantitative study of patient-provider communication. BMC Public Health. 2004;4:62.
38. Tenth Annual Report to Congress on High-Priority Evidence Gaps for Clinical Preventive Services | United States Preventive Services Taskforce [Internet]. [cited 2021 Oct 11]. https://www.uspreventiveservicestaskforce.org/uspstf/about-uspstf/reports-congress/tenth-annual-report-congress-high-priority-evidence-gaps-clinical-preventive-services.
39. Eighth Annual Report to Congress on High-Priority Evidence Gaps for Clinical Preventive Services | United States Preventive Services Taskforce [Internet]. [cited 2021 Oct 11]. https://www.uspreventiveservicestaskforce.org/uspstf/about-uspstf/reports-congress/eighth-annual-report-congress-high-priority-evidence-gaps-clinical-preventive-services.
40. Nelson HD, Cantor A, Humphrey L, Fu R, Pappas M, Daeges M, et al. Screening for breast cancer: a systematic review to update the 2009 U.S. preventive services task force recommendation. Rockville, MD: Agency for Healthcare Research and Quality (US); 2016.
41. Fenton JJ, Weyrich MS, Durbin S, Liu Y, Bang H, Melnikow J. Prostate-specific antigen-based screening for prostate cancer: a systematic evidence review for the U.S. Preventive Services Task Force. Rockville, MD: Agency for Healthcare Research and Quality (US); 2018.
42. Doubeni CA, Simon M, Krist AH. Addressing systemic racism through clinical preventive service recommendations from the US Preventive Services Task Force. JAMA. 2021;325(7):627–8.
43. NICE International | What we do | About | NICE [Internet]. [cited 2022 Feb 12]. https://www.nice.org.uk/about/what-we-do/nice-international.
44. Chalkidou K, Levine R, Dillon A. Helping poorer countries make locally informed health decisions. BMJ. 2010;341:c3651.
45. About us | Cochrane [Internet]. [cited 2022 Feb 5]. https://www.cochrane.org/about-us.
46. About the USPSTF | United States Preventive Services Taskforce [Internet]. [cited 2022 Jan 13]. https://www.uspreventiveservicestaskforce.org/uspstf/about-uspstf.
47. Procedure Manual Section 7. Formulation of Task Force Recommendations | United States Preventive Services Taskforce [Internet]. [cited 2021 Oct 11]. https://www.uspreventiveservicestaskforce.org/uspstf/about-uspstf/methods-and-processes/procedure-manual/procedure-manual-section-7-formulation-task-force-recommendations.
48. PDQ Adult Treatment Editorial Board. Non-small cell lung cancer treatment (PDQ®): health professional version. PDQ cancer information summaries. Bethesda, MD: National Cancer Institute (US); 2002.
49. Alberg AJ, Brock MV, Ford JG, Samet JM, Spivack SD. Epidemiology of lung cancer: diagnosis and management of lung cancer, 3rd ed: American College of Chest Physicians evidence-based clinical practice guidelines. Chest. 2013;143(5 Suppl):e1S–e29S.
50. US Preventive Services Task Force, Krist AH, Davidson KW, Mangione CM, Barry MJ, Cabana M, et al. Screening for lung cancer: US Preventive Services Task Force recommendation statement. JAMA. 2021;325(10):962–70.
51. Lung Cancer Statistics | How common is lung cancer? [Internet]. [cited 2021 Oct 8]. https://www.cancer.org/cancer/lung-cancer/about/key-statistics.html.
52. de Koning HJ, van der Aalst CM, de Jong PA, Scholten ET, Nackaerts K, Heuvelmans MA, et al. Reduced lung-cancer mortality with volume CT screening in a randomized trial. N Engl J Med. 2020;382(6):503–13.
53. Pinsky PF, Church TR, Izmirlian G, Kramer BS. The National Lung Screening Trial: results stratified by demographics, smoking history, and lung cancer histology. Cancer. 2013;119(22):3976–83.
54. Jonas DE, Reuland DS, Reddy SM, Nagle M, Clark SD, Weber RP, et al. Screening for lung cancer with low-dose computed tomography: updated evidence report and systematic review for the US Preventive Services Task Force. JAMA. 2021;325(10):971–87.
55. Zahnd WE, Eberth JM. Lung cancer screening utilization: a behavioral risk factor surveillance system analysis. Am J Prev Med. 2019;57(2):250–5.
56. Elwyn G, Frosch D, Thomson R, Joseph-Williams N, Lloyd A, Kinnersley P, et al. Shared decision making: a model for clinical practice. J Gen Intern Med. 2012;27(10):1361–7.
57. Breast cancer overtakes lung as most common cancer-WHO | Reuters [Internet]. [cited 2021 Oct 28]. https://www.reuters.com/article/health-cancer-int/breast-cancer-overtakes-lung-as-most-common-cancer-who-idUSKBN2A219B.
58. How common is breast cancer? | Breast Cancer Statistics [Internet]. [cited 2021 Oct 28]. https://www.cancer.org/cancer/breast-cancer/about/how-common-is-breast-cancer.html.
59. Siu AL, U.S. Preventive Services Task Force. Screening for breast cancer: U.S. Preventive Services Task Force recommendation statement. Ann Intern Med. 2016;164(4):279–96.
60. Tabár L, Dean PB, Chen TH-H, Yen AM-F, Chen SL-S, Fann JC-Y, et al. The incidence of fatal breast cancer measures the increased effectiveness of therapy in women participating in mammography screening. Cancer. 2019;125(4):515–23.
61. Collaborative Group on Hormonal Factors in Breast Cancer. Familial breast cancer: collaborative reanalysis of individual data from 52 epidemiological studies including 58,209 women with breast cancer and 101,986 women without the disease. Lancet. 2001;358(9291):1389–99.
62. van Ravesteyn NT, Miglioretti DL, Stout NK, Lee SJ, Schechter CB, Buist DSM, et al. Tipping the balance of benefits and harms to favor screening mammography starting at age 40 years: a comparative modeling study of risk. Ann Intern Med. 2012;156(9):609–17.
63. Hubbard RA, Kerlikowske K, Flowers CI, Yankaskas BC, Zhu W, Miglioretti DL. Cumulative probability of false-positive recall or biopsy recommendation after 10 years of screening mammography: a cohort study. Ann Intern Med. 2011;155(8):481–92.
64. Breast cancer risk factors | Breastcancer.org [Internet]. [cited 2021 Oct 28]. https://www.breastcancer.org/symptoms/understand_bc/risk/factors.
65. ACS breast cancer early detection recommendations [Internet]. [cited 2021 Oct 28]. https://www.cancer.org/cancer/breast-cancer/screening-tests-and-early-detection/american-cancer-society-recommendations-for-the-early-detection-of-breast-cancer.html.
66. ACOG revises breast cancer screening guidance: ob-gyns promote shared decision making | ACOG [Internet]. [cited 2021 Oct 28]. https://www.acog.org/news/news-releases/2017/06/acog-revises-breast-cancer-screening-guidance-ob-gyns-promote-shared-decision-making.
67. Monticciolo DL, Newell MS, Hendrick RE, Helvie MA, Moy L, Monsees B, et al. Breast cancer screening for average-risk women: recommendations from the ACR Commission on Breast Imaging. J Am Coll Radiol. 2017;14(9):1137–43.
68. FastStats – Leading causes of death [Internet]. [cited 2021 Oct 23]. https://www.cdc.gov/nchs/fastats/leading-causes-of-death.htm.
69. Meschia JF, Bushnell C, Boden-Albala B, Braun LT, Bravata DM, Chaturvedi S, et al. Guidelines for the primary prevention of stroke: a statement for healthcare professionals from the American Heart Association/American Stroke Association. Stroke. 2014;45(12):3754–832.

70. US Preventive Services Task Force, Krist AH, Davidson KW, Mangione CM, Barry MJ, Cabana M, et al. Screening for asymptomatic carotid artery stenosis: US Preventive Services Task Force recommendation statement. JAMA. 2021;325(5):476–81.
71. Jonas DE, Feltner C, Amick HR, Sheridan S, Zheng Z-J, Watford DJ, et al. Screening for asymptomatic carotid artery stenosis: a systematic review and meta-analysis for the U.S. Preventive Services Task Force. Rockville, MD: Agency for Healthcare Research and Quality (US); 2014.
72. Guirguis-Blake JM, Webber EM, Coppola EL. Screening for asymptomatic carotid artery stenosis in the general population: an evidence update for the U.S. Preventive Services Task Force. Rockville, MD: Agency for Healthcare Research and Quality (US); 2021.
73. Preventing stroke: healthy living habits | cdc.gov [Internet]. [cited 2022 Jan 7]. https://www.cdc.gov/stroke/healthy_living.htm.
74. Primary, secondary and tertiary prevention [Internet]. [cited 2022 Feb 6]. https://www.iwh.on.ca/what-researchers-mean-by/primary-secondary-and-tertiary-prevention.
75. Herman CR, Gill HK, Eng J, Fajardo LL. Screening for preclinical disease: test and disease characteristics. AJR Am J Roentgenol. 2002;179(4):825–31.
76. The top 10 causes of death [Internet]. [cited 2022 Feb 6]. https://www.who.int/news-room/fact-sheets/detail/the-top-10-causes-of-death.
77. Hobbs FDR. Cardiovascular disease: different strategies for primary and secondary prevention? Heart. 2004;90(10):1217–23.
78. Gómez CA, Kleinman DV, Pronk N, Wrenn Gordon GL, Ochiai E, Blakey C, et al. Addressing health equity and social determinants of health through healthy people 2030. J Public Health Manag Pract. 2021;27(Suppl 6):S249–57.
79. Gama e Colombo D. Closing the gap in a generation: health equity through action on the social determinants of health. Final report of the Commission on Social Determinants of Health. Rev Direito Sanit. 2010;10(3):253.
80. Davidson KW, Kemper AR, Doubeni CA, Tseng C-W, Simon MA, Kubik M, et al. Developing primary care-based recommendations for social determinants of health: methods of the U.S. Preventive Services Task Force. Ann Intern Med. 2020;173(6):461–7.
81. O'Gurek DT, Henke C. A practical approach to screening for social determinants of health. Fam Pract Manag. 2018;25(3):7–12.
82. Centers for Medicare and Medicaid Services, Billioux A, Verlander K, Anthony S, et al. Standardized screening for health-related social needs in clinical settings: the accountable health communities screening tool. NAM Perspect. 2017;7(5).
83. Centers for Medicare & Medicaid Services. The accountable health communities health-related social needs screening tool. Center for Medicare and Medicaid Innovation; 2017.
84. AAFP PATIENT FORM (short version) social needs screening tool. https://www.aafp.org/dam/AAFP/documents/patient_care/everyone_project/patient-short-print.pdf. Accessed 2 Dec 2022.

Vaccines and Immunization

Zachary J. Pettigrew, Min Kim, and Sylvia Becker-Dreps

Introduction

Since ancient times, humans have developed ways to stimulate the body's immune system to decrease future infectious disease burden. Records indicate variolation against smallpox—or inoculating individuals with scrapings of smallpox lesions—took place in China as early as 1000 CE in attempts to curb infection and prevent outbreaks [1]. However, individuals undergoing variolation could succumb to smallpox through this process and the procedure was associated with a 2–3% fatality rate [1]. Finding a way to prevent infection without the risk of causing disease would not occur until centuries later, when in 1796, Edward Jenner famously took exudates from the hand of a milkmaid with cowpox and scratched it into the skin of 8-year-old James Phipps. Six weeks later, Jenner exposed Phipps to smallpox, and the boy never succumbed to disease [2, 3]. This ushered in the modern *vaccine* era, named after the very *vaccinia* species of cowpox that Jenner used to confer protection.

Since the eighteenth century, vaccines have evolved to include a wide array of vaccine types and modes of delivery. These range from live attenuated vaccines to new mRNA-based vaccines in widespread use during the COVID-19 era. Regardless of the specific type, all vaccines serve the purpose of immunizing or stimulating the immune system to create a protective response against infectious diseases for either an individual or a group of individuals [4]. The ultimate goal of immunization is "control of infection transmission, elimination of disease, and eventually, eradication of the pathogen that causes the infection and disease" [4]. It is this process of immune system stimulation and subsequent creation of an immune memory that has led to dramatic decreases in the rates of burdensome infectious disease across the world [4–6].

Vaccines specifically stimulate the adaptive branch, as opposed to the innate branch, of the immune system by introducing all or part of a microorganism, or a modified part of a microorganism, into a person [4, 7]. After injection, ingestion, or inhalation of a vaccine, antigens from the pathogen of interest are presented to lymphocytes through a variety of antigen-presenting cells. This sparks an immune system cascade that results in the creation of long-lasting B-cells and/or T-cells that are able to recognize and act against a specific pathogen, via humoral (antibody) or cell-mediated immunity, respectively. More specifically, vaccines containing only polysaccharide moieties elicit B-cell responses in a T-cell-independent manner, while those containing protein components will stimulate CD4+ T-helper (Th) cells that then induce humoral and cell-mediated immunity in a T-cell-dependent manner [8]. T-cell-dependent vaccines in turn induce a more pronounced immune response, leading to higher-avidity antibodies, greater immunologic memory and duration of response, and greater reduction of pathogen carriage rates in the community compared to their T-cell-independent counterparts [9]. Though single vaccination may not always confer as robust of an immune response as infection by the pathogen of interest, repeated vaccination over time can prime the immune system to create sustained memory B-cells and T-cells that can fight future infection. As immunity then wanes with time, booster vaccines may be provided to re-stimulate the immune system and ensure continued protection, particularly for those with chronic disease that are predisposed to infections [7–9].

Although ever changing, there are currently vaccination recommendations that target 17 pathogens in the United States (US): *Corynebacterium diphtheriae*, *Clostridium tetani*, *Bordetella pertussis*, poliovirus, *Haemophilus influen-*

Z. J. Pettigrew
Pediatric Teaching Program, Cone Health, Greensboro, NC, USA
e-mail: zachary.pettigrew@conehealth.com

M. Kim
Division of Infectious Diseases, Department of Medicine, University of North Carolina at Chapel Hill, Chapel Hill, NC, USA
e-mail: min_kim@med.unc.edu

S. Becker-Dreps (✉)
Department of Family Medicine, University of North Carolina at Chapel Hill, Chapel Hill, NC, USA
e-mail: sbd@email.unc.edu

zae type B (Hib), hepatitis A virus, hepatitis B virus, measles virus, mumps virus, rubella virus, rotavirus, varicella zoster virus, pneumococcus, meningococcus, influenza virus, human papillomavirus (HPV), and SARS-CoV-2 [10]. Additional vaccines recommended in other global regions include those that target Japanese encephalitis virus, rabies virus, tick-borne encephalitis virus, *Mycobacterium tuberculosis*, *Salmonella typhi*, *Vibrio cholerae*, and yellow fever virus [8, 11], with vaccines against adenovirus, dengue fever virus, *Yersinia pestis*, and smallpox available for certain populations [1]. This chapter provides an overview of vaccines and immunization. The first section introduces different forms of vaccines that can be categorized into live attenuated versus inactivated forms, depending on the vaccine components which act as antigens [1, 7, 12]. The subsequent section reviews related concepts, immunization strategies, and recommended administration schedules from different countries. This is followed by vaccine and immunization considerations for subgroups of patients with chronic disease before the chapter closes with strategies for promoting vaccine uptake.

Vaccine Classes

Live Attenuated Vaccines

In live attenuated vaccines, living viruses or bacteria are introduced to the patient after an attenuation process aimed at decreasing the pathogenicity of the organism or its ability to create clinical disease [7]. Such vaccines contain sufficient antigenic components to stimulate a protective immune response in a T-cell-dependent manner [8]. However, the bacterial or viral vector is still able to replicate within the cells and, for those who may be immunocompromised, cause disease [7]. As such, special consideration should be taken prior to administration of live vaccines depending on the patients underlying chronic disease(s). Commonly used live attenuated viral vaccines include vaccines against varicella virus, measles, mumps, rubella, rotavirus, and yellow fever as well as oral poliovirus vaccine and the live attenuated influenza vaccine (LAIV). Live attenuated bacterial vaccines include the oral cholera, oral typhoid, and the Bacillus Calmette-Guérin (BCG) vaccines [4, 9, 10, 11].

Inactivated Vaccines

Whole-cell/killed antigen vaccines. Heat, chemicals, or other processes are used to weaken a pathogen's ability to replicate while leaving the antigens in the virus or bacteria itself—the components of the vaccine—intact [7] in order to stimulate T-cell-dependent immunologic responses [8]. Commonly used whole-cell-inactivated vaccines include the typhoid, hepatitis A virus, rabies virus, inactivated poliovirus (IPV), Japanese encephalitis virus, and tick-borne encephalitis virus vaccines [1, 4, 7, 10].

Protein subunit vaccines. Protein subunit vaccines use only part of a pathogen as the immunogenic stimulus for a T-cell-dependent response [8]. These are often produced through recombinant technologies that introduce genetic material into yeast, bacteria, or viral vectors which then synthesize the desired protein antigens [7]. Examples of subunit vaccines include the acellular pertussis, hepatitis B, recombinant zoster vaccine (RZV), and inactivated influenza vaccines [4, 7–9].

Toxoids. Toxoid vaccines use inactivated toxins from bacteria as the antigenic stimulus for a T-cell-dependent immunologic response [7, 8]. Commonly used toxoid vaccines include those against *Corynebacterium diphtheriae* and *Clostridium tetani* [4, 7, 8]. These are usually combined with the acellular pertussis vaccine [10, 11].

Polysaccharide vaccines. Polysaccharide vaccines contain purified polysaccharide antigens that induce antibody production in a T-cell-independent manner [8]. In general, they are not as immunogenic as their conjugated counterparts, and they are not effective in children under 2 years old [8, 9]. However, some vaccines, such as the pneumococcal polysaccharide vaccine (PPSV), still play a role in recommended vaccination schedules due to the greater amounts of serotypes covered when compared to conjugate vaccines [13]. Other commonly used polysaccharide vaccines include the meningococcal and typhoid polysaccharide vaccines [4, 7–9].

Protein-conjugated vaccines. Protein-conjugated, or conjugate, vaccines include polysaccharides bound to more immunogenic proteins due to the T-cell-dependent immunologic response they elicit [4, 8, 9]. Stimulation of CD4+ Th lymphocytes induces not only humoral immunity through activation of B lymphocytes, but also can lead to cytotoxic CD8+ Th lymphocytes activation that can help clear pathogens [8]. CD4+ Th lymphocytes also stimulate B-cell differentiation into plasma cells, leading to a more sustained humoral immunity compared to polysaccharide vaccines [8]. Because of their stronger activation of humoral and cell-mediated immunity, conjugated vaccines have better immunogenicity in children under the age of 2 years old and immunocompromised individuals [8, 9]. Commonly used conjugate vaccines include pneumococcal conjugate vaccine (PCV), meningococcal conjugate vaccine (MCV), and Hib vaccines [4, 7–9].

Virus-like particle vaccines. Virus-like particle (VLP) vaccines employ genetic engineering to introduce a gene or select genes from a pathogen into a carrier virus that is grown in cell culture [8]. The carrier virus in turn produces VLPs, typically containing antigenic capsid proteins that closely resemble viruses but do not contain genetic material and therefore cannot replicate [14]. The VLPs are then harvested and purified for use as the immunogenic antigen in a vaccine [14, 15]. Such vaccines typically confer long-lasting protection [8]. A commonly used VLP-based vaccine is the human papillomavirus vaccine [8, 14].

Vaccine types used against SARS-CoV-2. Recent development of new SARS-CoV-2 vaccines has demonstrated the success of burgeoning vaccination strategies. Two vaccine types have been in general use for prevention of SARS-CoV-2. The first is a messenger ribonucleic acid (mRNA)-based vaccine that uses a lipid nanoparticle delivery system to introduce mRNA coding for the SARS-CoV-2 spike protein into human host cells, which is then translated and presented through major histocompatibility complexes (MHCs) to subsequently stimulate a T-cell-mediated immune response [16]. The second SARS-CoV-2 vaccine type uses a non-replicating viral vector to introduce antigenic substrate to the host. In this strategy, replication-deficient viral vectors, such as adenovirus, carry the deoxyribonucleic acid (DNA) coding for SARS-CoV-2 antigenic proteins such as the spike protein. Once infected, a human host cell then transcribes and translates the genetic material into proteins that trigger the immune system in a T-cell-dependent manner [17]. Other vaccines in development are employing more traditional approaches, including inactivated virus vaccines and recombinant protein subunit vaccines to help limit the burden of disease and spread of infection [17, 18].

Passive Immunization

The aforementioned immunization mechanisms employ an active immunization strategy in which protection against disease is produced by a person's own immune system [7]. This contrasts with passive immunization, in which antibodies or antitoxins against a specific pathogen are directly administered to a human subject [8]. Passive immunization offers immediate protection against disease when a person most needs it. Such protection, however, is short-lived [9]. Examples of passive immunization include maternal antibodies transferred through the placenta before birth or in the breast milk during lactation; pooled community antibodies transferred through intravenous, intramuscular, or subcutaneous immunoglobulin or other blood products; hyperimmune serum or antitoxins produced in animals (e.g., those against botulism and diphtheria); and monoclonal antibodies engineered to target specific diseases, such as palivizumab for respiratory syncytial virus (RSV) in premature children with chronic pulmonary or cardiovascular disease [4, 7, 9].

Key Concepts

Cocooning

Although a consensus definition of "close contact" is lacking, the term generally includes household contacts and/or immediate family members and can be expanded to include others with whom an individual has frequent or prolonged contact, such as a coworkers [19, 20]. Vaccination of close contacts, often known as "cocooning" or "shielding," aims to protect at-risk populations by limiting exposure to vaccine-preventable diseases (VPDs) by decreasing their close contacts' chance of becoming infected (Fig. 12.1) [19, 20, 21, 22]. Consequentially, morbidity and mortality due to VPDs are theoretically decreased for those with chronic illness, particularly conditions that alter immunity and blunt vaccine response [20, 23].

Because of the theoretical reduced risk of VPD-related morbidity and mortality, guidelines in several countries encourage vaccination against influenza, measles, mumps, rubella, varicella/zoster, and rotavirus for household members and for long-term care facility personnel caring for those with immunocompromising conditions [21–24]. Further recommendations are emerging in support of Hib, pneumococcal, and pertussis vaccination for close contacts of immunocompromised persons [25–28] in addition to recommendations for vaccination against SARS-CoV-2 [29–32]. An increasing number of national health authorities and professional societies have recommended close contact vaccination for individuals with other chronic conditions leading to altered immunity, such as asthma, neurodegenerative disorders, and chronic lung and liver disease [21, 24, 33].

Close contact vaccination strategies are considered to be safe and carry little adverse consequence to the patient with chronic medical conditions [22, 34, 35]. Inactivated vaccines carry no transmissible disease, and live vaccines carry minimal risk of transmission from the immunocompetent to the immunocompromised host and subsequent development of vaccine-type disease—a risk many experts deem to be much less than that of succumbing to wild-type disease [22, 28]. To further minimize the risk of vaccine-type viral transmission, many countries' immunization guidelines recommend the following protective measures: (1) avoiding live attenuated influenza virus vaccination in close contacts of hematopoietic stem-cell transplant (HSCT) recipients in the months following transplant, in HSCT recipients with graft-versus-host disease (GVHD), and patients with primary severe combined immunodeficiency (SCID); (2) for those with rash after receiving varicella or zoster vaccines, avoiding close contact with immunocompromised persons until lesions have resolved; and (3) for the highly immunocompromised, avoiding handling of diapers in infants vaccinated with rotavirus for 4 weeks following vaccination. Furthermore, oral

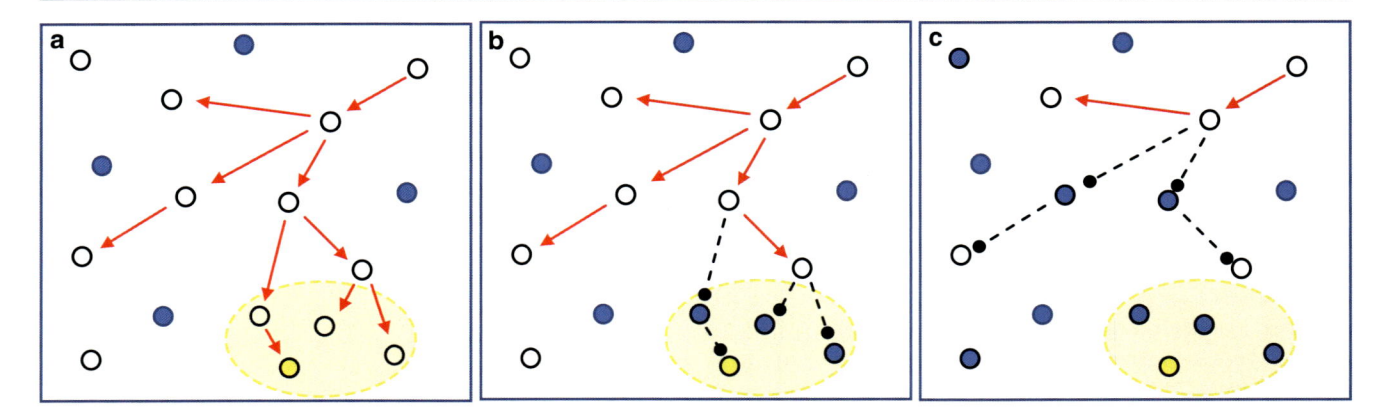

Fig. 12.1 Spread of infection in groups with varying vaccination rates. (**a**) Low community vaccination rates facilitate the spread of disease. (**b**) Close contact vaccination greatly decreased the risk of infection for a person with chronic disease. (**c**) High levels of community protection decrease the rates of disease transmission in a population, protecting some individuals who may not be vaccinated. Key: Blue dots = vaccinated person. White dots = unvaccinated person. Yellow dot = person with chronic illness. Red lines = spread of infection in the community. Black dotted lines = potential spread of disease that did not occur due to vaccination. Yellow region = close contacts of the individual with chronic illness

polio vaccine (OPV) should be avoided in all close contacts of immunocompromised persons; inactivated polio vaccines (IPV) should be given instead [4, 11, 22, 27, 28]. As OPVs are being phased out globally with a shift to IPV use, this should be less of a concern in the future.

Despite recommendations for household contact vaccination for at-risk populations, vaccination rates remain low [29, 36]. Isolated retrospective, survey-based studies from the Netherlands [37] and Greece [30] have demonstrated that most household contacts of those with chronic conditions do not receive yearly influenza vaccines, with 55% of adult solid tumor household contacts and up to 80% of pediatric asthma contacts lacking vaccination, respectively. One study looking at household contact vaccination status in children with solid organ tumors demonstrated that 50% of siblings had not completed their age-appropriate vaccination series. In the same study, none of the patient's parents had complete vaccination records and/or knew of their vaccination status [36]. Primary care providers are in a key position to help close such gaps between vaccination recommendations and reality by acting as reliable resources for open dialogue pertaining to recommendations for close contact vaccination.

Community Immunity

While cocooning aims to decrease rates of disease transmission by close household contacts of those with chronic illness, community protection—also known as herd immunity or community immunity—aims to limit disease transmission and further protect those with chronic illness on a larger scale [38]. By increasing the number of vaccinated members in the community or "herd," the transmissibility of pathogens greatly decreases [38, 39, 40]. Eventually, large enough community vaccination rates can eliminate local transmission, protecting unvaccinated and under-vaccinated individuals, as well as those who do not respond immunologically to vaccination, from infection and disease (see Fig. 12.1). Such "threshold" vaccination rates are typically calculated by using the R_0, or basic reproduction number of the pathogen, and varies based on pathogen and characteristics of local populations [41, 42].

Many studies have demonstrated the effectiveness of community protection in terms of decreasing incidence of disease. In the years after the introduction of 7-valent pneumococcal conjugate vaccine (PCV7) to US children in 2000, invasive pneumococcal disease (IPD) rates for children <2 months old (who were not yet vaccinated) decreased by 42% [43]. Similarly, introduction of the 13-valent vaccine (PCV13) into the US childhood vaccination schedule in 2010 led to a 58–72% reduction in rates of IPD due to PCV13-specific serotypes in adults by 2013 [44]. A study demonstrated similar findings across 10 European countries, with significant decreases in vaccine-serotype disease in adults after widespread childhood vaccination [45]. Other studies have demonstrated similar effects of community immunity in terms of reducing rates of Hib, HPV, meningococcus, and rotavirus infections in unvaccinated individuals after introduction of the corresponding vaccines into routine childhood immunization schedules [45, 46].

In contrast, sub-optimal community vaccination rates often result in disease breakouts and epidemics. Outbreaks of measles in New York [47] and southwestern France [48], pertussis in Kansas [49], varicella in North Carolina [50], and polio in the Netherlands [51] have occurred in largely unvaccinated communities, highlighting the threat of infection to those more susceptible to disease—including those with chronic illness—in such communities. This threat is arguably higher for those with chronic illness who have medical contraindications to vaccinations (as outlined elsewhere in this chapter) and are likely to experience greater morbidity and mortality from VPDs. Efforts to increase community vaccination rates can help further protect those with chronic disease by decreasing overall transmission rates—and thus both the incidence and prevalence of VPDs. As such, it is imperative for providers not only to offer but to encourage uptake of recommended vaccines to their patients, regardless of chronic illness status.

At a larger scale, national vaccination programs like the Vaccines for Children (VFC) program [52] promote vaccine access and, consequentially, improve community immunity. Partnerships between public and private stakeholders to facilitate strategic communication regarding vaccination recommendations, such as the ADVANCE Consortium in Europe and its successor, the Vaccine monitoring Collaboration for Europe (VAC4EU) [53], as well as support for local public health vaccination campaigns, may result in greater community vaccination and protection. Together with cocooning, community protection, through widespread vaccination, can help protect individuals with chronic illness.

Immunization Recommendations

United States

In the US, there is a formal process for establishing immunization recommendations that includes an ongoing evaluation of the health impact and safety of recommended vaccines [1, 54]. The first step in the process is vaccine licensure, which is the responsibility of the US Food and Drug Administration (FDA) [55]. The FDA bases this decision on safety and effectiveness data presented by entities seeking to market a vaccine in the US. The FDA also assures that the facility and manufacturing process maintain product quality and consistency [1, 56]. Approvals for licensure are made for specific indications and age groups, outlining specific vaccine schedules and dosages to be used as well as contraindications and precautions to the vaccine's use.

After FDA approval, recommendations for use of vaccines are made by the Centers for Disease Control and Prevention (CDC) with technical input from the Advisory Committee on Immunization Practices (ACIP) [57]. The ACIP is a group of 15 public health and medical experts who meet to review evidence and make decisions on each recommendation. These meetings are open to the public. During the meetings, ACIP members review scientific research on the vaccine's effectiveness and safety. The recommendations include who should receive the vaccine, vaccine schedules, precautions, and contraindications. The ACIP also provides specific vaccine indications for individuals with immunocompromising conditions or chronic illnesses [54, 57]. Only FDA-licensed or authorized vaccines are considered. Factors that are considered in the approval of vaccine recommendations include disease severity and incidence, vaccine efficacy in the intended target group, and factors that could impact the implementation of the recommendations, such as cost-effectiveness [54]. The ACIP also works closely with liaisons from groups such as the American Academy of Pediatrics, the American Academy of Family Physicians, and the American College of Obstetricians and Gynecologists to ensure that immunization recommendations are consistent across professional medical organizations [54, 57].

The CDC Director reviews the ACIP recommendations and then decides on their approval. Once these decisions are published in the CDC's Morbidity and Mortality Weekly Report, the recommendations become part of the official US immunization schedule [10, 57]. ACIP vaccine recommendations have important implications for coverage by private and public health insurance programs. For example, these recommendations determine which vaccines are provided through the VFC program, which provides free vaccines for uninsured and low-income children, including children receiving Medicaid [54]. Also, the Affordable Care Act requires private health insurance plans to cover ACIP-recommended vaccines without any patient cost-sharing [58]. Further, Medicare Part B covers the influenza, pneumococcal, hepatitis B, and COVID-19 vaccines, and Medicare Part D covers other vaccines indicated for adults that are recommended by the ACIP, such as Zoster and tetanus, diphtheria, and acellular pertussis (Tdap) vaccines [1, 54].

Europe, the United Kingdom, and Low- and Middle-Income Countries

The European Union does not support common immunization recommendations, but there is a shared process for vaccine licensing and testing [59]. European countries have national mechanisms in place for determining health policy, including immunization recommendations [59]. In some European countries, regional governments are permitted to decide on their own immunization policies, distinct from the national level. For example, in Germany, state governments are responsible for protecting public health and for making decisions on which vaccines are provided to their populations [59]. In Germany, recommendations for vaccine use are made by a national advisory committee, the *Ständige Impfkommission* (STIKO) [60]. However, these recommendations first need to be approved by individual states. Reimbursement for immunizations is made by individual health insurance plans, which are mostly publicly financed [60].

In the United Kingdom, immunization is administered through the centralized health system, the National Health Service (NHS), primarily through primary care providers but also in schools [59]. The Joint Committee on Vaccines and

Immunisation (JCVI) is an independent advisory committee that provides technical advice to the Secretary of State for Health on immunization policies [61]. In making immunization recommendations, the Committee considers the burden of disease, data on vaccine effectiveness and safety, and the implementation strategies that ensure the greatest benefit to public health [61]. The recommendations of the JCVI are published in a guide for clinicians, known as the "Green Book" [62]. Following approval by the Chief Medical Officers, the recommendations of the JCVI are required to be implemented by the Secretary of State for Health in England and Wales. As Scotland and Northern Ireland do not have independent advisory committees on immunization, they also rely on the JCVI's recommendations. Vaccines are procured on a national level, and all routine recommended vaccines are provided to the patient free of charge [59].

In most low- and middle-income countries, immunization programs are organized centrally and are typically administered through the public sector. Immunization strategies include both permanent immunization services, such as through health centers, and supplemental immunization activities, such as community outreach campaigns [63].

The World Health Organization (WHO) encourages all countries to have immunization advisory committees, which examine disease burden and make evidence-based recommendations for national immunization schedules. The WHO further encourages all countries to work toward high coverage rates and equitable access to vaccination, to ensure reach of immunization programs throughout all regions [64]. In 1974, the WHO established the Expanded Program on Immunization (EPI) to increase vaccination of children globally. Efforts first focused on establishing the infrastructure and appropriately trained personnel to deliver and monitor vaccination [63]. In 1984, the WHO established a standard schedule for the diphtheria-tetanus-pertussis (DTP), oral polio, measles, and BCG vaccines [63]. As new vaccines were developed, the WHO list of recommended vaccines was expanded to include others such as hepatitis B vaccines (HBV) and Hib conjugate vaccines. In 2008, the WHO further updated its list of recommended routine immunizations to include rotavirus, HPV, and pneumococcal conjugate vaccines [65]. In countries with the highest infant mortality, the primary series of pediatric vaccines start early, at 6, 10, and 14 weeks of age, with measles vaccination provided at 9 months of age. In Latin America, most primary pediatric vaccine schedules follow a 2, 4, 6 months schedule, with measles vaccination at 12 months of age. Information on all national immunization schedules for all countries is compiled by the WHO [66].

The Global Alliance for Vaccines and Immunization (Gavi), created in 1999, aims to extend the reach of the EPI in the world's lowest income countries. Gavi brings together United Nations (UN) Agencies, such as WHO and the United Nations Children's Fund (UNICEF), public health institutes, the vaccine industry, non-governmental organizations, and donors to achieve this goal [63]. Since its creation, the Gavi is responsible for providing over one billion vaccines, estimated to have averted 15 million deaths [67]. Immunization is estimated to prevent 4–5 million deaths each year; an additional 1.5 million deaths annually could be avoided if vaccine coverage improved [68]. Well-functioning immunization programs in both high- and low-income settings that address local disease priorities based on epidemiological data, include monitoring for impact, and generate trust with populations are essential to reduce vaccine-preventable disease burden.

Considerations for Chronic Illness and Associated Conditions

Vaccine recommendations for a variety of chronic illnesses are largely based on current immunization guidelines in the US at the time of this book's publication (Table 12.1) with

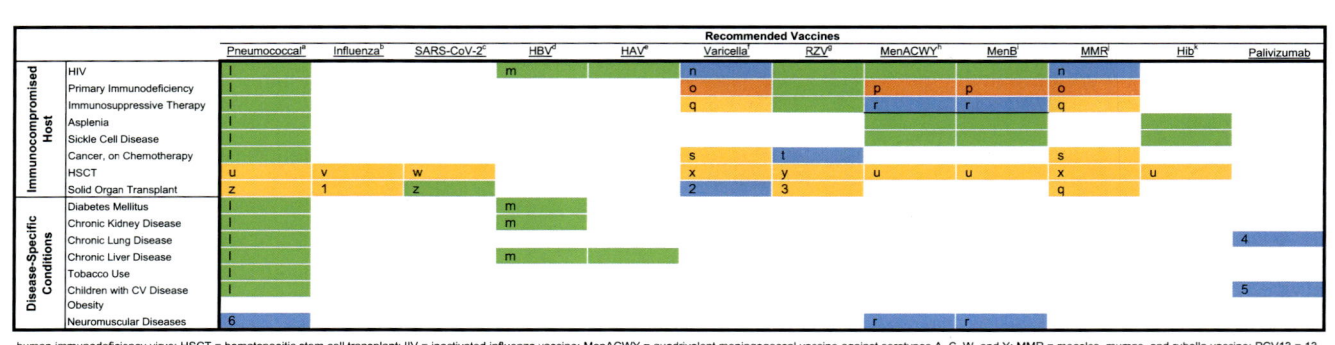

Table 12.1 US recommendations for vaccination, based on chronic conditions

		Recommended Vaccines											
		Pneumococcal[a]	Influenza[b]	SARS-CoV-2[c]	HBV[d]	HAV[e]	Varicella[f]	RZV[g]	MenACWY[h]	MenB[i]	MMR[j]	Hib[k]	Palivizumab
Immunocompromised Host	HIV	1		m			n				n		
	Primary Immunodeficiency	1					o		p	p	o		
	Immunosuppressive Therapy	1					q		r	r	q		
	Asplenia	1											
	Sickle Cell Disease	1											
	Cancer, on Chemotherapy	1					s	t			s		
	HSCT	u	v	w			x	y	u	u	x	u	
	Solid Organ Transplant	z	1	z			2	3			q		
Disease-Specific Conditions	Diabetes Mellitus	1			m								
	Chronic Kidney Disease	1			m								
	Chronic Lung Disease	1											4
	Chronic Liver Disease	1		m									
	Tobacco Use	1											
	Children with CV Disease	1											5
	Obesity												
	Neuromuscular Diseases	6						r	r				

human immunodeficiency virus; HSCT = hematopoietic stem cell transplant; IIV = inactivated influenza vaccine; MenACWY = quadrivalent meningococcal vaccine against serotypes A, C, W, and Y; MMR = measles, mumps, and rubella vaccine; PCV13 = 13-valent pneumococcal conjugate vaccine; PPSV23 = 23-valent pneumococcal polysaccharide vaccine; RZV = recombinant zoster vaccine

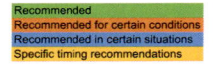

- Recommended
- Recommended for certain conditions
- Recommended in certain situations
- Specific timing recommendations

Table 12.1 (continued)

This table is based on CDC recommendations as of June 2022. Please refer your local public health agency for updated recommendations for your locale. Vaccine recommendations for the general population are shown in footnotes associated with each vaccine name

CV cardiovascular, *GVHD* graft-versus-host disease, *HAV* hepatitis A vaccine, *HBV* hepatitis B vaccine, *Hib Haemophilus influenzae* type B vaccine, *HIV* human immunodeficiency virus, *HSCT* hematopoietic stem-cell transplant, *IIV* inactivated influenza vaccine, *MenACWY* quadrivalent meningococcal vaccine against serotypes A, C, W, and Y, *MMR* measles, mumps, and rubella vaccine, *PCV13* 13-valent pneumococcal conjugate vaccine, *PPSV23* 23-valent pneumococcal polysaccharide vaccine, *RZV* recombinant zoster vaccine

[a] According to general vaccine recommendations, adults aged ≥65 should receive 1 dose of PCV (either PCV20 or PCV15); if PCV15 is used, it should be followed by a dose of PPSV23. All children should receive a primary series of PCV13 2, 4, and 6 months, and a booster at age 12–15 months. Specific recommendations for chronic conditions are shown in the table

[b] According to general vaccine recommendations, influenza vaccination is recommended for those aged ≥6 months who do not have contraindications to vaccination. The live influenza vaccine, LAIV4, should not be used in immunocompromised individuals

[c] COVID-19 vaccines are recommended for all individuals 5 years or older regardless of chronic condition as long as there are no other contraindications to COVID-19 vaccination

[d] According to general vaccine recommendations, immunization against hepatitis B is recommended for all individuals <60 years of age and for those ≥60 years old with risk factors for hepatitis B. Adults aged ≥60 years without known risk factors for hepatitis B may also receive HepB vaccines

[e] According to general vaccine recommendations, vaccination of children is recommended at 12–23 months of age, with catch-up for children up to age 18 years

[f] According to general vaccine recommendations, two doses of varicella vaccine are recommended for those without evidence of prior immunity and without contraindication to live vaccination

[g] According to general vaccine recommendations, vaccination with two doses of RZV is recommended for adults starting at 50 years of age

[h] According to general vaccine recommendations, recommended for adolescents aged 11–12 with a booster dose at age 16 years

[i] According to general vaccine recommendations, vaccination against meningococcus group B is not routinely recommended for all adolescents and young adults but can be provided following shared decision-making with individuals aged 16–23 years of age

[j] According to general vaccine recommendations, two doses of MMR vaccine should be provided to all children without a contraindication to live vaccination, with the first dose administered at age 12–15 months and the second dose administered at 4–6 years of age

[k] According to general vaccine recommendations, all infants should receive either two or three doses of a Hib vaccine (depending on the specific type of vaccine administered) between 2 and 6 months of age

[l] For adults, either (1) PCV20 or (2) PCV15 followed in 12 months by PPSV23. For children, PCV13 (for those who have not received this in the primary series) followed 8 weeks later by two doses of PPSV23, spaced 5 years apart, for immunocompromised hosts. Children with chronic lung disease, chronic CV disease, chronic liver disease, and tobacco use only require one dose of PPSV23

[m] In addition to the general recommendation for Hep B vaccination in all <60 years, this condition is considered a risk factor for acquiring hepatitis B in those ≥60 years

[n] May be given to children 1 year or older with CD4+ Th counts ≥15% or children 8 years or older with CD4+ Th cell counts of ≥200 cells/μL

[o] Children with certain immunodeficiencies, such as cyclic neutropenia, may still receive live vaccines, as can those with T-cell deficiencies meeting certain lymphocyte counts and those with impaired humoral immunity

[p] For patients with complement component deficiency

[q] Individuals should receive vaccination at least 4 weeks prior to the initiation of immunosuppression for this condition. In certain regions, vaccination may be recommended for those on stable doses of low-level immunosuppression. For other regions, consider live vaccination 1 month after discontinuing high-dose steroid therapy, 3 months after discontinuing other immunosuppressive therapy, and 6 months after discontinuing B-cell depletion therapy

[r] Recommended for those receiving a complement inhibitor such as eculizumab or ravulizumab

[s] May be given to those in remission who have not received chemotherapy for ≥3 months

[t] May be given to those in remission who have not received chemotherapy for ≥3 months. Can be considered for those at risk on continuous immunosuppressive therapy

[u] Recommended 6–12 months after HSCT

[v] Recommended at 6 months after HSCT; may be given as early as 4 months after HSCT if there is an outbreak in the community

[w] May be given before and post-transplant. If given prior to 3 months post-transplant, consider restarting the series to promote the development of post-transplant immunity

[x] Individuals should receive vaccination at least 4 weeks prior to the initiation of immunosuppression for this condition, based on current immune condition. May be given to those 24 months after transplant if they show no evidence of GVHD and/or are not on immunosuppressive therapy

[y] Should be administered 3–12 months after transplantation depending on type of HSCT and timing of antiviral therapy discontinuation

[z] Recommended to receive these vaccines at least 2 weeks prior to immunosuppression for this condition. May be given 2 or more months post-transplant

[1] IIV may be given as early as 1 month after transplant in cases of community outbreak

[2] Individuals should receive vaccination at least 4 weeks prior to the initiation of immunosuppression for this condition; in certain regions, vaccination may be recommended for those on stable doses of low-level immunosuppression. Vaccinate kidney or liver transplant recipients in the US without history of prior immunity with minimal to low immunosuppression and without recent history of graft rejection

[3] Preferable to give prior to transplantation; otherwise, administer at least 6–12 months after transplantation when there are no signs of graft rejection and patient is on maintenance immunosuppression

[4] Recommended for certain young children with chronic lung diseases

[5] Refer to local guidelines regarding indications for and timing of Palivizumab

[6] Recommended for certain conditions outside of the US

recommendations from different countries that are noted throughout. As recommendations vary by country or region, readers should refer to their local public health authority for the most up-to-date recommendations.

Vaccination of the Immunocompromised Host

General Principles

Vaccine recommendations for the immunocompromised host are largely guided by the state of host immune system, with special attention paid to the immunogenicity and safety of each vaccine. Key vaccines to consider for this population include pneumococcal vaccines, influenza vaccines, and zoster vaccines due to increased comorbidity from their associated illnesses, should one become infected [69]. However, providers should remember that patients, particularly children, should receive all routinely recommended vaccines if no contraindications to vaccination exist [4, 9]. Actual vaccination recommendations for different immunocompromised states vary by region and country.

In general, live vaccines are not recommended in immunocompromised hosts, except those with isolated IgA deficiency, immunoglobulin G (IgG) subclass deficiency, complement deficiency, or anatomical or functional asplenia, who may receive all recommended live and inactivated vaccines [4, 70]. Live vaccines should be avoided in immunocompromised hosts to decrease the risk of developing vaccine-type disease. There are certain circumstances in which the benefits of live vaccines outweigh the risks, such as in persons with human immunodeficiency virus (HIV) whose CD4 count is greater than 200 cells/μL [10, 11, 22]. Furthermore, a growing body of evidence suggests that it may be safe to administer certain live vaccines to those on low-level immunosuppressive therapy [71–75].

Vaccination guidelines continue to be updated as new evidence becomes available. Providers may refer to their respective country's vaccination guidelines or organizations such as the Infectious Diseases Society of America (IDSA), the CDC, the European Union League Against Rheumatism, and the European Centre for Disease Prevention and Control. Providers in regions where live vaccination is contraindicated while on immunosuppression may consider administering live vaccines 1 month after discontinuation of high-dose steroid therapy, 3 months after completion of other immunosuppressive or immunomodulatory therapy, or 6 months after completion of B-cell depletion therapy [70].

Recommendations for other key vaccine types follow general guiding principles. Increased rates of IPD in immunocompromised hosts have prompted recommendations for pneumococcal vaccination around the world [10, 27, 28]. In the US, for immunocompromised adults, the CDC recommends a single dose of 20-valent pneumococcal conjugate vaccine (PCV20), or alternately, 15-valent pneumococcal conjugate vaccine (PCV15) followed in 12 months by 23-valent pneumococcal polysaccharide vaccine (PPSV23) with an option to provide PPSV23 after a shorter interval of 8 weeks after PSV15 [76]. Recommendations for children with immunocompromising conditions in the US, for whom PCV20 and PCV15 are not yet approved at the time of this book's publication, are slightly different. Children over 2 years of age should receive two doses of 13-valent pneumococcal conjugate vaccine (PCV13) spaced by 8 weeks, if they have not received it as part of their primary series, followed 8 weeks later by a dose of PPSV23 and, for some, 5 years later by an additional dose of PPSV23, to provide coverage for additional pneumococcal serotypes [4, 22, 77, 78].

Influenza carries increased morbidity and mortality for immunocompromised patients, and annual receipt of inactivated influenza vaccine (IIV) as opposed to LAIV should be strongly encouraged [69]. Herpes zoster also confers higher disease burden for immunocompromised individuals when compared to their immunocompetent peers. While immunocompromised patients were excluded from two pivotal clinical trials of the recombinant zoster vaccine (RZV) [79, 80], there is not a true contraindication to administration. Subsequent clinical trials of RZV conducted in patients with solid tumors, hematological malignancies, renal transplants, and hematopoietic stem-cell transplantation (HSCT) [81] have demonstrated safety and efficacy of RZV in these patient groups. As such, current recommendations include a 2-dose RZV series for immunocompromised adults [82]. Finally, immunocompromised individuals are at increased risk of morbidity and mortality from SARS-CoV-2 infection and as such should receive vaccination according to local immunization guidelines and availability [62, 83].

Primary (Congenital) Immunodeficiencies

Inactivated vaccines are not contraindicated in individuals with primary immunodeficiencies, and these individuals should receive these vaccines per the CDC schedule for age-appropriate routine vaccination [10, 76]. Exceptions may be made for those receiving passive immunization through intravenous immunoglobulin (IVIG) replacement [4, 22]. Additional immunization recommendations for individual conditions depend on the specific defect in the immune system. For example, individuals with congenital or cyclic neutropenia are still able to receive live viral vaccines. Meanwhile, those with complement component deficiencies may require additional vaccines against encapsulated organisms, including pneumococcus, meningococcus, and *Haemophilus influenzae* [4, 22]. For those with primary immunodeficiencies resulting in T-cell deficiencies, the decision to use live vaccines depends on meeting certain CD3-

and CD8-cell counts levels and demonstration of an adequate mitogen response [4, 22]. In general, individuals with primary immunodeficiencies should also receive PPSV23 starting at 2 years of age, at least 8 weeks after the PCV series is completed, to provide additional protection against pneumococcal infections [22, 70, 76].

Patients on Immunosuppressive Therapy
Patients on immunosuppressive therapy should ideally receive any missing vaccines prior to initiation of immunosuppressive therapy. Generally, vaccination should occur at least 4 weeks prior to immunosuppression for live vaccines and 2 weeks for inactivated vaccines [4, 22, 70, 71, 84], though timelines may vary based on the specific drug being utilized. In such instances, it is recommended that providers refer to the associated disease society guidelines or drug reference to determine a safe and effective timeline for vaccination. Providers may also consider collecting vaccination titers for hepatitis B, measles, mumps, rubella, and varicella zoster viruses to determine the need for booster immunizations prior to immunosuppression [22, 84, 85]. Once immunosuppression has been initiated (or the immunocompromised status has been diagnosed), providers should continue to administer non-live vaccines, including annual influenza vaccines and additional pneumococcal, meningococcal (both ACWY beginning in infancy and B beginning at 10 years old), and Hib B vaccines as indicated per local schedules [4, 22, 28, 62, 77, 86, 87].

High-Level Immunosuppression
According to the 2013 IDSA guidelines, high-level immunosuppression can be defined by: (1) combined primary immunodeficiency disorder; (2) those receiving cancer chemotherapy; (3) solid organ transplant recipients within 2 months of transplantation; (4) people with HIV with CD4 Th lymphocyte counts less than 200 cells/µL for adults and adolescents and CD4 Th lymphocyte percentage less than 15% for infants and children; (5) those taking the equivalent of at least 2 mg/kg or 20 mg per day of prednisone, or its steroid equivalent, daily (whichever is the lesser) for greater than or equal to 14 days; or (6) those receiving certain biologic immune modulators such as TNF-alpha inhibitors or B-cell depleting therapies, such as rituximab [22]. Additionally, other chemotherapeutics and immunomodulators used for non-oncologic conditions, such as rheumatic disease, should be considered high-level immunosuppression, with special exceptions made for lower doses of methotrexate or azathioprine 6-mercaptopurine, as noted below [4, 22]. Biologics targeted at modifying allergic responses, such as targets of interleukin-5 (i.e., benralizumab, dupilumab, reslizumab, and mepolizumab) as well as the mast cell stabilizer, omalizumab, typically are not considered immunosuppressive in nature with respect to increasing the risk for infection or decreased immunogenicity of immunization [88–93]. However, no clear guidelines presently exist regarding additional vaccination or altered vaccination schedules for individuals receiving these drugs [22–28].

For adults on high-level immunosuppression, the CDC recommends administration of a single dose of PCV20, or alternately, PCV15 followed by PPSV23 in at least 8 weeks [76]. Immunosuppressed children should receive PCV13 (if not received during routine immunization) followed by PPSV23 in at least 8 weeks; for certain immunocompromising conditions, a second dose of PPSV23 should be administered 5 years after the first dose [77, 78]. The CDC and the IDSA also strongly recommend influenza vaccination with IIV annually for all immunosuppressed individuals 6 months of age and older [22, 76]. There are no contraindications to hepatitis A and B vaccines in immunocompromised individuals. Immunocompromised adults should also receive RZV [22, 69].

Low-Level Immunosuppression
The 2013 IDSA guidelines define low-level immunosuppression as (1) people with asymptomatic HIV infection with CD4 Th lymphocyte count 200–499 cells/µL for adults and adolescents and CD4 Th lymphocyte percentage of 15–24% for infants and children; (2) those receiving less than 20 mg/day or 2 mg/kg/day of systemic prednisone or steroid equivalent for 14 or more days; or (3) those receiving methotrexate therapy less than or equal to 0.4 mg/kg/week, azathioprine greater than or equal to 3 mg/kg/day, or 6-mercaptopurine less than or equal to 1.5 mg/kg/day [22]. The CDC and the IDSA recommend the same vaccines for those with high- and low-level immunosuppression. However, there is growing evidence demonstrating safety and efficacy of live vaccination in those with stable disease on low-level immunosuppression [73–75]. Refer to local guidelines for the most up-to-date recommendations. In general, live vaccines are not contraindicated in those on short-term corticosteroid therapy (i.e., under 14 days of therapy) or for those receiving topical, inhaled, or locally injected corticosteroids [22, 70, 94].

Adults with HIV
Both the CDC and the IDSA recommend a single dose of PCV20 or, alternatively, PCV15 followed by PPSV23 in people living with HIV who are at least 18 years of age [22, 76] and have not yet received a PCV series. PPSV23 is typically recommended at 12 months after PCV15 but could be given as early as 8 weeks after the administration of PCV15 if there is a benefit. In addition, annual flu vaccination with IIV is strongly recommended. Both the CDC and the IDSA recommend hepatitis A (HAV) and B (HBV) vaccines in people living with HIV with two possible pathways for hepatitis B immunization as described elsewhere [22].

Children with HIV
Children with HIV should receive all recommended inactivated vaccines based on local immunization schedules [4, 11, 22]. Meningococcal ACWY vaccination should be recommended for those living in or traveling to areas with a high risk of exposure. In terms of live vaccines, rotavirus may be given regardless of CD4 Th lymphocyte count or percentage. MMR and varicella vaccines may be given at or beyond 12 months of age to those with CD4 Th lymphocyte counts greater than 15% of all lymphocytes in children 1 to 7 years old or over 200 cells/µL for children 8 years or older [4]. Current recommendations in the US are to give the second dose of varicella vaccine 3 months after the first dose (as opposed waiting until the standard 4- to 6-year-old timeframe on traditional immunization schedules) [4, 22].

Similar recommendations have been made in Canada [95], Australia [27], and the United Kingdom [96], though the WHO and many other countries use a higher percent CD4 Th lymphocyte count of 25% or greater as the threshold for live vaccination [11]. Because of lack of safety data in patients with HIV, measles, mumps, rubella, and varicella (MMRV) combination vaccine and LAIV should not be administered to children with HIV [4, 27, 95]. Whereas the CDC does not recommend BCG vaccination for those living in the US, the WHO does recommend BCG vaccination for asymptomatic children with HIV living in endemic areas [11, 97]. For protection against pneumococcal disease, the CDC recommends that children with HIV receive a single PCV13 dose, followed in at least 8 weeks by a dose of PPSV23 and an additional dose of PPSV23 5 years later [77].

Asplenia or Sickle Cell Disease
Asplenia can be either structural or functional in nature. As the spleen not only filters the blood but also opsonizes bacteria, people with asplenia or sickle cell diseases are at greater risks for infections, particularly those caused by encapsulated bacteria such as *Streptococcus pneumoniae*, *Haemophilus influenzae*, and *Neisseria meningitidis* [98]. Patients with asplenia or sickle cell diseases have impaired serum opsonization against *Streptococcus pneumoniae*; therefore, they are at an increased risk for pneumococcal infections and IPD [78]. The CDC recommends PCV13 vaccines for children who are at least 2 years of age if they have not already been immunized with PCV13, followed by PPSV23 at least 8 weeks after the conjugate vaccine, and a second PPSV23 dose in 5 years [77]. According to the 2013 IDSA guideline, PPSV23 vaccines would be recommended for children whose splenectomy is planned at least 2 weeks prior to surgery or at least 2 weeks following surgery [22]. As for other immunocompromising conditions, both the CDC and IDSA strongly recommend inactivated influenza vaccines (IIV) annually. In addition, one dose of Hib vaccine in those who have not been previously vaccinated and are at least 5 years of age or older is recommended in people with anatomical or functional asplenia [22]. Children between 12 and 59 months of age who have received no prior Hib conjugate vaccine or one dose of vaccine before 12 months of age are recommended to receive two doses that are at least 8 weeks apart; children between 12 and 59 months of age who received two or more doses of Hib are recommended to receive one dose of Hib vaccine [99].

Quadrivalent meningococcal conjugate vaccines (MCV, or MenACWY) are recommended for those with anatomical or functional asplenia who are at least 2 months of age. The co-administration of MenACWY-D (Menactra®) and PCV vaccines may result in a reduction of antibody response to certain pneumococcal serotypes, so under the age of 2 years, MenACWY-CRM (Menveo®), which does not interfere with PCV seroconversion, should be used [100]. Even in older children, MenACWY-D should not be given within 4 weeks of completion of the PCV series. According to the CDC, adolescents with asplenia (and other immunocompromising conditions such as complement deficiency) should receive a two-dose primary series of MenACWY vaccine administered 8 weeks apart, as well as regular boosters [100]. A vaccine against meningitis serotype B (MenB) is approved for those 10 years of age and older. The CDC recommends this vaccine for those 10 and older with anatomic or functional asplenia, with periodic boosters [100]. For patients with anatomical or functional asplenia over 55 years of age and have not previously received MenACWY-D, then the quadrivalent meningococcal polysaccharide vaccine (MPSV-4) is recommended instead [22].

Patients with Cancer Receiving Chemotherapy
Per IDSA guidelines, live vaccines should *not* be given while patients are undergoing chemotherapy [22]. However, 3 months after chemotherapy is completed, inactivated vaccines should be given. Also, the live vaccines, varicella, measles, mumps, and rubella can be given for those in remission who have not received chemotherapy in greater than or equal to 3 months [22, 101]. All vaccines should be delayed at least 6 months if regimens included anti-B-cell therapies [22].

Hematopoietic Stem-Cell Transplant (HSCT) Recipients
Patients undergoing HSCT warrant additional vaccine administration due to two key mechanisms that increase their risk for VPDs. The first is the relatively immunosuppressed state caused by the primary underlying disease, which is further compounded by the conditioning process and ongoing maintenance immunosuppression. The second is the essential abolition of the host's current adaptive immune system, significantly decreasing one's prior immune memory including vaccine responses [69]. As such, the IDSA recommends

that candidates for HSCT follow standard vaccination schedules if they are considered immunocompetent at the time of vaccination [22]. Similar to vaccination recommendations prior to initiating immunosuppressive therapy, live vaccines (measles, mumps, rubella, and varicella) should not be given within 4 weeks of the initiation of the conditioning regimen, and inactivated vaccines should not be given within 2 weeks of the initiation of the conditioning regimen [22, 69].

IDSA recommend that post-HSCT, patients on ongoing immunosuppression or with active graft-versus-host disease (GVHD) should not be given live vaccines [22]. Annual IIV administration is recommended starting at 6 months after HSCT for anyone who is at least 6 months and older; it can be given earlier, at 4 months post-HSCT, if there is an influenza outbreak in the community in which patients reside [4, 22, 69]. In addition, the IDSA recommends that children and adults receive a three-dose series of PCV 3–6 months after HSCT. One dose of PPSV23 is recommended at 12 months after HSCT as long as there is no evidence of chronic graft-versus-host disease. In the presence of chronic GVHD, PCV can be given at 12 months after HSCT, however, the scientific evidence supporting this recommendation is weak. The IDSA further recommends that three doses of Hib vaccine, two doses of the quadrivalent meningococcal conjugate vaccine (MenACWY), three doses of tetanus-diphtheria (Td)-containing vaccines, three doses of IPV, and three doses of HBV be administered at 6–12 months after HSCT [22, 100].

For immunization against hepatitis B, measurement of a post-vaccination anti-HBs titer is recommended; if the anti-HBs titer is less than 10 mIU/mL, the three-dose series of HBV should be repeated. The IDSA also recommends a two-dose series of MMR vaccines in patients who are at least 24 months post-HSCT completion, based on moderate evidence for children, but low evidence for adolescents and adults [22]. To be considered for MMR vaccines, HSCT patients should not have active or chronic GVHD or ongoing immunosuppression. If intravenous immune globulin (IVIG) was given in the past, MMR vaccines should be deferred until at least 8–11 months after the last dose of IVIG was given, although the timing can be shortened in the case of a measles outbreak [4, 22, 74]. Administration of other live vaccines post-IVIG follow a similar schedule [22]. RZV should be administered to adults after transplant, with the timing of vaccination dependent on the type of HSCT performed (autologous vs allogeneic) and timing of antiviral therapy discontinuation [102].

Solid Organ Transplant (SOT) Recipients

The IDSA recommends that candidates for solid organ transplant (SOT) follow the vaccination schedules as outlined by CDC according to their immune status. Ideally, recommended vaccines are administered prior to transplantation. Live vaccines should be avoided within 4 years prior to transplantation [22]. For post-SOT patients, vaccination within 2 months of transplantation is not recommended as it is highly likely that there will be lack of adequate immune response while undergoing high-level immunosuppression [22]. However, in case of a community influenza outbreak, inactivated influenza vaccine (IIV) can be given at least 1 month after SOT. Two months after the time of transplantation, patients may again start receiving the recommended CDC vaccination schedule according to their immune status, with some notable modifications and exceptions. According to CDC guidelines, one dose of PCV is recommended in adults 2–6 months after SOT if there no prior PCV vaccination history [76]. For any SOT in children who are at least 2 years of age, one dose of PPSV23 should be given 2–6 months after SOT, and this would need to be administered at least 8 weeks after the most recent PCV13 dose. A booster PPSV23 dose should then be given 5 years later [4, 22, 77, 78]. In general, live vaccines including MMR and varicella are not recommended in SOT recipients, and efforts should be made to provide these vaccines to children at least 4 weeks prior to transplant [4, 22]. However, varicella vaccines are recommended in children who are kidney or liver transplant recipients and lack a prior varicella vaccination history, verified infection history, or serologic evidence of immunity if they are receiving minimal to no immunosuppression and have not had recent graft rejection [22]. For adults, RZV is recommended prior to transplantation when possible. For adults who did not receive it prior to transplantation, administration 6–12 months after transplantation is recommended for those on maintenance immunosuppressive therapy with stable graft function [102].

Immunocompromised Children with Chronic Illness

Chronically immunocompromised children require more vaccinations when compared to adults [86, 87]. For example, many young children with immunocompromising conditions or on immunosuppressive therapy may miss out on opportunities to receive their first doses of live attenuated vaccines such as MMR and varicella. Furthermore, these children are at increased risk of contracting VPDs and tend to have worse outcomes—as well as increased morbidity and mortality—compared to their immunocompetent counterparts [70, 103–105]. As a result, some will require extended vaccination beyond routine childhood vaccine series that may include (1) vaccines not typically given to children (such as PPSV23) and (2) vaccines not typically given beyond a certain age range (such as Hib) [70].

Obtaining accurate vaccine records, and perhaps vaccine titers, are keys to protecting this vulnerable population. Primary care and specialty providers should seek to obtain records from clinical sites and local immunization registries [4, 70, 103]. Once a child's immune status is clarified, provider teams may then develop a vaccination schedule to ensure that catch-up vaccines, and any supplementary vaccines, are given in a timely manner [4, 61]. This may include accelerated schedules that provide vaccines at ages younger than those recommended by local guidelines in order to confer additional protection [70, 104].

Special consideration should be given to each individual's anticipated disease course, as children may require or develop increased levels of immunosuppression or immunocompromise, respectively, as they age. Some conditions, particularly those that require initiation of immunosuppressive therapy, such as inflammatory bowel diseases, rheumatologic diseases, and other chronic inflammatory diseases, may necessitate an accelerated vaccination schedule prior to initiation of immunosuppressive therapy [69]. Once therapy has started, the child should continue to receive routine inactivated vaccination per routine local schedules [4]. Recommendations regarding administration of live vaccines, at present, are region-specific and largely apply to those with stable disease and low levels of immunocompromise [27, 28, 71, 86, 87]. Special attention should be paid to patients receiving chemotherapy or hematopoietic stem-cell transplants, as these individuals require re-vaccination after completion of therapy or transplant, respectively [103, 104].

Diabetes Mellitus

Diabetes mellitus is a condition caused by impaired insulin production that causes microvascular and macrovascular changes within the body, leading to various complications [106]. The host immune system is altered as a result of diabetes mellitus, which especially affects the innate immune system and phagocytic functions [107]. Uncontrolled hyperglycemia can increase the risk for infection, such as skin and soft tissue, ear, respiratory tract, and urinary tract infections caused by viral, bacterial, and fungal organisms [108, 109]. The mechanisms of impaired humoral immunity in the setting of hyperglycemia can include modification of the structure and functions of immunoglobulins which leads to decreased vaccine immunogenicity involving humoral immunity [108]. The glycated antibodies are not able to effectively neutralize viruses, thereby leading to increased infection risks. In addition, cellular immunity is also impaired as various components of cellular immunity are dysregulated leading to defective CD4 and CD8 cells [108].

Pneumococcal vaccines. The CDC recommends a dose of PCV-20 or, alternately, PCV-15 followed by PPSV23, in people with diabetes mellitus who are 19–64 years old [76]. Children of at least 2 years of age should receive a single dose of PPSV23 after completion of their PCV13 primary series [77, 78].

Influenza vaccines. The CDC recommends routine annual influenza vaccination. People with metabolic disorders including diabetes mellitus are at higher risk for complications of severe influenza [109]. There is some evidence of defective antibody response to influenza vaccine in individuals with diabetes, but in a systemic review the overall immunogenicity among people with diabetes mellitus was comparable to those without diabetes mellitus [110].

Hepatitis B vaccines. The CDC recommends hepatitis B immunization for all people under the age of 60 [111]. This recommendation is particularly important for people with diabetes, as they are at an increased risk of hepatitis B through blood glucose monitoring or other diabetes care equipment. For those who are 60 years of age or older, the decision to vaccinate would be based on shared decision-making with their health care providers [112].

Vaccines against SARS-CoV-2. Vaccines to prevent COVID-19 are recommended for people with Type 1 or Type 2 diabetes mellitus as these conditions increase the risk of developing severe COVID-19 [83, 113]. However, whether there are specific vaccine types or schedules that are more effective in individuals with diabetes mellitus has yet to be elucidated by the time of this chapters publication.

Chronic Kidney Disease (CKD)

Infection is among the leading causes of hospitalization in individuals with chronic kidney disease (CKD) and those on dialysis [114]. CKD is associated with chronic inflammation and alterations in adaptive and innate immunity, including diminished phagocytic capacity and antigen presentation, diminished function of B-cells and T-cells, and altered cytokine production, resulting in a higher burden of multiple infectious diseases [115–117]. For example, the mortality rate from pneumonia in patients with CKD is twice that of individuals without kidney disease [118], and influenza-like illness has been identified as an important contributor to mortality in individuals with end-stage renal disease (ESRD) [119]. Individuals with CKD also have a 20-fold higher rate of herpes zoster than the general population [120]. Although the prevalence of hepatitis B in the US is low [121], individuals with CKD who require dialysis are at high risk for developing chronic hepatitis B [122]. To reduce the burden of infectious diseases, the CDC provides specific recommendations for individuals with CKD [123], in addition to recommending age-appropriate immunization [124, 125].

Influenza vaccines. Immunization against influenza is especially important for individuals with CKD. However, vaccines are less immunogenic in this group, especially those with advanced disease requiring hemodialysis [126–128]. An active area of research is identifying ways to make influenza vaccines more efficacious in individuals with CKD. Among patients on hemodialysis, a clinical trial of an adjuvanted influenza vaccines showed improved immunogenicity as compared to a non-adjuvanted influenza vaccine [129]. Further, there is evidence that high-dose influenza vaccines are more effective than standard-dose vaccine in older adults [130]. A large observational study did not find a benefit of high-dose over standard-dose vaccine in adults undergoing hemodialysis [131]. The ACIP has not made a preferential recommendation for a specific type of influenza vaccine for individuals with CKD [130].

Pneumococcal vaccines. Pneumonia is a common cause of morbidity and mortality in patients with CKD, and *Streptococcus pneumoniae* is among the most common causes of pneumonia [132, 133]. The pneumococcal polysaccharide vaccine, PPSV23, has long been recommended for use in older and immunocompromised adults. However, recent studies raised questions about the benefit of PPSV23 in these high-risk populations, including individuals with CKD [134–136]. Pneumococcal conjugate vaccines evoke a more immunogenic T-cell dependent immune response and have higher immunogenicity in patients receiving hemodialysis [137]. Pneumococcal conjugate vaccines have been recommended for pediatric use since 2000 [138], resulting in substantial reductions in disease burden in children. Clinical trials in adults with HIV showed higher efficacy or non-inferior immune responses of conjugate vaccines as compared to polysaccharide vaccines [139, 140]. At present, the CDC recommends either PCV20 or, alternately, PCV15 followed by PPSV23, in adults ≥19 years with chronic kidney disease [76–78]. For children with CKD, PPSV23 should be given at 2 years of age, after the course of PCV13 has been completed, with a booster PPSV23 dose given 5 years later [77, 78, 141].

Hepatitis B vaccines. Occasional outbreaks of hepatitis B in hemodialysis centers highlight the need for hepatitis B immunization in individuals with CKD [122]. Unfortunately, seroconversion to the vaccine declines with renal disease progression [142, 143]. Despite lower seroconversion rates as compared to the general population, hepatitis B immunization still confers important benefits to individuals with CKD who progress to dialysis [144]. There are currently five hepatitis B vaccines recommended for use in the US. The most recently recommended vaccine, HepB-CpG, contains an adjuvant (1018 adjuvant) and has been found to induce seroconversion in 90–100% of subjects and is well tolerated [145]. For patients requiring dialysis, higher dose preparations in both three- and four-dose series are available, and guidelines recommend their use [146]. One to 2 months after series completion, testing of anti-HBs titers is recommended; those with levels less than 10 mIU/mL should receive a second series [146].

Pulmonary Disease

People with chronic respiratory conditions are at increased risk of exacerbations, hospitalizations, and mortality [147]. Vaccination against VPDs for those with chronic pulmonary conditions could reduce numbers of exacerbation episodes and associated complications, and providers should recommend them to optimize health outcomes [148].

Pneumococcal vaccines. Currently, pneumococcal vaccination is recommended for those with chronic lung conditions, including those with CF, chronic obstructive pulmonary disease (COPD), emphysema, and asthma [78, 149]. For adults with chronic lung conditions, the CDC recommends administration of PCV20 or, alternately, PCV15 followed by PPSV23 for those who have never before received PPSV23 [76]. In a Cochrane meta-analysis, people with COPD who had received either polysaccharide or conjugated pneumococcal vaccines had a lower chance of developing community-acquired pneumonia [150]. It is worth noting that antibody responses to PPSV23 in individuals with asthma were lower than those without asthma [78, 151]. Children with chronic lung conditions, including those with asthma treated with prolonged oral corticosteroids, should receive one dose of PPSV23 after completion of their PCV13 primary series [77, 78].

Influenza vaccines. The CDC recommends annual influenza vaccines for all individuals aged 6 months and older, including those with pulmonary conditions. For those who otherwise do not meet the criteria of immunocompromised hosts, both inactivated and live attenuated influenza vaccines can be given. A Cochrane Review found moderate evidence that influenza vaccines decreased the number of acute exacerbations of COPD [152]. Meanwhile, a systematic review found that influenza vaccination prevented between 59% and 78% of asthma exacerbations, significantly reducing related morbidity and mortality [153].

Chronic Liver Disease

Patients with advanced liver disease are at increased risk of bacterial infections, including spontaneous bacterial peritonitis, pneumonia, and bacteremia [154]. Immune dysfunction is thought to be caused by reduced production of innate immune proteins, the effect of hypersplenism on reducing leukocyte counts, and impaired phagocytic activity of neutrophils [155]. Also, viral infections, such as influenza and viral hepatitis, can cause decompensation of underlying liver disease. Vaccination with hepatitis A and B vaccines is important to mitigate the risk of superimposed hepatitis A and B in patients with chronic liver disease without prior immunity. Ideally, these vaccines are given early in the course of illness when immune responses to these vaccines are robust. Specific vaccine recommendations for children with chronic liver diseases, including non-alcoholic fatty liver disease, are available from the North American Society for Pediatric Gastroenterology, Hepatology, and Nutrition (NASPGHAN) [156].

Influenza vaccines. Several studies suggest that influenza immunization results in moderate to high seroconversion rates in patients with chronic liver disease [157–159]. While independent studies favor adequate seroconversion after influenza vaccination, a systematic review examining the effectiveness of influenza vaccines in patients with chronic liver disease found insufficient quantity and quality of studies to support such findings [160]. Since there are minimal serious adverse events following inactivated influenza immunization reported in patients with liver disease, including those receiving interferon-based treatment or those on immunosuppressants following liver transplantation, the influenza vaccine should be recommended in this group of patients.

Pneumococcal vaccines. Patients with chronic liver disease have twice the rate of IPD as compared to the general population [161]. In addition, pneumococcal bacteremia is known to carry a high case mortality rate in patients with cirrhosis [162]. There are limited studies on the effectiveness and immunogenicity of pneumococcal immunization in patients with chronic liver disease. In a clinical trial of PPSV23 in patients with end-stage liver disease being evaluated for liver transplantation, PPSV23 vaccination resulted in temporary increases in serum anti-pneumococcal polysaccharide antibodies. However, these antibody levels declined to at or below baseline levels by 3 months after liver transplantation [163]. This suggests that a booster dose would be warranted following liver transplantation; however, there have not been studies conducted to support this. Currently, the CDC recommends PCV20, or alternately, PCV15 followed by PPSV23 in adults with chronic liver diseases, and in patients with liver transplants on immunosuppressive medications [76]. Children with liver disease should receive a single dose of PPSV23 after completion of the PCV13 primary series [77, 78].

Hepatitis A and B vaccines. Hepatitis A or B infection in patients with chronic liver disease can cause further decompensation of liver disease or death [164] and hepatitis A and B vaccines are recommended in patients with chronic liver disease who do not have immunity. In the US, less than one-third of adult patients with chronic liver disease have been immunized against hepatitis A and B [165]. In contrast to hepatitis A immunogenicity, the immune response to the hepatitis B vaccine is much lower in patients with chronic liver disease as compared to healthy individuals [166, 167]. For example, one study examining patients with chronic liver disease awaiting liver transplant found only a 37% response rate after the three-dose series [168]. Therefore, it may be best to vaccinate patients with chronic liver disease before the onset of cirrhosis or advanced fibrosis. Some experts recommend high-dose or double-dose (40 μg) vaccine at standard intervals [169]. For patients with chronic hepatitis B infection, the American Association for the Study of Liver Diseases (AASLD) recommends that both household and sexual contacts who are negative for HBsAg and anti-HBs should receive HBV vaccination [169]. NASPGHAN recommends hepatitis A and B immunization for children with chronic liver disease, including non-alcoholic fatty liver disease, which has been increasing in prevalence in children [156].

Pregnancy

Immunization of pregnant patients protects both the mother and the child through the transfer of IgG antibodies across the placenta prior to delivery. After birth, primary vaccination does not yet provide adequate protection until after 6 months of age, at least based on standard US immunization schedules. Therefore, maternal immunization has the potential to close this "immunity gap" early in infancy [170]. While the altered immune state of pregnancy may result in slightly decreased vaccine-elicited immunity in pregnant women, these differences have not been found to be associated with decreased vaccine effectiveness [170]. Maternal immunization is especially important in pregnant women with chronic diseases, who may have an increased risk of infections or who are more likely to develop severe disease following infection.

Influenza vaccines. A systematic review following the 2009 influenza A pandemic found an increased risk of hospital and intensive care unit admission and death in pregnant women; pregnant women with additional risk factors were even more likely to develop severe disease [171]. In addition to pandemic influenza, seasonal influenza also causes a high burden of disease in pregnant women [172]. Influenza vaccines have been shown to be safe and effective in pregnancy, providing benefits both to mother and infant [173]. Therefore, to reduce the burden of influenza during pregnancy, the CDC, Public Health England, and the WHO all recommend influenza vaccines during pregnancy [11, 62, 65, 86]. The vaccine can be administered during any trimester of pregnancy and is especially important in women at higher risk for severe disease due to other chronic illnesses.

Other vaccines. In addition to influenza and COVID-19 immunization, maternal Tdap immunization is routinely recommended (optimal timing is between 27 and 36 weeks of gestation according to the CDC) to provide young infants with protection against pertussis infections during the first months of life [174]. While safety studies in pregnant women are limited, inactivated vaccines are considered safe in pregnancy. Live vaccines are generally avoided due to the theoretical risk of fetal infection. Common inactivated vaccines such as pneumococcal vaccines, hepatitis A and hepatitis B, should not be withheld from pregnant patients when the benefit outweighs the likely low risks of these inactivated vaccines [175].

Other considerations for maternal immunization. IgG antibodies are actively transported across the placenta into the fetal circulation, a process that begins at about 13 weeks of gestation and increases during the third trimester. Certain chronic maternal conditions can result in a decrease in transplacental transfer of IgG antibodies to the infant [176–178]. Conditions that cause placental pathology, such as HIV and placental malaria, can result in a decrease in maternal antibody transfer to the developing fetus [179].

Tobacco Use Disorder

Components of tobacco products, including nicotine, acrolein, and others, paralyze the respiratory cilia [180, 181]. This prevents the cilia from partaking in their normal upward sweeping pattern that clears infectious particles such as influenza virus and pneumococcus bacilli, and, more recently, SARS-CoV-2 virus from the respiratory tract [182, 183]. Toxins in the inhaled fumes also increase local inflammation and fibrosis, damage the underlying respiratory epithelial barrier, and alter immune cell activity (such as neutrophil chemotaxis and macrophage signaling), understandably increasing the rates of respiratory infection in chronic smokers [181].

Smokers are five times more likely to develop influenza infections compared to healthy peers [184] and are twice as likely to develop community-acquired pneumonia [181]. Smokers also demonstrate prolonged in vitro adherence of *Strep pneumoniae* to the buccal mucosa [185] which likely contributes to the higher rates of both pneumococcal pneumonia and invasive pneumococcal disease seen in this population [186, 187]. Early studies report that smoking increases the risk of hospitalization and death for individuals infected with SARS-COV-2 [188–190].

Because of increased morbidity and mortality risk [191–193], individuals who smoke should receive a yearly influenza vaccine, and adults who smoke should receive pneumococcal vaccinations in accordance with local immunization guidelines [94, 109]. For example, the current recommendation in the US is for current smokers to receive one dose of PCV20 or, alternately, PCV15 followed by PPSV23 [76]. US guidelines expanded to recommend vaccination against SARS-CoV-2 for smokers, both for primary vaccination and booster vaccination [10, 194]. Increased rates of vaping have raised questions as to whether those who vape—or use electronic cigarettes—should receive extended pneumococcal vaccination. Studies have shown that chemical components of vaping products including nicotine, cinnamaldehyde, and other oxidative components can lead to decreased ciliary clearance in a fashion not dissimilar to tobacco products [180]. Though the CDC does not recommend pneumococcal vaccination for those who use E-cigarette products at this time, it does recommend annual influenza vaccination [195]. Primary care and specialty providers should strongly encourage influenza immunization and should consider vaccinating such individuals against pneumococcus given their increased risk.

Children with Cardiovascular Disease

Children with cardiovascular disease should receive routine immunizations per local schedules, whether standard or catch-up, including at least two doses of the most current pneumococcal conjugate vaccine approved for use in children [77, 87, 196]. In addition, children with a history of chronic heart disease (including cyanotic congenital heart disease and chronic heart failure) should receive at least one additional dose of PPSV23 after the age of 2 years [77, 78, 87] due to their increased risk of invasive and non-invasive pneumococcal disease [196]. Annual influenza vaccine should be encouraged, as infection has been associated with increased in-hospital morbidity, mortality, and length of stay for those with severe and non-severe congenital heart disease [197] and heart failure. For infants with certain types of congenital heart disease, passive immunization with palivizumab or a humanized monoclonal antibody against the F glycoproteins of RSV should be given during RSV season, per local guidelines [198–201].

Obesity

Obesity may contribute to sub-optimal responses to some vaccines. There is a decreased response to hepatitis vaccines in obese individuals [202, 203], which is concerning given the higher risk of non-alcoholic steatohepatitis in obese individuals and the potential for viral hepatitis to further compromise hepatic function. Obese children also produce lower antibody levels after tetanus vaccination, as compared to children of normal weight [204]. Further, obesity is a risk factor for severe outcomes of influenza and SARS-CoV-2 infections [194, 205]. While obese individuals produced a similar antibody response to both H1N1 and seasonal influenza vaccines as compared to non-obese individuals [206, 207], obese individuals exhibited both lower levels of antibody 12 months after vaccination and decreased T-cell immunity, which may affect disease progression and cross-reactivity to related influenza strains [208].

The COVID-19 vaccines which have been approved by the US FDA [209, 210] show high efficacy in obese individuals. For example, a subgroup analysis of the Pfizer-BioNTech COVID-19 vaccine efficacy trial showed a vaccine efficacy similar to non-obese participants [211]. Similarly, the Moderna COVID-19 vaccine efficacy trial found an efficacy of 95% among its obese participants [212]. The available evidence supports high efficacy of COVID-19 vaccines in obese individuals, which is critical, given the higher risk of severe outcomes of SARS-CoV-2 infections experienced by obese individuals [213].

Neurodegenerative and Neuromuscular Disease

Neurodegenerative and neuromuscular diseases place individuals at increased risk of acquiring respiratory infections, including influenza and pneumonia, due to weakened respiratory effort and airway clearance. Immunosuppressive therapy used to treat some of these diseases can also place this population at higher risk for respiratory disease and related complications [33, 84, 214–216]. For most neurodegenerative and neuromuscular conditions that do not require immunosuppressive therapy, additional vaccination beyond routine vaccination and annual influenza vaccination has historically not been recommended. However, some countries, such as Canada [217], Ireland [218], and the United Kingdom [219, 220], as well as professional societies have started recommending additional pneumococcal vaccination for individuals with impaired clearance of oral secretions [221, 222]. Individuals with a history of neurosurgical intervention in the central nervous system, such as a ventriculoperitoneal shunt, or other conditions, such as skull fracture, that predispose to CSF leak should receive extra pneumococcal vaccination as well [4, 22, 217–219, 223]. Additionally, those with myasthenia gravis and other conditions being treated with eculizumab, a monoclonal antibody against terminal complement protein C5, are at increased risk of meningococcal meningitis and should receive meningococcal vaccination against serotypes A, C, W, Y, and B per local guidelines and vaccine availability [4, 22, 100, 224, 225].

Strategies to Promote Vaccine Uptake

Barriers to vaccine uptake include both difficulties in access and acceptance. Time constraints, childcare challenges, and transportation difficulties have been identified as important barriers to vaccination [226]. Vaccine hesitancy—a delay or refusal of vaccination despite vaccine availability—is a difficult problem for medical providers. Specific approaches to address vaccine hesitancy are provided in recent systematic reviews [227, 228].

Several evidence-based approaches have been shown to increase vaccination acceptance and administration. Studies have examined interventions implemented at the practice level and the provider level [229]. Immunization information systems (IIS) are an important tool for providing vaccination history and identifying recommended vaccines by age group [230]. IIS are electronic registries that record vaccines administered to individuals living in a geographic area. With the increasing numbers of vaccines recommended, the IIS provides a time-efficient method of identifying which vaccines are indicated at the point of clinical care. While the use of IIS has streamlined the identification of patients due for routine vaccines, they typically do not contain information on chronic illness to guide immunization for these subpopulations. Providers need to consider vaccine recommendations when providing medical care for these patients. Evidence-based recommendations on interventions to promote vaccine uptake are provided by the Community Preventive Services Task Force, an independent panel of public health and prevention experts in that provides recommendations about interventions at the community level to improve population health [231].

Communication Approaches

Providers frequently assume that patients or caregivers will opt for vaccination according to national guidelines. Statements such as "You are due for the pneumococcal vaccine today" should be used instead of "Are you interested in receiving the pneumococcal vaccine?" [232, 233]. In addition to providers, other clinical staff should be instructed to use comparable directive approaches when offering vaccination. If patients decline initial prompting, providers and clinical staff should address any concerns that patients voice in areas such as vaccine safety or effectiveness and use plain language that is accessible to the patient. For patients with chronic diseases, providers and staff can tailor conversations by explaining risk factors that place the patient at higher risk for disease burden. A motivational interviewing approach, which has been found to increase vaccine uptake in adolescent populations [234], is another strategy that can be employed to promote vaccination. Interventions that are multi-component and dialogue-based have been found to be most helpful in addressing continued vaccine hesitancy [235]. However, more evidence is needed to guide the choice of which specific interventions are likely to lead to greater vaccination [236].

Missed Opportunities

Patients with chronic illness generally have multiple encounters with their providers and other health care services. Unfortunately, patients and providers will often have multiple competing priorities in chronic illness management, which can result in delays in recommended vaccination. Vaccination can and should be offered at every visit [237, 238]. Providers should also be aware of contraindications to vaccination, which are limited.

Provider Reminders

Health information technologies and electronic tools can be used to prompt providers and clinical staff to provide vaccines to those who are due for vaccination. Electronic health record (EHR) notifications, such as pop-up "best-practice advisories," or daily lists of patients on the schedule who are due for vaccination are a few representative examples. Studies across multiple clinical settings have found that these approaches contribute to increased vaccine uptake, including among patients with chronic illness [239–241]. Standing orders and protocols can be developed and implemented to allow clinical staff ready administration of vaccines [242–244]. Protocols should clearly designate vaccination parameters, such as frequency, and reasons for non-administration.

Patient Reminders and Recall Systems

EHR queries can be performed to identify patients who are due for vaccines and can be contacted through electronic messaging, phone calls, or letters to inform them of their need for vaccination. Prior studies have shown that this approach increases vaccination rates across multiple settings and patient populations [245–247].

Data-Informed Feedback

Providing data on vaccination coverage can be integrated into larger quality improvement initiatives being implemented in practices. Strategies that provide data to providers and clinical staff on the vaccine coverage for patient panels have been reported [248–250]. Feedback can be provided to the entire practice, or to individual providers, to benchmark performance in comparison to other providers in the practice. Using EHR, data reports can identify variances in vaccine uptake and identify patients at greater risk who should be targeted for vaccination. In addition, data can be reported by different sociodemographic variables to identify disparities in care and potential interventions. These approaches tend to work best as part of multifaceted approaches to improve quality of health care delivery and increase vaccination [238].

Future Directions

Primary care physicians will continue to play an important role in providing vaccinations to patients with chronic illness, whether through individual patient interactions or as part of clinical teams. In the future, there will likely be increasing use of information technology tools, such as EHR prompts and patient panel reports from EHR data to support vaccine guideline adherence. Also, vaccine recommendations for patients with chronic illnesses will continue to change to reduce the existing burden of infectious diseases, incorporate new vaccines as they become available, and confront newly emerging pathogens. Vaccine classes that were advanced during the COVID-19 pandemic, such as mRNA vaccines, may accelerate the introduction of future vaccines and expand the benefits of vaccinations for patients with chronic illness.

References

1. Plotkin SA, Orenstein WA, Offit PA. Plotkin's vaccines. 7th ed. Elsevier Inc.; 2017. p. 1–1637.
2. Jenner E. Dr. Jenner, on the vaccine inoculation. Med Phys J [Internet]. 1800 Jun [cited 2021 Sep 29];3(16):502. https://www.ncbi.nlm.nih.gov/pmc/articles/PMC5659579/.
3. Sadanand S. Putting smallpox out to pasture. Nat Res 2021 [Internet]. 2020 Sep 28 [cited 2021 Sep 29]. https://www.nature.com/articles/d42859-020-00007-6.
4. AAP Committee on Infectious Diseases. Section 1: Active and passive immunization. In: Kimberlin DW, Barnett ED, Lynfield R, Sawyer MH, editors. The Red Book. 32nd ed. Itasca, IL: The American Academy of Pediatrics; 2021. p. 1–105.
5. World Health Organization Team on Immunization V and B. Global vaccine action plan monitoring, evaluation & accountability: Secretariat Annual Report 2020 [Internet]. Geneva; 2020 Jun [cited 2021 Oct 3]. https://www.who.int/publications/i/item/global-vaccine-action-plan-monitoring-evaluation-accountability-secretariat-annual-report-2020.
6. WHO Immunization Data portal [Internet]. World Health Organization. 2020 [cited 2021 Oct 3]. https://immunizationdata.who.int/.
7. Wodi AP, Morelli V. Principles of vaccination. In: Hall E, Wodi AP, Hamborsky J, Morelli V, Schillie S, editors. The Pink Book: epidemiology and prevention of vaccine-preventable diseases. 14th

ed. Washington, DC: Centers for Disease Control and Prevention; 2021. p. 1–8.
8. Siegrist CA. Vaccine immunology. In: Vaccines. 6th ed. W.B. Saunders; 2013. p. 14–32.
9. Bernstein HH, Kilinsky A, Orenstein WA. Immunization practices. In: Kliegman R, editor. Nelson textbook of pediatrics. 21st ed. Philadelphia: Elsevier; 2020. p. 1347–66.
10. National Center for Immunization and Respiratory Diseases. Immunization Schedules. Published February 17, 2022. https://www.cdc.gov/vaccines/schedules/index.html. Accessed 28 Mar 2022.
11. WHO recommendations for routine immunization - summary tables [Internet]. World Health Organization. 2021 [cited 2021 Sep 29]. https://www.who.int/teams/immunization-vaccines-and-biologicals/policies/who-recommendations-for-routine-immunization%2D%2D-summary-tables.
12. Different types of vaccines | History of vaccines [Internet]. The College of Physicians of Philadelphia. 2018 [cited 2021 Sep 29]. https://www.historyofvaccines.org/content/articles/different-types-vaccines.
13. Klugman KP, Black S, Dagan R, Malley R, Whitney CG. Pneumococcal conjugate vaccine and pneumococcal common protein vaccines. In: Vaccines. 6th ed. W.B. Saunders; 2013. p. 504–41.
14. Schiller JT, Lowy DR, Markowitz LE. Human papillomavirus vaccines. In: Plotkin SA, Orenstein WA, Offit PA, eds. Vaccines. 6th ed. Elsevier; 2013:235–256. doi:https://doi.org/10.1016/B978-1-4557-0090-5.00006-9.
15. Gomez PL, Robinson JM, Rogalewicz JA. Vaccine manufacturing. In: Plotkin SA, Orenstein WA, Offit PA, eds. Vaccines. 6th ed. Elsevier; 2013:44–57. doi:https://doi.org/10.1016/B978-1-4557-0090-5.00019-7.
16. Pardi N, Hogan MJ, Porter FW, Weissman D. mRNA vaccines — a new era in vaccinology. Nat Rev Drug Discov [Internet]. 2018 Mar 28 [cited 2021 Sep 29];17(4):261. https://www.ncbi.nlm.nih.gov/pmc/articles/PMC5906799/.
17. Zhao J, Zhao S, Ou J, Zhang J, Lan W, Guan W, et al. COVID-19: coronavirus vaccine development updates. Front Immunol [Internet]. 2020 Dec 23 [cited 2021 Oct 3];11. https://www.ncbi.nlm.nih.gov/pmc/articles/PMC7785583/.
18. Triggle CR, Bansal D, Ding H, Islam MM, Farag EABA, Hadi HA, et al. A comprehensive review of viral characteristics, transmission, pathophysiology, immune response, and management of SARS-CoV-2 and COVID-19 as a basis for controlling the pandemic. Front Immunol [Internet]. 2021 Feb 26 [cited 2021 Sep 29];12:631139. https://www.ncbi.nlm.nih.gov/pmc/articles/PMC7952616/.
19. Grizas AP, Camenga D, Vázquez M. Cocooning. Curr Opin Pediatr. 2012;24:1.
20. National Center for Immunization and Respiratory Diseases. Appendix A: Glossary of key terms. Interim Guidance on Developing a COVID-19 Case Investigation and Contact Tracing Plan: Overview. Published online January 4, 2022. https://www.cdc.gov/coronavirus/2019-ncov/php/contact-tracing/contact-tracing-plan/appendix.html#Key-Terms. Accessed 28 Mar 2022.
21. Health Information and Quality Authority of Ireland 2021. Protective measures for groups vulnerable to COVID-19 [Internet]. Dublin; 2021 Aug [cited 2021 Oct 3]. https://www.hiqa.ie/reports-and-publications/health-technology-assessment/protective-measures-groups-vulnerable-covid.
22. Rubin LG, Levin MJ, Ljungman P, Davies EG, Avery R, Tomblyn M, Bousvaros A, Dhanireddy S, Sung L, Keyserling H, Kang I, Infectious Diseases Society of America. 2013 IDSA clinical practice guideline for vaccination of the immunocompromised host. Clin Infect Dis. 2014;58(3):309–18.
23. Crawford NW, Bines JE, Royle J, Buttery JP. Optimizing immunization in pediatric special risk groups. Expert Rev Vaccines. 2011;10(2):175–86.
24. Immunization of persons with chronic diseases: Canadian Immunization Guide - Canada.ca [Internet]. Government of Canada. 2021 [cited 2021 Sep 16]. https://www.canada.ca/en/public-health/services/publications/healthy-living/canadian-immunization-guide-part-3-vaccination-specific-populations/page-7-immunization-persons-with-chronic-diseases.html.
25. Doherty M, Schmidt-Ott R, Santos JI, Stanberry LR, Hofstetter AM, Rosenthal SL, et al. Vaccination of special populations: protecting the vulnerable. Vaccine. 2016;34(52):6681–90.
26. Fernandes EG, Rodrigues CCM, Sartori AMC, de Soárez PC, Novaes HMD. Economic evaluation of adolescents and adults' pertussis vaccination: a systematic review of current strategies. Hum Vaccin Immunother. 2019;15(1):14–27.
27. Vaccination for people who are immunocompromised | The Australian Immunisation Handbook [Internet]. Australian Department of Health. 2020 [cited 2021 Sep 16]. https://immunisationhandbook.health.gov.au/vaccination-for-special-risk-groups/vaccination-for-people-who-are-immunocompromised.
28. Immunization of immunocompromised persons: Canadian Immunization Guide - Canada.ca. Government of Canada. Published December 24, 2020. https://www.canada.ca/en/public-health/services/publications/healthy-living/canadian-immunization-guide-part-3-vaccination-specific-populations/page-8-immunization-immunocompromised-persons.html#shr-pg0. Accessed 16 Sept 2021.
29. Yue X, Black CL, Williams WW, Lu P-J, Srivastav A, Amaya A, et al. Influenza vaccination among adults living with persons at high-risk for complications from influenza during early 2016–17 influenza season. Vaccine. 2018;36(52):7987–92.
30. Gkentzi D, Aggelopoulos K, Karatza A, Sinopidis X, Dimitriou G, Fouzas S. Influenza vaccination among caregivers and household contacts of children with asthma. Vaccine. 2021;39(17):2331–4.
31. National Center for Immunization and Respiratory Diseases. Interim clinical considerations for use of COVID-19 vaccines currently approved or authorized in the United States [Internet]. Centers for Disease Control and Prevention. 2021 [cited 2021 Nov 21]. https://www.cdc.gov/vaccines/covid-19/clinical-considerations/covid-19-vaccines-us.html.
32. Ramsay M, editor. COVID-19—SARS-CoV-2. In: Immunisation against infections disease: The Green Book [Internet]. London: Public Health England; 2021 [cited 2021 Nov 21]. p. 1–40. https://www.gov.uk/government/publications/covid-19-the-green-book-chapter-14a.
33. Esposito S, Bruno C, Berardinelli A, Filosto M, Mongini T, Morandi L, et al. Vaccination recommendations for patients with neuromuscular disease. Vaccine. 2014;32(45):5893–900.
34. Miller E, Wodi P. General best practice guidance for immunization. In: Hall E, Wodi AP, Hamborsky J, Morelli V, Schillie S, editors. The Pink Book: epidemiology and the prevention of vaccine-preventable diseases. Centers for Disease Control and Prevention; 2021. p. 9–28.
35. Kroger AT, Atkinson WL, Pickering LK. General immunization practices. In: Plotkin SA, Orenstein WA, Offit PA, editors. Vaccines. 6th ed. Elsevier; 2013. p. 88–112. https://doi.org/10.1016/B978-1-4557-0090-5.00002-1.
36. Cortina G, Ojinaga V, Zlamy M, Giner T, Riedl M, Rauchenzauner M, et al. Vaccination status in pediatric solid-organ transplant recipients and their household members. Exp Clin Transplant. 2019;17(4):429–34.
37. Rensink MJ, van Laarhoven HWM, Holleman F. Cocoon vaccination for influenza in patients with a solid tumor: a retrospective study. Support Care Cancer. 2021;29(7):3657–66.

38. Fine P, Eames K, Heymann DL. "Herd immunity": a rough guide. Clin Infect Dis. 2011;52(7):911–6.
39. Smith CE. Prospects for the control of infectious disease. Proc R Soc Med. 1970;63(11 Part 2):1181–90.
40. Anderson EJ, Daugherty MA, Pickering LK, Orenstein WA, Yogev R. Protecting the community through child vaccination. Clin Infect Dis. 2018;67(3):464–71.
41. Halloran ME. Overview of vaccine field studies: types of effects and designs. J Biopharm Stat. 2006;16(4):415–27.
42. Delamater PL, Street EJ, Leslie TF, Yang YT, Jacobsen KH. Complexity of the basic reproduction number (R 0). Emerg Infect Dis. 2019;25(1):1–4.
43. Poehling KA, Talbot TR, Griffin MR, Craig AS, Whitney CG, Zell E, et al. Invasive pneumococcal disease among infants before and after introduction of pneumococcal conjugate vaccine. JAMA. 2006;295(14):1668–74.
44. Moore MR, Link-Gelles R, Schaffner W, Lynfield R, Lexau C, Bennett NM, et al. Effect of use of 13-valent pneumococcal conjugate vaccine in children on invasive pneumococcal disease in children and adults in the USA: analysis of multisite, population-based surveillance. Lancet Infect Dis. 2015;15(3):301–9.
45. Hanquet G, Krizova P, Valentiner-Branth P, Ladhani SN, Nuorti JP, Lepoutre A, et al. Effect of childhood pneumococcal conjugate vaccination on invasive disease in older adults of 10 European countries: implications for adult vaccination. Thorax. 2019;74(5):473–82.
46. Kim TH, Johnstone J, Loeb M. Vaccine herd effect. Scand J Infect Dis. 2011;43(9):683–9.
47. Patel M, Lee AD, Redd SB, Clemmons NS, McNall RJ, Cohn AC, et al. Increase in measles cases—United States, January 1–April 26, 2019. MMWR Morb Mortal Wkly Rep. 2019;68(17):402–4.
48. Bernadou A, Astrugue C, Méchain M, le Galliard V, Verdun-Esquer C, Dupuy F, et al. Measles outbreak linked to insufficient vaccination coverage in Nouvelle-Aquitaine Region, France, October 2017 to July 2018. Eur Secur. 2018;23(30):1800373.
49. Raybern C, Fornshell S, DeWeese L. Community-wide outbreak of pertussis in a highly unvaccinated community—Pottawatomie County, June 2014 [Internet]. Westmoreland, KS; 2016 Aug [cited 2021 Aug 6]. https://www.kdheks.gov/epi/download/Pott_County_Pertussis_Outbreak_Report_final.pdf.
50. Caron C. Chickenpox outbreak at school linked to vaccine exemptions - The New York Times [Internet]. New York Times. 2018 [cited 2021 Sep 16]. https://www.nytimes.com/2018/11/20/health/chicken-pox-vaccine-asheville.html.
51. Oostvogel PM, van der Avoort HGAM, Mulders MN, van Loon AM, Conyn-van Spaendonck MAE, Rümke HC, et al. Poliomyelitis outbreak in an unvaccinated community in the Netherlands, 1992–93. Lancet. 1994;344(8923):665–70.
52. National Center for Immuization and Respiratory Diseases. Vaccines for Children Program (VFC). Centers for Disease Control and Prevention. Published February 18, 2016. https://www.cdc.gov/vaccines/programs/vfc. Accessed 28 Mar 2022.
53. Chevalier-Cottin E-P, Ashbaugh H, Brooke N, Gavazzi G, Santillana M, Burlet N, et al. Communicating benefits from vaccines beyond preventing infectious diseases. Infect Dis Ther. 2020;9(3):467–80.
54. Cohn A, Rodewald LE, Orenstein WA, Schuchat A. Immunization in the United States. In: Plotkin SA, Orenstein WA, Offit PA, Edwards KM, editors. Plotkin's vaccines. 7th ed. Elsevier; 2018. p. 1421–1440.e4. https://doi.org/10.1016/B978-0-323-35761-6.00073-0.
55. U.S. Food and Drug Administration. https://www.fda.gov/. Accessed 3 May 2022.
56. Gruber MF, Marshall VB. Regulation and testing of vaccines. In: Plotkin SA, Orenstein WA, Offit PA, Edwards KM, editors. Plotkin's vaccines. 7th ed. Elsevier; 2018. p. 1547–1565.e2. https://doi.org/10.1016/B978-0-323-35761-6.00079-1.
57. Advisory Committee on Immunization Practices. https://www.cdc.gov/vaccines/acip/index.html. Accessed 3 May 2022.
58. Patient Protection and Affordable Care Act of 2010, Pub. L. No. 111–148, 124 Stat. 119 (2010).
59. Johansen K, Pfeifer D, Salisbury D. Immunization in Europe. In: Plotkin SA, Orenstein WA, Offit PA, Edwards KM, editors. Plotkin's vaccines. 7th ed. Elsevier; 2018. p. 1441–1465.e7. https://doi.org/10.1016/B978-0-323-35761-6.00074-2.
60. Standing Committee on Vaccination. https://www.rki.de/EN/Content/infections/Vaccination/Vaccination_node.html. Accessed 3 May 2022.
61. Joint Committee on Vaccines and Immunisation. https://www.gov.uk/government/groups/joint-committee-on-vaccination-and-immunisation. Accessed 3 May 2022.
62. England PH. The Green Book [Internet]. 2020. https://www.gov.uk/government/collections/immunisation-against-infectious-disease-the-green-book#the-green-book.
63. Cherian T, Cutts F, Eggers R, Lydon P, Sodha SV, Okwo-Bele JM. Immunization in developing countries. In: Plotkin SA, Orenstein WA, Offit PA, Edwards KA, editors. Plotkin's vaccines. 7th ed. Elsevier; 2018. p. 1486–1511.e5. https://doi.org/10.1016/B978-0-323-35761-6.00076-6.
64. World Health Organization. Immunization Agenda 2030: a global strategy to leave no one behind. https://www.who.int/teams/immunization-vaccines-and-biologicals/strategies/ia2030. Accessed 3 May 2022.
65. World Health Organization (WHO). WHO recommendations for routine immunization [Internet]. 2020. https://www.who.int/publications/m/item/table-1-who-recommendations-for-routine-immunization.
66. World Health Organization (WHO). WHO vaccine-preventable diseases: monitoring system. 2020 global summary [Internet]. 2020. https://apps.who.int/immunization_monitoring/globalsummary/schedules.
67. GAVI_Alliance. GAVI Progress Report [Internet]. 2020. https://www.gavi.org/sites/default/files/programmes-impact/our-impact/apr/Gavi-Progress-Report-2020.pdf.
68. World Health Organization (WHO). Immunizations [Internet]. 2019. https://www.who.int/news-room/facts-in-pictures/detail/immunization.
69. Ljungman P. Vaccination of immunocompromised hosts. In: Plotkin SA, Orenstein WA, Offit PA, eds. Vaccines. 6th ed. Elsevier; 2013:1243–1256. doi:https://doi.org/10.1016/B978-1-4557-0090-5.00016-1.
70. Moore DL. Immunization of the immunocompromised child: key principles. Paediatr Child Health. 2018;23(3):203–5. https://doi.org/10.1093/pch/pxx180.
71. Furer V, Rondaan C, Heijstek MW, et al. 2019 update of EULAR recommendations for vaccination in adult patients with autoimmune inflammatory rheumatic diseases. Ann Rheum Dis. 2020;79(1):39–52.
72. Esposito S, Bruno C, Berardinelli A, et al. Vaccination recommendations for patients with neuromuscular disease. Vaccine. 2014;32(45):5893–900.
73. Pileggi GS, de Souza CBS, Ferriani VPL. Safety and immunogenicity of varicella vaccine in patients with juvenile rheumatic diseases receiving methotrexate and corticosteroids. Arthritis Care Res. 2010;62(7):1034–9.
74. Seitel T, Cagol L, Prelog M, et al. Varicella-zoster-virus vaccination of immunosuppressed children with inflammatory bowel disease or autoimmune hepatitis: a prospective observational study. Vaccine. 2020;38(50):8024–31.
75. Tse HN, Borrow R, Arkwright PD. Immune response and safety of viral vaccines in children with autoimmune diseases

76. Kobayashi M, Farrar JL, Gierke R, Britton A, Childs L, Leidner AJ, Campos-Outcalt D, Morgan RL, Long SS, Talbot HK, Poehling KA, Pilishvili T. Use of 15-valent pneumococcal conjugate vaccine and 20-valent pneumococcal conjugate vaccine among U.S. adults: updated recommendations of the Advisory Committee on Immunization Practices - United States, 2022. MMWR Morb Mortal Wkly Rep. 2022;71(4):109–17.
77. Centers for Disease Control and Prevention (CDC). Use of 13-valent pneumococcal conjugate vaccine and 23-valent pneumococcal polysaccharide vaccine among children aged 6–18 years with immunocompromising conditions: recommendations of the Advisory Committee on Immunization Practices (ACIP). MMWR Morb Mortal Wkly Rep. 2013;62(25):521–4. PMID: 23803961; PMCID: PMC4604951
78. Centers for Disease Control and Prevention (CDC). Pneumococcal vaccination: summary of who and when to vaccinate. Published January 24, 2022. https://www.cdc.gov/vaccines/vpd/pneumo/hcp/who-when-to-vaccinate.html. Accessed 10 May 2022.
79. Lal H, Cunningham AL, Godeaux O, Chlibek R, Diez-Domingo J, Hwang S-J, et al. Efficacy of an adjuvanted herpes zoster subunit vaccine in older adults. N Engl J Med. 2015;22:2087–96.
80. Cunningham AL, Lal H, Kovac M, Chlibek R, Hwang S-J, Díez-Domingo J, et al. Efficacy of the herpes zoster subunit vaccine in adults 70 years of age or older. N Engl J Med. 2016;375(11):1019–32.
81. Racine É, Gilca V, Amini R, Tunis M, Ismail S, Sauvageau C. A systematic literature review of the recombinant subunit herpes zoster vaccine use in immunocompromised 18–49 year old patients. Vaccine. 2020;38(40):6205–14.
82. Centers for Disease Control and Prevention (CDC). Shingrix recommendations. CDC. Published January 24, 2022. https://www.cdc.gov/vaccines/vpd/shingles/hcp/shingrix/recommendations.html#:~:text=CDC%20recommends%20Shingrix%20(recombinant%20zoster,prior%20episode%20of%20herpes%20zoster. Accessed 9 May 2022.
83. Centers for Disease Control and Prevention (CDC). Underlying medical conditions associated with higher risk for severe COVID-19: information for healthcare professionals. CDC. Published February 15, 2022. https://www.cdc.gov/coronavirus/2019-ncov/hcp/clinical-care/underlyingconditions.html. Accessed 11 May 2022.
84. Righi E, Gallo T, Azzini AM, et al. A review of vaccinations in adult patients with secondary immunodeficiency. Infect Dis Ther. 2021;10(2):637–61.
85. Kruk SK, Pacheco SE, Koenig MK, Bergerson JRE, Gordon-Lipkin E, McGuire PJ. Vulnerability of pediatric patients with mitochondrial disease to vaccine-preventable diseases. J Allerg Clin Immunol Pract. 2019;7(7):2415–2418.e3.
86. Centers for Disease Control and Prevention (CDC). Vaccines indicated for adults based on medical indications. CDC. Published February 12, 2021. https://www.cdc.gov/vaccines/schedules/hcp/imz/adult-conditions-shell.html. Accessed 16 Sept 2021.
87. Centers for Disease Control and Prevention (CDC). Vaccines indicated for persons aged 0 through 18 years based on medical indications. CDC. Published February 12, 2021. https://www.cdc.gov/vaccines/schedules/hcp/imz/child-indications.html. Accessed 16 Sept 2021.
88. Zeitlin PL, Leong M, Cole J, et al. Benralizumab does not impair antibody response to seasonal influenza vaccination in adolescent and young adult patients with moderate to severe asthma: results from the Phase IIIb ALIZE trial. J Asthma Allergy. 2018;11:181–92.
89. Tang YW, Graham BS. Anti-IL-4 treatment at immunization modulates cytokine expression, reduces illness, and increases cytotoxic T lymphocyte activity in mice challenged with respiratory syncytial virus. J Clin Investig. 1994;94(5):1953–8.
90. Cuellar-Barboza A, Zirwas M, Feldman SR. Is dupilumab an immunosuppressant? J Drugs Dermatol. 2020;19(2).
91. Deniz YM, Gupta N. Safety and tolerability of omalizumab (Xolair®), a recombinant humanized monoclonal anti-IgE antibody. Clin Rev Allergy Immunol. 2005;29(1):31–48.
92. Mepolizumab. LiverTox: clinical and research information on drug-induced liver injury. National Institute of Diabetes and Digestive and Kidney Diseases. Published online April 11, 2016. https://www.ncbi.nlm.nih.gov/books/NBK548052/. Accessed 16 Sept 2021.
93. Reslizumab. LiverTox: clinical and research information on drug-induced liver injury. National Institute of Diabetes and Digestive and Kidney Diseases. Published online March 14, 2017. https://www.ncbi.nlm.nih.gov/books/NBK548383/. Accessed 16 Sept 2021.
94. Mirsaeidi M, Ebrahimi G, Allen MB, Aliberti S. Pneumococcal vaccine and patients with pulmonary diseases. Am J Med. 2014;127(9):886.e1–8.
95. Tan B, Ismail S. Updated recommendations for the use of varicella and MMR vaccines in HIV-infected individuals. Can Commun Dis Rep. 2010;36(ACS-7):1–19.
96. Vaccination of HIV infected children (UK Schedule, 2018). Children's HIV Association. Published 2018. https://www.chiva.org.uk/infoprofessionals/guidelines/immunisation/. Accessed 16 Sept 2021.
97. World Health Organization. BCG vaccines: WHO position paper -- February 2018. Wkly Epidemiol Rec. 2018;93(8):73–96. https://apps.who.int/iris/handle/10665/260307. Accessed 8 Sept 2021
98. Lee GM. Preventing infections in children and adults with asplenia. Hematol Am Soc Hematol Educ Program. 2020;1:328–35.
99. Briere EC, Rubin L, Moro PL, et al. Prevention and control of Haemophilus influenzae type b disease: recommendations of the Advisory Committee on Immunization Practices (ACIP). MMWR Recomm Rep. 2014;63(RR-01):1–14.
100. Mbaeyi SA, Bozio CH, Duffy J, Rubin LG, Hariri S, Stephens DS, MacNeil JR. Meningococcal vaccination: recommendations of the Advisory Committee on Immunization Practices, United States, 2020. MMWR Recomm Rep. 2020;69(9):1–41.
101. Centers for Disease Control and Prevention (CDC). Varicella vaccine recommendations. CDC. Published April 28, 2021. https://www.cdc.gov/vaccines/vpd/varicella/hcp/recommendations.html. Accessed 9 May 2022.
102. National Center for Immunization and Respiratory Diseases. Clinical considerations for use of recombinant zoster vaccine (RZV, Shingrix) in immunocompromised adults aged >/=19 Years. Centers for Disease Control and Prevention (CDC). Published January 20, 2022. https://www.cdc.gov/shingles/vaccination/immunocompromised-adults.html. Accessed 9 May 2022.
103. Pittet LF, Posfay-Barbe KM. Vaccination of immune compromised children—an overview for physicians. Eur J Pediatr. 2021;180(7):2035–47.
104. MacDonald SE, Palichuk A, Slater L, Tripp H, Reifferscheid L, Burton C. Gaps in knowledge about the vaccine coverage of immunocompromised children: a scoping review. Hum Vaccin Immunother. 2021;16:1–16.
105. Hofstetter AM, Camargo S, Natarajan K, Rosenthal SL, Stockwell MS. Vaccination coverage of adolescents with chronic medical conditions. Am J Prev Med. 2017;53(5):680–8.
106. Berbudi A, Rahmadika N, Tjahjadi AI, Ruslami R. Type 2 diabetes and its impact on the immune system. Curr Diabetes Rev. 2020;16(5):442–9.
107. Peleg AY, Weerarathna T, McCarthy JS, Davis TM. Common infections in diabetes: pathogenesis, management and relationship to glycaemic control. Diabetes Metab Res Rev. 2007;23(1):3–13.

108. Daryabor G, Atashzar MR, Kabelitz D, Meri S, Kalantar K. The effects of type 2 diabetes mellitus on organ metabolism and the immune system. Front Immunol. 2020;11:1582.
109. Grohskopf LA, Alyanak E, Broder KR, Blanton LH, Fry AM, Jernigan DB, Atmar RL. Prevention and control of seasonal influenza with vaccines: recommendations of the Advisory Committee on Immunization Practices - United States, 2020–21 influenza season. MMWR Recomm Rep. 2020;69(8):1–24.
110. Dos Santos G, Tahrat H, Bekkat-Berkani R. Immunogenicity, safety, and effectiveness of seasonal influenza vaccination in patients with diabetes mellitus: a systematic review. Hum Vaccin Immunother. 2018;14(8):1853–66.
111. Weng MK, Doshani M, Khan MA, Frey S, Ault K, Moore KL, Hall EW, Morgan RL, Campos-Outcalt D, Wester C, Nelson NP. Universal hepatitis B vaccination in adults aged 19-59 years: updated recommendations of the Advisory Committee on Immunization Practices - United States, 2022. MMWR Morb Mortal Wkly Rep. 2022;71(13):477–83.
112. Centers for Diseases Control and Prevention (CDC). Use of hepatitis B vaccination for adults with diabetes mellitus: recommendations of the Advisory Committee on Immunization Practices (ACIP). MMWR Morb Mortal Wkly Rep. 2011;60(50):1709–11.
113. Pal R, Bhadada SK, Misra A. COVID-19 vaccination in patients with diabetes mellitus: current concepts, uncertainties and challenges. Diabetes Metab Syndr. 2021;15(2):505–8.
114. USRDS Annual Report: morbidity and mortality in patients with CKD [Internet]. [cited 2021 Jun 14]. https://adr.usrds.org/2020/chronic-kidney-disease/3-mobidity-and-mortality-in-patients-with-ckd.
115. Ishigami J, Matsushita K. Clinical epidemiology of infectious disease among patients with chronic kidney disease. Clin Exp Nephrol. 2019;23(4):437–47.
116. Kato S, Chmielewski M, Honda H, Pecoits-Filho R, Matsuo S, Yuzawa Y, Tranaeus A, Stenvinkel P, Lindholm B. Aspects of immune dysfunction in end-stage renal disease. Clin J Am Soc Nephrol. 2008;3(5):1526–33.
117. Vaziri ND, Pahl MV, Crum A, Norris K. Effect of uremia on structure and function of immune system. J Renal Nutr. 2012;22(1):149–56.
118. Su G, Iwagami M, Qin X, McDonald H, Liu X, Carrero JJ, et al. Kidney disease and mortality in patients with respiratory tract infections: a systematic review and meta-analysis. Clin Kidney J. 2021;14(2):602–11.
119. Gilbertson DT, Rothman KJ, Chertow GM, Bradbury BD, Brookhart MA, Liu J, et al. Excess deaths attributable to influenza-like illness in the ESRD population. J Am Soc Nephrol. 2019;30(2):346–53.
120. Marra F, Parhar K, Huang B, Vadlamudi N. Risk factors for herpes zoster infection: a meta-analysis. Open Forum Infect Dis. 2020;7(1):ofaa005.
121. Schweitzer A, Horn J, Mikolajczyk RT, Krause G, Ott JJ. Estimations of worldwide prevalence of chronic hepatitis B virus infection: a systematic review of data published between 1965 and 2013. Lancet (London, England). 2015;386(10003):1546–55.
122. Fabrizi F, Marzano A, Messa P, Martin P, Lampertico P. Hepatitis B virus infection in the dialysis population: current perspectives. Int J Artif Organs. 2008;31(5):386–94.
123. Advisory Committee on Immunization Practices. Recommended adult immunization schedule by medical condition and other indications, United States, 2021 [Internet]. [cited 2021 Jun 14]. https://www.cdc.gov/vaccines/schedules/hcp/imz/adult-conditions.html#notes.
124. Centers for Disease Control and Prevention (CDC). Recommended adult immunization schedule for ages 19 years or older: United States, 2021 [Internet]. Vol. 34. 2021 [cited 2021 Jun 15]. https://www.cdc.gov/vaccines/schedules/hcp/imz/adult.html#table-age.
125. Centers for Disease Control and Prevention (CDC). Recommended child and adolescent immunization schedule for ages 18 years or younger, United States, 2021 [Internet]. [cited 2021 Jun 15]. https://www.cdc.gov/vaccines/schedules/hcp/imz/child-adolescent.html#birth-15.
126. Watcharananan SP, Thakkinstian A, Srichunrasmee C, Chuntratita W, Sumethkul V. Comparison of the immunogenicity of a monovalent influenza A/H1N1 2009 vaccine between healthy individuals, patients with chronic renal failure, and immunocompromised populations. Transplant Proc. 2014;46(2):328–31.
127. Broeders NE, Hombrouck A, Lemy A, Wissing KM, Racapé J, Gastaldello K, et al. Influenza A/H1N1 vaccine in patients treated by kidney transplant or dialysis: a cohort study. Clin J Am Soc Nephrol. 2011;6(11):2573–8.
128. Ishigami J, Sang Y, Grams ME, Coresh J, Chang A, Matsushita K. Effectiveness of influenza vaccination among older adults across kidney function: pooled analysis of 2005–2006 through 2014–2015 influenza seasons. Am J Kidney Dis. 2020;75(6):887–96.
129. Noh JY, Song JY, Choi WS, Lee J, Bin SY, Kwon YJ, et al. Immunogenicity of trivalent influenza vaccines in patients with chronic kidney disease undergoing hemodialysis: MF59-adjuvanted versus non-adjuvanted vaccines. Hum Vaccin Immunother. 2016;12(11):2902–8.
130. Lee JKH, Lam GKL, Shin T, Kim J, Krishnan A, Greenberg DP, et al. Efficacy and effectiveness of high-dose versus standard-dose influenza vaccination for older adults: a systematic review and meta-analysis. Expert Rev Vaccines. 2018;17(5):435–43.
131. Butler AM, Layton JB, Dharnidharka VR, Sahrmann JM, Seamans MJ, Weber DJ, et al. Comparative effectiveness of high-dose versus standard-dose influenza vaccine among patients receiving maintenance hemodialysis. Am J Kidney Dis. 2020;75(1):72–83.
132. Weycker D, Farkouh RA, Strutton DR, Edelsberg J, Shea KM, Pelton SI. Rates and costs of invasive pneumococcal disease and pneumonia in persons with underlying medical conditions. BMC Health Serv Res. 2016;16:182.
133. Weycker D, Strutton D, Edelsberg J, Sato R, Jackson LA. Clinical and economic burden of pneumococcal disease in older US adults. Vaccine. 2010;28(31):4955–60.
134. Moberley S, Holden J, Tatham DP, Andrews RM. Vaccines for preventing pneumococcal infection in adults. Cochrane Database Syst Rev. 2013;(1):CD000422.
135. Huss A, Scott P, Stuck AE, Trotter C, Egger M. Efficacy of pneumococcal vaccination in adults: a meta-analysis. CMAJ. 2009;180(1):48–58.
136. Mahmoodi M, Aghamohammadi A, Rezaei N, Lessan-Pezeshki M, Pourmand G, Mohagheghi M-A, et al. Antibody response to pneumococcal capsular polysaccharide vaccination in patients with chronic kidney disease. Eur Cytokine Netw. 2009;20(2):69–74.
137. Vandecasteele SJ, De Bacquer D, Caluwe R, Ombelet S, Van Vlem B. Immunogenicity and safety of the 13-valent Pneumococcal Conjugate vaccine in 23-valent pneumococcal polysaccharide vaccine-naive and pre-immunized patients under treatment with chronic haemodialysis: a longitudinal quasi-experimental phase IV study. Clin Microbiol Infect. 2018;24(1):65–71.
138. Centers for Disease Control and Prevention (CDC). Preventing pneumococcal disease among infants and young children [Internet]. https://www.cdc.gov/mmwr/preview/mmwrhtml/rr4909a1.htm.
139. French N, Gordon SB, Mwalukomo T, White SA, Mwafulirwa G, Longwe H, et al. A trial of a 7-valent pneumococcal conjugate vaccine in HIV-infected adults. N Engl J Med. 2010;362(9):812–22.
140. Feikin DR, Elie CM, Goetz MB, Lennox JL, Carlone GM, Romero-Steiner S, et al. Randomized trial of the quantitative and functional antibody responses to a 7-valent pneumococcal conjugate vaccine and/or 23-valent polysaccharide vaccine among HIV-infected adults. Vaccine. 2001;20(3–4):545–53.

141. Nuorti JP, Whitney CG. Prevention of pneumococcal disease among infants and children - use of 13-valent pneumococcal conjugate vaccine and 23-valent pneumococcal polysaccharide vaccine - recommendations of the Advisory Committee on Immunization Practices (ACIP). MMWR Recomm Rep. 2010;59(RR-11):1–18.
142. Ghadiani MH, Besharati S, Mousavinasab N, Jalalzadeh M. Response rates to HB vaccine in CKD stages 3–4 and hemodialysis patients. J Res Med Sci. 2012;17(6):527–33.
143. DaRoza G, Loewen A, Djurdjev O, Love J, Kempston C, Burnett S, et al. Stage of chronic kidney disease predicts seroconversion after hepatitis B immunization: earlier is better. Am J Kidney Dis. 2003;42(6):1184–92.
144. Miller ER, Alter MJ, Tokars JI. Protective effect of hepatitis B vaccine in chronic hemodialysis patients. Am J Kidney Dis. 1999;33(2):356–60.
145. Schillie S, Harris A, Link-Gelles R, Romero J, Ward J, Nelson N. Recommendations of the Advisory Committee on Immunization Practices for use of a hepatitis B vaccine with a novel adjuvant. MMWR Morb Mortal Wkly Rep. 2018;67(15):455–8.
146. Centers for Disease Control and Prevention (CDC). Guidelines for vaccination renal dialysis patients and patients with chronic kidney disease. [Internet]. [cited 2021 Jun 14]. https://www.cdc.gov/dialysis/PDFs/Vaccinating_Dialysis_Patients_and_Patients_dec2012.pdf.
147. Froes F, Roche N, Blasi F. Pneumococcal vaccination and chronic respiratory diseases. Int J Chron Obstruct Pulmon Dis. 2017;12:3457–68. https://doi.org/10.2147/COPD.S140378.
148. Hewitt R, Farne H, Ritchie A, Luke E, Johnston SL, Mallia P. The role of viral infections in exacerbations of chronic obstructive pulmonary disease and asthma. Ther Adv Respir Dis. 2016;10(2):158–74.
149. BurgessL SK. Cochrane Library Cochrane Database of Systematic Reviews Pneumococcal vaccines for cystic fibrosis (Review). 2016.; www.cochranelibrary.com.
150. Walters JA, Tang JN, Poole P, Wood-Baker R. Pneumococcal vaccines for preventing pneumonia in chronic obstructive pulmonary disease. Cochrane Database Syst Rev. 2017;1(1):CD001390.
151. Sheen YH, Kizilbash S, Ryoo E, Wi C-I, Park M, Abraham RS, et al. Relationship between asthma status and antibody response pattern to 23-valent pneumococcal vaccination. J Asthma. 2020; Apr 2 [cited 2021 Oct 13];57(4):1. https://www.ncbi.nlm.nih.gov/pmc/articles/PMC6702096/
152. Cochrane Library Cochrane Database of Systematic Reviews. Influenza vaccine for chronic obstructive pulmonary disease (COPD) (Review) Influenza vaccine for chronic obstructive pulmonary disease (COPD) (Review). 2018. www.cochranelibrary.com.
153. Vasileiou E, Sheikh A, Butler C, El Ferkh K, von Wissmann B, McMenamin J, Ritchie L, Schwarze J, Papadopoulos NG, Johnston SL, Tian L, Simpson CR. Effectiveness of influenza vaccines in asthma: a systematic review and meta-analysis. Clin Infect Dis. 2017;65(8):1388–95.
154. Borzio M, Salerno F, Piantoni L, Cazzaniga M, Angeli P, Bissoli F, et al. Bacterial infection in patients with advanced cirrhosis: a multicentre prospective study. Dig Liver Dis. 2001;33(1):41–8.
155. Piano S, Tonon M, Angeli P. Changes in the epidemiology and management of bacterial infections in cirrhosis. Clin Mol Hepatol. 2021;27(3):437–45.
156. Vos MB, Abrams SH, Barlow SE, Caprio S, Daniels SR, Kohli R, et al. NASPGHAN clinical practice guideline for the diagnosis and treatment of nonalcoholic fatty liver disease in children: recommendations from the expert committee on NAFLD (ECON) and the North American Society of Pediatric Gastroenterology, Hepatology and Nutrition (NASPGHAN). J Pediatr Gastroenterol Nutr. 2017;64(2):319–34.
157. Su F-H, Huang Y-L, Sung F-C, Su C-T, Hsu W-H, Chang S-N, et al. Annual influenza vaccination reduces total hospitalization in patients with chronic hepatitis B virus infection: a population-based analysis. Vaccine. 2016;34(1):120–7.
158. Gaeta GB, Stornaiuolo G, Precone DF, Amendola A, Zanetti AR. Immunogenicity and safety of an adjuvanted influenza vaccine in patients with decompensated cirrhosis. Vaccine. 2002;20(Suppl 5):B33–5.
159. Gaeta GB, Pariani E, Amendola A, Brancaccio G, Cuomo G, Stornaiuolo G, et al. Influenza vaccination in patients with cirrhosis and in liver transplant recipients. Vaccine. 2009;27(25–26):3373–5.
160. Härmälä S, Parisinos CA, Shallcross L, O'Brien A, Hayward A. Effectiveness of influenza vaccines in adults with chronic liver disease: a systematic review and meta-analysis. BMJ Open. 2019;9(9):e031070.
161. Baxter R, Yee A, Aukes L, Snow V, Fireman B, Atkinson B, et al. Risk of underlying chronic medical conditions for invasive pneumococcal disease in adults. Vaccine. 2016;34(36):4293–7.
162. Gransden WR, Eykyn SJ, Phillips I. Pneumococcal bacteraemia: 325 episodes diagnosed at St Thomas's Hospital. Br Med J (Clin Res Ed). 1985;290(6467):505–8.
163. McCashland TM, Preheim LC, Gentry MJ. Pneumococcal vaccine response in cirrhosis and liver transplantation. J Infect Dis. 2000;181(2):757–60.
164. Vento S, Garofano T, Renzini C, Cainelli F, Casali F, Ghironzi G, et al. Fulminant hepatitis associated with hepatitis A virus superinfection in patients with chronic hepatitis C. N Engl J Med. 1998;338(5):286–90.
165. Younossi ZM, Stepanova M. Changes in hepatitis A and B vaccination rates in adult patients with chronic liver diseases and diabetes in the U.S. population. Hepatology (Baltimore, Md). 2011;54(4):1167–78.
166. Arguedas MR, Johnson A, Eloubeidi MA, Fallon MB. Immunogenicity of hepatitis A vaccination in decompensated cirrhotic patients. Hepatology (Baltimore, Md). 2001;34(1):28–31.
167. Leise MD, Talwalkar JA. Immunizations in chronic liver disease: what should be done and what is the evidence. Curr Gastroenterol Rep. 2013;15(1):300.
168. Horlander JC, Boyle N, Manam R, Schenk M, Herring S, Kwo PY, et al. Vaccination against hepatitis B in patients with chronic liver disease awaiting liver transplantation. Am J Med Sci. 1999;318(5):304–7.
169. Terrault NA, Lok ASF, McMahon BJ, Chang K-M, Hwang JP, Jonas MM, et al. Update on prevention, diagnosis, and treatment of chronic hepatitis B: AASLD 2018 Hepatitis B Guidance. Clin Liver Dis. 2018;12(1):33–4.
170. Omer SB. Maternal immunization. N Engl J Med. 2017;376(13):1256–67.
171. Mosby LG, Rasmussen SA, Jamieson DJ. 2009 pandemic influenza A (H1N1) in pregnancy: a systematic review of the literature. Am J Obstet Gynecol. 2011;205(1):10–8.
172. Martin A, Cox S, Jamieson DJ, Whiteman MK, Kulkarni A, Tepper NK. Respiratory illness hospitalizations among pregnant women during influenza season, 1998–2008. Matern Child Health J. 2013;17(7):1325–31.
173. Zaman K, Roy E, Arifeen SE, Rahman M, Raqib R, Wilson E, et al. Effectiveness of maternal influenza immunization in mothers and infants. N Engl J Med. 2008;359(15):1555–64.
174. Centers for Disease Control and Prevention (CDC). Updated recommendations for use of tetanus toxoid, reduced diphtheria toxoid, and acellular pertussis vaccine (Tdap) in pregnant women—Advisory Committee on Immunization Practices (ACIP), 2012. MMWR Morb Mortal Wkly Rep. 2013;62(7):131–5. PMID: 23425962; PMCID: PMC4604886

175. Munoz FM, Jamieson DJ. Maternal immunization. Obstet Gynecol. 2019;133(4):739–53.
176. Alonso S, Vidal M, Ruiz-Olalla G, González R, Manaca MN, Jairoce C, et al. Reduced placental transfer of antibodies against a wide range of microbial and vaccine antigens in HIV-infected women in Mozambique. Front Immunol. 2021;12:614246.
177. Cavalcante RS, Kopelman BI, Costa-Carvalho BT. Placental transfer of Haemophilus influenzae type b antibodies in malnourished pregnant women. Braz J Infect Dis. 2008;12(1):47–51.
178. de Souza EG, Hara CCP, Fagundes DLG, de Queiroz AA, Morceli G, Calderon IMP, et al. Maternal-foetal diabetes modifies neonatal Fc receptor expression on human leucocytes. Scand J Immunol. 2016;84(4):237–44.
179. Wilcox CR, Holder B, Jones CE. Factors affecting the FcRn-mediated transplacental transfer of antibodies and implications for vaccination in pregnancy. Front Immunol. 2017;8:1294.
180. Chung S, Baumlin N, Dennis JS, Moore R, Salathe SF, Whitney PL, et al. Electronic cigarette vapor with nicotine causes airway mucociliary dysfunction preferentially via TRPA1 receptors. Am J Respir Crit Care Med. 2019;200(9):1134–45.
181. Arcavi L, Benowitz NL. Cigarette smoking and infection. Arch Intern Med. 2004;164(20):2206–16.
182. Xavier RF, Ramos D, Ito JT, Rodrigues FMM, Bertolini GN, Macchione M, et al. Effects of cigarette smoking intensity on the mucociliary clearance of active smokers. Respiration. 2013;86(6):479–85.
183. Shastri MD, Shukla SD, Chong WC, Rajendra KC, Dua K, Patel RP, et al. Smoking and COVID-19: what we know so far. Respir Med. 2021;176:106237.
184. Lawrence H, Hunter A, Murray R, Lim WS, McKeever T. Cigarette smoking and the occurrence of influenza – systematic review. J Infect. 2019;79(5):401–6.
185. Raman AS, Swinburne AJ, Fedullo AJ. Pneumococcal adherence to the buccal epithelial cells of cigarette smokers. Chest. 1983;83(1):23–7.
186. Bello S, Menéndez R, Antoni T, Reyes S, Zalacain R, Capelastegui A, et al. Tobacco smoking increases the risk for death from pneumococcal pneumonia. Chest. 2014;146(4):1029–37.
187. Baskaran V, Murray RL, Hunter A, Lim WS, McKeever TM. Effect of tobacco smoking on the risk of developing community acquired pneumonia: a systematic review and meta-analysis. PLoS One. 2019;14(7):e0220204.
188. Lowe KE, Zein J, Hatipoglu U, Attaway A. Association of smoking and cumulative pack-year exposure with COVID-19 outcomes in the Cleveland Clinic COVID-19 Registry. JAMA Intern Med. 2021;181(5):709–11.
189. Espejo-Paeres C, Núñez-Gil IJ, Estrada V, Fernández-Pérez C, Uribe-Heredia G, Cabré-Verdiell C, et al. Impact of smoking on COVID-19 outcomes: a HOPE Registry subanalysis. BMJ Nutr Prev Health. 2021;4(1):285–92.
190. Mahabee-Gittens EM, Mendy A, Merianos AL. Assessment of severe COVID-19 outcomes using measures of smoking status and smoking intensity. Int J Environ Res Public Health. 2021;18(17):8939.
191. Han L, Ran J, Mak Y-W, Suen LK-P, Lee PH, Peiris JSM, et al. Smoking and influenza-associated morbidity and mortality. Epidemiology. 2019;30(3):405–17.
192. Godoy P, Castilla J, Mayoral JM, Delgado-Rodríguez M, Martín V, Astray J, et al. Smoking may increase the risk of hospitalization due to influenza. Eur J Public Health. 2016;26(5):882–7.
193. Torres A, Peetermans WE, Viegi G, Blasi F. Risk factors for community-acquired pneumonia in adults in Europe: a literature review. Thorax. 2013;68(11):1057–65.
194. Dooling K, Marin M, Wallace M, McClung N, Chamberland M, Lee GM, et al. The Advisory Committee on Immunization Practices' updated interim recommendation for allocation of COVID-19 vaccine—United States, December 2020. MMWR Morb Mortal Wkly Rep. 2021;69(5152):1657–60.
195. Centers for Disease Control and Prevention (CDC). Frequently asked questions: questions about flu season and the use of E-cigarette, or vaping, products [Internet]. CDC Office on Smoking and Tobacco Use. 2020 [cited 2021 Sep 16]. https://www.cdc.gov/tobacco/basic_information/e-cigarettes/severe-lung-disease/faq/index.html.
196. Solórzano-Santos F, Espinoza-García L, Aguilar-Martínez G, Beirana-Palencia L, Echániz-Avilés G, Miranda-Novales G. Pneumococcal conjugate vaccine and pneumonia prevention in children with congenital heart disease. Rev Investig Clin. 2017;69(5):270–3.
197. Ghimire LV, Chou F-S, Moon-Grady AJ. Impact of congenital heart disease on outcomes among pediatric patients hospitalized for influenza infection. BMC Pediatr. 2020;20(1):450.
198. Walmsley D. Routine pediatric immunization, special cases in pediatrics: prematurity, chronic disease, congenital heart disease: recent advancements/changes in pediatric vaccines. Prim Care. 2011;38(4):595–609.
199. Updated guidance for palivizumab prophylaxis among infants and young children at increased risk of hospitalization for respiratory syncytial virus infection. Pediatrics. 2014;134(2).
200. Respiratory syncytial virus prophylaxis for high-risk infants program reference manual [Internet]. Ottawa; 2021 Oct [cited 2021 Oct 14]. https://www.health.gov.on.ca/en/pro/programs/drugs/funded_drug/fund_respiratory.aspx.
201. Ramsay M. Respiratory syncytial virus. In: Ramsay M, editor. Immunisation against infectious disease: the Green Book. London: Public Health England; 2020.
202. Weber DJ, Rutala WA, Samsa GP, Santimaw JE, Lemon SM. Obesity as a predictor of poor antibody response to hepatitis B plasma vaccine. JAMA. 1985;254(22):3187–9.
203. Van der Wielen M, Van Damme P, Chlibek R, Smetana J, von Sonnenburg F. Hepatitis A/B vaccination of adults over 40 years old: comparison of three vaccine regimens and effect of influencing factors. Vaccine. 2006;24(26):5509–15.
204. Eliakim A, Schwindt C, Zaldivar F, Casali P, Cooper DM. Reduced tetanus antibody titers in overweight children. Autoimmunity. 2006;39(2):137–41.
205. Louie JK, Acosta M, Samuel MC, Schechter R, Vugia DJ, Harriman K, et al. A novel risk factor for a novel virus: obesity and 2009 pandemic influenza A (H1N1). Clin Infect Dis. 2011;52(3):301–12.
206. Callahan ST, Wolff M, Hill HR, Edwards KM. Impact of body mass index on immunogenicity of pandemic H1N1 vaccine in children and adults. J Infect Dis. 2014;210(8):1270–4.
207. Talbot HK, Coleman LA, Crimin K, Zhu Y, Rock MT, Meece J, et al. Association between obesity and vulnerability and serologic response to influenza vaccination in older adults. Vaccine. 2012;30(26):3937–43.
208. Sheridan PA, Paich HA, Handy J, Karlsson EA, Hudgens MG, Sammon AB, et al. Obesity is associated with impaired immune response to influenza vaccination in humans. Int J Obes (2005). 2012;36(8):1072–7.
209. U.S. Food and Drug Administration. Comirnaty and Pfizer-BioNTech COVID-19 vaccine. https://www.fda.gov/emergency-preparedness-and-response/coronavirus-disease-2019-covid-19/comirnaty-and-pfizer-biontech-covid-19-vaccine. Accessed 3 May 2022.
210. U.S. Food and Drug Administration. Spikevax and Moderna COVID-19 vaccine. https://www.fda.gov/emergency-preparedness-and-response/coronavirus-disease-2019-covid-19/spikevax-and-moderna-covid-19-vaccine#:~:text=On%20

January%2031%2C%202022%2C%20the,years%20of%20age%20and%20older. Accessed 3 May 2022.
211. Polack FP, Thomas SJ, Kitchin N, Absalon J, Gurtman A, Lockhart S, et al. Safety and efficacy of the BNT162b2 mRNA covid-19 vaccine. N Engl J Med. 2020;383(27):2603–15.
212. Baden LR, El Sahly HM, Essink B, Kotloff K, Frey S, Novak R, et al. Efficacy and safety of the mRNA-1273 SARS-CoV-2 vaccine. N Engl J Med. 2021;384(5):403–16.
213. Bennett TD, Moffitt RA, Hajagos JG, Amor B, Anand A, Bissell MM, et al. Clinical characterization and prediction of clinical severity of SARS-CoV-2 infection among US adults using data from the US National COVID Cohort Collaborative. JAMA Netw Open. 2021;4(7):e2116901.
214. Kondrich J, Rosenthal M. Influenza in children. Curr Opin Pediatr. 2017;29(3):297–302.
215. Keren R. Neurological and neuromuscular disease as a risk factor for respiratory failure in children hospitalized with influenza infection. JAMA. 2005;294(17):2188–94.
216. Shea KM, Edelsberg J, Weycker D, Farkouh RA, Strutton DR, Pelton SI. Rates of pneumococcal disease in adults with chronic medical conditions. Open Forum Infect Dis. 2014;1(1):ofu024.
217. Pneumococcal vaccine: Canadian Immunization Guide - Canada.ca [Internet]. Government of Canada. 2016 [cited 2021 Sep 16]. https://www.canada.ca/en/public-health/services/publications/healthy-living/canadian-immunization-guide-part-4-active-vaccines/page-16-pneumococcal-vaccine.html.
218. Pneumococcal vaccine [Internet]. Health Service Executive of Ireland National Immunisation Office. 2019 [cited 2021 Sep 16]. https://www.hse.ie/eng/health/immunisation/hcpinfo/othervaccines/pneumo/#Who%20is%20most%20at%20risk%20of%20pneumococcal%20disease?
219. Complete routine immunisation schedule [Internet]. Public Health England. 2020 [cited 2021 Sep 16]. https://www.gov.uk/government/publications/the-complete-routine-immunisation-schedule.
220. Ramsay M. Pneumococcal. In: Ramsay M, editor. Immunisation against infectious disease: the Green Book. London: Public Health England; 2020.
221. Kasarskis E. FYI: Influenza and ALS [Internet]. The ALS Association. 2020 [cited 2021 Sep 16]. https://www.als.org/navigating-als/resources/fyi-influenza-and-als.
222. Alkon C. Are vaccines safe? | Muscular Dystrophy Association. Quest Magazine of the Muscular Dystrophy Association [Internet]. 2021 Mar 4 [cited 2021 Sep 16]. https://www.mda.org/quest/article/are-vaccines-safe.
223. Gierke R, Wodi P, Kobayashi M. Pneumococcal disease. In: Hall E, Wodi AP, Hamborsky J, Morelli V, Schillie S, editors. The Pinkbook: epidemiology and prevention of vaccine-preventable diseases. 14th ed. Washington, DC: Centers for Disease Control and Prevention; 2021.
224. Narayanaswami P, Sanders DB, Wolfe G, Benatar M, Cea G, Evoli A, et al. International consensus guidance for management of myasthenia gravis. Neurology. 2021;96(3):114–22.
225. Centers for Disease Control and Prevention (CDC). Vaccines indicated for adults based on medical indications [Internet]. CDC. 2021 [cited 2021 Sep 16]. https://www.cdc.gov/vaccines/schedules/hcp/imz/adult-conditions-shell.html.
226. Kaufman J, Tuckerman J, Bonner C, Durrheim DN, Costa D, Trevena L, Thomas S, Danchin M. Parent-level barriers to uptake of childhood vaccination: a global overview of systematic reviews. BMJ Glob Health. 2021;6(9):e006860. https://doi.org/10.1136/bmjgh-2021-006860.
227. Jarrett C, Wilson R, O'Leary M, Eckersberger E, Larson HJ, SAGE Working Group on Vaccine Hesitancy. Strategies for addressing vaccine hesitancy - a systematic review. Vaccine. 2015;33(34):4180–90.
228. Singh P, Dhalaria P, Kashyap S, Soni GK, Nandi P, Ghosh S, Mohapatra MK, Rastogi A, Prakash D. Strategies to overcome vaccine hesitancy: a systematic review. Syst Rev. 2022;11(1):78.
229. Szilagyi P, Vann J, Bordley C, Chelminski A, Kraus R, Margolis P, Rodewald L. Interventions aimed at improving immunization rates. Cochrane Database Syst Rev. 2002;(4):CD003941. https://doi.org/10.1002/14651858.CD003941. Update in: Cochrane Database Syst Rev. 2005;(3):CD003941.
230. Groom H, Hopkins DP, Pabst LJ, Murphy Morgan J, Patel M, Calonge N, Coyle R, Dombkowski K, Groom AV, Kurilo MB, Rasulnia B, Shefer A, Town C, Wortley PM, Zucker J, Community Preventive Services Task Force. Immunization information systems to increase vaccination rates: a community guide systematic review. J Public Health Manag Pract. 2015;21(3):227–48.
231. Centers for Disease Control and Prevention (CDC). The community guide, vaccination [Internet]. 2015. https://www.thecommunityguide.org/topic/vaccination?page=1.
232. Brewer NT, Hall ME, Malo TL, Gilkey MB, Quinn B, Lathren C. Announcements versus conversations to improve HPV vaccination coverage: a randomized trial. Pediatrics. 2017;139(1):e20161764.
233. Opel DJ, Zhou C, Robinson JD, Henrikson N, Lepere K, Mangione-Smith R, et al. Impact of childhood vaccine discussion format over time on immunization status. Acad Pediatr. 2018;18(4):430–6.
234. Dempsey AF, Pyrznawoski J, Lockhart S, Barnard J, Campagna EJ, Garrett K, et al. Effect of a health care professional communication training intervention on adolescent human papillomavirus vaccination: a cluster randomized clinical trial. JAMA Pediatr. 2018;172(5):e180016.
235. Jarrett C, Wilson R, O'Leary M, Eckersberger E, Larson HJ. Strategies for addressing vaccine hesitancy - a systematic review. Vaccine. 2015;33(34):4180–90.
236. Dubé E, Gagnon D, MacDonald NE. Strategies intended to address vaccine hesitancy: review of published reviews. Vaccine. 2015;33(34):4191–203.
237. Vielot NA, Islam JY, Sanusi B, Myers J, Smith S, Meadows B, et al. Overcoming barriers to adolescent vaccination: perspectives from vaccine providers in North Carolina. Women Health. 2020;60(10):1129–40.
238. Sabnis SS, Pomeranz AJ, Amateau MM. The effect of education, feedback, and provider prompts on the rate of missed vaccine opportunities in a community health center. Clin Pediatr. 2003;42(2):147–51.
239. McAdam-Marx C, Tak C, Petigara T, Jones NW, Yoo M, Briley MS, et al. Impact of a guideline-based best practice alert on pneumococcal vaccination rates in adults in a primary care setting. BMC Health Serv Res. 2019;19(1):474.
240. Klatt TE, Hopp E. Effect of a best-practice alert on the rate of influenza vaccination of pregnant women. Obstet Gynecol. 2012;119(2 Pt 1):301–5.
241. Ledwich LJ, Harrington TM, Ayoub WT, Sartorius JA, Newman ED. Improved influenza and pneumococcal vaccination in rheumatology patients taking immunosuppressants using an electronic health record best practice alert. Arthritis Rheum. 2009;61(11):1505–10.
242. Bardenheier BH, Shefer AM, Lu P-J, Remsburg RE, Marsteller JA. Are standing order programs associated with influenza vaccination? - NNHS, 2004. J Am Med Dir Assoc. 2010;11(9):654–61.
243. Coyle CM, Currie BP. Improving the rates of inpatient pneumococcal vaccination: impact of standing orders versus computerized reminders to physicians. Infect Control Hosp Epidemiol. 2004;25(11):904–7.
244. Dexter PR, Perkins SM, Maharry KS, Jones K, McDonald CJ. Inpatient computer-based standing orders vs physician

reminders to increase influenza and pneumococcal vaccination rates: a randomized trial. JAMA. 2004;292(19):2366–71.

245. Daley MF, Barrow J, Pearson K, Crane LA, Gao D, Stevenson JM, et al. Identification and recall of children with chronic medical conditions for influenza vaccination. Pediatrics. 2004;113(1 Pt 1):e26–33.

246. Suh CA, Saville A, Daley MF, Glazner JE, Barrow J, Stokley S, et al. Effectiveness and net cost of reminder/recall for adolescent immunizations. Pediatrics. 2012;129(6):e1437–45.

247. Dini EF, Linkins RW, Sigafoos J. The impact of computer-generated messages on childhood immunization coverage. Am J Prev Med. 2000;18(2):132–9.

248. Bordley WC, Chelminski A, Margolis PA, Kraus R, Szilagyi PG, Vann JJ. The effect of audit and feedback on immunization delivery: a systematic review. Am J Prev Med. 2000;18(4):343–50.

249. Brousseau N, Sauvageau C, Ouakki M, Audet D, Kiely M, Couture C, et al. Feasibility and impact of providing feedback to vaccinating medical clinics: evaluating a public health intervention. BMC Public Health. 2010;10:750.

250. Kiefe CI, Allison JJ, Williams OD, Person SD, Weaver MT, Weissman NW. Improving quality improvement using achievable benchmarks for physician feedback: a randomized controlled trial. JAMA. 2001;285(22):2871–9.

Medication Management and Treatment Adherence

Emily M. Hawes and Kimberly A. Sanders

Introduction

It is estimated that 82% of adults in the United States take at least one medication (i.e., prescription drug, herbal supplement, or over-the-counter drug) and almost 30% take five or more medications [1]. In annual usage data, an estimated 45.8% of the US population used one or more prescription drugs in a 30-day period, and as high as 85% in adults over the age of 60 [2]. Errors can occur with any type of medication across all care settings, including long-term care facilities, hospitals, and ambulatory care clinics as well as home health care. The frequency of medication-related problems (MRPs), including medication errors and adverse drug events (ADEs), are a serious public health problem which contribute to morbidity and mortality [3]. Each year, 1.3 million emergency department (ED) visits and 350,000 hospitalizations are due to ADEs [4] and at least $3.5 billion is spent on medical treatment of ADEs annually. Approximately 8.3–16.2% of ED visits and 7% of hospitalizations are attributed to ADEs at a cost of more than $5.6 million per hospital per year [5]. One quarter of the ADEs are preventable, resulting in unnecessary cost and harm [3]. One study, for example, conservatively estimated 530,000 preventable ADEs in outpatient Medicare patients [3]. Additionally, the Institute of Medicine has reported that more than 40% of costs related to non-hospital ADEs might be preventable and $3.5 billion is spent on excess medical costs of ADEs annually [6]. Of note, cost of prescription drug-related morbidity and mortality have increased substantially over the past two decades. Approximately $200 billion worth of expenditures were attributed to MRPs in 2000, whereas in 2016 the annual cost from nonoptimized medication therapy was $528.6 billion (representing 16% of total health care expenditures that year) billion [7, 8]. Regrettably, the United States spends almost as much on complications associated with medications (e.g., adverse drug events) as it does for the medications itself [9].

Individuals 65 years and older continue to be the largest consumers of medications, with almost 20% taking at least ten drugs weekly [1, 10]. The greater number of medications, as well as age-related physiologic changes, contributes to a disproportionate effect of ADEs in this population. Unintentional overdoses are one of the most common causes of ADEs contributing to hospitalizations, with older adults being more than twice as likely to be treated emergently for an ADE and nearly seven times as likely to require hospitalization than individuals younger than 65 years [10]. In fact, two-thirds of unintentional overdoses and one-third of ED-treated ADEs in patients aged 65 years or older were due to toxicity associated with medications commonly used to treat chronic illnesses [10]. One study in 2019 found that outpatient ADE rates in Medicare beneficiaries were highest in those taking anticoagulants, opioids, and anti-diabetic agents [11] and another study evaluating ED data in 2013–2014 found those same drug classes implicated in 60% of ED visits for ADEs [4]. High-risk drugs used for chronic disease management (i.e., warfarin, insulin, and digoxin) are frequently associated with ADEs and require routine monitoring to prevent complications [12]. In review of younger populations, pediatric patients with complex chronic conditions also have a higher risk of ED visits related to ADEs compared to other children [13]. The highest rates are associated with drug classes including psychotropic agents, anticonvulsants, antimicrobial agents, hormones/steroids, and analgesics.

Medications prescribed in outpatient settings will continue to increase due to an aging population, the development of new drugs with more indications for approved

E. M. Hawes (✉)
Department of Family Medicine, University of North Carolina at Chapel Hill School of Medicine, Chapel Hill, NC, USA

University of North Carolina Eshelman School of Pharmacy, Chapel Hill, NC, USA
e-mail: emily_hawes@med.unc.edu

K. A. Sanders
University of North Carolina Eshelman School of Pharmacy, Chapel Hill, NC, USA

University of North Carolina Adams School of Dentistry, Chapel Hill, NC, USA
e-mail: kim.sanders@unc.edu

medications, the transition of prescription to OTC availability, enhanced coverage of medications, and more frequent use of medications for disease prevention [10, 14]. The greater quantity of medications used in the ambulatory setting increases the likelihood of MRPs, such as mixing problematic over-the-counter (OTC) and prescription medications, stopping a needed medication, administering the wrong dose, using incorrect technique, and consuming interacting foods and supplements with certain medications [3, 14].

People are living longer with chronic conditions which requires more time to discuss treatment options, greater complexity in coordinating care, and a higher risk of complications in a clinical environment that is moving to value-based care. Health care professionals and patients need to be trained and prepared to effectively manage medications [3], and although much attention has been focused on identifying, resolving, and preventing MRPs in hospitalized patients, less effort has been directed to MRPs occurring outside of hospital settings [10]. This chapter seeks to assist physicians and other care providers in a better understanding of medication management. The first section provides an overview to the nomenclature used in medication management, while the remainder of the chapter reviews applied strategies and approaches for effectively managing medications in multiple chronic conditions, especially in the ambulatory care setting [3].

Understanding Medication Management

Pharmacotherapy involves the provision of medication-based treatment for the purpose of achieving measurable therapeutic outcomes that improve a patient's quality of life. Such therapeutic outcomes include curing disease, eliminating or reducing symptoms, stopping or slowing disease progression, and preventing disease or symptomatology. Managing medication-related problems (MRPs) involves three major domains: (1) identifying potential and actual MRPs, (2) resolving actual MRPs, and (3) preventing potential MRPs [15].

Medication-Related Problems (MRPs)

An MRP, also known as a drug-related problem or drug-therapy problem, is an event or circumstance involving medication that actually or potentially interferes with an intended health outcome [15–17]. MRPs can include medication errors as well as ADEs, and these are described in Table 13.1 [3, 18, 19].

While determining the nature of the MRP is an important component of medication management, a universally accepted classification system has not been adopted though a couple exist including the Pharmaceutical Care Network Europe (PCNE) Classification for Drug-related Problems [19, 20]. Classification systems generally include at least the MRP categories in Table 13.2 [16, 19–22].

Table 13.1 Typology of medication-related problems

Medication-related problem (MRP)	An event or circumstance involving medication that actually or potentially interferes with a desired health outcome.
Error	The failure of a planned action to be completed as intended or the use of a wrong plan to achieve an aim.
Medication error	Any error occurring in the medication-use process.
Adverse drug event (ADE)	Any injury resulting from a medication.
High alert medications	Medications that have a higher risk of causing significant harm when used in error. Although mistakes may or may not be more likely with these medications, the consequences of an error are more devastating to patients.
Polypharmacy	The use of multiple medications by a patient, generally considered to be at least 5–10 medications. It can include not only prescriptions, but over-the-counter medications and herbal supplements.

Table 13.2 Common medication-related problems

Untreated indications	The patient has a medical problem that requires pharmacotherapy but is not receiving a drug for that indication.
Improper drug selection	The patient has an indication but is taking the wrong pharmacotherapy or has inappropriate duplication or combination of drugs of a therapeutic group.
Subtherapeutic dosage	The patient is being treated with too little of the correct medication.
Failure to receive medication	The patient has a medical problem that is the result of not receiving a medication.
Overdosage	The patient is being treated with too much of the correct medication.
Adverse reactions	The patient has a medical problem that is due to an adverse drug reaction or adverse effect.
Drug interactions	A drug–drug, drug–food, or drug–laboratory test interaction is present.
Medication use without indication	The patient is taking a medication for no valid indication.

Patient non-adherence is a key MRP factor that impacts chronic illness care. Less than half of patients actually remain adherent to their medications after 1 year [23–25] and non-adherence has been attributed to 125,000 deaths annually, 10% of hospitalizations, and an estimated $100 billion in direct and indirect costs [26]. In particular, cost-related non-adherence has been associated with 15–22% higher all-cause mortality rates for conditions of diabetes, cardiovascular disease, and hypertension [27]. Polypharmacy also contributes significantly to the likelihood of MRPs, especially adverse reactions and drug interactions, and subsequently, increased mortality [3, 28, 29]. Prescription and

OTC drug use are increasing, as is the growing prevalence of herbal supplements and alternative medications in the United States. Although more patients are requesting these agents as part of their therapy regimens, many of these products are not evaluated, monitored, and regulated to the same degree as prescription and OTC drugs. This can contribute to side effects that are exacerbated in those with renal and hepatic impairment, which is more common in older adults or those with chronic illnesses [3].

Effective Medication Management

The Institute of Medicine (IOM) advocates that health care should be safe, individualized, timely, and effective to meet the needs of patients and that patients should be actively involved in their health care to prevent MRPs [3]. Effective medication management consists of medication reconciliation, comprehensive medication review to identify and resolve MRPs, and patient education [3, 30–32]. A basic framework for medication management in patients with chronic diseases involves understanding the recommended components for medication reconciliation, a comprehensive medication review, and patient education.

Medication Reconciliation

Medication reconciliation is the process of creating and maintaining a valid and verified list of medications and using that list to guide therapy decisions and patient education. An up-to-date, accurate, and available medication list is critical to ensuring safe medication use across all health care settings [3, 30, 33]. Outpatient visits may result in no changes or modifications to the list, however after care transitions (e.g., hospital discharge), medication reconciliation can be time-consuming and often complicated. The goal in each setting is to provide a ledger of correct medications, including drug name, dosage, frequency, and route, with verified indication to the patient and other care providers.

It is critical to understand what medications the patient is actually taking to reconcile medications. Information sources can be obtained from patient report, medication refill history, as well as reviewing the patient's pill box and medication bottles. The Institute for Healthcare Improvement (IHI) has recommended a three-step process involving (1) Verification (i.e., obtaining the medication history); (2) Clarification (i.e., ensuring that the regimens are appropriate); and (3) Reconciliation (i.e., documentation of changes). At patient care encounters, every drug should be reviewed and noted as continued, discontinued, held, or modified (e.g., dose adjustment). Successful reconciliation also ensures that medication modifications, and ultimately an updated list, have been communicated to the patient as well as other providers [30].

Patients should be counseled to maintain an updated medication list in some proximity and to give a copy to their emergency contact. This list can be useful when picking up prescriptions at the pharmacy, as well as when attending health care appointments. The list should include allergies (such as drugs, food, dyes, and insects) and a description of the adverse reaction, if any, that the patient has experienced from prior medicines. The list should also document the patient's primary care provider name and phone number, as well as the pharmacy name, phone number, and location. The elements of the medication should include the brand and generic name of each medicine, dose, route (e.g., by mouth, under tongue, injection), frequency of administration, and indication. Over-the-counter, herbal, vitamin, and dietary supplement products as well as all formulations, such as tablets, patches, drops, ointments, and injections, should be included. "As needed" medications—even those taken only on an intermittent or periodic basis—should be included along with the frequency and situations when they are needed. Ideally, an updated medication list should accompany a patient when they leave a health care setting [33].

Comprehensive Medication Review

According to the Center for Medicare and Medicaid Services, a comprehensive medication review is composed of a detailed evaluation of a patient's medications, including prescriptions, OTC medications, herbal and dietary supplements, that guides pharmacotherapy and optimizes patient outcomes [31, 34]. The review is a systematic process of collecting patient-specific information, assessing medication therapies to identify MRPs, developing a prioritized list of MRPs, and creating a plan to mitigate MPRs. Medication reviews should be tailored to the individual needs of the patient and may include the following actions [31, 34, 35]:

- Obtaining patient data including demographic information, general health and activity status, past medical history, medication history (including adherence and past drug trials), allergy history, immunization history, and patient's thoughts or perceptions about their health conditions and medication use.
- Assessing medications according to relevant clinical indications, as well as the patient's physical and overall health status, including current and previous conditions.
- Understanding the patient's values, preferences, quality of life, and goals of therapy.
- Assessing the patient's cultural context, education level, language barriers, literacy level, and other communication factors.

- Interpreting signs and symptoms that could be due to adverse events from current medications.
- Interpreting, monitoring, and evaluating laboratory results.
- Identifying, evaluating, and prioritizing MRPs including but not limited: appropriateness of each medication, including efficacy, tolerability, safety, and ease of use; dosing, which includes consideration of indications, contraindications, potential side effects, and interactions; duplication or other unnecessary medications; adherence; untreated conditions; cost and access considerations.
- Developing a strategy to mitigate each MRP.
- Providing education and training on the appropriate use of medications and medication delivery devices.
- Coaching to empower patients to self-manage their medications.
- Monitoring and evaluating the response to therapy, including safety and efficacy.
- Communicating needed information to other health care professionals.

Assessing medication use and identifying MRPs "behind the scenes," sometimes involves calling the community pharmacy regarding refill histories, which can be a helpful piece of a comprehensive medication review. An interactive, face-to-face encounter with the patient can facilitate a comprehensive assessment of the patient's needs and goals and assess actual use and identify MRPs.

Patient Counseling

Effective education about medications can empower patients to be active partners in their care and promote treatment adherence. Establishing a therapeutic relationship built on trust is key to promoting learning and encouraging self-management. Counseling involves assessing the patient's understanding about his or her health problems and medications, the capacity to use the prescribed medications correctly, and attitudes toward the health-related issues and associated pharmacotherapy [3, 32].

Open-ended questioning is a strategy that can be used to gauge patient understanding, reinforce important concepts, and determine what information is required for patients [32]. For example, "what questions do you have for me?" instead of "do you have any questions?" can invite richer dialogue [36, 37]. When starting a new medication, an inquiry about each medication's purpose and the patient's expectations, as well as asking the patient to demonstrate self-administration through the method of "teach back," will facilitate the communication process. This approach can be repeated during follow-up visits to possibly uncover medication-related problems or concerns that arise.

Visual aids and demonstration devices can fill gaps in knowledge for patients and their caregivers. Opening medication bottles, for example, can visually display to patients the pill color, size, and shape. For injectable medications, this may involve showing patients the dosage marking on the measuring devices. Devices such as inhalers and pens may require a demonstration of the assembly of the device and the correct use of administration. The direct observation of medication use can also gauge correct usage and reinforce important concepts. Written handouts can supplement more complex medication regimens and help patients recall information.

The agenda for the counseling session may include the information listed below, which can be dependent on each patient's regimen and monitoring plan and based on the educator's professional judgment.

- The medication's brand and generic name, common synonym, or other descriptive name(s) and, when needed, its therapeutic class and efficacy.
- The medication's indication and expected benefits. This may include whether the medication is intended to cure a disease, eliminate, or reduce symptoms, arrest or slow the disease, or prevent the disease or symptom.
- The medication's anticipated onset of action and what steps to take if the expected result does not occur.
- The medication's route, dosage form, dose, and administration schedule.
- Directions for preparing and using the medication, which may include adapting to patients' schedule.
- Steps to take in case of a missed dose.
- Precautions to look for when using the medication and the potential risks in relation to benefits.
- Common side effects that may occur, actions to prevent or minimize their occurrence, and actions to take if they occur, including notifying the prescriber, pharmacist, or other health care provider.
- Strategies for self-monitoring.
- Potential drug–drug (including OTC), drug–food, and drug–disease interactions or contraindications.
- The medication's relationships to procedures, such as radiological, laboratory, or surgical.
- Prescription refills authorized and the process for getting refills.
- Proper storage and disposal.
- Any other helpful information unique to the specific patient or medication.

Understanding patients' cultural context, especially health and illness beliefs, attitudes, and practices can help individualize educational strategies. Culture, beliefs, religion, and ethnic customs can impact how patients comprehend health concepts, health care decisions, and their agency in taking care of their health [36]. Health care professionals should adapt their teaching content and style to patients' communication skills, often with the use of teaching aids, interpreters, or cultural guides. By failing to account for cultural practices, clinical providers may communicate medical advice without understanding how it may be received. Assessing a patient's cognitive abilities, health literacy, learning style, and physical status can also help tailor information and educational methods to meet the patient's needs. Some patients may learn best by listening to information, by seeing a picture or model, and/or by feeling the medications and devices [32, 37].

Some patients may lack the visual acuity to read prescription labels on bottles, find syringe markings, or follow written educational material. An impaired ability to read instructions printed on medication bottles or package inserts increases the likelihood for errors in self-managing medications. These patients may need special services such as blister packaging provided by a community pharmacy. In addition, they may rely on family members, friends, or care givers to read instructions on bottles or leaflets, memorize how the pill feels in their hand, or use enhanced lighting devices and magnifiers. Others may use technological devices (such as talking pill bottles, glucometers, or scales), smartphone devices and applications, or computer software that converts printed information to Braille.

Arthritis or other functional limitations can reduce patient dexterity or strength in a way that challenges the use of devices such as child-resistant containers and may require special lids for medication bottles. Patients may also have hearing impairments which can limit an understanding of oral instructions and force reliance on a written format. Challenges and limitations in verbal communication between health care professionals and patients can lead to misunderstandings in the execution of the prescribed regimen. Although approaches for meeting the medication safety needs of patients with hearing or visual impairment are challenging, efforts should be made to tailor self-management to each patient's limitations [3, 32].

For patients, medication management requires physical and cognitive skills, including higher level cortical processing and integration. With cognitive impairment, parts of the brain responsible for thinking and executive functions (such as memory, reasoning, learning) can be compromised and may interfere with daily activities including self-management of medications [38]. Even memory changes associated with normal aging can be an impediment to effective medication use, especially for chronic diseases such as type 2 diabetes that require problem-solving. Various interventions such as behavior modification, caregiver involvement, and utilizing weekly pill boxes can be helpful in managing medications in patients with cognitive impairment. These individuals may variably rely on informal caregivers for medication management and error prevention. Such caregivers require adequate training and emotional support to carry out this role for chronic conditions that are often long term. Given that caregiver burnout increases the risk for medication errors, efforts should be made to simplify the medication regimen for each patient and their support system [3, 38].

Assessment Tools for Non-adherence and Health Literacy

Non-adherence

Medication adherence is the extent to which patients take medications as prescribed by a health care provider [3, 39]. For many chronic medical conditions, medication adherence has been associated with enhanced disease control, reduced symptoms, and decreased hospitalizations and mortality. A review of over 500 studies of chronically ill patients reported a non-adherence rate of 24.8% [39, 40]. Studies in other populations have reported non-adherence rates of approximately 50%, suggesting that one in every two medication doses for chronic conditions is missed [39, 41]. Prevalence of cost-related non-adherence is high in the United States as well [27]. For example, two studies on patients with type 1 or type 2 diabetes reported 25% of patients rationing insulin in the previous year to manage costs and 40% of patients not discussing underuse of insulin with their physician [42, 43].

Both subjective and objective measures of adherence are useful in clinical practice. Objective measures, such as tracking clinical outcomes, pill counts, dispensing pharmacy records, electronic monitoring of pill administration (e.g., MEMS, the Medication Event Monitoring System), and drug concentrations, provide the most accurate measure of patient adherence. Subjective measures, including reports by family members and the patient as well as use of self-report adherence scales, have less accuracy but greater potential to gain understanding around the reasons for non-adherence. These measures are simple to use and are less expensive and time-consuming than objective assessments, but they are prone to recall bias and the potential that respondents may provide answers that conform to their perceived expectations of the interviewer [39, 41].

There are a large number of well-validated adherence scales, including the Brief Medication Questionnaire, Morisky Medication Adherence Scale (MMAS-8), Adherence Self-Report Questionnaire (ASRQ), Adherence Visual Analogue Scale (VAS), Self-Efficacy for Appropriate Medication Use Scale (SEAMS), and Medication Adherence Questionnaire (MAQ) [39, 41, 44–48]. The MMAS-8 remains one of the most widely used mechanisms to assess patient adherence for chronic illnesses.

Table 13.3 Morisky Medication Adherence Scale (MMAS-8) Questions used in the SPRINT trial

	Answer choices
Do you sometimes forget to take your high blood pressure pills?	Yes or No
Over the past 2 weeks, were there any days when you did not take your high blood pressure medicine?	Yes or No
Have you ever cut back or stopped taking your medication without telling your doctor because you felt worse when you took it?	Yes or No
When you travel or leave home, do you sometimes forget to bring along your medications?	Yes or No
Did you take your high blood pressure medicine yesterday?	Yes or No
When you feel like your blood pressure is under control, do you sometimes stop taking your medicine?	Yes or No
Do you ever feel hassled about sticking to your blood pressure treatment plan?	Yes or No
How often do you have difficulty remembering to take all your blood pressure medication?	Never; Almost never; Sometimes; Quite often; Always

Table 13.3 includes an example of the MMAS-8 questions used in the SPRINT trial, a landmark hypertension study [49].

Validated self-report measures are not routinely found in clinical practice to assess medication adherence, despite the capacity to provide actionable information for the medical team. One example of a validated self-report scale is the Medication Adherence Reasons Scale (MAR-Scale) that has been used to identify extent of non-adherence and reasons for non-adherence across multiple chronic disease conditions [50, 51]. Many clinicians believe they can accurately estimate medication adherence, but research demonstrates that clinician assumptions of adherence are often inaccurate [52]. In consequence, assessment of adherence is an important strategy for managing chronic illness and brief and validated self-report measures of adherence should be considered for use in clinical practice [39, 52].

Health Literacy

The definition of health literacy has been recently updated in the Healthy People 2030 initiative to be twofold in that there are personal and organizational roles [53, 54]. **Personal health literacy** is the degree to which individuals have the ability to find, understand, and use information and services to inform health-related decisions and actions for themselves and others. **Organizational health literacy** is the degree to which organizations equitably enable individuals to find, understand, and use information and services to inform health-related decisions and actions for themselves and others [53]. Health literacy has historically been classified by reading level as low or inadequate (i.e., sixth grade or less), marginal (i.e., seventh to eighth grade), or adequate (i.e., ninth grade and above) [37]. Almost half of high-school graduates have low health literacy and most people do not reveal this limitation to their health care providers [37, 55]. Additionally, more current adult literacy data from the Program for the International Assessment of Adult Competencies (PIAAC) found that on a scale of proficiency, only 12% of US adults scored in the highest literacy proficiency levels and only 9% in highest numeracy levels [56]. Low health literacy is frequently under-recognized in clinical practice since there is a common assumption for patients to accurately read and comprehend prescription labels, in addition to understanding medical information. Practice-level barriers include a compressed and busy work environment, which can compromise the ability of providers to gauge the health literacy of their patients.

Low health literacy results in worsened health outcomes and increased cost. It contributes to medication non-adherence via missed medication refills, problems understanding prescription instructions and warning labels, inappropriate dosing or administration times, and failure to recognize side effects or drug interactions [37, 57–59]. In a study enrolling 400 English-speaking patients across three large primary care clinics, patients with low literacy had difficulty understanding label instructions for the medications that they were prescribed. Although two-thirds of patients with low literacy correctly read the instructions, "Take two tablets by mouth twice daily," only one-third of those patients could show the correct number of pills to be taken in a day. Although this may reflect a deficiency in mathematical skills rather than reading proficiency, numeracy is an aspect of functional health literacy [59].

Functional literacy is the ability to use literacy to complete a task. It includes speaking and comprehension (such as reporting symptoms, describing medication use), reading and writing (such as reading and understanding a label on a prescription bottle, completing a questionnaire), and basic math skills (such as calibrating a medical device at home, calculating the correct dose of a drug) [3]. One study reported that almost half of the patients (including those with adequate skills) misunderstood one or more of the prescription label instructions and that lower literacy and a high number of medications are independently associated with misunderstanding of prescription instructions [59].

An additional study evaluated the impact of literacy in anticoagulated patients and found that low health literacy was associated with deficits in warfarin-related knowledge. Of those with limited health literacy, 70% of the patients understood that warfarin was a "blood thinner" and only half of these patients understood that bleeding and bruising were the most common side effects [41]. In addition to creating barriers in medication-related comprehension, low health literacy may contribute to non-prescribing of indicated therapy, such as anticoagulation [60, 61]. Helping address and improve health literacy can be a factor in mitigating health disparities among socially segmented subgroups in the United States including older adults and ethnic minorities [62, 63].

Signs of low health literacy can include patients who ask for instructions to be repeated, those who ask fewer questions overall, do not use medical terminology, do not know the name of the medications, rely on the shape, size, and color to identify their medication, "forget their glasses," are non-adherent, and have difficulty explaining their concerns [37, 64]. Objectively assessing health literacy is an important step in accurately gauging literacy level and better tailoring medication education for patients. The Rapid Estimate of Adult Literacy in Medicine (REALM), the most widely used measure of health literacy, is a 66-item word recognition and pronunciation test using common terms from the health care setting. Raw scores can be converted into 1 of 3 reading levels: sixth grade or less (score, 0–46, low literacy), seventh to eighth grade (score, 45–60, marginal literacy), and ninth grade and above (score, 61–66, adequate literacy) [37].

The REALM-Short Form (REALM-SF) is a 7-item word test that gives clinicians a quicker assessment of health literacy and has excellent agreement with the 66-item REALM test [65]. The interviewer prompts the REALM-SF test as follows [65]: "Providers often use words that patients don't understand. We are looking at words providers often use with their patients in order to improve communication between health care providers and patients. Here is a list of medical words. Starting at the top of the list, please read each word aloud to me. If you don't recognize a word, you can say 'pass' and move on to the next word." The interviewer than gives the participant the word list, which includes the following words: behavior, exercise, menopause, rectal, antibiotics, anemia, and jaundice. If the patient takes more than 5 s to respond to the word prompt, the interview moves on to the next word [37, 65–67]. Other validated literacy tools include the Short Assessment of Health Literacy—Spanish and English (SAHL—S & E) and Short Assessment of Health Literacy for Spanish Adults (SAHLSA-50) [37, 68, 69].

Communication Strategies

When interacting with patients, physicians and other health care providers should explain concepts plainly in nonmedical jargon. Terms such as use versus utilize, side effect versus adverse reaction, blood pressure versus hypertension, low sugar versus hypoglycemia, when you need it versus PRN, and on the skin versus topical are generally easier to understand for patients [37]. Standardized instructions about medication dosing schedules (e.g., morning, noon, night, and bedtime) improve patient understanding and reduce medication errors. Imprecise and vague information about dosing frequency (e.g., every 4–6 h) should be avoided for those patients with low health literacy. A prescription label that has explicit instructions such as "Take one tablet in the morning and one at 4 PM" instead of "Take one tablet twice daily" significantly reduces the possibility of improper dosing frequency and administration [37, 59].

Providers should be mindful of their pace of speech and content and volume of medical information, especially when communicating to patients with limited health literacy. For example, "take on an empty stomach" instead of "take 2 h before lunch or 2 h after lunch" may have greater relevance for patients. The communication focus should be on 1–3 key concepts and important information should be repeated with succinct explanations for common chronic disease and potential side effects [37, 59].

Patient-friendly educational material is an important adjunct to communicating medication administration. Unfortunately, drug information sources (e.g., pharmacy and package inserts) that are intended to supplement provider–patient communications and self-management are inadequate for this purpose since they are often inconsistent, complex, incomplete, and written at a college reading level [3]. Creation of a medication list, using graphics or simple phrases to show the medicine, its indication, how much to take, and when to take it can be useful resources. There are software and smartphone applications available, and Table 13.4 displays an example of a pill card [37, 70].

A "teach back" or "show me" technique is an effective strategy to evaluate patient understanding, clarify important points, and close any communication gaps between the patient and provider or health educator [36, 37, 53]. In this approach, patients are asked to repeat instructions to demonstrate their understanding. A provider, for example, may prompt by saying: "I want to make sure that I have explained everything clearly. If you were trying to explain to your partner how to take this medication, what would you say? I want to make sure that I mentioned the main side effects of this new medicine. Could you tell me what you plan to watch out for? Please show me how you would use this inhaler so I can make sure that I explained it well" [37].

The provider or health educator confirms understanding when the patient is able to correctly demonstrate use or explain how to use the medication with his or her own words. If a patient cannot remember or accurately repeat what was presented, the information is presented, clarified, and the patient is invited to teach back again. This process continues until the patient can adequately describe the directions. Misinformation and other errors can be corrected with further targeted teaching and/or reevaluating comprehension again [32, 37]. The teach back may be a valid approach to identify potential errors in medication administration, since

Table 13.4 Medication list image schedule card example

Name: Ana Martinez　　Date Created: 11/9/2021
Pharmacy phone number: 111-222-3344

Name	Used for	Instructions	Morning	Noon	Evening	Bedtime
Crestor 20 mg tablet	Heart Disease	Take 1 pill at bedtime				●
Metformin 500 mg tablet	Diabetes	Take 2 pills in the morning and 2 pills in the evening	⬭ ⬭		⬭ ⬭	
Chlorthalidone 25 mg tablet	High Blood Pressure	Take ½ (half) pill in the morning	◗			

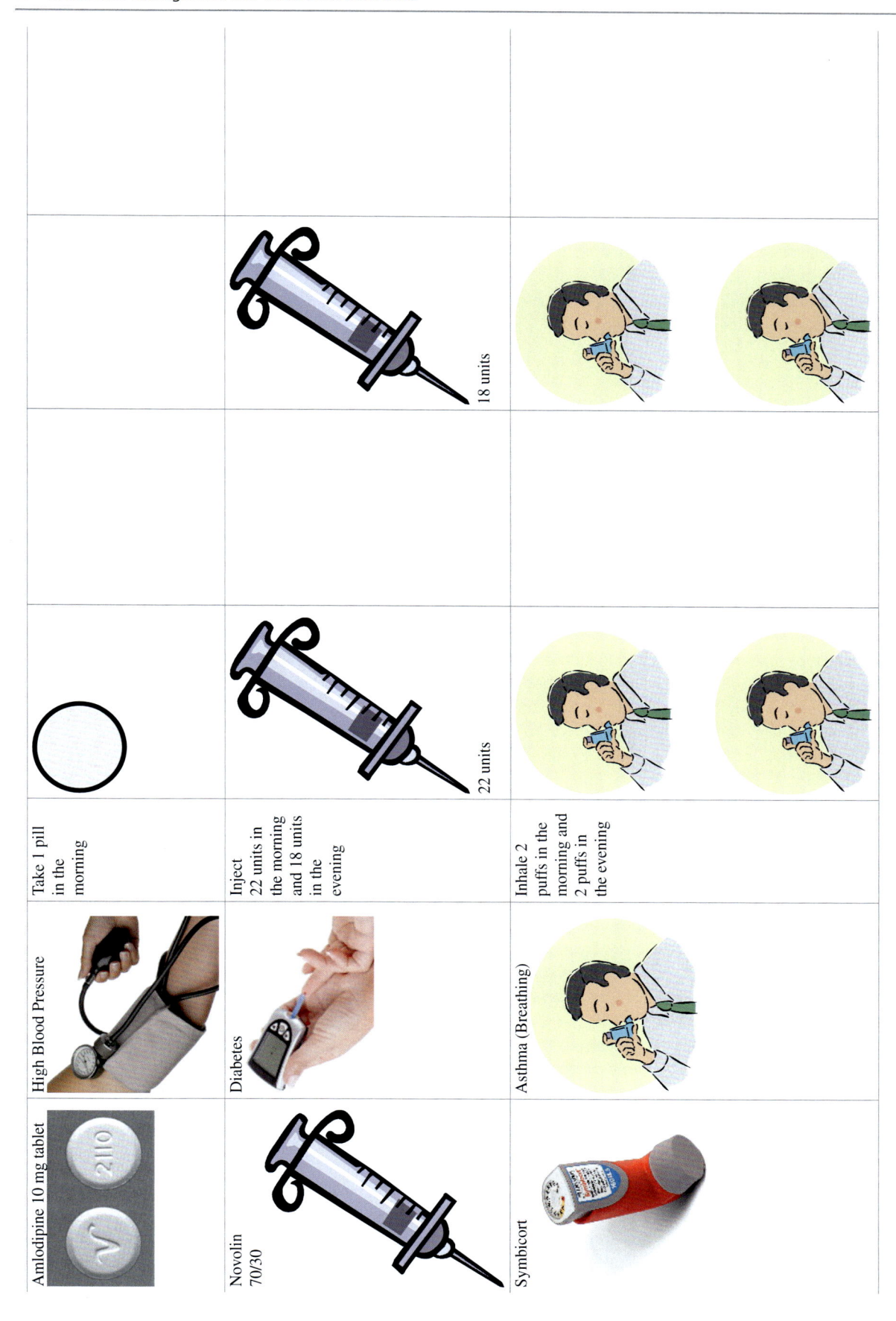

13 Medication Management and Treatment Adherence

	18 units	
○	22 units	
Take 1 pill in the morning	Inject 22 units in the morning and 18 units in the evening	Inhale 2 puffs in the morning and 2 puffs in the evening
High Blood Pressure	Diabetes	Asthma (Breathing)
Amlodipine 10 mg tablet	Novolin 70/30	Symbicort

studies have found a gap between a patient's ability to correctly verbalize instructions and his or her ability to correctly show the correct number of pills to be taken daily [37, 59].

Strategies to Promote Treatment Adherence and Medication Management

There are several principles that underline strategies to promote treatment adherence and medication management. One basic principle is that the patient should be incorporated in the decision-making and that family caregiver support needs to be encouraged to improve treatment adherence and effectively manage medications. Establishing a patient–provider relationship that is based on a mutually beneficial exchange in which the patient gives authority to the provider and the provider gives competence and commitment to the patient is fundamental to effective medication management and adherence [3, 15, 32]. Patients should be empowered as partners in their care, with appropriate communication, teaching, and resources in place to support them. In turn, health care professionals should engage in meaningful discussions regarding the safe and effective use of medications at multiple points in the medication-use process [3]. Finally, the health care environment should be representative of a patient-centered culture [3].

The largest barrier to patient education and adequate medication self-management is lack of knowledge about the safe and effective use of medications. Both prescribers and patients are often required to make decisions by weighing pros and cons of medication regimens with knowledge limitations in the context of real-time practice. Physicians and other health care providers are often under time constraints that limit time spent with patients and most prescriptions are written in the last minute of the encounter with limited time for counseling regarding the medication [3]. Prescribing requirements associated with various formularies are another practical barrier impacting providers in practice. Some aspects of managing different formulary requirements can be alleviated with the use of information technology and digital health but are not always accurate and comprehensive [3].

A rapidly growing strategy to promote medication management is found in health information technology applications and digital health that identify areas around medication safety and use this information to inform patients and providers. Many health care systems and institutions are seeking ways to implement and sustain these technologies in a way that enables providers to readily access evidenced-based resources, effectively communicate medication-related information to patients, use automated decision-support tools and best practice alerts, run drug–drug interaction screenings, and assess the safety of medication use through monitoring and reporting [3]. Medication reminders, such as smartphone apps, adherence aids (such as pill boxes or blister packages), medication calendars, as well as appointment reminders (text, telephone, or computer-based), are useful tools. Promoting the use of a weekly pill box and encouraging patients to bring it to clinic appointments can help improve adherence and can assist the provider in confirming that the patient is organizing medications as prescribed [26, 37, 71].

Patient access to the electronic medical record (EMR), which includes a medication list, and provider access to patient adherence data (including EMR alerts) can also increase compliance and helps empower patients to update their medication list more regularly. Telephone, mail, or video support and counseling has also been implemented throughout the United States with an increase in telehealth services particularly [26, 72]. Maintaining contact with patients improve adherence as well. This can include strategies of more frequent follow-up appointments; telephone calls encouraging self-reporting, such as daily weights, home blood pressure readings, blood sugar readings, and responding to the information; reaching out to patients who do not return to clinic; inquiring about adherence; and encounters with allied health professionals (such as pharmacists, nurses, and case managers) [26, 71].

Targeted patient education initiatives can significantly improve medication use and subsequently chronic disease outcomes [3]. For example, a nurse-led intervention that included medical detailing to patients about gout and its treatment options, as well as individualized lifestyle advice and pharmacotherapy modification, led to 91% adherence to allopurinol and 85% attainment of the goal uric acid to reduce gout flares [73, 74]. Information-grounded interventions such as disease state education (including the goal and anticipated outcomes of treatment), self-monitoring guidance, lifestyle modifications and counseling, and drug education and counseling have been found to promote adherence for patients [3, 26, 71].

Prescribers should be mindful of medication costs. Reducing medication copays through prescribing of generic brands, preferred low-cost drugs on insurance plans, and combination drugs is one of the most effective strategies to improve adherence [26, 27, 71]. Other approaches include ordering specific surveillance labs (e.g., serum potassium rather than chemistry profile), obtaining and recording home readings, such as blood glucose and blood pressure data, emphasizing non-pharmacologic therapies (e.g., exercise), and using daily versus multiple daily dosing. Standardizing workflows (e.g., lab draws at specific intervals), for drug monitoring and appropriate dose adjustments, as well as optimizing therapies in order to resolve adverse drug reactions, drug–drug interactions, and food–drug interactions are also important strategies [26, 71].

Case management is another strategy that seeks to create connectivity, alignment, and collaboration within and between the patient and the care providers as well as health care system. The goal is to improve quality of care, reduce barriers to care, and enhance patient experience. It often involves systematic monitoring of patients for non-adherence and clinical status, facilitation of guideline recommendations to providers, patient support for decisions, self-management and treatment, as well as appropriate follow-up [75, 76]. Case management can additionally be defined as "a collaborative approach to ensure, coordinate and integrate care and services for patients, in which a case manager evaluates, plans, implements, coordinates, and prioritizes services on the basis of patient's needs" [77]. Multidisciplinary case management has been found to improve patient outcomes across a spectrum of chronic diseases, including but not limited to asthma, COPD, hypertension, congestive heart failure, coronary artery disease, gout, depression, and HIV [78]. Individuals such as nurses, care managers, and pharmacists can serve as liaisons between primary care providers and patients to promote adherence [19]. For example, a nurse-administered phone intervention increased patient confidence in managing hypertension and a nurse-led face-to-face self-management program increased inhaler adherence in patients with asthma [79, 80]. A 2011 meta-analysis showed that pharmacist face-to-face interventions can significantly improve adherence and blood pressure control in patients with hypertension [71]. In patients receiving multiple medications, periodic telephone counseling by a pharmacist improved compliance and reduced mortality [28]. Although the majority of the literature highlights the significant impact of pharmacist involvement, health care assistants can also promote adherence to medications. Case management provided by primary care practice-based health care assistants conducting a structured phone interview to support adherence demonstrated a decrease in depression symptoms in patients with major depression [75].

Multidisciplinary chronic disease management program may especially benefit patients with low literacy. A prospective randomized clinical trial reported that diabetic patients with low literacy, who received a comprehensive disease management intervention, were more likely than control patients (i.e., usual care) to have better control of their diabetes [81]. Patients with higher literacy had a similar likelihood of achieving the goal levels regardless of intervention participation. Multifaceted interventions—those that included reduced copayments, case management, patient education with behavioral support—have shown to be effective strategies for enhancing adherence in patients with chronic conditions. In any intervention, efforts should be made to improve medication management and treatment adherence by meaningfully connecting with patients [26, 71].

Future Directions

Medication-related problems (MRPs) commonly occur in patients with chronic diseases and effective medication management consists of medication reconciliation, comprehensive medication review, and patient counseling. Direct integration of literacy and adherence assessment data from computer-based self-report measures into EMR should be developed further since this will allow information to be readily available for use by providers to improve care [39]. Finally, clinicians and health care settings should provide a patient-centered approach to medication-related care encompassing patients' individual cultural context with the overall purpose of improving patient outcomes.

References

1. Slone Epidemiology Center. Patterns of medication use in the United States, 2006: a report from the Slone Survey. Slone Epidemiology Center at Boston University. https://www.bu.edu/slone/files/2012/11/SloneSurveyReport2006.pdf. Accessed Oct 2021.
2. Martin CB, Hales CM, Gu Q, Ogden CL. Prescription drug use in the United States, 2015–2016. NCHS Data Brief, no 334. Hyattsville, MD: National Center for Health Statistics. p. 2019.
3. Institute of Medicine, Committee on Identifying and Preventing Medication Errors. Preventing medication errors. Washington, DC: The National Academies Press; 2006.
4. Shehab N, Lovegrove MC, Geller AI, Rose KO, Weidle NJ, Budnitz DS. US Emergency Department visits for outpatient adverse drug events, 2013–2014. JAMA. 2016;316(20):2115–25. https://doi.org/10.1001/jama.2016.16201.
5. Tamblyn R, Abrahamowicz M, Buckeridge DL, et al. Effect of an electronic medication reconciliation intervention on adverse drug events: a cluster randomized trial. JAMA Netw Open. 2019;2(9):e1910756. https://doi.org/10.1001/jamanetworkopen.2019.10756.
6. Gurwitz JH, Field TS, Harrold LR, Rothschild J, Debellis K, Seger AC, Cadoret C, Fish LS, Garber L, Kelleher M, Bates DW. Incidence and preventability of adverse drug events among older persons in the ambulatory setting. JAMA. 2003;289:1107–16.
7. Ernst FR, Grizzle AJ. Drug-related morbidity and mortality: updating the cost-of-illness model. J Am Pharm Assoc (Wash). 2001;41(2):192–9.
8. Watanabe JH, McInnis T, Hirsch JD. Cost of prescription drug-related morbidity and mortality. Ann Pharmacother. 2018;52(9):829–37. https://doi.org/10.1177/1060028018765159.
9. The Pharmacists' Role in the Patient-Centered Medical Home (PCMH): a white paper created by the Health Policy Committee of the Pennsylvania Pharmacists Association (PPA). Ann Pharmacother. 2012;46:723–50.
10. Budnitz DS, Pollock DA, Weidenbach KN, Mendelsohn AB, Schroeder TJ, Annest JL. National surveillance of emergency department visits for outpatient adverse drug events. JAMA. 2006;296:1858–66.
11. Digmann R, Thomas A, Peppercorn S, et al. Use of Medicare administrative claims to identify a population at high risk for adverse drug events and hospital use for quality improvement. J Manag Care Spec Pharm. 2019;25(3):402–10. https://doi.org/10.18553/jmcp.2019.25.3.402.

12. Budnitz DS, Shehab N, Kegler SR, Richards CL. Medication use leading to emergency department visits for adverse drug events in older adults. Ann Intern Med. 2007;147(11):755–65. https://doi.org/10.7326/0003-4819-147-11-200712040-00006.
13. Feinstein JA, Feudtner C, Kempe A. Adverse drug event-related emergency department visits associated with complex chronic conditions. Pediatrics. 2014;133(6):e1575–85. https://doi.org/10.1542/peds.2013-3060.
14. Medication Safety Basics. https://www.cdc.gov/medicationsafety/basics.html.
15. American Society of Hospital Pharmacists. ASHP statement on pharmaceutical care. Am J Hosp Pharm. 1993;50:1720–3. https://www.ashp.org/-/media/assets/policy-guidelines/docs/statements/pharmaceutical-care.ashx
16. Hepler CD, Strand LM. Opportunities and responsibilities in pharmaceutical care. Am J Hosp Pharm. 1990;47:533–43.
17. Adverse Drug Event Trigger Tool. https://www.cms.gov/Medicare/Provider-Enrollment-and-Certification/QAPI/downloads/adverse-drug-event-trigger-tool.pdf. Accessed 16 Oct 2021.
18. Institute for Healthcare Improvement. How-to guide: prevent harm from high-alert medications. Cambridge, MA: Institute for Healthcare Improvement; 2012. www.ihi.org. Accessed 16 Oct 2021
19. Basger BJ, Moles RJ, Chen TF. Application of drug related problem (DRP) classification systems: a review of the literature. Eur J Clin Pharmacol. 2014;70(7):799–815.
20. PCNE Classification for drug-related problems v9.1. Pharmaceutical Care Network Europe Association. 2020. https://www.pcne.org/upload/files/417_PCNE_classification_V9-1_final.pdf.
21. Strand LM, Morley PC, Cipolle RJ, Ramsey R, Lamsam GD. Drug-related problems: their structure and function. DICP. 1990;24(11):1093–7.
22. Van Mil JWF, Westerlund T, Hersberger T, Schaefer MA. Drug-related problem classification systems. Ann Pharmacother. 2004;38:859–67.
23. Benner JS, Glynn RJ, Mogun H, Neumann PJ, Weinstein MC, Avorn J. Long-term persistence in use of statin therapy in elderly patients. JAMA. 2002;288(4):455–61.
24. Cramer J, Rosenheck R, Kirk G, Krol W, Krystal J, VA Naltrexone Study Group 425. Medication compliance feedback and monitoring in a clinical trial: predictors and outcomes. Value Health. 2003;6(5):566–73.
25. Benjamin RM. Medication adherence: helping patients take their medicines as directed. Public Health Rep. 2012;127(1):2–3. https://doi.org/10.1177/003335491212700102.
26. Viswanathan M, Golin CE, Jones CD, Ashok M, Blalock SJ, Wines RC, Coker-Schwimmer EJ, Rosen DL, Sista P, Lohr KN. Interventions to improve adherence to self-administered medications for chronic diseases in the United States: a systematic review. Ann Intern Med. 2012;157(11):785–95.
27. Van Alsten SC, Harris JK. Cost-related nonadherence and mortality in patients with chronic disease: a multiyear investigation, National Health Interview Survey, 2000–2014. Prev Chronic Dis. 2020;17:200244. https://doi.org/10.5888/pcd17.200244.
28. Wu JY, Leung WY, Chang S, Lee B, Zee B, Tong PC, Chan JC. Effectiveness of telephone counselling by a pharmacist in reducing mortality in patients receiving polypharmacy: randomised controlled trial. BMJ. 2006;333(7567):522. Epub 2006 Aug 17
29. Rankin A, Cadogan CA, Patterson SM, et al. Interventions to improve the appropriate use of polypharmacy for older people. Cochrane Database Syst Rev. 2018;9(9):CD008165. https://doi.org/10.1002/14651858.CD008165.pub4.
30. Medication Reconciliation to Prevent Adverse Drug Events. http://www.ihi.org/Topics/ADEsMedicationReconciliation/Pages/default.aspx.
31. Medication Therapy Management in Pharmacy Practice: Core Elements of an MTM Service Model. https://aphanet.pharmacist.com/sites/default/files/files/core_elements_of_an_mtm_practice.pdf.
32. American Society of Health-System Pharmacy. ASHP guidelines on pharmacist-conducted patient education and counseling. https://www.ashp.org/-/media/assets/policy-guidelines/docs/guidelines/pharmacist-conducted-patient-education-counseling.ashx.
33. Universal Medication Form. http://www.ihi.org/resources/Pages/Tools/UniversalMedicationForm.aspx.
34. Hardin HC, Salo J. Conducting the comprehensive medication review. In: Whalen K, Hardin HC, editors. Medication therapy management: a comprehensive approach. 2nd ed. McGraw Hill; 2018. https://accesspharmacy.mhmedical.com/content.aspx?bookid=2319&sectionid=180048105. Accessed 16 Oct 2021.
35. Centers for Medicare & Medicaid Services. Medication therapy management. https://www-cms-gov.libproxy.lib.unc.edu/Medicare/Prescription-Drug-Coverage/PrescriptionDrugCovContra/MTM.
36. Agency for Healthcare Research and Quality. Health literacy tools for providers of medication therapy management. Rockville, MD: Agency for Healthcare Research and Quality; 2020. https://www.ahrq.gov/health-literacy/improve/pharmacy/medication-mgt.html
37. Health Literacy in pharmacy. Agency for Healthcare Research and Quality, Rockville, MD. http://www.ahrq.gov/professionals/education/curriculum-tools/pharmlitqi/ppt-slides.html.
38. Elliott RA, Goeman D, Beanland C, Koch S. Ability of older people with dementia or cognitive impairment to manage medicine regimens: a narrative review. Curr Clin Pharmacol. 2015;10(3):213–21. https://doi.org/10.2174/1574884710666150812141525.
39. Stirratt MJ, Dunbar-Jacob J, Crane HM, et al. Self-report measures of medication adherence behavior: recommendations on optimal use. Transl Behav Med. 2015;5(4):470–82.
40. DiMatteo MR. Variations inpatients' adherence to medical recommendations: a quantitative review of 50 years of research. Med Care. 2004;42:200–9.
41. Nguyen TM, La Caze A, Cottrell N. What are validated self-report adherence scales really measuring? A systematic review. Br J Clin Pharmacol. 2014;77(3):427–45.
42. T1International. Costs and rationing of insulin and diabetes supplies: findings from the 2018 T1International patient survey. https://www.t1international.com/media/assets/file/T1International_Report_-_Costs_and_Rationing_of_Insulin__Diabetes_Supplies_2.pdf. Accessed 17 Oct 2021.
43. Herkert D, Vijayakumar P, Luo J, Schwartz JI, Rabin TL, DeFilippo E, et al. Cost-related insulin underuse among patients with diabetes. JAMA Intern Med. 2019;179(1):112–4.
44. Svarstad BL, Chewning BA, Sleath BL, Claesson C. The Brief Medication Questionnaire: a tool for screening patient adherence and barriers to adherence. Patient Educ Couns. 1999;37(2):113–24.
45. Morisky DE, Green LW, Levine DM. Concurrent and predictive validity of a self-reported measure of medication adherence. Med Care. 1986;24(1):67–74.
46. Kalichman SC, Amaral CM, Swetzes C, et al. A simple single item rating scale to measure medication adherence: further evidence for convergent validity. J Int Assoc Physicians AIDS Care (Chic). 2009;8(6):367–74.
47. Zeller A, Schroeder K, Peters TJ. An adherence self-report questionnaire facilitated the differentiation between nonadherence and nonresponse to antihypertensive treatment. J Clin Epidemiol. 2008;61(3):282–8.
48. Risser J, Jacobson TA, Kripalani S. Development and psychometric evaluation of the Self-efficacy for Appropriate Medication Use Scale (SEAMS) in low-literacy patients with chronic disease. J Nurs Meas. 2007;15(3):203–19.
49. Haley WE, Gilbert ON, Riley RF, et al. The association between Self-Reported Medication Adherence scores and systolic blood

pressure control: a SPRINT baseline data study. J Am Soc Hypertens. 2016;10(11):857–864.e2. https://doi.org/10.1016/j.jash.2016.08.009.
50. Unni EJ, Sternbach N, Goren A. Using the Medication Adherence Reasons Scale (MAR-Scale) to identify the reasons for nonadherence across multiple disease conditions. Patient Prefer Adherence. 2019;13:993–1004. https://doi.org/10.2147/PPA.S205359.
51. Unni EJ, Olson JL, Farris KB. Revision and validation of Medication Adherence Reasons Scale (MAR-Scale). Curr Med Res Opin. 2014;30(2):211–21. https://doi.org/10.1185/03007995.2013.851075.
52. Miller LG, Liu H, Hays RD, et al. How well do clinicians estimate patients' adherence to combination antiretroviral therapy? J Gen Intern Med. 2002;17:1–11.
53. Agency for Healthcare Research and Quality. About health literacy. Rockville, MD: Agency for Healthcare Research and Quality; 2020. https://www.ahrq.gov/health-literacy/about/index.html
54. Santana S, Brach C, Harris L, et al. Updating health literacy for healthy people 2030: defining its importance for a new decade in public health. J Public Health Manag Pract. 2021;27:S258–64. https://doi.org/10.1097/PHH.0000000000001324.
55. Parikh NS, Parker RM, Nurss JR, Baker DW, Williams MV. Shame and health literacy: the unspoken connection. Patient Educ Couns. 1996;27(1):33–9.
56. Highlights of the 2017 U.S. PIAAC Results Web Report (NCES 2020–777). U.S. Department of Education, Institute of Education Sciences, National Center for Education Statistics. https://nces.ed.gov/surveys/piaac/current_results.asp.
57. American Medical Association Foundation. Health literacy and patient safety: help patients understand. 2007. https://psnet.ahrq.gov/resources/resource/5839/health-literacy-and-patient-safety-help-patients-understand-manual-for-clinicians-2nd-ed.
58. Berkman ND, Sheridan SL, Donahue KE, Halpern DJ, Viera A, Crotty K, Holland A, Brasure M, Lohr KN, Harden E, Tant E, Wallace I, Viswanathan M. Health literacy interventions and outcomes: an updated systematic review. Evid Rep Technol Assess (Full Rep). 2011;199:1–941.
59. Davis TC, Wolf MS, Bass PF III, et al. Literacy and misunderstanding prescription drug labels. Ann Intern Med. 2006;145(12):887–94.
60. Fang MC, Machtinger EL, Wang F, Schillinger D. Health literacy and anticoagulation-related outcomes among patients taking warfarin. J Gen Intern Med. 2006;21(8):841–6.
61. Man-Son-Hing M, Laupacis A, O'Connor AM, Biggs J, Drake E, Yetisir E, Hart RG. A patient decision aid regarding antithrombotic therapy for stroke prevention in atrial fibrillation: a randomized controlled trial. JAMA. 1999;282(8):737–43.
62. A Health Literacy Report: analysis of 2016 behavioral risk factor surveillance system health literacy data. Centers for Disease Control. 2016. https://www.cdc.gov/healthliteracy/pdf/Report-on-2016-BRFSS-Health-Literacy-Data-For-Web.pdf.
63. Scott TL, Paasche-Orlow MK, Wolf MS. Promoting health literacy research to reduce health disparities. J Health Commun. 2010;15(S2):34–41.
64. Katz MG, Jacobson TA, Veledar E, Kripalani S. Patient literacy and question-asking behavior during the medical encounter: a mixed-methods analysis. J Gen Intern Med. 2007;22(6):782–6.
65. REALM-SF Score Sheet. Health Literacy and how to assess it. http://www.ahrq.gov/sites/default/files/wysiwyg/professionals/quality-patient-safety/quality-resources/tools/literacy/realm.pdf.
66. Davis TC, Long SW, Jackson RH, Mayeaux EJ, George RB, Murphy PW, et al. Rapid estimate of adult literacy in medicine: a shortened screening instrument. Fam Med. 1993;25:391–5.
67. Arozullah AM, Yarnold PR, Bennett CL, Soltysik RC, Wolf MS, Ferreira RM, Lee SY, Costello S, Shakir A, Denwood C, Bryant FB, Davis T. Development and validation of a short-form, rapid estimate of adult literacy in medicine. Med Care. 2007;45(11):1026–33.
68. Lee SY, Stucky BD, Lee JY, Rozier RG, Bender DE. Short Assessment of Health Literacy-Spanish and English: a comparable test of health literacy for Spanish and English speakers. Health Serv Res. 2010;45(4):1105–20.
69. Lee SY, Bender DE, Ruiz RE, Cho YI. Development of an easy-to-use Spanish Health Literacy test. Health Serv Res. 2006;41(4 Pt 1):1392–412.
70. Kripalani S, Robertson R, Love-Ghaffari MH, Henderson LE, Praska J, Strawder A, Katz MG, Jacobson TA. Development of an illustrated medication schedule as a low-literacy patient education tool. Patient Educ Couns. 2007;66:368–77.
71. Morgado MP, Morgado SR, Mendes LC, Pereira LJ, Castelo-Branco M. Pharmacist interventions to enhance blood pressure control and adherence to antihypertensive therapy: review and meta-analysis. Am J Health Syst Pharm. 2011;68(3):–241.
72. Demeke HB, Merali S, Marks S, et al. Trends in use of telehealth among health centers during the COVID-19 pandemic—United States, June 26–November 6, 2020. MMWR Morb Mortal Wkly Rep. 2021;70:240–4. https://doi.org/10.15585/mmwr.mm7007a3.
73. Rees F, Jenkins W, Doherty M. Patients with gout adhere to curative treatment if informed appropriately: proof-of-concept observational study. Ann Rheum Dis. 2013;72(6):826–30.
74. Harrold LR, Andrade SE, Briesacher BA, Raebel MA, Fouayzi H, Yood RA, Ockene IS. Adherence with urate-lowering therapies for the treatment of gout. Arthritis Res Ther. 2009;11(2):R46.
75. Gensichen J, von Korff M, Peitz M, Muth C, Beyer M, Güthlin C, Torge M, Petersen JJ, Rosemann T, König J, Gerlach FM, PRoMPT (PRimary care Monitoring for depressive Patients Trial). Case management for depression by health care assistants in small primary care practices: a cluster randomized trial. Ann Intern Med. 2009;151(6):369–78.
76. Bogner HR, de Vries HF. Integrating type 2 diabetes mellitus and depression treatment among African Americans: a randomized controlled pilot trial. Diabetes Educ. 2010;36(2):284–92.
77. Hudon C, Chouinard MC, Pluye P, El Sherif R, Bush PL, Rihoux B, et al. Characteristics of case management in primary care associated with positive outcomes for frequent users of health care: a systematic review. Ann Fam Med. 2019;17(5):448–58.
78. Hudon C, Chouinard MC, Lambert M, Dufour I, Krieg C. Effectiveness of case management interventions for frequent users of healthcare services: a scoping review. BMJ Open. 2016;6(9):e012353. https://doi.org/10.1136/bmjopen-2016-012353.
79. Bosworth HB, Olsen MK, Gentry P, Orr M, Dudley T, McCant F, Oddone EZ. Nurse administered telephone intervention for blood pressure control: a patient-tailored multifactorial intervention. Patient Educ Couns. 2005;57(1):5–14.
80. Berg J, Dunbar-Jacob J, Sereika SM. An evaluation of a self-management program for adults with asthma. Clin Nurs Res. 1997;6(3):225–38.
81. Rothman RL, DeWalt DA, Malone R, Bryant B, Shintani A, Crigler B, Weinberger M, Pignone M. Influence of patient literacy on the effectiveness of a primary care-based diabetes disease management program. JAMA. 2004;292(14):1711–6.

Patient-Provider Communication and Interactions

14

Kelly Lacy Smith and Jennifer Martini

Introduction

In a letter to his new primary care physician John Steinbeck reflected, "What do I want in a doctor? Perhaps more than anything else—a friend with special knowledge" [1]. Steinbeck alluded not only to the importance of the relationships that develop between healthcare providers and their patients, but also to the key role that the communication of medical knowledge plays in fostering those relationships and facilitating care over time. Communication between healthcare providers and their patients, particularly during chronic illness, shapes a patient's healthcare experience. It influences information that is gathered from patients, informs an understanding and conceptualization of their illness, and provides a foundation for the collaborative work that patients and providers will engage in around disease management.

The Institute of Medicine highlighted six aims for improving healthcare in *Crossing the Quality Chasm* report, including the need for care to be patient-centered, responsive to individual patient preferences, needs, and values, to ensure that patient values guide clinical decisions [2]. The report further highlighted the essential role that patient-provider communication plays in achieving this aim, recommending that care be based on continuous healing relationships, that knowledge and information flow freely between providers and patients [2].

There is a substantial body of evidence that supports these recommendations, demonstrating an association between effective patient-provider communication and important health outcomes [3–6]. In addition, quality communication between patients and providers has been linked to patient satisfaction, which is important not for better health, an outcome in a value-based care environment [3, 4, 7]. Healthcare providers may also find greater professional satisfaction through care that involves effective communication, a quadruple aim that includes a patient-centered experience, quality improvement, reducing costs, and improving the work life of healthcare providers [8]. One plausible pathway that described the relationship of effective communication and health outcomes is the association of defined communication elements, such as emotional response and relationship building, as mediators of outcomes, such as disease resolution, survival, emotional well-being, and functionality [9]. Effective communication also impacts proximal patient-centered outcomes, such as satisfaction, trust, motivation, and clinician-patient rapport and agreement [9].

This chapter provides an overview of patient-provider communication in healthcare. The first section focuses on components, processes, and communication techniques in the provider-patient dyad, encounters that have historically been central to patient-provider communication. Understanding and developing communication competencies in this setting is key to the successful provision of chronic illness care. Next, communication within chronic illness care models is introduced and described in relation to health services. Team-based models of care, virtual and technology-based initiatives, and group care are representative of these trends. The chapter closes with future directions in patient-provider communications and interactions.

Communication in the Provider-Patient Dyad

Meaningful and effective provider-patient communication increases disease self-management and treatment adherence, promotes patient satisfaction, and improves quality of care and health outcomes [3, 4]. In face-to-face encounters, provider and patient personal identities and communication styles influence the information that is prioritized and shared [5, 6]. To optimize communication, understanding the patient-provider dyad interaction, and specific techniques,

K. L. Smith
School of Medicine, University of North Carolina at Chapel Hill, Chapel Hill, NC, USA
e-mail: Kelly_Smith@med.unc.edu

J. Martini (✉)
Department of Family Medicine, University of North Carolina at Chapel Hill School of Medicine, Chapel Hill, NC, USA
e-mail: jennifer_martini@med.unc.edu

knowledge, and skills, can facilitate patient health outcomes.

Goals of Patient-Provider Interactions

Patient communication is most effective when there are specific goals, which may be organized along six dimensions: (1) exploring the illness experience; (2) understanding the whole person; (3) finding common ground regarding management; (4) incorporating prevention and health promotion; (5) enhancing the doctor-patient relationship; and (6) being realistic about personal limitations [10]. This approach is informed by a biopsychosocial model, viewing the patient as a person, sharing power and responsibility, building effective relationships, maintaining and conveying positive regard for patients, and remaining aware of the doctor as person [11].

When considering communication approaches, providers should be aware of techniques that can promote goals of care. The patient-centered medical interview is an approach that views the patient as a unique human being with a life story, promoting trust by clarifying and characterizing the patient's symptoms and concerns in ways that may include biological and psychosocial dimensions of illness, and provides a foundation for an ongoing relationship [12]. Another strategy emphasizes establishing both traditional biomedical goals (e.g., blood pressure) and socioemotional goals (e.g., reduced depressive symptoms), using "2 F's" (Find the illness and Fix it) for the former as well as the "4 E's" for the latter (Engage patients via an interpersonal connection; Empathize with patients' illnesses and situation; Educate patients by effectively delivering information; and Enlist patients to actively participate in decision-making and disease management) [13, 14].

Communication Approaches and Techniques

Several organizing principles can orient providers to actionable communication concepts and skills. Seeing health and illness through patients' eyes allows providers to consider a more inclusive worldview [15]. The perspective of exploring the patient illness experience has been independently associated with increased patient trust [7]. This emotional activity is a central aspect of patient-centered communication [15, 16]. Additionally, provider introspection, self-awareness, and mindfulness are important since provider and patient character traits and personal beliefs strongly influence the communication styles, as well as the nature and content of information that is exchanged [3, 6, 7, 17, 18]. Providers may seek ways to reflect and maintain an awareness of their own traits, biases, beliefs, mannerisms, and reactions that influence their interactions. As providers progress in their communication strategies, they may find a deeper understanding of their patients and of themselves [7].

Several techniques and approaches can facilitate patient-centered communication. A curriculum for conducting medical interviews, for example, identifies knowledge, attitudinal, and skill components for patient-centered communication (Table 14.1) [12].

Table 14.1 Components of patient-centered communication

Knowledge	• Recognize different question types (e.g., open-ended, closed-ended, directive but nonbiased, directive and biased) • Understand the stages of an interview (e.g., opening, characterization of present illness and life setting, closing) • Understand interview functions (e.g., interest and commitment to patient, facilitating communication, calibrating and overcoming barriers in communication, surveying patient problems, selecting priorities and limitations, negotiating contract, use of self and helping skills, the avoidance of hindering skills) • Recognize forms of nonverbal behavior and understand communication patterns • Define transference and countertransference and explore how each effects medical relationships
Attitude	• Approach patients respectfully and nonjudgmentally • Respect patient autonomy and individuality • Willingness to see patients as partners by sharing diagnostic and treatment processes and decisions • Openness to work with and learn from patients with diverse backgrounds and personal styles

Skills	• Elicit illness narrative that includes a delineation of symptoms while pursuing contextual setting
	• Express interest in and commitment to the patient
	  – Verbal behaviors: introduce self; clarify patient's preferred name; attend to physical comfort; elicit patient's view of the problem; clarify extent of commitment; discuss questions
	  – Nonverbal behaviors: touch, get comfortable, eye contact
	• Facilitate communication
	  – Verbal behaviors: allow patient to narrate illness story; balance open-ended and closed-ended questions; use nonbiased questions; seek clarification of vague or ambiguous data; use empathy where appropriate; reflect back patient's words and affects; convey nonjudgmental, unconditional positive regard; define the patient's strengths; and utilize in the treatment plan
	  – Nonverbal behaviors: arrange space comfortably; nod, show affect, use posture that communicates interest; acknowledge patient's nonverbal behavior; quiet attention
	• Avoid hindering behavior
	  – Verbal behavior to be avoided: use of technical language, injecting biases, false or premature reassurance, noninteraction, discussion of fees first, frequent interruptions
	  – Nonverbal behavior to be avoided: posture communicates disinterest, not listening; reading chart or writing note during interview; allowing interruption

Table 14.2 Kalamazoo Consensus Statement Elements

Task	Technique
Open the Discussion	• Allow the patient to complete opening statement • Elicit that patient's full set of concerns • Establish/maintain a personal connection
Gather Information	• Use open-ended and closed-ended questions appropriately • Structure, clarify, and summarize information • Actively listen using nonverbal (e.g., eye contact) and verbal (e.g., words of encouragement) techniques
Understand the Patient's Perspective	• Explore contextual factors (e.g., family, culture, gender, age, socioeconomic status, spirituality) • Explore beliefs, concerns, and expectations about health and illness • Acknowledge and respond to the patient's ideas, feelings, and values
Share Information	• Use language the patient can understand • Check for understanding • Encourage questions
Reach Agreement on Problems and Plans	• Encourage the patient to participate in decisions to the extent he or she desires • Check the patient's willingness and ability to follow the plan • Identify and enlist resources and supports
Provide Closure	• Ask whether the patient has other issues or concerns • Summarize and affirm agreement with the plan of action • Discuss follow-up (e.g., next visit, plan for unexpected outcomes)

The Kalamazoo consensus statement has identified a framework and key elements of patient-provider communication. The statement is grounded in the assumption that a therapeutic relationship is the sine qua non of physician-patient communication; building this relationship is the fundamental communication task with which providers are charged [19] (Table 14.2).

Two sets of techniques can help foster effective, efficient relationship building and communication during patient interactions [20]. The first is rapport building and relationship maintenance, which can be accomplished through warm greetings, eye contact (when culturally appropriate), brief non-medical conversation during visits, acknowledging patient cues with empathetic responses, and checking in on important life events [20]. Additionally, providers can facilitate a mindful approach by being present and curious during patient interactions. Maintaining focus on mutually agreed-upon topics and discussing them in an organized fashion across encounters can help to further reinforce consistency and cohesiveness in the provider-patient relationship [20].

The second set of communication techniques involves partnering with patients to problem-solve and can be iterative utilized during follow-up encounters. An intentional, collaborative agenda focuses the work, which enables providers and patients to explore and prioritize the concerns [20]. Once established, patients' perspectives regarding their concerns and medical conditions are explored using open-ended questions and curious listening [20]. Providers and patients can collaborate to create a plan that incorporates patients' goals of care, gauges readiness to change, and clarifies the roles that the provider, patient, and family members or other supports will play [20].

Shared Decision-Making

Shared decision-making is a communication approach in which clinicians disclose information about alternative diagnostic and therapeutic options, and patients describe what matters to them regarding care choices [21, 22]. Patients with chronic illness often face complicated decisions that involve a complex interplay of personal priorities, changing risk/benefit ratios, and the overall impact of their choices on health. Historical communication models were often paternalistic and more contemporary approaches recognize the importance and value of engaging patients in shared decision-making that is meaningfully patient-centered [23, 24]. Effective shared decision-making is associated with improved patient satisfaction, reduced undesired care, and improved patient functioning [22, 24, 25]. In addition, providers prefer this approach since it can encourage patient understanding of risks and benefits of treatment plans [26]. Shared decision-making is often hindered by logistical, emotional, and knowledge barriers [21, 26, 27] and can be mitigated by the use of facilitative decision aids and tools [23, 28, 29].

Patient knowledge and perception of risk regarding medical treatments are more meaningful with decision aids since they report feeling more knowledgeable, better informed, and clearer about their values [29]. Decision aids come in several forms; however, there is limited evidence regarding the effectiveness of a particular aid [29]. Historically, decision aids were printed educational materials that were reviewed by patients prior to, or following, face-to-face visits with their providers; contemporary aids guide providers and patients through discussions [21, 22, 28, 29]. Information technology has a greater role in decision aids with multiple interactive online tools for patients that can gather and communicate patient preferences and concerns to providers via reports and/or electronic medical records [29, 30].

SHARE is a program developed by Agency for Healthcare Research and Quality to promote shared decision-making in clinical practice [31]. The SHARE approach facilitates productive discussions of the pros and cons of proposed interventions in the context of an individual patient's goals and priorities. Table 14.3 displays the SHARE steps and activities.

Table 14.3 SHARE Program Steps and Activities [31]

Step	Tasks and activities
Seek patient's participation in decision-making	Highlight the importance of patient engagement in decisions
	Summarize the health problems to be addressed
Help patient explore and compare treatment options	Communicate risks and benefits in patient-oriented terms
	Assess patient's pre-existing knowledge
	Use the "teach-back" technique to ensure understanding
Assess patient values and preferences	Ask open-ended questions
	Demonstrate empathy and interest in how treatments might impact patient's life
	Encourage a discussion of patient's goals and priorities
	Obtain agreement and shared understanding of the aspects of interventions that are most important to the patient
Reach decisions	Confirm that patient has had ample time and information to make a decision
Evaluate decisions and interventions	Ongoing assessment of barriers to implementation, impact of the decisions on patient's life, and evolving patient priorities
	This is particularly important in chronic care as intervention risks/benefits and patient status may change significantly during the disease process

Table 14.4 Best practices for working with interpreters

Introduce yourself to the interpreter	Acknowledge the interpreter as a professional in communication
Speak directly to the patient	
Speak more slowly rather than more loudly	
Speak at an even pace in relatively short segments	Pause so the interpreter can interpret
Assume and insist that everything you say, and everything the patient says, is interpreted	
Do not hold the interpreter responsible for what the patient does or does not say	The interpreter is the medium, not the source of the message. If you feel that you are not getting the type of response that you were expecting, restate the question or consult with the interpreter to better understand if there is a cultural barrier that is interfering with communication
Be aware that concepts you express may have no linguistic or conceptual equivalent in other languages	Conveying what you say may take longer or shorter than your original speech
Give the interpreter time to restructure information and present it in a culturally and linguistically appropriate manner	
Be conscious of asking personal or sensitive information	Explain to the patient that doing so is part of your evaluation and reiterate that information will remain confidential
Avoid highly idiomatic speech	Complicated sentence structure, sentence fragments, changing your idea in the middle of a sentence, and asking multiple questions at a time can also make communication more difficult
Encourage the interpreter to ask questions and alert you about potential cultural misunderstandings	
Avoid patronizing or infantilizing the patient	
Ask the patient to repeat back important information	
Be patient	Recognize that providing effective care and communication across a language barrier takes time
When possible, allow time for a pre-session with the interpreter	This provides an opportunity to be clear about the nature of the upcoming encounter and the information and type of communication it will involve

Acknowledging, Bridging, and Embracing Language, Identity, and Culture

Navigating Language Differences

The US Census Bureau's 2011 American Community Survey Report noted that 21% of the US population spoke a language other than English at home; of these individuals, only 58% spoke English "very well" [32]. Language discordance between patients and providers can adversely impact healthcare communication [33–35]. Providing care and communicating in a shared language is important. The prevalence and diversity of languages other than English create healthcare encounters in which providers and patients must bridge language gaps [33]. In these settings, in-person or telephonic professional interpreters are critical [34–36] and are associated with positive effects on communication, care plan comprehension, health resource utilization, clinical outcomes, mental illness management, and satisfaction with care [34–37]. Patients who receive care with interpreter assistance do not differ significantly from those who meet with language concordant providers in their propensity to rate the care they receive as "excellent" or "very good" but are more likely to have questions about their care after their visits [33].

Some best practices for working with interpreters, as outlined by the National Council on Interpreting in Healthcare, can be found in Table 14.4 [38].

The National Association for the Deaf's Position Statement on Health Care Access for Deaf patients is consistent with the interpreter principles described above [39]. It also emphasizes the importance of using visual aids when needed to enhance communication and of avoiding lip reading and written communication whenever possible when communicating with patients who speak American Sign Language [39].

Cultural Competence and Humility

Cultural humility and the provision of culturally competent care can promote patient-provider interactions in many ways [18, 40, 41]. The acknowledgment of, and willingness to embrace, health-associated cultural factors is essential to establishing trust and promoting effective communication. Medical cultural competence is the communication of diagnosis and treatment plans in ways that are acceptable to patients from different cultural backgrounds [42, 43]. Cultural humility reflects an interpersonal perspective that is other-oriented rather than self-focused, is characterized by respect and lack of superiority toward another's cultural background, and is positively associated with the establishment of strong working alliances between patients and providers [43].

There are several techniques that enhance culturally competent healthcare interactions and communication [11]. Providers can explore and acknowledge patient beliefs, values, their meaning of illness, preferences, and needs, which helps to bridge cultural differences and build relationships. To build rapport and find common ground with patients, providers need to be mindful of their own biases and assumptions and informed about cultures that are reflective of their patient populations [11]. Such awareness is essential; however, it is important that providers avoid cultural generalizations and communicate with each patient as individuals whose interactions with the healthcare system are shaped by a complex set of personal, cultural, socioeconomic, and situational factors [44].

Acknowledging Structural Racism

Practicing cultural humility and providing culturally competent care involves understanding and acknowledging the legacy of medical systems and structural racism, which has contributed to healthcare disparities among individuals of different races, ethnicities, sexual orientations, and other demographic characteristics [45–48]. There are documented examples of explicit injustice and violence by medical professionals directed at historically marginalized communities, including conversion therapy of LGBTQ+ patients, sterilization abuse of Native American women, and the medical experimentation on Black patients [49–51]. A systematic review of the effects of race and patient-provider racial concordance on physician-patient communication reported that Black patients consistently experienced poorer communication quality, information-giving, patient participation, and participatory decision-making than white patients during clinical encounters [52]. The review emphasized the importance of training physicians and patients to engage in meaningful communication with Black and racially discordant patients by focusing on improving patient-centeredness, information-giving, partnership building, and patient engagement in communication processes [52].

Intersectionality, Positionality, and Implicit Bias

Intersectionality refers to the complex and cumulative way in which multiple forms of discrimination, such as racism and sexism, accumulate and overlap in marginalized individuals or groups [53, 54]. Providers should consider how patients self-identify to inform the communication dynamics in clinical encounters. Positionality is a concept in which people are not defined by fixed identities (e.g., race, socioeconomic status), but by their location within shifting networks of relationships [55]. This concept can be relevant for providers during patient encounters, where there is a complex interplay between the identities, cultural connotations, and power dynamics of physician and patient. The concept of implicit bias is a bias or prejudice that is operative but not consciously recognized, often influencing the communications, perceptions, and interaction that occur during clinical encounters [55]. Patient-provider communication that is informed by an understanding of intersectionality, positionality, history, systemic racism, and implicit bias can promote strategies to mitigate healthcare disparities.

Communication in Chronic Care Models

Providing chronic illness care accounts for the contributions of an interdisciplinary team and is mindful of significant interactions that occur outside the context of a traditional face-to-face encounters. Multiple providers participate in healthcare teams that incorporate shared decision-making practices, group care models, and expanded communication channels via health information technology (HIT), expanding access and complexity to the dynamics of contemporary chronic care communication.

Healthcare Team Communication

Healthcare team communication is essential to providing efficient, comprehensive, chronic care and improves satisfaction for both patients and providers [21–24]. Healthcare teams may include physicians, nurse practitioners, physician assistants, nurses, care managers, dieticians, pharmacists, social workers, office staff, health coaches, and home health aides, who may work in different clinical settings and may be responsible for different aspects of patient care. An Agency for Healthcare Research and Quality (AHRQ) report on creating patient-centered team-based care highlights the centrality of good relationships among provider team members as the foundation for good relationships with patients and lays out several principles of quality team-based care [56].

A cohesive and high-performing team often reflects a larger organizational culture. The AHRQ report points out that traditional care models have been hierarchical with physicians taking the lead role; however, emerging approaches value the knowledge base and skills of each team member [56]. It is essential for all team members to develop and sustain communication tools for information gathering, synthesis, and reporting [56]. Electronic health records (EHRs) can facilitate synchronous and asynchronous communication across care team members. Other communication modes, such as secure text messaging or emails, allow for real-time updates on patient status and can streamline the process by which the care plan is adapted and advanced.

Introducing team members to patients using bio sheets, formal naming of teams, and visual cues facilitate cohesion and continuity [25]. Involving patients in interprofessional rounds has also been advocated [57]. In these settings, eliciting patient preferences on how, where, and when they would prefer to communicate with the team is critical since patients often have preferences on specific team members and the mode of communication [25, 58]. Warm hand-offs between providers, highlighting and reinforcing information from other team members, and signposting the roles of other team members can provide clear and consistent communication between the care team and the patient [25].

Real-time communication can be facilitated by co-locating team members in a proximate clinical space to promote team huddles or informal meetings develop rapport and share insights for care coordination [23, 56, 57]. Developing innovative workspaces for patient care, such as dedicated chronic care clinics with multiple co-located providers and resources, may help to improve patient communication and satisfaction [58]. Setting expectations and parameters for communication, such as modes and expected response time, can enhance team functioning and patient care. For example, verbal or face-to-face communication may be preferred for unclear or emotional content since it allows for more nuanced information exchange, while an email or text communication may be preferential for routine messages or those with a large amount of data to be assimilated [59].

Group Care Models

Group care has promise and adds complexity to healthcare communication. Ideally, group visits provide patient-centered care in a manner that optimizes quality and outcomes while decreasing access barriers for patients [60]. Chronic care group visits can occur as drop-in appointments, in which a small group of patients meet with the help of a provider facilitator, or as part of cooperative and interactive healthcare encounter with multiple providers to manage their chronic illnesses [61]. During group visits, providers should adopt an empathetic, open communication approach comparable to individual visits [62, 63]. Providers should direct patient-generated questions to the group for discussion and feedback, rather than providing answers directly, to leverage the perspectives and experience of group members [63]. Other approaches include using local subject matter experts and evidence-based educational materials and demonstrative learning environments such as cooking classes or grocery store visits, which can potentiate the group visit format [62].

Specific Challenges and Special Situations

Situations may arise during chronic care that require attention to communication dynamics. Early recognition of communication problems, advance planning, and using effective tools and strategies can avoid disruptions to the patient-provider relationships and maintain information flows.

Working with Family Members, Advocates, and Other Proxies

Patients with chronic illness often receive care in settings accompanied by family members, friends, and other advocates. The level of involvement and responsibility that these companions assume can vary depending upon the decision-making capacity, health and functional status, and social network of the patient. Patient companions/proxies can facilitate communication by assisting the patient in building rapport with providers, advocating for patients, and ensuring accurate and thorough information exchange [64–66]. Companions/proxies can also add important collateral information, such as a contextual understanding of patients' lives, symptoms, and living conditions. Interactions between providers and companions/proxies can be "autonomy enhancing" since they may encourage patients in self-management of their disease and promote personal agency. Companions/proxies can clarify background and presenting medical information, facilitate patient comprehension of treatment recommendations, and activate and prompt discussion of topics.

Although companion/proxies often have a positive impact on patient-provider communication, there may be challenges, including unclear, undisclosed, or competing agendas between patients and companions/proxies, incomplete and inconsistent information, and concerns of privacy and confidentiality, which impede information exchange and rapport building [64]. In addition, there is variation among patients of how involved they would like family members and companions to be in their care. Several autonomy-detracting behaviors, such as companions/proxies who interrupt patients, disclose irrelevant information about their personal health or that of a third party, correct or blame patients in front of providers, attempt to take on an expert role, or answer questions for patients without allowing them to respond, create communication difficulties [65, 66]. Other actions include companions/proxies who engage in inappropriate alliance building, intentionally or unintentionally attempting to persuade patients and/or providers to agree to agendas that are primarily based on the companions' opinions or preferences [65, 66].

Several techniques can maximize the positive contributions of companions/proxies have while mitigating potential pitfalls. The first involves encouraging and welcoming companions/proxies to the healthcare encounter, ascertaining reasons why companions are involved from both patients' and companions' perspectives, and clarifying the roles of patients and companions at the commencement of the visit [23]. Respecting patients' autonomy and preferences and attending to their communication preferences regarding sensitive information is important. A second approach recognizes value-added companion/proxy behaviors and reinforces strategies that companions can use to provide emotional, informational, and logistical support.

The use of communication tools before and during the encounter may foster the patient-companion-provider interactions [23, 67]. A checklist that is given to the patient/companion before the visit can elicit and organize a healthcare agenda and has been found to improve the experiences of patients and their providers [67]. These checklists, pictured below, prompt patients and companions/proxies to independently identify and prioritize medical concerns and prompt patients to designate the role that the companion/proxy is expected to play [67]. The use of a pre-visit checklist and modifying it during the encounter allows providers to leverage the contribution of the companion/proxy [67] (Fig. 14.1).

Giving Bad News

Chronic illness care is interwoven with the lived experience of patients, including moments of joy, sorrow, adjustment, and change. Bad news in healthcare settings is information which adversely affects an individual's view of their future health and well-being [68, 69]. Physicians and other providers sometimes provide clinical information that is disappointing, upsetting, or devastating to patients and their families. The communication of bad news is an area where many providers feel uncomfortable [17]. In addition to the task of informing patients of potentially distressing and life changing information, communicating bad news involves responding to patients' emotional responses, involving them in subsequent decision-making, and being available for concerns that arise as patients and their family members come to terms with the implications of information that has been conveyed [69].

Two sets of factors influence communication around delivering bad news [70]. One involves the provider assessment of the internal dynamics of patients; the attitudes, wishes, and needs that arise when bad news is delivered. Providers should seek a balance between accurately disclosing distressing news and sustaining hope, being mindful that patient and provider emotions play a significant role in the communication dynamics. The second set is external to the patient-provider dyad, such as family relationships, systematic and institutional factors such as the time available for conversations, the clinical settings in which news is delivered, and the cultural and socioeconomic contexts in which patients and their providers are situated. Family relationships are particularly powerful and providers should guide the level of involvement for family and other support system members. Each set of factors should be considered by providers in determining the time, location, and strategies to optimize a compassionate and effective communication of bad news.

The SPIKES algorithm, initially developed to assist oncology providers in delivering upsetting news to patients, and now widely utilized, provides a stepwise framework by which difficult news can be delivered effectively and in an empathetic, patient-centered manner (Table 14.5) [69].

Crucial Conversations and Conflict Management

Crucial conversations are communication events in which stakes are high, emotions are high, and/or opinions among the participants can differ [71]. The ongoing relationships between chronic care providers and their patients, and the emotionally charged situations that arise, set the stage for the crucial conversations during chronic care. Managing visible and unseen conflicts that often undergird these conversations requires specialized, intentional communication skills. Providers should be self-aware of their emotional states and those of their patients during a crucial conversation. Feeling states of anger or fear may manifest in some as physical cues of arousal, louder speech, or clenched muscles. In others, behaviors such as sarcasm, withdrawing from the conversation, and short answers reflect a silent response, while hyperbolic or threatening statements and aggressive posture reflect a violent response [71]. Acknowledging these cues allows providers to step back and meaningfully employ techniques to address arising conflict while managing their own emotions.

Several techniques can diffuse emotionally charged patient-provider conversations and manage arising conflict. Taking time to reflect on the goal of a conversation, and then planning a progression of talking points can facilitate an intentional and emotionally defused dialog [71]. Apologizing,

Common Concerns	Level of Concern			Discuss with Doctor
	Not at All	A Little	A Lot	
Shortness of breath	1	2	3	
Pain	1	2	3	
Falling or fear of falling	1	2	3	
Dizziness or balance	1	2	3	
Hearing or vision	1	2	3	
Trouble with sleep	1	2	3	
Lack of energy	1	2	3	
Incontinence/bladder problems	1	2	3	
Constipation or bowel problems	1	2	3	
Poor appetite or weight loss	1	2	3	
Concerns about driving	1	2	3	
Difficulty bathing, dressing, or walking	1	2	3	
Receiving the help I need	1	2	3	
Getting out to do the things I enjoy	1	2	3	
Regular exercise	1	2	3	
Stress or worry	1	2	3	
Feeling sad or blue	1	2	3	
Trouble concentrating or remembering	1	2	3	
Sexual function or sexuality	1	2	3	
Smoking or alcohol use	1	2	3	
Medication issues side effects	1	2	3	
Results from a lab test or consultation	1	2	3	
Keeping up with appointments	1	2	3	
Other issues/concerns	1	2	3	
	1	2	3	

I would like my companion to (check all that apply)
Listen to what the doctor says.
Take notes (for example, about your diagnosis, medications, diet, or referrals).
Remind me to ask my questions.
Ask the doctor questions directly, on my behalf.
Remind me to tell the doctor about my symptoms.
Provide information about my health to the doctor.
Make sure I understand what the doctor says.
Stay in the waiting room for part of the visit.
Stay in the waiting room for the entire visit so that I may talk to the doctor alone.
List other help you would like from your companion below:

Fig. 14.1 Patient checklists [67]

when appropriate, creates an atmosphere of mutual respect and helps identify a shared purpose that can maintain a safe environment for negotiation and exchange. Specific techniques such as reflecting observed emotions (e.g., "You seem angry to me. Did I misread you?"), paraphrasing what has been said (e.g., "Let me make sure I'm understanding this correctly…"), and actively soliciting others' viewpoints (e.g., "How do you see it? I'd really like to know your opinions

Table 14.5 The SPIKES Algorithm (from reference [69])

Set Up	Focus on encounter location and privacy
	Minimize disturbances or interruptions
	Gather appropriate medical team and family members
	Sit down and establish connection with patient
Perceptions	Ask open-ended questions to elicit what the patient knows
Invitation	Assess how and to what extent patient would like to be informed about the facts at hand
Knowledge	Begin with a "warning shot" that there is distressing information to deliver
	Share the news using nontechnical words
	Provide information in small increments with periodic checks on patient understanding
Emotions	Offer empathetic statements
	Use exploratory and validating responses
	Help patient connect and process thoughts
Summarize and Strategize	Discuss next steps
	Take the information and context elicited in the first five SPIKES steps into consideration

about this.") are often effective in diffusing and advancing difficult conversations in an open, respectful manner [71].

Communication regarding medical errors and unanticipated poor outcomes often generates crucial conversations with patients and can be difficult to navigate [13, 72, 73]. Patients may have powerful reactions to these situations since a trusting relationship with their medical providers may have been compromised [73]. Fear, loss of trust, and isolation are some of the complex emotions that patients may experience in these situations [73] Direct, clear communication, preparing for and openly acknowledging patients' emotional reactions, and summarizing an actionable plan are important elements in communicating medical errors to patients [13]. Patients who receive factual information about medical errors are less likely to dismiss their physicians and have greater overall satisfaction [72].

Health Information Technology

Health information technology (HIT) permeates all aspects of chronic care and has permanently altered patient-provider communication in both direct and indirect patient care. Telemedicine and asynchronous electronic communication via patient electronic health record platforms provide multiple portals for patients and providers to engage with one another beyond traditional office visits. In addition, the growth of health education information via websites and apps has introduced new opportunities and challenges to chronic illness care. The wide adoption of electronic health records (EHRs) and other HIT, such mobile devices and tablets examination rooms, has led to concerns about compromising the provider-patient relationship.

One study reported that the adoption of computers and the full implementation of the EHR fostered collaborative physician-patient relationships, contrary to prior expectations and fears [74]. Many physicians reported changing workflows from making unobtrusive entries in paper charts to using the EHR to collaborate with patients in making electronic chart entries and sharing chart information [74]. Physicians were more likely to share electronic health information with patients than with paper records. A systematic review on EHR use and patient-doctor relationships and communication reported no change in patient satisfaction [75]. In addition, several skills can promote patient-centered care including signposting computer use, inviting patients to look at the screen, maintaining eye contact, continuing verbal and nonverbal communication cues aloud, and making computer use less obvious [75] (Table 14.6).

The COVID-19 pandemic has highlighted the capacity and limitations of telehealth to increase healthcare access [80]. The major principles of in-person communication are applicable to telehealth encounters, however there are several considerations. Webside manner is a concept that illustrates a clinician's ability to transfer relational skills via HIT and telehealth [81]. During the initial phase of the telehealth visit, acknowledging the virtual nature of the interaction, smiling, looking at the camera and not the screen, and gathering names from everyone on camera and inquiring about their relationships with the patient are important behaviors for clinicians [81]. In addition, providers should be mindful of their talking speed, tone, body language, and nonverbal cues. Finally, components from the provider and patient communication environment, such as Internet connectivity, lighting, sound, background disruptions, and privacy impact the quality of the telehealth communication [82].

Patients expect to have access to their health information, be included with their providers in the healthcare decision-making process, and have their care be collaborative, convenient, and accessible [80]. Patient portals have emerged in healthcare and are a secure online platform that gives patients 24-h access to their personal health information [83]. Portals have basic features that enable patients to access information such as recent office visits, medications, immunizations, allergies, and lab results. More advanced features provide capacity for patients to request prescription refills, schedule non-urgent appointments, and exchange secure messaging with their providers [83].

Secure electronic messaging is often utilized by patients and providers to extend and/or augment the communication that occurs during office visits and is considered a key element of providing access [60]. A study in primary care practice reported that patients found the clinical notes relatively easy to understand, and access to these notes could help reduce confusion and enhance understanding of test results as well as the reasons behind tests [84].

Table 14.6 Health information technology strategies to promote patient-centered care [75]

Practice context	Study finding	Recommendation
Outpatient general practice [76]	Patients did not understand computer functions and preferred being able to see the computer screen.	Invite patients to look at the screen. For example, sharing results or imaging.
Outpatient general practice [77]	Clinicians have a difficult time with multi-tasking; for example, using the computer while interviewing the patient. To improve, clinicians can use specific communication skills to manage the visit.	• Consider position of provider, patient, and computer in the space. • Explain why the computer is being used. • Face patient when using computer. • Stop typing when the patient speaks.
Veteran Affairs (VA) internal medicine clinic [78]	"Open" office arrangement helped physicians improve physical orientation and eye contact than with the patient. Physicians who accessed the EMR and took breaks to sustain eye contact with patients used more nonverbal cues in communication. High EMR use interviews were associated with patients asking more questions than low EMR use interviews.	• Consider position of provider, patient, and computer in the space. • Take pauses from computer to engage in nonverbal communication such as eye contact and head nodding.
Academic primary care clinics [79]	EMR use interfered with patient-doctor communication. Example includes that the average screen gaze lasted from 25% to 55% of the visit time.	Separate EMR use from time spent communicating with patients: • Read aloud while typing. • Maintain eye contact. • Use body language to show attention and empathy. • Disengage from computer use for important or sensitive topics.

There are privacy, confidentiality, and end-user concerns with HIT, including the complexity of portal designs, the lack of guidance in how to use applications and portal, and the inability to understand the information presented [83]. Older patients are more likely to have trouble using technology than younger patients, a gap that has been described as the digital divide [83]. In addition, children, adolescents, and their parents are less likely to use patient portals for information or communication, compared to adults, due to the inadequate usability [83]. Healthcare providers are facing an increased volume of electronic messages, which can overwhelm clinical workflows [83]. There are currently no standards for proxy access and EHRs are not designed to allow care teams to filter sensitive versus non-sensitive data [80].

Healthcare providers should ideally discuss preferred modes and expectations regarding HIT communication for a shared understanding. Providers may also identify the characteristics that their patients operationalize as good communication. For example, some patients may place value on easy, direct access to providers, frequent communication, and the flexibility provided by asynchronous communication through messaging, while others may prioritize longer face-to-face encounters of greater depth.

Future Directions

Physicians and other healthcare providers are sharing a growing virtual communication space with their patients; however, there are significant gaps and growing disparities that will need to be addressed and mitigated. For example, patients with limited English language proficiency, low health and digital literacy, and residing in rural and inner-city locations with restricted access to high-speed Internet are limited in utilizing health information technology (HIT) [80]. Digital literacy (i.e., comfort with using web-based technology) is reduced among older Americans and those with limited health literacy [85]. HIT and telehealth will need to increase access, which may be achieved through large-scale expansion of broadband Internet and through distribution of secure mobile WiFi hotspots and video-compatible devices. Additionally, community-based telehealth educators can provide individual or group instruction for those with low digital literacy [85].

As health information technology and digital health applications grow, chronic care providers will still need to establish and sustain meaningful relationships with patients and seek to effectively impart the "special knowledge" that Steinbeck highlighted. Providers will face an ever-changing healthcare landscape and will need to optimize interactions and exchange information across several forums, ranging from the intimate conversations of patient-provider dyad to the more complicated choruses that characterize group and team-based care. While the goal and tasks of effective patient-provider communication in this landscape are daunting, it provides the foundation to the patient-provider relationships and enhances the lives of providers and the patients they serve.

References

1. Steinbeck J. What do I want in a doctor? 2012. http://www.lettersofnote.com/2012/09/what-do-i-want-in-doctor.html.
2. Briere R. Institute of Medicine: crossing the quality chasm. Washington, DC: National Academies Press; 2001.

3. Epstein RM, Franks P, Shields CG, Meldrum SC, Miller KN, Campbell TL, et al. Patient-centered communication and diagnostic testing. Ann Fam Med. 2005;3(5):415–21.
4. Ha JF, Longnecker N. Doctor-patient communication: a review. Ochsner J. 2010;10(1):38–43.
5. Street RL. Communicative styles and adaptations in physician parent consultations. Soc Sci Med. 1992;34(10):1155–63.
6. Chapman BP, Duberstein PR, Epstein R, Fiscella K, Kravitz RL. Patient centered communication during primary care visits for depressive symptoms: what is the role of physician personality? Med Care. 2008;46(8):806.
7. Fiscella K, Meldrum S, Franks P, Shields CG, Duberstein P, McDaniel SH, et al. Patient trust: is it related to patient-centered behavior of primary care physicians? Med Care. 2004;42(11):1049–55.
8. Bodenheimer T, Sinsky C. From triple to quadruple aim: care of the patient requires care of the provider. Ann Fam Med. 2014;12(6):573–6.
9. Street RL, Makoul G, Arora NK, Epstein RM. How does communication heal? Pathways linking clinician–patient communication to health outcomes. Patient Educ Couns. 2009;74(3):295–301.
10. Stewart MBJ, Weston W, et al. Patient-centered medicine: transforming the clinical method. London: Sage; 1995.
11. Saha S, Beach MC, Cooper LA. Patient centeredness, cultural competence and healthcare quality. J Natl Med Assoc. 2008;100(11):1275–85.
12. Lipkin M, Quill TE, Napodano RJ. The medical interview: a core curriculum for residencies in internal medicine. Ann Intern Med. 1984;100(2):277–84.
13. Tongue JR, Epps HR, Forese LL. Communication skills for patient-centered care: research-based, easily learned techniques for medical interviews that benefit orthopaedic surgeons and their patients. JBJS. 2005;87(3):652–8.
14. Keller VF, Carroll JG. A new model for physician-patient communication. Patient Educ Couns. 1994;23(2):131–40.
15. McWhinney I. The need for a transformed clinical method. London: Sage; 1989.
16. Levinson W, Lesser CS, Epstein RM. Developing physician communication skills for patient-centered care. Health Aff. 2010;29(7):1310–8.
17. Tesser A, Rosen S, Tesser M. On the reluctance to communicate undesirable messages (the MUM effect): a field study. Psychol Rep. 1971;29(2):651–4.
18. Van Ryn M. Research on the provider contribution to race/ethnicity disparities in medical care. Med Care. 2002;40(1):I-140–I-51.
19. Makoul G. Essential elements of communication in medical encounters: the Kalamazoo consensus statement. Acad Med. 2001;76(4):390–3.
20. Mauksch LB, Dugdale DC, Dodson S, Epstein R. Relationship, communication, and efficiency in the medical encounter: creating a clinical model from a literature review. Arch Intern Med. 2008;168(13):1387–95.
21. Agoritsas T, Heen AF, Brandt L, Alonso-Coello P, Kristiansen A, Akl EA, et al. Decision aids that really promote shared decision making: the pace quickens. BMJ. 2015;350:g7624.
22. Elwyn G, Lloyd A, May C, van der Weijden T, Stiggelbout A, Edwards A, et al. Collaborative deliberation: a model for patient care. Patient Educ Couns. 2014;97(2):158–64.
23. Barry MJ, Edgman-Levitan S. Shared decision making – the pinnacle of patient-centered care. N Engl J Med. 2012;366(9):780–1.
24. O'Connor A, Stacey D, Rovner D, Holmes-Rovner M, Tetroe J, Llewellyn-Thomas H, et al. Patient decision aids for balancing the benefits and harms of health care options: a systematic review and meta-analysis. 2004. http://www.ihi.org/resources/Pages/Publications/PatientDecisionAidsforBalancingBenefitsHarmsofHealthCareOptions.aspx.
25. Laidsaar-Powell R, Butow P, Bu S, Charles C, Gafni A, Lam W, et al. Physician–patient–companion communication and decision-making: a systematic review of triadic medical consultations. Patient Educ Couns. 2013;91(1):3–13.
26. Davis K, Haisfield L, Dorfman C, Krist A, Taylor KL. Physicians' attitudes about shared decision making for prostate cancer screening. Fam Med. 2011;43(4):260.
27. Wright AA, Zhang B, Ray A, Mack JW, Trice E, Balboni T, et al. Associations between end-of-life discussions, patient mental health, medical care near death, and caregiver bereavement adjustment. JAMA. 2008;300(14):1665–73.
28. Tai-Seale M, Elwyn G, Wilson CJ, Stults C, Dillon EC, Li M, et al. Enhancing shared decision making through carefully designed interventions that target patient and provider behavior. Health Aff. 2016;35(4):605–12.
29. Stacey D, Bennett CL, Barry MJ, Col NF, Eden KB, Holmes-Rovner M, et al. Decision aids for people facing health treatment or screening decisions. Cochrane Database Syst Rev. 2011;(10):CD001431.
30. Krist AH, Woolf SH, Rothemich SF, Johnson RE, Peele JE, Cunningham TD, et al. Interactive preventive health record to enhance delivery of recommended care: a randomized trial. Ann Fam Med. 2012;10(4):312–9.
31. Agency for Health Care Research and Quality. The SHARE approach—essential steps of shared decisionmaking: quick reference guide; 2014. 4 Apr 2017. http://www.ahrq.gov/professionals/education/curriculum-tools/shareddecisionmaking/tools/tool-1/index.html.
32. Ryan C. Language use in the United States: 2011. Am Commun Surv Rep. 2013;22:1–16.
33. Green AR, Ngo-Metzger Q, Legedza AT, Massagli MP, Phillips RS, Iezzoni LI. Interpreter services, language concordance, and health care quality. J Gen Intern Med. 2005;20(11):1050–6.
34. Karliner LS, Jacobs EA, Chen AH, Mutha S. Do professional interpreters improve clinical care for patients with limited English proficiency? A systematic review of the literature. Health Serv Res. 2007;42(2):727–54.
35. Flores G. The impact of medical interpreter services on the quality of health care: a systematic review. Med Care Res Rev. 2005;62(3):255–99.
36. Hampers LC, McNulty JE. Professional interpreters and bilingual physicians in a pediatric emergency department: effect on resource utilization. Arch Pediatr Adolesc Med. 2002;156(11):1108–13.
37. Kravitz RL, Helms LJ, Azari R, Antonius D, Melnikow J. Comparing the use of physician time and health care resources among patients speaking English, Spanish, and Russian. Med Care. 2000;38(7):728–38.
38. Best Practices for Communicating Through an Interpreter. Refugee Health Technical Assistance Center, contributed by the National Council on Interpreting in Healthcare. Updated January 2022. https://refugeehealthta.org/access-to-care/language-access/best-practices-communicating-through-an-interpreter/. Accessed 19 Feb 2022.
39. Position Statement on Health Care Access for Deaf Patients. National Association for the Deaf. Updated January 2022. https://www.nad.org/about-us/position-statements/position-statement-on-health-care-access-for-deaf-patients/. Accessed 19 Feb 2022.
40. Smedley BD, Stith AY, Nelson AR, Committee on Understanding and Eliminating Racial and Ethnic Disparities in Health Care, editors. Unequal treatment: confronting racial and ethnic disparities in health care. Washington, DC: National Academy of Science; 2003.
41. Agency for Healthcare Research and Quality. National healthcare disparities report. Rockville: Agency for Healthcare Research and Quality; 2003.
42. Misra-Hebert AD. Physician cultural competence: cross-cultural communication improves care. Cleve Clin J Med. 2003;70(4):289–93. 96–8 passim.
43. Hook JN, Davis DE, Owen J, Worthington EL Jr, Utsey SO. Cultural humility: measuring openness to culturally diverse clients. J Couns Psychol. 2013;60(3):353.

44. Carrillo JE, Green AR, Betancourt JR. Cross-cultural primary care: a patient-based approach. Ann Intern Med. 1999;130(10):829–34.
45. Institute of Medicine. Unequal treatment: confronting racial and ethnic disparities in healthcare. Washington, DC: Institute of Medicine; 2003.
46. Fiscella K, et al. Inequality in quality: addressing socioeconomic, racial, and ethnic disparities in health care. JAMA. 2000;283(19):2579–84.
47. Institute of Medicine Committee on Lesbian, Gay, Bisexual, and Transgender Health Issues and Research Gaps and Opportunities. The health of lesbian, gay, bisexual, and transgender people: building a foundation for better understanding. Washington, DC: National Academies Press; 2011.
48. Indian Health Service. IHS fact sheets—Indian Health Disparities 2011. http://www.ihs.gov/newsroom/factsheets/disparities. Accessed 12 Jul 2013.
49. Mallory C, Brown TN, Conron KJ. Conversion therapy and LGBT youth update. Los Angeles: The Williams Institute, UCLA School of Law; 2019.
50. Carpio MV. The lost generation: American Indian women and sterilization abuse. Social Justice. 2004;3(4):40–53.
51. Washington HA, editor. Medical Apartheid: the dark history of medical experimentation on Black Americans from colonial times to the present. New York: Random House, Inc; 2006.
52. Shen MJ, Peterson EB, Costas-Muñiz R, et al. The effects of race and racial concordance on patient-physician communication: a systematic review of the literature. J Racial Ethn Health Disparities. 2018;5(1):117–40. https://doi.org/10.1007/s40615-017-0350-4.
53. Crenshaw K. Demarginalizing the intersection of race and sex: a black feminist critique of antidiscrimination doctrine, feminist theory and antiracist politics. University of Chicago Legal Forum; 1989. p. Article 8.
54. Merriam-Webster. Intersectionality. In Merriam-Webster.com dictionary. n.d. https://www.merriam-webster.com/dictionary/intersectionality. Accessed 31 Oct 2021.
55. Maher FA, Tetreault MKT. The feminist classroom: dynamics of gender, race, and privilege. Expanded ed. New York: Rowman & Littlefield Publishers, Inc.; 2001.
56. Schottenfeld L, Petersen D, Peikes D, Ricciardi R, Burak H, McNellis R, et al. Creating patient-centered team-based primary care. Rockville: Agency for Healthcare Research and Quality; 2016.
57. Reeves S, Pelone F, Harrison R, Goldman J, Zwarenstein M. Interprofessional collaboration to improve professional practice and healthcare outcomes. Cochrane Database Syst Rev. 2017;6:CD000072.
58. Coleman E, Grothaus L, Sandhu N, Wagner E. Chronic care clinics: a randomized controlled trial of a new model of primary care for frail older adults. J Am Geriatr Soc. 1999;47(7):775–83.
59. Tallia AF, Lanham HJ, McDaniel RR Jr, Crabtree BF. Seven characteristics of successful work relationships. Fam Pract Manag. 2006;13(1):47.
60. Martin JC, Avant RF, Bowman MA, Bucholtz JR, Dickinson JR, Evans KL, et al. The future of family medicine: a collaborative project of the family medicine community. Ann Fam Med. 2004;2(Suppl 1):S3–32.
61. Jaber R, Braksmajer A, Trilling J. Group visits for chronic illness care: models, benefits and challenges. Fam Pract Manag. 2006;13(1):37.
62. Masley SC, Sokoloff J, Hawes C. Planning group visits for high-risk patients. Fam Pract Manag. 2000;7(6):33.
63. Houck S, Kilo C, Scott JC. Group visits 101. Fam Pract Manag. 2003;10(5):66.
64. Vick JB, Amjad H, Smith KC, Boyd CM, Gitlin LN, Roth DL, et al. "Let him speak:" a descriptive qualitative study of the roles and behaviors of family companions in primary care visits among older adults with cognitive impairment. Int J Geriatr Psychiatry. 2017; https://doi.org/10.1002/gps.4732.
65. Wolff JL, Guan Y, Boyd CM, Vick J, Amjad H, Roth DL, et al. Examining the context and helpfulness of family companion contributions to older adults' primary care visits. Patient Educ Couns. 2017;100(3):487–94.
66. Clayman ML, Roter D, Wissow LS, Bandeen-Roche K. Autonomy-related behaviors of patient companions and their effect on decision-making activity in geriatric primary care visits. Soc Sci Med. 2005;60(7):1583–91.
67. Wolff JL, Roter DL, Barron J, Boyd CM, Leff B, Finucane TE, et al. A tool to strengthen the older patient–companion partnership in primary care: results from a pilot study. J Am Geriatr Soc. 2014;62(2):312–9.
68. Buckman R. How to break bad news: a guide for health care professionals. Baltimore: JHU Press; 1992.
69. Baile WF, Buckman R, Lenzi R, Glober G, Beale EA, Kudelka AP. SPIKES – a six-step protocol for delivering bad news: application to the patient with cancer. Oncologist. 2000;5(4):302–11.
70. Bousquet G, Orri M, Winterman S, Brugière C, Verneuil L, Revah-Levy A. Breaking bad news in oncology: a metasynthesis. J Clin Oncol. 2015;33(22):2437–43.
71. Patterson K. Crucial conversations: tools for talking when stakes are high. New York: Tata McGraw-Hill Education; 2002.
72. Mazor KM, Simon SR, Yood RA, Martinson BC, Gunter MJ, Reed GW, et al. Health plan members' views about disclosure of medical errors. Ann Intern Med. 2004;140(6):409–18.
73. Vincent C. Understanding and responding to adverse events. N Engl J Med. 2003;348(11):1051–6.
74. Doyle RJ, Wang N, Anthony D, Borkan J, Shield RR, Goldman RE. Computers in the examination room and the electronic health record: physicians' perceived impact on clinical encounters before and after full installation and implementation. Fam Pract. 2012;29(5):601–8. https://doi.org/10.1093/fampra/cms015.
75. Alkureishi MA, Lee WW, Lyons M, et al. Impact of electronic medical record use on the patient-doctor-relationship and communication: a systematic review. J Gen Intern Med. 2016;31(5):548–60. https://doi.org/10.1007/s11606-015-3582-1.
76. Als AB. The desk-top computer as a magic box: patterns of behaviour connected with the desk-top computer; GPs' and patients' perceptions. Fam Pract. 1997;14(1):17–23. https://doi.org/10.1093/fampra/14.1.17. PMID: 9061339
77. Booth N, Robinson P, Kohannejad J. Identification of high-quality consultation practice in primary care: the effects of computer use on doctor-patient rapport. Inform Prim Care. 2004;12(2):75–83. https://doi.org/10.14236/jhi.v12i2.111. PMID: 15319059
78. McGrath JM, Arar NH, Pugh JA. The influence of electronic medical record usage on nonverbal communication in the medical interview. Health Informatics J. 2007;13(2):105–18. https://doi.org/10.1177/1460458207076466. PMID: 17510223
79. Shachak A, Hadas-Dayagi M, Ziv A, Reis S. Primary care physicians' use of an electronic medical record system: a cognitive task analysis. J Gen Intern Med. 2009;24(3):341–8. https://doi.org/10.1007/s11606-008-0892-6. Epub 2009 Jan 7. PMID: 19130148; PMCID: PMC2642564
80. Robinson SK, Meisnere M, Phillips RL, McCauley L, National Academies of Sciences, Engineering, and Medicine; Health and Medicine Division; Board on Health Care Services; Committee on Implementing High-Quality Primary Care. Implementing high-quality primary care: rebuilding the foundation of health care. National Academies Press (US); 2021. https://doi.org/10.17226/25983.
81. Modic MB, Neuendorf K, Windover AK. Enhancing your webside manner: optimizing opportunities for relationship-centered care in virtual visits. J Patient Exp. 2020;7(6):869–77. https://doi.org/10.1177/2374373520968975.

82. Brazelton T. STFM task force releases learning objectives for national telemedicine curriculum. Ann Fam Med. 2021;19(1):91. https://doi.org/10.1370/afm.2665.
83. Kruse CS, Argueta DA, Lopez L, Nair A. Patient and provider attitudes toward the use of patient portals for the management of chronic disease: a systematic review. J Med Internet Res. 2015;17(2):e40. https://doi.org/10.2196/jmir.3703.
84. van Kuppenveld SI, van Os-Medendorp H, Tiemessen NA, van Delden JJ. Real-time access to electronic health record via a patient portal: is it harmful? A retrospective observational study. J Med Internet Res. 2020;22(2):e13622. https://doi.org/10.2196/13622.
85. Kaplan B. Access, equity, and neutral space: telehealth beyond the pandemic. Ann Fam Med. 2021;19(1):75–8. https://doi.org/10.1370/afm.2633.

Ambulatory Primary Care and Urgent Care

15

Clark Denniston and LeRon Jackson

Defining Ambulatory Care, Ambulatory Primary Care, and Urgent Care

Ambulatory care is identified by medical care provided in any outpatient setting; the type of outpatient setting may include private offices, clinics, community health centers, retail pharmacies, or house calls in a person's home. The hallmark of these medical visits is that they are usually composed of single visits addressing a discreet selection of medical problems or concerns, as stand-alone visits, or performed in a longitudinal fashion. The type of issues addressed may include prevention, screening, health promotion, acute self-limited illnesses and injuries, and chronic disease management.

Ambulatory primary care is identified by medical services delivered by primary care clinicians. Primary care clinicians are defined by the Centers for Medicare and Medicaid Services (CMS) as physicians who have a primary specialty designation of family medicine, internal medicine, geriatric medicine, or pediatrics, or nurse practitioners, clinical nurse specialists, or physician assistants for whom primary care services account for at least 60% of their allowed charges [1].

The Institute of Medicine (IOM) defines primary care in the following manner:

> Primary care is the provision of integrated, accessible health care services by clinicians who are accountable for addressing a large majority of personal health care needs, developing a sustained partnership with patients, and practicing in the context of family and community. [2]

In the National Academies of Sciences, Engineering, and Medicine report *Implementing High-Quality Primary Care: Rebuilding the Foundation of Health Care (2021)*, hereafter referred to as the NASEM 2021 report, a more robust and compelling definition of high-quality primary care is offered:

> High-quality primary care is the provision of whole-person, integrated, accessible, and equitable health care by interprofessional teams that are accountable for addressing the majority of an individual's health and wellness needs across settings and through sustained relationships with patients, families, and communities. [3]

Urgent care, a subset of ambulatory care, is composed of outpatient visits that address issues requiring immediate attention at a level of seriousness that at least initially does not require an emergency department (ED) level of care. Urgent care situations can be influenced by underlying chronic illnesses so those nuances must be considered in discussing models of ambulatory urgent care. Urgent care may be provided in outpatient clinic settings or, increasingly, in stand-alone centers devoted exclusively to this type of ambulatory care [4–6].

It is through the lens of the re-imagined foundation of health care through high-quality primary care and the proposed necessary adaptations for our health care system offered in the NASEM 2021 report that anchors much of the context of this chapter as we explore the intersection of ambulatory primary care, urgent care, and chronic disease.

The Ecology of Medical Care

Before the COVID-19 pandemic, little had changed in the ecology of medical care in the US since 1961; most medical care is delivered in the ambulatory setting [7–9]. In the original publication exploring this concept in 1961 [9], in any given month, within a cohort of 1000 adult patients, 250 will consult a physician but only 9 people will be cared for in a community hospital and only 1 person will be hospitalized in an academic medical center. When examined again nearly four decades later, using similar comparative methodology, within a cohort of 1000 patients, 317 received care in ambulatory settings, 13 visited an emergency department, 8 were

C. Denniston · L. Jackson (✉)
Department of Family Medicine, University of North Carolina at Chapel Hill, Chapel Hill, NC, USA
e-mail: clark_denniston@med.unc.edu;
leron_jackson@med.unc.edu

hospitalized, and less than 1 person was admitted to an academic medical center [7]. Consistent with these long-term trends of the majority of medical care being delivered in the ambulatory setting, hospitalization rates did not increase with the implementation of the Affordable Care Act [8].

Regarding the specific ecology of ambulatory primary care, it is important to understand that over the last 25 years primary care visits have accounted for 35% of all health care visits in the US, hence the critical nature of ambulatory primary care's contribution to the health of our nation [3].

The full and enduring effects of the COVID-19 pandemic on the ecology of medical care remain to be seen. Given the severity of illness caused by the SARS-CoV2 virus, it is likely that once data is available, we will see a much larger percentage of medical care being delivered in hospital settings compared to the last 50 years. It is also likely that the data will show that far fewer people sought ambulatory medical care during the height of the pandemic and that many types of ambulatory medical care including routine childhood immunizations, other health maintenance, and chronic disease management were deferred or delayed with yet to be determined long-term harmful patient outcomes. The pandemic-driven rapid and transformative pivot to virtual medical care delivery mechanisms has likely altered the landscape of the ecology of medical care permanently [10].

Ambulatory Primary Care and Chronic Disease

Chronic illness care is a valuable and frequent function of the ambulatory primary care delivery systems currently in place in the US. In one analysis of 219 Accountable Care Organizations (ACOs), nearly 61% of ambulatory chronic disease visits were provided by primary care providers (PCPs) [11]. In one study involving prevalence of chronic disease and multimorbidity in 148 primary care practices across the US, 45% of patients cared for by those practices had more than one chronic illness [12]. Having a source of longitudinal primary care, compared to emergency department utilization for usual care, reduces adverse cardiovascular outcomes [13]. Clearly, chronic disease management is a cornerstone of high-quality ambulatory primary care.

Chronic Disease Care Quality in Ambulatory Primary Care

Different types of clinicians provide chronic disease care in the context of their ambulatory practices. The uniqueness of ambulatory primary care provided by family physicians, general internists, geriatricians, and primary care pediatricians is distinct from the chronic disease management provided by specialty clinicians with subspecialty fellowship training. In the debates that surround comparisons of chronic disease quality measures between primary care clinicians and specialty care clinicians, the focus is usually on disease-specific clinical parameters. For example, one study examining data from the National Ambulatory Medical Care Survey from the period 1997 to 2010 reported that cardiologists performed better than generalists in terms of cardiovascular quality metrics based on rates of medication prescribing for key cardiovascular diseases [14]. However, as pointed out in the NASEM 2021 report, these narrow disease-specific measures miss the mark for truly representing effective primary care quality measures because they fail to align with the purpose and function of primary care [3]. An example that comes closer to measuring the more holistic quality of coordination in primary care are studies demonstrating that primary care improves health through coordination of care following hospitalizations, by preventing readmissions and reducing the overall risk of hospitalization [15, 16]. However, demonstrating the prevention of readmissions or reduction in risk of hospitalization falls short of measuring the overarching value that primary care brings to patients through the primary care principles that have been proposed that are rooted in community, accessibility, longitudinal personal relationships, coordination and whole-person focus [17]. The NASEM 2021 report offers a compelling rationale for a completely redesigned paradigm to measure quality in primary care:

> The challenge, then, is to unhitch primary care from a subspecialty model that uses measures derived from partial representations or pieces of patients and instead link it to measures appropriate for its generalist, whole-person approach to medicine. [3]

With that future state of quality measurement yet to be realized, it is important to recognize that current and existing quality metrics still play an important role in the day-to-day operations of a primary care practice and may impact the financial bottom line through pay-for-performance metrics. These include data on disease-specific clinical measures, screening and prevention rates, utilization, access, and emerging health equity measures. The role that health information technology plays in quality measurement, access to care, communication between the health care system and patients, coordination of care, population health, chronic disease registries, and point-of-care decision support is an immense and evolving field.

It is also important to consider how quality can be affected if attention deviates from the *quadruple aim* [18], an aspirational extension of the *triple aim*. The *triple aim* is a concept widely adopted since 2008 [19, 20] that frames optimal health outcomes in terms of the need to improve the health of the population, enhance the patient experience, and reduce costs. The *quadruple aim* stresses that potential barriers to achieving those *triple aim* quality measures include factors that contribute to health care team dysfunction, stress, and burnout, and therefore adds as the fourth aim the need to improve working conditions for clinicians and other health care teammates [18].

Ambulatory Primary Care Chronic Care Models

The provision of high-quality ambulatory primary care for patients with chronic disease is promoted and supported with a theoretical framework and models of care that assist health care teams in the complex management of chronic illnesses, addressing not only the medical complexities but also the often-overlapping psychosocial needs and adverse social determinants of health that accompany chronic illness. While not an exhaustive list, four specific approaches/models are presented, along with a broader discussion of the need for an enhanced team-based approach to ambulatory primary care to people with chronic illness.

Starfield's 4 C's

Although not a discrete practice model, Barbara Starfield's 4 C's provide a foundational framework for a high-value approach to ambulatory primary care that includes the following attributes: (1) first Contact, (2) Continuity, (3) Comprehensiveness, and (4) Coordination, with each having a strong evidence base for enhancing the quality of care for people with chronic diseases [21]. This framework lends itself to application in all primary care disciplines, including family medicine, and is widely adopted as a vision for primary care.

First contact is the concept that for each new medical need, primary care is the entry point into the health care system. This first contact source, or access to the same entry point for all health needs, provides the patient with a medical home. *Continuity* is best achieved by having access to the same primary care provider over time. The continuity provider becomes known to the patient, knows the patient's history, needs, and health goals, and develops a partnership with the patient. *Comprehensiveness* means that all problems are cared for in the context of the patient's source of primary care, with short-term referrals as needed when medical issues are beyond the primary care clinician's expertise. *Coordination* means the primary care practice oversees and manages all aspects of the patient's health care. Applying this framework, any practice, clinic, or heath center in the primary care disciplines of family medicine, general internal medicine, geriatrics, and pediatrics should be able to provide high-quality ambulatory care to patients with chronic diseases.

Wagner's Chronic Care Model

Originally published in 1996, this model proposed a structure based on the extensive review of available literature at the time that identified five essential elements of an effective chronic care model (CCM) [22, 23]. These five elements include (1) evidence-based protocols, (2) practice redesign, (3) enhanced patient education, (4) expert systems, and (5) information systems. These elements of a chronic care model informed significant movement in primary care and prompted several adaptations and explorations of different approaches to delivering care for chronic illnesses [24–38].

This CCM was revised slightly in 1998 to emphasize that there are two distinct entities, the community and the health care system, that need to work in concert, with specific elements of the model now considered to be (1) self-management support, (2) delivery system design, (3) decision support, and (4) clinical information systems [39]. The vision for this revised model is an "informed active patient" productively engaged with a "prepared proactive practice team" [39] and remains a guiding force for the transformation of primary care chronic disease management.

Patient-Centered Medical Home

As asserted by Wagner, the concept of the patient-centered medical home (PCMH), first proposed in 2007, was essentially the combination of the CCM and the pediatric patient-centered medical home [39]. The PCMH concept was the joint vision of the American Academy of Family Physicians, the American Academy of Pediatrics, American College of Physicians, and the American Osteopathic Association [40]. The Agency for Healthcare Research and Quality (AHRQ) has fully adopted the crucial elements of the PCMH as defined by (1) comprehensive care, (2) patient-centered, (3) coordinated care, (4) accessible services, and (5) quality and safety [41]. Further, AHRQ has compiled a resource list of three foundational elements of the PCMH-health information technology, workforce, and finance—without which the full potential of the PCMH will not be realized [42].

The literature regarding implementation of the PCMH model is voluminous with some key learnings emerging. There are factors which contribute to the success of implementing the PCMH model [43], and there are different typologies that inform our understanding of the function and contribution of the PCMH model to outcomes [44]. Analyses of utilization and cost outcomes reveal a favorable impact of PCMH implementation, including enhanced patient outcomes in chronic disease care, including those with multi-morbidity [45–48].

While there are benefits to patients and society related to the adoption of the PCMH model, as pointed out in the NASEM 2021 report, the PCMH model lacks integration with public health and community-oriented primary care [3]. The foundation for addressing this exists within the PCMH model, but will require vision and will to advance further.

Direct Primary Care

Direct primary care (DPC), also known as cash-only care, concierge care, retainer care, or boutique care, is a model in which patients pay directly for some or all of the services provided by their medical practice, in lieu of or in addition to health insurance plans [49]. The original DPC practice called "MD^2" is attributed to Dr. Howard Mason, who in 1996 provided care to only 50 families [50]. Initially the model saw slow growth; in 2005, there were only 146 physicians providing DPC in the US, but within a few years there was exponential growth to 4400 physicians providing DPC [51].

With the growth of "concierge" practices, enthusiastically endorsed by many as providing greater provider satisfaction and better care, several articles were published describing and promoting the model [52–56]. With the growth of these models of care came questions about the legal, moral, and ethical implications [57–59]. By 2015, the growth and variability of DPC practices was such that the American College of Physicians saw the need to publish a policy position paper about the impact of DPC on access, cost, quality, and concerns that DPCs may cause access issues for underserved patients [49].

Acknowledging that the terms *direct primary care* and *concierge care* were becoming the most widely recognized terms, an important distinction emerged. The DPC model only charges a periodic fee without any third-party fee-for-service payments, while the typical concierge practice charges both periodic fees and continues to bill third parties in a traditional fee-for-service fashion. The distribution and costs of these models were examined in a large-scale study published in 2015, where DPC practices were found to charge lower fees than concierge practices, and when large established DPC practices were examined, there were cost savings, though it was pointed out that further study was necessary to generalize [60].

Questions remain regarding the ultimate role that DPC will play in the US health care system [61–64]. Whether DPC practices outperform other evolving models of primary care in terms of cost savings, provider and patient satisfaction, access, overcoming health care disparities, addressing adverse social determinants of health, integrating with public health, and improving overall health outcomes remains to be determined.

Enhanced Team-Based Ambulatory Primary Care Chronic Illness Care

Physicians and other primary care providers cannot alone accomplish optimum chronic illness care, which requires an interprofessional team. Borrowing a phrase from the NASEM 2021 report, the future of high-quality primary care depends on "primary care teams to care for people, not doctors to deliver service" [3].

The biomedical complexities of chronic diseases and the challenging interplay between individuals, families, communities, public health, social determinants of health, and health literacy all demand that each member of the interprofessional team work in concert with other team members. The various members of the enhanced primary care team, including the clinicians themselves as well as pharmacists, social workers, care managers, nurse educators, community health workers, mental health professionals, dentists, home health providers, and health information technology experts, all must contribute to the care of the person, in the context of their social milieu, working "to the top of their skills" [3]. Given the importance of complex interprofessional teams working effectively toward their common purpose, family medicine educators include formal experience in interprofessional practice during residency training [65].

Urgent Care

Urgent care is a subset of ambulatory care that is distinguished from primary care and defined as the treatment of minor acute illness and injury by a provider who is not the individual's primary care physician. Urgent care centers rose in popularity in the 1970s as a method of treating persons with non-critical illnesses and injuries outside of the emergency department to reduce overcrowding in that setting and foster appropriate use of emergency department resources. Since that time, urgent care centers have diversified in scope and remain a critical access point of acute ambulatory care for both insured and uninsured patients [6]. Many urgent care centers are stand-alone medical facilities with a client/consumer-driven focus of delivering care with an emphasis on convenience and efficiency of scale [66]. In addition to providing after hours acute care, urgent care centers provide health services that would typically be performed in a primary care setting, such as vaccinations, pre-employment examinations, and school/sports physicals. There exists great variability in the types of illnesses and injuries in patients presenting to the urgent care setting. The geographic location of urgent care facilities is often concentrated in high population, high traffic areas, urban to semi-urban. Rural areas remain underserved in this regard [67].

Acute Illnesses Superimposed on Chronic Disease in Urgent Care

According to the Center for Disease Control's National Center for Chronic Disease Prevention and Health Promotion, nearly 60% of adults in the US are diagnosed with at least one chronic disease; 40% of adults have two or more chronic conditions. Persons with chronic diseases may suffer a dual burden of acute exacerbations of their chronic condition as well as superimposed acute illness. Ambulatory care sensitive conditions are described as chronic diseases that can be managed in primary care settings, including angina, asthma, and diabetes, with hospitalizations for these conditions considered potentially avoidable with adequate primary care interventions [68]. Controlled trial evidence about chronic disease management in terms of mortality, morbidity, quality of care, and patient satisfaction of walk-in clinics is needed [5].

Currently there are limited data regarding best practices in the urgent care setting to reduce transfers to the emergency department (ED) [69]. Retrospective analysis suggests that nearly 36% of patient transfers from the urgent care setting to the emergency department are unnecessary and 64% of patients transferred are ultimately discharged home. An unnecessary transfer is defined as one where the ED provider does not order any advanced imaging tests, advanced procedures, or specialty consultations in the ED, and the patient is not admitted to hospital [69].

Choosing Urgent Care

Several distinct factors explain why patients choose to access emergency and urgent care services: limited access to or confidence in primary care; patient perceived urgency; convenience; views of family, friends, or other health professionals; and a belief that their condition required the resources and facilities offered by a particular health care provider [70]. Convenience and access for the delivery of health care are key factors in how individuals choose their usual source of care. Urgent care centers provide access outside of the traditional hours of the primary care office. To address this, many primary care offices offer open access scheduling and early morning and late evening appointments to allow persons to be seen within their medical home. A benefit of incorporating acute/urgent care into outpatient practice is that continuity of the individual's care within the medical home is maintained.

Coordinating Care with Primary Care Physicians

Timely coordination of care with the primary care physician or primary care provider (PCP) is essential to address chronic care gaps and identify medical concerns which warrant further evaluation. Prior to widespread adoption of the electronic health record (EHR), communication between urgent care centers and primary care offices was limited to facsimile or telephonic communications. Wide implementation of electronic medical records has improved information sharing. Suggested best practices for communication and coordination of care include asking patients for the name of their PCP and/or home health care providers, sending summary clinical information to the PCP and/or home health providers upon visit completion, sending summary clinical information to the ED physician upon patient referral, medication reconciliation, patient education, and providing written discharge instructions upon conclusion of the visit [71].

Addressing Chronic Disease Metrics in Urgent Care

Chronic care measures are defined as evidence-based metrics which, when completed, improve the effectiveness of care in patients with chronic diseases. Examples include hypertension control, diabetes management, screening for depression, and preventive care such as recommended immunizations. Care within stand-alone urgent care centers is usually provided by a physician or advance practice provider (physician assistant or nurse practitioner) who typically does not have access to the patient's complete medical history and is not the patient's PCP. As such, there has not been a concerted focus on addressing chronic care gaps in the context of the urgent care visit. Shared electronic medical records promote continuity of care and communication with the patient's medical home to follow-up and address these gaps. In urgent care centers that are linked to a larger health care system, potential exists for optimizing of the management of patients with chronic diseases [72].

Transitional Care

Transitional care is ambulatory care during the immediate post-hospitalization phase and is intended to reduce hospital readmissions for patients with chronic disease. Transitional care is generally team based and employs the interdisciplinary approach of physicians, pharmacists, nurses, and social workers. Commonly, transitional care includes patient education, discharge planning, follow-up telephone call, patient-centered discharge instructions, and discharge coaches or nurses who interact with the patient before and after discharge [73]. Transitional care services also include a review of discharge information, medication reconciliation, as well as coordinating community referrals. Ideally, transitional care is coordinated by a patient's medical home [74]. For patients without an identified medical home, urgent care centers may play a limited role in addressing patient transitional care needs.

Organizing Urgent Care

Urgent care centers have a variety of staffing models including physician-led teams or advanced practice provider (APP)-led teams which employ a supervising physician. The urgent care team may consist of medical assistants, nurses, and administrative staff. In many settings, staff members are cross trained to perform a variety of tasks including patient registration, phlebotomy, and performing radiographs. Stand-alone urgent cares must have the equipment and supplies to treat a wide range of conditions including fractures, foreign body removal, eye/skin procedures, and gynecologic examinations. Radiography equipment, electrocardiograms, supplemental oxygen, and nebulizing machines are standard needs, along with the ability to provide intravenous infusions. Point-of-care laboratory testing is a mainstay of urgent care including urinalysis, urine pregnancy tests, and testing for infections such as those caused by streptococcus influenza, SARS-CoV-2, and mononucleosis. Basic Life Support (BLS) may be needed in urgent care but not usually Advanced Cardiovascular Life Support (ACLS) or the higher levels of support provided in the ED. Urgent care usually has naloxone available for opioid overdose and epinephrine for treatment of anaphylaxis but generally does not have medications for cardiac arrest. Medication inventories are wide ranging and may include intramuscular analgesia, antiemetics, antibiotics, and oral medications for symptom management.

Access and Time Challenges in Ambulatory Care

Traditional ambulatory clinics only offered access for scheduled appointments through a clerk or registrar. Clinical administrators are tasked with the challenge of balancing the available scheduling template for continuity wellness visits, chronic illness care, and new patient appointments, while also providing same day access. Innovations in patient *direct* scheduling and patient portals have improved access to appointments in the ambulatory clinic setting. Early adopters of direct scheduling via a patient portal are more likely to be younger, white, and commercially insured. Direct scheduling visits are more likely to be for a general medical examination/physical and more likely to be scheduled with the patient's PCP than visits scheduled through traditional means [75]. Demographic and socioeconomic disparities in patient portal adoption have been described; nonusers are more likely to be male, on Medicaid, lack a regular provider, and have less than a college education [76]. Non-white persons were also less likely to report being offered access to a patient portal. In addition to socioeconomic differences, there may be individual factors that determine uptake of patient portal usage such as a desire to communicate in person.

Urgent care utilizes walk-in scheduling, which results in unpredictable peaks in clinic volume and prolonged patient wait times. Urgent care administrators utilize triage principles to prioritize which patients are seen first, based upon acuity of presenting illness. Lower patient satisfaction scores are associated with prolonged wait times; furthermore, confidence in the care by the provider and perceived quality of care are also correlated negatively with longer wait times [77]. To address this, many urgent cares have adopted strategies to reduce wait times and improve patient satisfaction, including online appointment scheduling, online visit pre-registration, and telehealth visits.

A major challenge facing ambulatory and urgent care settings is the conundrum of time restraints in the clinical encounter. Primary care physicians spend nearly 2 h on electronic health record (EHR) tasks per hour of direct patient care [78]. The use of medical scribes may lessen the burden of documentation on providers and improve efficiency in the clinical encounter. Medical scribes are associated with decreased physician EHR documentation burden, improved work efficiency, and improved visit interactions in primary care [79]. In the emergency department, use of medical scribes is associated with improved productivity per hour and per encounter, as measured by relative value units, patients per hour, provider satisfaction, and patient satisfaction [80].

Another challenge arises when providers must address the needs of patients with multiple comorbidities affected by social determinants of health. Access to social work team members is an invaluable resource in assisting patients with crisis and trauma management, housing insecurity, food insecurity, or interpersonal violence concerns. Access to a behavioral health team member for on-site consultation is also an important resource, as 75% of all visits to primary care physicians involve a behavioral health concern [81]. A multidisciplinary approach to care delivery is paramount as patients often present to the ambulatory and urgent care setting with a variety of needs that require coordination of care.

Payment Models and Financing

Payment for primary care is evolving, with ongoing urgent calls for payment reform that rewards physicians for keeping people healthy with focus on value rather than volume [82, 83]. There are currently several primary care payment models in existence, or in evolution, which will be reviewed and described in basic terms.

Fee for Service

The traditional payment model for primary care is fee for service, where each service provided for a patient is individually billed at a level determined by the complexity and scope of medical decision-making, face-to-face time spent with a patient, or by charges related to specific procedures performed or provided during that encounter. Another way to describe this model is one of volume-based payment, where reimbursement is based on the numbers of patients seen or procedures performed. For cognitive services provided in this model, documentation by the primary care clinician must support the level of billing. These Evaluation and Management (E&M) codes, with their associated documentation requirements, were overhauled by Centers for Medicare and Medicaid Services (CMS), with significant changes that went into effect January 1, 2021. These changes, the first in many years, allowed broader application of time-based codes to include not only time spent directly with the patient, but also time spent reviewing records and completing documentation, as well as changes in the criteria required to justify the billed level of complexity in medical decision-making [84–87]. These E&M changes were intended to increase reimbursement for ambulatory providers, but they did not alter the volume-based nature inherent in fee-for-service models. Further, Current Procedural Terminology (CPT) procedural codes, which can increase reimbursement, do not exist for many of the services provided by primary care clinicians and thus undervalue these necessary services [88]. Fee-for-service payment systems do allow for billing of chronic care management (CCM) for care of patients with multiple co-morbid conditions, though these codes are likely underutilized [89–91].

Capitation

This model is one in which a fixed amount of money is paid to an individual clinician, practice, or organization to cover the costs of the care of one person's health care needs over a particular unit of time. This *per member per month* reimbursement structure is intended to reduce wasteful health care expenditures by moving away from volume-based payment structures, but, when first introduced in the 1990s with the advent of Health Maintenance Organizations (HMOs), was met with dissatisfaction and placed the insurance companies in the position of care decision oversight [92]. Alternative visions that move to population-based capitation, with risk-adjusted payments, incentives based on meeting quality metrics, and a demonstrated track record of waste reduction, may be a viable alternative payment model (APM) [92].

Value-Based Payments

Value-based health care is a health care delivery framework that incentivizes physicians and other health care workers to focus on the quality of services rendered, as opposed to the quantity, with health care providers compensated based on health outcomes. The most applicable value-based payment models in primary care arose from CMS alternative payment models (APMs) that are designed to reduce cost and increase quality by incentivizing value-based care in defined populations. These APMs, a subgroup of which are referred to as population-based payment models, hold clinicians financially accountable for the cost and quality of care delivered to their specifically identified population [93]. These models are highlighted in accountable care organizations (ACOs) where a collection of physician groups, hospitals, and other providers form an entity that contracts with an insurer to coordinate the care for a defined population measured against cost and quality metrics. The ACOs assume financial risk if expenditures exceed contractual agreements or can share in cost savings as long as quality is not compromised [93].

Direct Primary Care

As previously described, these practices use models of payment where patients pay a fixed fee to cover their primary care medical services in lieu of, or in addition to, insurance payments. A direct primary care practice may operate with lower overhead costs, may provide more holistic and personalized care, and may have more predictable cash flow because they are not dependent on volume of visits to generate revenue. There are many proponents of this model, and these practices continue to grow.

Telehealth and Virtual Care

With the rapid pivot to telehealth services in response to the COVID-19 pandemic, previous restrictions on E&M billing for telehealth services were relaxed by Medicare, Medicaid, and private insurers [94]. This response to the pandemic public health emergency allowed full in-person equivalent E&M levels of coding, including time-based coding for visits conducted by video platform or telephone. Prior to the pandemic, telehealth services were used to provide access to care for rural and geographically distanced patients, access to regional specialty care without travel, virtual consultations for remote emergency departments, and offered the possibility of high-quality care at reduced cost [95]. Given the rapid adoption of virtual visits in response to the pandemic, it seems likely that the demand for telehealth visits will continue, with the role that virtual visits play in primary care and their associated payment models continuing to evolve [96].

Impact of COVID-19 Pandemic on Ambulatory Care

The emergence of the novel coronavirus in late 2019, and the pandemic which ensued, forced rapid change in access to and the delivery of health care across the globe. The number of affected persons seeking care increased to unprecedented numbers, resulting in emergency departments and intensive care units operating at or above capacity. To address the surge in persons seeking care, health care organizations developed contingency plans regarding allocation of health care resources, including the construction of overflow facilities. Innovative policies and procedures were adopted to address the ever-changing landscape of patient care during the pandemic. These organizational changes span every aspect of resource utilization and care delivery including supply chain management, deployment of critical personnel to areas of increased need, diversion of elective procedures, and creating best practices to mitigate risk of infection within facilities.

Ambulatory care providers witnessed a rapid upscaling of telehealth services with resulting legislative adaptations to deliver reimbursement. The effect of the coronavirus pandemic on chronic disease care in the ambulatory setting continues to unfold. As many as four in ten individuals delayed seeking in-person care for both routine and acute illness due to pandemic-related concerns [97].

Future Directions

The value that primary care brings to chronic care management, population health, community engagement, public health, and social justice is indisputable. Primary care has long been underfunded and underappreciated in the US health care system, but with the growing recognition that robust primary care is foundational to a functional health care system, the opportunity presents to develop best practices, which will include teaching and training, research, investment, and payment reform.

Teaching and Training in the Ambulatory Setting

If the vision of the future of high-quality primary care outlined in the NASEM 2021 report is to be realized, the training environment for primary care physicians must evolve [3]. Building on Starfield's 4 C's model, Neutze et al. propose a new training environment where the "practice is the curriculum" to teach family medicine residents the principles of effective primary care, adding Cost and Community to the 4 C's to reflect these two evolving imperatives of primary care [98]. Further proposals for family medicine residency redesign that build on the 4 C's includes the 7 C's model proposed by Bazemore et al., in which Community, patient-Centeredness, and Complexity are included in the foundational principles of residency education [99]. These models encourage primary care residency educators to use the learning laboratory of a high-functioning primary care clinical practice as the ideal place to ground the teaching of the expanding principles of primary care; ones that serve to cement our covenant with not only our patients, but their communities and society at large.

Payment Reform

The NASEM 2021 report describes the financial challenges that are responsible for the headwinds preventing viable fiscal stability of our primary care infrastructure and proposes payment reform that will deflect those headwinds. Objective One in the report's proposals is to *pay for primary care teams to care for people, not doctors to deliver services* [3]. To achieve this objective, payors must move to models that promote high-quality care, rather than those designed to achieve short-term cost savings and develop hybrid models (part fee-for-service, part capitated) that pay prospectively for team-based care that is risk adjusted for complexity and aligns with improving the health of the attributed population. Additionally, CMS and individual states should increase the overall portion of health care dollars spent on primary care [3]. Movement from fee-for-service payment models to value-based care will dramatically alter the financial and practice management of ambulatory care.

Research in Primary Care and Urgent Care

Further research and supporting research infrastructure will be crucial to the success of the evolving models of high-quality primary care. The NASEM 2021 report calls for the formation of an Office of Primary Care Research at the National Institutes of Health to prioritize funding for primary care research at the federal level [3]. As urgent care utilization continues to be an adjunct to the existing primary care landscape, further research must be devoted to understanding access patterns, developing best practices for coordination with primary care, measuring quality of care, and reducing unnecessary emergency department transfers.

References

1. CMS 1500 claim form and UB 04 form - Instruction and Guide. 2016 [October 7, 2021]. http://www.cms1500claimbilling.com/2016/07/definition-of-primary-care.html.
2. Primary care: America's health in a new era. 1996 [October 7, 2021]. http://nap.edu/5152.
3. Robinson SK, et al., editors. Implementing high-quality primary care: rebuilding the foundation of health care. Washington, DC: National Academies Press; 2021.
4. Burns J. The urgent care surge. Manag Care. 2019;28(5):38–43.
5. Chen CE, et al. Walk-in clinics versus physician offices and emergency rooms for urgent care and chronic disease management. Cochrane Database Syst Rev. 2017;2(2):Cd011774.
6. Weinick RM, Bristol SJ, DesRoches CM. Urgent care centers in the U.S.: findings from a national survey. BMC Health Serv Res. 2009;9:79.
7. Green LA, et al. The ecology of medical care revisited. N Engl J Med. 2001;344(26):2021–5.
8. Johansen ME, Richardson CR. The ecology of medical care before and after the affordable care act: trends from 2002 to 2016. Ann Fam Med. 2019;17(6):526–37.
9. White KL, Williams TF, Greenberg BG. The ecology of medical care. N Engl J Med. 1961;265:885–92.
10. Neves AL, et al. Virtual primary care in high-income countries during the COVID-19 pandemic: policy responses and lessons for the future. Eur J Gen Pract. 2021;27(1):241–7.
11. Cole ES, Leighton C, Zhang Y. Distribution of visits for chronic conditions between primary care and specialist providers in medicare shared savings accountable care organizations. Med Care. 2018;56(5):424–9.
12. Ornstein SM, et al. The prevalence of chronic diseases and multimorbidity in primary care practice: a PPRNet report. J Am Board Fam Med. 2013;26(5):518–24.
13. Ndumele CD, et al. Cardiovascular disease and risk in primary care settings in the United States. Am J Cardiol. 2012;109(4):521–6.
14. Edwards ST, Mafi JN, Landon BE. Trends and quality of care in outpatient visits to generalist and specialist physicians delivering primary care in the United States, 1997–2010. J Gen Intern Med. 2014;29(6):947–55.
15. Bricard D, Or Z. Impact of early primary care follow-up after discharge on hospital readmissions. Eur J Health Econ. 2019;20(4):611–23.
16. Einarsdóttir K, et al. Regular primary care lowers hospitalisation risk and mortality in seniors with chronic respiratory diseases. J Gen Intern Med. 2010;25(8):766–73.
17. Stange KC, et al. Metrics for assessing improvements in primary health care. Annu Rev Public Health. 2014;35:423–42.
18. Bodenheimer T, Sinsky C. From triple to quadruple aim: care of the patient requires care of the provider. Ann Fam Med. 2014;12(6):573–6.
19. Berwick DM, Nolan TW, Whittington J. The triple aim: care, health, and cost. Health Aff (Millwood). 2008;27(3):759–69.
20. Whittington JW, et al. Pursuing the triple aim: the first 7 years. Milbank Q. 2015;93(2):263–300.
21. Starfield B, Shi L, Macinko J. Contribution of primary care to health systems and health. Milbank Q. 2005;83(3):457–502.
22. Wagner EH, Austin BT, Von Korff M. Organizing care for patients with chronic illness. Milbank Q. 1996;74(4):511–44.
23. Wagner EH, Austin BT, Von Korff M. Improving outcomes in chronic illness. Manag Care Q. 1996;4(2):12–25.
24. Bodenheimer T, Wagner EH, Grumbach K. Improving primary care for patients with chronic illness. JAMA. 2002;288(14):1775–9.
25. Bodenheimer T, Wagner EH, Grumbach K. Improving primary care for patients with chronic illness: the chronic care model, Part 2. JAMA. 2002;288(15):1909–14.
26. Hooker RS, et al. Ambulatory and chronic disease care by physician assistants and nurse practitioners. J Ambul Care Manage. 2013;36(4):293–301.
27. Bayliss EA, et al. Perspectives in primary care: implementing patient-centered care coordination for individuals with multiple chronic medical conditions. Ann Fam Med. 2014;12(6):500–3.
28. Grembowski D, et al. A conceptual model of the role of complexity in the care of patients with multiple chronic conditions. Med Care. 2014;52(Suppl 3):S7–s14.
29. Milani RV, Lavie CJ. Health care 2020: reengineering health care delivery to combat chronic disease. Am J Med. 2015;128(4):337–43.
30. Smith SM, et al. Interventions for improving outcomes in patients with multimorbidity in primary care and community settings. Cochrane Database Syst Rev. 2016;3(3):Cd006560.
31. Bauer L, Bodenheimer T. Expanded roles of registered nurses in primary care delivery of the future. Nurs Outlook. 2017;65(5):624–32.
32. Yeoh EK, et al. Benefits and limitations of implementing Chronic Care Model (CCM) in primary care programs: a systematic review. Int J Cardiol. 2018;258:279–88.
33. Parker S, et al. Electronic, mobile and telehealth tools for vulnerable patients with chronic disease: a systematic review and realist synthesis. BMJ Open. 2018;8(8):e019192.
34. Leppin AL, et al. Integrating community-based health promotion programs and primary care: a mixed methods analysis of feasibility. BMC Health Serv Res. 2018;18(1):72.
35. Damian AJ, Gallo JJ. Models of care for populations with chronic conditions and mental/behavioral health comorbidity. Int Rev Psychiatry. 2018;30(6):157–69.
36. Stephen C, McInnes S, Halcomb E. The feasibility and acceptability of nurse-led chronic disease management interventions in primary care: an integrative review. J Adv Nurs. 2018;74(2):279–88.
37. Reynolds R, et al. A systematic review of chronic disease management interventions in primary care. BMC Fam Pract. 2018;19(1):11.
38. Garland-Baird L, Fraser K. Conceptualization of the chronic care model: implications for home care case manager practice. Home Healthc Now. 2018;36(6):379–85.
39. Wagner EH. Organizing care for patients with chronic illness revisited. Milbank Q. 2019;97(3):659–64.
40. Joint Principles of the Patient-Centered Medical Home. https://www.aafp.org/dam/AAFP/documents/practice_management/pcmh/initiatives/PCMHJoint.pdf.
41. Defining the PCMH. Content last reviewed September 2021. Agency for Healthcare Research and Quality, Rockville, MD [October 11, 2021]. https://www.ahrq.gov/ncepcr/tools/pcmh/defining/index.html.
42. PCMH Foundations. Content last reviewed September 2021. Agency for Healthcare Research and Quality, Rockville, MD [October 11, 2021]. https://www.ahrq.gov/ncepcr/tools/pcmh/implement/foundations.html.
43. Budgen J, Cantiello J. Advantages and disadvantages of the patient-centered medical home: a critical analysis and lessons learned. Health Care Manag (Frederick). 2017;36(4):357–63.
44. Kieber-Emmons AM, Miller WL. The Patient-Centered Medical Home (PCMH) framing typology for understanding the structure, function, and outcomes of PCMHs. J Am Board Fam Med. 2017;30(4):472–9.
45. Veet CA, et al. Impact of healthcare delivery system type on clinical, utilization, and cost outcomes of patient-centered medical homes: a systematic review. J Gen Intern Med. 2020;35(4):1276–84.
46. John JR, et al. The effectiveness of patient-centred medical home-based models of care versus standard primary care in chronic

disease management: a systematic review and meta-analysis of randomised and non-randomised controlled trials. Int J Environ Res Public Health. 2020;17(18):6886.
47. Pourat N, Charles SA, Snyder S. Availability of care concordant with patient-centered medical home principles among those with chronic conditions: measuring care outcomes. Med Care. 2016;54(3):262–8.
48. Schuttner L, et al. Association of the patient-centered medical home implementation with chronic disease quality in patients with multimorbidity. J Gen Intern Med. 2020;35(10):2932–8.
49. Doherty R. Assessing the patient care implications of "concierge" and other direct patient contracting practices: a policy position paper from the American College of Physicians. Ann Intern Med. 2015;163(12):949–52.
50. MD2: The Founders of Concierge Medicine in 1996 [October 12, 2021]. https://www.md2.com/our-story.
51. Direct primary care: an innovative alternative to convential health insurance [October 12, 2021]. http://report.heritage.org/bg2939.
52. Bowers J. Further perspectives on concierge medicine. Ann Intern Med. 2010;153(4):275.
53. Cascardo D. Concierge Medicine: is it becoming mainstream? Part II. Steps to developing a concierge practice. J Med Pract Manage. 2014;30(3):176–9.
54. Cascardo D. Concierge medicine: is it becoming mainstream? Part I. J Med Pract Manage. 2014;29(6):362–5.
55. Childs S. Direct Pay/Concierge/Blended Care: where is the sweet spot? Part II—Seen from your patients' perspective. J Med Pract Manage. 2015;31(1):50–3.
56. Dalen JE, Alpert JS. Concierge medicine is here and growing!! Am J Med. 2017;130(8):880–1.
57. Carnahan SJ. Law, medicine, and wealth: does concierge medicine promote health care choice, or is it a barrier to access? Stanford Law Pol Rev. 2006;17(1):121–63.
58. Eskew P. Direct primary care business of insurance and state law considerations. J Leg Med. 2017;37(1–2):145–54.
59. Chappell GE. Health care's other "big deal": direct primary care regulation in contemporary American Health Law. Duke Law J. 2017;66(6):1331–70.
60. Eskew PM, Klink K. Direct primary care: practice distribution and cost across the nation. J Am Board Fam Med. 2015;28(6):793–801.
61. Scherger JE. Direct primary care may become the norm. Med Econ. 2016;93(12):59.
62. Adashi EY, Clodfelter RP, George P. Direct primary care: one step forward, two steps back. JAMA. 2018;320(7):637–8.
63. Carlasare LE. Defining the place of direct primary care in a value-based care system. WMJ. 2018;117(3):106–10.
64. Rubin R. Is direct primary care a game changer? JAMA. 2018;319(20):2064–6.
65. Arenson C, Brandt BF. The importance of interprofessional practice in family medicine residency education. Fam Med. 2021;53(7):548–55.
66. Yee T, Lechner AE, Boukus ER. The surge in urgent care centers: emergency department alternative or costly convenience? Res Brief. 2013;26:1–6.
67. Le ST, Hsia RY. Community characteristics associated with where urgent care centers are located: a cross-sectional analysis. BMJ Open. 2016;6(4):e010663.
68. Wallar LE, De Prophetis E, Rosella LC. Socioeconomic inequalities in hospitalizations for chronic ambulatory care sensitive conditions: a systematic review of peer-reviewed literature, 1990–2018. Int J Equity Health. 2020;19(1):60.
69. Zitek T, et al. Most transfers from urgent care centers to emergency departments are discharged and many are unnecessary. J Emerg Med. 2018;54(6):882–8.
70. Coster JE, et al. Why do people choose emergency and urgent care services? A rapid review utilizing a systematic literature search and narrative synthesis. Acad Emerg Med. 2017;24(9):1137–49.
71. Shamji H, et al. Improving the quality of care and communication during patient transitions: best practices for urgent care centers. Jt Comm J Qual Patient Saf. 2014;40(7):319–24.
72. Barzin A, Seybold OC, Page C. Integrating an urgent care clinic into an academic family medicine practice. Fam Med. 2020;52(6):440–3.
73. Kripalani S, et al. Reducing hospital readmission rates: current strategies and future directions. Annu Rev Med. 2014;65:471–85.
74. Farrell TW, et al. Impact of an integrated transition management program in primary care on hospital readmissions. J Healthc Qual. 2015;37(1):81–92.
75. Ganguli I, et al. Patient and visit characteristics associated with use of direct scheduling in primary care practices. JAMA Netw Open. 2020;3(8):e209637.
76. Anthony DL, Campos-Castillo C, Lim PS. Who isn't using patient portals and why? Evidence and implications from a national sample of US adults. Health Aff (Millwood). 2018;37(12):1948–54.
77. Bleustein C, et al. Wait times, patient satisfaction scores, and the perception of care. Am J Manag Care. 2014;20(5):393–400.
78. Arndt BG, et al. Tethered to the EHR: primary care physician workload assessment using EHR event log data and time-motion observations. Ann Fam Med. 2017;15(5):419–26.
79. Mishra P, Kiang JC, Grant RW. Association of medical scribes in primary care with physician workflow and patient experience. JAMA Intern Med. 2018;178(11):1467–72.
80. Gottlieb M, et al. Effect of medical scribes on throughput, revenue, and patient and provider satisfaction: a systematic review and meta-analysis. Ann Emerg Med. 2021;77(2):180–9.
81. Robinson PJ, Reiter JT. Behavioral consultation and primary care: a guide to integrating services. New York: Springer; 2007.
82. Bazemore A, et al. Advancing primary care through alternative payment models: lessons from the United States & Canada. J Am Board Fam Med. 2018;31(3):322–7.
83. Gold SB, Green LA, Westfall JM. Heeding the call for urgent primary care payment reform: what do we know about how to get started? J Am Board Fam Med. 2021;34(2):424–9.
84. Flamm A, Bridges A, Siegel DM. E/M coding in 2021: the Times (and more) are a-changin'. Cutis. 2021;107(6):301–25.
85. Millette KW. Countdown to the E/M coding changes. Fam Pract Manag. 2020;27(5):29–36.
86. Peters SG. New billing rules for outpatient office visit codes. Chest. 2020;158(1):298–302.
87. Self C, Moore KJ, Church SL. The 2021 office visit coding changes: putting the pieces together. Fam Pract Manag. 2020;27(6):6–12.
88. Young RA, et al. The full scope of family physicians' work is not reflected by current procedural terminology codes. J Am Board Fam Med. 2017;30(6):724–32.
89. Fortin M, et al. Integration of chronic disease prevention and management services into primary care (PR1MaC): findings from an embedded qualitative study. BMC Fam Pract. 2019;20(1):7.
90. Gardner RL, et al. Use of chronic care management codes for medicare beneficiaries: a missed opportunity? J Gen Intern Med. 2018;33(11):1892–8.
91. Reddy A, et al. Use of chronic care management among primary care clinicians. Ann Fam Med. 2020;18(5):455–7.
92. James BC, Poulsen GP. The case for capitation. Harv Bus Rev. 2016;94(7–8):102–11, 34.
93. Liao JM, Navathe AS, Werner RM. The impact of Medicare's alternative payment models on the value of care. Annu Rev Public Health. 2020;41(1):551–65.

94. Brotman JJ, Kotloff RM. Providing outpatient telehealth services in the United States: before and during coronavirus disease 2019. Chest. 2021;159(4):1548–58.
95. Hare N, et al. Work group report: COVID-19: unmasking telemedicine. J Allergy Clin Immunol Pract. 2020;8(8):2461–2473.e3.
96. Jetty A, et al. Capacity of primary care to deliver telehealth in the United States. J Am Board Fam Med. 2021;34(Suppl):S48–s54.
97. Czeisler M, et al. Delay or avoidance of medical care because of COVID-19-related concerns - United States, June 2020. MMWR Morb Mortal Wkly Rep. 2020;69(36):1250–7.
98. Neutze D, et al. The practice is the curriculum. Fam Med. 2021;53(7):567–73.
99. Bazemore A, Grunert T. Sailing the 7C's: Starfield revisited as a Foundation of Family Medicine Residency Redesign. Fam Med. 2021;53(7):506–15.

Virtual Care

Vinay Reddy and Amir Barzin

Introduction

Telehealth encompasses the use of electronic information and telecommunication technologies to support remote clinical health care, patient and professional health-related education, public health, and health care administration [1]. Generally, telehealth denotes a broader set of services that are both clinical and non-clinical. Telemedicine has been used synonymously with telehealth and usually refers to the use of remote clinical services and medical information exchanged from one site to another via electronic communications to improve patient health [1]. Virtual care is a broader term that encompasses the many ways in which health care providers remotely interact with their patients [2]. This includes the practice of using remote technologies such as phone calls, video conferencing, connected devices, and online chats, to connect with patients [3].

Telehealth services has seen a steady rise over the last several decades and parallels the use of technology such as computers, mobile devices, and electronic forms of communication [4]. This chapter provides an overview of telehealth and virtual care. The first section introduces concepts, principles, and limitations of telehealth. Next, a history of key developments in telehealth is narrated and followed by organizational aspects of providing telehealth in different clinical settings. The subsequent section reviews important considerations regarding the management and operations of telehealth before the chapter closes with future directions.

Principles and Concepts of Telehealth

There are four main categories of telehealth, including synchronous communication through live video conferencing, asynchronous communication, remote patient monitoring (RPM), and mobile health (mhealth) [5]. Synchronous communication involves a two-way audio/video communication between health care providers or between patients and a provider that can be telephonic without video. Asynchronous communication is the exchange of recorded patient health information between providers or between a patient and a provider [5]. This type of communication is also known as store and forward and involves collecting information from the patient or provider and then sending it to another party for review [5]. Asynchronous communication is typically done through secure patient portals or from within the electronic health record (EHR) system and includes secure exchange of e-mails, sending and receiving e-consultations, and e-visits.

The use of secure email communication between providers and patients offers a mechanism for discussing non-urgent medical questions and patient health care concerns [6]. These exchanges are stored within the EHR. E-visits are a non-face-to-face evaluation and management service that typically involves the use of a standardized questionnaire designed for specific complaints such as sore throat, ear pain, and urinary symptoms [6]. It includes the collection of subjective information from the patient, often using a templated questionnaire, as well as documentation of the diagnosis and treatment plan [6]. E-visits provide capacity for providers to ask follow-up questions in an asynchronous manner.

E-consults are provider-to-provider electronic asynchronous exchanges that are generally utilized between primary care providers and specialists and involve clinical questions regarding diagnosis and treatment that do not require an in-person exam [6]. These encounters usually involve a review of labs, imaging, and previous clinic notes in the electronic chart linked to a specific clinical question. This approach can be efficient and timely when seeking advice from specialists who may have a long wait time for patient appointments.

Remote patient monitoring (RPM) includes the monitoring, collection, and sending of clinical data, such as blood pressure readings, blood glucose readings, heart rate/rhythm data, oxygen saturation, and weight readings [6]. Data can be

V. Reddy · A. Barzin (✉)
Department of Family Medicine, University of North Carolina at Chapel Hill, Chapel Hill, NC, USA
e-mail: vreddy@med.unc.edu; amir_barzin@med.unc.edu

self-collected by the patient through manual entry into a secure portal or recorded by autonomous devices that collect and transmit the data directly in the patient secure portal. These data become part of the medical record for review by member of their care team or by a central monitored dashboard [6]. RPM data can facilitate chronic disease management, such as hypertension and diabetes mellitus, by providing blood pressure and blood sugar information. In addition, RPM data provide collateral information that can reduce acute care use for patients with cardiovascular disease and COPD [7].

mHealth typically involves the monitoring and sharing of heath information via mobile technology such as wearables, health tracking apps tablets, and smartphones [6]. The World Health Organization (WHO) has defined mHealth as the "use of mobile and wireless technologies to support the achievement of health objectives" [8], while the National Institutes of Health defines mHealth as "the use of mobile and wireless devices (cell phones, tablets, etc.) to improve health outcomes, health care services, and health research" [9]. Wearable activity trackers and smartphone apps can record and report biometric data such as physical activity, sleep cycles, heart rate, and oxygen levels.

Mobile or electronic journaling tracks a patient's thoughts and associated symptoms, often with a goal to promote patient engagement in areas such as mindfulness and stress-mitigating exercises, and to develop healthy habits [10]. Journaling can assist patients in developing chronic disease self-management plans, whether through checklists, or by providing a reflective account of their daily experiences. Mobile journals are also effective as self-report measurement tools [10] and have been reported to mitigate stress by providing a forum for emotional disclosure [11].

The use of health chatbots is an emerging mHealth technology. Health chatbots are computer programs or smart algorithms that conduct a conversation with a patient via auditory or textual methods [12]. This technology can help patient care teams by triaging patients to appropriate care pathways, assisting with medication management, providing information for uncomplicated medical issues, and reporting test results and providing follow-up information [12].

Telemedicine in ambulatory settings is primarily in direct patient care (i.e., evaluation, diagnosis, treatment, and follow-up of illness) and consultations [13]. In 2016, 15% of physicians worked in practices that used telemedicine for patient interactions and 11% used it for communicating with other health care professionals [13]. Specialties that utilized telemedicine for direct patient care were radiology (40%), psychiatry (28%), pathology (23%), and emergency medicine (22%) while emergency medicine (39%), pathology (30%), and radiology (26%) were specialties that utilized telemedicine in a consultative capacity.

A systematic review and meta-analysis concluded the effectiveness of telehealth interventions for certain conditions and found that telehealth interventions appeared equivalent to in-person care [14]. Another review reported that telehealth can be equivalent or clinically more effective when compared to usual care but is discipline specific [15]. A third review noted that telehealth services via telephone or videoconferencing are effective alternatives to in-person visits for many patients needing primary care and mental health services [16].

Limitations of Telehealth

Telehealth services have many benefits; however, they should not be considered as a replacement for in-person visits and are not designed to be used for all patients or in all clinical situations. A significant limitation is the inability to conduct an in-person physical examination which may be required for certain clinical situations and patient concerns. Additionally, the components of an in-person visit, such as the development and maintenance of the patient-provider relationship, can be hindered by telehealth [17]. There is also variability regarding reimbursement for telehealth services as well as the inconsistency of broadband internet and computers/mobile devices, which often limit patient access.

In recent years, telehealth's growth has been incremental and reflects low levels of adoption prior to the COVID-19 pandemic. For example, a survey showed 8% of Americans have tried telehealth, while 66% of consumers are willing to use telehealth [18]. An earlier study reported that 15% of pediatricians reported having used telehealth [19]. A more representative study of adults found that more than half of the respondents had never used a non-telephone telehealth modality to discuss a health issue with a physician [20]. The most common reasons for not using telehealth included having no perceived need, that their physician did not offer it, and not feeling comfortable using the technology [20]. Other barriers to wider adoption have been identified as limited reimbursement, geographical restrictions of where the patient can be located, and lack of comfort with telemedicine technologies by patients and providers [21].

History of Telehealth

The technology supporting telehealth has existed for decades. The exchange of medical information to provide medical services over a landline phone has evolved to the use of video technologies. An early use of interactive health care video communications was at the University of Nebraska, where clinicians transmitted neurological examinations across campus to medical students in 1959 [22]. In subsequent years, a CCTV link was created between the Nebraska Psychiatric Institute and Norfolk State Hospital for virtual psychiatric and neurologic consultations [22]. During the 1960s, the National Aeronautics and Space Administration (NASA) began monitoring Mercury astronauts in flight by physicians and medical teams stationed around the world and continued testing and refining protocols for telehealth in communities located in Arizona and Alaska [23].

The use of teleradiology accelerated in the 1990s with the transmittal of images from one location to another for reading and interpretation; in 20 years, it accounted for more than half of all telemedicine services provided in the United States [24]. This timeframe also saw the development of the hub (i.e., medical center locations) and spoke (i.e., patient sites) model of telehealth and the expansion of inpatient and emergency telehealth (e.g., teleneurology and teleintensive care services) in rural and remote access areas. Emergency departments implemented telestroke programs to provide time sensitive and efficient stroke care in locations where neurologists were limited [25].

The American Recovery and Reinvestment Act (ARRA) of 2009 provided stimulus funding for health information technology and incentivized the use of electronic health records which further promoted the use of technology solutions in health care [26]. In subsequent years, there has been marked adoption of telehealth services with state and federal policy and regulatory advancements. During this time, telehealth expanded from acute hospital settings to the ambulatory environments. For example, in-home monitoring though remote patient monitoring systems and video conferencing systems began for monitoring chronic illnesses like diabetes, hypertension, congestive heart failure, and chronic obstructive pulmonary disease [7]. To offset financial disincentives for hospital readmissions, health care systems sought innovative ways to monitor and treat patients in less acute settings, such as programs targeting patients with congestive heart failure [27].

Despite many barriers, health care systems continued investing in building telehealth capacity [28], due to an assumption that these technologies could reduce cost and improve access to care, especially for underserved populations and residents of rural areas. The number of telehealth visits increased from just over 7000 in 2004 to 108,000 in 2013 among rural Medicare recipients [29]. The use of hospital-based telehealth has grown from 35% of hospitals using telehealth platforms in 2010 to 76% of hospitals in 2017 [30]. Videoconferencing, remote patient monitoring, and store-and-forward data have been the most favored telehealth modalities, as represented by telestroke programs that utilize a combination of video conferencing and review of stored and transmitted imaging, and teleradiology programs which use store and forward technology for review of diagnostic imaging [5]. Other programs such as teletrauma, teleburns, teledermatology, and teleintensive care units continue to be developed and implemented across the country, especially in areas that have a shortage of these services [5].

Impact of COVID-19 Pandemic

The growth and adoption of telehealth was incremental until the COVID-19 pandemic. In response to the pandemic, health systems quickly pivoted to telehealth platforms and technologies for patient care in March 2020 [31]. Simultaneously, US federal regulations and enacted polices that fast-tracked the implementation of telehealth tools and supported fiscal viability. Through a series of waivers and expanded reimbursement, location restrictions were removed, allowable video conferencing platforms were expanded, interstate licensure requirements were relaxed, and reimbursement policies changed [28]. The previously restrictive health care environment that were barriers to the dissemination of telehealth tools changed dramatically due to the COVID-19 pandemic, resulting in a skyrocketed increase in telehealth utilization [20]. The Centers for Disease Control and Prevention reported a 50% increase in the first quarter of 2020 of the four largest US telehealth service providers and a 154% increase in visits when compared to same period in 2019 [32]. Patient acceptance of telehealth increased, with 46% of patient reporting telehealth use for some of their visits compared to just 11% in 2019 [33].

The rapid acceptance of telehealth tools by patients and providers has evolved into an expectation of continuing these services after the pandemic. Since the COVID-19 pandemic, telehealth uptake has been the highest in psychiatry (50%), substance use disorder treatment (30%), endocrinology (17%), and rheumatology (17%) [33]. Virtual care was provided in a small number of outpatient practices prior to the COVID-19 pandemic [34], which has resulted in exponential growth [32]. While the pandemic increased the use of virtual care, the increase in utilization was not predominantly associated with COVID-19 complaints but with behavioral health concerns and chronic disease management [35].

Factors Influencing Telehealth Growth

There are several reasons for the initial and ongoing growth of telehealth. First, the increasing availability of digital patient information by conversion to electronic health record (EHR) platforms has made it easy to access and review patient information in secure ways [36]. The impetus to value-based care seeks to achieve cost saving and provide accessible and quality care. Telehealth modalities, such as video visits and electronic consults, are attractive solutions that have potential to increase access, encourage quality of care, while driving down costs. The lower overhead and capital costs that are associated with telehealth services are also aligned in value-based care. The COVID-19 pandemic revealed an acceptance of telehealth by the patients and other stakeholders [37]. For example, 65% of patients reported that they would be comfortable talking with a doctor or nurse practitioner online or over the phone instead of seeing them in person [37]. Finally, telehealth services are time efficient, potentially saving patients over 100 min of time spent in health care [38].

Organization of Telehealth Services

In traditional health care delivery, a patient receives care in a physical environment where a health care provider is located (i.e., originating site) such as an outpatient clinic, urgent care, and hospital, which has defined the services provided [39]. The patient location is the originating site in virtual care services. The provider may or may not be located in an originating site. Care can be provided to patients in the settings of their own choosing. For example, for those with sufficient IT capability, care can be provided in the patient's home. Patients who reside in areas with limited broadband or IT equipment may access virtual care through community access hubs [40]. These centers provide a safe, reliable locations to access care that is located usually in community centers or in public locations such as libraries.

Several models may be considered in organizing telehealth services. A co-located space in a traditional outpatient clinic can designate and upfit rooms for virtual care. Limitations of this model include potentially underutilized space is there lacks a capability to quickly adjust to in-person care depending on demand and patient preference. Another organizational model places health care providers in locations that are not originating sites, such as personal offices and residences. The information technology (IT) needs, including broadband access, video equipment, audio equipment, and support, need to be met. Although this model is not limited by space, capacity is limited by the number of patients requesting this type of care, scheduling support, and other administrative concerns. Finally, patients may utilize sites that connect to an off-site provider.

Primary Care

Virtual care in primary care offers advantages and opportunities. The American Hospital Association (AHA) reports that over 3.5 million patients in the United States do not access medical care due to transportation [41], a gap that virtual care can fill for those with transportation barriers. Primary care practices can expand their capacity by having providers utilize virtual platform from a remote location that is not co-located in a brick-and-mortar clinic. Such increased availability can improve health outcomes, particularly for patients that may not have had access to health care [42].

The use of e-visits in primary care allows for the asynchronous interactions between a patient and a provider through a secure portal that allows for exchange of information [43]. The diagnostic accuracy of e-visits for low-acuity illness is comparable to face-to-face visits [43]. For example, urinary tract symptoms is a common presenting concern in e-visits and there is no increased utilization of antimicrobials, follow-up, or adverse clinical outcomes when compared to in-person visits [44]. Primary care practices may also consider a mixed-model of care that accommodates higher acuity, more complex patients during in-person visits and lower risk, less acute care via virtual care.

Urgent Care

During the peak of the COVID-19 pandemic, virtual urgent care centers were scaled to manage a large volume of patients across a New York City catchment area, half of whom would have required care in a traditional health facility [45]. The advantages for virtual urgent care are comparable to primary care, which has been shown to decrease emergency department utilization and enhance primary care engagement [46]. Urgent care provides convenience and access but does not maintain a 24/7 model and expansion may be advanced through virtual care. The exchange of medical information between urgent care sites and primary care is an important consideration.

Specialty Care

The use of virtual platforms in specialty care has been associated with increased patient satisfaction when compared to in-person consultations [47, 48]. Access to specialty care can be limited due to provider availability and geographic constraints, and the use of telehealth can provide care to those who might not be able to seek in-person care [49, 50]. E-consults facilitate provider-to-provider communication of complex medical conditions by allowing referring providers the capability to ask diagnostic and management questions for non-emergent issues [48]. Improvements in virtual technology have allowed diagnostic studies to be performed remotely utilizing virtual platforms. For example, portable sleep monitoring devices have increased the availability of polysomnography for obstructive sleep apnea [51]. In addition, remote electroencephalogram (EEG) extends the diagnostic reach for patients with limited access [52].

Acute Hospital Care

Virtual care has been incorporated in acute hospital settings, particularly in connecting tertiary care centers to rural and resource-limited areas. This approach has the potential to increase bed capacity and improve patient satisfaction. A neonatal intensive care unit (NICU) telemedicine program connected a Level IV NICU to Level II NICU reported positive outcomes in length of stay, days on oxygen, days on non-invasive ventilation, and time to full enteral feeds [53]. Acute telepsychiatry services have been used to provide inpatient evaluation of patients requiring acute psychiatric services from a tertiary center to a community hospital [54]. The initial design of services focused on involuntarily detained patients; however, the program expanded to include additional psychiatric conditions and diagnoses [54].

Providing acute hospital care virtually in patients' homes is a novel service that has expanded the traditional approach to inpatient care [55]. In this model, a patient receives nursing, ancillary and support services, such as lab and imaging, in the home while the medical evaluation and management is provided virtually [55]. A virtual "hub" coordinates care and can utilize community paramedics and remote patient monitoring devices such as home blood pressure monitors and pulse oximetry that are remotely monitored. This approach was used to provide COVID-related to patients treated at home [56].

Post-acute Care

Post-acute virtual care can provide services as patients transition from inpatient care to home. Post hospitalization needs such as allied health services (physical, occupational, and speech) and ancillary supports (nutrition therapy, care management, and pharmacy services) are augmented in a virtual environment. For example, pharmacy services can achieve medication reconciliation through virtual platforms, providing education and teaching on vital medications and reporting concerns to the prescribing provider, which is a cost-effective model in rural areas [40]. Allied health services may also use this approach to facilitate treatment and connection to distribution centers for assistive devices to be delivered to the patient's home without disruption of care in the home setting.

Management and Operations of Telehealth Services

The successful adoption and sustained implementation of telehealth services is dependent upon managing and operating systems that provide reliable connectivity and a seamless end-user and provider experience. There are many stakeholders, including information technology (IT) specialists, physician champions and other operational leaders, legal and compliance representatives, and revenue cycle management teams [57].

Information Technology (IT) Infrastructure

A high performing IT infrastructure that meets the needs of virtual care is at the core of telehealth services. Well-maintained network, hardware, and software systems allow for audiovisual connection for both the provider and the patient. The use of cellular services via mobile applications can augment services areas where broadband coverage is limited. Telephonic coverage is also an option for those with limited IT capabilities and broadband coverage [58]. IT systems that provide reliable and timely internet services may be challenging in geographic areas that have limited access to broadband coverage [59]. The utilization of care hubs can mitigate these limitations, which are often in rural locations. Likewise, electronic medical records (EMR) that allow for bidirectional communication between a patient and care provider are essential to facilitating documentation and exchange of health information in a clinical setting.

The development of downtime/backup IT systems and workflows are required as contingency plans when the main operating system is malfunctioning. Strategies can include the utilization of a secondary system or temporary paper records until systems can be restored [60]. Backup and contingency systems and plans can add increased cost and redundancy.

System Oversight and Workflows

The administrative and IT requirements of virtual care require input and oversight by stakeholders, such as provider champions and technical support, to identify performance goals and measures, and to identify gaps in health care delivery. Health care system may convene oversight committees to standardize policies and protocols regarding the implementation and execution of virtual care services. Such committees and groups can inform goals and develop initiatives from operational leaders to promote care across the delivery system. A process that utilizes dynamic oversight and frequent surveys to assess the patient and provider experience can lead to improvements in virtual care [61].

In some health care systems, virtual care modalities and functional workflows are often driven within specific service units, departments, or sub-specialty groups. Other systems may utilize a designated provider pool to provide care in a designated virtual care center. These pools and service units may include primary care, urgent care, specialty, and hospital-based clinicians. The service sites may in a centralized virtual care centers or existing the clinical sites, such as outpatient clinics. A centralized model has capacity to expand specialty care access to inpatient and outpatient locations affiliate sites. In both centralized and decentralized models, standardized workflows and policies provide a more uniform approach to care and reduces inefficiencies.

A dyad that includes a medical director and technical director can promote the functionality of virtual care services. This leadership structure can provide operational and medical oversight for clinical care through reporting relationships with stakeholders, clinical champions, and operational leaders. High performing teams provide opportunities for individual and team growth and can ensure strategic alignment with the larger health care system.

Legal and Compliance Considerations

The growth of virtual care has broadened medical-legal and compliance issues associated with the delivery of health care, including licensure, state laws, billing, malpractice insurance, and HIPPA compliance [62]. These legal and regulatory challenges are important components that can lead to the successful implementation or failure of virtual care [63]. Historically, virtual care was limited due to restrictions in Section 1824(m) of the Social Security Act to approved areas, traditionally in rural communities [64]. As the COVID-19 pandemic worsened, these laws were modified to accommodate public health emergency (PHE) waivers, including permanent removal of geography as a limitation to care (e.g., the CONNECT Act) [65]. Since virtual care can provide care across state lines and large geographic locations, questions remain about licensure and credentialing of health care providers that are traditionally reviewed and granted at the local (i.e., state) level. There are additional concerns about the security and privacy of protected health information and regulation requirements such as the Health Insurance Portability and Accountability Act of 1996 (HIPAA) [66].

Health insurance regulations, including billing and coding, revenue cycle, and compliance, are important considerations in evolving virtual care services. Medicare, Medicaid, and many commercial insurance carriers changed their virtual care fee schedules and regulations in response to COVID-19 [31]. With these modifications, virtual care visits generally received reimbursement that was equivalent to in person care, particularly if live video was used. As the public health emergency (PHE) declaration is lifted, it will be important to monitor reimbursement and legal changes of providing services virtually.

The rapid expansion virtual care can be facilitated by utilizing legal and compliance subject matter experts. Ongoing communication that addresses the changing landscape of care and reviews new legislation, changes to compensation for care, and development of educational material is critical. Playbooks that provide providers and health care staff with protocols and workflows for medical conditions that are suited for virtual visits, information sources regarding documentation, compliance, and billing are also important [67].

Future Directions

The COVID-19 pandemic established telehealth as a core health service. Both patient and provider attitudes toward telehealth have been positive, with over 80% of patients reporting that they are likely to use telemedicine after the pandemic is over [68]. Easy to use technology, available services, online scheduling options, and immediate availability are the major reasons driving adoption by patients [68]. The exponential rise in telehealth utilization has leveled off to approximately 15% of office visits across all specialties [33]. This parallels capital and infrastructure investments in virtual care and digital health has with evolving business models [33].

Even with expansion, two challenges will hamper the growth of telehealth services. The first is the digital divide, or the gap between individuals and populations with access to technology, the internet, and digital literacy and those who do not. Digital literacy involves the delivery of information as well as the ability to understand the information being presented in a digital medium [69]. Reading online content or knowing how to send a text, or social media posting is not equivalent to digital literacy. A substantial number of lower income households in the United States do not own a smartphone, have broadband services, and/or have a desktop or laptop computer [70].

Health care systems may consider partnering with telecommunication companies and state and local governments to increase broadband internet access in low resource areas and in vulnerable populations. Other strategies may include providing culturally sensitive IT services, peer support, and training to use platforms such as portals, video conferencing, smartphone apps, and other mobile technologies [71]. The use of kiosk style video hubs in accessible locations, such as local churches or community centers, can mitigate barriers. The digital divide is also associated with socioeconomic status and the implementation of telehealth services may reinforce disparities in health access in marginalized and underserved communities [72]. To promote health equity, virtual care stakeholders may consider: simplifying complex interfaces and workflows to make to make it easier for patients to engage virtually; using supportive intermediaries to provide direct and immediate support to help navigate the telehealth visit; and creating mechanisms through which marginalized community members can provide immediate input into the planning and delivery of care [73].

The second challenge to telehealth growth is the potential for disrupting continuity and care coordination, which are hallmarks of primary care [74]. The convenience of telehealth may result in patients receiving care from multiple virtual providers, potentially leading to fragmented care. Telehealth services should not be viewed by patients, providers, and stakeholders as a replacement of in-person services, but as a complement. A hybrid model of care, one that uses a variety of telehealth modalities with in-person visits, has the potential to meaningfully engage patients with complex chronic conditions and improve their care [74]. Telehealth services should be aligned with in-person visits with a goal of enhancing continuity of care by providing communication between providers and patients across the care spectrum. It is important that telehealth services not operate independently from the continuity care a patient receives. An integrated services approach (i.e., in-person visits supplemented by telehealth) improves continuity of care, decreases geographical barriers, and increases access without negatively impacting quality of care or patient satisfaction [74].

COVID-19 has brought attitudinal, infrastructure, and regulatory changes to telehealth. For telehealth to be equitably responsive, after the pandemic has ended, health care systems will need to create and implement reliable technology platforms, programs, and strategies that are accessible to all patients and communities.

References

1. What is telehealth? How is telehealth different from telemedicine? | HealthIT.gov [Internet]. [cited 2021 Nov 7]. https://www.healthit.gov/faq/what-telehealth-how-telehealth-different-telemedicine.
2. Teledoc Health. Telemedicine vs. virtual care: defining the difference [Internet]. [cited 2022 Apr 18]. https://intouchhealth.com/finding-the-right-term-for-modern-digital-healthcare/.
3. Digital health vs. virtual care: what's the difference? – Qure4u [Internet]. [cited 2022 Apr 18]. https://www.qure4u.com/digital-health-vs-virtual-care-whats-the-difference/.
4. Kichloo A, Albosta M, Dettloff K, Wani F, El-Amir Z, Singh J, et al. Telemedicine, the current COVID-19 pandemic and the future: a narrative review and perspectives moving forward in the USA. Fam Med Commun Health. 2020;8(3):e000530.
5. Mechanic OJ, Persaud Y, Kimball AB. Telehealth systems. Treasure Island, FL: StatPearls Publishing; 2022.
6. Center for Connected Health Policy. What is telehealth? - CCHP [Internet]. [cited 2022 Apr 18]. https://www.cchpca.org/what-is-telehealth/.
7. Taylor ML, Thomas EE, Snoswell CL, Smith AC, Caffery LJ. Does remote patient monitoring reduce acute care use? A systematic review. BMJ Open. 2021;11(3):e040232.
8. World Health Organization. Mhealth: new horizons for health through mobile technologies [Internet]. [cited 2022 Mar 10]. https://www.who.int/goe/publications/goe_mhealth_web.pdf.
9. Mobile health—technology and outcomes in low- and middle-income countries (NIH). Federal Grants & Contracts. 2021;45(20):6.
10. O'Reilly GA, Spruijt-Metz D. Current mHealth technologies for physical activity assessment and promotion. Am J Prev Med. 2013;45(4):501–7.
11. Whitney RV, Smith G. Emotional disclosure through journal writing: telehealth intervention for maternal stress and mother-child relationships. J Autism Dev Disord. 2015;45(11):3735–45.
12. Dennis AR, Kim A, Rahimi M, Ayabakan S. User reactions to COVID-19 screening chatbots from reputable providers. J Am Med Inform Assoc. 2020;27(11):1727–31.
13. Kane CK, Gillis K. The use of telemedicine by physicians: still the exception rather than the rule. Health Aff (Millwood). 2018;37(12):1923–30.
14. Shigekawa E, Fix M, Corbett G, Roby DH, Coffman J. The current state of telehealth evidence: a rapid review. Health Aff (Millwood). 2018;37(12):1975–82.
15. Snoswell CL, Chelberg G, De Guzman KR, Haydon HH, Thomas EE, Caffery LJ, et al. The clinical effectiveness of telehealth: a systematic review of meta-analyses from 2010 to 2019. J Telemed Telecare. 2021; https://doi.org/10.1177/1357633X211022907.
16. Carrillo de Albornoz S, Sia K-L, Harris A. The effectiveness of teleconsultations in primary care: systematic review. Fam Pract. 2022;39(1):168–82.
17. Hjelm NM. Benefits and drawbacks of telemedicine. J Telemed Telecare. 2005;11(2):60–70.
18. Telehealth Index: 2019 Consumer Survey. [cited 2022 Apr 18]. https://static.americanwell.com/app/uploads/2019/07/American-Well-Telehealth-Index-2019-Consumer-Survey-eBook2.pdf.
19. Sisk B, Alexander J, Bodnar C, Curfman A, Garber K, McSwain SD, et al. Pediatrician attitudes toward and experiences with telehealth use: results from a national survey. Acad Pediatr. 2020;20(5):628–35.
20. Fischer SH, Ray KN, Mehrotra A, Bloom EL, Uscher-Pines L. Prevalence and characteristics of telehealth utilization in the united states. JAMA Netw Open. 2020;3(10):e2022302.
21. Dorsey ER, Topol EJ. State of telehealth. N Engl J Med. 2016;375(2):154–61.
22. Nesbitt TS. History of telehealth | Understanding telehealth | AccessMedicine | McGraw Hill Medical [Internet]. 2018 [cited 2021 Nov 8]. https://accessmedicine.mhmedical.com/content.aspx?bookid=2217&sectionid=187794434.
23. Link MM. Space medicine in project Mercury. NASA SP-4003. NASA Special Publication [Internet]. 1965 [cited 2021 Nov 8]. http://articles.adsabs.harvard.edu/full/1965NASSP4003.....L.
24. Weinstein RS, Lopez AM, Joseph BA, Erps KA, Holcomb M, Barker GP, et al. Telemedicine, telehealth, and mobile health applications that work: opportunities and barriers. Am J Med. 2014;127(3):183–7.
25. Aita MC, Nguyen K, Bacon R, Capuzzi KM. Obstacles and solutions in the implementation of telestroke: billing, licensing, and legislation. Stroke. 2013;44(12):3602–6.
26. Doarn CR, Pruitt S, Jacobs J, Harris Y, Bott DM, Riley W, et al. Federal efforts to define and advance telehealth—a work in progress. Telemed J E Health. 2014;20(5):409–18.
27. Kulshreshtha A, Kvedar JC, Goyal A, Halpern EF, Watson AJ. Use of remote monitoring to improve outcomes in patients with heart failure: a pilot trial. Int J Telemed Appl. 2010;2010:870959.
28. Mann DM, Chen J, Chunara R, Testa PA, Nov O. COVID-19 transforms health care through telemedicine: evidence from the field. J Am Med Inform Assoc. 2020;27(7):1132–5.
29. Mehrotra A, Jena AB, Busch AB, Souza J, Uscher-Pines L, Landon BE. Utilization of telemedicine among rural Medicare beneficiaries. JAMA. 2016;315(18):2015–6.
30. Fact Sheet: Telehealth | AHA [Internet]. [cited 2022 Apr 18]. https://www.aha.org/factsheet/telehealth.

31. HHS. Notification of enforcement discretion for telehealth | HHS.gov [Internet]. 2021 [cited 2021 Nov 8]. https://www.hhs.gov/hipaa/for-professionals/special-topics/emergency-preparedness/notification-enforcement-discretion-telehealth/index.html.
32. Koonin LM, Hoots B, Tsang CA, Leroy Z, Farris K, Jolly T, et al. Trends in the use of telehealth during the emergence of the COVID-19 pandemic - United States, January–March 2020. MMWR Morb Mortal Wkly Rep. 2020;69(43):1595–9.
33. Bestsennyy O. Telehealth: a post-COVID-19 reality? | McKinsey [Internet]. 2021 [cited 2022 Apr 18]. https://www.mckinsey.com/industries/healthcare-systems-and-services/our-insights/telehealth-a-quarter-trillion-dollar-post-covid-19-reality.
34. Cheung L, Leung TI, Ding VY, Wang JX, Norden J, Desai M, et al. Healthcare service utilization under a new virtual primary care delivery model. Telemed J E Health. 2019;25(7):551–9.
35. Uscher-Pines L, Thompson J, Taylor P, Dean K, Yuan T, Tong I, et al. Where virtual care was already a reality: experiences of a nationwide telehealth service provider during the COVID-19 pandemic. J Med Internet Res. 2020;22(12):e22727.
36. HealthIT.gov. What are the advantages of electronic health records? | HealthIT.gov [Internet]. [cited 2022 Apr 18]. https://www.healthit.gov/faq/what-are-advantages-electronic-health-records.
37. Johansson A. The 7 factors pushing for telemedicine growth | IEEE Computer Society [Internet]. 2020 [cited 2021 Nov 7]. https://www.computer.org/publications/tech-news/trends/the-7-factors-pushing-for-telemedicine-growth.
38. Ashford K. 1 In 5 people would switch doctors for video visits [Internet]. 2017 [cited 2021 Nov 7]. https://www.forbes.com/sites/kateashford/2017/01/30/videodoctor/?sh=36c26b0a10ce.
39. Federal Register [Internet]. 2020 [cited 2020 Apr 7]. https://www.govinfo.gov/content/pkg/FR-2020-04-06/pdf/2020-06990.pdf.
40. Perdew C, Erickson K, Litke J. Innovative models for providing clinical pharmacy services to remote locations using clinical video telehealth. Am J Health Syst Pharm. 2017;74(14):1093–8.
41. Wallace R, Hughes-Cromwick P, Mull H, Khasnabis S. Access to health care and nonemergency medical transportation: two missing links. Transport Res Record. 2005;1924:76–84.
42. Shi L. The impact of primary care: a focused review. Scientifica (Cairo). 2012;2012:432892.
43. Hertzog R, Johnson J, Smith J, McStay FW, da Graca B, Haneke T, et al. Diagnostic accuracy in primary care E-visits: evaluation of a large integrated health care delivery system's experience. Mayo Clin Proc. 2019;94(6):976–84.
44. Murray MA, Penza KS, Myers JF, Furst JW, Pecina JL. Comparison of eVisit management of urinary symptoms and urinary tract infections with standard care. Telemed J E Health. 2020;26(5):639–44.
45. Lovell T, Albritton J, Dalto J, Ledward C, Daines W. Virtual vs traditional care settings for low-acuity urgent conditions: an economic analysis of cost and utilization using claims data. J Telemed Telecare. 2021;27(1):59–65.
46. Barzin A, Seybold OC, Page C. Integrating an urgent care clinic into an academic family medicine practice. Fam Med. 2020;52(6):440–3.
47. Pflugeisen BM, Mou J. Patient satisfaction with virtual obstetric care. Matern Child Health J. 2017;21(7):1544–51.
48. Wasfy JH, Rao SK, Chittle MD, Gallen KM, Isselbacher EM, Ferris TG. Initial results of a cardiac E-consult pilot program. J Am Coll Cardiol. 2014;64(24):2706–7.
49. Roberts LJ, Lamont EG, Lim I, Sabesan S, Barrett C. Telerheumatology: an idea whose time has come. Intern Med J. 2012;42(10):1072–8.
50. Ketchell RI. Telemedicine is the way forward for the management of cystic fibrosis - the case in favour. Paediatr Respir Rev. 2018;26:19–21.
51. Su S, Baroody FM, Kohrman M, Suskind D. A comparison of polysomnography and a portable home sleep study in the diagnosis of obstructive sleep apnea syndrome. Otolaryngol Head Neck Surg. 2004;131(6):844–50.
52. Healy PD, O'Reilly RD, Boylan GB, Morrison JP. Web-based remote monitoring of live EEG. In: The 12th IEEE International Conference on e-Health Networking, Applications and Services. IEEE; 2010. p. 169–74.
53. Makkar A, McCoy M, Hallford G, Escobedo M, Szyld E. A hybrid form of telemedicine: a unique way to extend intensive care service to neonates in medically underserved areas. Telemed J E Health. 2018;24(9):717–21.
54. Kimmel RJ, Toor R. Telepsychiatry by a public, academic medical center for inpatient consults at an unaffiliated, community hospital. Psychosomatics. 2019;60(5):468–73.
55. Rosen JM, Adams LV, Geiling J, Curtis KM, Mosher RE, Ball PA, et al. Telehealth's new horizon: providing smart hospital-level care in the home. Telemed J E Health. 2021;27(11):1215–24.
56. Sitammagari K, Murphy S, Kowalkowski M, Chou S-H, Sullivan M, Taylor S, et al. Insights from rapid deployment of a "virtual hospital" as standard care during the COVID-19 pandemic. Ann Intern Med. 2021;174(2):192–9.
57. Rincon TA. How NPs can help expand telehealth services. Nurse Pract. 2019;44(11):30–5.
58. Webster P. Virtual health care in the era of COVID-19. Lancet. 2020;395(10231):1180–1.
59. Bauerly BC, McCord RF, Hulkower R, Pepin D. Broadband access as a public health issue: the role of law in expanding broadband access and connecting underserved communities for better health outcomes. J Law Med Ethics. 2019;47(2_suppl):39–42.
60. Kashiwagi DT, Sexton MD, Souchet Graves CE, Johnson JM, Callies BI, Yu RC, et al. All CLEAR? Preparing for IT downtime. Am J Med Qual. 2017;32(5):547–51.
61. Malathi S. Enhancing patient engagement during virtual care: a conceptual model and rapid implementation at an academic medical center [Internet]. 2020 [cited 2022 Apr 18]. https://catalyst.nejm.org/doi/pdf/10.1056/CAT.20.0262.
62. Cason J, Brannon JA. Telehealth regulatory and legal considerations: frequently asked questions. Int J Telerehabil. 2011;3(2):15–8.
63. Nittari G, Khuman R, Baldoni S, Pallotta G, Battineni G, Sirignano A, et al. Telemedicine practice: review of the current ethical and legal challenges. Telemed J E Health. 2020;26(12):1427–37.
64. CMS. [Internet]. [cited 2022 Apr 18]. https://www.cms.gov/About-CMS/Agency-Information/OMH/Downloads/Information-on-Medicare-Telehealth-Report.pdf.
65. Telehealth: the legal and regulatory issues amid the COVID-19 pandemic and the return to pre-pandemic life [Internet]. [cited 2022 Apr 18]. https://www.americanbar.org/groups/business_law/publications/blt/2022/04/telehealth/.
66. Young CJ. Telemedicine: patient privacy rights of electronic medical records. UMKC Law Rev. 1998;66(4):921–37.
67. Dosaj A, Thiyagarajan D, Ter Haar C, Cheng J, George J, Wheatley C, et al. Rapid implementation of telehealth services during the COVID-19 pandemic. Telemed J E Health. 2021;27(2):116–20.
68. Zimeles A. Four new statistics that prove that telemedicine isn't just a pandemic fad [Internet]. [cited 2021 Nov 13]. https://www.medicaleconomics.com/view/four-new-statistics-that-prove-that-telemedicine-isn-t-just-a-pandemic-fad.
69. Dunn P, Hazzard E. Technology approaches to digital health literacy. Int J Cardiol. 2019;293:294–6.
70. Vogels E. Lower-income Americans still less likely to have home broadband, smartphone | Pew Research Center [Internet]. [cited 2021 Nov 14]. https://www-pewresearch-org.libproxy.lib.unc.edu/

fact-tank/2021/06/22/digital-divide-persists-even-as-americans-with-lower-incomes-make-gains-in-tech-adoption.
71. Tierney AA. Tackling the digital divide by improving internet and telehealth access for low-income populations [Internet]. 2020 [cited 2022 Apr 18]. https://healthequity.berkeley.edu/sites/default/files/tacklingthedigitaldivide.pdf.
72. Chang JE, Lai AY, Gupta A, Nguyen AM, Berry CA, Shelley DR. Rapid transition to telehealth and the digital divide: implications for primary care access and equity in a post-COVID era. Milbank Q. 2021;99(2):340–68.
73. Shaw J, Brewer LC, Veinot T. Recommendations for health equity and virtual care arising from the COVID-19 pandemic: narrative review. JMIR Formativ Res. 2021;5(4):e23233.
74. Holyk T. The role of telehealth in improving continuity of care: the Carrier Sekani Family Services primary care model. BCMJ. 2017;59(9):459–64. https://bcmj.org/articles/role-telehealth-improving-continuity-care-carrier-sekani-family-services-primary-care-model

Acute Hospital Care

Amir Barzin, Yee Lam, and Matthew Zeitler

Introduction

Patients with chronic conditions contribute to a large portion of healthcare services and costs that are attributed to acute hospitalization. Among Americans, 25% have two or more chronic conditions and 68–80% of people aged 65 years or older have multiple chronic conditions [1]. In 2009, the Centers for Disease Control and Prevention (CDC) reported that 39% of all hospital admissions were associated with patients who had two to three chronic conditions, while 33% of admissions were tied to those who had four or more chronic conditions [2]. More than two-thirds of all hospital discharges in the United States are for individuals with multiple chronic conditions [1]. The aggregate number of chronic illnesses is associated with overall mortality, cost, and length of stay for hospitalized patients (Table 17.1) [1, 2].

Common chronic illnesses that are treated in acute hospital settings can broadly be classified into four categories: circulatory disorders (e.g., hypertension, congestive heart failure [CHF], stroke, coronary artery disease); respiratory disorders (e.g., asthma, chronic obstructive pulmonary disease [COPD]); endocrine disorders (e.g., diabetes mellitus); and mental health disorders (e.g., depression, anxiety, substance abuse, schizophrenia) [2]. Chronic diseases such as congestive heart failure (CHF) or chronic obstructive pulmonary disease (COPD) account for greater than 35% of admissions not related to surgery, obstetric care, newborn care, or psychiatric admission [3].

Each acute hospitalization is an opportunity to improve chronic disease management. This care goal starts with a structured, patient-centered approach at admission and ends with successful post-hospital planning. If hospital and transition care—from the inpatient to the outpatient setting—are well executed, there is great potential to improve outcomes, decrease inappropriate healthcare utilization, and reduce costs. This chapter addresses the unique challenges of providing hospital-based care for chronically ill patients. The first section directs attention to assessment and evaluation strategies, as well as admission workflows, for patients requiring hospital care. The next part addresses systems-level (e.g., antibiotic stewardship) and patient-level (e.g., advance care planning [ACP]) care principles for chronically ill patients who are hospitalized. The chapter then provides a review of discharge planning principles that are inclusive of transitional care and discusses the rapid changes in inpatient care during the global COVID-19 pandemic. The subsequent section highlights the unique impacts and challenges of comorbid mental health conditions on acute hospital care before closing with future directions in hospital care.

Table 17.1 Number of chronic diseases and mortality, inpatient service use, and cost for hospitalized patients (from Ref. [1])

	0–1 Chronic conditions	2–3 Chronic conditions	>4 Chronic conditions
Percent of discharges	28.81	38.56	32.64
Mortality rate	0.02	0.03	0.03
Mean length of stay (days)	4.46	5.21	5.42
Mean cost (USD)	10,544	11,180	11,095

Pre-admission Evaluation and Assessment

When evaluating a chronically ill patient for possible admission, it is important to address the patient's presenting complaints and gather collateral subjective and objective information regarding both the acute problem and the underlying chronic medical conditions.

A. Barzin · Y. Lam · M. Zeitler (✉)
Department of Family Medicine, University of North Carolina at Chapel Hill, Chapel Hill, NC, USA
e-mail: amir_barzin@med.unc.edu; yee_lam@med.unc.edu; mzeitler@med.unc.edu

History and Physical Examination

In an era of multiple information sources, a clear understanding of the patient's chief complaint and associated signs and symptoms is essential. This process begins with a detailed history of the events that contributed to a new or unexplained presenting symptom or to an acute exacerbation of the chronic illness. While gathering the history and developing a differential diagnosis, it is important to note the patient's main complaint, and the linkage of signs and symptoms with the underlying chronic disease. Understanding patient self-description and management of chronic conditions (e.g., glycemic control, home/clinic blood pressure readings), medication usage, and acute changes allows the provider to gauge insight into the patient's understanding of their chronic disease or gaps in current medical management. Communication techniques such active listening, rapport building, targeted open-ended and closed-ended questions, and non-verbal communication can be adapted to facilitate information gathering from the patient [4].

After the initial history taking and information gathering has been completed, a thorough physical examination can refine the differential diagnoses and guide next steps in ordering laboratory and other diagnostic testing. The physical examination should include a comprehensive inventory, as well as focused organ systems (e.g., heart and cardiovascular) that are guided by the history. Collateral information from family members or prior medical records can help distinguish physical findings (e.g., dependent edema, cardiac murmurs) that are stable and chronic versus those that are acute and decompensating. Biometric data, such as dry weight, blood pressure, and other vital signs, should be confirmed during the initial evaluation.

Collateral Information

As part of the American Recovery and Reinvestment Act, all public and private healthcare providers are required to adopt electronic medical records (EMRs) in order to participate in Medicaid and Medicare, a regulation that has promoted the widespread use of EMRs [5]. The patient's primary care physician (PCP) can be a key information source since most chronic disease management is provided in this setting [6]. In recent years, hospitalists have increased and fewer primary care physicians include hospital care in their scope of practice [7]. With this growing trend, many patients who have a long-established relationship with an outpatient provider are being cared for by hospital physicians who may not be familiar with their medical history. Effective and timely communication with the PCP and family members can improve the quality of care by gauging potential barriers to care, prior medication, and therapeutic regimens that have been ineffective and comorbid problems that may have contributed to hospitalization.

Medication Reconciliation

Medication reconciliation is a valuable component to the initial assessment since medication errors occur in 3.8 million inpatient admissions and 3.3 million outpatient visits a year, accounting for 7000 deaths annually [8, 9]. Several medication-related triggers can contribute to a hospitalization, including patient misunderstanding of medication instructions or misadministration. Ideally, medication reconciliation should be performed via direct visualization of pharmacy bottles or containers with the patient. However, this may not always be an option and reconciliation via an EMR report, a patient medication list, or verbally with the patient are alternative approaches. Other strategies include conversations with family members who have access to the patient's medications or confirmation of fill history with a patient's pharmacy.

Advance Care Planning

In chronically ill patients, advance care planning, discussions of resuscitation status, and surrogate decision-making should ideally occur prior to admission. Most healthcare costs are accrued in the last year of life and are often associated with unwanted and aggressive interventions with no defined endpoint [10]. Emergent procedures such as intubation and other resuscitation measures may not meaningfully contribute to the overall quality of life or functional status in chronically ill patients. Initiating discussions that are patient-centered and informed by evidence can guide goals of care discussions to identify the preferred level of care, and parameters around escalating medical management (e.g., intensive care) should the clinical condition worsen. These discussions and decisions should be clearly documented in the patient chart and be accessible to all members of the care team.

Admission

After the pre-admission assessment has been completed and the decision for hospitalization has been made, there are several areas to consider. These domains include determining the appropriate level of care (e.g., intensive care, step-down, acute, or observation bed) and a reasoned process for admitting orders that address active medical problems and limit the risk for iatrogenic error. At the time of admission, a rational approach to diagnostic testing and planned therapeutics should also consider discharge planning to facilitate transitional care once discharge goals have been met.

Level of Care

Patients who are admitted to the hospital in a non-surgical setting are generally designated as either inpatient or observation status. This classification impacts not only the level and intensity of care, but also the potential cost of care to the patient [11]. For example, there is variability among third-party payers regarding reimbursement for observation admissions, which are considered outpatient services. In some cases, the cost can fall to the patient (e.g., co-payment, deductible); in others, the hospital is the responsible party. The admitting physician should use clinical judgment to decide on the level of care that is the most appropriate for the patient. A discussion with the primary care physician at the time of admission may be informative, since early and reliable outpatient follow-up can often contribute to a shorter length of stay. Utilization management and physician advisors can help guide the appropriate admission level of care.

Admitting Orders

Admitting orders should be placed in an organized fashion that is responsive to the total care needs of the patient, and with attention to limiting unnecessary testing and prevention of nosocomial infections and iatrogenic errors. Many electronic health records include the capacity for provider order entry (POE), which is an electronic interface that allows clinicians to directly place orders [12]. POE programs were originally designed to identify and mitigate medication errors and have evolved with capacities to order laboratory tests, imaging, and hospital and outpatient consultations [13]. In addition, they often have functionalities for clinical decision support and evidence-based order sets that standardize workflows.

Patient mapping is an emerging practice that seeks to match and aggregate patients in specific hospital locations based on the clinical needs of the patient and the nursing and associated resources of the hospital. The process begins at admission when patient needs are identified, such as complicated medication regimens, frequent nursing assessments, or intensive biomonitoring (e.g., telemetry), and are then matched to the hospital location that can provide the level of care. Ideally, patient mapping has the potential to facilitate throughput from the emergency room to the hospital wards; however, bed availability is a rate-limiting step [14].

Preventing Iatrogenic Errors and Nosocomial Infections

Approximately 60% of hospitalized patients are at risk for developing venous thromboembolism (VTE) and nearly 275,000 new cases of VTE occur each year [15]. Despite evidence that a substantial proportion of hospitalized patients are at high risk for VTE, prophylaxis is underutilized [16]. Appropriate VTE prophylaxis can decrease VTE events by up to 63% and there are many approaches to prophylaxis, including both mechanical and pharmacologic prophylaxis [15]. The assessment of VTE risk at admission should be undertaken with consideration of existing chronic diseases to mitigate the potential risk for kidney damage or bleeding events. There are several validated risk assessment models, such as the Padua Prediction Score, that improve VTE risk stratification and aid in determining appropriateness of prophylaxis and account for underlying chronic comorbidities [16].

The prophylaxis modality is guided by an assessment of functional status, estimated length of stay, and risk of bleeding during admission. For those with limited mobility and longer lengths of stay or those at increased risk of VTE, pharmacologic prophylaxis such as subcutaneous heparin or low molecular-weight heparin is preferred [17]. Attention should be directed to patients with chronic kidney disease in dosing and medication selection. For those patients who are already on anticoagulation such as warfarin or direct oral anticoagulants (DOACs), continuation of these therapies is preferable if there are no contraindications [17]. Patients with anticipated shorter hospital stays may benefit from early ambulation or sequential compression devices (SCDs) if ambulation is not a limiting factor.

In addition to VTE prophylaxis, gastrointestinal (GI) prophylaxis should be considered in certain situations. The American Society of Health System Pharmacists recommends prophylaxis with a proton pump inhibitor (PPI) for patients with the following conditions in the intensive care unit (ICU): coagulopathy, mechanical ventilation longer than 48 h, GI ulcer or bleeding within the past year, sepsis, a stay longer than 1 week in the ICU, GI bleeding for 6 or more days, and steroid therapy with more than 250 mg of hydrocortisone daily, on nonsteroidal or antiplatelet medications [18]. Patients admitted to a general medical unit who are hemodynamically stable and not actively showing signs of GI hemorrhage do not require GI prophylaxis since this intervention does not significantly decrease the risk of GI bleeding [19]. However, the risks of continued or unnecessarily prolonged PPI use may lead to infections and complications, such as *Clostridium difficile* and community-acquired pneumonia, bone fracture, and reduced efficacy of medication absorption [20].

Nosocomial, or hospital-acquired, infections account for approximately 7 infections per 100 admissions [21]. Patients with chronic conditions are at increased risk for these infections, and hospital-wide protocols can limit the spread of existing infections and prevent outbreaks of new infections. At admission, providers should be aware of isolation/contact precaution guidelines, such as requirements for contact precautions in patients with a known history of resistant infection or respiratory precautions. Frequent handwashing or use of a sanitizing agent, and the use of sterile gowns, gloves, and masks in identified patients are hallmarks of such precautions. These measures have been shown to significantly reduce the risk of spreading nosocomial infections in healthcare settings [22, 23]. Additionally, safe injection and procedural techniques, as well as minimizing the duration of instrumentation such as central venous and urinary catheters, play an important role in nosocomial infection reduction.

Patients who are at risk for developing pressure ulcers (e.g., limited mobility, cognitive impairment) should be identified at admission and a prevention and treatment plan should be in place to reduce further progression. A thorough initial skin examination can target specific body locations (e.g., buttocks, heels) in patients who have decreased mobility or those with neuropathic conditions that limit their perception of pain. Risk factors for these patients include non-blanchable erythema, lymphopenia, immobility, dry skin, and decreased body weight [24]. Some current interventions to reduce the risk of skin ulcers and breakdown include the use of support surfaces, frequent repositioning by nursing or ancillary staff, and the use of nutritional support [25]. The evidence base around repositioning and nutritional support for mitigating skin breakdown is variable, while some studies support the use of technology-based support surfaces in the management and prevention of pressure ulcerations [25].

Laboratory and Diagnostic Testing

Laboratory and diagnostic testing can guide disease management during hospitalization. In patients with chronic conditions, laboratory values and radiographic studies should be compared to prior values if available. An elevated creatinine in a patient with chronic kidney disease, for example, may not reflect an acute event and needs to be placed within the context of a larger disease trajectory. Abnormal diagnostic values may trigger a cascade of unnecessary testing or duplicate. To limit unnecessary testing, collateral information from the electronic health record (EHR) and primary care physician, as well as the clinical history and physical exam findings, can reduce unnecessary phlebotomy draws and decrease hospital costs [26]. Less frequent testing can also be patient-centered via fewer patient interruptions and improvement in overall patient satisfaction.

Medication Management

Ongoing medication management is a foundation to quality hospital care. Providers should be attentive to the indication and selection of medications, and the potential interactions of new medications with existing chronic medications. For example, acute infections may require initial empiric antibiotic coverage which may have interactions with existing medications (e.g., fluoroquinolones and warfarin), or may predispose to iatrogenic complications (e.g., clindamycin and *C. diff* colitis). To mitigate this risk, a growing number of EMRs have the capacity to identify drug-drug interactions and reconcile medications.

Patients with chronic illness are generally maintained on long-term medications that reduce progression of their disease or improve their overall health status [27]. During admission, these medications may need to be titrated depending on the clinical status, a task that requires an understanding of attempted and failed therapies, and the therapeutic goals for treatment. Comprehensive changes to the medication regimen should weigh indications and benefits related to initiating a new drug and potential adverse effects, versus the proven track record of the long-term medication. It is also important to evaluate the efficacy and indications for new therapeutics after the acute phase of treatment.

Anti-hypertensive medications and heart failure regimens are frequently modified during acute hospitalization. A patient with hypertensive crisis in the hospital, for example, may need to have an increased dose of home medications to maximize therapy. For patients with preexisting heart failure or a heart failure exacerbation, evidence-based, goal-directed therapies may be added or titrated during hospitalization. When considering a medication change, the provider should consider how the presenting signs and symptoms—and the preliminary diagnosis—may impact the decision to increase or alter therapy. In a patient admitted with a COPD exacerbation, increasing the frequency of home medications (e.g., inhaled short-acting beta agonist) should be considered in the context of potential long-term therapy escalations to prevent future exacerbations, such as long-acting bronchodilators or combination therapies with antimuscarinic or corticosteroid-inhaled therapies [28]. As per the Global Initiative for Chronic Obstructive Lung Disease (GOLD), treatment pathways are guided by the patient's disease severity based on pulmonary function tests, symptoms, and frequency of exacerbations [28].

The management of fluids and electrolytes is another clinical consideration at admission. Maintaining overall fluid balance is important to prevent electrolyte abnormalities and to treat possible volume depletion states that can occur with acute illnesses. In some clinical settings (e.g., septic shock), timely fluid resuscitation is critical, and the immediate post-resuscitation period requires close monitoring of the patient.

Fluid and electrolyte management requires the appropriate selection of maintenance fluids and infusion rates. For hospitalized patients who require intravenous fluids, a combination of 5% dextrose in isotonic saline solutions is commonly used [29]. The infusion rates should be guided by the underlying disease process, ongoing fluid shifts or losses, and associated laboratory values. A commonly ordered rate in a euvolemic patient with no underlying illness is 100–120 cc/h [29].

Glucose management is critical in patients with diabetes mellitus. An informed understanding of the patient's medication regimen, current disease state, and nutritional status (e.g., nothing by mouth) leads to a structured approach to glucose management. Diabetic patients may require coverage with sliding-scale insulin or a higher dose of insulin to treat hyperglycemic states that are present in infection or acute illness. According to the American Diabetes Association (ADA), insulin should be administered using validated protocols that allow for predefined adjustments in the insulin dosage based on glycemic fluctuations [30]. Table 17.2 presents a sliding-scale insulin regimen for hospitalized patients.

There is increased risk of hypoglycemia in patients with acute illness with rigid glycemic control [31]. Patients who have limited or no oral intake require an adjustment in their home insulin dosing regimen, which is achieved by a reduction in the basal insulin requirement by approximately 50%, and by limiting bolus dosing and covering elevated glucose readings with sliding-scale parameters for testing and insulin administration [32]. Metformin has the potential to cause renal injury, particularly in patients with volume depleted states and those undergoing intravenous contrast studies.

The ADA recommends that all patients with diabetes or hyperglycemia (blood glucose >140 mg/dL/7.8–10.0 mmol/L) admitted to the hospital have A1C testing if not performed in the prior 3 months and consultation with a specialized diabetes or glucose management team if possible [30]. Insulin therapy should be initiated for treatment of persistent hyperglycemia starting at a threshold ≥180 mg/dL (10.0 mmol/L), with a target glucose range of 140–180 mg/dL (7.8–10.0 mmol/L) for the majority of critically ill and noncritically ill patients. More stringent goals, such as 110–140 mg/dL (6.1–7.8 mmol/L), may be appropriate for selected patients if they can be achieved without significant hypoglycemia [30].

Finally, acute hospitalization may present an opportunity for deprescribing of medications, such as aspirin and proton pump inhibitors that may no longer be indicated, potentially reducing polypharmacy in a monitored setting. Care should be taken when modifying a patient's chronic medication regimen and primary care physicians can be helpful in navigating changes.

Anticipated Length of Stay and Discharge Needs

The final component of the admission process is an estimation of the length of stay and the anticipated needs at hospital discharge. By identifying potential barriers to discharge at the time of admission, care teams can assess needs, such as occupational or physical therapy, or home health nursing care, or other community-based services. The early identification of discharge care needs has the potential to reduce length of stay, and subsequently decrease in-hospital mortality and 30-day mortality in chronic conditions such as congestive heart failure [33]. Although the anticipated length of stay may change due to progression of the index disease or new medical problems, the consideration of discharge planning at the time of admission can help optimize resource planning.

Acute Hospital Management

After admission, attention turns to hospital management of the patient. There are greater healthcare costs and increased morbidity associated with chronically ill patients who are hospitalized and a structured daily management plan must be utilized and adapted to maximize care.

Antibiotic and Medication Stewardship

With a rise in antibiotic resistance in the United States, the Center for Disease Control and Prevention (CDC) has identified antibiotic stewardship as a public health issue [34]. In acute hospital settings, more than half of the antibiotics pre-

Table 17.2 Suggested insulin protocol for hospitalized patients

Blood glucose level	51–70 mg/dL	71–150 mg/dL	151–200 mg/dL	201–250 mg/dL	251–300 mg/dL	301–350 mg/dL	351–400 mg/dL	>400 mg/dL
Units of aspart Insulin sensitive	Give juice	0	1	2	3	4	5	6
Units of aspart Standard	Give juice	0	2	4	6	8	10	12
Units of aspart Insulin resistant	Give juice	0	4	8	12	16	20	24

scribed are either not needed or inappropriate for patient care, which contributes to resistance or an increase in nosocomial infections such as *Clostridium difficile* [35–37]. For example, antibiotic prescribing was not supported in 79% of patients with community-acquired pneumonia, 77% of patients with urinary tract infections, 47% of patients prescribed with fluoroquinolone treatment, and 27% of patients prescribed with intravenous vancomycin [37]. Hospital care of the chronically ill patient should include measures to limit unnecessary or prolonged medication use through antibiotic stewardship programs [37].

According to the CDC, successful stewardship programs contain the following elements: leadership commitment, accountability, pharmacy expertise, action, tracking, reporting, and education [37]. Sustained implementation includes support from administrative and clinical champions, as well as securing institutional resources and removing barriers that impact the unnecessary use of antibiotics [37]. Implementation strategies include planning and execution approaches, as well as information technology (IT) systems that can provide tracking and reporting mechanisms for the care teams [37]. IT prompts and workflows that have been embedded in provider order entry (POE) systems have included required documentation of the antibiotic indication with clear start and stop dates, and prompts and flow charts to inform antibiotic coverage [37].

Both IT-based interventions and academic detailing by pharmacy specialists have been found to be effective strategies. For example, Doctor of Pharmacy (Pharm.D) programs include training in health improvement and outreach, an initiative that has increased the role of hospital pharmacists in promoting antibiotic management and diabetes care [38–40]. The responsible and evidence-based use of medications can reduce approximately 20,000 deaths that are attributed to antibiotic-resistant infections [41]. Additionally, structured antibiotic "time-outs" during acute hospitalization to review the dose, duration, and indication of antibiotics when cultures and new clinical information become available may help optimize appropriate antibiotic use and stewardship [42].

These system-level principles of active medication management can be applied to other hospital workflows. For example, the use of fixed order sets (i.e., bundles) for sepsis often includes rapid laboratory and other diagnostic tests and targeted antibiotics that are based on a presumed source of infection [43]. In addition, a patient at risk for VTE would have a bundle that includes laboratory and radiographic testing, nursing interventions, and a heparin nomogram based on whether treatment is indicated for a pulmonary embolism or deep vein thrombosis.

Changes in Patient Status

The clinical course of the hospitalized patient changes, which guides the level of surveillance, nursing, and ancillary care, such as a medical unit bed or higher level of care (i.e., ICU or intermediate care unit). Medical unit beds are generally indicated for stable hospitalized patients who require structured surveillance (e.g., vital signs, biometrics) and a standardized level of nursing and ancillary care (e.g., intravenous medication administration, wound care, respiratory therapy).

The staffing requirements for medical beds can vary by hospital; however, there are common guidelines which include the nursing to patient ratio and frequency of patient assessments [44]. Intensive care units (ICU) typically have an individualized nurse to patient ratio and greater resources to care for critically ill patients, such as the capacity for patients requiring mechanical ventilation. This level of care is generally managed by a team of specialists, led by an intensivist, and is usually limited to a finite number of patients. Hospitals may have an intermediate care or step-down unit, which is a hybrid between the medical floor and ICU. These units have a reduced nursing staff model when compared to an ICU setting, but they provide a more closely monitored environment than a medical floor. For example, patients who are transitioning out of the ICU are often transferred to a step-down unit for closer monitoring. Others patient subgroups who are candidates for step-down units include those who require closer monitoring for conditions such as alcohol withdrawal or patients that are not critically ill but are unstable and require advanced therapies such as continuous respiratory support with bilevel positive airway pressure (BIPAP).

Chronically ill patients may acutely decompensate in hospital settings and these situations require a timely assessment, expedited treatment, and possible escalation in their care. Prompt evaluation of such patients can be achieved through a rapid response or code team [45]. The rapid response or code can be initiated by any member of the hospital staff and activation results in a structured and timely evaluation of the patient, and mobilization of resources to promote care. These teams can be composed of a physician, a senior nurse, and if available a pharmacist, a security officer, and a patient transport technician. Common conditions for evaluation of such patients include low blood pressure, rapid heart rate, respiratory distress, and altered mental status [46]. After the arrival of the team, stabilization of the patient is performed, and a rapid assessment process allows for administration of medications and bedside testing. Once the patient is stabilized, the care team decides on the subsequent level of care.

Care Teams

Acute hospital service lines are utilizing multi-disciplinary teams, which have improved quality of care and decreased length of stay [47]. These teams are generally composed of physicians or advanced practice providers (APPs), nurses, therapists (speech, occupational, and physical), pharmacists, care managers, and chaplains. Within this structure, each provider works at the top of his or her license to complement the skill set of each team member. Physicians and APPs may direct the team and are directly accountable for the overall care provided to the patient. However, information about the patient and care duties—such as daily care plans, medication management, and assessment for discharge—can be delegated to respective members. Input across all team members is vital for effective patient management. Activities and tasks include ongoing nursing discussions regarding changes in patient status, vital signs, or overall medical condition [47]. Allied health therapists (e.g., OT, PT) provide functional assessments and treatments that inform discharge planning.

Medical specialists (e.g., cardiology, nephrology) and/or surgical specialists (e.g., general surgery, orthopedics) may be requested to consult on the patient's acute presentation and/or their underlying chronic condition(s). Consultations may take place in-person or through virtual platforms including telephone, video, or electronic consultation (e-consultation) that involve extensive chart review followed by recommendations without in-person contact [48]. Consulting teams provide recommendations to the patient's primary medical or surgical team and may lead to transfer of care to subspecialty teams, depending on the patient's medical or surgical needs.

Care managers are an important complement to the hospital care team and are traditionally either social work or nursing trained. They are available to patients and their families for facilitating discharge planning and coordinating care across healthcare environments, as well as in the home or long-term care setting [49]. Care management functions may include identifying resources to help with chronic disease management, assisting families in outreach to community-based organizations, or by serving as a line of communication between the patient and the physician [49]. Care managers can also provide patients with resources regarding government and private agencies in areas such as housing, legal aid, and securing health insurance.

Multi-disciplinary rounding (MDR) or communication and patient planning (CAPP) rounds is a process that involves a discussion among all members of the patient care team about patient care, including progress, barriers, and disposition [50]. Physicians, nurses, and other members of the care team may address the hospital course while ancillary staff cover social and other resource needs that impact discharge, such as durable medical equipment, transitional care to a skilled nursing facility (SNF), or referral to other providers if indicated. Afternoon CAPP rounds to identify early patient discharges the following day have been shown to increase electronic discharge orders and patient discharges by noon without an adverse change in readmission rates and length of stay (LOS) [50].

Quality Improvement and Patient Safety

Healthcare systems strive to provide safe and high-quality care to patients. Many hospitals have defined quality improvement metrics and performance measures that are actively tracked, acted on, reevaluated, and modified over time [51]. These performance measures may include outcomes such as inpatient falls, venous thromboembolic events, catheter-associated urinary tract infections (CAUTIs), surgical site infections, and readmission rates. Most healthcare systems engage in ongoing quality improvement, patient safety, and track morbidity and mortality to identify gaps in patient safety and opportunities for improvement [51]. Hospitals have patient reporting systems for adverse events and mechanisms for patients and caregivers to identify care gaps and areas of improvement [52].

Advance Care Planning

Advance care planning should ideally be undertaken during each hospital admission for chronically ill patients. Advance care planning (ACP) has shown to improve the quality of end-of-life care and decrease unnecessary hospitalizations, although there is variability in the number and types of frequently hospitalized patients with chronic diseases who have considered ACP [53–55]. Several principles can help guide effective ACP: (a) there is an overall intent to improve communication with patients, caregivers, and providers; (b) the process seeks to identify and clarify goals of care; (c) care teams and providers should prepare patient and family caregivers for the functional limitations and overall health declines that may occur at the end of life; and (d) the ACP process should seek to mitigate family member or surrogate burden [56]. Particularly among chronically ill patients with end-stage disease, providers can promote ACP discussions when patients are clinically stable and have decisional capacity. Family members and other stakeholders should also be involved in the discussion and ongoing decision-making process [56]. In cases where there is a lack of patient decisional capacity, the provider and care team should seek to facilitate the appointment of a surrogate.

There are many resources to help with ACP. Some organizations have trained and certified staff workers to assist in locating documents (e.g., living wills) and in the process of appointing decision-makers and healthcare powers of attorney [57]. In some states, a medical orders for scope of treatment (MOST) form can tailor specific care plans, such as the initiation or withholding of antibiotic therapy [58]. Do not resuscitate (DNR) orders and information placards that specify no further hospitalizations provide visual reminders to providers of patient directives. ACP should be viewed as an ongoing, iterative process and it is important to review prior discussions and documents to promote an active dialogue with the patient and surrogate decision-makers.

Family members and patient surrogate decision-makers may request a meeting with the care team to clarify ACP. Standardized documentation of the meeting's outcome in the medical record is recommended to communicate the care plan to all members of the hospital team. Elements of the meeting might include documentation of the meeting's date; the stakeholders who were involved and their role in the patient's care; the disease process and patient and stakeholder understanding of the disease trajectory; treatment options; and prior discussions and current decisions regarding care planning. Closed-loop communication between providers and both inpatient and outpatient care team members (i.e., nurses, therapists, primary care physician) can promote an understanding of the care plan to all members.

Discharge

Discharge planning should not wait until the day of discharge but should be part of the ongoing workflow in daily inpatient care to facilitate a timely and effective transition after acute hospitalization.

Post-discharge Location

Table 17.3 displays post-hospitalization care sites and associated services which include home healthcare, skilled nursing facility care, and hospice care. Many chronically ill patients who are stable after an acute hospitalization can safely be discharged to home with early follow-up with their primary care physician. Other patients may have nursing or other needs at discharge that require sub-acute care.

Home healthcare services are resources for patients who may require a basic level of nursing care, such as wound care or intravenous antibiotic therapy, or allied healthcare services such as physical, occupational, or speech therapy. Home health agencies provide patient education around medication management and self-monitoring of chronic diseases, such as congestive heart failure. Family and other caregivers are generally required to be available to assist patients in their care [59]. In general, to be eligible for home health services by Medicare, the patient must be confined to the home, under the care of a physician, have a prescribed plan of care, and need skilled nursing on an intermittent (i.e., approximately three times a week) basis or require physical, speech, or continued occupational therapy [60]. Information regarding the patient's progress and care plan is reported to the primary care physician.

Table 17.3 Post-hospitalization care sites and associated services

	Home with no home health	Home with home health	Skilled nursing facility	Home hospice
Nursing services	None	Medication reconciliation and management Wound care IV therapy Chronic disease teaching	Provided on site at facility for oversight of care of the patient	Provided on intake and an on-call basis
Medication management	Patient administers own medications	Patient administers own medications	Administered by facility staff	Review of medications with family and emphasis on pain and symptom control
Physical therapy	Not provided	Provided at a maximum of three times a week	Provided up to five times a week	Provided as needed
Occupational therapy	Not provided	Provided at a maximum of three times a week	Provided up to five times a week	Provided as needed
Speech therapy	Not provided	Provided at a maximum of three times a week	Provided up to five times a week	Provided as needed
Responsible physician	Primary care physician	Initial orders usually signed by hospital physician with subsequent orders by primary care physician	Facility medical director	Hospice medical director or primary care physician

Skilled nursing facilities (SNFs) may be considered in patients who require more intense or prolonged therapy that cannot be provided in the home. SNFs are licensed facilities that provide onsite nursing and allied health services with medical oversight; the average length of stay is about 26 days [61]. If a patient is a candidate for a SNF, the patient or family caregivers work with ancillary team members (e.g., care manager or discharge planner) to identify a facility that will accept the patient for admission. Once identified, the discharging physician prepares a discharge summary with an accurate medication list and care plan to the facility. Upon transfer to the SNF, the receiving physician (i.e., the medical director) reviews the orders and assumes care of the patient while they are in the SNF. The Centers for Medicare and Medicaid Services (CMS) has developed a five-star quality rating system for nursing homes that is indexed to quality of care [62].

Acute inpatient rehabilitation and long-term acute care hospitals are additional post-hospital settings that have functional criteria, such as the capacity to participate in therapy, for admission [63, 64]. Hospice care, either at home or in an inpatient facility, is an option for chronically ill patients if they have a life expectancy of less than 6 months [65]. The hospice model offers patients and families a patient-centered approach to care where a family member serves as the primary caregiver. The hospice care team develops an individualized plan to meet the needs of the patient based on managing symptoms and provides on-call staff to manage acute symptoms or other problems [65]. Over 75% of those entering hospice care, the primary diagnosis is cancer, dementia, heart disease, or lung disease [66]. Inpatient hospice is generally considered for patients with sustained nursing care needs, such as pain and symptom management, which cannot be managed in other settings. The quality of life for patients who are in hospice remains relatively stable throughout their terminal illness course and at the end of life [67].

Medication Reconciliation

Medication reconciliation is a vital part of the discharge process since medications often change during hospitalization. The patient's medication list should be reviewed and updated to reflect for what will be prescribed during post-hospital care. This list should also identify medications that the patient is no longer taking, as well as the duration of medicines that have a defined timeframe, such as antibiotic therapy. Medication adherence and compliance can be enhanced after discharge with the use of a pillbox or blister packaging dispensed by pharmacies [68].

Patient Education

Patient education should include information about the underlying disease processes, treatment instructions, an inventory of warning signs and symptoms, and guidelines and locations for seeking emergency care for worsening conditions. Unfortunately, patient discharge information is generally provided at a level that is higher than the reading level of the average patient, overestimating patient's cognitive function and health literacy [69]. The provider or health educator should identify any functional, cognitive, or educational limitations to how patients process information and consider strategies to mitigate these challenges.

Patient education can be facilitated by several members of the hospital care team; nursing or pharmacy staff can complement and enhance patient understanding. Teach back is one strategy in which the patient educator provides the patient with specific information items, such as how to limit future exacerbations, and then asks the patient to instruct the provider in their own words [70]. Multi-disciplinary approaches and strategies that use detailed information sources can improve outcomes as much as 50–80% [71]. Patients and their support systems should ideally be discharged with a clear understanding of the reasons for hospitalization, their medications, follow-up plans, and red flag or alarm symptoms.

Discharge Summary

After a hospitalization, communication with primary care providers (PCP) and other treating clinicians can be achieved through a structured and well-documented discharge summary. There is no standard format for information components in the discharge summary in the United States; however, other countries have required specific elements. In the United Kingdom, for example, discharge summaries include complete patient details (e.g., name, date of birth, admission date, discharge date); admitting diagnosis and any comorbidities, procedures; prescribed medications and dosing and frequency of all medications; description of why a medication was started or stopped; length of course for medications (i.e., antibiotics); allergies and health and treatment information that was provided to the patient [72].

The hospital course should accurately describe the patient's clinical problems and associated treatment plan. A clear and succinct narrative allows the follow-up physician to grasp the differential diagnosis for nonspecific presenting symptoms (e.g., chest pain) and follow the clinical logic flow of a patient's hospitalization. The discharge summary should also include relevant laboratory values that informed treatment, as well as those that are still pending at the time of discharge and require follow up. Any diagnostic tests or therapeutic procedures or operations should also be included to limit duplicate testing.

Finally, the discharge summary should include any clinical complications that occurred or new diagnoses that will require follow-up items after discharge. Documentation of advanced care planning should also be included. Social determinants that were identified during the hospitalization, such as poverty, should be included since these factors may impact the capacity of the patient to receive medications or follow-up care.

Transitional Care

Transitional care focuses on the care processes that occur when a patient moves between healthcare settings, such as from hospital or skilled nursing facility to home. The Coleman Model is well recognized and seeks to engage patients with multiple care needs and improve the quality of the care they receive at the time they are being discharged from hospitalization [73]. There are four pillars in the model: assistance with medication self-management; a patient-centered record owned and maintained by the patient; timely follow-up with primary or specialty care (within 7–14 days); and a list of "red flags" indicative of a worsening condition and instructions on how to respond to them [73]. The model has demonstrated that engaging chronically ill patients with a transition coach helps reduce hospital readmissions and has associated cost savings [73]. In this approach, patients take ownership in their disease process and the coaches provide the capacity for ongoing assessments in the critical timeframe immediately after discharge [73].

Special Considerations

Hospital medicine is constantly adapting to patient and community needs, integrating new technologies and innovating new strategies to improve care.

COVID-19 Pandemic

In early 2020, the landscape of hospital care was changed by the COVID-19 pandemic, as the medical and scientific community adapted and responded to adverse health and health service impacts of this new virus [74]. Hospital teams worked to care for patients in multiple inpatient units that were at or over capacity, often with inadequate supplies of personal protective equipment (PPE). Teams huddled daily within and across healthcare systems, sharing information about new therapies and novel uses for established therapies.

As the PPE supply chain stabilized, healthcare systems adopted universal precautions (e.g., masking, face shield) and symptom screening precautions. Donning and doffing monitors observed healthcare staff putting on and taking off PPE from gloves to respirators to avoid contamination. Patients requiring care ranging from observation to intensive care were interacting with team members often without seeing their faces, highlighting even more the importance of clear communication and empathic care [75, 76]. Hospital staffing shortages reflected long hours of emotionally and physically draining work [77]. Patient visitation was restricted in the hospital across all patient care areas, such as laboring mothers and patients receiving cancer treatment [78, 79]. These restrictions impacted family members' ability to advocate and understand the care of their loved ones [80].

Behavioral Health

Behavioral health disorders are among the costliest conditions and poor mental health has profound consequences [81–83]. Mental health disorders, such as depression, impact the etiology, course, and outcomes associated with chronic disease while different mental health conditions may increase risk for chronic disease and disability [84]. Chronically ill patients may be admitted to the hospital for acute or unstable mental illness or behavioral health disturbances may manifest or exacerbate during acute hospitalizations. Consultation with a psychiatrist may be helpful and patient-centered depending on the mental health condition and the comfort level of the inpatient care team. On the other hand, unstable patients admitted to a psychiatric hospital or facility may have chronic diseases that complicate their hospitalization, sometimes necessitating medical consultation [85]. Several innovative models have emerged that integrate mental health and medical care, including virtual or digitally enabled care, and inpatient collaborative care with consultation-liaison psychiatry [86, 87].

Patients with Limited Decision-Making Capacity

The patient capacity for medical decision-making is an important consideration during hospitalization. Medical decision-making capacity is the ability of a patient to understand the benefits, risks, and the alternatives to a proposed treatment or intervention including no treatment [88]. Capacity is the basis of informed consent. Patients have medical decision-making capacity if they can demonstrate understanding of the situation, appreciation of the consequences of their decision, reasoning in their thought process, and if they can communicate their wishes [88]. Sometimes, a formal capacity evaluation should be considered if there is reason to question a patient's decision-making abilities, including an acute change in mental status, refusal of a clearly beneficial recommended treatment, risk factors for impaired decision-making, or readily agreeing to an invasive or risky procedure without adequately considering the risks and benefits. Psychiatrists may be helpful in formally evaluating a patient's capacity and there are several validated assessment tools. Ultimately, final determination on capacity is made by the treating physician [88].

Patients with mental illness who pose a danger to self or others may be admitted to a psychiatric hospital involuntarily through a process called involuntary civil commitment (IVC). IVC is enacted either over a patient's objection or where it's felt that they are so incapacitated that they're not able to provide informed consent for a voluntary hospitalization for the purpose of stabilizing a mental illness and treating the symptoms that led to them being admitted to the hospital on an involuntary basis. Laws, policies, and procedures for IVC vary by state in the United States [89].

Future Directions

There is an ongoing movement to value-base healthcare and the US Center for Medicare and Medicaid Services (CMS) has established reimbursement and penalty guidelines around hospital readmission [90]. In consequence, hospitals and healthcare systems will be looking at ways to decrease inappropriate readmissions and improve the care of those with chronic disease. Many hospital systems are looking at extensivist model. In general, extensivists are physicians or care providers who provide comprehensive, coordinated care to a limited number of high-risk chronically ill patients [91]. The small panel size facilitates a focus on managing complex medical conditions and coordinating care. This innovation seeks to place patients at the center of a complex medical system and work with them to improve care. Many variations of extensivist models are beginning to appear across the country and the impact of this staffing approach on chronic disease management is uncertain [91].

Transition clinic models are another development. In these settings, high-risk and medically complex patients receive care in outpatient primary and specialty care settings by a team that includes a physician, a pharmacist, and a care manager [92]. This model has shown benefit, especially when performed within 7 days of discharge and can lead to a 20% reduction in readmission for patients with multiple chronic conditions [92]. The COVID-19 pandemic has also revitalized telehealth innovation. Electronic inpatient consults are much more widely available now, with associated payment models in place [93].

CMS has rolled out the Hospital Without Walls program, which was expanded to Acute Hospital Care at Home in November 2020 [94, 95]. These models utilize a remote virtual provider who is linked with an augmented home healthcare team. These teams provide inpatient level care in patients' homes with intravenous diuresis, antibiotics, and other services. The ultimate goal for these and other innovations is to increase access and optimize hospitalize resource utilization while maintaining high-quality and compassionate patient care.

References

1. Skinner HG, Coffey R, Jones J, Heslin KC, Moy E. The effects of multiple chronic conditions on hospitalization costs and utilization for ambulatory care sensitive conditions in the United States: a nationally representative cross-sectional study. BMC Health Serv Res. 2016;16:77.
2. Steiner CA, Friedman B. Hospital utilization, costs, and mortality for adults with multiple chronic conditions, Nationwide Inpatient Sample, 2009. Prev Chronic Dis. 2013;10:E62.
3. Pfuntner A, Wier LM, Stocks C. Most frequent conditions in U.S. hospitals, 2010: statistical brief #148. Healthcare Cost and Utilization Project (HCUP) Statistical Briefs. Rockville, MD: Agency for Healthcare Research and Quality (US); 2006.
4. Lauster CD, Srivastava SB. Fundamental skills for patient care in pharmacy practice. Burlington, MA: Jones & Bartlett Learning; 2013.
5. GovInfo [Internet]. [cited 2022 May 1]. https://www.govinfo.gov/content/pkg/PLAW-111publ5/pdf/PLAW-111publ5.pdf.
6. CDC [Internet]. [cited 2022 Apr 7]. https://www.cdc.gov/nchs/data/ahcd/namcs_summary/2018-namcs-web-tables-508.pdf.
7. Hospitalists: a growing part of the primary care workforce [Internet]. [cited 2022 May 1]. https://www.aamc.org/media/8316/download.
8. Mehi [Internet]. [cited 2022 May 1]. https://mehi.masstech.org/sites/mehi/files/documents/cpoe2008.pdf.
9. Institute of Medicine (US) Committee on Quality of Health Care in America. In: Kohn LT, Corrigan JM, Donaldson MS, editors. To err is human: building a safer health system. Washington, DC: National Academies Press; 2000.
10. Hogan C, Lunney J, Gabel J, Lynn J. Medicare beneficiaries' costs of care in the last year of life. Health Aff (Millwood). 2001;20(4):188–95.
11. Clevelandclinic [Internet]. [cited 2022 Apr 7]. https://my.clevelandclinic.org/-/scassets/files/org/locations/price-lists/main-campus-hospital-patient-price-list.pdf.
12. Aarts J, Koppel R. Implementation of computerized physician order entry in seven countries. Health Aff (Millwood). 2009;28(2):404–14.
13. Agency for Healthcare Research and Quality. Inpatient computerized provider order entry: findings from the AHRQ Health IT Portfolio (Prepared by the AHRQ National Resource Center for Health IT). AHRQ Publication No. 09-0031-EF. Rockville, MD: Agency for Healthcare Research and Quality; 2009. [Internet]. [cited 2022 May 1]. https://digital.ahrq.gov/sites/default/files/docs/page/09-0031-EF_cpoe.pdf.

14. Martin M, Champion R, Kinsman L, Masman K. Mapping patient flow in a regional Australian emergency department: a model driven approach. Int Emerg Nurs. 2011;19(2):75–85.
15. Qazizada M, McKaba J, Roe M. Hospital-acquired venous thromboembolism: a retrospective analysis of risk factor screening and prophylactic therapy. Hosp Pharm. 2010;45(2):122–8.
16. Barbar S, Noventa F, Rossetto V, Ferrari A, Brandolin B, Perlati M, et al. A risk assessment model for the identification of hospitalized medical patients at risk for venous thromboembolism: the Padua Prediction Score. J Thromb Haemost. 2010;8(11):2450–7.
17. Guyatt GH, Akl EA, Crowther M, Gutterman DD, Schuünemann HJ, American College of Chest Physicians Antithrombotic Therapy and Prevention of Thrombosis Panel. Executive summary: Antithrombotic therapy and prevention of thrombosis, 9th ed: American college of chest physicians evidence-based clinical practice guidelines. Chest. 2012;141(2 Suppl):7S–47S.
18. Barkun AN, Bardou M, Pham CQD, Martel M. Proton pump inhibitors vs. histamine 2 receptor antagonists for stress-related mucosal bleeding prophylaxis in critically ill patients: a meta-analysis. Am J Gastroenterol. 2012;107(4):507–20; quiz 521.
19. Herzig SJ, Vaughn BP, Howell MD, Ngo LH, Marcantonio ER. Acid-suppressive medication use and the risk for nosocomial gastrointestinal tract bleeding. Arch Intern Med. 2011;171(11):991–7.
20. Moayyedi P, Leontiadis GI. The risks of PPI therapy. Nat Rev Gastroenterol Hepatol. 2012;9(3):132–9.
21. Haley RW, Hooton TM, Culver DH, Stanley RC, Emori TG, Hardison CD, et al. Nosocomial infections in U.S. hospitals, 1975–1976: estimated frequency by selected characteristics of patients. Am J Med. 1981;70(4):947–59.
22. Safdar N, Marx J, Meyer NA, Maki DG. Effectiveness of preemptive barrier precautions in controlling nosocomial colonization and infection by methicillin-resistant Staphylococcus aureus in a burn unit. Am J Infect Control. 2006;34(8):476–83.
23. Seto WH, Tsang D, Yung RWH, Ching TY, Ng TK, Ho M, et al. Effectiveness of precautions against droplets and contact in prevention of nosocomial transmission of severe acute respiratory syndrome (SARS). Lancet. 2003;361(9368):1519–20.
24. Allman RM, Goode PS, Patrick MM, Burst N, Bartolucci AA. Pressure ulcer risk factors among hospitalized patients with activity limitation. JAMA. 1995;273(11):865–70.
25. Lozano-Montoya I, Vélez-Díaz-Pallarés M, Abraha I, Cherubini A, Soiza RL, O'Mahony D, et al. Nonpharmacologic interventions to prevent pressure ulcers in older patients: an overview of systematic reviews (The Software ENgine for the Assessment and optimization of drug and non-drug Therapy in Older peRsons [SENATOR] definition of Optimal Evidence-Based Non-drug Therapies in Older People [ONTOP] Series). J Am Med Dir Assoc. 2016;17(4):370.e1–10.
26. May TA, Clancy M, Critchfield J, Ebeling F, Enriquez A, Gallagher C, et al. Reducing unnecessary inpatient laboratory testing in a teaching hospital. Am J Clin Pathol. 2006;126(2):200–6.
27. Bauer UE, Briss PA, Goodman RA, Bowman BA. Prevention of chronic disease in the 21st century: elimination of the leading preventable causes of premature death and disability in the USA. Lancet. 2014;384(9937):45–52.
28. 2022 GOLD reports - global initiative for chronic obstructive lung disease - GOLD [Internet]. [cited 2022 Apr 7]. https://goldcopd.org/2022-gold-reports-2/.
29. Moritz ML, Ayus JC. Maintenance intravenous fluids in acutely ill patients. N Engl J Med. 2015;373(14):1350–60.
30. American Diabetes Association. 15. Diabetes Care in the hospital: standards of medical care in diabetes-2021. Diabetes Care. 2021;44(Suppl 1):S211–20.
31. Wiener RS, Wiener DC, Larson RJ. Benefits and risks of tight glucose control in critically ill adults: a meta-analysis. JAMA. 2008;300(8):933–44.
32. Schnipper JL, Ndumele CD, Liang CL, Pendergrass ML. Effects of a subcutaneous insulin protocol, clinical education, and computerized order set on the quality of inpatient management of hyperglycemia: results of a clinical trial. J Hosp Med. 2009;4(1):16–27.
33. Bueno H, Ross JS, Wang Y, Chen J, Vidán MT, Normand S-LT, et al. Trends in length of stay and short-term outcomes among Medicare patients hospitalized for heart failure, 1993–2006. JAMA. 2010;303(21):2141–7.
34. CDC looks back at 2013 health challenges, ahead to 2014 health worries | Press Release | CDC Online Newsroom | CDC [Internet]. [cited 2022 May 1]. https://www.cdc.gov/media/releases/2013/p1216-eoy2013.html.
35. Ingram PR, Seet JM, Budgeon CA, Murray R. Point-prevalence study of inappropriate antibiotic use at a tertiary Australian hospital. Intern Med J. 2012;42(6):719–21.
36. Fridkin S, Baggs J, Fagan R, Magill S, Pollack LA, Malpiedi P, et al. Vital signs: improving antibiotic use among hospitalized patients. MMWR Morb Mortal Wkly Rep. 2014;63(9):194–200.
37. Core elements of hospital antibiotic stewardship programs | Antibiotic use | CDC [Internet]. [cited 2021 Dec 1]. https://www.cdc.gov/antibiotic-use/core-elements/hospital.html.
38. ACPE [Internet]. [cited 2022 May 3]. https://www.acpe-accredit.org/pdf/Standards2016FINAL.pdf.
39. Zenzano T, Allan JD, Bigley MB, Bushardt RL, Garr DR, Johnson K, et al. The roles of healthcare professionals in implementing clinical prevention and population health. Am J Prev Med. 2011;40(2):261–7.
40. Cranor CW, Christensen DB. The Asheville Project: factors associated with outcomes of a community pharmacy diabetes care program. J Am Pharm Assoc (Wash). 2003;43(2):160–72.
41. CDC [Internet]. [cited 2022 May 3]. https://www.cdc.gov/drugresistance/pdf/ar-threats-2013-508.pdf.
42. Lee TC, Frenette C, Jayaraman D, Green L, Pilote L. Antibiotic self-stewardship: trainee-led structured antibiotic time-outs to improve antimicrobial use. Ann Intern Med. 2014;161(10 Suppl):S53–8.
43. Armen SB, Freer CV, Showalter JW, Crook T, Whitener CJ, West C, et al. Improving outcomes in patients with sepsis. Am J Med Qual. 2016;31(1):56–63.
44. Nurse staffing | American Nurses Association | ANA [Internet]. [cited 2022 May 3]. https://www.nursingworld.org/practice-policy/nurse-staffing/.
45. Beitler JR, Link N, Bails DB, Hurdle K, Chong DH. Reduction in hospital-wide mortality after implementation of a rapid response team: a long-term cohort study. Crit Care. 2011;15(6):R269.
46. Jones DA, DeVita MA, Bellomo R. Rapid-response teams. N Engl J Med. 2011;365(2):139–46.
47. O'Mahony S, Mazur E, Charney P, Wang Y, Fine J. Use of multidisciplinary rounds to simultaneously improve quality outcomes, enhance resident education, and shorten length of stay. J Gen Intern Med. 2007;22(8):1073–9.
48. Serling-Boyd N, Miloslavsky EM. Enhancing the inpatient consultation learning environment to optimize teaching and learning. Rheum Dis Clin N Am. 2020;46(1):73–83.
49. Bindman AB, Cox DF. Changes in health care costs and mortality associated with transitional care management services after a discharge among Medicare beneficiaries. JAMA Intern Med. 2018;178(9):1165–71.
50. Kher S, Haas M, Schelling K, Wright S, Allison H, Poutsiaka DD, et al. Late-afternoon communication and patient planning (CAPP) rounds: an intervention to allow early patient discharges. Hosp Pract (Minneap). 2021;49(1):56–61.
51. Vaughan Sarrazin MS, Girotra S. Exact science and the art of approximating quality in hospital performance metrics. JAMA Netw Open. 2019;2(7):e197321.
52. Moureaud C, Hertig JB, Weber RJ. Guidelines for leading a safe medication error reporting culture. Hosp Pharm. 2020;2020:001857872093175.

53. Brinkman-Stoppelenburg A, Rietjens JAC, van der Heide A. The effects of advance care planning on end-of-life care: a systematic review. Palliat Med. 2014;28(8):1000–25.
54. Heyland DK, Barwich D, Pichora D, Dodek P, Lamontagne F, You JJ, et al. Failure to engage hospitalized elderly patients and their families in advance care planning. JAMA Intern Med. 2013;173(9):778–87.
55. Sam M, Singer PA. Canadian outpatients and advance directives: poor knowledge and little experience but positive attitudes. Can Med Assoc J. 1993;148(9):1497–502.
56. Fried TR, Redding CA, Robbins ML, Paiva A, O'Leary JR, Iannone L. Stages of change for the component behaviors of advance care planning. J Am Geriatr Soc. 2010;58(12):2329–36.
57. Advance Care Planning-general [Internet]. [cited 2022 May 3]. https://coalitionccc.org/CCCC/Our-Work/Advance-Care-Planning/CCCC/Our-Work/Advance-Care-Planning-general.aspx?hkey=a1277e14-9608-4c20-b90e-0706babfda36.
58. Caprio AJ. Medical Orders for Scope of Treatment (MOST): honoring patient preferences across the continuum of care. N C Med J. 2014;75(5):349–50.
59. Nadarević-Stefanec V, Malatestinić D, Mataija-Redzović A, Nadarević T. Patient satisfaction and quality in home health care of elderly islanders. Coll Antropol. 2011;35(Suppl 2):213–6.
60. CMS [Internet]. [cited 2022 Apr 11]. https://www.cms.gov/medicare/medicare-fee-for-service-payment/homehealthpps/downloads/face-to-face-requirement-powerpoint.pdf.
61. DaVanzo JE [Internet]. [cited 2022 May 3]. https://www.aopanet.org/wp-content/uploads/2014/07/Dobson-DaVanzo-Final-Report-Patient-Outcomes.pdf.
62. Five-star quality rating system | CMS [Internet]. [cited 2022 May 3]. https://www.cms.gov/Medicare/Provider-Enrollment-and-Certification/CertificationandComplianc/FSQRS.
63. Inpatient rehabilitation facilities | CMS [Internet]. [cited 2022 May 3]. https://www.cms.gov/Medicare/Provider-Enrollment-and-Certification/CertificationandComplianc/InpatientRehab.
64. CMS [Internet]. [cited 2022 May 3]. https://www.cms.gov/medicare/medicare-fee-for-service-payment/longtermcarehospitalpps/downloads/rti_ltchpps_final_rpt.pdf.
65. Hospice care coverage [Internet]. [cited 2022 Apr 7]. https://www.medicare.gov/coverage/hospice-care.
66. NHPCO [Internet]. [cited 2022 May 3]. https://www.nhpco.org/wp-content/uploads/NHPCO-Facts-Figures-2020-edition.pdf.
67. Bretscher M, Rummans T, Sloan J, Kaur J, Bartlett A, Borkenhagen L, et al. Quality of life in hospice patients. A pilot study. Psychosomatics. 1999;40(4):309–13.
68. Petersen ML, Wang Y, van der Laan MJ, Guzman D, Riley E, Bangsberg DR. Pillbox organizers are associated with improved adherence to HIV antiretroviral therapy and viral suppression: a marginal structural model analysis. Clin Infect Dis. 2007;45(7):908–15.
69. Williams DM, Counselman FL, Caggiano CD. Emergency department discharge instructions and patient literacy: a problem of disparity. Am J Emerg Med. 1996;14(1):19–22.
70. Scott C, Andrews D, Bulla S, Loerzel V. Teach-back method: using a nursing education intervention to improve discharge instructions on an adult oncology unit. Clin J Oncol Nurs. 2019;23(3):288–94.
71. Lagger G, Pataky Z, Golay A. Efficacy of therapeutic patient education in chronic diseases and obesity. Patient Educ Couns. 2010;79(3):283–6.
72. Hammad EA, Wright DJ, Walton C, Nunney I, Bhattacharya D. Adherence to UK national guidance for discharge information: an audit in primary care. Br J Clin Pharmacol. 2014;78(6):1453–64.
73. Coleman EA, Parry C, Chalmers S, Min S-J. The care transitions intervention: results of a randomized controlled trial. Arch Intern Med. 2006;166(17):1822–8.
74. U.S. Department of Health and Human Services [Internet]. [cited 2022 May 3]. https://oig.hhs.gov/oei/reports/oei-06-20-00300.pdf.
75. Houchens N, Tipirneni R. Compassionate communication amid the COVID-19 pandemic. J Hosp Med. 2020;15(7):437–9.
76. Knollman-Porter K, Burshnic VL. Optimizing effective communication while wearing a mask during the COVID-19 pandemic. J Gerontol Nurs. 2020;46(11):7–11.
77. HealthData.gov [Internet]. [cited 2022 May 3]. https://healthdata.gov.
78. Arora KS, Mauch JT, Gibson KS. Labor and delivery visitor policies during the COVID-19 pandemic: balancing risks and benefits. JAMA. 2020;323(24):2468–9.
79. Schrag D, Hershman DL, Basch E. Oncology practice during the COVID-19 pandemic. JAMA. 2020;323(20):2005–6.
80. Hugelius K, Harada N, Marutani M. Consequences of visiting restrictions during the COVID-19 pandemic: an integrative review. Int J Nurs Stud. 2021;121:104000.
81. Figueroa JF, Phelan J, Orav EJ, Patel V, Jha AK. Association of mental health disorders with health care spending in the Medicare population. JAMA Netw Open. 2020;3(3):e201210.
82. Roehrig C. Mental disorders top the list of the most costly conditions in the United States: $201 billion. Health Aff (Millwood). 2016;35(6):1130–5.
83. McDaid D, Park A-L, Wahlbeck K. The economic case for the prevention of mental illness. Annu Rev Public Health. 2019;40:373–89.
84. Chapman DP, Perry GS, Strine TW. The vital link between chronic disease and depressive disorders. Prev Chronic Dis. 2005;2(1):A14.
85. Levenson JL. The American Psychiatric Association Publishing textbook of psychosomatic medicine and consultation-Liaison psychiatry. American Psychiatric Association Publishing; 2018.
86. Rebello TJ, Marques A, Gureje O, Pike KM. Innovative strategies for closing the mental health treatment gap globally. Curr Opin Psychiatry. 2014;27(4):308–14.
87. Thorpe K, Jain S, Joski P. Prevalence and spending associated with patients who have a behavioral health disorder and other conditions. Health Aff (Millwood). 2017;36(1):124–32.
88. Barstow C, Shahan B, Roberts M. Evaluating medical decision-making capacity in practice. Am Fam Physician. 2018;98(1):40–6.
89. Testa M, West SG. Civil commitment in the United States. Psychiatry (Edgmont). 2010;7(10):30–40.
90. The 2,597 hospitals facing readmissions penalties this year [Internet]. [cited 2022 May 3]. https://www.advisory.com/daily-briefing/2016/08/04/hospitals-facing-readmission-penalties.
91. Powers BW, Milstein A, Jain SH. Delivery models for high-risk older patients: back to the future? JAMA. 2016;315(1):23–4.
92. Jackson C, Shahsahebi M, Wedlake T, DuBard CA. Timeliness of outpatient follow-up: an evidence-based approach for planning after hospital discharge. Ann Fam Med. 2015;13(2):115–22.
93. Rikin S, Epstein EJ, Gendlina I. Rapid implementation of Inpatient eConsult Programme addresses new challenges for patient care during COVID-19 pandemic. BMJ Innov. 2021;7(2):271–7.
94. CMS [Internet]. [cited 2022 May 3]. https://www.cms.gov/newsroom/fact-sheets/additional-backgroundsweeping-regulatory-changes-help-us-healthcare-system-address-covid-19-patient.
95. CMS [Internet]. [cited 2022 May 3]. https://www.cms.gov/newsroom/press-releases/cms-announces-comprehensive-strategy-enhance-hospital-capacity-amid-covid-19-surge.

Emergency Care

Ryan M. Finn, Mary Mulcare, and Christina Shenvi

Introduction

Emergency care is defined as "any healthcare service provided to evaluate and/or treat any medical condition such that a prudent layperson possessing an average level of knowledge of medicine and health, believes that immediate unscheduled medical care is required" [1]. This care may be provided in the field (i.e., non-health care settings) by emergency medical services (EMS) personnel or in an emergency facility. Emergency medicine (EM) is the practice of assessing, treating, and stabilizing the signs and symptoms of serious medical illness and acute injuries, as well as the care coordination with other health care providers and services [2].

The need for emergency care services has increased over the years in the United States, which is due to the increased medical complexity of patients seeking care in emergency departments (EDs), the lack of access to health care services, and barriers to primary care [3–5]. From 2018 to 2060, the population of adults 65 years of age and older is expected to more than double to 95 million [6], increasing the number of older adults with chronic medical diseases and further burdening an already overcrowded emergency care system [6]. Individuals with chronic illness utilize health care services, including emergency care, at a high rate [7] which is a significant driver of health care costs [8].

Although most patients can be managed in ambulatory care and lower acuity settings [9], many opt for emergency care due to a lack of health insurance; the recommendations of friends, family, and other informal health advisors [9]; the patient's perception of symptom severity; the availability of diagnostic services; and the lack of after-hours primary care [10, 11]. Patients' expectations of care when presenting for emergency care include expedited wait times and facilitated communication with physicians or other health care providers [12]; however, these expectations vary based on an individual's understanding of their illness, their cultural background, health beliefs, and ability to comprehend their current situation [13].

For patients with chronic illness, emergency care is available 24 h a day, 7 days a week, and 365 days a year. Emergency medicine physicians are trained to handle life-threatening emergencies and other sequelae that are associated with an acute or chronic illness or injury [14]. The goals of emergency care are to stabilize the patient, identify and manage acute health concerns, and coordinate the admission, discharge, or transfer of care to other providers [14]. Whether an acute problem or an exacerbation of a chronic disease, emergency care is enhanced when communication between physicians and other providers is facilitated in the prehospital setting and after discharge [15]. This chapter will provide an overview of emergency care services, an outline of the processes of care in this setting, and considerations of providing emergency care in the context of chronic illness.

Organization of Emergency Care Services

In the United States, emergency care is provided through a complex network of public and private organizations and agencies, designed to evaluate, treat, and transport a patient from the location of occurrence to the appropriate facility for definitive care [16]. For example, the evaluation and treatment in the emergency setting may identify the need for acute hospitalization, which may be followed by discharge to a long-term care facility before returning home [17]. In other scenarios, a patient may be safely discharged home directly from the emergency facility.

R. M. Finn
Rayus Radiology, Mayo Clinic and University of Minnesota, Minneapolis, MN, USA
e-mail: finn.ryan@mayo.edu

M. Mulcare
Weill Cornell Medical College, New York, NY, USA
e-mail: mrm9006@med.cornell.edu

C. Shenvi (✉)
University of North Carolina at Chapel Hill School of Medicine, Chapel Hill, NC, USA
e-mail: cshenvi@med.unc.edu

Table 18.1 Emergency care designations

Emergency care setting	Capabilities
Emergency department affiliated with and located in a medical center or hospital	24/7 physician and nursing care and ability to assess and stabilize patients and either admit or transfer them if needed.
Free-standing emergency departments	A licensed facility providing emergency care but structurally separate from a hospital. It may be owned and operated with a hospital or may be independent. Must be able to assess and provide initial stabilization and care for all emergency conditions. Available 24/7.
Urgent care center	These centers are not licensed as emergency departments. They can provide care for a restricted number of low-acuity conditions. They are often available for limited hours of the day.
Level 1 Trauma Center—determined by individual state laws	Can provide comprehensive trauma care including general surgery and surgical subspecialty care. Serves as a regional resource and engages in leadership, teaching, and research activities with a minimum volume of severely injured patients.
Level 2 Trauma Center	Can initiate definitive care, with 24/7 availability of general surgery, critical care, and some surgical subspecialties.
Level 3 Trauma Center	Able to provide initial assessment and resuscitation with 24/7 availability of emergency physicians, general surgeons, and anesthesiologists.
Primary stroke center certification designated by the Joint Commission	Able to provide comprehensive care for patients with a stroke, with 24/7 acute stroke team availability and ability to provide endovascular therapy and neurosurgery.
Comprehensive cardiac center designated by the Joint Commission	Designation indicates the facility can provide comprehensive care for cardiac conditions and emergencies such as STEMI, valve replacement and repair, diagnostic cardiac catheterizations, coronary artery bypass, cardiac arrest. It requires a standardized use of practice guidelines and evidence-based medicine and achievement of specific performance metrics.

Emergency care is provided in a variety of settings that have different capabilities and designations that are usually regulated by state law (Table 18.1). The traditional and most comprehensive type of facility is an emergency department (ED) affiliated with and located in a medical center or hospital and open 24 h a day every day of the year. These EDs are subject to the rules and regulations of the Centers for Medicare and Medicaid Services (CMS), as well as other state rules and regulations that apply to the facility within which they are located. The Emergency Medicine Treatment & Labor Act (EMTALA) [18] was enacted in 1986 as part of the Social Security Act to ensure that anyone seeking emergency medical treatment in the United States is seen, regardless of ability to pay. This act requires hospitals to provide an appropriate medical screening examination to determine whether a medically emergent condition exists in any person who presents for care in the ED [18]. If a patient is found to have an emergent medical condition, they must be stabilized and treated within the capabilities of the facility [19]. This legislation was created to ensure that an expectation of service is met at a minimum uniform standard at institutions receiving public support.

Acute care can be provided in hospital-based or free-standing EDs, or in urgent care centers. Based on their capabilities and staffing, hospitals can apply for varied accreditations or certifications. Three of the most significant are trauma center designation, stroke center certification, and cardiac care designations. There are multiple different certifying or accrediting bodies for these designations.

EDs associated with larger hospitals usually have access to a broad range of services, including procedural interventions such as a cardiac catheterization, operating rooms, subspecialty consultation, and pharmacologic therapy. These settings may also have access to case management and social workers who can facilitate care plans, including home services or placement in a skilled nursing facility (SNF). Larger hospitals are typically staffed by physicians trained in emergency medicine, while smaller hospitals and rural critical access hospitals are usually staffed by general internists, family physicians, and advanced practice providers (APPs), such as physician assistants or nurse practitioners.

Emergency medical services (EMS) are usually the first responders after the 911 system is activated [20]. EMS units can be volunteer or salaried and are staffed by four levels of providers: Emergency Medical Responder (EMR), Emergency Medicine Technician-Basic (EMT-B), Advanced Emergency Medical Technician (AEMT), and Paramedic (EMT-P) [20]. The scope of these providers is state-regulated and can vary considerably between jurisdictions [21]. All EMS providers are trained in basic resuscitation and can take a comprehensive history, including gathering information from bystanders at the scene, to convey accurate and contextual information to receiving providers in the ED.

EMS information collected in the field is the first step in a triage system that is designed to determine the acuity of illness, and the appropriate cadence for transportation, and diagnostic and treatment services, especially if multiple patients are involved. EMS personnel provide out-of-hospital acute care and transportation to EDs for illness and injury that can be associated with a medical problem or trauma. Depending on location, EMS systems may have ambulances as well as other forms of emergency transportation including helicopters or fixed-wing planes [21].

Since up to two-thirds of care rendered in the ED can be provided in a less resource-intensive setting [9], alternative settings and facilities have been evolving. Free-standing emergency departments (FSEDs) are facilities that are physically separate from acute hospitals and inpatient services

[22, 23], and as of 2016 account for approximately 11% of EDs in the United States [24]. These facilities have grown in popularity since 2004 in response to Medicare reimbursement policy, as well as the growing demand for emergency or "convenience" care [25]. Some FSEDs are owned and operated by a hospital or hospital system and are bound by the same regulatory rules as the sponsoring institution, while others operate independently [26]. The care services, regulatory statutes, and reimbursement models vary. Only hospital-affiliated FSEDs are reimbursed by CMS. [23].

Telemedicine is evolving in emergency care. Telemedicine uses video technology that allows communication between a patient and a health care provider who is not in the same place, allowing for face-to-face interaction but without physical contact [27]. This technology has expanded access for patients in areas that lack health care services, or who are without transportation, and can determine if ambulatory or emergency care is needed. In addition, some EDs rely on telemedicine providers to triage and evaluate patients during surges in patient visits [28]. Telemedicine has also expanded access to subspecialty consultation services within the ED, such as acute stroke care and psychiatric evaluation [29, 30].

Some critical access hospitals are staffed by APPs and rely on telemedicine consultation with an emergency physician available to assist with medical and trauma care, as well as management decisions for complex patients [28]. These remote physicians have the capacity to document, place orders, call consultations, and arrange admissions. During the COVID-19 pandemic, use of telemedicine expanded rapidly to mitigate health care worker exposure [31]. CMS waived the EMTALA requirement of a medical screening examination to be performed in-person during the pandemic and allowed telemedicine to charge for critical care services [31], a factor that has historically limited the adoption of this technology [32].

Processes of Emergency Care

In the Field/Pre-arrival

Patients or bystanders who call 911 or activate an EMS system are connected to a dispatch center. The emergency medical dispatcher asks a series of questions to determine the acuity and condition of the patient, the mechanism of injury, and the safety of the scene [33]. This exchange can be particularly challenging when the clinical situation precipitates emotional stress among patients and bystanders. Based on this information, the dispatcher will then deploy the appropriate EMS unit and provide instructions for basic life support or first aid, if necessary. Some EMS services are adding live video to emergency calls from bystanders' smartphones to improve the emergency triage process and to better utilize emergency resources [34]. The receiving hospital for EMS transport is determined by geographic location, the nature of the injury or illness, and the services of the receiving facility. For example, patients with significant trauma are transported to a designated regional trauma center and may bypass other EDs that do not have the same level of services. Patients presenting with a concern for stroke may be transported to the nearest stroke center [35].

EMS will transport patients from any location that they are called to, within a given radius of care, including private dwellings, skilled nursing facilities, ambulatory care centers, and outpatient settings. Patients can also be transported from hospitals to other facilities, including other hospitals, skilled nursing homes, or private homes; however, this may strain already scarce resources for emergency calls [36]. EMS providers can communicate with a "medical control" physician, who provides real-time consultation in areas such as clinical decisions and medication management [37]. Prior to ED arrival, EMS personnel will relay patient information and clinical status to facilitate the transfer of care and to prepare for anticipated patient resuscitation or other critical treatment.

Arrival at the Emergency Department

Upon arrival at the receiving ED, EMS usually hands-off care of the patient to a nurse or physician as the patient is roomed. To facilitate appropriate triage, the nurse assigns the patient an Emergency Severity Index (ESI) score. The ESI score is a validated tool that assesses patient acuity and resource needs and helps the charge nurse direct the patient to the appropriate area of the ED [38–40]. ESI is rooted in military and mass-casualty incidents and utilizes a five-point scale. A score of 1 represents a patient who most acutely needs care while a score of 5 represents a patient with minimal acuity. While the ESI system is useful, its utility in older adults and among those who are chronically ill remains unclear. For example, because older patients often present with nonspecific complaints, or atypical symptoms in common diseases, the ESI triage score has been shown to under-identify older adults who need life-saving care [41]. In some cases, an underlying chronic illness may mask an acute serious problem, particularly in older adults, and providers need to have a high level of suspicion for serious illness when treating patients with chronic disease.

There are other components of the intake or triage process that can facilitate the care of chronically ill patients including identifying advance directives and health care powers of attorney, determining functional status and the risk of falls in their home environment, and assessing the level of pain and other symptom distress since this will reduce under-triage in the elderly [42]. For a subset of homebound and vulnerable patients, an ED encounter can represent an opportunity to evaluate and screen for needed preventive services or provide education and support in chronic disease management.

Assessment and Treatment

A thorough history, physical examination, and review of available records are critical components in the patient assessment. For chronically ill and older patients, ascertaining the patient's baseline health status, acute changes in mental status, ambulatory capabilities, and ability for self-care is important and can help guide diagnostic testing, treatment options, and disposition [43]. In addition to the medical and surgical history, medical records can also provide information regarding family history, which may help to stratify a patient's risk of disease [43]. All prescribed and over-the-counter medications and allergies need to be reviewed since accurate medication lists may not be provided by the patient [44].

A social history and the identification of social determinants of health (SDOH) can be key information sources for patients with chronic illness, particularly geographic location, the patient's social support, and the availability of home and community-based services [45]. These resources are important for a safe disposition from the ED should the patient be medically cleared to go home. SDOH can also provide insight to the worsening of a chronic condition due to housing or food insecurity, intimate partner violence, or the lack of transportation for medical care [45].

The absence of an integrated electronic health record in the United States limits the provision of efficient care in emergency settings. For example, many ambulatory care practices do not share the same electronic medical record (EMR) platform as the hospital system in their area, and many hospitals in the same geographic region lack EMR integration. The lack of integrated health care information across systems and hospitals significantly hampers care for patients with chronic illnesses, many of whom see a variety of providers and can present for emergency care [46].

Health information exchange (HIE) between hospitals reduces the need for laboratory and imaging studies to be repeated; it has been shown to improve quality, enhance patient safety, increase efficiency, and result in cost savings [46]. In regards to integrated health care information across systems, a Picture Archiving and Communication System (PACS) and EMR integration significantly improves efficiency for radiologists in accessing clinical data [47]. This improved efficiency is thought to translate to a more accurate diagnosis in an average of 8.1 cases per radiologist per year [47]. In addition to integrated documentation, EDs rely on integrated communication between providers. Among patients who are referred to the ED, the referring provider should ideally communicate the pertinent medical history and relevant physical exam findings, the reasons for referral, and the desired plan of care either by phone or by documentation in the patient's EMR.

Clinical algorithms are standardized protocols usually based on expert consensus that describe a step-by-step approach to a specific medical problem that guides clinical decision-making and management [48]. Clinical algorithms are important tools in emergency care settings, providing an expedited diagnostic and treatment approach to undifferentiated symptoms that may have high potential for morbidity and mortality [49]. Symptom-specific algorithms can combine clinical interventions and diagnostic testing to assist providers in their clinical decision-making regarding disposition to hospital admission for further care or safe discharge with appropriate follow-up.

Disposition

After a patient is evaluated, assessed, stabilized, and received a preliminary diagnosis, the ED provider must determine the appropriate disposition. This may include continued observation, admission, transfer, or discharge to home or another facility. Some patients may need continued observation in the ED, admission to an ED observation unit, admission to an inpatient unit, or transfer to a different health care facility, such as a nursing home or psychiatric facility. Some EDs have capacity for observation units, which are not considered inpatient admissions [50] and is an option when a disposition decision cannot be determined within 6 h of presentation to the ED [51].

An ED observation unit (EDOU) can be considered for patients who require monitoring and/or treatment for more than 8 h, but less than 24 h. Institutional guidelines often dictate which patients are candidates, which conditions can be managed, and the staffing requirements in an EDOU [52]. Depending on the condition managed in the EDOU, diagnosis-driven protocols are often implemented to guide care. These protocols, selected by the admitting provider, detail frequency of vital signs, monitoring, nursing orders, diet, activity, labs, fluids, medications, when to page the physician, as well as anticipated time and requirement for discharge [52]. The Centers for Medicare and Medicaid Services (CMS) specifies the "Two-Midnight Rule," which notes that patients who are expected to stay less than two midnights should be assigned observation status; patient should be assigned inpatient status if the care timeframe is projected to be longer [53]. Some patients who have an acute change in functional status are admitted with the anticipation of placement in a subacute nursing facility (SNF). Under traditional Medicare, patients must be hospitalized for three consecutive midnights for SNF benefit coverage. Unfortunately, if a patient is upgraded from observation status to inpatient status, the observation days do not count toward this benefit. In addition, there is variation in insurance coverage for observation unit stays, which are subject to Medicare Part B copays and can be associated with greater out-of-pocket expenses [51].

Some chronically ill or elderly patients are brought to the ED from home when family members are no longer able to care for them. In many cases, patients are admitted because of safety concerns; however, without a qualifying medical diagnosis for hospital admission, the patient will not be eligible for the three-day qualifying stay that would activate Medicare coverage for skilled nursing home services. Some patients may need nursing home level of care, but EDs do not have the capacity to admit patients directly to long-term care. Patient disposition in these scenarios can be challenging and requires the involvement of care managers who can facilitate home care services for patients who need additional assistance at home.

Advance care planning and goals of care discussions are important, especially for chronically ill patients who may be presenting to the ED with an acute problem. There are several types of documents that can inform these discussions including Durable Powers of Attorney for Health Care (DPAHC), Living Wills (LW), and Physician Orders for Life-Sustaining Treatment (POLST) [54]. A DPAHC is a signed legal document in which a patient designates a health care proxy to make medical decisions for them if they lose decision-making capacity. A LW usually designates code status, including specifications for cardiopulmonary resuscitation and ventilatory support; however, it may also address preferences for hospitalization, nutrition, dialysis, chemotherapy, and other specific interventions.

A POLST is not a legal document, but a physician order that details a patient's resuscitation status, goals of care, and preferences regarding antibiotics, disposition, intravenous fluids, non-invasive ventilation, and medically assisted nutrition. This document can be updated during a patient's chronic illness course and can provide critical information regarding treatment decisions. If a patient has a POLST or LW, the wishes of the patient are known and should be honored. In acute, unanticipated situations, patient care goals and treatment decisions may change, which highlights the importance of goals of care conversations with the patient or the health care proxy during the emergency department visit. It is important to note that ED providers generally defer to life-sustaining interventions based on the principle of beneficence if a patient's advance care plans are uncertain [55].

Quality of Care

As the demand for emergency care has increased and patients with chronic illness become more complex, quality improvement strategies have been expanding to optimize efficiency and improve health outcomes. From prehospital to post-discharge, there are multiple quality domains including safety, performance, patient experience, timeliness, appropriateness of resource utilization, and equity [56]. Safety review is performed through root cause analysis in areas such as hospital-acquired infections, medication errors, as well as other adverse incidents [57]. Evidence-based guidelines and protocols are other quality improvement tools. Emergency departments (EDs) are often evaluated based on their compliance with recognized standards in areas such as trauma, sepsis, stroke, acute coronary syndromes, as well as morbidity and mortality [58]. Many EDs have specific protocols that promote more timely diagnostic testing and treatment, which contributes to quality control. For example, a decision algorithm regarding urinary catheter placement can reduce overutilization and prevent unintended consequences such as catheter-associated urinary tract infections, falls, and urethral trauma [59].

Efficiency and throughput are other quality indicators since EDs are expected to deliver care in a timely manner. To promote care efficiency, predictive modeling is used to analyze historical patterns of patient volume and modify staffing to projected demand [60]. EDs can employ backup call systems to ensure adequate staffing during peak hours and surge patient volumes. Third-party payers are promoting quality care by using these and other metrics that promote transparency and value-driven health care [61].

Patient experience and care satisfaction are other quality domains, which are tied to Medicare and other commercial insurance reimbursement. The Hospital Outpatient Quality Reporting Program (Hospital OQR) is a CMS program with a goal to create a standardized data reporting portal that can provide information regarding quality indicators for hospital outpatient settings, including EDs [61]. This initiative seeks to promote standards of care and the resultant data is available to consumers. Figure 18.1 shows examples of CMS quality measures, which include domains such as mortality and complications, health care-associated infections, patient safety, patient experience, and efficiency and cost reduction.

CMS guidelines have attempted to reduce hospital readmission rates within 30 days of discharge. In the early 2000s, this was noted to be as high as 20% [62]. Readmission rates are being tied to reimbursement penalties and have promoted a focus on outpatient disposition planning in ED patients rather than readmitting a returning patient [63]. Some mitigation strategies to reduce readmission rates include ensuring a timely follow-up appointment with an outpatient provider either through direct communication with a provider or through referral to a post-ED visit scheduling department [64]. Other strategies include designating nursing or other dedicated clinical staff follow-up with patients after the emergency department visit [64]. These follow-up calls may communicate information such as follow-up instructions, diagnostic, imaging, or laboratory results from the visit,

Outpatient Delivery Settings

		Acute Myocardinal Infarction(AMI)
Measures	OP-2	Fibrinolytic Therapy Received Within 30 Minutes of ED Arrival
	OP-3	Median Time to Transfer to Another Facility for Acute Coronary Intervention

		ED-Throughput
Measures	OP-18	Median Time from ED Arrival to ED Departure for Discharged ED Patients
	OP-22	Left Without Being Seen

		Stroke
Measures	OP-23	Head CT or MRI Scan Results for Acute Ischemic Stroke or Hemorrhagic Stroke Patients who Received Head CT or MRI Scan Interpretation Within 45 Minutes of ED Arrival

		Imaging Efficiency
Measures	OP-8	MRI Lumbar Spine for Low Back Pain
	OP-10	Abdomen CT – Use of Contrast Material
	OP-13	Cardiac Imaging for Preoperative Risk Assessment for Non-Cardiac Low-Risk Surgery

		Measures Submitted via a Web-Based Tool
Measures	OP-29	Appropriate Follow-up Interval for Normal Colonoscopy in Average Risk Patients
	OP-31	Cataracts – Improvement in Patient's Visual Function within 90 Days Following Cataract Surgery

		Outcome
Measures	OP-32	Facility 7-Day Risk-Standardized Hospital Visit Rate after Outpatient Colonoscopy
	OP-35	Admissions and Emergency Department (ED) Visits for Patients Receiving Outpatient Chemotherapy
	OP-36	Hospital Visits after Hospital Outpatient Surgery

Fig. 18.1 Outpatient CMS quality measures 2020. (Adapted from the Hospital Outpatient Quality Reporting Specifications Manual Version 14.0, accessed 6/29/2021 [61])

reassess patient safety, treatment adherence, and symptom severity [65].

Special Considerations

Older Adults

Chronic illness is more common in older patients and as the population ages, increased ED visits by older patients will place greater stress on the emergency health care system [66, 67]. Older adults with chronic illness account for over 20% of ED presentations [44], represent 43% of admissions, and 48% of intensive care admissions [68]. Compared to younger patients, older adults stay in the ED 20% longer, use 50% more imaging studies, and require 400% more social services [69]. When these patients are hospitalized, they tend to have longer lengths of stay and are at increased risk of delirium, hospital-acquired infections, medication errors, and general functional decline [68].

Older adults usually present to the ED from either a community dwelling or a skilled nursing facility (SNF) [69]. More than 25% of SNF residents present to the ED at least once annually [70] and often have several comorbid conditions, are on multiple medications, may be cognitively impaired, and are at greater risk of falls [71]. Patients who reside in a SNF and are hospitalized are at significant risk of iatrogenic complications [72].

Significant barriers to ED care for SNF patients include lack of access to medical information [72] and ineffective communication between the ED providers, emergency medical services, and the SNF care team [73]. SNF patients often arrive at the ED without records or without collateral information that can inform patient care [74, 75]. For example, 94% of patient transfers from SNFs had information gaps including code status, the reason for transfer, and current medications [74].

The American College of Emergency Physicians (ACEP), the American Geriatric Society (AGS), the Emergency Nurses Association (ENA), and the Society for Academic Emergency Medicine (SAEM) recognize the need for better protocols for triage, care, and coordination to improve acute care for older adults which led to the Geriatric Emergency Department Guidelines [68]. The guidelines recommend specific protocols around staffing, transitions of care, equipment and supplies, infection prevention, falls, delirium, polypharmacy, as well as palliative and end of life.

ACEP has also created a system of accreditation of EDs as Level 1, 2, or 3 Geriatric EDs (GEDs). The accreditation is based on the implementation of certain protocols focused on geriatric care (Table 18.2), staffing by geriatric EM-trained nurses or at least general education of nursing and physician staff on geriatric care principles, and availability of geriatric-focused resources such as canes or walkers.

Table 18.2 Protocols for Geriatric emergency department accreditation (www.acep.org/geda). For accreditation, EDs must demonstrate implementation and monitoring of 20, 10, or 1 protocol(s) for Levels 1, 2, and 3 accreditations, respectively

Category or focus	Protocol
Staffing	Access to palliative care
	Geriatric psychiatry access
	Guideline for volunteer engagement
Medication safety	Medication reconciliation with a pharmacist
	Guideline to minimize potentially inappropriate medications
	Pain control guidelines
ED screening	Delirium screening
	Dementia screening
	Standard assessment of function and appropriate follow-up
	Elder abuse identification
Care processes	Falls risk assessment guideline
	Guideline to promote mobility
	Three order sets for common Geriatric ED presentations
	Protocol to minimize urinary catheter use
	Protocol to minimize NPO designations and provide access to food and water
	Guideline to minimize physical restraints
	Transportation services from the ED to the patient's home or facility
Transitions of care	Guideline for PCP notification
	Guideline for transitions of care
	Access to geriatric-specific follow-up clinics
	Guideline for post-discharge follow-up
	Access to short- or long-term rehab services
	Outreach program for home assessments
	Access to community paramedicine follow-up services
	Outreach to residential care homes to improve transitions
	Standardized discharge instructions

Pain Management

Pain is the most common presentation in the emergency department, and it is a complaint associated with chronically ill patients [76]. Many patients presenting to the ED have an acute exacerbation of chronic pain or are experiencing acute pain from an underlying clinical problem. The proliferation of opioid prescription use has led to a public health emergency [77], and a marked rise in the number of persons dying from an opioid overdose [78]. With increasing rates of addiction and diversion [79], the opioid epidemic has challenged physicians to treat pain in a responsible and evidence-based way. Creative solutions to manage pain in the emergency department have included instituting opioid-sparing protocols for acute or chronic pain that utilize analgesic adjunctive therapies [80, 81]. Other opioid-sparing protocols for musculoskeletal concerns include early involvement of physical therapy to reduce the amount of opioids administered [82].

Given that most acute pain is first seen in the emergency department, these visits present a unique opportunity to prevent the development of chronic pain from acute pain. The main targets to prevent chronic pain include reducing peripheral sensitization (increased nociceptor responsiveness), reducing central sensitization (increased responsiveness to nociceptor neurons within the spinal cord or within the brain), and increasing descending inhibitory modulation [83–85].

Peripheral sensitization can be prevented by reducing nociceptor activation in the tissue, reducing nociceptor signaling, and preventing neurogenic inflammation [83]. Some therapies to reduce peripheral sensitization include topical medications (8% capsaicin patch, topical lidocaine), regional anesthesia, opioids, nonsteroidal anti-inflammatory drugs (NSAIDs), acetaminophen, and anticonvulsants. Non-pharmacologic interventions to reduce peripheral sensitization include transcutaneous electrical nerve stimulation, acupuncture, and massage [86].

Central sensitization often occurs when a repeated stimulus causes a progressively lower threshold for the afferent neuron to synapse within the dorsal horn of the spinal cord, or for the signal to reach the brain. Interventions to prevent central sensitization include neuraxial analgesia, opioids, anticonvulsants (gabapentin, pregabalin), alpha-2 adrenergic agonist (clonidine, dexmedetomidine), NMDA antagonist (ketamine), acetaminophen, and spinal cord stimulation [87].

Descending inhibitory pathways within the spinal cord can inhibit central sensitization as well through their effects on interneurons and glial cells. Pharmacologic mechanisms that modulate these pathways include opioids, serotonergic and noradrenergic agonists, tricyclic antidepressants (nortriptyline), serotonin-norepinephrine reuptake inhibitors (duloxetine), and anticonvulsants (gabapentin, pregabalin) [88]. Non-pharmacologic treatments to prevent central sensitization via descending inhibitory pathways include cognitive-behavioral therapy and biofeedback, which engage supraspinal modulating centers [89].

Acute pain management in older patients can be challenging due to the side effects of systemic analgesic medications, including altered mental status, respiratory depression, and hemodynamic compromise. To minimize these potential adverse events, some EDs employ regional anesthesia techniques to manage localized pain. For example, there are emergency departments that have instituted geriatric hip fracture and rib fracture protocols [90, 91]. These programs have shown to decrease opioid utilization, rates of delirium, and overall pain scores compared to standard care [90].

Future Directions

Emergency care use by patients with chronic illness deserves additional research and process improvement given how costly and resource-intensive it is. Interventions to reduce emergency department utilization have typically focused on patients with specific chronic diseases such as congestive heart failure or chronic obstructive pulmonary disease, but few studies have demonstrated success in reducing emergency department use by patients with chronic illness [92].

One major area of opportunity is research into and implementation of alternate models or locations of care. For example, some clinics have implemented treatment modalities such as IV diuresis or administration of IV antibiotics, which typically require an ED visit or hospital admission. There is also evidence that home-based primary care can reduce ED visits and hospitalization rates [93, 94]. By providing assessment and treatment in the home or clinic setting, patients may be able to avoid an ED visit.

A second area of needed research is prevention of chronic disease. The morbidity associated with largely preventable conditions such as diabetes, obesity, and smoking is enormous and prevention efforts have had limited effects. However, to ultimately improve care and reduce costs, prevention of their development and severity are key. Efforts could include access to primary and preventative care, medication access, and education as well as more holistic health and fitness programs.

A third opportunity is more advanced coordination of care. Once a patient arrives in the ED, the options are typically to either admit the patient or discharge them. However, many patients fall into a gray area in which they do not require hospitalization but are not safe for discharge to their current living situation. Alternatives such as hospital at home, observation settings, or discharge with coordinated follow-up could reduce unnecessary, recurrent admissions. Coordination of care could also involve home visits, coordination of access for treatment, or addressing financial concerns or medication access.

The ED provides a key site of acute care and care coordination for patients with chronic diseases. There are many more opportunities to develop and enhance the acute and emergency care for patients with chronic diseases, from prevention to hospitalization. In the coming decades, the ED will likely play an even greater role given the aging population and their care needs.

References

1. Definition of an emergency service. 2015. https://www.acep.org/Clinical%2D%2D-Practice-Management/Definition-of-an-Emergency-Service/.
2. Schneider SM, Hamilton GC, Moyer P, Stapczynski JS. Definition of emergency medicine. Acad Emerg Med. 1998;5(4):348–51. https://doi.org/10.1111/j.1553-2712.1998.tb02720.
3. Grumbach K, Keane D, Bindman A. Primary care and public emergency department overcrowding. Am J Public Health. 1993;83(3):372–8.
4. Institute NEH. A matter of urgency: reducing emergency department overuse - an NEHI research brief. Institute NEH; 2010.
5. Nawar EW, Niska RW, Xu J. National Hospital Ambulatory Medical Care Survey: 2005 emergency department summary. Adv Data. 2007:1–32.
6. Mather M, Scommegna P, Kilduff L. Fact sheet: aging in the United States. Population Reference Bureau; 2019. http://www.prb.org/Publications/Media-Guides/2016/aging-unitedstates-fact-sheet.aspx.
7. Coster JE, Turner JK, Bradbury D, Cantrell A. Why do people choose emergency and urgent care services? A rapid review utilizing a systematic literature search and narrative synthesis. Acad Emerg Med. 2017;24(9):1137–49.
8. Zuckerman S, Shen YC. Characteristics of occasional and frequent emergency department users: do insurance coverage and access to care matter? Med Care. 2004;42:176–82.
9. Penson R, Coleman P, Mason S, Nicholl J. Why do patients with minor or moderate conditions that could be managed in other settings attend the emergency department? Emerg Med J. 2012;29:487–91.
10. O'Neill Hayes T. PRIMER: examining trends in emergency department utilization and costs. American Action Forum; 2018.

11. Byrne M, Murphy AW, Plunkett PK, McGee HM, Murray A, Bury G. Frequent attenders to an emergency department: a study of primary health care use, medical profile, and psychosocial characteristics. Ann Emerg Med. 2003;41:309–18.
12. Cooke T, Watt D, Wertzler W, Quan H. Patient expectations of emergency department care: phase II–a cross-sectional survey. Can J Emerg Med. 2006;8(3):148–57.
13. Lateef F. Patient expectations and the paradigm shift of care in emergency medicine. J Emerg Trauma Shock. 2011;4:163–7.
14. Suter RE. Emergency medicine in the United States: a systemic review. World J Emerg Med. 2012;3(1):5–10. https://doi.org/10.5847/wjem.j.issn.1920-8642.2012.01.001.
15. Bost N, Crilly J, Wallis M, Patterson E, Chaboyer W. Clinical handover of patients arriving by ambulance to the emergency department - a literature review. Int Emerg Nurs. 2010;18(4):210–20. https://doi.org/10.1016/j.ienj.2009.11.006.
16. Atkins JM, Wainscott MP. Role of emergency medical services. Heart Lung. 1991;20(5 Pt 2):576–81.
17. Calder LA, Forster AJ, Stiell IG, et al. Mapping out the emergency department disposition decision for high-acuity patients. Ann Emerg Med. 2012;60(5):567–576.e4. https://doi.org/10.1016/j.annemergmed.2012.04.013.
18. Emergency Medical Treatment and Active Labor Act. In: U.S.C., ed. 421986.
19. Lulla A, Svancarek B. EMS USA Emergency Medical Treatment and Active Labor Act. 2020.
20. National Association of State EMS Officials. National EMS scope of practice model 2019: including change notices 1.0 and 2.0. United States. Department of Transportation, National Highway Traffic Safety Administration; 2021.
21. Reed-Schrader E, Mohney S. EMS, scope of practice. 2020.
22. American College of Emergency Physicians. Freestanding emergency departments and urgent care centers: an information paper. http://www.acep.org2015.
23. Herscovici DM, Boggs KM, Sullivan AF, Camargo CA Jr. What is a freestanding emergency department? Definitions differ across major United States data sources. Western J Emerg Med. 2020;21(3):660.
24. Medicare Payment Advisory Commission (MEDPAC). Report to the congress: Medicare and the Health Care Delivery System. Washington, DC: Medicare Payment Advisory Commission (MEDPAC); 2017.
25. Gutierrez C, Lindor RA, Baker O, Cutler D, Schuur JD. State regulation of freestanding emergency departments varies widely, affecting location, growth, and services provided. Health Aff. 2016;35(10):1857–66.
26. Sullivan AF, Bachireddy C, Steptoe AP, Oldfield J, Wilson T, Camargo CA Jr. A profile of freestanding emergency departments in the United States, 2007. J Emerg Med. 2012;43:1175–80.
27. Teoli D, Aeddula NR. Telemedicine. [Updated 2021 Sep 8]. In: StatPearls [Internet]. Treasure Island (FL): StatPearls Publishing; 2021. https://www.ncbi.nlm.nih.gov/books/NBK535343/
28. Rademacher NJ, Cole G, Psoter KJ, Kelen G, Fan JW, Gordon D, Razzak J. Use of telemedicine to screen patients in the emergency department: matched cohort study evaluating efficiency and patient safety of telemedicine. JMIR Med Inform. 2019;7(2):e11233.
29. Demaerschalk BM, Levine SR. Telestroke: solid support for virtual acute stroke care. Neurology. 2016;87(13):1314–5.
30. Hubley S, Lynch SB, Schneck C, Thomas M, Shore J. Review of key telepsychiatry outcomes. World J Psychiatry. 2016;6(2):269.
31. Hamm JM, Greene C, Sweeney M, Mohammadie S, Thompson LB, Wallace E, Schrading W. Telemedicine in the emergency department in the era of COVID-19: front-line experiences from 2 institutions. J Am Coll Emerg Physicians Open. 2020;1(6):1630–6.
32. Neufeld JD, Doarn CR, Aly R. State policies influence medicare telemedicine utilization. Telemed J E Health. 2016;22:70–4.
33. McQueen C, Smyth M, Fisher J, Perkins G. Does the use of dedicated dispatch criteria by Emergency Medical Services optimise appropriate allocation of advanced care resources in cases of high severity trauma? A systematic review. Injury. 2015;46(7):1197–206.
34. Linderoth G, Lippert F, Østergaard D, Ersbøll AK, Meyhoff CS, Folke F, Christensen HC. Live video from bystanders' smartphones to medical dispatchers in real emergencies. BMC Emerg Med. 2021;21(1):1.
35. Prabhakaran S, O'Neill K, Stein-Spencer L, Walter J, Alberts MJ. Prehospital triage to primary stroke centers and rate of stroke thrombolysis. JAMA Neurol. 2013;70:1126–32.
36. Heaton J, Kohn MD. EMS inter-facility transport. StatPearls. 2020.
37. Benitez FL, Pepe PE. Role of the physician in prehospital management of trauma: North American perspective. Curr Opin Crit Care. 2002;8(6):551–8.
38. Tanabe P, Travers D, Gilboy N, et al. Refining Emergency Severity Index triage criteria. Acad Emerg Med. 2005;12:497–501.
39. Tanabe P, Gimbel R, Yarnold PR, Kyriacou DN, Adams JG. Reliability and validity of scores on The Emergency Severity Index version 3. Acad Emerg Med. 2004;11:59–65.
40. Tanabe P, Gimbel R, Yarnold PR, Adams JG. The Emergency Severity Index (version 3) 5-level triage system scores predict ED resource consumption. J Emerg Nurs. 2004;30:22–9.
41. Platts-Mills TF, Travers D, Biese K, et al. Accuracy of the Emergency Severity Index triage instrument for identifying elder emergency department patients receiving an immediate life-saving intervention. Acad Emerg Med. 2010;17:238–43.
42. Malinovska A, Pitasch L, Geigy N, Nickel CH, Bingisser R. Modification of the emergency severity index improves mortality prediction in older patients. Western J Emerg Med. 2019;20(4):633.
43. Ellis G, Marshall T, Ritchie C. Comprehensive geriatric assessment in the emergency department. Clin Interv Aging. 2014;9:2033.
44. McCabe JJ, Kennelly SP. Acute care of older patients in the emergency department: strategies to improve patient outcomes. Open Access Emerg Med. 2015;7:45.
45. Axelson DJ, Stull MJ, Coates WC. Social determinants of health: a missing link in emergency medicine training. AEM Educ Training. 2018;2(1):66–8.
46. Winden TJ, Boland LL, Frey NG, Satterlee PA, Hokanson JS. Care everywhere, a point-to-point HIE tool. Appl Clin Inform. 2014;5(02):388–401.
47. Mongan J, Avrin D. Impact of PACS-EMR integration on radiologist usage of the EMR. J Digit Imaging. 2018;31(5):611–4.
48. Margolis CZ. Uses of clinical algorithms. JAMA. 1983;249(5):627–32.
49. Khalil PN, Kleespies A, Angele MK, et al. The formal requirements of algorithms and their implications in clinical medicine and quality management. Langenbecks Arch Surg. 2011;396:31–40.
50. American College of Emergency Physicians. State of the art: observation units in the emergency department. Policy Resource and Education Paper. American College of Emergency Physicians; 2011. http://www.acep.org.
51. Feng Z, Wright B, Mor V. Sharp rise in Medicare enrollees being held in hospitals for observation raises concerns about causes and consequences. Health Aff. 2012;31:1251–9.
52. Wiler JL, Ross MA, Ginde AA. National study of emergency department observation services. Acad Emerg Med. 2011;18(9):959–65.
53. Wright B, Zhang X, Rahman M, Kocher K. Informing Medicare's two-midnight rule policy with an analysis of hospital-based long observation stays. Ann Emerg Med. 2018;72(2):166–70.
54. Silveira M. Advance Care Planning and Advance Directives. 2020. https://www.uptodate.com/contents/advance-care-planning-and-advance-directives. Accessed 29 Jun 2021.
55. Mohr M, Kettler D. Ethical conflicts in emergency medicine. Anaesthesist. 1997;46(4):275–81.

56. Atkinson S, Ingham J, Cheshire M, Went S. Defining quality and quality improvement. Clin Med. 2010;10(6):537.
57. Charles R, Hood B, Derosier JM, Gosbee JW, Li Y, Caird MS, Biermann JS, Hake ME. How to perform a root cause analysis for workup and future prevention of medical errors: a review. Patient Saf Surg. 2016;10(1):1–5.
58. Section 3. Measuring Emergency Department Performance. Content last reviewed April 2020. Rockville, MD: Agency for Healthcare Research and Quality. https://www.ahrq.gov/research/findings/final-reports/ptflow/section3.html.
59. Mulcare MR, Rosen T, Clark S, et al. A novel clinical protocol for placement and management of indwelling urinary catheters in older adults in the emergency department. Acad Emerg Med. 2015;22:1056–66.
60. Jilani T, Housley G, Figueredo G, Tang PS, Hatton J, Shaw D. Short and long term predictions of hospital emergency department attendances. Int J Med Inform. 2019;129:167–74.
61. Services CfMM. Hospital outpatient quality reporting specifications manual: encounter dates 01-01-2021 (1Q21) through 12-31-2021 (4Q21) v 14.0. In: Association AM, editor. The hospital outpatient quality reporting specifications manual is periodically updated by the Centers for Medicare & Medicaid Services. Users of the Hospital Outpatient Quality Reporting Specifications Manual must update their software and associated documentation based on the published manual production timelines; 2020.
62. Jencks SF, Williams MV, Coleman EA. Rehospitalizations among patients in the Medicare fee-for-service program. N Engl J Med. 2009;360(14):1418–28.
63. McIlvennan CK, Eapen ZJ, Allen LA. Hospital readmissions reduction program. Circulation. 2015;131(20):1796–803.
64. Kripalani S, Theobald CN, Anctil B, Vasilevskis EE. Reducing hospital readmission rates: current strategies and future directions. Annu Rev Med. 2014;65:471–85.
65. Luciani-McGillivray I, Cushing J, Klug R, Lee H, Cahill JE. Nurse-led call back program to improve patient follow-up with providers after discharge from the emergency department. J Patient Experience. 2020;7(6):1349–56.
66. Lowenstein SR, Crescenzi CA, Kern DC, Steel K. Care of the elderly in the emergency department. Ann Emerg Med. 1986;15:528–35.
67. McCusker J, Healey E, Bellavance F, Connolly B. Predictors of repeat emergency department visits by elders. Acad Emerg Med. 1997;4:581–8.
68. American College of Emergency Physicians, Emergency Nurses Association. Geriatric emergency department guidelines. Ann Emerg Med. 2014;63(5):e7–25.
69. Brownell J, Wang J, Smith A, Stephens C, Hsia RY. Trends in emergency department visits for ambulatory care sensitive conditions by elderly nursing home residents, 2001 to 2010. JAMA Intern Med. 2014;174(1):156–8.
70. Terrell KM, Miller DK. Challenges in transitional care between nursing homes and emergency departments. J Am Med Dir Assoc. 2006;7:499–505.
71. Briggs R, Coughlan T, Collins R, O'Neill D, Kennelly SP. Nursing home residents attending the emergency department: clinical characteristics and outcomes. QJM. 2013;106:803–8.
72. Platts-Mills TF, Biese K, LaMantia M, et al. Nursing home revenue source and information availability during the emergency department evaluation of nursing home residents. J Am Med Dir Assoc. 2012;13:332–6.
73. Hsiao CJ, Hing E. Emergency department visits and resulting hospitalizations by elderly nursing home residents, 2001–2008. Res Aging. 2014;36:207–27.
74. Terrell KM, Brizendine EJ, Bean WF, et al. An extended care facility-to-emergency department transfer form improves communication. Acad Emerg Med. 2005;12:114–8.
75. Jones JS, Dwyer PR, White LJ, Firman R. Patient transfer from nursing home to emergency department: outcomes and policy implications. Acad Emerg Med. 1997;4:908–15.
76. Tyler KR, Hullick C, Newton BA, Adams CB, Arendts G. Emergency department pain management in older patients. Emerg Med Australas. 2020;32(5):840–6.
77. What is the U.S. Opioid Epidemic? https://www.hhs.gov/opioids/about-the-epidemic/index.html. Accessed 1 Jul 2021.
78. Understanding the epidemic. https://www.cdc.gov/opioids/basics/epidemic.html. Accessed 1 Jul 2021.
79. Schiller EY, Goyal A, Mechanic OJ. Opioid overdose. Treasure Island, FL: StatPearls Publishing; 2021.
80. Cohen V, Motov S, Rockoff B, et al. Development of an opioid reduction protocol in an emergency department. Am J Health Syst Pharm. 2015;72(23):2080–6. https://doi.org/10.2146/ajhp140903.
81. Strauss DH, Santhanam DR, McLean SA, Beaudoin FL. Study protocol for a randomised, double-blind, placebo-controlled clinical trial of duloxetine for the treatment and prevention of musculoskeletal pain: altering the transition from acute to chronic pain (ATTAC pain). BMJ Open. 2019;9(3):e025002.
82. Pugh A, Roper K, Magel J, Fritz J, Colon N, Robinson S, Cooper C, Peterson J, Kareem A, Madsen T. Dedicated emergency department physical therapy is associated with reduced imaging, opioid administration, and length of stay: a prospective observational study. PLoS One. 2020;15(4):e0231476.
83. McGreevy K, Bottros MM, Raja SN. Preventing chronic pain following acute pain: risk factors, preventive strategies, and their efficacy. Eur J Pain Suppl. 2011;5(2):365–72. https://doi.org/10.1016/j.eujps.2011.08.013.
84. Basbaum AI, Bautista DM, Scherrer G, Julius D. Cellular and molecular mechanisms of pain. Cell. 2009;139(2):267–84. https://doi.org/10.1016/j.cell.2009.09.028.
85. Spiegel DR, Pattison A, Lyons A, et al. The role and treatment implications of peripheral and central processing of pain, pruritus, and nausea in heightened somatic awareness: a review. Innov Clin Neurosci. 2017;14(5–6):11–20.
86. Beckwée D, De Hertogh W, Lievens P, Bautmans I, Vaes P. Effect of TENS on pain in relation to central sensitization in patients with osteoarthritis of the knee: study protocol of a randomized controlled trial. Trials. 2012;13(1):1–7.
87. Goldberg ME, Torjman MC, Schwartzman RJ, Mager DE, Wainer IW. Pharmacodynamic profiles of ketamine (R)- and (S)- with 5-day inpatient infusion for the treatment of complex regional pain syndrome. Pain Physician. 2010;13(4):379–87.
88. Bannister K, Dickenson AH. What do monoamines do in pain modulation? Curr Opin Support Palliat Care. 2016;10(2):143–8. https://doi.org/10.1097/SPC.0000000000000207.
89. Bushnell MC, Ceko M, Low LA. Cognitive and emotional control of pain and its disruption in chronic pain. Nat Rev Neurosci. 2013;14(7):502–11. https://doi.org/10.1038/nrn3516.
90. Casey SD, Stevenson DE, Mumma BE, Slee C, Wolinsky PR, Hirsch CH, Tyler K. Emergency department pain management following implementation of a geriatric hip fracture program. Western J Emerg Med. 2017;18(4):585.
91. Kumar R, Sharma A, Bansal R, Kamal M, Sharma L. Ultrasound-guided continuous erector spinae plane block in a patient with multiple rib fractures. Turk J Anaesthesiol Reanim. 2019;47(3):235–7. https://doi.org/10.5152/TJAR.2018.46794.
92. Moe J, Kirkland S, Rawe E, et al. Effectiveness of interventions to decrease emergency department visits by adult frequent users: a systematic review. Acad Emerg Med. 2017;24(1):40–52.
93. Kim CO, Jang SN. Home-based primary care for homebound older adults: literature review. Ann Geriatr Med Res. 2018;22(2):62.
94. Chiang JK, Kao YH. Quality of end-of-life care of home-based care with or without palliative services for patients with advanced illnesses. Medicine. 2021;100(18):e25841.

Post-Acute and Long-Term Care

Karen Halpert and Margaret R. Helton

Introduction

Residential care has evolved from the almshouses for the poor and elderly of medieval England to the modern skilled nursing facility that employs health care professionals who provide care to patients with increasingly complex needs. In the US, the number of nursing homes increased in the 1950's after Congress approved the construction of hospitals and related health care facilities in response to President Harry Truman's call to improve the health and health care of Americans [1]. The US has 15,600 certified nursing facilities with 1.7 million licensed beds [2]. The average number of nursing facility beds is 109 with an 82% occupancy rate [3]. Nursing homes can be classified as either for-profit, non-profit, or government-owned. Sixty-nine percent of nursing homes are for-profit entities, and nearly 60% are affiliated with companies that own or operate more than one nursing home (chain ownership) [4].

Nursing home care is generally classified as acute rehabilitation (short-stay patients) or long-term care (residence), both of which can occur in the same facility (Fig. 19.1) [5]. Short-stay care has grown significantly over the past decades and provides subacute (post-acute) rehabilitation, usually after hospitalization. Long-stay residents have care needs that can no longer be met independently or by family members, usually requiring assistance with activities of daily living and close supervision of location and behavior. Nearly half of these residents have dementia, and nearly a third have psychiatric conditions such as schizophrenia or other mental health problems [3]. Nearly 65% of residents depend on a wheelchair for mobility or are unable to walk without constant support from others. Four percent are bed-bound. Behavior problems such as wandering, hitting, yelling, and disinhibition are common, making this a challenging population for caregivers.

Fig. 19.1 Types of patients residing in nursing homes. (Modified from Ouslander JG, Grabowski DC. Rehabbed to Death Reframed: In Response to "Rehabbed to Death: Breaking the Cycle." J Am Geriatr Soc. 2019;67(11):2225–8)

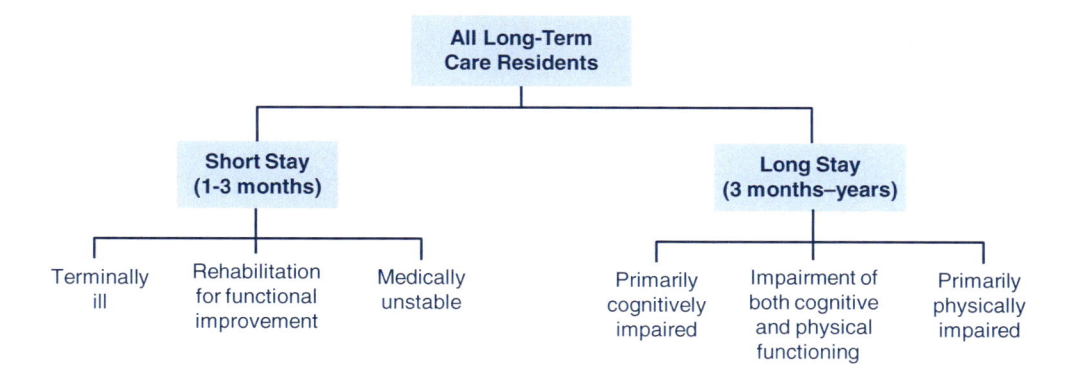

K. Halpert · M. R. Helton (✉)
Department of Family Medicine, University of North Carolina at Chapel Hill, Chapel Hill, NC, USA
e-mail: karen_halpert@med.unc.edu;
Margaret_helton@med.unc.edu

Short-Term or Post-Acute Care

Acute rehabilitation is also known as subacute, post-acute, or short-stay care, and usually follows hospitalization and for the purpose of rehabilitation or reconditioning, with the intention that the patient will recover and transition back to independent living. The most common medical conditions treated in acute rehabilitation are stroke, acute hip fracture, and elective joint replacement.

Common Conditions in Acute Rehabilitation

Stroke

Strokes are the fifth leading cause of death in the US [6, 7]. Between 2015 and 2035, total direct medical stroke-related costs are projected to more than double, from $37 billion to $94 billion, with much of the projected increase in costs arising from those ≥80 years of age [8]. Stroke is a major cause of disability and reduces mobility in more than half of stroke survivors who are older than 65 years of age [7]. Of stroke patients with Medicare admitted to a hospital, 19% were discharged to inpatient rehabilitation facilities, 25% were discharged to skilled nursing facilities, and 12% received home health care [9]. As more people survive strokes, rehabilitation is essential for restoring function as well as helping to compensate or adapt to permanent changes in physical, mental, or intellectual abilities.

Evaluation by a multidisciplinary team after a stroke determines rehabilitation needs and develops an appropriate care plan. Patients should initially be evaluated by physical, occupational, and speech therapists. Early evaluation and initiation of therapy is important to decrease the risk of medical complications and improve functional outcomes [10]. Evaluation for therapy starts within 48 h of hospitalization with the goal of managing comorbid diseases, facilitating the patient's and family's psychological state and coping skills, and maximizing the patient's ability to fully engage in therapy [11].

Post-stroke management is complex and involves a multi-disciplinary team to manage multiple medical issues, whether the treatment is in the acute inpatient rehabilitation or outpatient setting. Guidelines for rehabilitation after a stroke are available through the Department of Veteran Affairs or the American Heart Association/American Stroke Association [12, 13]. These guidelines emphasize coordinated care which reduces complications and one-year mortality rates and improves functional independence. Medical complications frequently occur during the post-acute phase of rehabilitation affecting as many as 60% of patients, with higher rates in those with severe injuries [14].

Common conditions following stroke include dysphagia (difficulty swallowing), aspiration, malnutrition, pneumonia, neurogenic bladder with urinary incontinence or retention, constipation, and fecal incontinence. Depression after a stroke is common, with 29% prevalence persisting up to 10 years [15]. There is limited evidence supporting pharmacologic intervention or psychological therapy as effective treatments for post-stroke depression [16].

Hip Fracture

Each year more than 300,000 people aged 65 years and older are hospitalized for hip fractures [17]. Most patients with hip fractures receive post-acute hospital care either in acute inpatient rehabilitation or in skilled nursing facilities (SNF), especially as hospital length of stay shortens. Effective rehabilitation prevents complications, assists in regaining function, and aims to return patients to their pre-fracture level of function. Successful discharge to home from a SNF varies substantially based on SNF provider volume and staffing characteristics [18]. The mortality rate after 1 year ranges from 14% to 58%, and can be improved with comprehensive programs involving collaborative care between orthopedic surgeons and physicians trained in the care of older adults [19]. Some older adults with multiple comorbidities may not be surgical candidates and have limited rehabilitation potential, so care is focused on pain control [20].

Total Joint Arthroplasty

There are more than one million total joint arthroplasties (mostly hip and knee) performed in the US annually [21, 22]. Rehabilitation seeks to restore mobility, range of motion, weight bearing, strength, and flexibility while preventing deep vein thrombosis and other post-operative complications. Common milestones in recovery include ability to ambulate with an assistive device, balance, and functional independence with transfers, bed mobility, toileting, and activities of daily living. Physical therapy facilitates these goals after both knee and hip replacement surgery [23, 24]. The site of rehabilitation depends on the functional status of the patient and the safety of the home environment. The most common place for post-surgery rehabilitation is at a SNF. Patients with Medicare have longer lengths of stays than those with private health coverage, which is likely related to slower progress in recovery but also influenced by insurance reimbursement policies [25]. Stays range from a few days to several weeks or even months, usually related to pre-surgery functional status.

Acute Rehabilitation Sites of Care

Acute Inpatient Rehabilitation

Acute inpatient rehabilitation (AIR) in a free-standing rehabilitation hospital or a rehabilitation unit in an acute care hospital is the most intensive type of rehabilitation.

To qualify for AIR, patients must have complex needs requiring an inter-professional team and be able to participate in at least 3 h of rehabilitation per day for at least 5 days per week (15 h per week) [26]. To assess appropriateness for this level of care, patients are screened to evaluate their condition, need for services, prior level of function, motivation, and physical and cognitive ability and motivation to participate in the intensive nature of this type of rehabilitation. Admission to these services is limited by the selective admission criteria and the limited number of AIR beds.

Patients in AIR have close medical supervision by a physician with special training or experience in rehabilitation, 24-h rehabilitation nursing care, and the services of an interdisciplinary team of skilled nurses and physical, occupational, recreational, and respiratory therapists. Psychologists, social workers, dieticians, and designers of orthotics and prosthetics are also available, all of whom contribute to ongoing assessment and discharge planning with the goal of helping medically complex patients transition to their home or community. Families are routinely involved in these discussions.

Long-Term Acute Care Hospitals

Long-term acute care hospitals (LTACHs) provide extended medical and rehabilitative care for patients who are clinically complex or have multiple acute or chronic conditions [27]. Patients admitted to these facilities are often transferred from an intensive or critical care unit with medically complex needs and an average length of stay of more than 25 days [28]. Generally, appropriate patients require at least eight or more hours of direct skilled nursing care per day which can include ventilator weaning, daily wound care, or dialysis. Patients may also qualify if they need four or more hours of direct skilled nursing care a day due to complex airway management due to a ventilator or tracheostomy. LTACHs vary in specialty and in most regions of the country may be primarily respiratory in nature [28, 29]. These facilities may be difficult to qualify for and are not available in many regions of the country. They are often the only option for patients who are medically complex with limited prospects for meaningful rehabilitation, but it is provided with the goal of transferring the patient to home or to a skilled nursing facility.

Skilled Nursing Facility

Skilled nursing facilities provide a steppingstone from hospital-level care to home, providing skilled nursing care and therapy when home services are not sufficient or safe for the patient. They are appropriate for patients who need rehabilitation but are unable to tolerate the more intense therapy of an AIR. Patients must have a qualifying hospital stay which is defined by Medicare as a medically necessary 3-day-consecutive inpatient stay that does not include day of discharge or time spent in the emergency room or outpatient observation [30]. The patient must require daily skilled nursing services or skilled rehabilitation services (physical or occupational therapy) for conditions treated during the hospitalization or that arose in the SNF while being treated for a condition previously treated in the hospital [31]. The patient must have been transferred to the subacute facility within 30 days of discharge from the hospital and is medically stable so that the focus can be on rehabilitation and returning to functional baseline.

Qualifying skilled nursing needs include injectable medications, tube feeding for new g-tubes, and wound care (wound vacuums, severe pressure ulcers). Skilled physical therapy addresses loss of function due to illness or injury where significant improvement would not be expected to occur spontaneously and requires professional therapy. Occupational therapy includes teaching compensatory techniques to improve independence in activities of daily living (ADLs), as well as designing, fabricating, and fitting orthotic and self-help devices. Speech therapy includes improving voice production and patient's ability to communicate, and training family to help augment, treat, and perform maintenance program. Dietary, pharmacy, and social work services are also available.

Nursing care in SNFs is less intensive than in acute care hospitals and one nurse may be responsible for 12–20 patients simultaneously. Patients undergoing rehabilitation in the SNF tend to be younger than the long-term care SNF residents (average age in their 70s vs. 80s in long-term care) [4]. The SNF must provide 24 h a day nursing care and clinician access for urgent or emergent needs, and provide daily therapy at least 5 days a week for up to 3 h a day as tolerated by the patient. Physicians must complete a comprehensive history and physical examination within 48 h of the patient's arrival to the SNF, then weekly and on an as-needed basis.

Subacute care facilities are licensed under the same regulations as nursing homes under the directives of the Omnibus Budget Reconciliation Act (OBRA) of 1987 [32]. These regulations are comprehensive and address medical regimens interdisciplinary care plans, patients' physical and mental well-being, and restraints, among many other areas of concerns.

Transitions Across Care Sites During Rehabilitation

Transitions between health care settings are a vulnerable time for patients with multiple comorbidities, complicated treatment regimens, or limited caregiver support, and 23% of patients admitted to a skilled nursing facility after hospitalization have at least one hospital readmission [33]. Medication errors due to poor communication between facilities are common, occurring in 75% of SNF admissions [34, 35]. Delays in treatment occur as long-term care facilities wait to obtain medications from their pharmacies.

Readmissions to an acute care hospital are associated with complications and increased morbidity and account for more than $17 billion in what are considered avoidable Medicare expenditures [36]. To address this, the Affordable Care Act of 2010 created the Hospital Readmissions Reduction Program which since 2013 penalizes hospitals with higher-than-expected 30-day readmission rates for selected clinical conditions, including acute rehabilitation conditions such as total hip or knee replacement. Improved communication, early interventions to stabilize and treat conditions that cause functional decline, and other interventions have successfully reduced readmission rates [37–39].

Long-Term Care

Nursing homes have long been viewed negatively by the public, with people claiming they would "rather die" than live in a nursing home. Alarmed by ongoing reports of fraud, neglect, abuse, fires, and "shockingly deficient" care in nursing homes, the Institute of Medicine in 1986 released a report proposing regulation to improve care [40]. In response, the federal Omnibus Budget Reconciliation Act (OBRA) of 1987 included requirements to improve the physical, mental, and psychosocial well-being of residents in what were now termed "skilled nursing facilities" [32]. The disproportionate number of nursing home residents who suffered and died in the COVID-19 pandemic showed that care in these facilities remains deficient, with inadequate staffing and poor infection control that fails to protect vulnerable older adults. In response to this toll, the National Academies of Sciences, Engineering, and Medicine convened a group of experts to conduct a comprehensive study of all aspects of long-term care in the US. This extraordinary report was released in 2022 and provides a thorough review of the current state and provides specific recommendations for improvement [41].

Quality of Care

Nursing home quality means *residents of nursing homes receive care in a safe environment that honors their values and preferences, addresses goals of care, promotes equity, and assesses benefits and risks of care and treatments* [41]. Reaching this goal requires establishment of quality metrics, accurate and timely measurement of those indicators of quality care, accountability and regulatory oversight.

As part of the federal Nursing Home Reform Act part of OBRA-87, a resident-assessment instrument known as the Minimum Data Set (MDS) was developed and remains the foundation of clinical assessment and function for individual residents [42]. The 230-item MDS collects information on each resident of the nursing home and is used for quality, care planning, payment, and research purposes. Soon thereafter, the federal government mandated public reporting on quality with the website Nursing Home Compare, whose name was changed to Care Compare in 2020 [43]. The site provides a five-star rating system based on quality, staffing, inspections, complaints, and other measures, which provide a reasonable reflection of the care provided with room for improvement [44]. As part of the Agency for Healthcare Research and Quality's (AHRQ) Consumer Assessment of Healthcare Providers and Systems (CAHPS®) program, the Centers for Medicaid and Medicare Services (CMS) mandates that nursing homes survey long-stay residents, discharged residents, and family members [45].

The 2010 Affordable Care Act (ACA) furthered quality of care efforts for nursing facilities that participate in Medicare and Medicaid by requiring nursing homes to be transparent in disclosing financial relationships and costs and imposing monetary penalties for lack of compliance with federal regulations [46]. The ACA requires all nursing homes to implement Quality Assurance Performance Improvement (QAPI) programs including quarterly meetings to identify and address any quality concerns. The ACA also incorporated the Elder Justice Act and the Patient Safety and Abuse Prevention Act, which protect nursing facility residents from abuse and other crimes and require that staff undergo background checks. CMS has other initiatives underway to address quality, including the Interventions to Reduce Acute Care Transfers (INTERACT) program that aims to reduce patient transfers to hospital [38, 47].

State and Federal Government Oversight

States license facilities and are primarily responsible for ensuring that nursing homes meet federal and state regulations. The federal government standardizes care expectations with the State Operations Manual and has the ultimate authority and can audit or sanction facilities [48]. State surveyors visit nursing homes roughly once every 12–15 months and review patient care and overall functioning of the facility and assess both process and outcome measures for almost 200 individual requirements across 8 areas (Table 19.1).

Table 19.1 State surveyors assess and measure both the process and outcomes of nursing home care in eight categories. Each category includes numerous federal regulations known as "F-tags"

Administration
Environment
Mistreatment
Nutrition
Pharmacy
Quality of care
Resident assessment
Resident rights

Each specific requirement has a description, measurement, and identifying number known as a federal tag (F-tag). Failure to meet a requirement results in a citation.

In addition to formal federal regulation, long-term care ombudsman programs exist in all 50 states and serve to advocate for residents and ensure their rights are met [49]. These programs are administered by the Administration on Aging within the Administration for Community Living of the US Department of Health and Human Services (DHHS).

Despite decades of regulation since the implementation of OBRA-87, there is only modest evidence of effectiveness in ensuring a minimum standard of quality [41]. Advocates for better care and well-being for nursing home residents recognize the ongoing shortcomings but there is little consensus on how to improve the system.

Common Conditions in Long-Term Care

Dementia is the most common diagnosis among long-stay residents in nursing facilities (59%). Other common chronic diagnoses include arthritis (30%), depression (53%), and diabetes (32%) [4]. Most residents need assistance with one or more activities of daily living (ADLs), such as bathing (97%), dressing (93%), toileting (90%), transferring (87%), and eating (60%).

Behavioral issues, particularly in patients with dementia, are common and difficult problems and may have been the reason for long-term care placement in the first place. These behavioral problems range from anxiety and depression to psychosis, agitation, aggression, and wandering, which can be dangerous to the patient as well as other residents and staff. Antipsychotics are modestly effective in reducing these behaviors in people with dementia but have adverse effects including extrapyramidal symptoms, worsened cognitive function, and an increase in cerebrovascular events and overall mortality; hence, their use should be reserved for severe symptoms that have not responded to nonpharmacologic management strategies [50].

The use of anti-psychotic medications is included in the Five-Star Quality Rating System that is available to the public. Physical restraints for aggressive behavior are now subject to federal law and ongoing education about the negative effects of this practice, which has reduced the share of residents in physical restraints to 2% in 2014 [3]. An F-tag (F221) requires residents to be free of physical restraints imposed for purposes of discipline or convenience and not required to treat medical symptoms. Non-pharmaceutical interventions for behavior issues such as patient-centered care, dementia care mapping, music therapy, exercise, and other methods show promise but have limited proven effectiveness [51, 52].

Urinary incontinence is a leading cause of long-term care placement. This and other pre-disposing conditions lead to urinary tract infections (UTIs) which, while common, are overdiagnosed in the nursing home population and bacteriuria is often treated without evidence of clinically significant infection. Overuse of antibiotics can lead to side effects, resistant bacteria, and other infections such as candidiasis and *Clostridium difficile* colitis. Despite this, the use of antibiotics in long-term care is substantial and antibiotic resistance is common and affects morbidity, mortality, and health care costs [53]. Infection control measures and antibiotic stewardship may help. Indwelling urinary catheter (Foley) use is historically high in nursing home residents and increases the risk of UTI, morbidity, and mortality. A CMS F-tag (F315) has prioritized interventions to reduce infections and overprescribing [54, 55].

The frailty and cognitive and functional impairment that is characteristic of nursing home residents lead to high frequency of falls, which can lead to a fracture, hospitalization, and mortality. There is little evidence that exercise, medication review, or Vitamin D supplementation reduces the frequency of falls [56].

Pressure ulcers (bedsores) are found in 22% of residents in long-term care [57]. These wounds can be complex and slow to heal. The National Quality Forum has declared pressure ulcers to be a "never event" and since 2008 Medicare considers pressure ulcers preventable and does not pay hospitals for hospital-acquired pressure ulcers [58, 59]. Whether changes in the way care is delivered, a team-based approach, or nursing expertise improve prevention or treatment of these wounds is not clear [60].

Polypharmacy is another common challenge in the nursing home population and is driven by multimorbidity, multiple prescribers, hospitalization, multiple new medications for conditions such as diabetes, and the cascade of treating symptoms that are due to medication side effects with other medications [61, 62]. Polypharmacy is associated with increased risk of adverse drug reactions and interactions, functional decline, as well as geriatric syndromes such as incontinence, falls, and delirium. Generally defined as the use of five or more medications, the rate of polypharmacy is high in the US and guidelines exist to encourage safe deprescribing [63, 64]. One widely used reference is the American Geriatrics Society's Beers Criteria for potentially inappropriate medication use in older adults [65].

The practice of bringing hospice agencies into the nursing home more than doubled in frequency between 1999 and 2006, with 80% of SNFs now offering hospice services for end-of-life care [4, 66]. This increase is due to the use of hospice for non-cancer diagnoses as well as an increase in hospice providers. The increasingly long stays of nursing home patients in hospice care have raised concern about higher Medicare hospice expenditures. The challenge is how to rein in the costs of long hospice stays without removing the accessibility of a comfort care approach to dying patients in nursing homes. Proposals to vary payments based on length of enrollment in hospice may address this. Experienced physicians who work in nursing homes can effectively provide comfort to dying patients without outside hospice care and most patients who die there are perceived to do so quietly and without suffering [67]. New models that increase physician presence in nursing homes would likely increase physician engagement and expertise in end-of-life care, improve care, and decrease costs [68].

Financing of Acute Rehabilitation and Long-Term Care

Payment and financing of acute rehabilitation and long-term care is poorly understood by the public, who often learn the rules and regulations when a loved one enters the system. The US health care system still primarily uses a fee-for-service payment model which is poorly suited for the type of chronic care rendered in skilled nursing facilities and does not support or incentivize access, quality, efficiency, or equity. Payment models differ for patients receiving post-acute care versus those who are long-stay residents of a nursing home.

Financing of Acute Rehabilitation

Medicare, the federal health insurance program for people who are aged 65 years or older, is the payer for most post-acute care in skilled nursing facilities. Medicare requires a 3-day qualifying stay in the hospital (cannot be on observation status) with a discharging physician ordering care that requires the skills of a professional staff of nurses and therapists for a condition for which the patient was hospitalized or for a new condition that started during the stay in the nursing home. Medicare fully covers the first 20 days of rehabilitation in the nursing home, after Part A deductible is met, and partially covers days 21 through 100. Medicare does not cover a nursing home stay beyond 100 days [69].

Medicare Part A covers inpatient rehabilitation in free-standing rehabilitation hospitals and rehabilitation units in acute care hospitals, provided a physician certifies that the patient has a medical condition that requires intensive rehabilitation, medical supervision, and coordinated care from physicians and therapists [70]. No initial deductible is required if the patient is transferred to inpatient rehabilitation directly from an acute care hospital or within 60 days of discharge from such a hospital. As with skilled nursing facilities, Medicare Part A fully covers days 1–20 in inpatient rehabilitation, partially covers days 21–100 (co-payment required), and will not cover care beyond 100 days. Private insurance pays depending on the patient's status and improvement during rehabilitation.

Long-term acute care hospitals are paid on a prospective payment system (PPS) which classifies patients into long-term care diagnosis-related groups (LTC-DRGs) based on clinical characteristics and expected resource needs. These are the same diagnoses used in hospital inpatient PPS but are weighted to reflect the resources needed to treat the medically complex patients at LTACHs [71].

Financing of Long-Term Care

Spending on nursing homes and continuing care retirement communities reached $196.8 billion in 2020, representing 5% of total health expenditures [72]. Three main payers cover nursing home services: the federal Medicare program, the federal–state Medicaid program, and private payers. In 2020, Medicaid paid for the care of 62% of all nursing home residents, Medicare for 12% of all nursing home residents, and private payers for the remaining 26% [73]. Medicare has higher payment rates than Medicaid, leading facilities to prefer short-stay nursing home patients for financial reasons [74].

A year's worth of care in a US nursing home for an individual averaged $108,405 in 2020 [75]. This is clearly out of reach for most individuals and their families which is why Medicaid, the jointly funded federal and state health insurance program for low-income and needy people, is the primary payer source for long-term care and serves as the safety net for millions of people who can no longer be cared for at home. Individuals must first exhaust or spend down all their personal assets before they qualify for Medicaid. Eligibility is determined by the individual states, but in general people must reduce their assets to less than $2000 to qualify, with a monthly income less than $2500. Medicaid pays about 70% of what private insurance pays.

Licensed nursing facilities must be certified for participation in the Medicare and/or Medicaid program. The vast majority (96%) of beds are dually certified though Medicaid is the primary payer for most residents in SNFs. In 2015, 62% of total residents in SNF had Medicaid as their primary payer, which represents more than 830,000 people at any given time [3].

Multidisciplinary Care Team

Working as a team is imperative to meeting the complex needs of patients in rehabilitation and long-term care facilities, addressing not only medical and personal care needs, but also keeping pace with the demands of new technology, delivering care across settings, and managing the complex payment structure [76]. Brief descriptions of the roles or scope of practice of team members are described in Table 19.2. Features of successful interdisciplinary interac-

Table 19.2 Roles of team members in effective and comprehensive rehabilitation, which depends on multiple professionals who communicate well and work cohesively

Role	Responsibilities
Physician	Lead the multidisciplinary team, working collegially with other team members
	Ensure the rehabilitation program is safe, appropriate, comprehensive, and cost-effective
	Certify the need for rehabilitation
	Evaluate and treat medical comorbidities
	Direct program evaluation, ongoing quality improvement
Advance practice providers	Partner with physicians to deliver care
	May provide medically necessary visits prior to and after the physician's initial comprehensive visit. Ongoing required visits may alternate between physician and advance practice provider
Administrator	Proficient in both business management and health care
	Oversee operation of the facilities including supervision of staff and personnel management
	Financial planning and budgeting
	Ensure compliance with state and federal regulations
	Handle grievances of employees, patients, and families
Physical therapist	Assess the patient's pain, ability to move, and function, and develop a treatment plan
	Instruct physical exercise to improve and restore range of motion, strength, endurance, balance, coordination, and gait
	Provide appropriate assistive devices
Occupational therapist	Evaluate self-care skills and ability to conduct activities of daily living (ADLs)
	Provide training that helps the patients return to participation in activities that they need and want to do
	Make recommendation and train in use of assistive technology
	Fabricate splints
Speech therapist	Evaluate and treat patients regarding communication ability such as language comprehension, verbal expression, and auditory comprehension
	Address cognitive function such as attention, memory, thought organization, reasoning, and problem solving
	Assess swallowing disorders and recommend dietary or positioning changes to treat dysphagia
Recreation therapist	Meet patients' individual interests to help them reach their physical, cognitive, emotional, social, and leisure needs
	Assist in developing skills, knowledge, and behaviors for daily living and community involvement
	Use of recreational modalities to improve function
Social worker	Advocate for the patients and promote their dignity and intrinsic worth
	Assess psychosocial factors and address uncertainty, anxiety, depression
	Help patients adjust to changes such as increased dependency, loss, grief
	Support patient and family in adapting to changed roles or relationships
	Address financial and social stressors related to disability and help with medical expenses
	Find resources needed in home environment or transportation
Pharmacist	Monthly medication review; monitor for polypharmacy
	Make recommendations about tapering or discontinuing medications
Nurse	Monitor for signs and symptoms of medical conditions
	Administer medications
	Care for wounds
	Assist patient with tasks of bathing, dressing, and other ADLs
Nutritionist	Assess nutritional status, eating patterns, and dietary issues associated with medical conditions
	Create and support individual plan for sustained healthy eating
Family caregivers	Involvement may vary among patients
	Support patient and team
Support	Food preparation, building and grounds keepers, transportation, security, technical support, business and financial staff, administrative support, chaplains

tions include formal team-based care, communication, coordination, and leadership [77]. The interdisciplinary approach for assessing and planning care contributes to the psychological well-being of residents, earlier intervention of patients' medical conditions, lower costs, reduced staff turnover, and increased satisfaction [78–81].

Although the physician role in short-term rehabilitation or long-term care is important, in the US physicians are not usually the most present members of the patient care team as they maintain office and hospital-based practices, meaning much of the care plan is implemented by others [82]. Worldwide, only the Netherlands has special training programs to become a qualified nursing home physician [83]. In the US, most physicians are family physicians, geriatricians, or internists who round in the nursing home on a part-time basis, though there is a growing trend of nursing home specialists who work exclusively in the facility [84]. Federal regulations dictate the frequency with which physicians must see patients and they must also be available for acute issues. CMS also requires that all nursing homes have one physician who serves as the medical director [85]. The American Medical Directors Association (AMDA) has a certification program for this role, although this is not a requirement to be a medical director. Other leaders include a Director of Nursing and a lead administrator who oversees compliance with federal and state regulations, resident care, human resources, financial stewardship, and maintainence of the physical environment.

Many physicians partner with advanced practice providers to deliver care in nursing facilities. Nurse practitioners have been authorized to provide Medicare services to residents in long-term care facilities for 40 years and serve as an important and growing foundation of skilled nursing home care and rehabilitative care. Their presence is associated with decreased unnecessary hospitalizations and emergency room use, improved health outcomes, and increased family satisfaction [86, 87].

Most direct care in the nursing home is performed by nursing assistants [88]. More than 90% of these workers are women, 58% are people of color, and 21% were born outside of the US [89]. The demand for direct-care workers will grow over the next decades and filling those roles will be challenging due to low wages and lack of respect or recognition, much of which reflects the legacy of longstanding institutional racism, sexism, and ageism [90].

Racial Disparities in Long-Term Care

Skilled nursing and long-term care services in the US are provided in a complex, racially segregated system. Disparities have been documented in access, process, and outcomes of care for patients and residents. Systemic racism has perpetuated these disparities with inherent biases built within the long-term care system's organization, administration, regulations, and human services [90].

Black Americans are more likely to use nursing home care than White Americans and are concentrated in a relatively small number of homes that are largely for-profit organizations, serve primarily patients with Medicaid, have lower levels of nurse staffing, and overall have worse resident outcomes regardless of race [91–93]. Racial segregation of nursing homes mirrors residential segregation with 14% of nursing home residents who are Black concentrated in a small number of homes (17%) that are majority Black. Nearly half of nursing homes (43%) have fewer than 2% minority residents [4, 94]. In addition to the segregation, Black residents are more often physically restrained, more frequently develop pressure ulcers, are less likely to have effective treatment for pain, and are more likely to be hospitalized and report lower quality of life compared to white residents [92, 95–98]. A key factor leading to the concentration of Black individuals in low-quality nursing homes is the payment system. Medicare and most private insurance contracts only pay for post-acute, rehabilitative care. Most long-term care residents and their families pay out of pocket if they are able to and the longstanding discriminatory policies of the US make it less likely that Black individuals have been able to accumulate this level of wealth [90]. Persons who have few assets, or have spent them down, are eligible for Medicaid to cover long-term care; however, these payment rates are much lower than those of other payers. This leads to inherently discriminatory situations where residential long-term care settings compete for non-Medicaid (disproportionately non-Black) patients [99].

Addressing the impact of systemic racism on long-term care requires significant reforms, including changing the current financing model for nursing home care [100]. The marked difference between Medicaid reimbursement and that provided by other payers is a key factor leading to the stratification of long-term care settings by race and resources [101]. Increasing Medicaid payment reduces disparities and reduces the incentive to avoid serving patients whose care is covered by Medicaid [94]. Major reform for how long-term care is funded is required along with societal agreement that long-term care is a right, as is the case in other countries where the quality of care is not linked to race and class [102, 103].

COVID-19 and Infection Prevention

The age and health status of nursing home residents, the congregate setting that creates many resident-to-resident interactions, large facilities, inherent health inequities, and frequent staff and patient interactions make residents of nursing homes vulnerable to transmitted infections, which was made dramatically obvious to the public by the disproportionate number of deaths of nursing home residents during the COVID-19 pandemic [104, 105]. As of May 2022, more than 152,000 residents and more than 2300 staff members had died of COVID-19 [106]. Inadequate supplies of personal protection equipment, communication challenges between nursing homes and public health departments, systematic health care disparities, and staffing shortages fueled the spread of the infection in facilities [41]. The introduction of vaccines and prioritizing their distribution to nursing homes in December 2020 greatly reduced the impact of the pandemic on these residents, as it has for all populations [107].

Though the impact of COVID-19 was dramatic, respiratory and gastrointestinal infections like influenza and norovirus have long been a source of outbreaks in nursing homes, and lead to higher rates of hospitalization and death than in the community [108]. CMS requires nursing homes to have a comprehensive infection control program that includes surveillance of infections, rapid implementation of preventative measures and isolation measures when needed, and employee health guidelines including hand hygiene and the importance of staff vaccinations.

Emerging as another vital role for infection control programs is antibiotic stewardship, especially with the increase in antibiotic resistant bacteria. Educational initiatives that distinguish between bacterial colonization (in chronic wounds and urine) and infection, and collaborations with pharmacy on appropriate duration of therapy may decrease complications such as *Clostridium difficile* colitis and the development and spread of multi-drug resistant organisms, although whether these interventions have a lasting effect on prescribing practices is uncertain [109].

Future Directions

The Committee on the Quality of Care in Nursing Homes is a group of experts in long-term care who put together an extraordinary report that examines how the US currently delivers, staffs, finances, and regulates nursing home care, with the conclusion that the current system is ineffective, inefficient, fragmented, and unsustainable [41]. They call for immediate action from state and federal governments, health care systems, payers, regulators, and researchers to create a shared vision of high-quality nursing home care. They emphasize that quality improvement initiatives must not exacerbate disparities in care, including racial and ethnic disparities. Low wages, lack of transparency regarding nursing home finances and operations, and perverse incentives in payment models are only some of the issues that will need to be addressed. A summary of the committee's goals is presented in Table 19.3.

Given the aging of the population and the growth in need for rehabilitative services and long-term care and the billions of dollars that this will cost, innovative models are needed to improve the quality of care, improve the health of the population, reduce costs, and provide professional health and satisfaction to the people who work in the system. If these goals are met, nursing homes will transform from being dreaded institutions to places where chronically ill people with significant care needs can be treated with quality care in a dignified manner by staff who are compassionate and competent.

Table 19.3 The Committee on the Quality of Care in Nursing Homes: goals and recommendations [41]

Goals	Recommendation
Deliver comprehensive, person-centered, equitable care that ensures residents' health, quality of life, and safety; promotes autonomy; and manages risks	• Shared decision-making • Identify, document, implement, and monitor patient preferences • Fund translational research on best care models • Ensure emergency services ensure the safety of nursing home residents in public health emergencies and natural disasters • Renovate nursing homes to provide smaller, more home-like environments or units
Ensure a well-prepared, empowered, and appropriately compensated workforce	• Ensure competitive wages and benefits to recruit and retain nursing home staff • Enhance the current minimum staffing requirements • Fund research to identify optimum staffing standards, based on resident case mix • Enhance expertise of professional staff in the nursing home • Advance and empower the role of the nursing assistants • Establish minimum education and competency requirements for staff, including administrators and clinical staff • Proving ongoing diversity and inclusion training • Fund research on systemic barriers and opportunities to improve recruitment, training, and advancement of nursing home workers
Increase the transparency and accountability of finances, operations, and ownership	• Make publicly available facility-level data on ownership, finances, and operations of nursing homes • Assess the relationship of quality of care to ownership patterns
Create a more rational and robust financing system	• Establish a federal long-term care benefit to expand access and advance equity for all adults who need long-term care • CMS should ensure that payments are adequate to cover comprehensive, high-quality, and equitable care to all nursing home residents • Extend bundled payments to all conditions, holding hospitals financially accountable for Medicare post-acute care spending and outcomes • Explore alternative payment models for long-term care, separate from bundled payments for post-acute care, such as global capitated budgets

(continued)

Table 19.3 (continued)

Goals	Recommendation
Design a more effective and responsive system of quality assurance	• CMS should ensure that state survey agencies have adequate resources to fulfill their nursing home oversight responsibilities • Make quality assurance efforts more effective, efficient, and responsive • Increase funding to the Long-Term Care Ombudsman Program • Poor performing facilities should be subject to oversight and enforcement actions • States should eliminate certificate-of-need requirements and construction moratoria for nursing homes to encourage innovation and competition
Expand and enhance quality measurement and continuous quality improvement	• Add Consumer Assessment of Healthcare Providers and Systems (CAHPS) surveys to the Care Compare website • Expand and enhance the quality measures on the Care Compare website, including data on multi-facility chains, risk-adjusted clinical quality, more weight to staffing ratios, palliative care and end-of-life care, implementation of resident care plans, staff well-being • Define and measure disparities in care, including those related to race, ethnicity, LGBTQ+ populations, and sources of payment
Adopt health information technology in all nursing homes	• Provide financial incentives for facilities to adopt certified electronic medical records • Train workers on core health information technology competency • Research on the relationship between health information technology and resident outcomes, innovation, and staff, family, and resident perceptions

CMS = Centers for Medicare & Medicaid Services

References

1. Peters G, Woolley JT. Harry S Truman's special message to the congress recommending a comprehensive health program. The American Presidency Project. www.presidency.ucsb.edu/node/230961.
2. CDC, National Center for Health Statistics. Nursing home care [Internet]. https://www.cdc.gov/nchs/fastats/nursing-home-care.htm.
3. Harrington C, Carrillo H, Garfield R. Nursing facilities, staffing, residents and facility deficiencies, 2009–2015. https://files.kff.org/attachment/REPORT-Nursing-Facilities-Staffing-Residents-and-Facility-Deficiencies-2009-2015.
4. Harris-Kojetin L, Sengupta M, Lendon JP, Rome V, Valverde R, Caffrey C. Long-term care providers and services users in the United States, 2015–2016 Natl Cent Health Stat Vital Health Stat. 2019;3(43).
5. Ouslander JG, Grabowski DC. Rehabbed to death reframed: in response to "Rehabbed to death: breaking the cycle". J Am Geriatr Soc. 2019;67(11):2225–8.
6. Heron M. Deaths: leading causes for 2018 [Internet]. National Center for Health Statistics; 2021 May [cited 2022 Mar 5]. https://stacks.cdc.gov/view/cdc/104186.
7. Benjamin EJ, Virani SS, Callaway CW, Chamberlain AM, Chang AR, Cheng S, et al. Heart disease and stroke statistics-2018 update: a report from the American Heart Association. Circulation. 2018;137(12):e67–492.
8. Nelson S, Whitsel L. Projections of cardiovascular disease prevalence and costs: 2015–2035. Technical Report [prepared for the American Heart Association]. Res Triangle Park NC [Internet]. https://www.heart.org/idc/groups/heart-public/@wcm/@adv/documents/downloadable/ucm_491513.pdf.
9. Commission MPA. Report to the Congress: Medicare payment policy Washington. DC Medicare Paym Advis Comm. 2013.
10. Musicco M, Emberti L, Nappi G, Caltagirone C, Italian Multicenter Study on Outcomes of Rehabilitation of Neurological Patients. Early and long-term outcome of rehabilitation in stroke patients: the role of patient characteristics, time of initiation, and duration of interventions. Arch Phys Med Rehabil. 2003;84(4):551–8.
11. National Institute of Neurologic Disorders and Stroke. Post-stroke rehabilitation fact sheet [Internet]. https://www.ninds.nih.gov/Disorders/Patient-Caregiver-Education/Fact-Sheets/Post-Stroke-Rehabilitation-Fact-Sheet.
12. Winstein CJ, Stein J, Arena R, Bates B, Cherney LR, Cramer SC, et al. Guidelines for adult stroke rehabilitation and recovery: a guideline for healthcare professionals from the American Heart Association/American Stroke Association. Stroke. 2016;47(6):e98–169.
13. Department of Veterans Affairs. VA/DoD clinical practice guidelines for the management of stroke rehabilitations. https://www.healthquality.va.gov/guidelines/Rehab/stroke/VADoDStrokeRehabCPGFinal8292019.pdf.
14. Kalra L, Yu G, Wilson K, Roots P. Medical complications during stroke rehabilitation. Stroke. 1995;26(6):990–4.
15. Ayerbe L, Ayis S, Wolfe CDA, Rudd AG. Natural history, predictors and outcomes of depression after stroke: systematic review and meta-analysis. Br J Psychiatry J Ment Sci. 2013;202(1):14–21.
16. Allida S, Cox KL, Hsieh C-F, House A, Hackett ML. Interventions for preventing depression after stroke [Internet]. [cited 2022 Mar 19]. https://www.cochrane.org/CD003689/interventions-preventing-depression-after-stroke.
17. Agency for Healthcare Research and Quality. Hip fractures among older adults. HCUPnet. Healthcare Cost and Utilization Project (HCUP). Rockville, MD. 2012 [cited 2022 Mar 19]. http://hcupnet.ahrq.gov.
18. Gozalo P, Leland NE, Christian TJ, Mor V, Teno JM. Volume matters: returning home after hip fracture. J Am Geriatr Soc. 2015;63(10):2043–51.
19. Schnell S, Friedman SM, Mendelson DA, Bingham KW, Kates SL. The 1-year mortality of patients treated in a hip fracture program for elders. Geriatr Orthop Surg Rehabil. 2010;1(1):6–14.
20. Roche JJW, Wenn RT, Sahota O, Moran CG. Effect of comorbidities and postoperative complications on mortality after hip fracture in elderly people: prospective observational cohort study. BMJ. 2005;331(7529):1374.
21. Williams SN, Wolford ML, Bercovitz A. Hospitalization for total knee replacement among inpatients aged 45 and over: United States, 2000–2010. NCHS Data Brief. 2015;(210):1–8.

22. Wolford WM, Palso K, Bercovitz A. Hospitalization for total hip replacement among inpatients aged 45 and over: United States, 2000–2010. NCHS Data Brief. 2015;(186):1–8.
23. Doma K, Grant A, Morris J. The effects of balance training on balance performance and functional outcome measures following total knee arthroplasty: a systematic review and meta-analysis. Sports Med Auckl NZ. 2018;48(10):2367–85.
24. Wu JQ, Mao LB, Wu J. Efficacy of exercise for improving functional outcomes for patients undergoing total hip arthroplasty: a meta-analysis. Medicine (Baltimore). 2019;98(10):e14591.
25. Haghverdian BA, Wright DJ, Schwarzkopf R. Length of stay in skilled nursing facilities following total joint arthroplasty. J Arthroplast. 2017;32(2):367–74.
26. CMS. Medicare Claims Processing Manual (Pub. 100-04), Chapter 3, Section 140, "Criteria that must be met by inpatient rehabilitation facilities" [Internet]. https://www.cms.gov/Regulations-and-Guidance/Guidance/Manuals/Downloads/clm104c03.pdf.
27. Dalton K, Kandilov AM, Kennell DK, Wright A. Determining medical necessity and appropriateness of care for Medicare long-term care hospitals. Falls Church, VA: Kennell and Associates Inc and RTI International; 2012.
28. Makam AN, Nguyen OK, Xuan L, Miller ME, Goodwin JS, Halm EA. Factors associated with variation in long-term acute care hospital vs skilled nursing facility use among hospitalized older adults. JAMA Intern Med. 2018;178(3):399–405.
29. Eskildsen MA. Long-term acute care: a review of the literature. J Am Geriatr Soc. 2007;55(5):775–9.
30. CMS. Skilled nursing facility 3-day rule billing [Internet]. 2021. https://www.cms.gov/Outreach-and-Education/Medicare-Learning-Network-MLN/MLNProducts/Downloads/SNF3DayRule-MLN9730256.pdf.
31. CMS. Medicare Benefit Policy Manual. Chapter 8 - Coverage of extended care (SNF) services under hospital insurance. [Internet]. 2021. https://www.cms.gov/regulations-and-guidance/guidance/manuals/downloads/bp102c08pdf.pdf.
32. H.R.3545 - 100th Congress (1987–1988): Omnibus Budget Reconciliation Act of 1987 [Internet]. 1987 [cited 2021 Nov 6]. https://www.congress.gov/bill/100th-congress/house-bill/3545.
33. Burke RE, Whitfield EA, Hittle D, Joon MS, Levy C, Prochazka AV, et al. Hospital readmission from post-acute care facilities: risk factors, timing, and outcomes. J Am Med Dir Assoc. 2016;17(3):249–55.
34. Tjia J, Bonner A, Briesacher BA, McGee S, Terrill E, Miller K. Medication discrepancies upon hospital to skilled nursing facility transitions. J Gen Intern Med. 2009;24(5):630–5.
35. Kerstenetzky L, Birschbach MJ, Beach KF, Hager DR, Kennelty KA. Improving medication information transfer between hospitals, skilled-nursing facilities, and long-term-care pharmacies for hospital discharge transitions of care: a targeted needs assessment using the Intervention Mapping framework. Res Soc Adm Pharm RSAP. 2018;14(2):138–45.
36. Jencks SF, Williams MV, Coleman EA. Rehospitalizations among patients in the Medicare fee-for-service program. N Engl J Med. 2009;360(14):1418–28.
37. Rantz MJ, Popejoy L, Vogelsmeier A, Galambos C, Alexander G, Flesner M, et al. Successfully reducing hospitalizations of nursing home residents: results of the Missouri quality initiative. J Am Med Dir Assoc. 2017;18(11):960–6.
38. Ouslander JG, Bonner A, Herndon L, Shutes J. The Interventions to Reduce Acute Care Transfers (INTERACT) quality improvement program: an overview for medical directors and primary care clinicians in long term care. J Am Med Dir Assoc. 2014;15(3):162–70.
39. Zuckerman RB, Sheingold SH, Orav EJ, Ruhter J, Epstein AM. Readmissions, observation, and the hospital readmissions reduction program. N Engl J Med. 2016;374(16):1543–51.
40. Institute of Medicine (US) Committee on Nursing Home Regulation. Improving the quality of care in nursing homes [Internet]. Washington, DC: National Academies Press (US); 1986 [cited 2021 Nov 6]. http://www.ncbi.nlm.nih.gov/books/NBK217556/.
41. National Academies of Sciences, Engineering, and Medicine. The national imperative to improve nursing home quality: honoring our commitment to residents, families, and staff [Internet]. Washington, DC: The National Academies Press; 2022. https://doi.org/10.17226/26526.
42. CMS. Minimum data set 3.0 public-reports [Internet]. https://www.cms.gov/Research-Statistics-Data-and-Systems/Computer-Data-and-Systems/Minimum-Data-Set-3-0-Public-Reports.
43. CMS. Compare nursing home quality [Internet]. https://www.cdc.gov/nchs/fastats/nursing-home-care.htm.
44. Konetzka TR, Yan K, Werner RM. Two decades of nursing home compare: what have we learned? Med Care Res Rev. 2021;78(4):295–310.
45. Agency for Healthcare Research and Quality. Nursing homes [Internet]. https://www.ahrq.gov/topics/nursing-homes.html.
46. Wells J, Harrington C. Implementation of affordable care act provisions to improve nursing home transparency, care quality, and abuse prevention [Internet]. Washington, DC: Kaiser Family Foundation; 2013. https://www.kff.org/medicaid/report/implementation-of-affordable-care-act-provisions-to-improve-nursing-home-transparency-care-quality-and-abuse-prevention/
47. CMS. Nursing home quality initiatives [Internet]. 2017. https://www.cms.gov/Medicare/Provider-Enrollment-and-Certification/QAPI/Downloads/Nursing-Home-Quality-Initiatives-FAQ.pdf.
48. CMS. State operations manual appendix PP - guidance to surveyors for long term care facilities [Internet]. 2017. https://www.cms.gov/medicare/provider-enrollment-and-certification/guidanceforlawsandregulations/downloads/appendix-pp-state-operations-manual.pdf.
49. NORC (NORC at the University of Chicago). Final report: Process evaluation of the Long-Term Care Ombudsman Program (LTCOP) [Internet]. 2019. https://acl.gov/sites/default/files/programs/2020-10/LTCOPProcessEvaluationFinalReport_2.pdf.
50. Tampi RR, Tampi DJ, Balachandran S, Srinivasan S. Antipsychotic use in dementia: a systematic review of benefits and risks from meta-analyses. Ther Adv Chronic Dis. 2016;7(5):229–45.
51. Livingston G, Kelly L, Lewis-Holmes E, Baio G, Morris S, Patel N, et al. Non-pharmacological interventions for agitation in dementia: systematic review of randomised controlled trials. Br J Psychiatry J Ment Sci. 2014;205(6):436–42.
52. Jutkowitz E, Brasure M, Fuchs E, Shippee T, Kane RA, Fink HA, et al. Care-delivery interventions to manage agitation and aggression in dementia nursing home and assisted living residents: a systematic review and meta-analysis. J Am Geriatr Soc. 2016;64(3):477–88.
53. van Buul LW, van der Steen JT, Veenhuizen RB, Achterberg WP, Schellevis FG, Essink RTGM, et al. Antibiotic use and resistance in long term care facilities. J Am Med Dir Assoc. 2012;13(6):568.e1–568.e13.
54. Johnson TM. The newly revised F-Tag 315 and surveyor guidance for urinary incontinence in long-term care. JAMDA. 2006;7(9):594–600.
55. Smith PW, Bennett G, Bradley S, Drinka P, Lautenbach E, Marx J, et al. SHEA/APIC guideline: infection prevention and control in the long-term care facility. Infect Control Hosp Epidemiol. 2008;29(9):785–814.
56. Cameron ID, Dyer SM, Panagoda CE, Murray GR, Hill KD, Cumming RG, et al. Interventions for preventing falls in older people in care facilities and hospitals. Cochrane Database Syst

57. VanGilder C, Amlung S, Harrison P, Meyer S. Results of the 2008–2009 International Pressure Ulcer Prevalence™ survey and a 3-year, acute care, unit-specific analysis. Ostomy Wound Manag. 2009;55(11):39–45.
58. CMS. Hospital acquired conditions [Internet]. https://www.cms.gov/Medicare/Medicare-Fee-for-Service-Payment/HospitalAcqCond.
59. AHRQ. Patient safety network never events [Internet]. 2019. https://psnet.ahrq.gov/primer/never-events.
60. Joyce P, Moore ZE, Christie J. Organisation of health services for preventing and treating pressure ulcers. Cochrane Database Syst Rev [Internet]. 2018 [cited 2022 Apr 24];2018(12). https://www.readcube.com/articles/10.1002%2F14651858.cd012132.pub2.
61. Tamura BK, Bell CL, Inaba M, Masaki KH. Factors associated with polypharmacy in nursing home residents. Clin Geriatr Med. 2012;28(2):199–216.
62. Messinger-Rapport BJ, Little MO, Morley JE, Gammack JK. Clinical update on nursing home medicine: 2016. J Am Med Dir Assoc. 2016;17(11):978–93.
63. Jokanovic N, Tan ECK, Dooley MJ, Kirkpatrick CM, Bell JS. Prevalence and factors associated with polypharmacy in long-term care facilities: a systematic review. J Am Med Dir Assoc. 2015;16(6):535.e1–12.
64. Linda M Liu DNP, Irene G, Campbell MSN. Tips for deprescribing in the nursing home. Ann Long-Term Care [Internet]. 2016 [cited 2022 Apr 24];24(9). https://www.hmpgloballearningnetwork.com/site/altc/articles/tips-deprescribing-nursing-home.
65. American Geriatrics Society. Updated AGS Beers Criteria® for potentially inappropriate medication use in older adults. J Am Geriatr Soc. 2019;67(4):674–94.
66. Miller SC, Lima J, Gozalo PL, Mor V. The growth of hospice care in U.S. nursing homes. J Am Geriatr Soc. 2010;58(8):1481–8.
67. van der Steen JT, Deliens L, Koopmans RTCM, Onwuteaka-Philipsen BD. Physicians' perceptions of suffering in people with dementia at the end of life. Palliat Support Care. 2017;15(5):587–99.
68. Katz PR, Ryskina K, Saliba D, Costa A, Jung HY, Wagner LM, et al. Medical care delivery in U.S. nursing homes: current and future practice. Gerontologist. 2021;61(4):595–604.
69. CMS. Skilled nursing care [Internet]. https://www.medicare.gov/coverage/skilled-nursing-facility-snf-care.
70. CMS. Inpatient rehabilitation care [Internet]. https://www.medicare.gov/coverage/inpatient-rehabilitation-care.
71. CMS. Long-term care hospital PPS [Internet]. 2021. https://www.cms.gov/Medicare/Medicare-Fee-for-Service-Payment/LongTermCareHospitalPPS/elements_ltch.
72. CMS. National Health Expenditures 2020 highlights [Internet]. [cited 2022 Apr 10]. https://www.cms.gov/files/document/highlights.pdf.
73. Distribution of certified nursing facility residents by primary payer source [Internet]. KFF. 2021 [cited 2022 Apr 10]. https://www.kff.org/other/state-indicator/distribution-of-certified-nursing-facilities-by-primary-payer-source/.
74. Grabowski DC. Medicare and Medicaid: conflicting incentives for long-term care. Milbank Q. 2007;85(4):579–610.
75. American Council on Aging. 2021 Nursing home costs by state and region [Internet]. https://www.medicaidplanningassistance.org/nursing-home-costs/.
76. Institute of Medicine, Committee on the Health Professions Education Summit. Health professions education: a bridge to quality institute of medicine (US). Washington, DC: National Academies Press (US); 2003.
77. Nazir A, Unroe K, Tegeler M, Khan B, Azar J, Boustani M. Systematic review of interdisciplinary interventions in nursing homes. J Am Med Dir Assoc. 2013;14(7):471–8.
78. Institute of Medicine (US) Committee on the Adequacy of Nursing Staff in Hospitals and Nursing Homes. Nursing staff in hospitals and nursing homes: is it adequate? Washington, DC: National Academies Press (US); 1996.
79. Mukamel DB, Cai S, Temkin-Greener H. Cost implications of organizing nursing home workforce in teams. Health Serv Res. 2009;44(4):1309–25.
80. Temkin-Greener H, Cai S, Katz P, Zhao H, Mukamel DB. Daily practice teams in nursing homes: evidence from New York state. Gerontologist. 2009;49(1):68–80.
81. Zimmerman S, Bowers BJ, Cohen LW, Grabowski DC, Horn SD, Kemper P, et al. New evidence on the green house model of nursing home care: synthesis of findings and implications for policy, practice, and research. Health Serv Res. 2016;51(Suppl 1):475–96.
82. Levy C, Palat SIT, Kramer AM. Physician practice patterns in nursing homes. J Am Med Dir Assoc. 2007;8(9):558–67.
83. Hoek JF, Ribbe MW, Hertogh CMPM, van der Vleuten CPM. The role of the specialist physician in nursing homes: the Netherlands' experience. Int J Geriatr Psychiatry. 2003;18(3):244–9.
84. Ryskina KL, Polsky D, Werner RM. Physicians and advanced practitioners specializing in nursing home care, 2012–2015. JAMA. 2017;318(20):2040–2.
85. AMDA. White Paper on the Nursing Home Medical Director: Leader & Manager. Teh Soc Post-Acute Long-Term Care Med. 2011.
86. Donald F, Martin-Misener R, Carter N, Donald EE, Kaasalainen S, Wickson-Griffiths A, et al. A systematic review of the effectiveness of advanced practice nurses in long-term care. J Adv Nurs. 2013;69(10):2148–61.
87. Mileski M, Pannu U, Payne B, Sterling E, McClay R. The impact of nurse practitioners on hospitalizations and discharges from long-term nursing facilities: a systematic review. Healthc Basel Switz. 2020;8(2):E114.
88. Campbell S, Drake ADR, Espinoza R, Scales K. Caring for the future: the power and potential of America's direct care workforce. New York: PHI; 2021.
89. PHI. Direct care workers in the United States: key facts. 2021. https://www.phinational.org/resource/direct-care-workers-in-the-united-states-key-facts-2/.
90. Sloane PD, Yearby R, Konetzka RT, Li Y, Espinoza R, Zimmerman S. Addressing systemic racism in nursing homes: a time for action. J Am Med Dir Assoc. 2021;22(4):886–92.
91. Li Y, Yin J, Cai X, Temkin-Greener H, Mukamel DB. Association of race and sites of care with pressure ulcers in high-risk nursing home residents. JAMA. 2011;306(2):179–86.
92. Gruneir A, Miller SC, Feng Z, Intrator O, Mor V. Relationship between State Medicaid Policies, Nursing Home Racial Composition, and the Risk of Hospitalization for Black and White residents. Health Serv Res. 2008;43(3):869–81.
93. Yearby R. African Americans can't win, break even, or get out of the system: the persistence of "unequal treatment" in nursing home care. 2010. https://scholarship.law.slu.edu/faculty/87.
94. Li Y, Harrington C, Temkin-Greener H, You K, Cai X, Cen X, et al. Deficiencies in care at nursing homes and racial/ethnic disparities across homes fell, 2006–11. Health Aff Proj Hope. 2015;34(7):1139–46.
95. Cassie KM, Cassie W. Racial disparities in the use of physical restraints in U.S. nursing homes. Health Soc Work. 2013;38(4):207–13.
96. Cai S, Mukamel DB, Temkin-Greener H. Pressure ulcer prevalence among black and white nursing home residents in New York state: evidence of racial disparity? Med Care. 2010;48(3):233–9.

97. Mack DS, Hunnicutt JN, Jesdale BM, Lapane KL. Non-Hispanic Black-White disparities in pain and pain management among newly admitted nursing home residents with cancer. J Pain Res. 2018;11:753–61.
98. Shippee TP, Ng W, Bowblis JR. Does living in a higher proportion minority facility improve quality of life for racial/ethnic minority residents in nursing homes? Innov Aging. 2020;4(3):igaa014.
99. Mor V, Zinn J, Angelelli J, Teno JM, Miller SC. Driven to tiers: socioeconomic and racial disparities in the quality of nursing home care. Milbank Q. 2004;82(2):227–56.
100. Dowling MK, Kelly RL. Policy solutions for reversing the color-blind public health response to COVID-19 in the US. JAMA. 2020;324(3):229–30.
101. Smith DB, Feng Z, Fennell ML, Zinn JS, Mor V. Separate and unequal: racial segregation and disparities in quality across U.S. nursing homes. Health Aff Proj Hope. 2007;26(5):1448–58.
102. Feagin J, Bennefield Z. Systemic racism and U.S. health care. Soc Sci Med. 2014;103:7–14.
103. Vighte BW, Bradley AL, Cohen M, Hartmann H. Designing universal family care: state-based social insurance programs for early child care and education, paid family and medical leave, and long-term services and supports. National Academy of Social Insurance. Natl Acad Soc Insur [Internet]. https://www.nasi.org/research/2019/designing-universal-family-care-state-based-social-insurance. Accessed 27 Oct 2020.
104. Abrams HR, Loomer L, Gandhi A, Grabowski DC. Characteristics of U.S. nursing homes with COVID-19 cases. J Am Geriatr Soc. 2020;68(8):1653–6.
105. Konetzka RT, White EM, Pralea A, Grabowski DC, Mor V. A systematic review of long-term care facility characteristics associated with COVID-19 outcomes. J Am Geriatr Soc. 2021;69(10):2766–77.
106. CDC. COVID-19 nursing home data. 2022 [cited 2022 May 14]. https://data.cms.gov/covid-19/covid-19-nursing-home-data.
107. CDC. Covid data tracker. [cited 2022 May 14]. https://covid.cdc.gov/covid-data-tracker/#datatracker-home.
108. Utsumi M, Makimoto K, Quroshi N, Ashida N. Types of infectious outbreaks and their impact in elderly care facilities: a review of the literature. Age Ageing. 2010;39(3):299–305.
109. Fleming A, Browne J, Byrne S. The effect of interventions to reduce potentially inappropriate antibiotic prescribing in long-term care facilities: a systematic review of randomised controlled trials. Drugs Aging. 2013;30(6):401–8.

Home- and Community-Based Care

Amy C. Denham and Christine E. Kistler

Introduction

Care for older adults and individuals with disabilities living in the community is complex and must balance acute care, preventive services, management of chronic diseases, and sometimes custodial care. More than half of Americans aged 65 years or older have three or more chronic diseases, often with cognitive or functional impairments [1]. Approximately 8% of community-dwelling adults aged 65 years and older have dementia, with higher prevalence in older age groups, and more than a third have functional limitations such visual and hearing impairment, mobility limitations, challenges with communication, and inability to perform activities of daily living (ADLs) or instrumental activities of daily living (IADLs) independently [2]. In younger populations, 4% of noninstitutionalized adults aged 18–65 years have cognitive disabilities and 6% have disabilities that affect their ability to live independently [3].

The US faces multiple challenges in meeting the healthcare needs of its population, especially since there are proportionally fewer younger adults to meet the care needs of an aging population [4]. Institutional settings such as nursing homes can manage the care of medically complex adults, but it is expensive and of varying quality, evidenced by the deficiencies in staffing and infection control that contributed to nursing home residents disproportionately dying from COVID-19 [5]. Most Americans prefer care in community-based settings, with most expressing a preference to remain in their own homes [6]. There is therefore a need for high-quality, cost-effective, community-based health care to meet the needs of an aging population.

Much of the care provided to older and disabled adults in the community is provided by family and friends, most commonly adult children and spouses [7]. About 90% of older adults who need help with ADLs or IADLs receive assistance from unpaid caregivers, and about two thirds receive assistance solely from unpaid caregivers [8]. Older adults perceive the care provided by family as high-quality and more responsive than that of paid caregivers [9]. Family caregivers, however, report high levels of emotional and physical stress, financial strain, and difficulty meeting their own healthcare needs because of their caregiving responsibilities, indicating a need for community-based care to augment the care from family [7].

Financing Community-Based Long-Term Care

Community-based care is financed through a patchwork of out-of-pocket payments and in-kind contributions by the individual older adults and their informal caregivers, Medicaid, Medicare, and other public sources (e.g., the Department of Veterans Affairs). Private medical insurance generally does not pay for institutional or community-based long-term care services. Private long-term care insurance is expensive, and few people have it [10].

Although Medicare is the main payer for *medical* services for older adults in the US, it has a limited role in paying for *custodial* care. Medicare pays for short-term skilled care in home or institutional settings, for example, following discharge from the hospital, and covers services for patients enrolled in hospice, but otherwise does not cover personal care costs. Medicare does pay in part for enrollment in Programs of All-Inclusive Care for the Elderly (PACE).

Medicaid is the main payer for long-term care services and is the source of over half of national spending on long-term care [11]. Medicaid is funded jointly by the federal government and states but is administered at the state level. While nursing home care is mandated by federal law, home- and community-based personal care services are optional, and states vary considerably in how they proportion Medicaid dollars between institutions and home- and community-based services (HCBS). Half of seniors and 80% of non-

A. C. Denham (✉) · C. E. Kistler
Department of Family Medicine, University of North Carolina at Chapel Hill, School of Medicine, Chapel Hill, NC, USA
e-mail: amy_denham@med.unc.edu;
christine_kistler@med.unc.edu

elderly disabled individuals who receive long-term care services through Medicaid receive those services in the community rather than in institutions [10]. In recent decades the proportion of Medicaid spending on HCBS has increased relative to spending on institutional long-term care [11]. In some states, Medicaid will pay a family member or an independent personal care agency to provide direct assistance to homebound patients [12].

Although the original Medicaid legislation was biased toward institutional care, newer legislation expands states' options for covering HCBS, with expansion of such since 2010, under the Affordable Care Act (ACA) [10, 11, 13, 14]. For example, the Balancing Incentive Program provides matching federal funds to states that spend less than 50% of their Medicaid dollars on HCBS [15], with the goal of shifting long-term care spending from institutional care to HCBS. The Personal and Home Care Aide State Training (PHCAST) Program is an ACA-funded demonstration project to develop career ladders for workforce training and development [16].

After Medicaid, the second largest source of funding for long-term care services is out-of-pocket payments. Medicaid only covers individuals with low incomes, so a large segment of the population is not Medicaid eligible and must pay out of pocket, with the median cost of these services in 2021 at $27 per hour for home health aides or $78 per day for adult day care [17]. Often individuals deplete their resources and become Medicaid eligible, making Medicaid the payer of last resort.

Most older adults living at home who need care receive at least some of that assistance from unpaid caregivers [7]. If these informal caregivers were reimbursed at market rates, the cost of their care would far exceed that provided by paid caregivers [9]. In addition, there is an opportunity cost when unpaid caregivers reduce or leave their employment. Community-based care alternatives are generally less expensive than nursing home care in part because they rely on unpaid caregivers filling in the gaps not covered by paid caregivers.

Emerging Payment Models

Innovations in healthcare financing have emerged that may alter how long-term care is organized and delivered. Although health care and long-term care are still largely paid for on a fee-for-service basis, the Centers for Medicare & Medicaid Services (CMS) is increasingly emphasizing value-based payments and capitation, a trend that was accelerated with the passage of the Affordable Care Act in 2010 [18].

Arrangements such as Accountable Care Organizations (ACOs) encourage physicians and healthcare organizations to build collaborative relationships in which they share responsibility for cost and quality of care, aligning incentives between primary care, specialty care, hospitals, and long-term care, with the potential to bring long-term care programs under the same umbrella as medical care. In older patients, medical illness and functional impairments are intertwined and treating them separately can lead to inefficiencies and increased cost. For example, acute hospitalizations may be due to unmet custodial care needs rather than medical illness. If ACOs bring providers of long-term care into their organization, they will have both the incentive and the mechanism to provide the right care in the right setting.

Capitated payment models that focus on overall cost rather than on payment for specific services offer healthcare systems the flexibility to deliver care in a way that is efficient and effective, without silos between medical and custodial care. Programs of All-Inclusive Care for the Elderly (PACE), described later, have demonstrated on a small scale how capitated payments can integrate medical and long-term care, and may model a way to replicate similar systems on a larger scale.

Home-Based Clinical Care

Home health care includes home health agencies, hospice, home-based medical care, and the emerging model of hospital-at-home and is usually time limited, addressing post-acute medical needs that are expected to resolve. In contrast, home-based personal care services or custodial care may be long term and are described later in this chapter.

Home Services by Allied Health Professionals

Home health agencies (HHAs) provide time-limited, skilled services that focus on recovery from reversible conditions. Discrete episodes of care, lasting no more than 4–6 weeks, are reimbursed by Medicare and require demonstrable improvement to continue service. They do not provide 24-h care or homemaker services. An episode of care may include home visits by nurses, physical therapists, occupational therapists, speech therapists, nutritionists, social workers, and home aides. Home health nurses may be registered nurses (RNs), with 2–4 years of training, or licensed practical nurses (LPNs), who typically have about one year of training. LPNs can provide education, medication reconciliation, wound care, and dressing changes [19], while RNs can perform higher order nursing such as physical assessments, triage, and administration of intramuscular or intravenous medications.

Home-based physical therapy focuses on mobility and may be complemented by occupational therapy, which addresses activities of daily living such as feeding, dressing, toileting, and bathing. Speech therapists address feeding and swallowing, speech, and cognition. Nutritionists address weight loss and healthy eating. Social workers provide a range of social, financial, and emotional support, including accessing resources in the community for transportation, meals, or aide personal care, as well as crisis intervention and direct counseling [20]. Home health agencies also coordinate medication and durable medical equipment (DME) delivery.

To be eligible for a HHA, a patient must be under the care of a physician who will guide the treatment plan, must have either nursing or physical therapy needs, and must be homebound [14], meaning they cannot leave their homes for anything other than medical appointments or religious services. Continuity of care from a small team of consistent providers decreases the risk of hospitalization and emergency department visits and increases the chances of improved functioning in ADLs [21].

Home-Based Medical Care by Physicians and Advance Practice Providers

Home-based medical care (HBMC) is the provision of care from physicians or advance practice providers. It includes primary care, consultative assessments, specialty and disease-specific care, and palliative care, and meets the healthcare needs of homebound patients with serious medical illness [22–25].

Home-Based Primary Care

Home-based primary care (HBPC) with a familiar clinician reduces costs and improves the quality of care when provided to frail patients with multimorbidity, along with desired impacts on patient satisfaction, care quality, hospitalizations, and emergency room visits [26–28]. One of the first of these programs was the Veterans' Affairs Home-based Primary Care (HBPC) program [29], which targets frail, chronically ill older veterans who have difficulty traveling to outpatient appointments, though may otherwise not be strictly homebound. The interdisciplinary program typically includes a physician, advance practice providers such as nurse practitioners and physician assistants, nurses, social workers, dieticians, pharmacists, and physical or rehabilitation therapists and focuses on longitudinal, comprehensive care of patients who have, on average, eight chronic diseases. The program remains involved if it is helping to maintain the person in the home environment. The HBPC model decreases hospitalization, nursing home placement, and costs while increasing satisfaction [24].

Independence at Home, a HBPC demonstration program funded by the Affordable Care Act (ACA), targets post-acute care patients who have two or more chronic conditions, have had a hospital admission in the last 12 months, need assistance with two or more ADLs, and have received subacute rehabilitation services in the last 12 months [25, 30, 31]. Participating sites, which vary in their organizational model, may be able to share in cost savings, which is intended to create incentives for clinicians to provide longitudinal home-based care for a high-cost population. Successful features include access, affordability, coordinated care, and patient-oriented goal alignment [32]. At the end of year 2 of this 3-year project, overall savings compared to a control group was $7.8 million for 10,000 beneficiaries, with reductions in hospitalization, nursing home placement, and emergency department visits with increased documentation of patient preferences, clinician contact within 48 h of a hospitalization, and medication reconciliation. This program's success demonstrates that home care for complex chronically ill individuals can save money and provide quality care.

Consultative Visits and Specialty Care

Specialty consultations in the home may happen after a hospitalization as part of transitions of care, with recommendations sent to the primary care clinician. The Community-Based Care Transition Programs, created under the ACA, funds pilot transitional care models at more than 100 participating sites, providing short-term assistance to manage the patient's transition from the hospital to the community-based setting, with improved outcomes and decreased costs [33].

Home-based medical care can include podiatry and dental care, though these services are generally not covered by insurers, require private payment, and are of variable quality. Care (or case) management refers to social workers or nurses who coordinate the homebound patient's medical care such as monitoring in-home aides and providing "eyes-on-the-ground" for out-of-town relatives. The National Association of Professional Geriatric Care Managers maintains a list of all accredited members (http://www.aginglifecare.org/), who may work for a health system or for the growing private sector. Costs of these services vary based on the level and frequency of the services provided.

Home-based medical care can positively impact specific chronic illnesses, such as lung disease, diabetes, and hypertension [28, 34–36]. Home-based medical care for adults with severe cognitive or mental illness, such as dementia or schizophrenia, may effectively manage behaviors and address safety concerns, and may prevent the need to live in a facility [28]. Some complex treatments can be provided in the home, such as peritoneal dialysis, ventilator care, left ventricular assist devices, total parenteral nutrition, and continuous inotrope infusions, with coordination and communication between the home care clinician and specialists.

Palliative Care

Home-based palliative care providers focus on symptom control for homebound patients with serious illnesses, prioritizing the relief of suffering, either physical or emotional, with the goal of maximizing quality of life for patients and families, avoiding hospitalization but still rendering appropriate treatments, such as palliative chemotherapy. Appropriate patients are seriously ill and functionally limited but not yet ready or eligible for hospice [37]. This care is covered under traditional Medicare services rather than the Medicare hospice benefit.

Hospital-at-Home

The hospital-at-home model reduces the use of limited hospital resources and provides an inpatient level of service in the home. Hospitalizations can be associated with adverse events and functional decline for older patients, and hospital-at-home programs may avoid some of this iatrogenic harm. These programs vary in the intensity of services they provide, the patients served, and can focus on supporting recent discharges or admission avoidance [38]. Hospital-at-home is associated with increased patient and caregiver satisfaction and reduced mortality and readmissions [39]. In 2020, CMS issued a "Hospitals Without Walls" regulatory guidance that led to many large hospitals developing programs, although less so in rural and small hospitals [40]. Programs that focus on admission avoidance are more cost-effective and have better outcomes than programs supporting recent discharge [41]. This care may not be useful for patients with intensive care needs or those without caregivers in the home. Future work may define best care team composition, number of visits needed, implementation, payment structures, and quality metrics as the use of hospital-at-home increases.

Evaluation and Assessment in the Home

Home care clinicians should develop skills in key domains of geriatric medicine, including palliative care, dementia, delirium, urinary incontinence, constipation, weight loss, hearing and vision impairment, pressure ulcers, and falls [42]. They need to understand rehabilitation modalities and be versed in prognosticating, clarifying goals of care, assessing decisional capacity, and reviewing advance directives. The cornerstone of home visits is trust between the provider, patient, family, and caregivers. While a clinic or hospital is the domain of doctors and nurses, the home is the patient's environment. The act of coming to the home tells the caregivers and patients that the provider sees them as individuals and is willing to put forth effort on their behalf. The clinician learns a great deal by seeing the patient at home, where the patient can demonstrate both the strengths and challenges of home, with solutions discussed in a pragmatic manner.

Home safety assessments aim to reduce falls and other injuries due to worsening cognitive impairment and functional decline and involve looking for safety concerns such as low lighting, clutter, throw rugs, electrical cords, stairs, and bathroom accessibility. Improving safety might include installing an alert system, placing locks on doors, and removing fall hazards. A home safety evaluation also looks for neglect, elder abuse, and caregiver fatigue. Other home-based programs that reduce falls and improve safety in the home environment include home intervention teams (HITs) [43] and the Community Aging in Place, Advancing Better Living for Elders (CAPABLE) program [44], which consists of a 10-session, home-based inter-professional intervention involving occupational therapists, nurses, and handymen.

Evaluation in the home gives a better sense of a patient's function than evaluation in clinical settings and includes assessing gait, balance, and ability to perform ADLs and IADLs [45–48]. Assistive devices or physical therapy may improve functional status. Medicare will cover one walker every 5 years, and prior authorization of durable medical equipment is usually required, given concerns about over-utilization [49]. There are specific requirements for power wheelchairs and scooters.

Reviewing how medications are administered, stored, dispensed, whether there are duplications, and what over-the-counter medications and supplements are being used allows the clinician to recommend practices that maximize adherence and limit adverse effects.

Homebound adults are at risk for malnutrition and limited access to food, which can lead to the frailty cascade of weight loss, muscle atrophy, exhaustion, inactivity, and increased mortality [50]. Home care clinicians can evaluate the availability of food in the home and observe for evidence that patients with dementia need assistance with meal preparation and eating. Food access problems can be addressed through Meals on Wheels or other local agencies that supply food to patients at home. Social support should also be assessed, with evidence of companionship and conversation from family members, friends, paid aides and attendants, and volunteers from local community organizations. Social workers help homebound patients complete applications for benefits such as pharmacy assistance, food stamps, or housing vouchers, and contact adult protective services agencies if indicated.

A thorough home visit by a clinician includes a comprehensive physical examination of the patient, including assessing hearing aids and glasses, and testing memory and cognition with screening tools such as the Veteran's Affairs St. Louis University Mental Status (VA-SLUMS) test or the Montreal Cognitive Assessment (MoCA) [51, 52].

Telehealth and Virtual Care

Telehealth improves the ability to manage medically complex adults at home and its use was accelerated by the COVID-19 pandemic when Congress lifted many limitations on telehealth services [53]. Barriers to telehealth include lack of financial reimbursement, lack of internet access, discomfort with telehealth visits, training, and deviations in standards of care, such as lack of vital sign assessment [54]. Telehealth requires web cameras and monitors, training, and the development of operational guidelines [55]. Alternative payment models may support more use of telehealth [56]. Successful implementation depends on preparation, innovation, standardization, technology, and communication [57].

Telehealth home care requires devices that monitor weight, vital signs, and glucose, and technologies such as sensors or cameras to monitor the patient, all of which improve outcomes for patients with complex illnesses [14, 58–60].

Telehealth for caregivers of patients living with dementia may improve caregivers' depression and sense of competence, although no improvements in caregiver burden or sleep disturbance have been observed [61, 62]. Veterans Administration home telehealth programs reduce hospitalizations for veterans with schizophrenia and other psychiatric conditions [63, 64]. Telehealth improves the management of patients with heart failure and reduces emergency department utilization [60].

Nonresidential Community-Based Care

Community-based care services for adults with chronic illness can be provided in patients' homes, facilities that patients visit during the day but return to their own home at night, or in residential facilities. There is some overlap between these models, and patients may receive care from more than one model simultaneously.

Home-Based Personal Care Services

Personal care provided by home aides is the most common form of home care [2]. This care may be provided through licensed home care agencies or through direct arrangements with independent caregivers, and may include assistance with IADLs, such as housekeeping or meal preparation; hands-on assistance with bathing and dressing; or supervision for patients with cognitive impairment. Licensing for home care agencies occurs at the state level, so there is state-to-state variability in how home care services are organized and what training and licensing is required. Home care aides or personal care attendants may have limited education, training, and supervision and are paid low wages, contributing to problems with recruitment and retention of workers [65].

Area Agencies on Aging and Senior Centers

Established by the Older Americans Act of 1965, Area Agencies on Aging coordinate services for older adults at the local level, providing information on community-based supports, case management, and counseling to help connect older adults and their families with long-term care services. Area Agencies on Aging may operate as branches of state, county, or local government, or states may contract with nonprofit organizations to fulfill these services. Senior centers, often the focal point of services provided by Area Agencies on Aging, are community centers financed through a combination of federal, state, local, and private funds. Senior centers provide social and recreational activities, as well as congregate meals and transportation services. They may provide health and wellness activities such as exercise programs or health screenings. They are an appropriate setting for daytime activities and meals for older adults who have mild functional or cognitive impairments but do not need significant supervision or assistance with personal care.

Adult Day Services Centers

Adult day services (ADS) centers, also referred to as adult day care or adult day health programs, provide care during daytime hours for community-dwelling chronically ill people, allowing them to live at home with caregivers but receive support during the day, giving respite to caregivers, or allowing them to remain in the workforce. Although the majority of participants are aged 65 years and older, ADS also serves younger adults with intellectual or developmental disabilities or severe mental health concerns, so the average age of participants is younger than users of other long-term care services [66, 67]. About a quarter to half of ADS participants have dementia, most need assistance with three or more ADLs, and about a quarter have chronic mental health conditions [67, 68]. The patient population served tends to be more racially and ethnically diverse than that of other types of long-term care services [66].

Although there is heterogeneity in the services provided by ADS, typically programs include recreation and social engagement, supervision, assistance with personal care, and meals. Although it is not typical for ADS centers to have physician services on site, the majority have nurses on staff, with about half providing complex nursing services such as wound, ostomy, or catheter care. Other common health-related services include health education, blood pressure or blood sugar monitoring, medication management, and foot care [68]. ADS may also provide social work services, skilled therapy services such as physical or occupational therapy, mental health counseling, caregiver support, and dietary and pharmacy services [66, 69].

There are currently approximately 4800 ADS centers in the US, serving more than 286,300 people with increasing enrollment as home- and community-based options for long-term care increase [66, 68]. Although historically provided by non-profit organizations, sometimes in association with larger organizations such as hospitals and nursing homes, for-profit businesses now account for 44% of ADS. The average size of ADS facilities is also increasing, with about half of the centers serving greater than 25 participants, and most are in metropolitan areas [66]. Funding for ADS comes mostly from public sources such as Medicaid or the Department of Veterans Affairs, with a smaller portion coming from privately paid participant fees, with centers varying in the proportion of public versus private funding [68].

Enrollment in ADS programs appears to lower caregivers' levels of stress and burden, reducing the amount of time caregivers spend addressing behavior problems, reducing the level of hostility caregivers feel from their loved ones, and allowing caregivers to attend to their own medical needs [70–74]. Participants may also experience benefits, including improved cognition, decreased agitation, improved sleep patterns, and lower rates of hospitalizations and emergency department visits [70, 71, 75–78]. ADS programs may delay institutionalization [79], but the research is mixed with some studies suggesting that ADS attendance has no effect or even increases nursing home placement [76, 80–82]. Severe illness or caregiver stress might result in both increased ADS attendance and increased risk for nursing home placement, so it cannot be inferred that ADS attendance *causes* nursing home placement. In many cases, ADS may serve as a steppingstone toward nursing home care, as caregivers transition from providing all care in the home to a greater level of reliance on institutional care.

Programs of All-Inclusive Care for the Elderly

Programs of All-inclusive Care for the Elderly (PACE) are an innovative model for community-based care, serving as an alternative to nursing home care for frail, functionally, and/or cognitively impaired older adults. The PACE model originated in San Francisco in 1971 and has evolved and spread nationally in the subsequent decades. PACE services are typically based at an adult day services center, with a primary care clinic and rehabilitation services on site, with the interdisciplinary PACE care team coordinating medical care and long-term services across settings, including home, hospital, clinics, and nursing homes. To be eligible for PACE, individuals must be aged 55 years or older and must be impaired enough to be nursing home eligible in their state of residence but still able to be safely supported in the community at the time of enrollment. The average PACE participant is 77 years old and has 5.8 chronic medical conditions. Most (57%) are dependent in three or more ADLs and 46% have dementia [83].

The first PACE program, On-Lok Senior Health Services, was created in San Francisco's Chinatown in 1971 as a culturally acceptable alternative to nursing home care in the Chinese immigrant community. On-Lok is Cantonese for "peaceful, happy abode." When On-Lok demonstrated success in providing coordinated support services for individuals with long-term care needs, the organization was provided Medicare and Medicaid waivers to allow it to receive a monthly fixed payment for each enrolled individual to deliver full medical services, while assuming full risk for the cost of that individual's medical care. In 1986, ten additional waivers were provided by the federal government to replicate and disseminate the On-Lok model to other areas of the country, and in 1997 PACE was recognized as a permanent provider type to receive Medicare and Medicaid funding. In 2005, more grants were awarded to expand the PACE model to rural areas of the US [84]. The PACE model continued to expand and in 2022 there are 272 PACE centers in 30 states, serving approximately 60,000 participants [83]. PACE organizations are typically operated by non-profit organizations, although in 2019 CMS adjusted regulations to allow for-profit companies to operate PACE centers [85].

Most PACE participants are dually eligible for both Medicare and Medicaid, which fund PACE through capitated payments, although some PACE organizations also enroll participants who do not have Medicaid and who pay privately for a portion of PACE fees. Medicaid pays PACE organizations a fixed per-member-per-month fee that is set at the state level. Medicare pays a risk-adjusted per-member-per-month fee that varies at the individual participant level, based on demographics, frailty, and medical diagnoses [84]. In exchange for these capitated payments, PACE organizations assume full risk for the cost of medical and custodial care for their participants. The PACE organization assumes the cost not only for the services provided at the PACE center but also for subspecialty medical care, hospitalizations, emergency care, short- and long-term nursing home placement, home care, and durable medical equipment.

The PACE financing model allows individual PACE organizations flexibility in what services to deliver, allowing coverage for some services that might not be typically covered under fee-for-service Medicare or Medicaid. This flexibility results in variability in services among PACE organization, but there are several common features to the care provided. Care is coordinated by an interdisciplinary team, typically consisting of a primary care clinician, nurse, social worker, physical therapist, occupational therapist, dietician, recreational therapist, home care coordinator, aide, driver, and PACE center supervisor. This team assesses the medical, functional, nutritional, and psychosocial needs of each participant on enrollment and at least every 6 months thereafter to create an interdisciplinary plan of care. Participants attend an adult day health center, generally from 1 to 5 days a week, that provides primary medical care, rehabilitation services, socialization, recreational activities, exercise, meals, daily transportation, and personal care services. Occasionally a PACE organization partners with primary care physicians in the community. Personal care assistance in the home may also be provided outside the hours of PACE attendance, either by PACE staff or on a contract basis with home care agencies in the community. The PACE team follows each participant across sites of care, including if the person is ultimately placed in a nursing home, through the end of life.

Outcomes for PACE participants are positive, as measured by quality of care, functional status, mortality, and health services utilization. Satisfaction with PACE is high, evidenced by low disenrollment rates and participate and caregiver satisfaction [86, 87]. Participants in PACE have better control of pain, higher receipt of preventive services, and higher rates of completion of advance directives [88, 89]. Some research suggests that PACE participants have lower mortality [90, 91], while other research suggests similar mortality to comparable patients [92, 93].

Rates of hospitalization, preventable hospitalization, readmission, and emergency department use are lower for PACE participants than for similar individuals dually eligible for Medicare and Medicaid [90, 92–95]. All PACE enrollees are nursing home eligible at the time of enrollment, reflecting a high risk for nursing home placement. Although early research suggested higher rates of nursing home admissions among PACE participants as compared to other community-based populations, these studies did not distinguish between short- and long-term nursing home placements [88]. More recent research has suggested lower rates of long-term nursing home placements compared with participants in other Medicaid HCBS waiver programs [96] and beneficiaries of dually eligible integrated care programs [92]. These data may reflect that PACE programs make use of short-term nursing home placements for respite or to avoid unnecessary hospitalizations for unmet custodial care needs, but that they are still able to minimize long-term nursing home placements.

Further research is needed to address whether PACE services are more cost-effective than other models of HCBS for dually eligible Medicare and Medicaid beneficiaries, who comprise less than 20% of Medicare and Medicaid beneficiaries, but account for a third of Medicare and Medicaid spending [92]. There is active interest in finding models for cost-effective care for this population. Although PACE does appear to decrease utilization of some costly services, the cost of PACE services overall may be greater than other HCBS, though lower than nursing home care [93]. Medicare costs are similar between PACE participants and individuals enrolled in other HCBS models. Although Medicaid costs are similar to comparison populations living in nursing homes, they are higher than those of individuals enrolled in other HCBS funding models [88, 90].

Aging in Place and the Villages Movement

Aging in place "villages" are an emerging model that organizes neighborhoods to support older adults living in their own homes. Modern families are often widely dispersed and the informal networks that support older adults in their homes and neighborhoods may not be present. Individuals pay to participate in a village, which then provides some of that informal support. This model originated in the Beacon Hill neighborhood of Boston in 2002 and has grown to over 300 community-based villages nationally [97]. The village may have one or two paid staff to organize community members or other community-based organizations to provide needed services on a voluntary basis when needed. Village staff also maintain lists of resources for paid assistance, in some cases at a reduced fee negotiated on behalf of the village.

The village model can help members with minor tasks such as shopping, transportation, or household maintenance stay in their own homes longer than they might have otherwise been able to. However, it is typically not adequate to meet the needs of older adults with more significant cognitive and functional impairments, who need supervision or daily assistance with their ADLs.

Technologies to Facilitate Aging in Place

Smart home and robotic technologies are increasingly used to assist older adults to age in place in their own homes and aim to promote safety and social connections without the physical presence of another person. Simple call buttons to summon help in the event of a fall have advanced to more sophisticated devices such as remote sensors that can measure and transmit blood sugar or vital signs to healthcare providers. Pill boxes can provide medication reminders and monitor adherence. Smart devices can sense and report falls or turn off stoves if they are left unattended. GPS monitors can track and report wandering. There are even robotic technologies in development that assist with tasks such as toileting or transfers. Although none of these technologies fully substitutes for hands-on care or supervision from another person, they may contribute to keeping older individuals in their homes.

Residential Options for Community-Based Care

For people no longer able to live independently, there is a wide array of residential care options with varying degrees of support. Approximately 2% of people aged 65 years and older in the US live in community housing with services such as meals, personal care, housekeeping, or medication management in approximately 28,900 licensed residential care communities [2]. Most of these facilities are run by for-profit companies, and less than half participate in Medicaid [66]. As opposed to nursing homes, residential options do not provide clinical, skilled nursing, or rehabilitative services, rather are intended to meet social and custodial needs.

Senior Housing

Senior housing is independent living geared toward older adults who do not need supervision or assistance with personal care and usually includes freestanding homes or apartments that are set up to be accessible for people who are beginning to experience mobility limitations. These communities might provide some supports, such as congregate meals, activities, transportation, or housekeeping, but they do not provide personal care or supervision.

The cost of senior housing varies widely, depending on the type of housing and amenities provided, and might include both an initial investment and monthly fees. The cost of independent living is not covered by Medicaid or long-term care insurance. Senior housing subsidized by the US Department of Housing and Urban Development (HUD) is an option for low-income seniors, although waiting lists are often long.

Assisted Living

Assisted living describes a residential model of care that provides care in a home-like setting, emphasizing the privacy, dignity, and autonomy of residents, with private sleeping quarters that can be locked, bathrooms, small kitchens, and individual temperature controls [98]. Since the 1980s, *assisted living* has evolved to mean residential facilities that provide assistance with ADLs or IADLs but not skilled nursing care. Because there is no clear definition, there is wide variation in what types of facilities are marketed as assisted living [98–101].

Assisted living facilities aim to provide a homelike environment, although some are large and have an institutional feel. Residents generally live in private units furnished with their personal belongings with common dining and living areas. Assisted living facilities typically offer medication reminders or administration, but other health-related services are limited. They are generally staffed by aides trained to provide personal care assistance, but may not have nurses on-site or only present for limited hours [66, 99]. Many assisted living facilities offer a care unit for individuals with dementia, usually including restricted doors to manage residents who wander [66]. These units may also offer specialized programing for residents with cognitive impairment. Some research suggests that segregated care for residents with dementia may result in higher resident-to-resident aggression and higher use of antipsychotic medications [99, 102, 103].

Assisted living grew rapidly in the 1990s, and by 2007 there were 838,746 units in 11,276 facilities nationally [104]. There is no national regulatory structure, so how assisted living is defined and regulated varies from state to state [105]. Unlike nursing homes and home health agencies, which have national quality standards and measures, assisted living lacks quality accountability, making it harder for families to compare facilities. The Agency for Healthcare Research and Quality (AHRQ) has recommended use of a standardized reporting tool, but this has not been widely adopted [99]. The lack of consensus on what defines assisted living and how to measure quality limits the ability to interpret research comparing assisted living to other community-based models of care [101, 104, 106].

Assisted living is generally paid out of pocket by residents or their family members. In some states Medicaid pays for the personal care services provided in assisted living facilities, but not room and board. The median monthly cost of assisted living in the US is $4300, with annual cost increases outpacing rising costs in other health and long-term care sectors [99]. Assisted living is therefore out of reach for many low- and moderate-income older adults. The availability of assisted living is generally highest in areas with greater educational attainment, income, and wealth, with lower access in rural areas, geographic areas with lower incomes, and minority communities [99, 104].

Adult Foster Care

Adult foster care is another residential option for meeting the care needs of adults who have some functional impairments but do not need skilled nursing care. Adult foster care may be referred to by a variety of names, including family care homes, adult family homes, or elder group homes, all of which provide a home-like residence that serves a small number of individuals, generally up to six residents.

In some states, adult foster care is licensed and regulated in the same manner as assisted living, but in other states these smaller care settings have their own regulatory structure. Requirements for staffing ratios, staff training, and provision of services vary by state [107]. Individuals usually pay privately for the adult foster care services, but in some states Medicaid pays for the personal care services, but not room and board, in the context of HCBS waiver programs [108].

Individuals in adult foster care show greater improvements in self-care skills and mobility at a lower cost than nursing home residents and experience greater levels of social activity, though there has not been updated research on this in recent years [109, 110].

Medical Foster Home Care

The US Department of Veterans Affairs (VA) Medical Foster Home (MFH) is a program for veterans who have disabilities that qualify them for nursing home care and whose needs cannot be met by caregivers at home. In an MFH, caregivers with experience in nursing homes or with disabled persons care for up to three veterans, providing 24-h services including personal needs, supervision, meals, and medication management. Caregivers and homes are screened for suitability by a social worker and occupational therapist associated with the MFH program, and home safety is monitored through monthly unannounced visits by program staff. Veterans or their family members pay the caregiver a negotiated out-of-pocket rate for what is usually a long-term arrangement, often until the end of life [111–114]. The MFH program works collaboratively with the VA's home-based primary care (HBPC), in which medical care for homebound veterans is provided by a coordinated team of physicians, nurses, social workers, dieticians, pharmacists, and rehabilitation professionals.

The MFH program was established in 2008, and as of 2016, there were 117 MFH programs nationally, with a total of 693 homes serving 992 veterans [111]. Residents of MFHs have a similar level of frailty, comorbidity, and functional dependencies as veterans living in VA nursing homes, but at a lower cost of care with lower mortality rates and fewer hospitalizations for COPD, heart failure, diabetic crises, dehydration, pressure ulcers, skin infections, and mental health conditions [112–116].

The Green House Model

Models of long-term care are typically divided into nursing home care and home- and community-based care, but these divisions are not always distinct. Some community-based independent living and assisted living facilities may feel large and institutional while some nursing homes try to replicate home-like environments. The Green House model strives to make nursing homes feel home like and person-centered, with small units that house 10–12 residents in private rooms, with a shared living and dining area. Staff provide care, including meals, housekeeping, personal care, and medication management, with residents free to set their own schedules for meals and activities. Most Green House homes are licensed as skilled nursing homes, certified by Medicare and Medicaid, with a few licensed as assisted living facilities [117, 118]. The Green House model is trademarked, but some other nursing homes incorporate principles of the Green House "household model." Some evidence suggests that nursing home residents in a household model experience lower hospitalization, lower staff turnover, greater psychosocial well-being, and lower rates of COVID-19 deaths as compared with residents of conventional nursing homes [119, 120, 121].

Continuing Care Retirement Communities

Continuing Care Retirement Communities (CCRCs) provide progressive levels of care, from independent living to assisted living to nursing home care, so that individuals can remain in the same community through the end of life, regardless of their care needs. Usually, CCRCs require that individuals are healthy and functional enough to live independently upon joining the community and do not accept as new residents people who already have significant functional or cognitive impairments. CCRCs often have waiting lists, so older adults interested in CCRCs must plan for their care needs well in advance.

CCRCs vary in size, cost, and services offered, and can offer a range of independent living options, from freestanding homes or cottages to small apartments. They offer dining, social, and recreational activities, and many provide medical clinics on site. Some CCRCs now offer a "CCRC at home" or "CCRC without walls" option, meaning people pay an entrance fee and/or monthly fees to the CCRC and may access their services while remaining in their own homes, with an option to enter at a higher level of care in the future.

The high cost of CCRCs limits their accessibility to many people, with entry fees of tens to hundreds of thousands of dollars and monthly fees that increase as the level of care advances. Prior to joining a community, applicants must show they have the assets to sustain the fees over the many years. No licensing or regulatory agency oversees CCRCs, so it is difficult to determine how many there are or how many people live there. However, the assisted living and nursing home portions of CCRCs are regulated by state and federal agencies. CCRCs may be run by non-profit or for-profit organizations.

Principles of Care of the Community-Dwelling Older Patient

There is limited high-quality evidence that any one model of community-based care is superior to another, or to nursing home care, regarding quality of care, patient outcomes, or cost [106]. Patients and their caregivers can use shared decision-making with their primary care clinician to choose the most appropriate setting based on the person's needs and familiarity with local options. Function, cognition, behavior, and medical complexity are factors to consider in selecting a community option. The patient and family goals of care should be explored, including the tradeoffs between independence and safety. Depending on the patient's state of health and prognosis, the time of transition to more care may be an opportunity to discuss the patient's perspective on quality versus quantity of life.

Coordinating Care Across Settings of Care

Caring for medically complex adults living in the community can be challenging, with the need to address both acute and chronic illnesses and manage cognitive and functional limitations while navigating a complex web of community-based agencies and programs. Which clinicians are providing care and how do they communicate? Several models strive to provide coordinated quality care in the community. The Geriatric Resources for Assessment and Care of Elders (GRACE) model pairs primary care physicians practicing in community health centers with off-site geriatrics interdisciplinary teams who provide quarterly reviews and input on patient management. The Guided Care model partners primary care physicians with registered nurses who provide care management and self-management support for older patients who are at risk for high healthcare utilization. The CAPABLE program, in which a nurse, occupational therapist, and handy worker team assess function and symptom burden and implement strategies to facilitate patient goals, has demonstrated reductions in disability and hospitalizations in a broad range of settings [44]. These successful models use an interdisciplinary team to carry out medical and functional assessment of the patient, followed by the development of a comprehensive, evidence-based plan of care, which they then monitor for adherence. They coordinate care across and between settings and facilitate access to community-based resources [122].

Elements of team-based care for community-dwelling older patients can be provided by primary care clinicians through the Patient Centered Medical Home, which includes care coordination outside of face-to-face encounters in the office. The Center for Medicare and Medicaid Innovation (CMMI) is funding Primary Care Transformation demonstration projects which pilot practice and payment models that develop care management and coordination across disciplines, which assess medical and functional needs, collaborate with community-based care providers, and coordinate care across office, hospital, and long-term care settings [123].

Administrative and Regulatory Issues

Physicians generally need to complete forms before patients can enter long-term care, attesting to any functional impairments and suggesting the level of care to meet the patient's needs. Eligibility requirements for HCBS services or nursing home care are determined at the state level. For skilled home health care such as nursing or physical therapy, CMS requires that physicians (or nurse practitioners, certified nurse midwives, or physicians' assistants) attest to and date a face-to-face evaluation within 90 days before or 30 days after the initiation of services. This documentation must describe the clinical status of the patient, the reason the patient is homebound, and the conditions necessitating skilled services. The plan of care is reviewed and signed, and if home health services are still needed at the end of the initial 60 days, the clinician must review the plan of care, attest to the need for ongoing services, and estimate the length of time that services will be needed [124]. Medicare pays clinicians for certifying and recertifying home health plans of care, given the oversight requirements, if the requisite reimbursement codes are submitted.

Home- and Community-Based Services and Health Equity

Disparities in health care access and outcomes among older and disabled populations are well documented. Older patients who are members of racial and ethnic minority groups or are of low socioeconomic status (SES) have shorter life expectancies, greater levels of disability at younger ages, and higher burdens of serious illness, resulting in disproportionate need for long-term care services and supports [125–127]. Older patients who are racial and ethnic minorities have a cumulative lifetime exposure to the root causes of health disparities, including discrimination, environmental hazards, residential segregation, disparities in healthcare access and quality, and other structural factors that affect access to social and economic resources. Rural/urban disparities also exist in access to long-term care services. Gender and sexual minorities—including lesbian, gay, bisexual, transgender, or queer (LGBTQ) patients—may face particular vulnerabilities. The design and delivery of long-term care services should ameliorate rather than exacerbate health disparities.

Disparities in Access

Vulnerable populations such as those identified as racial and ethnic minorities, low socioeconomic status, rural, and LGBTQ may have disproportionate need for long-term care services but may be challenged to find high-quality community-based care. People of color or those with low incomes have greater concern than whites and those with higher incomes regarding their community's ability to support older people living at home [128]. Long-term care models such as CCRCs and assisted living are prohibitively expensive for many, reflected in those communities being disproportionately white and high income [99].

Although Blacks and other people of color have higher use of HCBS and informal support in the home and lower use of nursing home care than Whites, it is unclear whether this is due to preferences or an inability to secure institutional long-term care services, as Blacks report higher rates of unmet long-term care needs [129, 130]. For users of home health and other HCBS, racial and ethnic minorities and those living in low-income areas tend to receive services from agencies with lower quality-of-care ratings, and have higher rates of unplanned hospitalizations, readmissions, and emergency care, even when adjusting for comorbidities and baseline functional dependencies, raising concerns about quality of care [129–132].

There are also disparities between rural and urban areas and access to HCBS. Medicaid funding for long term is shifting to HCBS rather than institutional care, but rural areas often lack the infrastructure to make this shift. Limited transportation options, geographic dispersal of patients resulting in longer travel times, and lack of trained workforce often make HCBS in rural areas expensive and logistically difficult [133].

Specific challenges may also exist for LGBTQ populations seeking long-term care services. The current cohort of older LGBTQ patients has lived most of their lives without the social and economic benefits of marriage. They may be less likely to have adult children who can assist with caregiving and may be estranged from family due to homophobia and transphobia. Informal networks of same-age peers who are part of these individuals' "chosen family" may be unable to support long-term care needs [134]. LGBTQ individuals may feel vulnerable in bringing paid caregivers into their homes, fearing discrimination, which appears to be well-founded based on data on older LGBTQ individuals living in long-term care facilities [135]. Some resort to a phenomenon described as "going back in the closet" to hide one's sexuality or gender identity in order to feel safe and accepted in receiving long-term care services [136].

Table 20.1 Proposed strategies to address disparities in long-term care

- Ensure equitable access to public quality reporting through outreach to underserved populations and making materials easily navigable for low-literacy and low-English-proficiency populations [130]
- Include health equity measures in quality-of-care reporting [132]
- Ensure that pay-for-performance initiatives adequately adjust for the effects of social determinants of health and provide subsidies and technical support for low-resource settings to engage in quality improvement [130]
- Direct resources toward integrated care models that have a proven track record of providing equitable long-term care services, such as PACE and CAPABLE [132]
- Allow Medicaid payments for HCBS to go to informal and family caregivers, reducing dependence on home care agency infrastructure in rural and other under-resourced settings [130]
- Enhance reimbursement to long-term care providers who serve a disproportionate share of Medicaid insured individuals [132]
- Invest in training and support for long-term care providers to deliver care that is culturally and linguistically appropriate, including requiring training in care that meets the needs of LGBTQ communities [99, 132]
- Roll long-term care coverage into an entitlement program such as Medicare rather than a means-tested program such as Medicaid [137]

Strategies for Improving Equity

Initiatives to improve quality of care in long-term care can exacerbate disparities, increasing quality in higher-resource settings while leaving the most vulnerable patients behind. For example, consumer information about quality, such as CMS's Care Compare website (https://www.medicare.gov/care-compare/), is most accessible to individuals with high health literacy and internet skills. Pay-for-performance programs that direct resources toward long-term care programs that are providing the highest quality care end up diverting resources away from programs that have the lowest resources to pursue quality improvement initiatives [130, 132]. Proposed strategies for addressing disparities in long-term care are listed in Table 20.1.

Conclusion

Much of the complexity of caring for chronically ill older and disabled patients is due to the presence of medical illness, functional impairments, and cognitive deficits. Healthcare providers must attend to not only the medical needs but also the personal care needs of their patients. Although institutional care may seem to be the most straightforward way to meet functionally impaired adults' care needs, most patients prefer to remain in the community. There are a variety of community-based options that allow people to remain in their homes or in home-like settings, spanning the continuum from independence to complete functional dependency. The primary care clinician is a key resource in helping patients and families anticipate care needs and select the most appropriate setting of care.

References

1. Ornstein SM, Nietert PJ, Jenkins RG, Litvin CB. The prevalence of chronic diseases and multimorbidity in primary care practice: a PPRNet report. J Am Board Fam Med. 2013;26(5):518–24.
2. Federal Interagency Forum on Aging-Related Statistics. Older Americans 2020: key indicators of well-being. Washington, DC: U.S. Government Printing Office; 2020.
3. U.S. Census Bureau. American Community Survey S1810 DISABILITY CHARACTERISTICS [Internet]. 2020 [cited 2022 Apr 15]. https://data.census.gov/cedsci/table?t=Disability&tid=ACSST5Y2020.S1810.
4. Roberts AW, Ogunwole SU, Blakeslee L, Rabe MA. The population 65 years and older in the United States: 2016. Washington, DC: U.S. Census Bureau; 2018.
5. Committee on the Quality of Care in Nursing Homes (Washington, District of Columbia). The national imperative to improve nursing home quality: honoring our commitment to residents, families, and staff. Washington, DC: The National Academies Press; 2022.
6. The AP-NORC Center for Public Affairs Research. Long-term care in America: Americans want to age at home [Internet]. 2021 [cited 2022 Apr 15]. https://www.longtermcarepoll.org/project/long-term-care-in-america-americans-want-to-age-at-home/.
7. AARP. Caregiving in the United States 2020 [Internet]. 2020 [cited 2022 Apr 15]. https://www.aarp.org/ppi/info-2020/caregiving-in-the-united-states.html.
8. Federal Interagency Forum on Aging-Related Statistics. Older Americans 2016: key indicators of well-being. Washington, DC: U.S. Government Printing Office; 2016.
9. Institute of Medicine (US) Committee on the Future Health Care Workforce for Older Americans. Retooling for an aging America: building the health care workforce. Washington, DC: National Academies Press; 2008.
10. Reaves EL, Musumeci M. Medicaid and long-term services and supports: a primer [Internet]. 2015 [cited 2022 Apr 13]. https://www.kff.org/medicaid/report/medicaid-and-long-term-services-and-supports-a-primer/.
11. O'Malley Watts M, Musumeci M, Chidambaram PC. Medicaid home and community-based services: enrollment and spending [Internet]. 2020 [cited 2022 Apr 12]. https://www.kff.org/report-section/medicaid-home-and-community-based-services-enrollment-and-spending-issue-brief/.
12. Doty P, Mahoney KJ, Sciegaj M. New state strategies to meet long-term care needs. Health Aff (Millwood). 2010;29(1):49–56.
13. Martin EJ. Healthcare policy legislation and administration: patient protection and affordable care act of 2010. J Health Hum Serv Adm. 2015;37(4):407–11.
14. Weisfeld V, Lustig TA. The future of home health care: workshop summary. Washington, DC: National Academies Press; 2015.
15. Lustig TA, Olson S. Financing long-term services and supports for individuals with disabilities and older adults: workshop summary. Washington, DC: National Academies Press; 2014.
16. Health Resources and Services Administration. Report to Congress: Personal and Home Care Aide State Training (PHCAST) demonstration program evaluation [Internet]. [cited 2022 Apr 21]. https://www.hrsa.gov/sites/default/files/about/organization/bureaus/bhw/reportstocongress/phcastreport.pdf.
17. Genworth Financial Inc. Genworth cost of care survey: summary and methodology [Internet]. 2022 [cited 2022 Apr 15]. https://pro.genworth.com/riiproweb/productinfo/pdf/131168.pdf.
18. Blumenthal D, Abrams M. The affordable care act at 10 years - payment and delivery system reforms. N Engl J Med. 2020;382(11):1057–63.
19. Spector N. Practical nurse scope of practice white paper. Chicago, IL: National Council of State Boards of Nursing; 2005.
20. Koru G, Alhuwail D, Rosati RJ. Identifying the key performance improvement domains for home health agencies. SAGE Open Med. 2015;3:2050312115621924.
21. Russell D, Rosati RJ, Rosenfeld P, Marren JM. Continuity in home health care: is consistency in nursing personnel associated with better patient outcomes? J Healthc Qual. 2011;33(6):33–9.
22. Stall N, Nowaczynski M, Sinha SK. Systematic review of outcomes from home-based primary care programs for homebound older adults. J Am Geriatr Soc. 2014;62(12):2243–51.
23. Brian Cassel J, Kerr KM, McClish DK, Skoro N, Johnson S, Wanke C, et al. Effect of a home-based palliative care program on healthcare use and costs. J Am Geriatr Soc. 2016;64(11):2288–95.
24. Edes T, Kinosian B, Vuckovic NH, Nichols LO, Becker MM, Hossain M. Better access, quality, and cost for clinically complex veterans with home-based primary care. J Am Geriatr Soc. 2014;62(10):1954–61.
25. Kinosian B, Taler G, Boling P, Gilden D, Independence at Home Learning Collaborative Writing Group. Projected savings and workforce transformation from converting independence at home to a Medicare benefit. J Am Geriatr Soc. 2016;64(8):1531–6.
26. Totten AM, White-Chu EF, Wasson N, Morgan E, Kansagara D, Davis-O'Reilly C, et al. Home-based primary care interventions. Rockville, MD: Agency for Healthcare Research and Quality (US); 2016.
27. De Jonge KE, Jamshed N, Gilden D, Kubisiak J, Bruce SR, Taler G. Effects of home-based primary care on Medicare costs in high-risk elders. J Am Geriatr Soc. 2014;62(10):1825–31.
28. Zimbroff RM, Ornstein KA, Sheehan OC. Home-based primary care: a systematic review of the literature, 2010–2020. J Am Geriatr Soc. 2021;69(10):2963–72.
29. Cooper DF, Granadillo OR, Stacey CM. Home-based primary care: the care of the veteran at home. Home Healthc Nurse. 2007;25(5):315–22.
30. Centers for Medicare and Medicaid Services CMS. Independence at home demonstration [Internet]. 2017. https://innovation.cms.gov/initiatives/independence-at-home.
31. DeJonge KE, Taler G, Boling PA. Independence at home: community-based care for older adults with severe chronic illness. Clin Geriatr Med. 2009;25(1):155–69, ix.
32. Shafir A, Garrigues SK, Schenker Y, Leff B, Neil J, Ritchie C. Homebound patient and caregiver perceptions of quality of care in home-based primary care: a qualitative study. J Am Geriatr Soc. 2016;64(8):1622–7.
33. Centers for Medicare and Medicaid Services CMS. Community-based care transitions program [Internet]. 2016 [cited 2022 Apr 21]. http://innovation.cms.gov/initiatives/CCTP.
34. Michaelchuk W, Oliveira A, Marzolini S, Nonoyama M, Maybank A, Goldstein R, et al. Design and delivery of home-based telehealth pulmonary rehabilitation programs in COPD: a systematic review and meta-analysis. Int J Med Inform. 2022;162:104754.
35. Fernando ME, Seng L, Drovandi A, Crowley BJ, Golledge J. Effectiveness of remotely delivered interventions to simultaneously optimize management of hypertension, hyperglycemia and

36. Mabeza RMS, Maynard K, Tarn DM. Influence of synchronous primary care telemedicine versus in-person visits on diabetes, hypertension, and hyperlipidemia outcomes: a systematic review. BMC Prim Care. 2022;23(1):52.
37. Kamal AH, Currow DC, Ritchie CS, Bull J, Abernethy AP. Community-based palliative care: the natural evolution for palliative care delivery in the U.S. J Pain Symptom Manage. 2013;46(2):254–64.
38. Shepperd S, Iliffe S. Hospital at home versus in-patient hospital care. Cochrane Database Syst Rev. 2005;(3):CD000356.
39. Caplan GA, Sulaiman NS, Mangin DA, Aimonino Ricauda N, Wilson AD, Barclay L. A meta-analysis of "hospital in the home". Med J Aust. 2012;197(9):512–9.
40. Levine DM, DeCherrie LV, Siu AL, Leff B. Early uptake of the acute hospital care at home waiver. Ann Intern Med. 2021;174(12):1772–4.
41. Leong MQ, Lim CW, Lai YF. Comparison of Hospital-at-Home models: a systematic review of reviews. BMJ Open. 2021;11(1):e043285.
42. Parks SM, Harper GM, Fernandez H, Sauvigne K, Leipzig RM. American Geriatrics Society/Association of Directors of Geriatric Academic Programs curricular milestones for graduating geriatric fellows. J Am Geriatr Soc. 2014;62(5):930–5.
43. Nikolaus T, Bach M. Preventing falls in community-dwelling frail older people using a home intervention team (HIT): results from the randomized Falls-HIT trial. J Am Geriatr Soc. 2003;51(3):300–5.
44. Szanton SL, Leff B, Li Q, Breysse J, Spoelstra S, Kell J, et al. CAPABLE program improves disability in multiple randomized trials. J Am Geriatr Soc. 2021;69(12):3631–40.
45. Steffen TM, Hacker TA, Mollinger L. Age- and gender-related test performance in community-dwelling elderly people: Six-Minute Walk Test, Berg Balance Scale, Timed Up & Go Test, and gait speeds. Phys Ther. 2002;82(2):128–37.
46. Podsiadlo D. The timed "Up & Go": a test of basic functional mobility for frail elderly persons. J Am Geriatr Soc. 1991;39(2):142–8.
47. Lawton MP, Brody EM. Assessment of older people: self-maintaining and instrumental activities of daily living. Gerontologist. 1969;9(3):179–86.
48. Katz S, Downs TD, Cash HR, Grotz RC. Progress in development of the index of ADL. Gerontologist. 1970;10(1):20–30.
49. Centers for Medicare & Medicaid Services (CMS), HHS. Medicare Program; Prior authorization process for certain durable medical equipment, prosthetics, orthotics, and supplies. Final rule. Fed Regist. 2015;80(250):81673–707.
50. Fried LP, Tangen CM, Walston J, Newman AB, Hirsch C, Gottdiener J, et al. Frailty in older adults: evidence for a phenotype. J Gerontol A Biol Sci Med Sci. 2001;56(3):M146–56.
51. Nasreddine ZS, Phillips NA, Bédirian V, Charbonneau S, Whitehead V, Collin I, et al. The Montreal Cognitive Assessment, MoCA: a brief screening tool for mild cognitive impairment. J Am Geriatr Soc. 2005;53(4):695–9.
52. Tariq SH, Tumosa N, Chibnall JT, Perry MH, Morley JE. Comparison of the Saint Louis University mental status examination and the mini-mental state examination for detecting dementia and mild neurocognitive disorder—a pilot study. Am J Geriatr Psychiatry. 2006;14(11):900–10.
53. US Congress. Public Law 116–123: Making emergency supplemental appropriations for the fiscal year ending September 30, 2020, and for other purposes. [Internet]. 2020 [cited 2022 Apr 22]. https://www.congress.gov/116/plaws/publ123/PLAW-116publ123.pdf.
54. Omboni S, Padwal RS, Alessa T, Benczúr B, Green BB, Hubbard I, et al. The worldwide impact of telemedicine during COVID-19: current evidence and recommendations for the future. Connect Health. 2022;1:7–35.
55. Greenhalgh T, Wherton J, Shaw S, Morrison C. Video consultations for covid-19. BMJ. 2020;368:m998.
56. Zhao M, Hamadi H, Haley DR, Xu J, White-Williams C, Park S. Telehealth: advances in alternative payment models. Telemed J E Health. 2020;26(12):1492–9.
57. Knierim K, Palmer C, Kramer ES, Rodriguez RS, VanWyk J, Shmerling A, et al. Lessons learned during COVID-19 that can move telehealth in primary care forward. J Am Board Fam Med. 2021;34(Suppl):S196–202.
58. Rantz MJ, Skubic M, Miller SJ, Galambos C, Alexander G, Keller J, et al. Sensor technology to support Aging in Place. J Am Med Dir Assoc. 2013;14(6):386–91.
59. Flodgren G, Rachas A, Farmer AJ, Inzitari M, Shepperd S. Interactive telemedicine: effects on professional practice and health care outcomes. Cochrane Database Syst Rev. 2015;(9):CD002098.
60. Posadzki P, Mastellos N, Ryan R, Gunn LH, Felix LM, Pappas Y, et al. Automated telephone communication systems for preventive healthcare and management of long-term conditions. Cochrane Database Syst Rev. 2016;12:CD009921.
61. Williams KN, Perkhounkova Y, Shaw CA, Hein M, Vidoni ED, Coleman CK. Supporting family caregivers with technology for dementia home care: a randomized controlled trial. Innov Aging. 2019;3(3):igz037.
62. Gathercole R, Bradley R, Harper E, Davies L, Pank L, Lam N, et al. Assistive technology and telecare to maintain independent living at home for people with dementia: the ATTILA RCT. Health Technol Assess. 2021;25(19):1–156.
63. Flaherty LR, Daniels K, Luther J, Haas GL, Kasckow J. Reduction of medical hospitalizations in veterans with schizophrenia using home telehealth. Psychiatry Res. 2017;255:153–5.
64. Karlin BE, Karel MJ. National integration of mental health providers in VA home-based primary care: an innovative model for mental health care delivery with older adults. Gerontologist. 2014;54(5):868–79.
65. LeBlanc AJ, Tonner MC, Harrington C. State Medicaid programs offering personal care services. Health Care Financ Rev. 2001;22(4):155–73.
66. Harris-Kojetin L, Sengupta M, Lendon JP, Rome V, Valverde R, Caffrey C. Long-term care providers and services users in the United States, 2015–2016. Washington, DC: U.S. Department of Health and Human Services, Centers for Disease Control and Prevention, National Center for Health Statistics; 2019.
67. Lendon JP, Singh P. Adult day services center participant characteristics: United States, 2018. NCHS Data Brief. 2021;(411):1–8.
68. Anderson KA, Dabelko-Schoeny H, Johnson TD. The state of adult day services: findings and implications from the MetLife National Study of Adult Day Services. J Appl Gerontol. 2013;32(6):729–48.
69. Caffrey C, Lendon JP. Service provision, hospitalizations, and chronic conditions in adult day services centers: findings from the 2016 National Study of Long-Term Care Providers. Natl Health Stat Rep. 2019;(124):1–9.
70. Fields NL, Anderson KA, Dabelko-Schoeny H. The effectiveness of adult day services for older adults: a review of the literature from 2000 to 2011. J Appl Gerontol. 2014;33(2):130–63.
71. Zarit SH, Kim K, Femia EE, Almeida DM, Savla J, Molenaar PCM. Effects of adult day care on daily stress of caregivers: a within-person approach. J Gerontol B Psychol Sci Soc Sci. 2011;66(5):538–46.
72. Gaugler JE, Jarrott SE, Zarit SH, Stephens M-AP, Townsend A, Greene R. Respite for dementia caregivers: the effects of adult

72. day service use on caregiving hours and care demands. Int Psychogeriatr. 2003;15(1):37–58.
73. Gaugler JE, Jarrott SE, Zarit SH, Stephens M-AP, Townsend A, Greene R. Adult day service use and reductions in caregiving hours: effects on stress and psychological well-being for dementia caregivers. Int J Geriatr Psychiatry. 2003;18(1):55–62.
74. Parker LJ, Gaugler JE, Samus Q, Gitlin LN. Adult day service use decreases likelihood of a missed physician's appointment among dementia caregivers. J Am Geriatr Soc. 2019;67(7):1467–71.
75. Femia EE, Zarit SH, Stephens MAP, Greene R. Impact of adult day services on behavioral and psychological symptoms of dementia. Gerontologist. 2007;47(6):775–88.
76. Ellen ME, Demaio P, Lange A, Wilson MG. Adult day center programs and their associated outcomes on clients, caregivers, and the health system: a scoping review. Gerontologist. 2017;57(6):e85–94.
77. Honjo Y, Ide K, Takechi H. Use of day services improved cognitive function in patients with Alzheimer's disease. Psychogeriatrics. 2020;20(5):620–4.
78. Kelly R. The effect of adult day program attendance on emergency room registrations, hospital admissions, and days in hospital: a propensity-matching study. Gerontologist. 2017;57(3):552–62.
79. Kelly R, Puurveen G, Gill R. The effect of adult day services on delay to institutional placement. J Appl Gerontol. 2016;35(8):814–35.
80. Vandepitte S, Van Den Noortgate N, Putman K, Verhaeghe S, Verdonck C, Annemans L. Effectiveness of respite care in supporting informal caregivers of persons with dementia: a systematic review. Int J Geriatr Psychiatry. 2016;31(12):1277–88.
81. McCann JJ, Hebert LE, Li Y, Wolinsky FD, Gilley DW, Aggarwal NT, et al. The effect of adult day care services on time to nursing home placement in older adults with Alzheimer's disease. Gerontologist. 2005;45(6):754–63.
82. Rokstad AMM, Engedal K, Kirkevold Ø, Benth JŠ, Selbæk G. The impact of attending day care designed for home-dwelling people with dementia on nursing home admission: a 24-month controlled study. BMC Health Serv Res. 2018;18(1):864.
83. National PACE Association. PACE facts and trends [Internet]. 2022 [cited 2022 Apr 16]. https://www.npaonline.org/policy-and-advocacy/pace-facts-and-trends-0.
84. Hirth V, Baskins J, Dever-Bumba M. Program of all-inclusive care (PACE): past, present, and future. J Am Med Dir Assoc. 2009;10(3):155–60.
85. Gonzalez L. Will for-profits keep up the pace in the United States? The future of the program of all-inclusive care for the elderly and implications for other programs serving medically vulnerable populations. Int J Health Serv. 2021;51(2):195–202.
86. Temkin-Greener H, Bajorska A, Mukamel DB. Disenrollment from an acute/long-term managed care program (PACE). Med Care. 2006;44(1):31–8.
87. National PACE Association. PACE reduces burden of family caregivers [Internet]. 2018 [cited 2022 Apr 16]. https://www.npaonline.org/about-npa/press-releases/pace-reduces-burden-family-caregivers.
88. Ghosh A, Orfield C, Schmitz R. Evaluating PACE: a review of the literature [Internet]. 2013 [cited 2022 Apr 16]. https://aspe.hhs.gov/reports/evaluating-pace-review-literature-0.
89. Leavitt MO. Interim report to congress: the quality and cost of the Program of All-inclusive Care for the Elderly (PACE) [Internet]. 2009 [cited 2022 Apr 16]. https://www.cms.gov/Medicare/Health-Plans/PACE/Downloads/Report-to-Congress.pdf.
90. Ghosh G, Schmitz R, Brown R. Effect of PACE on costs, nursing home admissions, and mortality: 2006–2011 [Internet]. 2015 [cited 2022 Apr 16]. https://aspe.hhs.gov/reports/effect-pace-costs-nursing-home-admissions-mortality-2006-2011-0.
91. Wieland D, Boland R, Baskins J, Kinosian B. Five-year survival in a Program of All-inclusive Care for Elderly compared with alternative institutional and home- and community-based care. J Gerontol A Biol Sci Med Sci. 2010;65(7):721–6.
92. Feng Z, Wang J, Gadaska A, Knowles M, Haber S, Ingber MJ, et al. Comparing outcomes for dual eligible beneficiaries in integrated care: final report. Washington, DC: U.S. Department of Health and Human Services; 2021.
93. Arku D, Felix M, Warholak T, Axon DR. Program of All-Inclusive Care for the Elderly (PACE) versus other programs: a scoping review of health outcomes. Geriatrics (Basel). 2022;7(2):31.
94. Meret-Hanke LA. Effects of the Program of All-inclusive Care for the Elderly on hospital use. Gerontologist. 2011;51(6):774–85.
95. Segelman M, Szydlowski J, Kinosian B, McNabney M, Raziano DB, Eng C, et al. Hospitalizations in the Program of All-Inclusive Care for the Elderly. J Am Geriatr Soc. 2014;62(2):320–4.
96. Segelman M, Cai X, van Reenen C, Temkin-Greener H. Transitioning from community-based to institutional long-term care: comparing 1915(c) Waiver and PACE enrollees. Gerontologist. 2017;57(2):300–8.
97. Village to Village Network [Internet]. 2022 [cited 2022 Apr 17]. https://www.vtvnetwork.org/.
98. Zimmerman S, Sloane PD. Definition and classification of assisted living. Gerontologist. 2007;47 Spec No 3:33–9.
99. Zimmerman S, Carder P, Schwartz L, Silbersack J, Temkin-Greener H, Thomas KS, et al. The imperative to reimagine assisted living. J Am Med Dir Assoc. 2022;23(2):225–34.
100. Kane RL. Finding the right level of posthospital care: "We didn't realize there was any other option for him". JAMA. 2011;305(3):284–93.
101. Kane RA, Chan J, Kane RL. Assisted living literature through May 2004: taking stock. Gerontologist. 2007;47 Spec No 3:125–40.
102. Zimmerman S, Anderson WL, Brode S, Jonas D, Lux L, Beeber AS, et al. Systematic review: Effective characteristics of nursing homes and other residential long-term care settings for people with dementia. J Am Geriatr Soc. 2013;61(8):1399–409.
103. Calkins MP. From research to application: supportive and therapeutic environments for people living with dementia. Gerontologist. 2018;58(Suppl_1):S114–28.
104. Stevenson DG, Grabowski DC. Sizing up the market for assisted living. Health Aff (Millwood). 2010;29(1):35–43.
105. Temkin-Greener H, Mao Y, Ladwig S, Cai X, Zimmerman S, Li Y. Variability and potential determinants of assisted living state regulatory stringency. J Am Med Dir Assoc. 2021;22(8):1714–1719.e2.
106. Wysocki A, Butler M, Kane RL, Kane RA, Shippee T, Sainfort F. Long-term services and supports for older adults: a review of home and community-based services versus institutional care. J Aging Soc Policy. 2015;27(3):255–79.
107. Carder P, O'Keeffe J, O'Keeffe C. Compendium of residential care and assisted living regulations and policy: 2015 Edition [Internet]. 2015 [cited 2022 Apr 16]. https://aspe.hhs.gov/sites/default/files/migrated_legacy_files//73501/15alcom.pdf.
108. Mollica M, Booth M, Gray C, Sims-Kastelein K. Adult foster care: a resource for older adults [Internet]. 2008 [cited 2022 Apr 16]. https://www.nashp.org/wp-content/uploads/2009/03/AFC_resource.pdf.
109. Braun KL, Rose CL. Geriatric patient outcomes and costs in three settings: nursing home, foster family, and own home. J Am Geriatr Soc. 1987;35(5):387–97.
110. Kane RA, Kane RL, Illston LH, Nyman JA, Finch MD. Adult foster care for the elderly in Oregon: a mainstream alternative to nursing homes? Am J Public Health. 1991;81(9):1113–20.
111. Haverhals LM, Manheim CE, Gilman CV, Jones J, Levy C. Caregivers create a veteran-centric community in VHA medical foster homes. J Gerontol Soc Work. 2016;59(6):441–57.

112. Magid KH, Manheim C, Haverhals LM, Thomas KS, Saliba D, Levy C. Who receives care in VA medical foster homes? Fed Pract. 2021;38(3):102–9.
113. Levy C, Whitfield EA. Medical foster homes: can the adult foster care model substitute for nursing home care? J Am Geriatr Soc. 2016;64(12):2585–92.
114. Levy CR, Alemi F, Williams AE, Williams AR, Wojtusiak J, Sutton B, et al. Shared homes as an alternative to nursing home care: impact of VA's medical foster home program on hospitalization. Gerontologist. 2016;56(1):62–71.
115. Levy C, Whitfield EA, Gutman R. Medical foster home is less costly than traditional nursing home care. Health Serv Res. 2019;54(6):1346–56.
116. Pracht EE, Levy CR, Williams A, Alemi F, Williams AE. The VA medical foster home program, ambulatory care sensitive conditions, and avoidable hospitalizations. Am J Med Qual. 2016;31(6):536–40.
117. Waters R. The big idea behind A new model of small nursing homes. Health Aff (Millwood). 2021;40(3):378–83.
118. Cohen LW, Zimmerman S, Reed D, Brown P, Bowers BJ, Nolet K, et al. The green house model of nursing home care in design and implementation. Health Serv Res. 2016;51(Suppl 1):352–77.
119. Zimmerman S, Bowers BJ, Cohen LW, Grabowski DC, Horn SD, Kemper P, et al. New evidence on the green house model of nursing home care: synthesis of findings and implications for policy, practice, and research. Health Serv Res. 2016;51(Suppl 1):475–96.
120. Hermer L, Bryant NS, Pucciarello M, Mlynarczyk C, Zhong B. Does comprehensive culture change adoption via the household model enhance nursing home residents' psychosocial well-being? Innov Aging. 2017;1(2):igx033.
121. Zimmerman S, Dumond-Stryker C, Tandan M, Preisser JS, Wretman CJ, Howell A, et al. Nontraditional small house nursing homes have fewer COVID-19 cases and deaths. J Am Med Dir Assoc. 2021;22(3):489–93.
122. Boult C, Wieland GD. Comprehensive primary care for older patients with multiple chronic conditions: "Nobody rushes you through". JAMA. 2010;304(17):1936–43.
123. The CMS Innovation Center [Internet]. [cited 2022 Apr 22]. https://innovation.cms.gov/.
124. Centers for Medicare & Medicaid Services. CMS Home Health Agency (HHA) Center [Internet]. 2022 [cited 2022 Apr 17]. https://www.cms.gov/Center/Provider-Type/Home-Health-Agency-HHA-Center?redirect=/center/hha.asp.
125. Hill CV, Pérez-Stable EJ, Anderson NA, Bernard MA. The National Institute on Aging health disparities research framework. Ethn Dis. 2015;25(3):245–54.
126. Ferraro KF, Kemp BR, Williams MM. Diverse aging and health inequality by race and ethnicity. Innov Aging. 2017;1(1):igx002.
127. Forrester SN, Taylor JL, Whitfield KE, Thorpe RJ. Advances in understanding the causes and consequences of health disparities in aging minorities. Curr Epidemiol Rep. 2020;7(2):59–67.
128. The AP-NORC Center for Public Affairs Research. Long-term care in America: how well can communities support aging at home? [Internet]. 2021 [cited 2022 Apr 21]. https://apnorc.org/projects/long-term-care-in-america-how-well-can-communities-support-aging-at-home/.
129. Gorges RJ, Sanghavi P, Konetzka RT. A national examination of long-term care setting, outcomes, and disparities among elderly dual eligibles. Health Aff (Millwood). 2019;38(7):1110–8.
130. Konetzka RT, Werner RM. Disparities in long-term care: building equity into market-based reforms. Med Care Res Rev. 2009;66(5):491–521.
131. Joynt Maddox KE, Chen LM, Zuckerman R, Epstein AM. Association between race, neighborhood, and Medicaid enrollment and outcomes in Medicare home health care. J Am Geriatr Soc. 2018;66(2):239–46.
132. Shippee TP, Fabius CD, Fashaw-Walters S, Bowblis JR, Nkimbeng M, Bucy TI, et al. Evidence for action: addressing systemic racism across long-term services and supports. J Am Med Dir Assoc. 2022;23(2):214–9.
133. Siconolfi D, Shih RA, Friedman EM, Kotzias VI, Ahluwalia SC, Phillips JL, et al. Rural-urban disparities in access to home- and community-based services and supports: stakeholder perspectives from 14 states. J Am Med Dir Assoc. 2019;20(4):503–508.e1.
134. Movement Advancement Project (MAP), SAGE Advocacy and Services for LGBT Elders. Understanding issues facing LGBT older adults. Boulder, CO: Movement Advancement Project; 2017.
135. The National Senior Citizens Law Center, The National Gay and Lesbian Task Force, SAGE (Services and Advocacy for LGBT Elders), Lambda Legal, The National Center for Lesbian Rights, The National Center for Transgender Equality. LGBT older adults in long-term care facilities: stories from the field [Internet]. [cited 2022 Apr 21]. https://www.lgbtagingcenter.org/resources/pdfs/NSCLC_LGBT_report.pdf.
136. SAGE Advocacy and Services for LGBTQ+ Elders. LGBTQ+ seniors fear having to go back in closet for the care they need [Internet]. [cited 2022 Apr 21]. https://www.sageusa.org/news--posts/lgbtq-seniors-fear-having-to-go-back-in-closet-for-the-care-they-need/.
137. Werner RM, Konetzka RT. Reimagining financing and payment of long-term care. J Am Med Dir Assoc. 2022;23(2):220–4.

End-of-Life Care

Margaret R. Helton and Jenny T. van der Steen

Chronic Disease and the Change in How People Die

Throughout human history, death was an unpredictable and often random event that could strike anyone at any time at any age. People were used to being around death, which was usually due to infection, injury, starvation, or childbirth. In the last century, with the dramatic increase in life expectancy, the experience and expectations around death have changed. Advances in science have medicalized death to the point where it is seen as a failure of the system and something to be fought all the way to intensive care, if needed, and with aggressive therapies such as chemotherapy and life support, even if these interventions provide little if any chance of restoring meaningful life. The experience of death had been taken out of the home and placed in hospitals.

As the population ages and medical technology continues to develop, people question the utility and morality of prolonging life at all costs, especially when their loved one is not restored to health and has poor quality of life. Along with these concerns comes the advent of new attitudes such as increased intolerance of pain and suffering and the right to personal autonomy and self-determination. These demographic and cultural trends have brought awareness and preferences for a "good death" to the forefront and the experience and circumstances of how people die is seen as a significant issue in health care for society and a crucial aspect of population health [1].

Most people now die from chronic diseases such as heart disease, stroke, cancer, and diabetes, all of which are treatable at some stage. It is often not clear when it is time to stop treatment and the default has been to keep going. Death from chronic disease is rarely sudden and tends to follow one of three trajectories [1]. Those with cancer tend to be relatively stable and then enter a period of rapid decline. Those with organ failure tend to have ups and downs against a background of steadily declining function, while people with frailty and dementia tend to slowly dwindle (Fig. 21.1). These trajectories occur in the background of emotional, physical, and spiritual changes for the patient and the family. Addressing these issues through compassionate palliative care is considered by many governing, legal, and religious organizations to be a human right [2].

M. R. Helton (✉)
Department of Family Medicine, University of North Carolina at Chapel Hill, Chapel Hill, NC, USA
e-mail: margaret_helton@med.unc.edu

J. T. van der Steen
Department of Public Health and Primary Care, Leiden University Medical Center, Leiden, the Netherlands

Radboudumc Alzheimer Center and Department of Primary and Community Care, Radboud University Medical Center, Nijmegen, the Netherlands
e-mail: jtvandersteen@lumc.nl; Jenny.vandersteen@radboudumc.nl

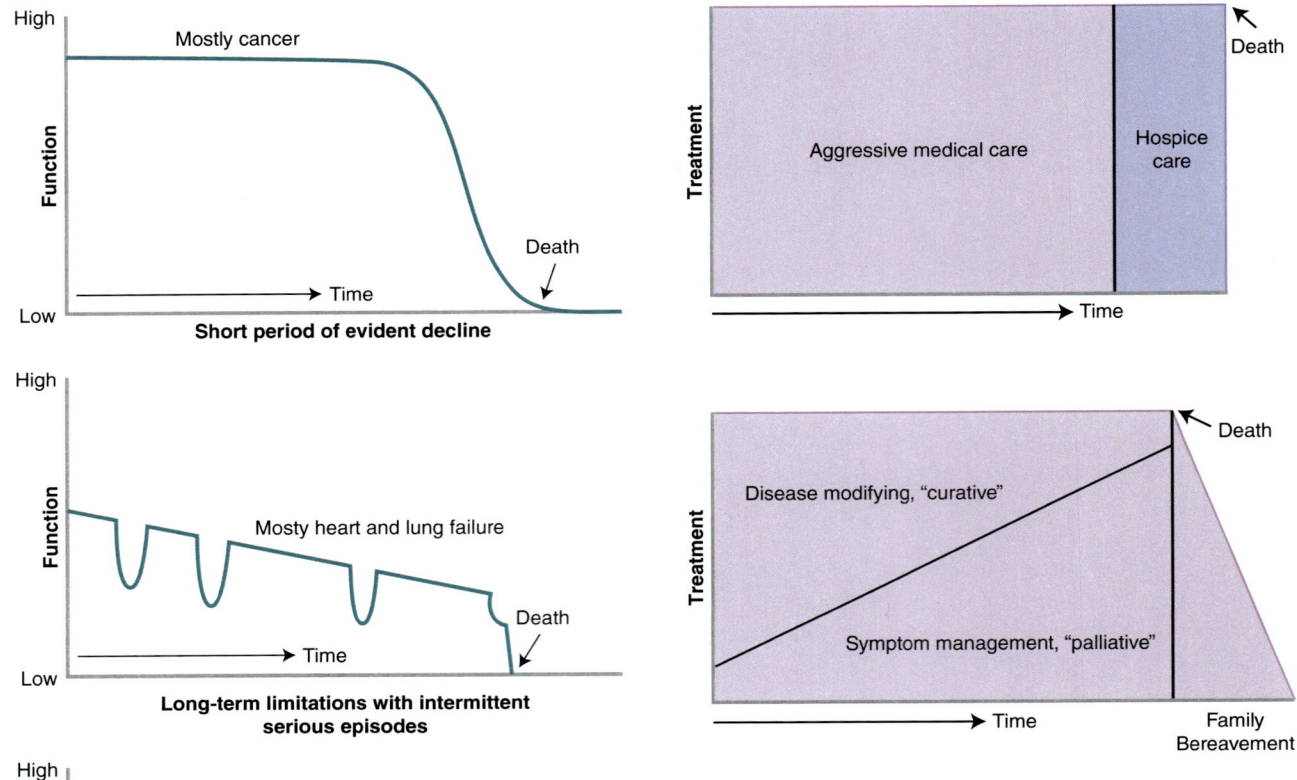

Fig. 21.1 Trajectories of death. (From Lynn J, Adamson DM. Living well at the end of life. Adapting health care to serious chronic illness in old age. RAND Health. DTIC Document; 2003)

Fig. 21.2 An older model (top) drew a sharp distinction between curative care and hospice, a line that patients and families were often reluctant to cross. A newer model (bottom) allows the integration of palliative care into the care continuum earlier in the disease process. (From Lynn J, Adamson DM. Living well at the end of life [1])

Birth of Modern Hospice and Palliative Care Movement

The modern hospice movement began with three women who brought public and professional attention to the plight of dying people and their families [3]. Cicely Saunders, considered the founder of the modern hospice movement, promoted teaching and research on the dying based on her clinical work at St. Christopher's Hospice in London, which she established in 1967. One of her protégés was Florence Wald, then dean of Yale's School of Nursing, who studied with Saunders and launched the American hospice movement, establishing Connecticut Hospice in 1974. Elisabeth Kübler-Ross brought the concept of death with dignity and her theory of the five stages of grief to the attention of the public with her international bestseller *On Death and Dying*, published in 1965 [4].

Awareness of the tension between what technology is capable of and what is ethical caused further reflection in the American public by highly publicized cases such as that of Karen Ann Quinlan, a young woman in a vegetative state who was granted the right to have life support withdrawn based on evidence of what her personal wishes had been, leading to the widespread use of advance care planning. In 1990, the US Supreme Court affirmed the right of a patient to refuse unwanted treatment in the case of Nancy Cruzan, another young woman in a persistent vegetative state. This led to a federal law, the patient Self-Determination Act, which requires medical institutions to counsel patients about their right to state their wishes regarding end-of-life care, should they become unable to do so themselves. Congress further advanced the discipline with the passage of a Medicare hospice benefit in 1982, made permanent in 1986. While well-intended, this provision drew a sharp distinction between curative care and comfort care, as patients crossed from one payment program to the other. Patients and their families were reluctant to cross that line and usually did so late in the course of the illness. This led to growth in palliative care which attends to patient suffering across the disease spectrum and allows for the integration of care that manages distressing symptoms while curative care efforts are still ongoing, whether the patient is expected to live days or years (Fig. 21.2) [1].

Table 21.1 Distinction between palliative care and hospice (adapted from Kelley AS, Morrison RS. Palliative Care for the Seriously Ill. The New England Journal of Medicine. 2015;373(8):747–55 [6])

	Palliative care	Hospice
Providers	Multidisciplinary team of physicians, nurses, social workers, chaplains	Multidisciplinary team of physicians, nurses, social workers, chaplains, volunteers
Goal	Improve quality of life through the prevention and relief of suffering related to physical, psychosocial, and spiritual issues, including pain.	Improve quality of life, relieve suffering, address emotional and spiritual issues of dying
Eligibility	Patients of all ages with any chronic illness; life-prolonging and disease-related treatments may continue. Family needs are considered, too.	Patients of all ages who are expected to live less than 6 months; curative treatments are foregone.
Place of care	Hospitals, outpatient, nursing homes, home	Home, assisted-living facilities, nursing homes, residential hospice facilities, inpatient hospice units
Payment	Provider fees covered by Medicare Part B; hospital care covered by Medicare Part A or commercial insurance; flexible bundled payments under Medicare Advantage, Managed Medicaid, Accountable Care Organizations, and other commercial payers	Medicare hospice benefit; standard hospice benefit from commercial payers is usually modeled after Medicare; Medicaid (varies by state); medications and supplies are covered for illnesses related to the terminal illness

In 2006, The American Board of Medical Specialties approved Hospice and Palliative Medicine as a subspecialty with the first board-certification examination offered in 2008. The Accreditation Council for Graduate Medical Education (ACGME) standardizes the program requirements for fellowship training with an emphasis on compassion, guidance in decision making, competence in reducing the burden of serious illness, and supporting the best quality of life possible for the patient and the family through the course of the disease [5].

Palliative care and hospice have evolved into distinct roles (Table 21.1). Palliative care is the provision of active holistic care that focuses on improving quality of life for people, and their families and caregivers, who are living with any serious illness, using a multidisciplinary approach that addresses pain, other symptoms, and psychological and spiritual distress [6]. It has evolved to include care to all individuals who suffer, not just those with a limited life span [7].

It is provided in addition to any ongoing curative treatments. Hospice is more specific in that it provides palliative care to dying patients in the last months of life. Patients are eligible and appropriate for hospice care if their prognosis of survival is 6 months or less and no further curative treatments will be sought. When hospice care was established in the US in the 1970s, most of the enrolled patients had cancer. Today, cancer diagnoses account for 30% of hospice admissions with the majority now due to other diseases, with the top four non-cancer diagnoses being cardiovascular disease (17%), dementia (16%), lung disease (11%), and stroke (10%) [8].

Decisions and Communication

Healthcare providers must determine which patients are suitable for palliative care or hospice and then support patients and families with an approach that allows for management of difficult symptoms, limitation of futile medical procedures and practices, psychosocial support, and assistance with decision making. Timely transition to palliative care optimizes the likelihood of appropriate care but often does not occur until late in the disease process without time to allow for the full provision of supportive services [9]. Almost a third of patients referred to hospice use those services for 3 days or less, and 40% of these late hospice referrals were preceded by hospitalization with a stay in intensive care with 14% of patients experiencing a transition in the place of care in the last 3 days of life [10]. While some late referrals to hospice occur because physicians did not communicate this option or prognostication is difficult, a third of patients who were referred for short stays in hospice had a sudden change in their medical condition or had previously refused hospice so were not able to be referred to hospice at an earlier point in time [11]. A few days of hospice care before death may not be consistent with patient preference, improved quality of life, or a reduction in resource utilization, but may be viewed as beneficial by the family of a dying patient and the healthcare system should be prepared and able to provide short-term hospice care.

Timely referral to end-of-life care is dependent on the establishment of a prognosis, which will always be an inexact science. Identifying who is suitable for palliative care can be challenging even for physicians with years of clinical experience. Though disease trajectories are better understood, there is uncertainty in predicting what will happen to an individual patient. Some have proposed that providers ask themselves "Would I be surprised if my patient were to die in the next 12 months?" as a guidepost as to whether a discussion of palliative care should be initiated [12]. The introduction of palliative care should not be seen as an abrupt cessation of curative treatment, rather it is an approach that is gradually adopted as the disease progresses [13]. Given the challenge of predicting life expectancy, palliative care should be offered based on a desire for comfort care, rather than on prognostication. Estimating life expectancy in people with advanced dementia is particularly challenging [14–16]. Patients with dementia who are reasonably functional and patients with strokes are especially likely to survive more than 6 months after enrollment in hospice [17]. These cases contribute to the significant minority of patients (10–15%)

referred to hospice who survive for more than 6 months with nearly 40% of those with dementia having a live discharge from hospice or a long enrollment in hospice (>180 days) [17–19]. In 2011, the US Center for Medicare and Medicaid Services (CMS) required that patients who have been enrolled long term in hospice have a face-to-face visit by a physician or nurse practitioner to ensure that they continue to meet eligibility criteria. These visits must occur to determine the continued eligibility of that patient prior to the 180-day recertification. This requirement for more scrutiny has not enhanced care or increased hospice discharges [20].

Physicians should not feel like they are abandoning patients when they consider palliative care, rather they are fulfilling their responsibility to provide compassionate, sensitive, and timely care for patients who are hopelessly ill or dying [21]. Provision of end-of-life care that is consistent with a patient's goals and values is an important part of high-quality care and a priority for the healthcare system [22].

Once a physician identifies the patient who is likely to benefit from palliative care, the next step is to effectively communicate with patients and families. While this may be uncomfortable for physicians, it is a skill that can be taught [23]. A structured approach may be helpful, with clinicians trained to identify patients with serious illnesses who are appropriate for palliative care and taught to use a guide for advance care planning conversations with the patient and family that can then be documented [24].

There is a range of styles in decision making, from paternalism, where the doctor knows best and makes the decisions, to a merely informative model, where the physician objectively provides information but otherwise plays a relatively passive role, leaving the decisions to the patient and family [25]. Neither of these styles is ideal. The medical evolution away from a physician-centered style toward patient-centered care, where the patient's perspective is considered, is applicable [26]. The best approach is usually a shared decision-making process using "enhanced autonomy," where deliberation and negotiation occur and include the physician's expertise and experience while also considering patient and family preferences and perspectives [27]. Still, there are times when a physician may override expressed values and use reasonable medical judgment when an intervention such as cardiopulmonary resuscitation is futile [28]. A special model of supportive decision making is ideal for people with cognitive and functional impairments that place them at the margins of autonomy [29].

Advance Care Planning

The consensus of experts in the field is that *Advance care planning is a process that supports adults at any age or stage of health in understanding and sharing their personal values, life goals, and preferences regarding future medical care. The goal of advance care planning is to help ensure that people receive medical care that is consistent with their values, goals, and preferences during serious and chronic illness* [30].

Explaining complicated medical information and dealing with the emotions involved in contemplating death, all in the setting of uncertainty, is challenging for clinicians, families, and patients. Since the default is care that is often undesired, aggressive, and nonbeneficial, the Institute of Medicine in *Dying in America* emphasizes the need to enhance advance care planning and improve decision making for patients with serious illness [22].

Decision Aids and Documentation

Discussions regarding palliation, hospice, and goals of care can be assisted by decision support tools [31]. Decision aids provide a framework for truthful discussions that help people feel more knowledgeable, better informed, clearer about their values, more accurate with risk perceptions and understanding of choices, less likely to receive futile care, more likely to receive comfort care, and more likely to play an active role in decision making [32, 33].

Most states provide forms that are variably known as Medical or Physician Orders indicating Scope of Treatment (MOST or POLST) and Do Not Resuscitate (DNR), which document treatment preferences. The state of Oregon reduced hospitalization rates and intensive care use in the last 30 days of life and increased the likelihood of death at home since initiating its POLST program, though this is attributable not only to the form but also to educational efforts, a statewide registry, regulation that allows EMS providers to honor the POLST form, and readily available home hospice services [34]. Other materials are available on-line at www.agingwithdignity.org/five-wishes and www.acpdecisions.org.

Patients should be encouraged to name a healthcare power of attorney, also known as surrogate decision maker or healthcare proxy, and ensure that person is aware of care preferences for medical treatment, which can be conveyed through a living will which spells out a person's directives regarding medical treatment should he or she become incapacitated. If a situation arises where the patient is incapacitated, the proxy will follow the wishes or use substituted judgment according to what they think the patient would want or decide based on what they perceive as being in the patient's best interest. This can be challenging as unanticipated, emotionally complex circumstances may arise and other considerations outweigh patient autonomy.

ACP documents are ineffective if they are not readily accessible when needed. Care plans are not consistently documented in the electronic medical record (EMR) nor are they necessarily available when needed, such as in the emergency room [35]. EMR-based reminders may somewhat improve advance directive documentation, but it is unclear if this impacts management or costs of care [36, 37].

Ethical Issues

The right of an individual to refuse care is well established and based on the principle of autonomy and the right of self-governance. Many landmark cases in the legal system have confirmed this based on ethics and constitutional law.

Withdrawing, Withholding, and Refusing Care

Withdrawal of life-sustaining medical support is a common event in the intensive care unit and guidelines have been developed that address the medical, legal, cultural, and ethical considerations that are involved [38–40]. This can be morally justified as omission rather than an act meaning that the practice lets someone die and is not an active act of killing [41]. There is general legal and ethical consensus that withdrawal is equivalent to withholding treatment. In practice, they are different in that doctors may withhold information about interventions they judge to be futile while withdrawal of care requires a discussion with patients and families [42].

Physician Assisted Death

When asked about end-of-life decisions for other people, two-thirds of Americans (66%) say there are at least some situations in which a patient should be allowed to die, while nearly a third (31%) say that medical professionals should always do everything possible to save a patient's life [43]. Though most Americans believe individuals have a right to end their own lives in the face of suffering and pain with no hope of improvement, the public is about equally divided on the issue of physician-assisted suicide, which is the practice where a doctor is aware of the patient's desire to end his or her life and provides that patient with the means (usually a medication) to do so. Euthanasia is the act of ending the life of a hopelessly sick and suffering individual at the patient's request. Currently, euthanasia or physician-assisted suicide is legal in the Netherlands, Belgium, Luxembourg, Canada, New Zealand, Spain, Switzerland, and parts of Australia [44]. As of 2021, physician-assisted suicide, excluding euthanasia, is legal in 11 US jurisdictions (Oregon, Washington, Montana, Vermont, California, Colorado, District of Columbia, Hawai'i, New Jersey, Maine, and New Mexico) [45]. In none of these jurisdictions is there evidence that vulnerable patients are more likely to die in this manner compared to the general population.

Palliative Sedation

The concept of terminal sedation was first described in 1990 as sedation-inducing sleep and is the practice of drug-induced sedation for painful or burdensome symptoms that are difficult to control [46]. When introduced, many expressed concern that this practice was "slow euthanasia" or mercy killing [47, 48]. Others are concerned that this practice is a diminishment of the hospice philosophy of a holistic and caring approach to human suffering and a turn toward the medicalization of end-of-life care. To clarify that the intent is not to end the life of the patient but to provide medications for the express purpose of limiting awareness of intractable and intolerable suffering in a patient who is dying, the term palliative sedation is now widely accepted. Multiple national organizations, or regional in the US and Canada, have issued guidelines that state that palliative sedation is different from euthanasia [49–52]. Research on the practice and agreement on the principles is limited by inconsistency regarding definitions, evidenced by a review of 29 guidelines in 14 countries [53]. While reduced consciousness is part of all guidelines, intention is not, and the goal in some is to relieve suffering and in others to relieve symptoms. Research on the practice of palliative sedation—mostly from Europe—indicates it is increasingly being used for non-physical symptoms including fear, anxiety, and psycho-existential distress [54]. There is ongoing controversy about the practice. While it is often acknowledged that the intent is sedation, there may be "mission creep" based on beliefs regarding aging, dependence, suffering, and dying [55]. Lay persons often do not distinguish between different intent with euthanasia and palliative sedation: in a study from the UK, one-third considered these practices as equivalent or somewhat similar [56]. However, there is no evidence that it hastens death [57].

Quality of Care

The Study to Understand Prognoses and Preferences for Outcomes and Risks of Treatment (SUPPORT) documented many shortcomings in end-of-life care, including poor communication and misunderstanding between physicians and patients regarding resuscitation preferences, which led to increased consumption of hospital resources [58, 59]. These findings fostered efforts to improve care of seriously ill and dying patients including in the public arena where written advance directives are widely accepted. The medical community has responded in kind and the maturation of palliative care as a medical specialty has created a growing evidence base for practices that improve care. The National Consensus Project (NCP) for Quality Palliative Care espouses the value of high-quality palliative care and the

Table 21.2 Domains of questions in the Centers for Medicare & Medicaid Services (CMS) Consumer Assessment of Healthcare Providers and Systems (CAHPS) Hospice Survey. Available at https://hospicecahpssurvey.org/

Communication with family
Getting timely help
Treating patient with respect
Emotional and spiritual support
Help for pain and symptoms
Training family to care for patient
Rating of this hospice
Willingness to recommend this hospice

importance of delivering it in an organized manner [60]. The NCP consists of multidisciplinary organizations with professional roles in hospice and palliative care and uses consensus to address policy and quality issues for end-of-life providers, caregivers, consumers, and payers. Their guidelines are available at www.nationalcoalitionhpc.org.

The Affordable Care Act of 2010 mandated the creation of the Hospice Quality Reporting Program (HQRP) website for which the Centers for Medicare & Medicaid Services (CMS) developed the Consumer Assessment of Healthcare Providers and Systems (CAHPS) 47-question hospice survey in several domains to measure the experiences of patients who died while receiving hospice care, as well as the experiences of their caregivers (Table 21.2) [61]. Medicare-certified hospices must complete the survey quarterly or face a payment penalty, with certain exemptions for smaller size or newness. The Hospice Item Set (HIS) is a standardized set of questions that measure patient-level data such as s symptom management, discussion of treatment preferences and addressing beliefs/values, and is gathered at the time of admission to hospice. Both surveys are available to the public at Care Compare on Medicare.gov.

High-performing hospices in the CAHPS survey tend to be smaller, non-profit agencies in rural areas while those doing well on the HIS measure were typically for-profit, larger, and with <40% of patients in nursing homes. Providing professional staff visits in the last 2 days of life to a higher proportion of patients was associated with hospices being in the top quartile of both HIS and CAHPS [62].

Financial Reimbursement and Cost Savings

The Medicare hospice benefit was created in 1983 with the dual intent of providing compassionate and quality end-of-life care while simultaneously reducing costs, hospitalization, intensive care use, and in-hospital deaths [63]. Palliative care consultation in the hospital reduces direct costs per admission to an average hospital [64]. The public has accepted that hospice improves the quality of care to both the patient and family at the end of life. In 2018, 1.55 million Medicare beneficiaries received hospice care, and 50.7% of Medicare decedents were enrolled in hospice at the time of death [65]. Hospice programs are available to almost all Americans and the number of hospice programs, including those that are for-profit, has risen substantially over the past 20 years [66].

Though hospice improves care at the end of life, the well-documented savings in the last months before death may diminish as hospice stays increase beyond 180 days after which the costs of prolonged care exceed the potential savings from hospitalizations. Due to concern that the flat per diem payment structure incentivized the recruitment of more stable patients, the Centers for Medicare and Medicaid Services (CMS) changed the payment model effective January 1, 2016, to a two-tiered per diem payment practice where hospice services are reimbursed at a higher rate for the first 60 days of care with a lower rate for subsequent days as patients are potentially relatively stable, with an allowance for increased payments in the last week of life as acuity of symptoms and need for care increases [67]. A provision for the payment for advanced care planning discussions between physicians, patients, and families was also added. Studies remain mixed on whether hospice saves money compared with conventional care.

Provision and Place of End-of-Life Care

Palliative care should be available to all sick and dying patients where they are, including homes, assisted living and rehabilitation facilities, skilled and intermediate care facilities, acute and long-term care hospitals, clinics, community health centers, hospice residences, correctional facilities, and homeless shelters [60]. Community-based care to seriously ill patients has generally only been available through hospice programs and, therefore, only available to patients with a prognosis of survival of 6 months or less [6]. Palliative care programs that can seamlessly link inpatient and outpatient settings, providing longitudinal care that is consistent, continuous, coordinated, collaborative, and fully integrated into the healthcare system, prevent gaps in care [68] (Fig. 21.3).

Primary care physicians, specialists, and other healthcare providers should be proficient at managing the common symptoms of dying patients and references are widely available to help them do so [69]. In addition to the management of physical symptoms, interdisciplinary care teams must address the emotional and spiritual issues of patients and their caregivers. Even if people can find meaning in the death of a chronically ill loved one, family caregivers may be anxious, depressed, feel exhausted, or even develop an existential crisis. Emotional support of family caregivers and the

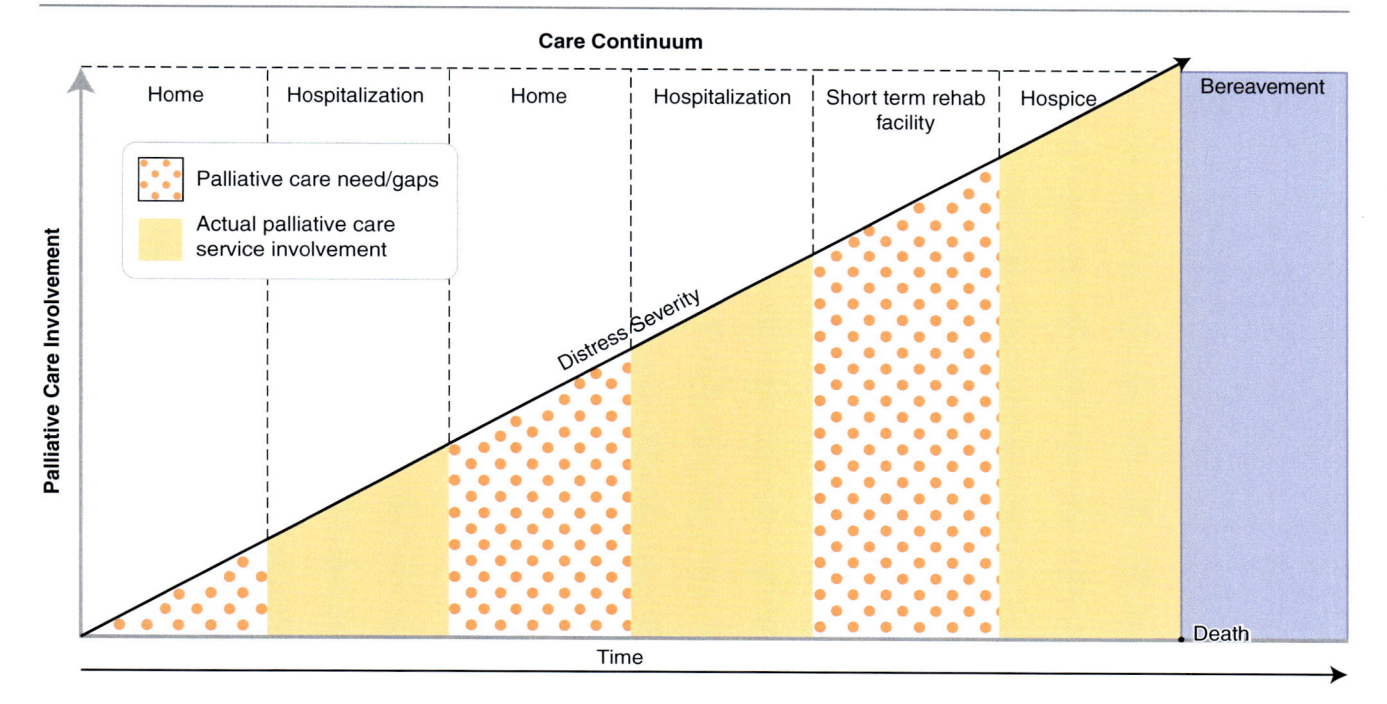

Fig. 21.3 Community based palliative care creates a continuum of care for a patient, regardless of location, linking home, institutional care, and hospice. Such a continuum ensures there are no gaps in palliative care delivery, especially during periods of worsening illness and deterioration. (Adapted from Kamal AH, Currow DC, Ritchie CS, Bull J, Abernethy AP. Community-based palliative care: the natural evolution for palliative care delivery in the U.S. Journal of pain and symptom management. 2013;46(2):254–64)

care team may lower levels of grief, improve psychological and physical health, and increase the chance that the patients may die at home [70].

Home

Many people, whether healthy or chronically ill, indicate that they would prefer to die at home and find nursing homes the least preferred place of death [71]. The relatively new Hospital at Home movement includes home-based end-of-life care which increases the number of people who die at home. Home-based end-of-life care in any form will continue to grow given the aging population and will need an adequate workforce and payment structure to support it. More research is needed to study the effect on patients' symptoms, quality of life, costs, and caregivers compared with inpatient hospital or hospice care [72]. Patterns and predictors of home death vary between countries likely due to policy and cultural differences.

Hospitals

Although many people express a wish to die at home, it cannot be assumed that *most* patients have this preference. Some prefer the hospital for safety and effective symptom control or do not want to be a burden for their family. Family members may not be comfortable with medicalizing the home environment with equipment and outside staff or may worry about exchanging the good memories associated with home with the legacy of a death at home. Given these feelings, it is likely that hospitals will continue to be the place of death for many and should be prepared to support dying patients and their families [73].

Hospitalizations of people with dementia in the last weeks of life may be medically unnecessary or discordant with the patients' preferences, yet still occur in up to 20% of nursing home patients with advanced dementia, a rate that can be lowered with advance care planning in the form of a do-not-hospitalize order [74, 75]. To address situations like this, or to care for patients with life-limiting chronic diseases that require symptom management or goals-of-care conversations, many hospitals have inpatient palliative care specialist consultation. In 2019, 72% of hospitals with 50 or more beds reported an interdisciplinary palliative care team, up from 67% in 2015 and 7% in 2001 [76]. These hospitals currently serve 87% of all hospitalized patients in the US. Inpatient palliative care consultation increases the likelihood of death at home, and likely improves patient and caregiver quality of life, satisfaction with care, and end-of-life care communication and care planning, as well as reduced costs, length of stay, and unwanted care among a range of conditions and settings [64, 77].

Nursing Homes

Rates of nursing home hospice use have increased over the past decades [78]. This increase is due to use of hospice for non-cancer diagnoses as well as to an increase in hospice providers. The increasingly long stays of nursing home patients in hospice care have raised concern about higher Medicare hospice expenditures. The challenge is how to rein in the costs of long hospice stays without removing the accessibility of a comfort care approach to dying patients in nursing homes. This can be addressed by varying payments based on length of enrollment in hospice (see "Financial" section below). Experienced physicians who work in nursing homes can effectively provide comfort to dying patients without outside hospice care and most patients who die there are perceived to do so quietly and without suffering [79]. New models that increase physician presence in nursing homes would likely increase physician engagement and expertise in end-of-life care, improve care, and decrease costs [80]. Physicians and advance practice providers are not likely to fill the needs of the burgeoning population of older adults in nursing homes without system and payment reform.

The global COVID-19 pandemic has had a significant impact on residents living in nursing homes. The practice of banning visitors was seen by some as reducing quality of life for individuals in their last phase of life, many of whom missed the family visits. As of the end of 2021, 142,405 residents in US nursing homes had died from COVID-19 infection, with 2256 deaths of nursing home staff members [81].

Special Populations

Dementia

Dementia is chronic, progressive, and incurable. People with dementia often die from complications such as pneumonia due to swallowing problems or, even more typically, from food and fluid intake problems [82–84]. These problems can begin when people have moderate dementia and continue until they are in the advanced stages where they can die from these complications or can continue to live for a surprisingly long time. Prognostication is difficult because it is hard to predict when a fatal infection or intake problem will develop [85, 86]. As a result, live discharge of patients with dementia from hospice programs or prolonged duration is common [19].

Caring for people with dementia is often burdensome for families who grieve while watching their loved one decline both cognitively and physically, and then may have to manage challenging behavior. Admission to a facility is sometimes unavoidable and in western countries many people with dementia spend the last part of their life in a nursing home [87]. However, home deaths are increasing in people with confirmed or suspected dementia in the US and other western countries, making high-quality home care relevant [88, 89]. People with dementia and their families have variable needs along the disease trajectory, and may benefit from palliative care, which is aimed at maintaining or improving quality of life. With advancing dementia, communication and shared decision making often established comfort as the goal of care rather than life prolongation [85]. Palliative care in dementia is distinct from palliative care in cancer. Because of the inevitable cognitive decline along with an uncertain trajectory, early advance care planning with the patient and the family is important. However, advance care planning in dementia is complicated and may raise moral dilemmas related to diminishing capacity and communication, and involvement of family [90, 91]. This can place people with dementia at risk for over-treatment with burdensome interventions and under-treatment of pain and other symptoms because of their difficulty verbalizing complaints [85]. Palliative care monitoring of symptoms should include observational scales that assess facial expressions and body language to recognize pain, discomfort, or other problems [92].

About three-quarters to nearly 90% of patients who die with advanced dementia and one-third to half of patients who die with mild to moderate dementia develop eating problems at the end of life [82–84]. This can be distressing for family caregivers and providers alike who may believe that providing artificial feeding through a percutaneous endoscopic gastrostomy (PEG) feeding tube will prolong life [93]. However, this is probably not the case regardless of the timing of the placement (early or late after the development of feeding problems) [94]. Feeding tubes neither prolong survival nor prevent aspiration in persons with advanced dementia [95, 96]. They do, however, increase healthcare costs [97]. By the time chronically ill persons are unable to eat, the quality of their life is so poor that insertion of a feeding tube likely just prolongs the dying process without the addition of days of meaningful life. However, persons with mild dementia may feel problems with food and fluid intake are irrelevant and unanticipated, leaving this distressing and common issue undiscussed in advance care planning conversations [98, 99]. Several organizations recommend against tube feeding in patients with advanced dementia [85, 100]. These messages seem effective as the proportion of US nursing home residents with advanced dementia and inability to eat who receive feeding tubes decreased by 50% between 2000 and 2014 [101].

Dementia-specific hospice programs that emphasize comfort rather than maximal survival time were first proposed in 1986 [102]. Over time, many western countries have expanded hospice and palliative care programs to include people with dementia. Medicare beneficiaries with dementia who sign up for the Medicare hospice benefit receive less aggressive care at the end of life, such as fewer feeding tubes, and are less likely to die in hospitals [103]. Raising awareness that dementia is a terminal disease to which palliative or hospice care applies is important in the education and training of healthcare professionals, families, and the general public [104].

People with Intellectual Disabilities or Mental Illness

An intellectual disability is usually a permanent condition while a mental illness may be temporary, but both bring special challenges in communication and ethics when it comes to end-of-life care.

Intellectual Disability

In the US and other countries, about 1% of people of all ages have an intellectual disability (ID), though the prevalence rates vary based on definition [105, 106]. The percentages of affected individuals are higher in children owing to a shorter life span. Though life expectancy for people with ID has increased due to improved health and social care, it remains below that of the general population with a life expectancy at birth that is 20 years lower than for people without ID, mainly due to circulatory and respiratory diseases and malignancy [107]. The difference may be attributed to genetic causes but health inequalities also play a role [108]. Still, the overall increase in life expectancy for people chronically affected by ID increases their chance of developing a life-limiting condition. People with intellectual disabilities are especially at increased risk of developing dementia [109]. People with intellectual disability are at risk of being under-referred including to palliative care or hospice. The American Association on Intellectual and Developmental Disabilities (AAIDD) calls for access to high-quality end-of-life care for people with intellectual disability that includes dignity, respect for autonomy, protection of life, and equality [110]. AAIDD and the European Association for Palliative Care recommend that discussions about the end of life begin before the anticipated last 6 months of life or before the need for palliative care [108, 110].

Some people with intellectual disability may not have a chance to contribute to advance care planning discussions or in-the-moment decisions, but others are able to communicate about death and dying and indicate preferences including a desire to be involved in their own care, have friends and family around, stay occupied, and be physically comfortable [111, 112]. Special communication and assessment skills are particularly relevant with these patients [113]. This can also prevent the well-intended but sometimes inappropriate tendency for relatives or others to protect people with intellectual disability from hearing bad news [114]. Unless it is demonstrated otherwise, people with intellectual disabilities should be assumed to have capacity to make decisions around their care and treatment and provided with support in end-of-life decision making. For some persons with intellectual disability who have had health problems since birth, advance care planning is relevant at an early age, and discussions of goals of care are part of building a trusting relationship between the family and healthcare professionals [112].

Symptom management in end-of-life care in people with intellectual disability requires special skill as it may not be clear whether a symptom is behavioral or reflects pain. Assessment tools such as the Disability Distress Assessment Tool (DisDAT) use baseline mapping of usual behaviors so that changes to that pattern can be recognized as a sign of distress [115]. Early referral to palliative care services is helpful so that the team can learn about the patient's usual behavior and build familiarity and trust with the patient, the family, and all members of the care team. People with intellectual disabilities have often been at the center of the family and caregivers' lives and they can be deeply affected by the loss of this beloved person and often need support in grief and bereavement [108].

Mental Illness

People with severe persistent mental illness including schizophrenia, bipolar disorder, and major depression have more and greater severity of chronic diseases, later diagnosis, and premature death compared to the general population [116]. In the US, nearly one in five adults live with a mental illness (52 million in 2019) [117]. Shortening of expected life span can be substantial for illness such as schizophrenia and anorexia, and palliative care and psychiatric care share many treatment approaches, such as communication of diagnosis and prognosis, symptom assessment and management, care planning, and assessment of caregiver needs [116, 118]. Mental illness increases risk of additional life-threatening physical illness for several reasons, including not attending cancer screening, unhealthy lifestyles, and physical complaints that are not well examined, rather ascribed to the mental illness, or are self-medicated rather than evaluated by a physician [116, 119, 120]. Late presentation can be due to both disease and system issues, resulting in overlapping and interacting health effects with high symptom burden. Social disadvantages include discrimination, isolation, poverty, and stigma while healthcare providers may be subject to internalized stigma [116, 120]. People with psychiatric illness and palliative conditions therefore often do not receive the care they need including at the end of life. Family caregivers may also have special needs as many have been lifelong caregivers, or may be suffering from strained relationships [116]. Similar to intellectual disability, psychiatric disease increases the risk of impaired decision-making capacity. Good communication, collaboration, and multidisciplinary teamwork are essential in providing good end-of-life care. This may be facilitated through a liaison who acts as a bridge between mental health and palliative care services [116, 118, 119].

Children

In the US, unintentional injury is the leading cause of death in children after the first year of life with congenital anomalies being the leading cause of death in infants under the age of 1 [121]. Malignant neoplasms are the second most frequent cause of death among those aged 5–9 years and can also cause death in toddlers and preschoolers. Although most children die in the hospital, an increasing number of children, even those under age 1, now die at home [18]. This normalizes the concept of palliative care and supports continuity of care and a continued focus on quality of life [122]. The focus may change depending on the location in the disease trajectory (whether far from or close to the end of life), but at any point managing and clarifying goals of care are important.

Assessing the pain and suffering of children can be challenging in both the physical and mental aspects. Psychosocial suffering and symptom burden are high in children with cancer [122, 123]. Symptom assessment and management is particularly challenging in caring for dying neonates, who are at risk of suffering due to under-detection of pain, dyspnea, and agitation [124]. The use of validated observational tools is pertinent when unable to self-report and parental perceptions of suffering are extremely important. Heart disease and chronic respiratory disease are other progressive conditions that can affect children. While any of these conditions can cause death, medical advances and better care allow many children with chronic, life-shortening illnesses to live into adolescence and young adulthood. An integrated model of palliative care for children with high-risk cancer and other life-threatening conditions is advocated by the American Pediatrics Society [125]. Integration of palliative care with intensive care rather than waiting until a neonate is imminently dying is encouraged, with palliative care provided by neonatologists and their teams [126].

Palliative care in pediatrics involves a broad target population of those involved in the child's social and relational spheres, such as parents, siblings, grandparents, and extended relatives. Parents or guardians need support in living with the prospect of a premature death and in subsequent bereavement, given the general expectation that children outlive their parents. Parents are distressed by seeing their children in pain, and patients may experience complex psychosocial symptoms with exponentiation of these symptoms at the end of life. Parents would like to know if professional caregivers are uncertain about the best treatment or prognosis, although not all wish to be responsible for end-of-life decision making [127]. Parents faced with difficult and stressful decisions regarding long-term ventilation want comprehensive information with medical providers being honest, tactful, patient, and supportive, and willing to discuss the option of not initiating long-term ventilation [128].

Professional caregivers can improve their comfort level regarding their responsibility to have these emotional conversations by preparing ahead of time and providing accurate and honest information while avoiding medical jargon [125, 127, 129]. Parents may be ambivalent about advance care planning and a sensitive and gradual approach with the same trusted professional with whom there is also room to discuss non-medical concerns may accommodate such ambivalence [130]. Young people may prefer not to discuss end-of-life care and prefer that advance care planning focuses on their individual needs and preferences, quality of care, emotional well-being, and living as a young person, with less emphasis on where care happens but who provides it [131].

Excellent interpersonal and communication skill is one of the six core competencies for all trainees in US residency programs, including those who will practice pediatric hospice and palliative medicine [132]. Conflict management skills may be particularly useful, given the emotional context of families dealing with very ill children [133]. Different settings and location in the disease trajectory (whether far from or close to the end of life) require different conversations, but typically patients and families simultaneously pursue disease-modifying therapies and palliative care, known as *parallel planning*, and managing and clarifying goals of care is of utmost importance [129]. Communication with children must be adapted to their cognitive ability. Symptom management is similar regardless of age, though dose adjustment and other treatments must consider the different physiology of a child in the context of growth. Perinatal palliative care is a special form of support directed to families preparing for bereavement in case of pregnancy loss or life-limiting fetal condition [134, 135].

The increasing prevalence in the number of children living with medically complex diseases, and the many family members who serve as caregivers, make it imperative that research and professional training in pediatric palliative care continue to develop to meet the rising demand for compassionate end-of-life care to support infants, children, and families across all care settings and transitions [136]. Pediatric palliative care is under-resourced and often misunderstood, with little evidence available regarding treatment of symptoms, which means that guidelines are mostly based on expert views [137]. There are efforts to improve and extend the provision of children's palliative care. The International Children's Palliative Care Network (ICPCN) provides a global network of advocacy (www.icpcn.org). There are pediatric networks such as that within the European

Association for Palliative Care which provide a platform to share knowledge and expertise between resource-rich and resource-poor countries in Europe as well as pediatric standards available through the National Hospice and Palliative Care Organization and the American Academy of Pediatrics [125, 138].

Future Directions

Changing the Focus

Despite the assumption that ACP will result in goal-directed care at the end-of-life, and the selection of a trusted medical decision maker, some thought leaders in this field feel it falls short, and that it only has a modest effect on the use of health care, emergency department visits, and hospitalization [139]. ACP discussions and the drawing up of living wills and advance directives often occur in times of good health and involve hypothetical future scenarios that do not anticipate how complex, uncertain, and emotionally laden a medical crisis can be. Sometimes living wills and advance directives are completed with attorneys and never communicated with healthcare providers. Other failures include lack of documentation, or access to it, substituted judgment invoked by the surrogate, or a healthcare system that does not commit resources and care delivery to support goal-concordant care. It may be that time, resources, and research are better directed to the improvement of shared decision-making skills between the surrogate decision maker (healthcare proxy) and clinicians at the time when actual (not hypothetical) decisions must be made.

Racial Disparities and Cultural Diversity

As western democracies grow increasing diverse, an understanding of racial, ethnic, or cultural variation in end-of-life decision making will allow for more culturally sensitive approaches to care. By 2050 there is estimated to be 33 million Black American, Hispanic, Asian, American Indian, or Alaskan Native individuals aged 65 years and older, representing nearly 40% of the population of this age group [140]. At this time, there are significant disparities in end-of-life care and planning, with racial and ethnic minorities more likely to die in hospital and less likely to engage in end-of-life planning activities [141]. Black individuals are significantly less likely to use hospice and more likely to have multiple emergency department visits and hospitalizations and undergo intensive treatment in the last 6 months of life compared with White individuals, regardless of cause of death [142]. Interdisciplinary end-of-life care teams must assess and respect values, beliefs, and traditions related to health, illness, family caregiver roles and decision making, and continually expand awareness of their own biases and perceptions about race, ethnicity, gender identity and gender expression, sexual orientation, immigration and refugee status, social class, religion, spirituality, physical appearance, and abilities [60].

Value-Based Payment Models

Alternative payment models are methods of paying for health care which reward quality and cost-effectiveness over the volume of services provided. This is rapidly evolving among US payors and given the complex care needs and costs of caring for a rapidly aging population, value-based payments will likely accelerate emphasis on palliative services. A growing number of Medicare payments are value-based, which is expected to continue to rise. Accountable care organizations, population health management, and the growing market share of Medicare Advantage plans will incentivize systems and providers to find ways to reduce costs. Many innovations are underway, including hospital care at home, virtual visits, telemedicine, and e-consults, all of which are likely to play a role in end-of-life care.

Workforce and Wellbeing

Effective end-of-life care requires an interdisciplinary team care, which ensures the delivery of holistic, patient-centered services and leads to positive outcomes related to quality of life, advance care planning, death at home, and patient/family satisfaction with care [77]. Given the significant growth in the number of patients in need of palliative care, a major challenge will be the provision of an adequately trained workforce. While physicians trained in the specialty of palliative care have expertise and comfort in such conversations, there are not nearly enough of them to meet the needs of the population [143]. It is critical that primary care physicians are trained and comfortable with end-of-life care. Graduate medical education should teach palliative medicine to all clinicians who serve patients with serious chronic illness. Practicing physicians should be provided opportunities for professional development in end-of-life care. The ongoing involvement of the patient's primary care physician can reduce the intensity and cost of end-of-life care [144]. Similar staffing challenges are likely to arise in the nursing, social work, pharmacy, and behavioral health professions, all of which play critical roles in end-of-life care. The quadruple aim in health care includes enhancing patient experience, improving population health, reducing costs, and ensuring a professionally and personally thriving healthcare workforce [145]. Providers who work in end-of-life care are vulnerable to burnout due to chronic stress from working with terminally ill patients with the associated frequent exposure to death and loss, physical and emotional suffering, increasing workloads, and competing role demands. The work also can lead palliative and hospice care professionals to develop a deep appreciation for life in the present moment and a perspective on love and family that enriches their own lives. Finding a balance will ensure that human beings will continue to work in a field that is valued and rewarding.

References

1. Lynn J, Adamson D. Living well at the end of life: adapting health care to serious chronic illness in old age. RAND Corporation; 2003 [cited 2021 Nov 6]. Available from: https://www.rand.org/pubs/white_papers/WP137.html.
2. Brennan F. Palliative care as an international human right. J Pain Symptom Manag. 2007;33(5):494–9.
3. Meier DE, Isaacs SL, Hughes R. Palliative care: transforming the care of serious illness. John Wiley & Sons; 2011.
4. Kűbler-Ross E. On death and dying. London: Tavistock Publications; 1969.
5. Accreditation Council for Graduate Medical Education (ACGME). Program requirements for graduate medical education in hospice and palliative medicine. 2020. Available from: https://www.acgme.org/globalassets/PFAssets/ProgramRequirements/540_HospicePalliativeMedicine_2020.pdf?ver=2020-06-29-164052-453&ver=2020-06-29-164052-453.
6. Kelley AS, Morrison RS. Palliative care for the seriously ill. N Engl J Med. 2015;373(8):747–55.
7. Radbruch L, De Lima L, Knaul F, Wenk R, Ali Z, Bhatnaghar S, et al. Redefining palliative care—a new consensus-based definition. J Pain Symptom Manag. 2020;60(4):754–64.
8. National Hospice and Palliative Care Organization. 2020 Edition: hospice facts and figures. Alexandria, VA: National Hospice and Palliative Care Organization; 2020. Available from: www.nhpco.org/factsfigures.
9. Zimmermann C, Riechelmann R, Krzyzanowska M, Rodin G, Tannock I. Effectiveness of specialized palliative care: a systematic review. JAMA. 2008;299(14):1698–709.
10. Teno JM, Gozalo P, Trivedi AN, Bunker J, Lima J, Ogarek J, et al. Site of death, place of care, and health care transitions among US Medicare beneficiaries, 2000-2015. JAMA. 2018;320(3):264–71.
11. Teno JM, Casarett D, Spence C, Connor S. It is "too late" or is it? Bereaved family member perceptions of hospice referral when their family member was on hospice for seven days or less. J Pain Symptom Manag. 2012;43(4):732–8.
12. Murray SA, Kendall M, Boyd K, Sheikh A. Illness trajectories and palliative care. BMJ. 2005;330(7498):1007–11.
13. Schofield P, Carey M, Love A, Nehill C, Wein S. "Would you like to talk about your future treatment options"? Discussing the transition from curative cancer treatment to palliative care. Palliat Med. 2006;20(4):397–406.
14. Jayes RL, Arnold RM, Fromme EK. Does this dementia patient meet the prognosis eligibility requirements for hospice enrollment? J Pain Symptom Manag. 2012;44(5):750–6.
15. Mitchell SL, Miller SC, Teno JM, Kiely DK, Davis RB, Shaffer ML. Prediction of 6-month survival of nursing home residents with advanced dementia using ADEPT vs hospice eligibility guidelines. JAMA. 2010;304(17):1929–35.
16. Mueller C, Ballard C, Corbett A, Aarsland D. The prognosis of dementia with Lewy bodies. Lancet Neurol. 2017;16(5):390–8.
17. Harris PS, Stalam T, Ache KA, Harrold JE, Craig T, Teno J, et al. Can hospices predict which patients will die within six months? J Palliat Med. 2014;17(8):894–8.
18. National Hospice and Palliative Care Organization. NHPCO facts and figures: pediatric palliative and hospice care in America. 2014. Available from: www.nhpco.org/factsfigures.
19. Luth EA, Russell DJ, Xu JC, Lauder B, Ryvicker MB, Dignam RR, et al. Survival in hospice patients with dementia: the effect of home hospice and nurse visits. J Am Geriatr Soc. 2021;69(6):1529–38.
20. Harrold J, Harris P, Green D, Craig T, Casarett DJ. Effect of the Medicare face-to-face visit requirement on hospice utilization. J Palliat Med. 2013;16(2):163–6.
21. Wanzer SH, Federman DD, Adelstein SJ, Cassel CK, Cassem EH, Cranford RE, et al. The physician's responsibility toward hopelessly ill patients. A second look. N Engl J Med. 1989;320(13):844–9.
22. Institute of Medicine. Dying in America: improving quality and honoring individual preferences near the end of life. Washington, DC: The National Academies Press; 2015 [cited 2022 Jan 17]. 638 p. Available from: https://www.nap.edu/catalog/18748/dying-in-america-improving-quality-and-honoring-individual-preferences-near.
23. Sullivan AM, Lakoma MD, Billings JA, Peters AS, Block SD, Core PCEP, Faculty. Teaching and learning end-of-life care: evaluation of a faculty development program in palliative care. Acad Med. 2005;80(7):657–68.
24. Bernacki R, Hutchings M, Vick J, Smith G, Paladino J, Lipsitz S, et al. Development of the Serious Illness Care Program: a randomised controlled trial of a palliative care communication intervention. BMJ Open. 2015;5(10):e009032.
25. Emanuel EJ, Emanuel LL. Four models of the physician-patient relationship. JAMA. 1992;267(16):2221–6.
26. Laine C, Davidoff F. Patient-centered medicine. A professional evolution. JAMA. 1996;275(2):152–6.
27. Quill TE, Brody H. Physician recommendations and patient autonomy: finding a balance between physician power and patient choice. Ann Intern Med. 1996;125(9):763–9.
28. Tomlinson T, Brody H. Futility and the ethics of resuscitation. JAMA. 1990;264(10):1276–80.
29. Peterson A, Karlawish J, Largent E. Supported decision making with people at the margins of autonomy. Am J Bioethics. 2021;21(11):4–18.
30. Sudore RL, Lum HD, You JJ, Hanson LC, Meier DE, Pantilat SZ, et al. Defining advance care planning for adults: a consensus definition from a multidisciplinary Delphi panel. J Pain Symptom Manag. 2017;53(5):821–832.e1.
31. Butler M, Ratner E, McCreedy E, Shippee N, Kane RL. Decision aids for advance care planning: an overview of the state of the science. Ann Intern Med. 2014;161(6):408–18.
32. Stacey D, Légaré F, Lewis K, Barry MJ, Bennett CL, Eden KB, et al. Decision aids for people facing health treatment or screening decisions. Cochrane Database Syst Rev. 2017;(4) [cited 2022 Jan 17]. Available from: https://www.cochranelibrary.com/cdsr/doi/10.1002/14651858.CD001431.pub5/full?highlightAbstract=treatment%7Cscreening%7Cdecision%7Cfor%7Cfacing%7Cscreen%7Chealth%7Cpeople%7Cpeopl%7Cpersons%7Cface%7Cfour%7Cperson%7Caids%7Cdecis%7Caid.
33. Austin CA, Mohottige D, Sudore RL, Smith AK, Hanson LC. Tools to promote shared decision making in serious illness: a systematic review. JAMA Intern Med. 2015;175(7):1213–21.
34. Tolle SW, Teno JM. Lessons from Oregon in embracing complexity in end-of-life care. N Engl J Med. 2017;376(11):1078–82.
35. Grudzen CR, Buonocore P, Steinberg J, Ortiz JM, Richardson LD, AAHPM Research Committee Writing Group. Concordance of advance care plans with inpatient directives in the electronic medical record for older patients admitted from the emergency department. J Pain Symptom Manag. 2016;51(4):647–51.

36. Hayek S, Nieva R, Corrigan F, Zhou A, Mudaliar U, Mays D, et al. End-of-life care planning: improving documentation of advance directives in the outpatient clinic using electronic medical records. J Palliat Med. 2014;17(12):1348–52.
37. Halpert KD, Ward K, Sloane PD. Improving advance care planning documentation using reminders to patients and physicians: a longitudinal study in primary care. Am J Hosp Palliat Care. 2022;39(1):62–7.
38. Truog RD, Campbell ML, Curtis JR, Haas CE, Luce JM, Rubenfeld GD, et al. Recommendations for end-of-life care in the intensive care unit: a consensus statement by the American College [corrected] of Critical Care Medicine. Crit Care Med. 2008;36(3):953–63.
39. Jensen HI, Halvorsen K, Jerpseth H, Fridh I, Lind R. Practice recommendations for end-of-life care in the intensive care unit. Crit Care Nurse. 2020;40(3):14–22.
40. Downar J, Delaney JW, Hawryluck L, Kenny L. Guidelines for the withdrawal of life-sustaining measures. Intensive Care Med. 2016;42(6):1003–17.
41. McGee A. Acting to let someone die. Bioethics. 2015;29(2):74–81.
42. Gedge E, Giacomini M, Cook D. Withholding and withdrawing life support in critical care settings: ethical issues concerning consent. J Med Ethics. 2007;33(4):215–8.
43. Pew Research Center. Views on end-of-life medical treatments. Pew Research Center's Religion & Public Life Project. 2013 [cited 2022 Jan 17]. Available from: https://www.pewforum.org/2013/11/21/views-on-end-of-life-medical-treatments/.
44. Rada AG. Spain will become the sixth country worldwide to allow euthanasia and assisted suicide. BMJ. 2021;372:n147.
45. Death with Dignity Acts—states that allow assisted death. Death with dignity. [cited 2022 Jan 17]. Available from: https://deathwithdignity.org/learn/death-with-dignity-acts/.
46. Ventafridda V, Ripamonti C, De Conno F, Tamburini M, Cassileth BR. Symptom prevalence and control during cancer patients' last days of life. J Palliat Care. 1990 Autumn;6(3):7–11.
47. Howland J. Questions about palliative sedation: an act of mercy or mercy killing? Ethics Medics. 2005;30(8):1–2.
48. Billings JA, Block SD. Slow euthanasia. J Palliat Care. 1996;12(4):21–30.
49. Kirk TW, Mahon MM, Palliative Sedation Task Force of the National Hospice and Palliative Care Organization Ethics Committee. National Hospice and Palliative Care Organization (NHPCO) position statement and commentary on the use of palliative sedation in imminently dying terminally ill patients. J Pain Symptom Manag. 2010;39(5):914–23.
50. Verkerk M, van Wijlick E, Legemaate J, de Graeff A. A national guideline for palliative sedation in the Netherlands. J Pain Symptom Manag. 2007;34(6):666–70.
51. National Ethics Committee, Veterans Health Administration. The ethics of palliative sedation as a therapy of last resort. Am J Hosp Palliat Care. 2006;23(6):483–91.
52. Cherny NI, Radbruch L, Board of the European Association for Palliative Care. European Association for Palliative Care (EAPC) recommended framework for the use of sedation in palliative care. Palliat Med. 2009;23(7):581–93.
53. Kremling A, Schildmann J. What do you mean by "palliative sedation"? BMC Palliat Care. 2020;19(1):147.
54. Heijltjes MT, van Thiel GJMW, Rietjens JAC, van der Heide A, de Graeff A, van Delden JJM. Changing practices in the use of continuous sedation at the end of life: a systematic review of the literature. J Pain Symptom Manag. 2020;60(4):828–846.e3.
55. ten Have H, Welie JVM. Palliative sedation versus euthanasia: an ethical assessment. J Pain Symptom Manag. 2014;47(1):123–36.
56. Takla A, Savulescu J, Kappes A, Wilkinson DJC. British laypeople's attitudes towards gradual sedation, sedation to unconsciousness and euthanasia at the end of life. PLoS One. 2021;16(3):e0247193.
57. Beller EM, van Driel ML, McGregor L, Truong S, Mitchell G. Palliative pharmacological sedation for terminally ill adults. Cochrane Database Syst Rev. 2015;1(1):CD010206.
58. Teno JM, Lynn J, Phillips RS, Murphy D, Youngner SJ, Bellamy P, et al. Do formal advance directives affect resuscitation decisions and the use of resources for seriously ill patients? SUPPORT Investigators. Study to understand prognoses and preferences for outcomes and risks of treatments. J Clin Ethics. 1994;5(1):23–30.
59. Teno JM, Hakim RB, Knaus WA, Wenger NS, Phillips RS, Wu AW, et al. Preferences for cardiopulmonary resuscitation: physician-patient agreement and hospital resource use. The SUPPORT Investigators. J Gen Intern Med. 1995;10(4):179–86.
60. National Consensus Project for Quality Palliative Care. Clinical practice guidelines for quality palliative care. 4th ed. Richmond, VA: National Coalition for Hospice and Palliative Care; 2018. https://www.nationalcoalitionhpc.org/ncp.
61. Centers for Medicare & Medicaid Services. Baltimore, MD; 2022. www.hospicecahpssurvey.org.
62. Anhang Price R, Tolpadi A, Schlang D, Bradley MA, Parast L, Teno JM, et al. Characteristics of hospices providing high-quality care. J Palliat Med. 2020;23(12):1639–43.
63. Kelley A, Deb P, Du Q, Aldridge M, Morrison R. Hospice enrollment saves money for Medicare and improves care quality across a number of different lengths-of-stay. Health Affairs (Project Hope). 2013;32:552–61.
64. Morrison RS, Penrod JD, Cassel JB, Caust-Ellenbogen M, Litke A, Spragens L, et al. Cost savings associated with US hospital palliative care consultation programs. Arch Intern Med. 2008;168(16):1783–90.
65. National Hospice and Palliative Care Organization 2020 edition: hospice facts & figures. NHPCO. 2020 [cited 2022 Jan 17]. Available from: https://www.nhpco.org/hospice-facts-figures/.
66. Thompson JW, Carlson MDA, Bradley EH. US hospice industry experienced considerable turbulence from changes in ownership, growth, and shift to for-profit status. Health Aff (Millwood). 2012;31(6):1286–93.
67. Center for Medicare & Medicaid Services. Medicare program; FY 2015 hospice wage index and payment rate update; hospice quality reporting requirements and process and appeals for part D payment for drugs for beneficiaries enrolled in hospice. Fed Regist. 2014;79(163):50451.
68. Kamal AH, Currow DC, Ritchie CS, Bull J, Abernethy AP. Community-based palliative care: the natural evolution for palliative care delivery in the U.S. J Pain Symptom Manag. 2013;46(2):254–64.
69. Albert RH. End-of-life care: managing common symptoms. Am Fam Physician. 2017;95(6):356–61.
70. Grande GE, Austin L, Ewing G, O'Leary N, Roberts C. Assessing the impact of a Carer Support Needs Assessment Tool (CSNAT) intervention in palliative home care: a stepped wedge cluster trial. BMJ Support Palliat Care. 2017;7(3):326–34.
71. Higginson IJ, Sarmento VP, Calanzani N, Benalia H, Gomes B. Dying at home—is it better: a narrative appraisal of the state of the science. Palliat Med. 2013;27(10):918–24.
72. Shepperd S, Gonçalves-Bradley DC, Straus SE, Wee B. Hospital at home: home-based end-of-life care. Cochrane Database Syst Rev 2021;3 [cited 2022 Jan 16]. Available from: https://www.cochranelibrary.com/cdsr/doi/10.1002/14651858.CD009231.pub3/full.
73. Pollock K. Is home always the best and preferred place of death? BMJ. 2015;351:h4855.
74. Givens JL, Selby K, Goldfeld KS, Mitchell SL. Hospital transfers of nursing home residents with advanced dementia. J Am Geriatr Soc. 2012;60(5):905–9.

75. Gozalo P, Teno JM, Mitchell SL, Skinner J, Bynum J, Tyler D, et al. End-of-life transitions among nursing home residents with cognitive issues. N Engl J Med. 2011;365(13):1212–21.
76. Center to Advance Palliative Care and the National Palliative Care Research Center. America's care of serious illness: a state-by-state report card on access to palliative care in our nation's hospitals. 2019. Available from: https://reportcard.capc.org/.
77. Ahluwalia SC, Chen C, Raaen L, Motala A, Walling AM, Chamberlin M, et al. A systematic review in support of the national consensus project clinical practice guidelines for quality palliative care, fourth edition. J Pain Symptom Manag. 2018;56(6):831–70.
78. Miller SC, Lima J, Gozalo PL, Mor V. The growth of hospice care in U.S. nursing homes. J Am Geriatr Soc. 2010;58(8):1481–8.
79. van der Steen JT, Deliens L, Koopmans RTCM, Onwuteaka-Philipsen BD. Physicians' perceptions of suffering in people with dementia at the end of life. Palliat Support Care. 2017;15(5):587–99.
80. Katz PR, Ryskina K, Saliba D, Costa A, Jung H-Y, Wagner LM, et al. Medical care delivery in U.S. nursing homes: current and future practice. Gerontologist. 2020;61(4):595–604.
81. Center for Medicare and Medicaid Services. COVID-19 nursing home data. [cited 2022 Jan 17]. Available from: https://data.cms.gov/covid-19/covid-19-nursing-home-data.
82. Hendriks SA, Smalbrugge M, Gageldonk-Lafeber ABV, Galindo-Garre F, Schipper M, Hertogh CMPM, et al. Pneumonia, intake problems, and survival among nursing home residents with variable stages of dementia in the Netherlands: results from a prospective observational study. Alzheimer Dis Assoc Disord. 2017;31(3):200–8.
83. Miranda R, van der Steen JT, Smets T, Van den Noortgate N, Deliens L, Payne S, et al. Comfort and clinical events at the end of life of nursing home residents with and without dementia: the six-country epidemiological PACE study. Int J Geriatr Psychiatr. 2020 [cited 2022 Jan 8]. https://doi.org/10.1002/gps.5290.
84. Mitchell SL, Teno JM, Kiely DK, Shaffer ML, Jones RN, Prigerson HG, et al. The clinical course of advanced dementia. N Engl J Med. 2009;361(16):1529–38.
85. van der Steen JT, Radbruch L, Hertogh CMPM, de Boer ME, Hughes JC, Larkin P, et al. White paper defining optimal palliative care in older people with dementia: a Delphi study and recommendations from the European Association for Palliative Care. Palliat Med. 2014;28(3):197–209.
86. Gill TM, Gahbauer EA, Han L, Allore HG. Trajectories of disability in the last year of life. N Engl J Med. 2010;362(13):1173–80.
87. Reyniers T, Deliens L, Pasman HR, Morin L, Addington-Hall J, Frova L, et al. International variation in place of death of older people who died from dementia in 14 European and non-European countries. J Am Med Dir Assoc. 2015;16(2):165–71.
88. Regier NG, Cotter VT, Hansen BR, Taylor JL, Wright RJ. Place of death for persons with and without cognitive impairment in the United States. J Am Geriatr Soc. 2021;69(4):924–31.
89. Xu W, Wu C, Fletcher J. Assessment of changes in place of death of older adults who died from dementia in the United States, 2000-2014: a time-series cross-sectional analysis. BMC Public Health. 2020;20(1):765.
90. Wendrich-van Dael A, Bunn F, Lynch J, Pivodic L, Van den Block L, Goodman C. Advance care planning for people living with dementia: an umbrella review of effectiveness and experiences. Int J Nurs Stud. 2020;107:103576.
91. Keijzer-van Laarhoven AJ, Touwen DP, Tilburgs B, van Tilborgden BM, Pees C, Achterberg WP, et al. Which moral barriers and facilitators do physicians encounter in advance care planning conversations about the end of life of persons with dementia? A meta-review of systematic reviews and primary studies. BMJ Open. 2020;10(11):e038528.
92. Ellis-Smith C, Evans CJ, Bone AE, Henson LA, Dzingina M, Kane PM, et al. Measures to assess commonly experienced symptoms for people with dementia in long-term care settings: a systematic review. BMC Med. 2016;14(1):38.
93. Carey TS, Hanson L, Garrett JM, Lewis C, Phifer N, Cox CE, et al. Expectations and outcomes of gastric feeding tubes. Am J Med. 2006;119(6):527.e11–6.
94. Teno JM, Gozalo PL, Mitchell SL, Kuo S, Rhodes RL, Bynum JPW, et al. Does feeding tube insertion and its timing improve survival? J Am Geriatr Soc. 2012;60(10):1918–21.
95. Gillick MR. Rethinking the role of tube feeding in patients with advanced dementia. N Engl J Med. 2000;342(3):206–10.
96. Davies N, Barrado-Martin Y, Rait G, Fukui A, Candy B, Smith CH, et al. Enteral tube feeding for people with severe dementia. Cochrane Database Syst Rev. 2019;2019(12):CD013503.
97. Hwang D, Teno JM, Gozalo P, Mitchell S. Feeding tubes and health costs postinsertion in nursing home residents with advanced dementia. J Pain Symptom Manag. 2014;47(6):1116–20.
98. Anantapong K, Barrado-Martín Y, Nair P, Rait G, Smith CH, Moore KJ, et al. How do people living with dementia perceive eating and drinking difficulties? A qualitative study. Age Ageing. 2021;50(5):1820–8.
99. Barrado-Martín Y, Hatter L, Moore KJ, Sampson EL, Rait G, Manthorpe J, et al. Nutrition and hydration for people living with dementia near the end of life: a qualitative systematic review. J Adv Nurs. 2021;77(2):664–80.
100. American Geriatrics Society Ethics Committee and Clinical Practice and Models of Care Committee. American Geriatrics Society feeding tubes in advanced dementia position statement. J Am Geriatr Soc. 2014;62(8):1590–3.
101. Mitchell SL, Mor V, Gozalo PL, Servadio JL, Teno JM. Tube feeding in US nursing home residents with advanced dementia, 2000-2014. JAMA. 2016;316(7):769–70.
102. Volicer L, Rheaume Y, Brown J, Fabiszewski K, Brady R. Hospice approach to the treatment of patients with advanced dementia of the Alzheimer type. JAMA. 1986;256(16):2210–3.
103. Miller SC, Lima JC, Mitchell SL. Influence of hospice on nursing home residents with advanced dementia who received Medicare-skilled nursing facility care near the end of life. J Am Geriatr Soc. 2012;60(11):2035–41.
104. Brazil K, Galway K, Carter G, van der Steen JT. Providing optimal palliative care for persons living with dementia: a comparison of physician perceptions in the Netherlands and the United Kingdom. J Palliat Med. 2017;20(5):473–7.
105. Anderson LL, Larson SA, MapelLentz S, Hall-Lande J. A systematic review of U.S. studies on the prevalence of intellectual or developmental disabilities since 2000. Intellect Dev Disabil. 2019;57(5):421–38.
106. McKenzie K, Milton M, Smith G, Ouellette-Kuntz H. Systematic review of the prevalence and incidence of intellectual disabilities: current trends and issues. Curr Dev Disord Rep. 2016;3(2):104–15.
107. Glover G, Williams R, Heslop P, Oyinlola J, Grey J. Mortality in people with intellectual disabilities in England. J Intellect Disabil Res. 2017;61(1):62–74.
108. Tuffrey-Wijne I, McLaughlin D, Curfs L, Dusart A, Hoenger C, McEnhill L, et al. Defining consensus norms for palliative care of people with intellectual disabilities in Europe, using Delphi methods: a white paper from the European Association of Palliative Care. Palliat Med. 2016;30(5):446–55.
109. Evans E, Bhardwaj A, Brodaty H, Sachdev P, Draper B, Trollor JN. Dementia in people with intellectual disability: insights and challenges in epidemiological research with an at-risk population. Int Rev Psychiatry. 2013;25(6):755–63.
110. American Association on Intellectual and Developmental Disabilities. Caring at the end of life. 2020 [cited 2022 Jan 9].

Available from: https://www.aaidd.org/news-policy/policy/position-statements/caring-at-the-end-of-life.
111. Tuffrey-Wijne I, Bernal J, Butler G, Hollins S, Curfs L. Using Nominal Group Technique to investigate the views of people with intellectual disabilities on end-of-life care provision. J Adv Nurs. 2007;58(1):80–9.
112. Voss H, Vogel A, Wagemans AMA, Francke AL, Metsemakers JFM, Courtens AM, et al. Advance care planning in palliative care for people with intellectual disabilities: a systematic review. J Pain Symptom Manag. 2017;54(6):938–960.e1.
113. Dunkley S, Sales R. The challenges of providing palliative care for people with intellectual disabilities: a literature review. Int J Palliat Nurs. 2014;20(6):279–84.
114. Ryan K, Guerin S, Dodd P, McEvoy J. Communication contexts about illness, death and dying for people with intellectual disabilities and life-limiting illness. Palliat Support Care. 2011;9(2):201–8.
115. Regnard C, Reynolds J, Watson B, Matthews D, Gibson L, Clarke C. Understanding distress in people with severe communication difficulties: developing and assessing the Disability Distress Assessment Tool (DisDAT). J Intellect Disabil Res. 2007;51(Pt 4):277–92.
116. Donald EE, Stajduhar KI. A scoping review of palliative care for persons with severe persistent mental illness. Palliat Support Care. 2019;17(4):479–87.
117. National Institute of Mental Health. Mental illness. National Institute of Mental Health (NIMH). [cited 2022 Jan 9]. Available from: https://www.nimh.nih.gov/health/statistics/mental-illness.
118. Trachsel M, Irwin SA, Biller-Andorno N, Hoff P, Riese F. Palliative psychiatry for severe persistent mental illness as a new approach to psychiatry? Definition, scope, benefits, and risks. BMC Psychiatry. 2016;16(1):260.
119. Ellison, N. Mental health and palliative care: literature review—The British Library. 2008 [cited 2022 Jan 9]. Available from: https://www.bl.uk/collection-items/mental-health-and-palliative-care-literature-review.
120. Grassi L, Riba M. Cancer and severe mental illness: bi-directional problems and potential solutions. Psychooncology. 2020;29(10):1445–51.
121. Murphy SL, Xu JQ, Kochanek KD, Arias E, Tejada-Vera B. Deaths: final data for 2018. National vital statistics reports, vol. 69(13). Hyattsville, MD: National Center for Health Statistics; 2020.
122. Kaye EC, Friebert S, Baker JN. Early integration of palliative care for children with high-risk cancer and their families. Pediatr Blood Cancer. 2016;63(4):593–7.
123. Weaver MS, Heinze KE, Kelly KP, Wiener L, Casey RL, Bell CJ, et al. Palliative care as a standard of care in pediatric oncology. Pediatr Blood Cancer. 2015;62(Suppl 5):S829–33.
124. Cortezzo DE, Meyer M. Neonatal end-of-life symptom management. Front Pediatr. 2020;8:574121.
125. American Academy of Pediatrics, Section on Hospice and Palliative Care and Committee on Hospital Care, Feudtner C, Friebert S, Jewell J, Friebert S, Carter B, et al. Pediatric palliative care and hospice care commitments, guidelines, and recommendations. Pediatrics. 2013;132(5):966–72.
126. Carter BS. Pediatric palliative care in infants and neonates. Children (Basel). 2018;5(2):E21.
127. Xafis V, Gillam L, Hynson J, Sullivan J, Cossich M, Wilkinson D. Caring decisions: the development of a written resource for parents facing end-of-life decisions. J Palliat Med. 2015;18(11):945–55.
128. Edwards JD, Panitch HB, Nelson JE, Miller RL, Morris MC. Decisions for long-term ventilation for children. perspectives of family members. Ann Am Thorac Soc. 2020;17(1):72–80.
129. Wolff T, Browne J. Organizing end of life care: parallel planning. Paediatr Child Health. 2011;21(8):378–84.
130. Lotz JD, Daxer M, Jox RJ, Borasio GD, Führer M. "Hope for the best, prepare for the worst": a qualitative interview study on parents' needs and fears in pediatric advance care planning. Palliat Med. 2017;31(8):764–71.
131. Taylor J, Murphy S, Chambers L, Aldridge J. Consulting with young people: informing guidelines for children's palliative care. Arch Dis Child. 2021;106(7):693–7.
132. Klick JC, Friebert S, Hutton N, Osenga K, Pituch KJ, Vesel T, et al. Developing competencies for pediatric hospice and palliative medicine. Pediatrics. 2014;134(6):e1670–7.
133. Lyons O, Forbat L, Menson E, Chisholm JC, Pryde K, Conlin S, et al. Transforming training into practice with the conflict management framework: a mixed methods study. BMJ Paediatr Open. 2021;5(1):e001088.
134. Wool C, Catlin A. Perinatal bereavement and palliative care offered throughout the healthcare system. Ann Palliat Med. 2019;8(1):S22–9.
135. Cortezzo DE, Ellis K, Schlegel A. Perinatal palliative care birth planning as advance care planning. Front Pediatr. 2020;8:556.
136. Center to Advance Palliative Care. Pediatric palliative care field guide. 2019 [cited 2021 Dec 30]. Available from: https://www.capc.org/documents/257/.
137. Knops RRG, Kremer LCM, Verhagen AAE, Dutch Paediatric Palliative Care Guideline Group for Symptoms. Paediatric palliative care: recommendations for treatment of symptoms in the Netherlands. BMC Palliat Care. 2015;14:57.
138. Arias-Casais N, Garralda E, Pons JJ, Marston J, Chambers L, Downing J, et al. Mapping pediatric palliative care development in the WHO-European Region: children living in low-to-middle-income countries are less likely to access it. J Pain Symptom Manag. 2020;60(4):746–53.
139. Morrison RS, Meier DE, Arnold RM. What's wrong with advance care planning? JAMA. 2021;326(16):1575–6.
140. Ortman JM, Velkoff VA, Hogan H UC. An aging nation: the older population in the United States. Census.gov [cited 2022 Jan 17]. Available from: https://www.census.gov/library/publications/2014/demo/p25-1140.html.
141. Orlovic M, Smith K, Mossialos E. Racial and ethnic differences in end-of-life care in the United States: evidence from the Health and Retirement Study (HRS). SSM Popul Health. 2018;7:100331.
142. Ornstein KA, Roth DL, Huang J, Levitan EB, Rhodes JD, Fabius CD, et al. Evaluation of racial disparities in hospice use and end-of-life treatment intensity in the REGARDS cohort. JAMA Netw Open. 2020;3(8):e2014639.
143. Lupu D, Quigley L, Mehfoud N, Salsberg ES. The growing demand for hospice and palliative medicine physicians: will the supply keep up? J Pain Symptom Manag. 2018;55(4):1216–23.
144. Ankuda CK, Petterson SM, Wingrove P, Bazemore AW. Regional variation in primary care involvement at the end of life. Ann Fam Med. 2017;15(1):63–7.
145. Bodenheimer T, Sinsky C. From triple to quadruple aim: care of the patient requires care of the provider. Ann Fam Med. 2014;12(6):573–6.

Special Population: Children and Adolescents

Morgan A. McEachern, Ashley Rietz, and Cristy Page

Definitions and Demographics

Chronic illness in childhood is defined as any biological, psychological, or cognitive condition expected to persist for at least 12 months that either necessitates health care and related services or leads to functional or cognitive limitations of the child compared to peers [1–3]. Conditions may result from genetic variations, environmental factors, or a combination of both, and are listed in Table 22.1. Multimorbidity refers to the co-occurrence of two or more chronic illnesses and physical-mental multimorbidity is further delineated as the co-occurrence of at least one chronic physical illness and one chronic psychological disorder [4]. Children with medical complexity include children with multimorbidity as well as children with singular chronic illnesses that require multidisciplinary and long-term care. Identifying children with medical complexity can be challenging at the population level as no singular definition or list of diagnosis codes exists that uniformly describe this group [5].

An estimated 25% of children in the United States (US) have at least one chronic illness and the prevalence of chronic illnesses in childhood has steadily increased over recent decades [6]. This is attributable to several factors. First, advances in medical care for many chronic conditions have increased life expectancies. For example, in the 1940s, children with cystic fibrosis had a life expectancy of less than 2 years of age but now have an average life expectancy exceeding 45 years of age [7]. Children can now live with their chronic disease well into adulthood. Secondly, dramatic increases in the incidence of chronic conditions such as obesity, asthma, and attention deficit disorder (ADD) contribute to the increasing prevalence of childhood chronic illness. Nearly 20% of children and adolescents in the US now meet clinical criteria for obesity compared with less than 5% of children and adolescents in the 1970s [8, 9]. The prevalence of asthma in children and adolescents in the US has nearly doubled since the 1980s, though the rise has slowed in recent years and rates have remained stable at nearly 10% [10, 11]. Rates of diagnosis are increasing also due to increased screening and greater awareness of diseases, as well as changes in childhood social environments, technology exposure, diet, and exercise [6]. Finally, while only 7% of children and adolescents have multimorbidity, this subset contributes to the greater burden of disease and accounts for a larger percentage of total healthcare expenditures [12].

Table 22.1 Common chronic diseases in children and adolescents

Anxiety
Asthma
Attention deficit disorder
Autism spectrum disorders
Cancer
Cerebral palsy
Congenital heart disease
Cystic fibrosis
Depression
Diabetes
Developmental disabilities
Immune deficiency
Inflammatory bowel disease
Learning and language disorders
Migraine headaches
Mood disorders
Obesity
Seizure disorder
Consequences of low birthweight and prematurity (chronic lung disease, developmental delays)

M. A. McEachern (✉)
Department of Family Medicine, University of North Carolina at Chapel Hill, Chapel Hill, NC, USA
e-mail: morgan_mceachern@med.unc.edu

A. Rietz
Department of Family Medicine, University of North Carolina School of Medicine, Chapel Hill, NC, USA
e-mail: ashley_rietz@med.unc.edu

C. Page
University of North Carolina at Chapel Hill School of Medicine, Chapel Hill, NC, USA
e-mail: CRISTY_PAGE@MED.UNC.EDU

Sites of Care for Children with Chronic Illness

Caring for a child with chronic illness is complex and requires a multidisciplinary approach involving caregivers and providers in a variety of settings. Comprehensive care for these children goes beyond traditional outpatient and inpatient settings into homes, schools, and the community.

Hospitals

There are over 250 children's hospitals in the US providing over 95% of cancer and tertiary care to children and adolescents in this country [13]. These unique hospitals provide multidisciplinary, comprehensive general and subspecialty care for children and adolescents. They offer expertise and provide resources in the care of children with medical complexity. Most of these hospitals are affiliated with academic medical centers located in urban or suburban areas.

In 2018, there were 5.3 million child and adolescent hospitalizations in the US, 71% of which were related to conditions in the newborn and infant period [14]. Depressive disorders now outrank asthma exacerbation as the most common chronic disease requiring admission in children over 1 year of age, with 91,000 hospital admissions in 2018 compared with 72,000 hospital admissions for asthma exacerbation in the same year. Other chronic illnesses that account for a significant number of hospitalizations in children and adolescents include epilepsy, diabetes, and cancer. Preliminary data from 2020 suggest an overall decrease in child and adolescent hospitalizations during the COVID-19 pandemic although the factors contributing to this remain unclear [15].

Prolonged or frequent hospitalizations can negatively affect a child's physical, cognitive, emotional, and psychological development. In addition to the provision of medical care, the hospital environment must support the child's growth and development. Parents must be allowed to stay with their children, and trained health professionals must provide programs that use age-appropriate therapeutic play to address the social, emotional, and developmental needs of hospitalized children [16]. Daily discussions regarding the plan of care should include the family, other caregivers, and the child when developmentally appropriate. Routine involvement of nurses and caregivers in daily bedside rounds improves communication, increases employee and patient satisfaction, and is highly recommended [17–19]. Expectations regarding behavior discussed early in the hospitalization and efforts to minimize fear and pain during procedures enhance care.

The Outpatient Medical Home

Poor communication between the inpatient and outpatient setting leads to fragmentation of care, hospital readmission, and poorer health outcomes in patients with chronic illness [20, 21]. The patient-centered medical home (PCMH) model of care addresses this problem and improves care for the child with chronic illness by providing patient-centered, comprehensive, team-based, coordinated, and accessible care that is focused on quality and safety [22]. In the PCMH model, the primary care physician coordinates the comprehensive care of children with complex medical conditions while addressing the patient's biopsychosocial concerns. Optimal management of chronic illness through the PCMH includes collaboration with children, families, and the entire care team and individualization of care to meet personal needs [21]. Co-located care management by a social worker is an especially important component of care to children with chronic disease and a cornerstone of the PCMH. Care managers identify barriers to care and provide connections to community resources [21, 23]. Using the population health principles of the PCMH, practices create disease registries that organize and track care and ensure evidence-based guidelines are followed. These registries can identify children who have missed appointments or who have had emergency room visits, alerting a care manager for outreach to the patient and family, which can improve outcomes.

Many communities outside of urban or suburban areas may have limited access to subspeciality care. Project Extension for Community Healthcare Outcomes (ECHO) is a collaborative medical education and care management model that allows primary care physicians and other healthcare providers to access regional subspecialists via regular virtual seminars and direct consultation, bringing evidence-based care to their home practices and communities [24].

Home

A comprehensive understanding of the home environment allows clinicians to better care for the child with chronic illness. For example, indoor pollutants and allergens are known triggers for asthma and disproportionately affect urban minority youth [25]. Clinicians and care managers can identify these problems and seek modifications, which could involve asking a landlord to remove mold or seeking help from legal services. Comprehensive medical care and support services can be provided in the home and are most successful when individualized for the child and their caregivers [26]. The home is usually a nurturing environment that best supports ongoing growth and development. Home care is expensive but potentially offsets higher healthcare costs by decreasing hospital admission rates and length of hospitalization [27]. Home care increases caregiver satisfaction, decreases parental anxiety, and improves behavior in children with chronic illness [28].

Telehealth has the potential to enhance the PCMH model, increasing care and convenience for caregivers and families while providing clinicians with invaluable information about the home environment. Prior to the COVID-19 pandemic, only 15% of pediatric providers provided telehealth services as part of their practice [29]. Shortly after COVID-19 cases were reported in the US, the Centers for Medicare & Medicaid Services (CMS) and other major insurers implemented waivers to expand coverage for a range of telehealth services which subsequently led to a 154% increase in the number of telehealth visits [30, 31]. While increases in telehealth have the potential to expand access to care, inconsistency in reimbursement as well as inequities in access to reliable internet and devices capable of accessing various telehealth platforms may limit benefits.

Family members and caregivers are active participants in a child's care in the inpatient and outpatient setting, but it is at home that family life can provide structure and stability. Empowering families and caregivers with the knowledge and tools to actively participate in the child's medical management improves adherence and outcomes for children with chronic illness [21, 23, 32]. Evidence-based care plans can help families and caregivers become informed partners in care and follow through on recommendations given by healthcare providers. Asthma action plans are an example where family members and caregivers learn to recognize the symptoms and severity of an asthma exacerbation, initiate appropriate treatment, and identify when the child needs care in the clinic or hospital setting [10, 20]. Caregivers and families can benefit from anticipatory guidance about the challenges of caring for a child with chronic illness at various stages in a child's development [16]. Telehealth can also be utilized to provide additional support and education to families and caregivers around chronic illness management [33].

Family structure and support systems play a critical role in the health of children with chronic illness. Children in single-parent or single-caregiver households tend to have poorer health outcomes and an increased number of unmet health needs compared to children in two-parent or multiple-caregiver households [34]. Decreased time and resources as well as increased stress are likely contributors to this disparity. Interventions aimed at providing additional support and resources may help improve outcomes.

Schools

Schools are an important care setting for children with chronic illness, as most children spend nearly as much time at school as they do at home. School-based health programs are integral to managing chronic illness and allow the child to pursue an education. Most publicly funded schools in the US include some level of nursing services and care management, although services vary widely among school systems based on community needs and financial support [35]. Schools with higher nurse-to-student ratios are associated with lower absenteeism rates and higher graduation rates [36]. As an example, the School Nurse Demonstration Project placed full-time nurses in individual schools and placed one full-time nurse practitioner over the system for follow-up and chronic care management [37]. All nurses in the project received standardized training on asthma management and rates of absenteeism. Emergency room visits for patients with asthma subsequently declined, which translated to decreased healthcare costs and decreased parental absenteeism and lost wages. Project ECHO models and school-based telehealth programs are examples of ways in which technology has been employed to expand access to school-based health services in lower resourced communities [38, 39].

School-based health centers provide primary care and mental health services to schools in high-risk communities [35]. Bringing health care to the school may decrease health disparities and improve the overall well-being of communities, including children with chronic disease. The Centers for Disease Control and Prevention (CDC) and ASCD (formerly known as the Association for Supervision and Curriculum Development) have developed the Whole School, Whole Community, Whole Child (WSCC) model, which is a framework for school-based health interventions [40–42]. This model of care aims to strengthen the collaboration between health and education by maximizing limited resources to address health-related barriers to learning. Embedded mental health services improve access for high-risk children and adolescents and are correlated with improved attendance, behavior, and test scores [41]. The connections between health and education makes school-based interventions important in improving health outcomes for children with chronic illness.

Community

The community in which one lives influences beliefs and attitudes about health, increases or decreases one's risk for certain health conditions, and impacts one's behavior [20, 43]. The condition of the community and its surrounding resources can have a dramatic impact on the health of children and their families. Improving the health of a community and those who live there requires more than simply embedding health services in the neighborhood. The social determinants of health that put individuals at increased risk of poor health outcomes must also be addressed. With the direct input of community members, community leaders and public health officials should work together to identify needs and decide which interventions are most likely to improve health in a particular community. Community-level interventions aimed at improving the health of children with chronic illness are highly varied. Successful interventions that have decreased childhood obesity rates in high-risk communities include improving access to outdoor recreational facilities, installing sidewalks to improve walkability, and embedding community gardens and farmer's markets [44]. Several community-level interventions reduce asthma exacerbations by promoting construction that reduces allergens and pollutants in public spaces and by conducting educational campaigns to promote flu vaccination [45, 46]. Care managers provide a link to appropriate community-based resources that can both improve the child's health and provide support to families and caregivers [23]. Community-based youth development programs and support groups that focus on children with chronic illness can not only improve health outcomes now, but also help children develop strategies to promote well-being as they transition to adulthood [47].

Quality of Care and Population Health

Quality improvement (QI) metrics for children and adolescents are not as well established as those for adults. However, attention to healthcare metrics for these populations increased with national funding from the Children's Health Insurance Program Reauthorization Act (CHIPRA) in 2009 and the creation of the Pediatric Quality Measures Program (PQMP) [48]. Many of these metrics focus on preventive care which is important for children with chronic illness. Primary metrics include the *Child Core Set*, used by Medicaid and the Children's Health Insurance Program (CHIP), but there are also multiple metrics that specifically address chronic illness [49]. Synergy between evidence-based interventions and quality measures is evident upon review of these core metrics. For example, the CDC created a framework for high yield interventions for asthma called EXHALE [50]. This is a broad approach that touches on multiple aspects of care. Specific quality metrics were identified to improve the impact of this framework, including a core asthma metric for children ages 5–18 years. It uses frequency of visits for asthma treatment in different care settings, along with dispensing data for controller and reliever medications, to measure medication adherence and reliever overuse in this population [51]. In addition to development and evaluation of pediatric quality measures, the PQMP also has created resources to help with implementation including a roadmap and toolkits for specific metrics [52].

Health Disparities in Care and Research

Significant disparities exist in the prevalence, morbidity, and mortality rates for children with chronic illnesses, based on race and ethnicity. The current overall prevalence rate of asthma in children under 18 years of age in the US is 5.8%, however there are disparities with 12% of Black children suffering from asthma, compared to 5.5% of White children, 7% of Hispanic children, 9% of Native American children, and 4% of children of Asian heritage [53]. In 2016, asthma mortality rates were more than nine times higher for Black children and adolescents than White children and adolescents [54]. Historical, institutional, structural, and environmental factors rather than individual or genetic factors explain and often perpetuate these disparities.

Race is socially constructed and is considered a social determinant of health, defined as a non-medical factor that influences health [55, 56]. It intersects with other social determinants of health such as housing, transportation, language, education level, literacy, income, and access to food and clean water, all of which can exacerbate health disparities. Within the PCMH, all staff should be trained in culturally competent care, the environment should be culturally safe for all patients, and questions about social determinants of health should be part of the routine screening for all children and families in the practice [55, 57, 58]. Care managers can assess social determinants of health and connect children and families to resources. Outside of the PCMH, strategies and interventions must be aimed at addressing other social determinants of health, as well as racism within larger systems, before significant improvements in these health disparities can be expected [55, 59]. Interventions aimed at individuals and groups are valuable but less likely to have a widespread and lasting impact unless the root causes of health disparities are also addressed.

COVID-19 and Chronic Illness in Children

The effect of COVID-19 on children and adolescents with chronic illnesses is multifactorial and will become more apparent with time. Similar to adults, children with pre-existing chronic illness are more likely to have severe disease or be hospitalized due to COVID-19 [60]. Caregivers of children with chronic disease were more likely to delay evaluation in an emergency department due to fear of contracting COVID-19 [61]. The disruptions in family life, school, and social functioning caused by the pandemic have had profound impacts on children, which is likely to be even more challenging for families and children dealing with chronic disease.

Medicaid and Financing

Chronic illnesses in childhood and adolescence contribute significantly to overall healthcare costs in the US. Total direct costs of pediatric asthma in the US in 2013 were

$5.92 billion [62]. Children receive financing for healthcare costs through several different sources. In 2019, 50% of US children under 18 years of age had employer-sponsored insurance, 39.5% had public insurance, 4.9% had individual coverage, and 5.6% were uninsured [63]. In the US, public insurance includes both Medicaid and the Children's Health Insurance Program (CHIP). Medicaid was established in 1965 and is jointly funded by state and federal governments and managed by the states. Established in 1997, CHIP is administered by the US Department of Health and Human Services and provides funds to states that cover uninsured children in low- and middle-income families whose incomes are slightly above the level at which they would qualify for Medicaid [64]. States have flexibility in how they use the CHIP funds, including using it to expand their Medicaid programs. The CHIP Reauthorization Act (CHIPRA) in 2009 increased appropriations to the program. As of May 2022, 41 million children were enrolled in CHIP or Medicaid, representing 46% of total Medicaid and CHIP enrollees [65].

This public insurance is a financial lifeline for vulnerable children with health needs and most children in these programs are economically disadvantaged and many have special needs. Health outcomes for children are similar regardless of whether they have public or private insurance, as long as coverage is continuous [66, 67]. Gaps in insurance coverage, whether public or private, can adversely affect a child's access to quality health care such as delaying necessary care or reliably filling prescriptions for recommended medications, compared to children with continuous health coverage [67]. More than 80% of children with gaps in insurance coverage had working parents at the time of the insurance lapse. Children without insurance or with gaps in insurance are less likely to have a primary care physician and less likely to receive necessary medical care [68]. While these realities are problematic for all children, those with chronic illness are at higher risk for worse health outcomes when appropriate access to care is limited.

The Affordable Care Act (ACA), which was implemented in 2010, includes provisions to improve the health of children and families by increasing access to quality covered health care and has increased the number of children with health insurance. The ACA expands Medicaid to families with incomes of up to 138% of the federal poverty limit, creates a health insurance marketplace where families can shop for plans, and allows young adults to remain on their parent's insurance plan until 26 years of age [64]. It also bars insurance companies from using pre-existing conditions as a means of denying coverage to individuals. The ACA provides a higher federal match for states that implement PCMHs for children with chronic illness, although many states have not implemented this provision [64]. While the future of the ACA is politically uncertain, it has resulted in improved access to care for US children.

Impact of Chronic Disease on Children

Chronic illness and frequent or prolonged hospitalizations can have a negative effect on a child's physical, cognitive, emotional, and psychological development. Early recognition and appropriate support and intervention may mitigate these effects.

Growth and Development

Chronic illness in childhood can affect normal patterns of growth and development, such as growth failure and decreased growth velocity. For example, delayed skeletal maturation and delayed puberty may be the presenting symptom in adolescents with inflammatory bowel disease [69]. Poor absorption of nutrients and prolonged steroid use can further complicate growth and lead to a reduced adult height in individuals with inflammatory bowel disease. Growth failure is also commonly seen in childhood chronic kidney disease and is associated with increased mortality rates, likely due to abnormalities in the growth hormone—insulin like growth factor axis [70]. Childhood obesity is associated with early pubertal onset and menarche in girls [71]. In boys this association with early puberty is not as clear [72].

Adolescents with chronic illness often define themselves by their disease and can have difficulty developing their identity and forming a sense of confidence [73]. This can lead to difficulty forming social relationships with healthy peers. Many adolescents with chronic illness report a higher rate of body dissatisfaction as they enter puberty. Healthcare providers may not provide age-appropriate anticipatory guidance on puberty and sexuality as they are focused on managing the child's chronic illness, even though adolescents with chronic illness report higher rates of sexual intercourse and unsafe sexual practice compared to healthy peers [74]. It is important that providers normalize sexuality and provide age-appropriate anticipatory guidance about sexual development for all children, including those with chronic illness [75]. This includes counseling on puberty, sexual identity, safe sexual practices, sexually transmitted infections, and contraception. For a subset of children with chronic illness, especially those with severe health impairment, their ability to engage in developmentally appropriate activities is disrupted leading to lifelong impacts [76]. The Academy of Pediatrics devised the term "children with medical complexity" (CMC) for this population, indicating chronic illness with

Education

Chronic illness can negatively impact a child's education, reduce academic achievement, and hinder learning. Frequent outpatient visits and hospitalizations can interfere with school and cause children to fall behind compared to their peers. In 2013, there were almost 14 million missed school days due to asthma alone [76]. Asthma accounts for 14–18% of student absenteeism [78]. The association between asthma, increased absenteeism, and poor academic achievement is well established [41, 79, 80]. Children with poorly controlled asthma exhibit lower performance on cognitive tasks, particularly those that assess concentration and memory. Uncontrolled nighttime symptoms may contribute to this educational gap given the importance of uninterrupted sleep for the cognitive development in children. Given that asthma is more prevalent among urban and low-income children, these problems further exacerbate educational disparities [79].

Children with chronic illness may be subject to bullying and are more likely to report feeling unsafe at school, which is associated with lower grades and increased absenteeism [41, 81]. Obesity is associated with poor academic performance, possibly due to increased rates of bullying but also to high rates of psychosocial comorbidities such as depression and anxiety [82]. Mild cognitive delays, decreased academic achievement, and increased rates of absenteeism are also seen in patients with sickle cell disease [83]. Children with sickle cell disease may develop neurocognitive deficits due to both silent and overt cerebral infarcts.

Creating a safe and supportive educational environment as well as promoting healthy behaviors for all children, including those with chronic illness, improves academic achievement [43, 81, 84]. This is a goal of the Whole School, Whole Community, Whole Child (WSCC) educational model developed by the CDC and ASCD [40].

Family Role and Socialization

Parents and caregivers play a crucial role in the emotional development of children and adolescents with chronic illness [85]. Parents and caregivers can foster independence by encouraging the child to assume increasing responsibility in the management of the disease. Parents who are overprotective and interfere with the child's ability to develop autonomy may foster *vulnerable child syndrome,* which is a phenomenon where parents and caregivers treat children with chronic illness differently than healthy children due to subconscious perceptions of increased vulnerability [86]. This can hinder a child's emotional development and delay their ability to function independently, making it difficult for the child to transition to self-management and leading to poorer long-term health outcomes. Providers should promote an encouraging family environment, which is associated with better adherence to medical treatment [87].

Psychological Consequences

Behavioral disorders resulted in almost 500,000 pediatric hospitalizations in 2012, 7.3% of which documented a primary or secondary behavioral disorder diagnosis [88]. Hospitalizations with secondary mental health diagnoses often resulted in longer stays and higher costs. Children with chronic illness and comorbid behavioral conditions are at increased risk of developing depression, anxiety, and post-traumatic stress disorder. However, children with chronic illness and their families can be resilient and learn to overcome adversity. The family's ability to cope with and manage the chronic illness is an important predictor of psychological outcomes for the child [89]. Factors associated with poor coping and increased risk of psychological comorbidities for the adolescent with chronic illness include dependence on others for daily activities, inability to engage in activities with peers, and social stigma [90]. Peer relationships are particularly important for the health and well-being of adolescents. Those who feel excluded from their peer group or who miss big events, such as prom or graduation, are at increased risk for poorer mental health outcomes. Adolescents with chronic illness have an increased risk of depression, low self-esteem, and suicidal ideation [73, 87, 89]. Obese and overweight children and adolescents are more likely to have low self-esteem and associated mental health conditions including depression and anxiety [82]. Signs of psychological distress include medical symptoms not explained by organic disease, nonadherence, poor educational achievement, or engagement in risky behavior including unsafe sexual practices and substance use [89]. Recognizing psychological distress can promote effective interventions such as cognitive behavioral therapy, biofeedback, and guided imagery. Interventions should be aimed at a child's mental age rather than chronological age, given the possibility of discrepancies between the two [91].

Transition to Adulthood

Over 90% of children with chronic illness born in the 1990s or later are expected to survive into adulthood, when they will continue to deal with the effects of the disease [92]. The American Academy of Pediatrics, the American Academy of

Family Physicians, the American College of Physicians, and the American Society of Internal Medicine agree that transitioning a young adult with special healthcare needs to adult care requires healthcare professionals to understand and assume responsibility for that transition, ensuring that high-quality, developmentally appropriate health care continues uninterrupted as the individual moves from adolescence to adulthood [93].

For primary care, the patient may continue to see a familiar family physician who is trained to provide care to persons of all ages or may transition from a general pediatrician to an adult clinician. For specialty care, the patient is likely to transition from pediatric to adult specialists. Components of a successful transition include current medical record, a comprehensive transition plan (in place by age 14 years), and continuous healthcare coverage [93]. Young adults are at risk of a gap in insurance coverage as they transition to adulthood, a problem largely addressed by the ACA's provision allowing young adults to remain on their parents' health plan until the age of 26 years [94]. The steady transition of disease management from the parent to the adolescent is important and ensures a foundation for independent disease management in adulthood. Lack of this transition can lead to persistence of unmanaged disease into adulthood. For example, childhood obesity often persists into adulthood and is associated with type II diabetes, hypertension, hyperlipidemia, obstructive sleep apnea, orthopedic complications, nonalcoholic fatty liver disease, and cardiovascular complications [82, 95].

Young adults with a history of childhood chronic illness often fare well socially and are as likely to get married and have children as healthy peers, but they have lower annual incomes and are less likely to graduate from college [91, 93, 96]. Children with developmental arrest due to disease may not have the life skills needed to operate independently in a complex medical system and are at higher risk of nonadherence, poor health outcomes, and comorbid mental health conditions [91]. As these individuals transition from the pediatric medical system to the adult medical system, they are sometimes labeled as "difficult patients," which may further impede their care. One recommendation to improve this transition is to help children with disabilities obtain specific foundational skills earlier in life [76].

Future Directions

With the shift in disease burden from acute to chronic illness over the last decades, new models of care are essential to maximizing the health potential of children and adolescents with chronic illness. PCMH models focus on individual patient needs and population health and can provide effective primary care, but many communities lack access to subspecialty care. Health systems must support effective collaboration and communication between patients and providers in underserved communities and specialists who are often found in academic health centers. Telemedicine may play a significant role in system improvement in this regard, and this should be studied.

There is a need for more research into the causes of increased rates of chronic disease in children, as well as factors that prevent or6 exacerbate illness. Unless social ecology factors are addressed, the same conditions that contributed to diseases in childhood will likely predispose these same children to adult diseases. Further research on the disparities in chronic disease between populations and the effect of the COVID-19 pandemic will identify factors that impact and exacerbate chronic illness in children. As child enrollment in managed Medicaid increases, it will be important to understand the effect on health outcomes for chronically ill children in this new payment program.

References

1. McPherson M, Arango P, Fox H, Lauver C, McManus M, Newacheck PW, et al. A new definition of children with special health care needs. Pediatrics. 1998;102:137–40.
2. Stein RE, Bauman LJ, Westbrook LE, Coupey SM, Ireys HT. Framework for identifying children who have chronic conditions: the case for a new definition. J Pediatr. 1993;122(3):342–7.
3. van der Lee JH, Mokkink LB, Grootenhuis MA, Heymans HS, Offringa M. Definitions and measurement of chronic health conditions in childhood: a systematic review. JAMA. 2007;297(24):2741–51.
4. Romano I, Buchan C, Baiocco-Romano L, Ferro MA. Physical-mental multimorbidity in children and youth: a scoping review. BMJ Open. 2021;11(5):e043124.
5. Berry JG, Hall M, Cohen E, O'Neill M, Feudtner C. Ways to identify children with medical complexity and the importance of why. J Pediatr. 2015;167(2):229–37.
6. Van Cleave J, Gortmaker SL, Perrin JM. Dynamics of obesity and chronic health conditions among children and youth. JAMA. 2010;303(7):623–30.
7. Dickinson KM, Collaco JM. Cystic fibrosis. Pediatr Rev. 2021;42(2):55–6.
8. Hales CM, Carroll MD, Fryar CD, Ogden CL. Prevalence of obesity and severe obesity among adults: United States, 2017–2018. NCHS Data Brief. 2020;360:1–8.
9. Ogden CL, Fryar CD, Martin CB, Freedman DS, Carroll MD, Gu Q, et al. Trends in obesity prevalence by race and Hispanic origin-1999-2000 to 2017-2018. JAMA. 2020;324(12):1208–10.
10. Patel SJ, Teach SJ. Asthma. Pediatr Rev. 2019;40(11):549–67.
11. Centers for Disease Control and Prevention. 2019 National Health Interview Survey data. Department of Health & Human Services; 2020. Retrieved from: https://www.cdc.gov/asthma/nhis/2019/data.htm.
12. Gerteis J, Izrael D, Deitz D, LeRoy L, Ricciardi R, Miller T, Basu J. Multiple chronic conditions chartbook. AHRQ publications no, Q14-0038. Agency for Healthcare Research and Quality: Rockville, MD; 2014.
13. Casimir G. Why children's hospitals are unique and so essential. Front Pediatr. 2019;7:305.

14. Agency for Healthcare Research and Quality. HCUPnet, healthcare cost and utilization project. Rockville, MD: Agency for Healthcare Research and Quality [cited 2021 Oct 4]. Available from: http://www.hcup-us.ahrq.gov/.
15. Reid LD, Fang Z. Changes in pediatric hospitalizations and in-hospital deaths in the initial period of the COVID-19 pandemic (April–September 2020), 13 States. HCUP Statistical Brief #283. Rockville, MD: Agency for Healthcare Research and Quality; 2021.
16. Pao M, Ballard ED, Rosenstein DL. Growing up in the hospital. JAMA. 2007;297(24):2752–5.
17. Committee on Hospital Care and Institute for Patient- and Family-Centered Care. Patient- and family-centered care and the pediatrician's role. Pediatrics. 2012;129(2):394–404.
18. Destino LA, Shah SS, Good B. Family-centered rounds: past, present, and future. Pediatr Clin N Am. 2019;66(4):827–37.
19. Knighton AJ, Bass EJ. Implementing family-centered rounds in hospital pediatric settings: a scoping review. Hosp Pediatr. 2021;11(7):679–91.
20. Rosenthal MP. Childhood asthma: considerations for primary care practice and chronic disease management in the village of care. Prim Care. 2012;39(2):381–91.
21. Wagner EH, Austin BT, Davis C, Hindmarsh M, Schaefer J, Bonomi A. Improving chronic illness care: translating evidence into action. Health Aff (Millwood). 2001;20(6):64–78.
22. Patient-Centered Primary Care Collaborative. [cited 2021 Oct 4]. Available from: http://www.pcpcc.org.
23. Bodenheimer T, Wagner EH, Grumbach K. Improving primary care for patients with chronic illness. JAMA. 2002;288(14):1775–9.
24. Lalloo C, Diskin C, Ho M, Orkin J, Cohen E, Osei-Twum J-A, et al. Pediatric project ECHO: implementation of a virtual medical education program to support community management of children with medical complexity. Hosp Pediatr. 2020;10(12):1044–52.
25. Gergen PJ, Teach SJ, Togias A, Busse WW. Reducing exacerbations in the Inner City: lessons from the Inner-City Asthma Consortium (ICAC). J Allergy Clin Immunol Pract. 2016;4(1):22–6.
26. Guidelines for home care of infants, children, and adolescents with chronic disease. American Academy of Pediatrics Committee on Children with Disabilities. Pediatrics. 1995;96(1 Pt 1):161–4.
27. Gay JC, Thurm CW, Hall M, Fassino MJ, Fowler L, Palusci JV, et al. Home health nursing care and hospital use for medically complex children. Pediatrics. 2016;138(5):e20160530.
28. Parab CS, Cooper C, Woolfenden S, Piper SM. Specialist home-based nursing services for children with acute and chronic illnesses. Cochrane Database Syst Rev. 2013;(6):CD004383.
29. Sisk B, Alexander J, Bodnar C, Curfman A, Garber K, McSwain SD, et al. Pediatrician attitudes toward and experiences with telehealth use: results from a national survey. Acad Pediatr. 2020;20(5):628–35.
30. Koonin LM, Hoots B, Tsang CA, Leroy Z, Farris K, Jolly T, et al. Trends in the use of telehealth during the emergence of the COVID-19 pandemic—United States, January-March 2020. MMWR Morb Mortal Wkly Rep. 2020;69(43):1595–9.
31. Curfman A, McSwain SD, Chuo J, Yeager-McSwain B, Schinasi DA, Marcin J, et al. Pediatric telehealth in the COVID-19 pandemic era and beyond. Pediatrics. 2021;148(3):e2020047795.
32. Fiese BH, Everhart RS. Medical adherence and childhood chronic illness: family daily management skills and emotional climate as emerging contributors. Curr Opin Pediatr. 2006;18(5):551–7.
33. Chi N-C, Demiris G. A systematic review of telehealth tools and interventions to support family caregivers. J Telemed Telecare. 2015;21(1):37–44.
34. Irvin K, Fahim F, Alshehri S, Kitsantas P. Family structure and children's unmet health-care needs. J Child Health Care. 2018;22(1):57–67.
35. Lear JG. Health at school: a hidden health care system emerges from the shadows. Health Aff (Millwood). 2007;26(2):409–19.
36. Maughan E. The impact of school nursing on school performance: a research synthesis. J Sch Nurs. 2003;19(3):163–71.
37. Rodriguez E, Rivera DA, Perlroth D, Becker E, Wang NE, Landau M. School nurses' role in asthma management, school absenteeism, and cost savings: a demonstration project. J Sch Health. 2013;83(12):842–50.
38. Sanchez D, Reiner JF, Sadlon R, Price OA, Long MW. Systematic review of school telehealth evaluations. J Sch Nurs. 2019;35(1):61–76.
39. Shimasaki S, Brunner Nii P, Davis L, Bishop E, Berget C, Perreault C, et al. A school nurse application of the ECHO model. J Sch Nurs. 2021;37(4):306–15.
40. Whole School, Whole Community, Whole Child (WSCC) overview. [cited 2021 Oct 11]. Available from: https://www.cdc.gov/healthyschools/wscc/WSCCmodel_update_508tagged.pdf.
41. Michael SL, Merlo CL, Basch CE, Wentzel KR, Wechsler H. Critical connections: health and academics. J Sch Health. 2015;85(11):740–58.
42. Basch CE. Healthier students are better learners. J Sch Health. 2011;81(10):591–2.
43. Jutte DP, Miller JL, Erickson DJ. Neighborhood adversity, child health, and the role for community development. Pediatrics. 2015;135(Suppl 2):S48–57.
44. Foltz JL, May AL, Belay B, Nihiser AJ, Dooyema CA, Blanck HM. Population-level intervention strategies and examples for obesity prevention in children. Annu Rev Nutr. 2012;32:391–415.
45. Labre MP, Herman EJ, Dumitru GG, Valenzuela KA, Cechman CL. Public health interventions for asthma: an umbrella review, 1990-2010. Am J Prev Med. 2012;42(4):403–10.
46. Clark NM. Community-based approaches to controlling childhood asthma. Annu Rev Public Health. 2012;33:193–208.
47. Maslow GR, Chung RJ. Systematic review of positive youth development programs for adolescents with chronic illness. Pediatrics. 2013;131(5):e1605–18.
48. The importance of pediatric quality measurement and improvement: the role of the PQMP I Agency for Healthcare Research and Quality. [cited 2021 Sep 13]. Available from: https://www.ahrq.gov/pqmp/about/pediatric-quality-measurement-importance.html.
49. Center for Medicaid & CHIP Services. 2021 Core set of children's health care quality measures for Medicaid and CHIP (child core set). [cited 2021 Oct 11]. Available from: https://www.medicaid.gov/medicaid/quality-of-care/downloads/2021-child-core-set.pdf.
50. Centers for Disease Control and Prevention. Review and selection of core asthma quality measures. [cited 2021 Oct 15]. Available from: https://www.cdc.gov/asthma/pdfs/White_paper_508.pdf.
51. Centers for Medicaid and Medicare Services. Asthma medication ratio: ages 5–18 (AMR-CH). [cited 2021 Oct 15]. Available from: https://www.medicaid.gov/state-overviews/scorecard/asthma-medication-ratio-ages-5-18/index.html.
52. PQMP measure implementation and quality improvement I Agency for Healthcare Research and Quality. [cited 2021 Oct 13]. Available from: https://www.ahrq.gov/pqmp/implementation-qi/index.html.
53. Centers for Disease Control and Prevention. Most recent national asthma data. https://www.cdc.gov/asthma/most_recent_national_asthma_data.htm. Accessed 4 Sept 2022.
54. Centers for Disease Control and Prevention. Asthma as the underlying cause of death. [cited 2021 Oct 10]. Available from: https://www-cdc-gov.libproxy.lib.unc.edu/asthma/asthma_stats/asthma_underlying_death.html.
55. Trent M, Dooley DG, Dougé J, Section on Adolescent Health, Council on Community Pediatrics, Committee on Adolescence. The impact of racism on child and adolescent health. Pediatrics. 2019;144(2)
56. World Health Organization. Social determinants of health. [cited 2021 Oct 11]. Available from: https://www.who.int/health-topics/social-determinants-of-health#tab=tab_1.

57. Garg A, Homer CJ, Dworkin PH. Addressing social determinants of health: challenges and opportunities in a value-based model. Pediatrics. 2019;143(4)
58. Cohen AJ, De Marchis EH. Building an evidence base for integration of social care into health care: our collective path ahead. Ann Fam Med. 2021;19(4):290–2.
59. Thornton RLJ, Glover CM, Cené CW, Glik DC, Henderson JA, Williams DR. Evaluating strategies for reducing health disparities by addressing the social determinants of health. Health Aff (Millwood). 2016;35(8):1416–23.
60. Kompaniyets L, Agathis NT, Nelson JM, Preston LE, Ko JY, Belay B, et al. Underlying medical conditions associated with severe COVID-19 illness among children. JAMA Netw Open. 2021;4(6):e2111182.
61. Davis AL, Sunderji A, Marneni SR, et al., International COVID-19 Parental Attitude Study (COVIPAS) Group. Caregiver-reported delay in presentation to pediatric emergency departments for fear of contracting COVID-19: a multi-national cross-sectional study. CJEM. 2021;23(6):778–86.
62. Perry R, Braileanu G, Palmer T, Stevens P. The economic burden of pediatric asthma in the United States: literature review of current evidence. PharmacoEconomics. 2019;37(2):155–67.
63. Kaiser Family Foundation. Health insurance coverage of children 0–18. [cited 2021 Oct 15]. Available from: https://www.kff.org/other/state-indicator/children-0-18/?currentTimeframe=0&sortModel=%7B%22colId%22:%22Location%22,%22sort%22:%22asc%22%7D.
64. Grace AM, Horn I, Hall R, Cheng TL. Children, families, and disparities: pediatric provisions in the affordable care act. Pediatr Clin N Am. 2015;62(5):1297–311.
65. April 2021 Medicaid & CHIP enrollment data highlights | Medicaid. [cited 2021 Oct 11]. Available from: https://www.medicaid.gov/medicaid/program-information/medicaid-and-chip-enrollment-data/report-highlights/index.html.
66. Dubay L, Guyer J, Mann C, Odeh M. Medicaid at the ten-year anniversary of SCHIP: looking back and moving forward. Health Aff (Millwood). 2007;26(2):370–81.
67. Olson LM, Tang SS, Newacheck PW. Children in the United States with discontinuous health insurance coverage. N Engl J Med. 2005;353(4):382–91.
68. Newacheck PW, Stoddard JJ, Hughes DC, Pearl M. Health insurance and access to primary care for children. N Engl J Med. 1998;338(8):513–9.
69. Heuschkel R, Salvestrini C, Beattie RM, Hildebrand H, Walters T, Griffiths A. Guidelines for the management of growth failure in childhood inflammatory bowel disease. Inflamm Bowel Dis. 2008;14(6):839–49.
70. Mahan JD, Warady BA, Consensus Committee. Assessment and treatment of short stature in pediatric patients with chronic kidney disease: a consensus statement. Pediatr Nephrol. 2006;21(7):917–30.
71. Kaplowitz PB. Link between body fat and the timing of puberty. Pediatrics. 2008;121(Suppl 3):S208–17.
72. Lee JM, Wasserman R, Kaciroti N, Gebremariam A, Steffes J, Dowshen S, et al. Timing of puberty in overweight versus obese boys. Pediatrics. 2016;137(2):e20150164.
73. Suris JC, Michaud PA, Viner R. The adolescent with a chronic condition. Part I: developmental issues. Arch Dis Child. 2004;89(10):938–42.
74. Tulloch T, Kaufman M. Adolescent sexuality. Pediatr Rev. 2013;34(1):29–37; quiz 38.
75. Fegran L, Hall EOC, Uhrenfeldt L, Aagaard H, Ludvigsen MS. Adolescents' and young adults' transition experiences when transferring from paediatric to adult care: a qualitative metasynthesis. Int J Nurs Stud. 2014;51(1):123–35.
76. National Academies of Sciences, Engineering, and Medicine, Health and Medicine Division, Board on Health Care Services, Committee on Improving Health Outcomes for Children with Disabilities. In: Byers E, Valliere FR, Houtrow AJ, editors. Opportunities for improving programs and services for children with disabilities. Washington, DC: National Academies Press (US); 2018.
77. Cohen E, Kuo DZ, Agrawal R, Berry JG, Bhagat SKM, Simon TD, et al. Children with medical complexity: an emerging population for clinical and research initiatives. Pediatrics. 2011;127(3):529–38.
78. Johnson SB, Spin P, Connolly F, Stein M, Cheng TL, Connor K. Asthma and attendance in urban schools. Prev Chronic Dis. 2019;16:190074.
79. Basch CE. Asthma and the achievement gap among urban minority youth. J Sch Health. 2011;81(10):606–13.
80. Taras H, Potts-Datema W. Childhood asthma and student performance at school. J Sch Health. 2005;75(8):296–312.
81. Basch CE. Healthier students are better learners: high-quality, strategically planned, and effectively coordinated school health programs must be a fundamental mission of schools to help close the achievement gap. J Sch Health. 2011;81(10):650–62.
82. Taras H, Potts-Datema W. Obesity and student performance at school. J Sch Health. 2005;75(8):291–5.
83. Kral MC, Brown RT, Hynd GW. Neuropsychological aspects of pediatric sickle cell disease. Neuropsychol Rev. 2001;11(4):179–96.
84. Centers for Disease Control and Prevention. Health and academic achievement. https://www.cdc.gov/healthyschools/health_and_academics/pdf/health-academic-achievement.pdf. Accessed 4 Sept 2022.
85. Law EF, Fisher E, Fales J, Noel M, Eccleston C. Systematic review and meta-analysis of parent and family-based interventions for children and adolescents with chronic medical conditions. J Pediatr Psychol. 2014;39(8):866–86.
86. Thomasgard M, Metz WP. The vulnerable child syndrome revisited. J Dev Behav Pediatr. 1995;16(1):47–53.
87. Christin A, Akre C, Berchtold A, Suris JC. Parent-adolescent relationship in youths with a chronic condition. Child Care Health Dev. 2016;42(1):36–41.
88. Witt WP, Weiss AJ, Elixhauser A. Overview of hospital stays for children in the United States, 2012: statistical brief #187. Healthcare cost and utilization project (HCUP) statistical briefs. Rockville, MD: Agency for Healthcare Research and Quality (US); 2006.
89. Geist R, Grdisa V, Otley A. Psychosocial issues in the child with chronic conditions. Best Pract Res Clin Gastroenterol. 2003;17(2):141–52.
90. American Academy of Pediatrics Committee on Children with Disabilities and Committee on Psychosocial Aspects of Child and Family Health: psychosocial risks of chronic health conditions in childhood and adolescence. Pediatrics. 1993;92(6):876–8.
91. Turkel S, Pao M. Late consequences of chronic pediatric illness. Psychiatr Clin North Am. 2007;30(4):819–35.
92. Shaw TM, Delaet DE. Transition of adolescents to young adulthood for vulnerable populations. Pediatr Rev. 2010;31(12):497–504; quiz 505.
93. American Academy of Pediatrics, American Academy of Family Physicians, American College of Physicians-American Society of Internal Medicine. A consensus statement on health care transitions for young adults with special health care needs. Pediatrics. 2002;110(6 Pt 2):1304–6.
94. https://www.healthcare.gov/young-adults/children-under-26/.
95. Friedlander SL, Larkin EK, Rosen CL, Palermo TM, Redline S. Decreased quality of life associated with obesity in school-aged children. Arch Pediatr Adolesc Med. 2003;157(12):1206–11.
96. Maslow GR, Haydon A, McRee A-L, Ford CA, Halpern CT. Growing up with a chronic illness: social success, educational/vocational distress. J Adolesc Health. 2011;49(2):206–12.

Special Population: Older Adults

Collin Burks and Mallory McClester Brown

Epidemiology of Chronic Disease in Older Adults

Adults are living longer lives due to public health measures, treatment for infectious diseases, and other medical advancements. Currently, approximately 49 million Americans are aged 65 or over [1]. By 2040, 20% of the population will be aged 65 and above, growing to 88 million people by 2050, more than double the number in 2008 (38 million). The number of U.S. residents aged 85 or over is projected to grow by more than 300% over the next 40 years [2].

The tradeoff for living longer lives is the likelihood of developing one or more chronic conditions. Eighty-five percent of adults aged 70 or over have at least one chronic condition, and nearly 70% of Medicare beneficiaries have two or more [2]. Science and technology have made the survival of acute issues such as myocardial infarction more likely, making the treatment of chronic conditions of our aging population a significant health, societal, and financial challenge. The most common chronic conditions in adults aged 55 and above include diabetes, cardiovascular disease, chronic obstructive pulmonary disease (COPD), asthma, cancer, stroke, dementia, and arthritis. These conditions require ongoing medical attention and can limit activities of daily living, day-to-day functioning, and quality of life [3, 4]. The treatment goal is slowing disease progression and addressing functional limitations. The burden of chronic illness on the individual, families, and society is significant. Chronic illness over many years can result in chronic pain, loss of function and independence, and increased reliance on family and friends for support. As the number of chronic conditions increases, the prevalence of functional limitations rises.

The care of individuals with chronic disease and functional limitations is expensive and largely covered by Medicare and Medicaid, as well as costly out-of-pocket expenses to the family. In the most basic of terms, 71 cents of every dollar spent on healthcare goes toward treating people with multiple chronic conditions [5]. Not surprisingly, people with multiple chronic conditions account for the majority of clinician visits, prescriptions, home health visits, and hospitalizations. For example, a 75-year-old patient with coronary artery disease, hypertension, diabetes, depression, and diabetes (or any combination of five or more chronic conditions) would see on average 14 different physicians, make 37 physician office visits, and fill 50 prescriptions in the course of 1 year [6].

Ageism

The aging of society brings with it the necessity of confronting the subject of biases against older adults. Ageism is the stereotyping, prejudice, and discrimination against people on the basis of their age and is highly prevalent [7, 8]. Ageism influences society's attitudes regarding older adults, which has consequences on health outcomes [9]. Data show that negative attitudes toward aging pose a significant risk to the health and well-being of older adults, contributing to mortality, poor functional health, slower recovery from illness, and poor mental health [10–12]. Ageism bias from healthcare professionals can result in discriminatory practices toward older adults [13]. For instance, if a medical provider carries an assumption regarding the functional or cognitive abilities of older adults, they may practice with a more limited scope of thought, withhold treatment options, and exclude individuals from clinical trials [14]. In a similar vein, practitioners who assume diagnoses like depression are "normal" for an older adult can limit that individual's treatment [15].

Ageism impacts not only the physical and medical care provided to patients but also their social engagement, employment, health policy, and general involvement in soci-

C. Burks
Division of Geriatrics, Duke University, Durham, NC, USA
e-mail: collin.burks@duke.edu

M. M. Brown (✉)
Department of Family Medicine, University of North Carolina at Chapel Hill, Chapel Hill, NC, USA
e-mail: mallory_mcclester@med.unc.edu

ety. Recurrent experiences with negative stereotypes combined with discrimination may make ageism a chronic stressor in the lives of older adults leading to accelerated physical deterioration and associated chronic disease [16].

Strategies that combat ageism improve the overall well-being of our older adults [7]. Effective interventions are inexpensive and include education and cross-generational contact.

The Impact of COVID-19 on Chronically Ill Older Adults

Adults aged 65 and above represent up to 80% of COVID-19 hospitalizations to date with 25 times the risk of death than those under age 65 [17]. Comorbidities such as cardiovascular disease, diabetes, and obesity increase the mortality, but age is an independent risk factor. During the peaks of the pandemic, older adults often did not survive, especially if decisions were required about medical care, triage, and life-saving therapies [18].

COVID-19 has affected the economic security of older adults as well as their access to healthcare and supportive services for chronic conditions [19]. Older adults with chronic comorbidities were among the most likely to have their healthcare delayed or canceled in the setting of the pandemic. Older adults with a need for help with activities of daily living were often left without support from both professional and informal caregivers. The spread of COVID-19 in care homes and institutions took a devastating toll on older people's lives, with distressing reports of neglect or mistreatment. Older persons who are quarantined or locked down with family members or caregivers faced higher risks of violence, abuse, and neglect [18]. Older adults in the United States have suffered the most economically from the COVID-19 pandemic, with many losing a job or using up all or most of their savings [19]. Black and Latino/Hispanic older adults were more likely than White older adults to suffer economic hardship in this pandemic, the impact of which will continue for years, influencing health and lifestyle choices.

Social Determinants of Health for Older Adults

Social determinants of health (SDOHs), as broadly defined by the World Health Organization, are the "non-medical factors that influence health outcomes….The conditions in which people are born, grow, work, live, and age" [20]. SDOHs have a considerable impact on the health and well-being of people of all ages and can especially impact older adults in ways that are unique to this population and are associated with and predictive of poorer outcomes. Data from the National Health and Nutrition Examination Survey showed that older adults with three or more SDOHs risk factors had more functional limitations, rated their general health to be worse, and were less likely to have a usual source of care, as compared to older adults who had two or fewer SDOHs risk factors [21]. This section reviews several SDOHs and introduces considerations specific to older adults; however, it is not a conclusive list or discussion of all categories of SDOHs.

Health Literacy

The 2003 National Assessment of Adult Literacy in the United States revealed that 59% of adults aged 65 and older have below basic or basic health literacy and only 3% have proficiency in health literacy [22]. Many factors contribute to low health literacy in older adults, including lower educational levels and age-related changes such as hearing loss, vision loss, and cognitive decline. Low health literacy in all ages is associated with and likely contributes to worse health outcomes, including in older adults where it contributes to poorer cognitive functioning [23, 24]. Low health literacy may be a barrier to effective provider–patient communication and the ability to actively participate in and follow a plan for chronic illness care, with mixed data on whether it affects medication adherence [23]. The assessment of health literacy is valuable in the clinical setting, particularly in older adults who have multiple chronic conditions and are expected to manage their care at home.

Social Support and Access to Community Resources

For many older adults with chronic illness and physical and/or cognitive decline, the presence of a caregiver, paid or unpaid, is essential to meet their daily needs and assist with or manage various aspects of chronic illness care. In 2020, there were an estimated 42 million people acting as caregivers for adults aged 50+ in the United States [25]. Despite this high number, there is a substantial group of older adults referred to as "elder orphans," meaning older adults who are aging alone and do not have a caregiver, making them vulnerable to medical and social stressors. Social isolation and loneliness are correlated with poorer health outcomes [26]. Conversely, the diversity of an older adult's social network is associated with higher health-related quality of life scores [27]. An assessment of social support provides valuable information and helps patients and clinicians more effectively manage chronic illnesses.

In addition to a caregiver, many older adults benefit from and even rely on access to community resources for their health and livelihood. Community resources for older adults include transportation services, food delivery, and caregiver support programs. Of the older adults who received community-based services from Title III programs supported by the Older Americans Act Funds, 90% were living with multiple chronic illnesses [28]. Healthcare providers should be aware of community programs in their geographic areas and help older adults engage with these resources if needed.

Elder Abuse

The prevalence of elder abuse is high, with 16% or more of older adults experiencing some form of abuse or neglect [29–31]. Elder abuse is categorized into five areas: physical, psychological/verbal, sexual, financial exploitation, and neglect. Younger age, lower income, isolation, and lack of social support are several of the risk factors for elder abuse [32–34]. Dementia, poor physical health, and functional impairment are all associated with a higher risk of abuse [29]. The consequences of elder abuse include increased rates of hospitalization, placement in nursing homes, and death. Healthcare providers should be aware of the possible manifestations of abuse and how to further inquire when abuse is suspected, as well as know how to make appropriate referrals when indicated.

Access to Food

Access to food is an SDOHs that has considerable impact on the lives of older adults, especially those who live with chronic illness. Millions of older adults in the United States experience food insecurity [35]. The lack of consistent access to adequate food is associated with a higher prevalence of chronic disease [36]. The interplay between food insecurity and chronic disease is complicated, with both potentially exacerbating the other. Many clinics and health systems screen their patients for food insecurity and then link patients and families to community resources that address this issue; this is an example of the trend of screening for SDOHs in the healthcare setting. There is much more work that needs to be done around appropriate screening and subsequent follow-through for addressing SDOHs in healthcare.

Health Disparities

Older adults are a heterogeneous population, and as with other age groups, there is an unequal distribution of chronic disease and poor health outcomes among older adults of different races, ethnicities, and sexual orientations, among other characteristics. It is imperative to acknowledge and understand that these health disparities exist and impact older adults.

In the United States, non-White older adults have higher numbers of chronic conditions than their non-Hispanic White counterparts. Mortality rates for chronic conditions, including diabetes, chronic kidney disease, and COPD, are highest among Native Americans and Indigenous Alaskans followed by Black individuals [37].

In addition to race and ethnicity, health disparities for older adults are influenced by sexual orientation and gender identity. Although there may not be significant differences in rates of chronic diseases such as diabetes or hypertension, lesbian, gay, bisexual, transgender, and queer (LGBTQ) older adults are more likely to have higher rates of poor mental health and disability [38]. LGBTQ older adults are more likely to live alone, experience financial insecurity, and have faced discrimination in the healthcare system [38]. Significant differences in health behaviors and disparities exist between the various subgroups within the LGBTQ population, as they do within racial and ethnic subgroups. Healthcare providers should be aware of the broader trends that affect their patients while treating each patient as a distinct individual with their own unique strengths and challenges.

Objectives of Care in Older Adults with Chronic Illness

Caring for older adults with chronic illness requires careful consideration of the individual's current state, the potential for improvement, and the patient and family's overall goals of care. Key objectives in caring for older adults with chronic health conditions include (1) attention to quality of life, (2) slowing the rate of functional decline, (3) consideration of life expectancy and prognosis, (4) advance care planning (ACP), and (5) the development of systems of support for the individual and their caregivers.

Quality of Life

Quality of life can be defined in several ways. For an individual, it may be defined as a sense of well-being, meaning, and value, or the subjective fulfillment of the dimensions of human life. Evaluating and understanding an individual's sense of their own quality of life helps determine needed resources and unmet needs as a medical care plan is determined [39]. Interpretation of an individual's quality of life includes the assessment of their own health, functional capacity, coping mechanisms, and how biophysical and sociocultural environmental factors contribute [40].

Function

Maintenance of physical function permits independence of older adults with chronic illness. This is important for those individuals who wish to remain in their own home, continue to drive their car, and complete their own daily tasks.

Table 23.1 Activities of daily living

Activities of daily living (ADLs)	Independent activities of daily living (IADLs)
Bathing	Transportation independence
Dressing	Medication management
Toileting	Meal preparation
Grooming	Managing finances
Transferring	Laundry
Feeding oneself	Keeping a tidy home

Assessment of an individual's ability to complete their own activities of daily living (ADLs) as well as independent activities of daily living (IADLs) is imperative in the routine assessment of patients living with chronic disease. While direct observation is best, asking about ADLs and IADLs to the patient and their families is also very useful (Table 23.1). An awareness of an individual's ability or failure to complete these tasks guides the treatment plan. Physical and occupational therapy and other rehabilitative services may help to reverse or slow loss of function. Social supports can also slow the loss of independence.

Life Expectancy and Prognosis

Older age logically shortens life expectancy, as does the presence of one or more chronic conditions. Estimating a patient's life expectancy can help determine the likelihood that certain treatments will be effective, helping to guide a patient-centered plan of care. Consideration of one's prognosis, based on age and health condition, is particularly important in clinical decision making for older adults [41]. Failure to include the discussion of poor prognosis leads to inappropriate medical care, such as delay in referral to hospice or unnecessary cancer screening. Conversely, underestimating a positive prognosis can lead to delayed treatment or testing [42].

Clinical practice guidelines increasingly consider life expectancy and function when determining the risks and benefits of intervention. For example, the American Geriatrics Society recommends a target goal for glycosylated hemoglobin (HgbA1c) in older adults with diabetes of 7.5–8%, which is more relaxed than the goal in younger adults. A HgbA1c goal of 7–7.5% may be appropriate in healthy older adults with few comorbidities and good functional status. Higher HbA1c targets of 8–9% are appropriate for older adults with multiple comorbidities, poor health, and limited life expectancy [43].

Actuarial tables estimate mean life expectancies but do not consider the presence of chronic diseases (Table 23.2). Several tools exist to more accurately predict an individual's life expectancy by taking into account the patient's health condition. These tools consider a patient's age, gender, weight, medical history, recent hospitalization, physical function, and other factors. One such tool, *ePrognosis*, is a repository of published evidence-based geriatric prognostic indices, which aid in formulating an individualized care plan for patients with chronic conditions [44].

Table 23.2 Mean life expectancy

	Mean remaining life expectancy (years)	
Current age	Men	Women
65	18	21
70	15	17
75	11	13
80	8	10
85	6	7
90	4	5
95	3	3
100	2	2
105	2	2

Adapted from Actuarial Life Table. Ssa.gov. 2019 [cited December 2, 2021]. Available from: https://www.ssa.gov/oact/STATS/table4c6.html

Advance Care Planning

Advance care planning (ACP) is a process that documents the patient's values and priorities about care at the end of life [45]. This is important in the care of older adults with chronic diseases and should be done while a patient still has decision-making autonomy. Advance care planning, which includes the patient and their loved ones, decreases caregiver burden and dissatisfaction with end-of-life care [46]. It is also imperative to document the patient's healthcare proxy, who will make healthcare decisions on the patient's behalf, should they no longer be able to do so themselves.

Systems of Support

Healthcare can be challenging to navigate at all ages, even more so for older adults with chronic illness. Functional limitations such as decreased mobility, hearing, and vision can further interfere with one's ability to obtain and follow through on adequate healthcare. In addition, as one ages, the likelihood of being widowed and therefore living alone is more likely. Since women tend to live longer than men, on average, they are particularly impacted and more likely to require support from a child or other caregiver.

It can be a challenge to serve as a caregiver. Spouses supporting loved ones with chronic illness may suffer from aging-related changes limiting function and making it harder to keep the household together, safely support the needy partner, and adequately care for themselves. Children and other family member caregivers may not live with the older adult, may work full time, or may have children who require care. These challenges are common and increase the stress of providing support to an aging loved one.

Caregiver support groups are available locally and nationally. These groups help individual caregivers think about new and different ways of providing support. Physicians should utilize the help of social workers or be aware of groups locally to whom they can refer families. Asking the caregiver how they are doing is an important part of the care a physician provides.

Each Individual Is Unique

Caring for older adults with chronic disease requires consideration of the varying components of the chronic diseases, even when the recommendations and guidelines for the different conditions can be contradictory. Care can be fragmented, inefficient, and ineffective, especially with multiple chronic conditions and treatment by multiple subspecialists. Effective primary care includes the provision of comprehensive assessments, evidence-based care planning and monitoring, patients' and family caregivers' active engagement, and coordination of care among the healthcare team and specialists, all tailored to the patient's goals and preferences.

Geriatric Syndromes

Geriatric syndromes are not part of the traditional disease model of care nor considered comorbidities but are as prevalent as chronic disease in older adults and are associated with functional disability [47]. Geriatric syndromes often co-occur or are exacerbated by chronic conditions in older adults [48]. Common geriatric syndromes include incontinence, cognitive impairment, delirium, frailty, falls, anorexia, and pressure ulcers. These geriatric syndromes reduce independence, function, and ability to provide self-care and lead to an increased rate of disability, hospitalization, institutionalization, and mortality, particularly for patients with chronic conditions.

By identifying and evaluating for geriatric syndromes and providing support and therapeutic intervention for those conditions, a physician may improve the patient's function and overall health. Rather than considering one condition or syndrome at a time, quality indicators and care guidelines should address comprehensive and coordinated management of co-occurring diseases and geriatric syndromes [48].

Organization of Care for Older Adults with Chronic Illness

From hospital medicine to home-based services, models of care for older adults aim to improve care for the patients who are most at risk, including those with multiple chronic illnesses. This section provides an overview of several of these models.

Hospital

In the 1990s, the *Acute Care for Elders (ACE)* model was designed to help prevent functional decline and associated complications in hospitalized older adults. Components of the ACE model include medical review, early rehabilitation, early discharge planning, prepared environment, and patient-centered care. The hospital units in which this model is implemented are referred to as ACE units. Since its inception, the ACE model has been implemented in over 200 hospitals and are associated with a reduction in falls, delirium, functional decline, length of hospital stay, and discharges to nursing homes [49].

The *Hospital Elder Life Program (HELP)* is another model designed to promote independence among hospitalized older adults and to prevent complications of hospitalization, with a focus on delirium. Like the ACE model, it was developed in the 1990s and has been implemented in numerous hospitals across the United States. HELP uses an interdisciplinary team, including volunteers, to work within existing hospital units to provide care to older adults at risk of functional decline [50]. HELP reduces the incidence of delirium and falls in hospitalized older adults who receive the intervention [51].

The *Nurses Improving Care for Healthsystem Elders (NICHE)* program focuses on improving nurses' knowledge and skills in care of geriatric patients while also providing institutions with tools to implement system-wide changes in their care of older adults. Founded in New York in 1992, the program has been implemented in hundreds of sites across the United States and several international sites [52]. The NICHE program is associated with a reduction in the incidence of delirium, the use of physical restraints, and rates of infection including urinary tract infections and pneumonia [52, 53].

Hospital at Home (HaH) is an emerging model of care in which individuals receive hospital-level services in their home. In this model, patients may never need to be hospitalized, or they may be discharged early to complete a course of hospital-level care at home. While not specifically designed for older adults, it holds greater benefits for older adults than other populations. Several healthcare systems in the United States have successfully implemented HaH programs; however, the challenges associated with the COVID-19 pandemic have spurred an increasing number of systems to develop their own HaH programs. In 2020, the Centers for Medicare & Medicaid Services (CMS) announced their Acute Hospital Care at Home program, providing a structure for Medicare reimbursement for HaH models. This model holds great promise for safer and more effective care for older adults, and we expect reimbursement mechanisms to grow and be refined over time.

Care Transitions

For older adults with chronic illness, transitions of care from hospital to home or other post-acute facility occur frequently due to exacerbations of chronic disease or acute illnesses. Older adults are particularly vulnerable in times of transitions. Several models of transitional care improve these transitions by increasing communication between providers, decreasing medication errors, and providing information and support to patients and families as they transition between different settings. While many of these models focus on supporting the transition between acute care and skilled nursing facilities (SNF), there are programs that support the SNF-to-home transition as well. The chapter in this book dedicated to Care Transitions includes a more thorough review of this topic.

Nursing Home Care

The Interventions to Reduce Acute Care Transfers (INTERACT) program was piloted in 2007 to help nursing homes reduce potentially avoidable hospitalization among their residents [54]. The INTERACT program provides nursing homes with tools to improve communication, evaluate and manage acute changes in a patient's condition, and perform advance care planning [55]. While initial non-randomized studies demonstrated a reduction in all-cause hospitalizations for nursing homes that implemented the INTERACT program [55], a later randomized implementation trial found no effect on hospitalization rates [56].

Institutional Special Needs Plans (I-SNPs), offered by Medicare Advantage plans using managed care, render a model in which advanced practitioners provide additional medical care as well as care coordination to patients in nursing homes. In this model, an advanced practitioner has frequent visits with patients in the long-term care setting and works with the patient's PCPs and nursing home staff to carry out a plan of care. I-SNPs and the original model from which they developed, the Evercare model, are associated with fewer ED visits and hospitalizations [57, 58].

Like the HaH model, an SNF-at-home model has garnered interest during the COVID-19 pandemic. In this model, rather than the provision of post-acute care at an SNF, those skilled nursing and rehabilitative services are moved to the home. Mount Sinai's Rehabilitation at Home (RaH) program is such a program, and it is likely that others will develop [59].

Outpatient and Community Care

The *Geriatrics Resources for Assessment and Care of Elders (GRACE)* model was implemented in 2002 as an additional service in primary care for low-income older adults. This model consists of a support team, a nurse practitioner and social worker, who perform in-home geriatric-focused assessments and then work with an interdisciplinary team to formulate a care plan for the older adult. The support team then reviews their assessment with the patient's PCP and carries out the care plan. In addition to the assessment and management of geriatric syndromes, the support team provides ongoing care coordination for the patient. Patients who receive GRACE services in addition to their primary care have fewer hospital admissions and a lower readmission rate than patients who receive usual primary care services [60].

Home-based primary care (HBPC) is the provision of in-home primary medical care and care management services to adults with chronic illness. This model was developed by the Department of Veterans Affairs in the 1970s and has expanded to other healthcare systems and free-standing HBPC programs. These programs rely on an interdisciplinary team to provide comprehensive care and are associated with a reduction in total inpatient days and readmission rates [61, 62].

The *Program of All-inclusive Care for the Elderly (PACE)* is a comprehensive program in which older adults who are typically nursing home-eligible receive a range of medical and social services from an interdisciplinary team. Most of these services are provided at the PACE site, which is an adult day center where the program's participants spend up to 5 days a week. The overarching aim of this program is to help older adults with chronic conditions and functional limitations remain in their homes for as long as possible by providing wrap-around support. The PACE model includes managed care, through which the sites receive capitated payments from Medicare and Medicaid (dual-eligible beneficiaries are the majority of enrollees in these programs) to cover the participant's expenses. This model began at a single site in 1973 and has expanded to over 200 centers in dozens of states. It is associated with fewer hospital admissions and readmissions as compared to the rates for dual-eligible beneficiaries who are not in a PACE program [63].

Telehealth

While there is not a unique, widely implemented telehealth model of care for older adults with chronic illness, telehealth certainly holds promise as a tool to improve the care of this population. Telehealth can be used to provide both standard chronic illness care and more comprehensive interventions to older adults living with chronic illness. Numerous studies have evaluated the benefits of various telehealth interventions in small groups of older adults, often focused on one specific chronic disease such as diabetes or heart failure. These interventions have targeted a variety of topics, including improving knowledge, self-care, and/or medication adherence, and in general do show improvements in older adults' self-management, among other positive outcomes [64]. Although telehealth in various forms has existed for several years, the COVID-19 pandemic spurred the widespread implementation of telehealth in the United States, and new models of telehealth care will likely arise in the coming years.

Future Directions

With a growing population of older adults in the United States with a growing burden of chronic disease, the provision of care for older adults living with chronic illnesses will continue to evolve. Increasing recognition of the role of caregivers will be paramount, including systematically ensuring that caregiver assessments are performed and reimbursed. Additionally, there must be ongoing efforts to teach geriatric principles and combat ageism in medical education. Health systems may choose to adopt the *Age-Friendly Health Systems* initiative, in which health systems commit to providing specific components of evidence-based care to older adults, or otherwise become more geriatric-friendly. New models of care may develop, and existing models of care will evolve to better serve the needs of older adults, including better incorporation of screening and care coordination around SDOHs. Research on these models must be prioritized, as should payment models to support the most effective models. As technology and precision medicine evolve with the goal of improving healthcare, it is imperative that older adults are uniquely considered in the design and implementation of such advances. Primary care providers and specialty providers who treat older adults with chronic illness must advocate locally, statewide, and nationally for efficient, effective, and affordable systems of care that best support these patients.

References

1. Administration on Aging. 2017 Profile of older Americans. Administration on Aging; 2018 [cited 2021 Nov 10]. 16 p. Available from: https://acl.gov/sites/default/files/Aging%20and%20Disability%20in%20America/2017OlderAmericansProfile.pdf.
2. Anderson, G. Chronic care: making the case for ongoing care. Robert Wood Johnson Foundation; 2010 [cited 2021 Nov 9]. 43 p. Available from: https://www.rwjf.org/en/library/research/2010/01/chronic-care.html.
3. Centers for Disease Control and Prevention. About chronic diseases. Centers for Disease Control and Prevention [updated 2021 Apr 28; cited 2021 Nov 9]. Available from: https://www.cdc.gov/chronicdisease/about/index.htm.
4. Martín Lesende I, Mendibil Crespo LI, Castaño Manzanares S, Otter AD, Garaizar Bilbao I, Pisón Rodríguez J, et al. Functional decline and associated factors in patients with multimorbidity at 8 months of follow-up in primary care: the functionality in pluripathological patients (FUNCIPLUR) longitudinal descriptive study. BMJ Open. 2018;8(7):e022377.
5. Gerteis J, Izrael D, Deitz D, LeRoy L, Ricciardi R, Miller T, Basu J. Multiple chronic conditions chartbook. Rockville, MD: Agency for Healthcare Research and Quality; 2014 [cited 2021 Nov 9]. 46 p. Available from: https://www.ahrq.gov/sites/default/files/wysiwyg/professionals/prevention-chronic-care/decision/mcc/mccchartbook.pdf.
6. Anderson GF. Medicare and chronic conditions. N Engl J Med. 2005;353(3):305–9.
7. Burnes D, Sheppard C, Henderson CR Jr, Wassel M, Cope R, Barber C, et al. Interventions to reduce ageism against older adults: a systematic review and meta-analysis. Am J Public Health. 2019;109(8):e1–9.
8. North MS, Fiske ST. Modern attitudes toward older adults in the aging world: a cross-cultural meta-analysis. Psychol Bull. 2015;141(5):993–1021.
9. Donizzetti AR. Ageism in an aging society: the role of knowledge, anxiety about aging, and stereotypes in young people and adults. Int J Environ Res Public Health. 2019;16(8):1329.
10. Meisner BA. A meta-analysis of positive and negative age stereotype priming effects on behavior among older adults. J Gerontol B Psychol Sci Soc Sci. 2012;67(1):13–7.
11. Bryant C, Bei B, Gilson K, Komiti A, Jackson H, Judd F. The relationship between attitudes to aging and physical and mental health in older adults. Int Psychogeriatr. 2012;24(10):1674–83.
12. Lamont RA, Swift HJ, Abrams D. A review and meta-analysis of age-based stereotype threat: negative stereotypes, not facts, do the damage. Psychol Aging. 2015;30(1):180–93.
13. Chrisler JC, Barney A, Palatino B. Ageism can be hazardous to women's health: ageism, sexism, and stereotypes of older women in the healthcare system. J Soc Issues. 2016;72(1):86–104.
14. Buttigieg SC, Ilinca S, de Sao Jose JMS, Larsson AT. Researching ageism in health-care and long term care. In: Ayalon L, Tesch-Römer C, editors. Contemporary perspectives on ageism. Cham: Springer International Publishing; 2018. p. 493–515.
15. Bodner E, Palgi Y, Wyman MF. Ageism in mental health assessment and treatment of older adults. In: Ayalon L, Tesch-Römer C, editors. Contemporary perspectives on ageism. Cham: Springer International Publishing; 2018. p. 241–62.
16. Allen JO. Ageism as a risk factor for chronic disease. Gerontologist. 2016;56(4):610–4.
17. Mueller AL, McNamara MS, Sinclair DA. Why does COVID-19 disproportionately affect older people? Aging (Albany NY). 2020;12(10):9959–81.

18. United Nations. Policy brief: the impact of COVID-19 on older persons. United Nations; 2020 [cited 2021 Nov 9]. 16 p. Available from: https://www.un.org/development/desa/ageing/wp-content/uploads/sites/24/2020/05/COVID-Older-persons.pdf
19. Williams RD, Shah A, Doty MM, Fields K, FitzGerald M. The impact of COVID-19 on older adults: findings from the 2021 International Health Policy Survey of Older Adults. Commonwealth Fund; 2021 [cited 2021 Nov 10]. Available from: https://www.commonwealthfund.org/publications/surveys/2021/sep/impact-covid-19-older-adults.
20. World Health Organization. World Health Organization. Social determinants of health [cited 2021 Nov 1]. Available from: https://www.who.int/health-topics/social-determinants-of-health#tab=tab_1.
21. Rhee TG, Marottoli RA, Cooney LM Jr, Fortinsky RH. Associations of social and behavioral determinants of health index with self-rated health, functional limitations, and health services use in older adults. J Am Geriatr Soc. 2020;68(8):1731–8.
22. Kutner M, Greenberg R, Jin Y, Paulsen C. The health literacy of America's adults: results from the 2003 national assessment of adult literacy. Washington, DC: National Center for Education Statistics; 2006 [cited 2021 Nov 1]. 60 p. Report No.: NCES 2006-483. Available from: https://nces.ed.gov/pubs2006/2006483.pdf.
23. Chesser AK, Keene Woods N, Smothers K, Rogers N. Health literacy and older adults: a systematic review. Gerontol Geriatr Med. 2016;2:2333721416630492.
24. Geboers B, Uiters E, Reijneveld SA, Jansen CJM, Almansa J, Nooyens ACJ, et al. Health literacy among older adults is associated with their 10-years' cognitive functioning and decline—the Doetinchem Cohort Study. BMC Geriatr. 2018;18(1):77.
25. AARP and National Alliance for Caregiving. Caregiving in the U.S. Washington, DC: AARP; 2020 [cited 2021 Nov 1]. Available from: https://www.caregiving.org/wp-content/uploads/2021/01/full-report-caregiving-in-the-united-states-01-21.pdf.
26. Carney MT, Fujiwara J, Emmert BE Jr, Liberman TA, Paris B. Elder orphans hiding in plain sight: a growing vulnerable population. Curr Gerontol Geriatr Res. 2016;2016:4723250.
27. Rhee TG, Marottoli RA, Monin JK. Diversity of social networks versus quality of social support: which is more protective for health-related quality of life among older adults? Prev Med. 2021;145:106440.
28. Kleinman R, Foster L. Multiple chronic conditions among OAA title III program participants. Administrating on Aging; 2011 [cited 2021 Nov 9]. Available from: https://www.mathematica.org/publications/multiple-chronic-conditions-among-oaa-title-iii-program-participants.
29. Lachs MS, Pillemer KA. Elder abuse. N Engl J Med. 2015;373(20):1947–56.
30. Yon Y, Mikton CR, Gassoumis ZD, Wilber KH. Elder abuse prevalence in community settings: a systematic review and meta-analysis. Lancet Glob Health. 2017;5(2):e147–56.
31. Yon Y, Mikton C, Gassoumis ZD, Wilber KH. The prevalence of self-reported elder abuse among older women in community settings: a systematic review and meta-analysis. Trauma Violence Abuse. 2019;20(2):245–59.
32. Laumann EO, Leitsch SA, Waite LJ. Elder mistreatment in the United States: prevalence estimates from a nationally representative study. J Gerontol B Psychol Sci Soc Sci. 2008;63(4):S248–s54.
33. Burnes D, Pillemer K, Caccamise PL, Mason A, Henderson CR Jr, Berman J, et al. Prevalence of and risk factors for elder abuse and neglect in the community: a population-based study. J Am Geriatr Soc. 2015;63(9):1906–12.
34. Acierno R, Hernandez MA, Amstadter AB, Resnick HS, Steve K, Muzzy W, et al. Prevalence and correlates of emotional, physical, sexual, and financial abuse and potential neglect in the United States: the National Elder Mistreatment Study. Am J Public Health. 2010;100(2):292–7.
35. James P. Ziliak CG. The state of senior hunger in America in 2019. 2021.
36. Laraia BA. Food insecurity and chronic disease. Adv Nutr. 2013;4(2):203–12.
37. Raghupathi W, Raghupathi V. An empirical study of chronic diseases in the United States: a visual analytics approach. Int J Environ Res Public Health. 2018;15(3):431.
38. Emlet CA. Social, economic, and health disparities among LGBT older adults. Generations. 2016;40(2):16–22.
39. Boggatz T. Quality of life in old age—a concept analysis. Int J Older People Nursing. 2016;11(1):55–69.
40. Sarvimäki A, Stenbock-Hult B. Quality of life in old age described as a sense of well-being, meaning and value. J Adv Nurs. 2000;32(4):1025–33.
41. Gill TM. The central role of prognosis in clinical decision making. JAMA. 2012;307(2):199–200.
42. Yourman LC, Lee SJ, Schonberg MA, Widera EW, Smith AK. Prognostic indices for older adults: a systematic review. JAMA. 2012;307(2):182–92.
43. Moreno G, Mangione CM, Kimbro L, Vaisberg E. Guidelines abstracted from the American Geriatrics Society guidelines for improving the care of older adults with diabetes mellitus: 2013 update. J Am Geriatr Soc. 2013;61(11):2020–6.
44. University of California San Francisco. ePrognosis. University of California San Francisco [cited 2021 Nov 9]. Available from: https://eprognosis.ucsf.edu.
45. Sedini C, Biotto M, Crespi Bel'skij LM, Moroni Grandini RE, Cesari M. Advance care planning and advance directives: an overview of the main critical issues. Aging Clin Exp Res. 2021;34:325.
46. McMahan RD, Tellez I, Sudore RL. Deconstructing the complexities of advance care planning outcomes: what do we know and where do we go? A scoping review. J Am Geriatr Soc. 2021;69(1):234–44.
47. Cigolle CT, Langa KM, Kabeto MU, Tian Z, Blaum CS. Geriatric conditions and disability: the health and retirement study. Ann Intern Med. 2007;147(3):156–64.
48. Lee PG, Cigolle C, Blaum C. The co-occurrence of chronic diseases and geriatric syndromes: the health and retirement study. J Am Geriatr Soc. 2009;57(3):511–6.
49. Fox MT, Persaud M, Maimets I, O'Brien K, Brooks D, Tregunno D, et al. Effectiveness of acute geriatric unit care using acute care for elders components: a systematic review and meta-analysis. J Am Geriatr Soc. 2012;60(12):2237–45.
50. Inouye SK, Baker DI, Fugal P, Bradley EH. Dissemination of the hospital elder life program: implementation, adaptation, and successes. J Am Geriatr Soc. 2006;54(10):1492–9.
51. Hshieh TT, Yang T, Gartaganis SL, Yue J, Inouye SK. Hospital elder life program: systematic review and meta-analysis of effectiveness. Am J Geriatr Psychiatry. 2018;26(10):1015–33.
52. Squires A, Murali KP, Greenberg SA, Herrmann LL, D'Amico CO. A scoping review of the evidence about the nurses improving care for healthsystem elders (NICHE) program. Gerontologist. 2021;61(3):e75–84.
53. Capezuti E, Boltz M, Cline D, Dickson VV, Rosenberg MC, Wagner L, et al. Nurses improving care for healthsystem elders—a model for optimising the geriatric nursing practice environment. J Clin Nurs. 2012;21(21–22):3117–25.
54. Ouslander JG, Perloe M, Givens JH, Kluge L, Rutland T, Lamb G. Reducing potentially avoidable hospitalizations of nursing home residents: results of a pilot quality improvement project. J Am Med Dir Assoc. 2009;10(9):644–52.
55. Ouslander JG, Bonner A, Herndon L, Shutes J. The Interventions to Reduce Acute Care Transfers (INTERACT) quality improvement program: an overview for medical directors and primary care clinicians in long term care. J Am Med Dir Assoc. 2014;15(3):162–70.
56. Kane RL, Huckfeldt P, Tappen R, Engstrom G, Rojido C, Newman D, et al. Effects of an intervention to reduce hospitalizations

from nursing homes: a randomized implementation trial of the INTERACT program. JAMA Intern Med. 2017;177(9):1257–64.
57. Kane RL, Keckhafer G, Flood S, Bershadsky B, Siadaty MS. The effect of Evercare on hospital use. J Am Geriatr Soc. 2003;51(10):1427–34.
58. McGarry BE, Grabowski DC. Managed care for long-stay nursing home residents: an evaluation of institutional special needs plans. Am J Manag Care. 2019;25(9):438–43.
59. Augustine MR, Davenport C, Ornstein KA, Cuan M, Saenger P, Lubetsky S, et al. Implementation of post-acute rehabilitation at home: a skilled nursing facility-substitutive model. J Am Geriatr Soc. 2020;68(7):1584–93.
60. Schubert CC, Myers LJ, Allen K, Counsell SR. Implementing geriatric resources for assessment and care of elders team care in a veterans affairs medical center: lessons learned and effects observed. J Am Geriatr Soc. 2016;64(7):1503–9.
61. Beales JL, Edes T. Veteran's affairs home based primary care. Clin Geriatr Med. 2009;25(1):149–54, viii–ix.
62. Totten AM, White-Chu EF, Wasson N, Morgan E, Kansagara D, Davis-O'Reilly C, et al. AHRQ comparative effectiveness reviews. Home-based primary care interventions. Rockville, MD: Agency for Healthcare Research and Quality (US); 2016.
63. Segelman M, Szydlowski J, Kinosian B, McNabney M, Raziano DB, Eng C, et al. Hospitalizations in the program of all-inclusive care for the elderly. J Am Geriatr Soc. 2014;62(2):320–4.
64. Guo Y, Albright D. The effectiveness of telehealth on self-management for older adults with a chronic condition: a comprehensive narrative review of the literature. J Telemed Telecare. 2018;24(6):392–403.

Special Population: Adults with Intellectual and Developmental Disabilities

Victoria L. Boggiano and Timothy P. Daaleman

Introduction

Adults with intellectual and developmental disabilities (IDD) encompass individuals who have a range of diagnoses (e.g., autism spectrum disorder) and designations (e.g., mental retardation) [1, 2]. An intellectual disability is characterized by significant limitations in both intellectual functioning, such as learning and problem-solving, and adaptive behaviors that generally include social and other everyday skills [3]. These limitations are typically made manifest before the age of 18 [3], and children who experience adverse childhood experiences (ACEs) are more likely to develop IDD as adults [4]. The term "developmental disabilities" is inclusive of intellectual disabilities and typically is used with individuals who: (1) have a severe, chronic disability that is due to a mental and/or physical impairment; (2) are diagnosed with the disability before age 22, and; (3) have substantial functional limitations in their activities of daily living [3, 5]. There are multiple causes of IDD which are attributable to different types of risk factors (e.g., biomedical, behavioral, social, educational) and the timing of the exposure to these factors [3, 4]. The most common cause of IDD is the genetic disorder Downs syndrome or trisomy 21 [6]. Some individuals may be identified as having intellectual disability but not developmental disability, and although there are a myriad of IDD causes, biological factors are identified only about 50% of the time [7].

In 2017, there were more than 7 million adults with IDD in the United States [8], encompassing approximately 1–3% of the population. There were an estimated 850,000 people with IDD who are age 60 years and older and who live in the community [9]. The number in this age group is projected to double over the next two decades, reaching 1.2 million in 2030 [10], which is a remarkable development since the average life expectancy of persons with IDD was 59 years in 1976, and 66 years in 1993 [9]. Currently, the causes of death for individuals with IDD are comparable to the general population (i.e., coronary artery disease, cancer, respiratory disease, type 2 diabetes mellitus); however, these individuals are more likely to have multiple comorbidities when compared to the general population [11, 12]. Increased life expectancy is due to improved living conditions as well as better access to medical care [13]. The genetic link between trisomy 21 and Alzheimer's disease has been clearly established, and at least 50% of adults who are aged 60 years and older will have clinical evidence of cognitive impairment and a lower life expectancy due to dementia-associated causes [14].

Persons with IDD unfortunately experience considerable health disparities throughout their lifetime, including decreased life expectancy and greater comorbidities [15–17]. Individuals with IDD experience poorer health outcomes and greater variation in the quality of their health care when compared to the general population for reasons that go beyond having more than one disease process [18, 19]. Patients can have cognitive challenges in recognizing and reporting symptoms, as well as in comprehending and adhering to treatment recommendations [20]. At the provider level, the lack of formal training in the healthcare needs of adults with IDD has resulted in many physicians and care providers lacking experience and may be uncomfortable in providing care to this population [19, 21]. Within outpatient practice and other healthcare settings, there can be barriers and varying degrees of access to primary care for chronic disease management and access to preventive services, such as cancer screening and immunizations [20].

Adults with IDD are at greater risk of having their symptoms go unrecognized, leading to several negative sequelae such as greater cancer burden at diagnosis [17]. Organizational barriers and implicit policies may be reflective of larger social and cultural attitudes, which can be seen in the biases and misconceptions of healthcare providers [20]. The

V. L. Boggiano (✉) · T. P. Daaleman
Department of Family Medicine, University of North Carolina at Chapel Hill, School of Medicine, Chapel Hill, NC, USA
e-mail: Victoria.boggiano@unchealth.unc.edu;
tim_daaleman@med.unc.edu

COVID-19 pandemic highlighted these challenges and placed a disproportionate burden on individuals with IDD and their caregivers [22]. Adults with IDD were uniquely affected by the pandemic, highlighting the need for greater attention to this vulnerable population.

The tenth anniversary of the United Nations Convention on Rights of Persons with Disabilities was recognized in 2016, a gathering which declared the right of persons with disabilities to "the highest attainable standard of health without discrimination on the basis of disability" [23]. In the United States, the American Association on Intellectual and Developmental Disabilities (AAIDD) also advocated that all persons with IDD should have timely access to high-quality, comprehensive, accessible, affordable, and appropriate health care that meets their individual needs, maximizes health, well-being and function, and increases independence and community participation (see Table 24.1) [24]. As adults with IDD are integrated into community-based settings to live and work [25], providers must develop patient-centered strategies to provide physical and mental health care.

This chapter provides an introduction to the principles and practice approaches of providing health care to adults with IDD and draws upon recommendations and consensus guidelines developed by the Massachusetts Department of Developmental Services [26], a Canadian guideline working group [27], the International Review of Research in Developmental Disabilities, Cochrane reviews [16], and other research. The first section reviews clinical assessment and management approaches to the general medical care of these vulnerable patients. The second section offers preventive services guidelines and is followed by strategies for managing behavioral and mental health conditions that can arise. The chapter closes with an examination of the organization and delivery of healthcare services and the unique healthcare challenges that individuals with IDD face during pandemics such as COVID-19.

Clinical Assessment and Management

General Principles

Scheduled and timely well maintenance visits, which include a structured physical examination, have been demonstrated to improve health and functional outcomes and can be responsive to the unique care needs of adults with IDD [12, 28]. Individuals with IDD may have more complex physical and mental healthcare needs [12], and a baseline assessment of intellectual and physical functioning is recommended [17]. Physicians should do complete physical exams during initial visits to avoid missing subtle clues that may reveal underlying health conditions [29]. This assessment may be aided by consultation with a psychologist, physical therapist, and/or occupational therapist [27]. Table 24.2 provides an inventory of functional areas and domains which can organize the assessment [30]. For providers who are seeing patients for the first time, the etiology of the IDD is important to verify since it often guides healthcare services that

Table 24.1 Key elements of joint position statement by American Association on Intellectual and Developmental Disabilities and The Arc on Health, Mental Health, Vision, and Dental Care (adapted from Ref. [24])

Access to care
• Healthcare systems must be accessible to individuals with intellectual and developmental disabilities (IDD) with respect to facilities and equipment, as well as communication needs and associated accommodations such as sufficient time and interpreters when necessary.
• Wellness, prevention, health promotion, and a robust public health infrastructure are essential components of health care for persons with IDD.
• Healthcare providers for persons with IDD must meet the highest standards of quality, including a comprehensive approach to treatment, disease prevention, and health maintenance.
• People with IDD need access to effective strategies to manage their care including care coordination, referral processes, transition assistance, and health promotion efforts in community settings.
Nondiscrimination
• Individuals with IDD must not experience disability-related discrimination in their health care.
• There should be parity between mental health and medical care in health insurance benefits.
Communication and decision making
• Individuals with IDD have a right to information with appropriate accommodations to assure informed consent including a process that allows an individual, or under appropriate legal conditions, a guardian, a healthcare power of attorney, or a surrogate decision maker of the individual's choice to accept or refuse healthcare services.
• For any procedure for which consent is sought, sufficient information to understand the benefits and risks should be provided in ways that accommodate reading, language, and other limitations that are common among persons with IDD.
• Individuals with IDD may temporarily or permanently lack the capacity to make some or all healthcare decisions. This lack of capacity may not be global, and the individual should always be assisted in making those decisions, for which they can participate in decisions.
• When an individual has been determined to lack capacity to make healthcare decisions and does not have an advance directive, a surrogate decision maker should be identified to make these decisions, whenever possible before a crisis arises. When the individual's wishes are not known, the surrogate must follow the person's probable wishes, taking into account the person's known values, and, as a fall back, act in the person's best interests.

Table 24.2 Functional domains for adults with intellectual and developmental disabilities (adapted from Ref. [30])

	Domains	Assessment modalities
Cognitive	Language, attentional, memory, literacy, problem-solving, social skills, self-direction.	Neuropsychiatric or special education assessments
Neuromuscular	Gait, posture, muscle tone, fine and gross motor control, range of motion, sensory processing, swallow. If applicable, seizure characteristics, type, length, and frequency.	Physical therapy, occupational therapy, speech therapy, neurology, physical medicine and rehabilitation, orthopedics. Patient and caregiver video documentation.
Sensory	Hearing and vision testing; sensitivity to light, sounds, odors, foods, or proprioception.	Audiometry and visual acuity; detailed visual exam.
Behavioral/Mental health	Mood, affect, disordered/ordered thinking, agitation, and other signs of distress.	Neuropsychiatric assessment Note: 1. Stereotyped behavior or emotion lasting less than 3 min (possible seizure). 2. Patient's usual behaviors when in pain or agitated. 3. Strategies for managing distress and other escalating behavior.

should be offered [31]. In patients who have an uncertain etiology to their IDD, or if there is a change in global functioning that is identified during the healthcare visit, referral to genetic counseling should be considered [32, 33].

Adults with IDD can vary in how they adapt to their functioning, and assessments of intellectual and adaptive functioning (Table 24.2) can establish a baseline and help gauge both acute and chronic changes that can inform care planning [34]. If the patient has had a comprehensive assessment during early life or adolescence, or if a life transition is anticipated, such as the cessation of school, a functional assessment with an occupational therapist, psychologist, or other specialist familiar with IDD, should be considered. Adults with IDD have a higher likelihood of experiencing pain than other patient populations [35]. Pain and distress are challenging symptoms and signs that often go unrecognized by caregivers and clinicians, and can present atypically, especially for patients who have difficulty communicating [36]. Moreover, adults with IDD may have less autonomic response to pain but instead represent experiences of pain by facial expressions and other signs and symptoms [35]. Atypical presentations of pain and distress can be assessed using tools that have been adapted for adults with IDD, such as the Non-Communicating Adult Pain Checklist (NCAPC) [37]. Table 24.3 contains domains and symptoms from the NCAPC. In patients who present with pain and distress, consideration should be given to some common underlying medical causes that may be found in this population, such as infection, constipation, and dental caries. Although it requires specialized training, the Pain and Discomfort Scale (PADS) can also be utilized by providers during an examination to determine whether a person with IDD is experiencing acute pain or discomfort [38, 39].

The limited life experiences of some adults with IDD, the level of intellectual functioning, learned helplessness, and cognitive impairment can compromise the capacity to give informed or voluntary consent. As a result, the capacity for informed consent varies among adults with IDD and it is important to assess capacity when proposing diagnostic studies or treatments in which consent is required [40]. For example, a patient who is determined to be incapable of some aspects of decision making, such as understanding consequences, might still be able to convey their wishes to a surrogate [40]. Caregivers can meaningfully contribute to decision making and may consent to or refuse treatment on behalf of an adult with IDD who is assessed to be incapable

Table 24.3 Domains and symptoms from the non-communicating adults pain checklist (adapted from Ref. [37])

Domain	Symptom
Vocal reaction	Moaning, whining, whimpering
	Crying
	Loud screaming or yelling
	A specific sound or word for pain
Emotional reaction	Not cooperating, cranky, irritable, unhappy
	Agitated, difficult to distract, not able to satisfy or pacify
Facial expression	Furrowed eyebrows, raising eyebrows
	Eye squinting, eyes opened wide, frowning
	Turning down of mouth, not smiling
	Movements of the lips and tongue, such as teeth grinding or tongue pushing
Body language	Moving more or less
	Stiff spastic, tense, rigid
Protective reaction	Gesturing to or touching part of the body that hurts
	Protecting, defending, or guarding part of the body that hurts
	Flinching or moving the body part away, being sensitive to touch
	Moving the body in a specific way to show pain, such as curls up
Physiological reaction	Change in facial color
	Respiratory irregular responses, such as breath holding

of providing informed consent [40]. Moreover, many patients with IDD live with family caregivers who become tasked with navigating the healthcare system on their behalf [41]. For all patients, it is important to treat adults with IDD with dignity in discussions about their health and well-being [42].

A key component of effective decision making is appropriate communication, and the level and means of communication (e.g., non-verbal cues) should be adapted to the patient's level of intellectual and physical functioning [43]. It is important to consider the best interests of the adult with IDD, including his or her perspective in pursuing or forgoing any healthcare intervention. This process is particularly important around advance care planning (ACP), which can help guide treatment decisions at the end-of-life, such as initiating palliative care [43]. ACP should be considered during primary care encounters, although research suggests that the rate at which this occurs can vary significantly within and among geographic regions [44]. ACP can positively impact the outcome of end-of-life care, a longitudinal process that ideally begins in the outpatient setting should seek to set goals of care and offer treatment options that are responsive to patient and caregiver's wishes. Advance care planning should be recorded early in a disease course and reviewed annually with the patient and caregiver, or within the context of a hospitalization or significant change in health or functional status [44].

Medical Conditions and Disorders

There are several medical conditions and disorders that are more commonly seen in adults with IDD. Dental disease is among the most common problems since patients and caregivers can have difficulty in maintaining oral hygiene routines and accessing dental care. Changes in behavior, as noted earlier, can be the result of pain and discomfort from dental disease [45]. Physicians and other healthcare providers should promote daily oral hygiene practices via individualized care plans [46] as well as scheduled preventive care, such as periodic examinations and fluoride applications by dental professionals [45, 46].

Swallowing difficulties may be associated with dental disease and are not uncommon, particularly among individuals with neuromuscular dysfunction and those taking medications with anticholinergic side effects. These populations are at risk for developing respiratory disorders, particularly asthma [12] and aspiration pneumonia [47]. Physicians and other providers should be alert for possible signs of aspiration, such as throat clearing after swallowing, coughing, choking, drooling, long mealtimes, aversion to food, weight loss, and should screen at least annually for signs and symptoms indicating respiratory disorders [26, 27].

Gastrointestinal problems, such as gastroesophageal reflux disease (GERD), are common among adults with IDD and can present more atypically than in the general population [48, 49]. These patients have an increased risk of Helicobacter pylori infection due to group home living, rumination, or exposure to saliva or feces [50]. Physicians should screen for H pylori infection in symptomatic adults with IDD or asymptomatic patients who have lived in institutions or group homes, and consider retesting at regular intervals [50]. The choice of urea breath testing, fecal antigen testing, or serologic testing should depend on the pre-test probability of the infection, the availability of the test, and tolerability of the test by the patient [50]. Symptomatic patients, or those taking medications that can aggravate GERD, or asymptomatic patients who have lived in institutions or group homes, should be screened annually for GERD [26, 27]. Constipation, GERD, peptic ulcer disease, and pica should also be considered if there are unexplained gastrointestinal findings or if there are changes in behavior or weight [27]. Individuals with IDD have a higher rate of gallbladder cancer, possibly because of higher rates of gallstones [12, 51].

Musculoskeletal disorders, such as scoliosis, contractures, and spasticity, can be possible sources of unrecognized pain and occur frequently among adults with IDD, resulting in reduced mobility and activity [29, 52]. These disorders, including osteoporosis and osteoporotic fractures, are more prevalent and tend to occur earlier in adults with IDD than in the general population [52, 53]. Risk factors for these conditions include reduced mobility, increased risk of falls, malnutrition, the presence of genetic syndromes (e.g., Down's Syndrome), and long-term medication use that may contribute to gait instability [54, 55]. For those patients at high risk of developing osteoporosis (e.g., medications such as antiepileptic drugs, immobility), bone mineral density testing should be considered beginning at age 19 [26, 27]. Osteoarthritis is also becoming more common in this population due to increased life expectancy and patients and caregivers should receive advice and information that promotes regular physical activity [56]. Physicians and other healthcare providers should promote regular physical activity, adequate calcium and vitamin D intake, smoking and alcohol cessation, and consider consulting a physical or occupational therapist if there is need for mobility adaptations, such as a wheelchair, modified splints, or orthotic device [53].

Epilepsy is more common among adults with IDD compared with the general population [12, 57] and the severity of condition increases with the underlying disability [58]. This disorder can be difficult to evaluate and control, and it has long-term effects on the lives of affected adults and their caregivers. A consensus set of guidelines for the management of epilepsy in adults with IDD noted that there was a paucity of high-quality evidence but issued several recommendations that were Grade B (i.e., based on hierarchy II evidence or extrapolated from hierarchy I) or higher. Individuals with IDD are more likely to experience side effects from anti-epileptic drugs and less likely to mention these effects, thus requiring close monitoring [59]. New prescriptions of phenobarbital are discouraged because of the high incidence of behavioral side effects; however, it may be used as a third-line agent if other, more suitable options have been used without success [2].

Topiramate can be considered add-on therapy since it demonstrates no significant behavior side effects [3]. In general, no recommendation can be given for a specific drug of choice in patients with epilepsy and IDD [4]. Next, patients on phenytoin need regular, at least yearly, serum drug concentration measurement; drug monitoring must be combined with clinical examination for side effects [5]. Finally, there is no comparative evidence for the treatment of adults with seizures in Lennox–Gastaut syndrome; however, evidence does exist for the impact of lamotrigine and topiramate on drop attacks [58]. Consideration should be given to specialty consultation regarding alternative medications when seizures persist, and possible discontinuation of medications for patients who become seizure-free [58].

Metabolic disorders have a greater prevalence in some subpopulations of adults with IDD [12, 60]. For example, there is a higher incidence of hypogonadism associated with Prader-Willi syndrome [60]. In these and other at-risk patients, laboratory screening for hypogonadism and testosterone may be considered at least once after full puberty is achieved [27]. Regarding routine screening for diabetes mellitus (DM), there are inconsistent data that support the increased prevalence of DM among adults with IDD, with the exception of persons with Down's Syndrome [61]. Screening for thyroid disease, however, should be considered in patients who are symptomatic (e.g., fatigue, progressive weight gain), have hyperlipidemia, are obese, or who have sedentary lifestyle [27]. In addition, for patients who are prescribed lithium or atypical or second-generation antipsychotic medications, a baseline thyroid function should be measured and tested at lease annually [27].

Cardiac disorders are prevalent among adults with IDD, due to risk factors such as physical inactivity, obesity, and prolonged use of some psychotropic medications [12, 62]. When any risk factor is present, physicians should consider screening for cardiovascular disease earlier than in the general population and initiate primary prevention strategies (e.g., encouraging physical activity, weight management) [62]. Some adults with DD have congenital heart disease and are susceptible to bacterial endocarditis. Antibiotic prophylaxis guidelines for patients who meet criteria or consultation with a cardiologist can help inform treatment decisions [63].

Polypharmacy is not uncommon among adults with IDD, especially those who have medical comorbidities. Adults with IDD tend to have more complex medication regimens compared to their counterparts, increasing the risk of adverse medication side effects [59, 64]. A medication review should be conducted at regular intervals to determine patient adherence, and to monitor for adverse side effects and medication interactions [27]. In general, medications not prescribed for a specific diagnosis should undergo a trial of reduction and cessation, with timely communication from patients and their caregivers during medication trials to monitor safety, side effects, and effectiveness [65]. The review should target psychotropic medications since they are regularly prescribed to adults in this population—despite the lack of evidence—and are often used in response to problem behaviors [27, 66, 67].

Preventive Services

Guidelines for preventive health services (e.g., US Preventive Services Task Force-USPSTF) should be applied to adults with IDD as in the general population with consideration to some modifications [26, 27]. Maintaining up-to-date immunizations are important since adult patients and their caregivers may have a reduced awareness of the importance of vaccines beyond childhood. To begin, both annual influenza and pneumococcal series vaccinations should be current and offered when appropriate. Due to an increased risk of exposure, the need for hepatitis A & B screening and vaccination should be determined [68] and this may include annual screening in high-risk patients (e.g., those with blood exposures) and periodic monitoring of liver function in hepatitis B carriers [26, 27]. Shared decision making about HPV vaccination should be initiated between patients who are in the preadolescent to early adult age group, their caregivers, and healthcare providers. Finally, COVID-19 vaccines should be given with the appropriate guidance from the Food and Drug Administration including booster shots when appropriate [69].

Cancer screening is an essential preventive service; however, adults with IDD are less likely than those in the general population to receive these services. Recommendations for cancer screening generally follow guidelines established for adults in the general population however there are practical and logistical issues when considering invasive testing [26, 70]. Colon cancer is slightly more prevalent in adults with IDD and constipation a common problem, which makes evaluating the onset of colon cancer symptoms challenging to determine [70]. Providers who care for women with IDD do not uniformly encourage mammography for their patients who are in the targeted age groups as recommended by the USPSTF [70]. Cervical cancer screening is controversial since fewer women with IDD are sexually active, when compared to the general population, and many have difficulty communicating their sexual history [70]. The decision and time interval to conduct cervical cancer screening should be individualized based on the patient's risk factors [70]. Women with IDD are more likely to undergo routine mammography and cervical cancer screening if they live in a supervised community-based living setting, group home, or medical facility [71]. Finally, prostate and skin cancer screening is routinely performed by many primary care physicians despite the lack of evidence [70]. As noted earlier, adults with IDD are less likely to have their symptoms recognized, leading to a higher cancer burden, which encourages primary care providers to be vigilant in their cancer screening and diagnosis [17].

Physical inactivity and obesity are more prevalent among adults with IDD and are associated with cardiovascular disease, diabetes, osteoporosis, and early mortality [72]. Physical strength and functional fitness may decline more quickly for individuals with IDD as compared to the general population [73]. Weight and height need to be monitored regularly, and body mass index and other biometric indices should be used to stratify cardiovascular risk [74]. Patients and their caregivers should be counseled annually, or more frequently if indicated, regarding strategies for maintaining healthy nutrition and physical fitness. Among adults who are significantly obese (e.g., BMI > 30), more intensive counseling (e.g., referral to dietitian) should be offered [26, 27]. Yoga and other functional fitness interventions have been demonstrated to improve strength and balance for individuals with IDD [73].

Vision and hearing impairments are often underdiagnosed in the IDD population and these limitations can impair behavior and adaptive functioning [75]. As adults with IDD age, they are more likely to develop hearing or vision problems [13]. Office-based vision and hearing screening should be part of the annual exam with the same frequency as recommended for average-risk adults, or when symptoms or signs of visual or hearing problems are identified [26, 27]. Hearing impairment due to cerumen impaction is not uncommon. All patients with IDD should be considered for glaucoma assessment beginning in early adulthood (e.g., age 21) with follow-up examinations every 2–3 years up to age 39, and 1–2 years for ages 40 and older [26].

Sexuality is an important, but frequently undiscussed area in the care of adults with IDD [76, 77]. Sexual health education is often overlooked in young adults with IDD [77, 78]. Open and patient-centered communication can facilitate understanding about patient or caregiver concerns regarding sexual health issues, such as menstruation, masturbation, contraception, and menopause. Physicians should work to connect their adult patients with IDD to education programs that will provide information about sexual health education in an unbiased, non-judgmental manner [77]. Women with IDD often experience hardships when trying to access information about contraception, for example [79], and providers should seek to provide this information in an easily accessible manner. All methods of contraception, including long-acting reversible contraception, should be offered to women with IDD [80]. In addition, adults with IDD should be able to discuss sexual health with their providers [81] and have appropriate testing for sexually transmitted infections when applicable.

Using an unbiased and non-judgmental communication approach may also help healthcare providers identify abuse and neglect, which occur frequently in adults with IDD and are often perpetrated by people known to them [82]. There are several behavioral signs and symptoms that may suggest abuse and neglect including: unexpected weight changes, aggression, withdrawal or noncompliance with treatment plans, depressive symptoms including sleep or eating problems, poor self-esteem, and inappropriate attachment or sexualized behavior [82]. Caregivers of adults with IDD are at risk for caregiver stress and burnout and should be screened at regular intervals. If abuse or neglect is suspected, physicians and other care providers are generally mandated to report to responsible authorities (e.g., social service or law enforcement) and address any associated physical or mental health issues, such as posttraumatic stress. Finally, inappropriate sexual behavior is more common among adults with IDD due to lack of sexual health education and primary care providers should screen for this and link patients with appropriate community-based interventions when necessary [83].

Managing Behavioral and Mental Health Conditions

Diagnosing Psychiatric Conditions and Mental Health Disorders

Psychiatric disorders and emotional disturbances are more prevalent among adults with IDD [84]; however, some behaviors are normalized or overlooked (i.e., diagnostic overshadowing) in these patients, resulting in delayed diagnoses and treatments [27]. Despite the prevalence, establishing or verifying a psychiatric diagnosis can be complex and difficult; mood, anxiety, and adjustment disorders are often underdiagnosed and psychotic disorders are over diagnosed [85]. As adults with IDD age, they are more likely to be diagnosed with anxiety or mood disorders [13]. However, notably, psychotic disorders can be difficult to diagnose when delusions and hallucinations cannot be expressed verbally, and in cases where developmentally appropriate fantasies (e.g., imaginary friends) might be mistaken for delusional ideation [86].

Alcohol or substance use is less common among adults with IDD than in the general population, but these individuals can have more difficulty moderating their intake and experience more barriers to treatment and rehabilitation services. Those that engage in substance or alcohol use are often more likely to have coexisting psychiatric morbidity and may be more likely to have negative consequences from this behavior such as aggression, risk-taking, or involvement in the criminal justice system [87]. Young adults with IDD often feel socially excluded even if they are engaged in community-based services, making it challenging to diagnose and treat psychiatric and mood disorders [88]. The COVID-19 pandemic posed a unique risk to adults with IDD and their caregivers, leading to higher rates of anxiety, isolation, agitation, and distress [89].

When screening for psychiatric conditions or mental health disorders, providers should use validated tools that have been developed for adults with IDD according to their functional level. The Aberrant Behavior Checklist-Community [ABC-C] is a rating scale that is designed to be used with community dwelling individuals with IDD and can be completed by caregivers, teachers, or others who have directly observed the patient's behavior [90]. The instrument asks observers to rate the level of problem behavior (e.g., not at all, slight, moderately serious, severe) across several domains, including physical body movements, social interactions, and mood and affect [90].

The Psychiatric Assessment Schedules for Adults with Developmental Disabilities Checklist (PAS-ADD) is a validated 25-item questionnaire that is designed for caregivers, family members, and others who have direct knowledge of behavior changes of individuals with IDD [91]. The Checklist is a screening tool that can determine if a more complete further assessment is needed, and it can be used to screen groups of individuals, or to monitor at-risk individuals [91]. The tool generates three scores relating to affective or neurotic disorders, neurodegenerative conditions, including dementia, and psychotic disorder [91].

Diagnosing attention deficit and hyperactivity disorder (ADHD) in adults with IDD is often difficult due to challenges with screening, as the validated instruments to screen for ADHD in the general adult population are often not useful for adults with IDD [92]. The Diagnostic Interview for ADHD in adults with intellectual disability (DIVA-5-ID) is one validated screening tool, although it is resource and time intensive [92]. There is ongoing work to create more streamlined screening tools as precursors to the DIVA-5-ID to properly identify ADHD in this patient population.

Screening instruments and tools are important; however, meaningful input and assistance from adults with IDD and their caregivers are vital for a more comprehensive understanding and determination of root causes to the problem behavior or emotional disturbances [88]. At the outset, establishing a collaborative approach of working with patients and caregivers that seeks input, agreement, and assistance, can help identify target symptoms and behavior [27]. Pain and other physical symptoms are often unrecognized and can present atypically, particularly for those patients who have difficulty communicating. Assessment tools adapted for adults with IDD, as noted earlier, can help identify uncharacteristic cues of pain and physical symptoms; collateral information from caregivers is highly useful [27].

Underlying medical causes (e.g., occult infection, constipation, dental disease) may be manifesting as behavioral changes and musculoskeletal disorders, such as scoliosis, contractures, and spasticity, can be sources of unrecognized pain and other physical symptoms [93]. Screening for underlying alcohol or substance use is important. Finally, unexplained changes in weight, noncompliance, aggression, withdrawal, depression, avoidance, poor self-esteem, sexualized behavior, sleep or eating disorders, and substance abuse might also be signals of abuse or neglect, which occur more frequently in this population and are often perpetrated by people known to adults with IDD [40]. In adults with Down Syndrome, early screening for cognitive impairment and dementia is suggested since the diagnosis can be overlooked [27, 94]. Differentiating dementia from depression and other behavioral disorders can be especially challenging among some adults with IDD, and referral for psychological testing that is inclusive of cognitive, adaptive, and communicative functioning can help clarify the underlying diagnosis [27]. If an underlying psychiatric disorder is suspected, interdisciplinary consultation from clinicians knowledgeable and experienced in IDD is recommended [27]. Collateral information and support from caregivers can effectively help develop and implement treatment plans [27]. Addressing sensory (e.g., overstimulation) and environmental (e.g., lack of space for physical activity) factors are important parts of care planning and there is increasing evidence of the efficacy of psychotherapy (i.e., cognitive behavioral therapy) for specific emotional problems that might be contributing to aggressive or anxious behavior [95].

Managing Acute Problem Behaviors

In an acute setting, problem behaviors can manifest as aggression, agitation, or self-injury and may be indicative of an underlying medical disorder or disruption in social or emotional supports [96]. Self-harm and other behaviors can also be a sign of physical pain or discomfort that may go unrecognized for providers and caregivers who may lack training [38]. As noted earlier, physicians and other providers should establish trust and a functional working relationship with patients and caregivers in order to gather information, determine safety, and gain agreement and assistance in developing treatments that can be implemented and monitored. Non-pharmaceutical behavioral approaches have proven efficacy for alleviating acute problem behaviors, and home and community-based resources are an additional benefit [16, 97]. Providers should actively involve other stakeholders, including community mental health agencies and emergency department staff, in order to develop a proactive, integrated response plan for patients at high risk of injury, and those with recurrent behavioral crises [27].

If there are new problem behaviors, other etiologies such as medical conditions, environmental changes, and emotional factors should be thoroughly assessed [27]. It is important to note that problem behaviors, such as aggression and self-injury, are not psychiatric disorders but might be a symptom of an underlying medical disorder or other social circumstance, such as insufficient support in the home environment [98]. Acute pain may manifest itself as a behavioral condition. Problem behaviors can occur because environments do not meet the developmental needs of adults with IDD and providers should seek to promote "enabling environments" with family members and caregivers to address unique developmental needs since this approach can markedly reduce problem behaviors [99].

Providers can consider a functional assessment in nonemergent situations when safety and reliable follow-up can be assured. This type of assessment is usually conducted by a mental healthcare professional, and an interdisciplinary understanding of problem behaviors can benefit from occupational therapists as well. Advancements in technology, including readily accessible telehealth services, can assist providers in conducting assessments in real time [100], which may reduce unnecessary emergency department visits and acute hospitalizations. Consideration should be given to reducing and stopping medications not prescribed for a specific psychiatric diagnosis [65]. If the problem behavior escalates into a crisis, psychotropic medications can be used to ensure safety, ideally as a temporary intervention [27]. Antipsychotic medications are often inappropriately prescribed for behavior problems and in the absence of a clinical indication, this class of medications should not be considered as first-line treatment [27, 66, 67]. However, when psychotropic medications are used to ensure safety during a behavioral crisis, there should be parameters for earlier follow-up—ideally no longer than 72 h—and possible discontinuation [27, 66, 67].

Behavioral crises can occasionally escalate and not be managed in outpatient or community-based settings which subsequently require management in an emergency department [101]. The presenting problem, collateral information, and outpatient interventions that have been tried should be accurately communicated to the emergency department staff prior to the patient's arrival. Across all care settings, it is important to debrief the crisis with care providers in order to minimize the likelihood of recurrence. The debriefing process should include a review of events that led to the crisis events, interventions, and responses, such as behavioral approaches and medications, and the identification of possible triggers and underlying causes [101].

Use of Psychotropic Medications

As noted earlier, psychotropic medications are regularly used to manage problem behaviors in adults with IDD, despite the lack of an evidence base [27, 66, 67]. Psychotropic medications are, however, equally effective in these individuals, as in the general population, for confirmed psychiatric disorders [102]. There is increased risk of polypharmacy in this population and concomitant adverse medication interactions [102]. As a result, adults with IDD are more likely to be hospitalized for adverse medication effects than the general population [64]. Some adults with IDD may have atypical responses or side effects at low doses, while others are limited in their ability to describe side effects of the medications that they are taking. Some classes of antipsychotic medications increase the risk of metabolic syndrome and can trigger other effects, such as akathisia, cardiac conduction problems, swallowing difficulties, and bowel dysfunction [102].

Table 24.4 displays the "10 Dos and 4 Don'ts" principle that was developed by a 1995 consensus conference on psychopharmacology and has undergone several iterations [102].

Table 24.4 Principles for psychotropic medication prescribing for adults with IDD (adapted from Ref. [102])

Do:
1. Treat any drug that is used to modify behavior (e.g., OTC sleep agent) as a psychotropic drug.
2. Use psychotropic medications within a coordinated care plan.
3. Base treatment decisions on a diagnosis or clinical indication.
4. Obtain consent.
5. Track efficacy by using validated scales and instruments.
6. Monitor side effects using rating instruments.
7. Monitor for tardive dyskinesia, metabolic syndrome, and other serious side effects.
8. Review all medications systematically and regularly.
9. Always seek to prescribe the lowest effective dose.
10. Monitor medication adherence by patients and caregivers.

Don't:
1. Do not use psychotropic drugs for convenience or as a substitute for behaviorally intensive activity or the need for changes in physical environment.
2. Avoid frequent drug and dose changes.
3. Avoid intra-class polypharmacy.
4. Seek to minimize:
   - Long-term as needed (i.e., PRN) medications
   - Long-acting sedative/hypnotics
   - Long-term hypnotics or anxiolytics
   - High-dose antipsychotic doses
   - Long-term anticholinergics

In addition to these principles, there are other practices that can promote the safe prescribing of psychotropic medications. Physicians should "start low and go slow" in initiating, increasing, or decreasing doses of medications, carefully monitoring for side effects, including metabolic syndrome [102]. The need for ongoing antipsychotic medications should be reassessed at regular intervals with consideration given to dose reduction or discontinuation when indicated [102]. Whenever there is a behavioral change, the psychiatric diagnosis and the appropriateness of the prescribed medications for this diagnosis should be reviewed. Prescribing physicians should also arrange to receive regular reports from patients and their caregivers during medication trials in order to monitor safety, side effects, and treatment effectiveness [102].

The Impact of COVID-19 on Individuals with IDD

The COVID-19 pandemic caused by the novel Sars-CoV-2 Coronavirus has led to significant morbidity and mortality in populations across the United States, including adults with IDD [103, 104]. Many individuals with IDD live in congregate care settings, where infection prevention is more challenging [103]. In addition, individuals with IDD rely on community-based educational and health services that were often less accessible during the height of the pandemic [22, 104, 105]. While signs and symptoms of COVID-19 are similar for adults with IDD compared to the general population, they are more at risk of severe infection particularly as they age [106].

The alteration of daily structure and routine caused by the pandemic was also particularly challenging for adults with IDD [22]. Family and other social support became an even more important resource for the health and wellbeing of individuals with IDD during the pandemic [22]. A coordinated, team-based approach to infection prevention (Table 24.5) facilitated the ongoing care for adults with IDD while preventing the spread of COVID-19 [103].

Organization and Delivery of Healthcare Services

Primary care providers are often the first point of contact for adults with IDD; if they are skilled in providing care to this patient population, emergency room and hospital visits decrease significantly [25]. Healthcare systems are moving to value-based care, which should provide a foundation for the development of integrated networks of primary care, specialized care, and ancillary services that can work on behalf of adults with IDD [107]. The patient-centered medical home (PCMH) model provides an organizational platform for addressing the healthcare needs of adults with IDD since it tailors and individualizes healthcare services by increasing access, managing all aspects of care, and through a team-based approach that is led by the patient's personal physician [108]. For example, the Healthy Outcomes Medical Excellence (HOME) project was developed to provide comprehensive care to adults and children with IDD [109]. Since its founding in 2000, the HOME project has resulted in decreased acute hospital utilization and readmissions and has improved quality outcomes such as vaccination rates and compliance with diabetes care management [109].

Interdisciplinary health care has been found to be an effective approach in addressing the complex needs of adults with IDD [16]. Operationally, this strategy involves the patient's primary care physician and other health providers as required (e.g., mental healthcare provider, physical therapy, occupational therapy), in addition to a care manager who is responsible for coordinating care across providers and service locations [110, 111]. Care managers are playing an increasingly major role in the redesign of primary care and in the evolution of PCMH by providing patient education in disease self-management skills, coordinating services across a continuum of care providers, and by linking patients to community and social services [112]. Indeed, home and community-based services that provide more intense services have been found to add benefit when compared to stan-

Table 24.5 Basic hygiene practices for residential settings (adapted from Ref. [105])

Recommendation 1	Hand hygiene	One of the most effective infection control tools is proper hand hygiene, which caregivers can model and reinforce for adults with IDD. Keep alcohol-based hand sanitizers available and accessible. Use soap to wash hands if visibly soiled.
Recommendation 2	Respiratory etiquette	Adults with IDD should be taught appropriate respiratory etiquette. Caregivers should model this. Tissues and masks should be easily accessible.
Recommendation 3	Environmental cleaning	Shared spaces, shared objects, such as remote controls for televisions or other household equipment, and eating utensils, should all be cleaned using appropriate disinfectants.
Recommendation 4	Oral hygiene	Because office dental care is limited in situations like the COVID-19 pandemic, home-based dental care should be emphasized. Caregivers assisting adults with IDD in their oral care should wear PPE to prevent infection spread.

dard medical services alone [16]. Peer-led community-based outreach programs that engage individuals with IDD via technology, such as text messages, have been shown to improve health outcomes [113]. As adults with IDD age, they tend to become more socially isolated, making this type of outreach work even more important [13].

There is growing interest in telemedicine and other health information technologies (HIT) as strategies that can expand the reach of services for adults with IDD into home and community-based settings [100]. A Cochrane review that explored the effectiveness of HIT for people with physical or learning disability, or cognitive impairment found a lack of empirical evidence to support or refute the use of these technologies [114]. Among individuals with autism spectrum disorders, one systematic review reported that telemedicine was used in a variety of ways, including diagnostic assessments and consulting, supervision of interventions and training, and program implementation [115]. Telehealth can be used to assist adults with IDD in learning new life and self-care skills that are sustained over time, increasing access to important services for patients and their caregivers [116]. Having access to iPhones, iPads, and other smart devices can help adults with IDD in medication adherence and in providing reminders about upcoming appointments [13]. Finally, telehealth has the potential to be used in group homes and other residential settings to improve care, reduce caregiver burden, provide greater access to providers, and screen for possible abuse or improper care [100].

Adults with IDD living in the United States can utilize community-based support services that are largely funded through Medicaid [25]. Currently, a large portion of expenditures from the Centers for Medicare and Medicaid Cervices (CMS) that is allocated toward adults with IDD is for emergency room visits and hospitalization reimbursement, costs that are largely preventable [25]. Greater emphasis and initiatives on integrative outpatient care models that provide holistic services have been highlighted by the National Council on Disability [117].

UCare Complete is a program for Twin Cities (Minnesota) area residents with physical disabilities who are between the ages of 18 and 64, which combines physician, hospital, home care, nursing, home and community-based services, an integrated care system. The program seeks to maximize independence while providing person-centered care and was designed in response to poor access to healthcare services, the lack of accommodations in healthcare settings, and the paucity of healthcare providers with skills in caring for this population [117]. Program participants work with a nurse to develop individualized care plans that are inclusive of services, such as personal care services to accompany diagnostic procedures or other clinical services, and home or worksite visits instead to promote access to health care [117].

Premier HealthCare provides health care for Medicaid and Medicare individuals who have developmental, physical, and learning disabilities throughout New York City [117]. The program has a comprehensive care practice model, which provides primary care and ready access to specialty and ancillary care offering a variety of services, such as dental, social work, and nutrition. Premier also engages in community outreach projects, and seeks to empower patients and family members by providing a community of support and understanding [117].

The Center for Development and Disability (CDD) at the University of New Mexico is a statewide organization that provides a range of individual and family-centered healthcare services for individuals with IDD [117]. CDD's work includes coordinating a statewide disability and health alliance, building community groups, running conferences and leadership trainings, and maintaining an inventory of disability resources in New Mexico [117]. There are technical assistance and trainings that are offered, including at-home online trainings for individuals with IDD. Some programs are embedded in hospital-based settings and provide care for subgroups of individuals with IDD (e.g., visually or hearing impaired) rather than more diverse population [117].

The Westchester (New York) Institute for Human Development (WIHD) is a former affiliate of the Westchester Medical Center, and is an institute that coordinates comprehensive health care and provides training and technical assistance for individuals with IDD, caregivers, family members, and healthcare professionals [117]. WIHD provides specialized outpatient health care for children and adults with developmental and other disabilities who reside in the metropolitan New York area [117]. Services include primary care, specialty care, and allied health services through a coordinated model that is designed to respond to the complex and chronic health problems of these individuals. Preventive services include health promotion and self-management programs, including nutrition, exercise, hygiene, and tobacco control [117].

Finally, efforts to engage adults with IDD in community-based and civic activities such as voting are very beneficial for this patient population [118]. To the extent that medical providers are able, working with caregivers, social workers, and community members to help patients with IDD engage in these types of activities is likely to have longstanding beneficial health effects [119].

Final Comments

Adults with intellectual and developmental disabilities (IDD) continue to bear a disproportionate burden of poor health and access preventive and healthcare services at a lower rate than people who do not have disabilities [117]. The lack of provider education and disability cultural awareness and competency creates significant barriers for people with disabilities to receive high-quality care [117]. Stereotypes and bias can lead to ineffective and inappropriate care, either through the lack of accessible equipment, or ineffective provider-patient communication or inadequate time to communicate effectively with a patients and caregivers. Adults with IDD receive most of their health care through the primary care providers in the communities in which they live [21]. These providers and innovative comprehensive care models need to take on greater responsibility for providing care that is marked by accessibility, continuity, and comprehensiveness [27]. The advent and expansion of telehealth should be explored as an avenue to increase access to healthcare services for adults with IDD [115], particularly during global crises such as the COVID-19 pandemic [120].

References

1. Ervin DA, Hennen B, Merrick J, Morad M. Healthcare for persons with intellectual and developmental disability in the community. Front Public Health. 2014;2:1–8.
2. Anderson LH, Humpries K, McDermott S, et al. The state of the science of health and wellness for adults with intellectual and developmental disabilities. Intellect Dev Disabil. 2013;51:385–98.
3. AAIDD. FAQs on intellectual disability: American Association on Intellectual and Developmental Disabilities (AAIDD). 2013. Available from: https://aaidd.org/intellectual-disability/definition/faqs-on-intellectual-disability#.V_VDcY8rKUk.
4. Morgart K, Harrison JN, Hoon AH Jr, Wilms Floet AM. Adverse childhood experiences and developmental disabilities: risks, resiliency, and policy. Dev Med Child Neurol. 2021;63(10):1129–60.
5. North Carolina Council on Developmental Disabilities. Definition of intellectual disability and developmental disabilities (I/DD). Raleigh, NC; 2015. Available from: http://www.nc-ddc.org/home/definition.html.
6. Carmeli E, Imam B. Health promotion and disease prevention strategies in older adults with intellectual and developmental disabilities. Front Public Health. 2014;2:1–7.
7. Polloway EA, Bouck EC, Patton JR, Lubin J. Intellectual and developmental disabilities. In: Kauffman JM, Hallahan DP, Pullen PC, editors. Handbook of special education. New York: Routledge; 2017. p. 265–85.
8. Zablotsky B, Black LI, Maenner MJ, Schieve LA, Blumberg SJ. Estimated prevalence of autism and other developmental disabilities following questionnaire changes in the 2014 national health interview survey. Hyattsville, MD: National Center for Health Statistics; 2015.
9. Ervin DA, Williams A, Merrick J. Primary care: mental and behavioral health and persons with intellectual and developmental disabilities. Front Public Health. 2014;2(76):1–5.
10. Videlefsky AS, Reznik JM, Nodvin JT, Heiman HJ. Addressing health disparities in adults with developmental disabilities. Ethn Dis. 2019;29:355.
11. Hsieh K, Rimmer J, Heller T. Prevalence of falls and risk factors in adults with intellectual disability. Am J Intellect Dev Disabil. 2012;117:442–54.
12. Liao P, Vajdic C, Trollor J, Reppermund S. Prevalence and incidence of physical health conditions in people with intellectual disability—a systematic review. PLoS One. 2021;16(8):e0256294.
13. Bradley VJ, Hiersteiner D, Li H, Bonardi A, Vegas L. What do NCI data tell us about the characteristics and outcomes of older adults with IDD? Dev Disabil Network J. 2020;1(1):6.
14. Moran JA, Rafii MS, Keller SM, et al. The National Task Group on intellectual and dementia practices consensus recommendations for the evaluation and management of dementia in adults with intellectual disabilities. Mayo Clin Proc. 2013;88(8):831–40.
15. Scepters M, Keer M, O'Hara D, et al. Reducing health disparity in people with intellectual disabilities: a report from the health issues special interest group of the International Association of Intellectual Disability. J Policy Pract Intellect Disabil. 2005;2:249–55.
16. Balogh R, Ouelette-Kuntz H, Bourne L, et al. Organising health care services for persons with an intellectual disability. Cochrane Database Syst Rev. 2016;4:CD007492.
17. Stirling M, Anderson A, Ouellette-Kuntz H, Hallet J, Shooshtari S, Kelly C, et al. A scoping review documenting cancer outcomes and inequities for adults living with intellectual and/or developmental disabilities. Eur J Oncol Nurs. 2021;54:102011.
18. Havercamp SM, Scott HM. National health surveillance of adults with disabilities, adults with intellectual and developmental disabilities, and adults with no disabilities. Disabil Health J. 2015;8:165–72.
19. Pinals DA, Hovermale L, Mauch D, Anacker L. Persons with intellectual and developmental disabilities in the mental health system: part 1. Clinical considerations. Psychiatr Serv. 2021;73:313.
20. US Public Health Service. Closing the gap: a national blueprint for improving the health of individuals with mental retardation. Washington, DC: US Public Health Service; 2001.
21. Wilkinson J, Dreyfus D, Cerreto M, Bokhour B. "Sometimes I feel overwhelmed": educational needs of family physicians caring for people with intellectual disability. Intellect Dev Disabil. 2012;50(3):243–50.
22. Redquest BK, Tint A, Ries H, Lunsky Y. Exploring the experiences of siblings of adults with intellectual/developmental disabilities during the COVID-19 pandemic. J Intellect Disabil Res. 2021;65(1):1–10.
23. United Nations. Convention on the rights of persons with disabilities. 2006.
24. American Association on Intellectual and Developmental Disabilities. Joint position statement of AAIDD and the arc on health, mental health, vision, and dental care. Washington, DC; 2013. Available from: http://aaidd.org/news-policy/policy/position-statements/health-mental-health-vision-and-dental-care#.VL01zkfF93M.
25. Blaskowitz MG, Hernandez B, Scott PW. Predictors of emergency room and hospital utilization among adults with intellectual and developmental disabilities (IDD). Intellect Dev Disabil. 2019;57(2):127–45.
26. Massachusetts Department of Developmental Services. Massachusetts Department of Developmental Services adult screening recommendations. Boston: Massachusetts Department of Developmental Services; 2012.
27. Sullivan WF, Berg JM, Bradley E, et al. Primary care of adults with developmental disabilities. Can Fam Physician. 2011;57:541–53.
28. Lennox N, Bain C, Rey-Conde T, Purdie D, Bush R, Pandeya N. Effects of a comprehensive health assessment programme for Australian adults with intellectual disability: a cluster randomized trial. Int J Epidemiol. 2007;36(1):139–46.
29. Amin MR, Gentile JP, Edwards B, Davis M. Evaluation of health care disparities for individuals with intellectual and developmental disabilities in Ohio. Community Ment Health J. 2021;57:482–9.
30. Kripke CC. Primary care for adolescents with developmental disabilities. Prim Care. 2014;41(3):507–18.
31. Cassidy SB, Allanson JE. Management of genetic syndromes. 3rd ed. Hoboken, NJ: Wiley-Blackwell; 2010. p. xxii, 962 p.

32. The AAIDD Ad Hoc Committee on Terminology and Classification. Intellectual disability, definition, classification, and systems of supports. Washington, DC: American Association on Intellectual and Developmental Disabilities; 2010.
33. Curry CJ, Stevenson RE, Aughton D, Byrne J, Carey JC, Cassidy S, et al. Evaluation of mental retardation: recommendations of a consensus conference: American College of Medical Genetics. Am J Med Genet. 1997;72(4):468–77.
34. Fletcher RJ, National Association for the Dually Diagnosed, American Psychiatric Association. DM-ID: diagnostic manual-intellectual disability: a clinical guide for diagnosis of mental disorders in persons with intellectual disability. Kingston, NY: NADD Press; 2007. p. xxxi, 351 p.
35. Defrin R, Benromano T, Pick CG. Specific behavioral responses rather than autonomic responses can indicate and quantify acute pain among individuals with intellectual and developmental disabilities. Brain Sci. 2021;11(2):253.
36. Oberlander TF, Symons FJ. Pain in children and adults with developmental disabilities. Baltimore: Paul H. Brookes Pub; 2006. p. xviii, 246 p.
37. Lotan M, Ljunggren EA, Johnsen TB, Defrin R, Pick CG, Strand LI. A modified version of the non-communicating children pain checklist-revised, adapted to adults with intellectual and developmental disabilities: sensitivity to pain and internal consistency. J Pain. 2009;10(4):398–407.
38. Rothschild AW, Ricciardi JN, Luiselli JK. Assessing pain in adults with intellectual disability: a descriptive and qualitative evaluation of ratings and impressions among care-providers. J Dev Phys Disabil. 2019;31:219–30.
39. Bodfish JW, Harper VN, Deacon JR, Symons FJ. Identifying and measuring pain in persons with developmental disabilities: a manual for the pain and discomfort scale (PADS). Morganton: Western Carolina Center Research Reports; 2001.
40. Brown I, Percy ME. A comprehensive guide to intellectual and developmental disabilities, vol. xxv. Baltimore, MD: P. H. Brookes; 2007, 768 p.
41. Holingue C, Kalb LG, Klein A, Beasley JB. Experiences with the mental health service system of family caregivers of individuals with an intellectual/developmental disability referred to START. Intellect Dev Disabil. 2020;58(5):379–92.
42. Reid DH, Rosswurm M, Rotholz DA. No less worthy: recommendations for behavior analysts treating adults with intellectual and developmental disabilities with dignity. Behav Anal Pract. 2018;11:71–9.
43. van Schrojenstein Lantman-de Valk HM, Walsh PN. Managing health problems in people with intellectual disabilities. BMJ. 2008;337:a2507.
44. McGinley J, Marsack-Topolewski CN, Church HL, Knoke V. Advance care planning for individuals with intellectual and developmental disabilities: a state-by-state content analysis of person-centered service plans. Intellect Dev Disabil. 2021;59(4):352–64.
45. Owens PL, Kerker BD, Zigler E, Horwitz SM. Vision and oral health needs of individuals with intellectual disability. Ment Retard Dev Disabil Res Rev. 2006;12(1):28–40.
46. Mac Giolla Phadraig C, Farag M, McCallion P, Waldron C, McCarron M. The complexity of tooth brushing among older adults with intellectual disabilities: findings from a nationally representative survey. Disabil Health J. 2020;13(4):100935.
47. Patja K, Molsa P, Iivanainen M. Cause-specific mortality of people with intellectual disability in a population-based, 35-year follow-up study. J Intellect Disabil Res. 2001;45(Pt 1):30–40.
48. Morad M, Nelson NP, Merrick J, Davidson PW, Carmeli E. Prevalence and risk factors of constipation in adults with intellectual disability in residential care centers in Israel. Res Dev Disabil. 2007;28(6):580–6.
49. Bohmer CJ, Klinkenberg-Knol EC, Niezen-de Boer MC, Meuwissen SG. Gastroesophageal reflux disease in intellectually disabled individuals: how often, how serious, how manageable? Am J Gastroenterol. 2000;95(8):1868–72.
50. Kitchens DH, Binkley CJ, Wallace DL, Darling D. Helicobacter pylori infection in people who are intellectually and developmentally disabled: a review. Spec Care Dentist. 2007;27(4):127–33.
51. Patja K, Eero P, Iivanainen M. Cancer incidence among people with intellectual disability. J Intellect Disabil Res. 2001;45(4):300–7.
52. Leslie WD, Pahlavan PS, Roe EB, Dittberner K. Bone density and fragility fractures in patients with developmental disabilities. Osteoporos Int. 2009;20(3):379–83.
53. Fritz R, Edwards L, Jacob R. Osteoporosis in adult patients with intellectual and developmental disabilities: special considerations for diagnosis, prevention, and management. South Med Assoc. 2021;114(4):246–51.
54. Jaffe JS, Timell AM, Elolia R, Thatcher SS. Risk factors for low bone mineral density in individuals residing in a facility for the people with intellectual disability. J Intellect Disabil Res. 2005;49(Pt 6):457–62.
55. Zylstra RG, Porter LL, Shapiro JL, Prater CD. Prevalence of osteoporosis in community-dwelling individuals with intellectual and/or developmental disabilities. J Am Med Dir Assoc. 2008;9(2):109–13.
56. Janicki MP, Davidson PW, Henderson CM, McCallion P, Taets JD, Force LT, et al. Health characteristics and health services utilization in older adults with intellectual disability living in community residences. J Intellect Disabil Res. 2002;46(Pt 4):287–98.
57. Robertson J, Hatton C, Baines S, Emerson E. Systematic reviews of the health or health care of people with intellectual disabilities: a systematic review to identify gaps in the evidence base. J Appl Res Intellect Disabil. 2015;28(6):455–523.
58. Kerr M, Guidelines Working G, Scheepers M, Arvio M, Beavis J, Brandt C, et al. Consensus guidelines into the management of epilepsy in adults with an intellectual disability. J Intellect Disabil Res. 2009;53(8):687–94.
59. Charlot LR, Doerfler LA, McLaren JL. Psychotropic medications use and side effects of individuals with intellectual and developmental disabilities. J Intellect Disabil Res. 2020;64(11):852–63.
60. Kapell D, Nightingale B, Rodriguez A, Lee JH, Zigman WB, Schupf N. Prevalence of chronic medical conditions in adults with mental retardation: comparison with the general population. Ment Retard. 1998;36(4):269–79.
61. McDermott S, Moran RR, Platt T. The epidemiology of common health conditions among adults with developmental disabilities in primary care. New York: Nova Biomedical Books; 2008. p. 140.
62. Wallace RA, Schluter P. Audit of cardiovascular disease risk factors among supported adults with intellectual disability attending an ageing clinic. J Intellect Dev Disabil. 2008;33(1):48–58.
63. Wilson W, Taubert KA, Gewitz M, Lockhart PB, Baddour LM, Levison M, et al. Prevention of infective endocarditis: guidelines from the American Heart Association: a guideline from the American Heart Association Rheumatic Fever, Endocarditis and Kawasaki Disease Committee, Council on Cardiovascular Disease in the Young, and the Council on Clinical Cardiology, Council on Cardiovascular Surgery and Anesthesia, and the Quality of Care and Outcomes Research Interdisciplinary Working Group. J Am Dent Assoc. 2008;139(Suppl):3S–24S.
64. Erickson SR, Kamdar N, Wu CH. Adverse medication events related to hospitalization in the United States: a comparison between adults with intellectual and developmental disabilities and those without. Am J Intellect Dev Disabil. 2020;125(1):37–48.
65. Deb S, Kwok H, Bertelli M, Salvador-Carulla L, Bradley E, Torr J, et al. International guide to prescribing psychotropic medication

66. Tsiouris JA. Pharmacotherapy for aggressive behaviours in persons with intellectual disabilities: treatment or mistreatment? J Intellect Disabil Res. 2010;54(1):1–16.
67. Tyrer P, Oliver-Africano PC, Ahmed Z, Bouras N, Cooray S, Deb S, et al. Risperidone, haloperidol, and placebo in the treatment of aggressive challenging behaviour in patients with intellectual disability: a randomised controlled trial. Lancet. 2008;371(9606):57–63.
68. Lewis MA, Lewis CE, Leake B, King BH, Lindemann R. The quality of health care for adults with developmental disabilities. Public Health Rep. 2002;117(2):174–84.
69. Centers for Disease Control and Prevention. COVID-19 vaccine booster shots. 2021. Available from: https://www.cdc.gov/coronavirus/2019-ncov/vaccines/booster-shot.html.
70. Wilkinson JE, Culpepper L, Cerreto M. Screening tests for adults with intellectual disabilities. J Am Board Fam Med. 2007;20:399–407.
71. Xu X, McDermott SW, Mann JR, Hardin JW, Deroche CB, Carroll DD, et al. A longitudinal assessment of adherence to breast and cervical cancer screening recommendations among women with and without intellectual disability. Prev Med. 2017;100:167–72.
72. Rimmer JH, Yamaki K. Obesity and intellectual disability. Ment Retard Dev Disabil Res Rev. 2006;12(1):22–7.
73. Reina AM, Adams EV, Allison CK, Mueller KE, Crowe BM, van Puymbroeck M, et al. Yoga for functional fitness in adults with intellectual and developmental disabilities. Int J Yoga. 2020;13(2):156–9.
74. Bhaumik S, Watson JM, Thorp CF, Tyrer F, McGrother CW. Body mass index in adults with intellectual disability: distribution, associations and service implications: a population-based prevalence study. J Intellect Disabil Res. 2008;52(Pt 4):287–98.
75. Evenhuis HM, Sjoukes L, Koot HM, Kooijman AC. Does visual impairment lead to additional disability in adults with intellectual disabilities? J Intellect Disabil Res. 2009;53(1):19–28.
76. Wilkinson JE, Cerreto MC. Primary care for women with intellectual disabilities. J Am Board Fam Med. 2008;21(3):215–22.
77. Kammes RR, Black RS, Easley T. A community-engaged project discovering the sexuality questions of adults with intellectual and developmental disabilities. Inclusion. 2021;9(1):2–16.
78. Treacy AC, Taylor SS, Abernathy TV. Sexual health education for individuals with disabilities: a call to action. Am J Sexual Educ. 2018;13(1):65–93.
79. Horner-Johnson W, Klein KA, Campbell J, Guise JM. Experiences of women with disabilities in accessing and receiving contraceptive care. J Obstet Gynecol Neonatal Nurs. 2021;50:732.
80. Wu J, Zhang J, Mitra M, Parish SL, Minama Reddy GK. Provision of moderately and highly effective reversible contraception to insured women with intellectual and developmental disabilities. Obstet Gynecol. 2018;132(3):565–74.
81. Walters FP, Gray SH. Addressing sexual and reproductive health in adolescents and young adults with intellectual and developmental disabilities. Curr Opin Pediatr. 2018;30(4):451–8.
82. Wehmeyer ML. A comprehensive guide to intellectual and developmental disabilities. 2nd ed. Baltimore: Paul H. Brookes Publishing, Co.; 2017.
83. Clay CJ, Bloom SE, Lambert JM. Behavioral interventions for inappropriate sexual behavior in individuals with developmental disabilities and acquired brain injury: a review. Am J Intellect Dev Disabil. 2018;123(3):254–82.
84. Lin E, Balogh R, Chung H, Dobranowski K, Durbin A, Volpe T, et al. Looking across health and healthcare outcomes for people with intellectual and developmental disabilities and psychiatric disorders: population-based longitudinal study. Br J Psychiatry. 2021;218(1):51–7.
85. Hassiotis A, Barron DA, Hall IP. Intellectual disability psychiatry: a practical handbook. Chichester: Wiley; 2009.
86. Deb S, Thomas M, Bright C. Mental disorder in adults with intellectual disability. 1: prevalence of functional psychiatric illness among a community-based population aged between 16 and 64 years. J Intellect Disabil Res. 2001;45(Pt 6):495–505.
87. Lin E, Balogh R, McGarry C, Selick A, Dobranowski K, Wilton AS, et al. Substance-related and addictive disorders among adults with intellectual and developmental disabilities (IDD): an Ontario population cohort study. BMJ Open. 2016;6(9):e011638.
88. Merrells J, Buchanan A, Waters R. "We feel left out": experiences of social inclusion from the perspective of young adults with intellectual disability. J Intellect Dev Disabil. 2019;44(1):13–22.
89. Doody O, Keenan PM. The reported effects of the COVID-19 pandemic on people with intellectual disability and their carers: a scoping review. Ann Med. 2021;53(1):786–804.
90. Aman MG, Singh NN, Stewart AW, Field CJ. Psychometric characteristics of the aberrant behavior checklist. Am J Ment Defic. 1985;89(5):492–502.
91. Taylor JL, Hatton C, Dixon L, Douglas C. Screening for psychiatric symptoms: PAS-ADD checklist norms for adults with intellectual disabilities. J Intellect Disabil Res. 2004;48(1):37–41.
92. Sawhney I, Perera B, Bassett P, Zia A, Alexander RT, Shankar R. Attention-deficit hyperactivity disorder in people with intellectual disability: statistical approach to developing a bespoke screening tool. BJPsych Open. 2021;7(6):e187.
93. Pfister AA, Roberts AG, Taylor HM, Noel-Spaudling S, Damian MM, Charles PD. Spasticity in adults living in a developmental center. Arch Phys Med Rehabil. 2003;84(12):1808–12.
94. Ball SL, Holland AJ, Treppner P, Watson PC, Huppert FA. Executive dysfunction and its association with personality and behaviour changes in the development of Alzheimer's disease in adults with Down syndrome and mild to moderate learning disabilities. Br J Clin Psychol. 2008;47(Pt 1):1–29.
95. McCabe MP, McGillivray JA, Newton DC. Effectiveness of treatment programmes for depression among adults with mild/moderate intellectual disability. J Intellect Disabil Res. 2006;50(Pt 4):239–47.
96. Hemmings CP, Gravestock S, Pickard M, Bouras N. Psychiatric symptoms and problem behaviours in people with intellectual disabilities. J Intellect Disabil Res. 2006;50(Pt 4):269–76.
97. Dosen A, Day K. Treating mental illness and behavior disorders in children and adults with mental retardation. 1st ed. Washington, DC: American Psychiatric Press; 2001. p. xv, 561 p.
98. Jones S, Cooper SA, Smiley E, Allan L, Williamson A, Morrison J. Prevalence of, and factors associated with, problem behaviors in adults with intellectual disabilities. J Nerv Ment Dis. 2008;196(9):678–86.
99. Jones RSP, Eayrs C. Challenging behaviour and intellectual disability: a psychological perspective. Philadelphia: BILD Publications; 1993. p. ix, 267 p.
100. Friedman C, Rizzolo MC. Electronic video monitoring in Medicaid home and community-based services waivers for people with intellectual and developmental disabilities. J Policy Pract Intellect Disabil. 2017;14(4):279–84.
101. Sullivan W, Berg JM, Bradley EA, Brooks-Hill RW, Goldfarb CE, Lovering JS, et al. Enhancing the emergency department outcomes of patients with mental retardation. Ann Emerg Med. 2000;36(4):399–400.
102. Bhaumik S, Branford D, Barrett M, Gangadharan SK. The Frith prescribing guidelines for people with intellectual disability. 3rd ed. Chichester: John Wiley & Sons Inc.; 2015.
103. Mills WR, Sender S, Lichtefeld J, Romano N, Reynolds K, Price M, et al. Supporting individuals with intellectual and developmental disability during the first 100 days of the COVID-19 outbreak in the USA. J Intellect Disabil Res. 2020;64(7):489–96.

104. Jeste S, Hyde C, Distefano C, Halladay A, Ray S, Porath M, et al. Changes in access to educational and healthcare services for individuals with intellectual and developmental disabilities during COVID-19 restrictions. J Intellect Disabil Res. 2020;64(11):825–33.
105. Johnson E, Ervin DA, Fray D, Keller S, Margolis B, Rader R, et al. COVID-19 support guidelines for individuals with IDD during the pandemic. American Academy of Developmental Medicine & Dentistry; 2020.
106. Huls A, Costa ACS, Dierssen M, Baksh RA, Bargagna S, Baumer NT, et al. Medical vulnerability of individuals with Down syndrome to severe COVID-19-data from the Trisomy 21 Research Society and the UK ISARIC4C survey. EClinicalMedicine. 2021;33:100769.
107. Ervin DA, Hennen B, Merrick J, Morad M. Healthcare for persons with intellectual and developmental disability in the community. Front Public Health. 2014;2:83.
108. Grumbach K, Bodenheimer T. A primary care home for Americans: putting the house in order. JAMA. 2002;288:889–93.
109. Weedon D, Carbone P, Bilder D, O'Brien S, Dorius J. Building a person-centered medical home: lessons from a program for people with developmental disabilities. J Health Care Poor Underserved. 2012;23(4):1600–8.
110. Drotar DD, Strum LA. Interdisciplinary collaboration in the practice of mental retardation. In: Jacobson JW, Mulick DC, editors. Manual of diagnosis and professional practice in mental retardation. Washington, DC: American Psychological Association; 1996.
111. Rich E, Lipson D, Libersky J, et al. Coordinating care for adults with complex care needs in the patient-centered medical home: challenges and solutions. Rockville, MD: AHRQ; 2012.
112. Taylor EF, Machta RM, Meyers DS, Et a. Enhancing the primary care team to provide redesigned care: the roles of practice facilitators and care managers. Ann Fam Med. 2013;11:80–3.
113. Marks B, Sisirak J, Magallanes R, Krok K, Donohue-Chase D. Effectiveness of a health messages peer-to-peer program for people with intellectual and developmental disabilities. Intellect Dev Disabil. 2019;57(3):242–58.
114. Martin S, Kelly G, Kernohan W, McCreight B, Nugent C. Smart home technologies for health and social care support. Cochrane Database Syst Rev. 2008;(4):CD006412.
115. Boisvert M, Lang R, Andrianopoulos M, Boscarin ML. Telepractice in the assessment and treatment of individuals with autism spectrum disorders: a systematic review. Dev Neurorehabil. 2010;13(6):423–32.
116. Pellegrino AJ, DiGennaro Reed FD. Using telehealth to teach valued skills to adults with intellectual and developmental disabilities. J Appl Behav Anal. 2020;53(3):1276–89.
117. National Council on Disability (U.S.). The current state of health care for people with disabilities. Washington, DC: National Council on Disability; 2009, 454 p.
118. Argan M, MacLean WE Jr, Kitchen Andren KA. "My Voice Counts, Too": voting participation among individuals with intellectual disability. Intellect Dev Disabil. 2016;54(4):285–94.
119. Schalock RL, Luckasson R, Tasse MJ. Ongoing transformation in the field of intellectual and developmental disabilities: taking action for future progress. Intellect Dev Disabil. 2021;59(5):380–91.
120. Zaagsma M, Volkers KM, Swart EAK, Schippers AP, Van Hove G. The use of online support by people with intellectual disabilities living independently during COVID-19. J Intellect Disabil Res. 2020;64(10):750–6.

Special Population: Adults with Severe and Persistent Mental Health Disorders

Kathleen Barnhouse, Sandra Clark, and Jessica Waters Davis

Introduction

Providing care for patients with serious mental illness (SMI) is both challenging and rewarding, and increased attention to whole-person care, through the integration of primary care with behavioral health and mental health services, enables persons diagnosed with SMI to live independent and productive lives in the community. Serious mental illness (SMI) is defined as a diagnosable mental, behavioral, or emotional disorder that is accompanied by functional impairment that substantially limits major life activities [1]. The terms "serious mental illness," "severe mental illness," and "severe and persistent mental illness" have often been used interchangeably and, while all forms of SMI impact functioning and are considered serious, the manifestation varies across individuals and is not always persistent, chronic, or severe [2]. There are several diagnoses that are considered SMI, including schizophrenia, schizoaffective disorder, bipolar disorder, and major depressive disorder [2]. Personality disorders and anxiety disorders resulting in significant disability may also fall under the category of SMI [2]. Persons with developmental disorders and substance use disorders are not usually considered to have SMI unless the diagnosis is comorbid with an SMI diagnosis [2].

The prevalence of SMI in the adult population is reported to be 4%, with a higher prevalence in women and the nonminority population [1]. A diagnosis of SMI carries with it a significant increase in morbidity and mortality. Estimates for years of life lost due to SMI vary with some estimates of increased mortality as high as 25 years [3]. Although some increased risk is related to suicide and accidental death, up to 85% of the differential is attributable to physical illness including cardiovascular disease, cancer, pulmonary disease, diabetes, and infection [4], i.e. conditions associated with preventable risk factors such as tobacco use, substance abuse, and obesity. The increase in mortality is associated with socioeconomic factors such as education and income level, access to housing, and employment [5]. Access to healthcare services and insurance status are also important factors since uninsured persons with an SMI diagnosis are less likely to access mental health services when compared to those with insurance [6].

This chapter is a primer to the care of persons with SMI. The first section provides an overview of the spectrum of SMI and associated comorbidities since an accurate diagnosis is critical to addressing care needs. Persons with SMI generally receive care from psychiatrists, primary care physicians, social workers, and occupational therapists, and the second section outlines management principles and strategies of care. Next, program-level strategies that highlight interdisciplinary teams and community-based services will be reviewed before the chapter closes with future directions.

The Spectrum of Serious Mental Illness

Psychosis is a constellation of symptoms characterized by abnormalities in thought processing and perception manifesting as hallucinations, delusions, and/or disorganized thinking [7]. Psychotic disorders are heterogeneous in their phenotypic expression as well as the severity of symptoms. The lifetime prevalence is 3% for primary psychosis, and less than 1% for psychosis due to a medical condition [8]. Primary psychosis refers to psychosis in the context of a psychiatric disorder, whereas secondary psychosis refers to psychosis secondary to a medical condition or substance [8].

K. Barnhouse (✉)
Department of Family Medicine, University of North Carolina at Chapel Hill, Chapel Hill, NC, USA
e-mail: kathleen_barnhouse@med.unc.edu

S. Clark · J. Waters Davis
Department of Family Medicine, University of North Carolina at Chapel Hill, Chapel Hill, NC, USA

Department of Psychiatry, University of North Carolina at Chapel Hill, Chapel Hill, NC, USA
e-mail: sandy_clark@med.unc.edu; jswaters@med.unc.edu

Persons with psychotic disorders and a higher burden of depressive symptoms suffer from impaired global functioning, which contributes to a lower quality of life [9, 10]. The individual and societal financial burden of psychotic disorders is attributable to direct healthcare costs, and to the loss of economic productivity due to functional impairment [11]. SMI care strategies should include multiple modalities to target global functioning and quality of life. Schizophrenia, schizoaffective disorder, and bipolar disorder are major psychotic disorders. Disorders within the schizophrenia spectrum are defined by abnormalities in at least one of five specific domains including delusions, hallucinations, disorganized thinking, grossly disorganized behavior, and negative symptoms [7].

Schizophrenia

Schizophrenia is a debilitating illness that causes degrees of psychosocial impairment, chronic psychotic symptoms, and cognitive impairment and has a lifetime prevalence of less than 1% [12]. The duration of symptoms is part of the diagnostic criteria and individuals must display continuous symptoms for at least 6 months [13]. Within that timeframe, individuals must display also a specific set of symptoms for at least 1 month, such as delusions, hallucinations, disorganized speech, grossly disorganized or catatonic behavior [13]. Delusions, hallucinations, and/or disorganized speech must be present in the absence of mood symptoms, which differentiates schizophrenia from schizoaffective disorder [7]. Schizophrenia is unique in that individuals often have more than one psychotic symptom (e.g., hallucinations and delusions) and the level of functioning in one or more major areas is significantly lower than prior to the onset of symptoms [12]. Other causes of hallucinations, delusions, and disorganized speech need to be excluded, including alterations due to a medical condition or substance use.

Schizophrenia often presents between late adolescence to early adulthood [7]. Children who later develop schizophrenia may have non-specific language, intellectual, or motor delay in addition to behavioral and emotional dysregulation [14]. There is no clear recessive or dominant genetic pattern and multiple genes are likely involved [13, 15]. A combination of genetic and environmental insults that occur early in life may result in abnormal neurodevelopmental processes that precede the onset of clinical symptoms by many years [13, 15]. Environmental factors may play a role in susceptibility to the development of psychotic disorders including urbanization, social disadvantage, and isolation [13]. Childhood trauma may also play a role in some who develop schizophrenia [12, 14], however there are many unknown factors that contribute to susceptibility and resiliency [14].

Schizoaffective Disorder

Schizoaffective disorder bridges mood and psychotic disorders and includes symptoms of schizophrenia in addition to a diagnosis of either major depressive disorder or mania [7]. It is less common than schizophrenia and patients must both meet the primary criteria for schizophrenia, and have symptoms of a major mood disorder for the majority of the symptomatic period [7]. It commonly presents in early adulthood, but may present as early as adolescence and into later adult life [16]. Sometimes individuals are diagnosed earlier with another disorder but the diagnosis of schizoaffective disorder is clarified as they develop more prominent mood symptoms. While the clinical presentation varies between individuals, many patients initially develop psychotic symptoms such as auditory hallucinations, and then develop major depressive symptoms which occur concurrently [16]. Schizoaffective disorder is more common in women than in men and has high heritability, but there are not specific genetic markers unique to schizoaffective disorder [16]. The clinical course is variable, but more favorable than that of schizophrenia.

Bipolar Disorder

Individuals with bipolar disorder report recurrent changes in mood, energy, and activity levels that are manifested as manic or hypomanic episodes, and depressive episodes [7]. Mania and hypomania are characterized by persistently and abnormally elevated or irritable mood and persistently and abnormally increased activity or energy [7]. Suicide rates are disturbingly high with almost 8% of males and almost 5% of females reported to die by suicide in the first 18 years of diagnosis [17]. Almost half of individuals diagnosed with bipolar depression at an early age attempt suicide [18]. Bipolar I and bipolar II differ in the degree and severity of mania that is present; those diagnosed with bipolar II disorder report hypomanic episodes rather than full-blown manic episodes [7]. Episodes of mania and depression may occur together, resulting in "mixed states." In addition, some patients with bipolar disorder may also experience psychotic symptoms, which can make distinguishing bipolar disorder from schizophrenia and schizoaffective disorder challenging at initial presentation. During manic episodes, individuals may have poor insight into their condition and may resist treatment or intervention [7, 17]. The clinical course of bipolar disorder is variable. Individuals with a predominance of depressive symptoms may have a greater duration of illness while persons with mania predominance have increased hospitalization [19, 20].

The diagnosis of bipolar I disorder requires a defined period of mania lasting at least 1 week in duration or any duration requiring hospitalization. Mania is defined by grandiosity, decreased need for sleep, pressured speech, flight of ideas, psychomotor agitation, or significant commitment to activities with negative consequences (e.g., spending sprees, gambling, sexual encounters). Manic episodes need to be severe enough to cause hospitalization, marked impairment in functioning, or be accompanied by psychotic features [7]. Individuals with bipolar I disorder must also have an episode of major depression, which generally lasts longer than the manic episode [17]. Bipolar I disorder can further be characterized as bipolar I with "rapid cycling" if an individual has four or more mood episodes within a year [7].

The diagnosis of bipolar II disorder requires a distinct period of hypomania and an episode of major depressive disorder. A hypomanic episode is characterized by mania lasting four or more days, with a change in functioning that is observable by others but not severe enough to cause marked impairment in functioning or to result in hospitalization. In order to establish the diagnosis of either bipolar I or bipolar II, the depressive, manic, or hypomanic episodes cannot be attributed to a substance or medical condition [7].

Medical Comorbidities

Although individuals with SMI are at risk of medical comorbidities that are comparable to the general US population, their life expectancy is dramatically less, which may be due to higher rates of homelessness, unemployment, and other social determinants of health [21]. Health behaviors such as sedentary lifestyle and tobacco use are associated with greater mortality risk. Antipsychotic medications that are often used in SMI treatment contribute to obesity, hypertension, hyperlipidemia, and diabetes [22]. In addition, patients with SMI are less likely to receive optimized treatment for these comorbidities [22].

Cardiovascular Disease

The relative risk of hypertension in individuals with schizophrenia and bipolar disorder is 2–3 times that of the general US adult population [23]. Ambulatory and home blood pressure monitoring should be considered in diagnosing hypertension, since the white coat effect may be more pronounced in individuals with underlying anxiety, mania, or paranoia [24]. Treatment principles for hypertension include diet modifications, increased physical activity, weight management for patients who are overweight or obese, moderation of or abstinence from alcohol, and pharmacotherapy. When prescribing medications, drug-drug interactions with psychiatric medications need to be considered. For instance, concurrent use of a thiazide diuretic, ACE inhibitor, or angiotensin receptor blocker with lithium, which is employed as a mood stabilizer in many patients with affective disorders, can increase the concentration of lithium by 25–50%, thus increasing the risk of lithium toxicity [25].

Several psychiatric medications prolong electrocardiographic QT intervals (e.g., haloperidol, thioridazine, and tricyclic antidepressants), and as such require regular monitoring and surveillance of serum electrolytes to minimize the risk of cardiac arrhythmia [26]. Notably, the risk of sudden cardiac death in patients taking an antipsychotic is twice than observed in the general population, although the absolute risk remains small (10–15 events per 10,000 person-years of observation) [27]. Patients with SMI have increased risk of death from all cardiovascular disease, including ischemic heart disease, nonischemic heart disease, cerebrovascular disease, and other circulatory disease [28]. For example, a cohort study of individuals with schizophrenia who were Medicaid beneficiaries reported that the observed mortality rate due to cardiovascular disease in this population was 3.6 times greater compared to the general population [28].

Metabolic Disorders

Approximately one-third of individuals with schizophrenia have metabolic syndrome and the mortality secondary to cardiovascular disease in patients with schizophrenia is 3–5 times higher than the general population [29, 30]. Some patient characteristics, such as non-white ethnicity, male sex, higher weight prior to starting medications, and multi-episode schizophrenia, are predictors of increased risk of metabolic syndrome [29, 30]. The use of antipsychotic medications increases the risk of metabolic syndrome and is associated with weight gain, insulin resistance, and dyslipidemia, particularly elevated LDL and triglyceride levels [29]. There is a differential effect between psychotropic medications, with the second-generation antipsychotics olanzapine and clozapine demonstrating the most adverse metabolic profiles, and aripiprazole, brexpiprazole, cariprazine, lurasidone, and ziprasidone having more favorable profiles [29]. Primary care and psychiatric providers should work together to determine an optimal medication regimen through individualized consideration.

Monitoring for metabolic syndrome in persons prescribed antipsychotic medications is an integral part of care. Interestingly, the degree of metabolic disturbances seems to correlate with improvement of symptoms so that individuals who develop higher degrees of metabolic syndrome also have the most marked improvement in psychotic symptoms [29]. Despite the metabolic risks, persons with schizophrenia who are treated with antipsychotics have a lower all-cause and cardiovascular mortality than those not treated with antipsychotic therapy; while this seems to be true with all antipsychotics, data suggests the effect is most pronounced with clozapine therapy [29, 31].

Table 25.1 Metabolic risk factor monitoring for patients with SMI or on an antipsychotic medication

Risk factor	First year of antipsychotic			Ongoing monitoring		
	Baseline	6 weeks	3 months	12 months	Quarterly	Annually
Personal and family history of CV risk factors	x					x
Smoking, physical activity, diet	x	x	x		x	
Weight/BMI	x	x	x		x	
Blood pressure	x	x	x		x	
Fasting glucose or A1c	x	x	x	x		x
Lipid profile	x		x	x		x

Reproduced with permission from De Hert M, Detraux J, van Winkel R, Yu W, Correll CU. Metabolic and cardiovascular adverse effects associated with antipsychotic drugs. Nat Rev Endocrinol. 2011;8(2):114–126. https://doi.org/10.1038/nrendo.2011.156

Note: More frequent monitoring is indicated when health indicators are out of the normal range

Lifestyle and socioeconomic factors including lack of physical activity, dietary choices, food insecurity, and poverty may also contribute to the increased prevalence of obesity and insulin resistance in patients with SMI, but research in these areas has been lacking [32]. What is known is that lifestyle interventions including dietary counseling, physical activity, and health coaching can be effective in helping individuals with SMI to meet their own health goals, including but not limited to weight loss [33]. There may additionally be a genetic predisposition or shared pathophysiology that contributes to the linkage between SMI and diabetes [34, 35]. Because of the increased risk of metabolic disorder in patients with SMI and antipsychotic medication usage, experts agree that body-mass index (BMI), blood pressure, lipid profile, and glucose should be monitored more frequently than in the general population [36]. Table 25.1 summarizes general monitoring guidelines.[1]

Patients with SMI should receive counseling on healthy diet and physical activity, with increased attention to patients with higher risk [37]. A team-based approach including clinicians, dietitians, social workers, and peer support specialists can increase the scope and intensity of services offered. Several evidence-based medications are indicated for the treatment of antipsychotic-associated weight gain. Metformin, topiramate, liraglutide, and aripiprazole have been shown to slow weight gain and contribute to weight loss [37]. The initiation and rationale for these medications should be discussed with the patient and guardian, when applicable, to facilitate informed and shared decision-making about the risks and benefits. Metformin may mitigate antipsychotic-associated weight gain and clinicians may consider starting this pharmacotherapy for weight management and diabetes prevention even in patients with normal glucose levels [37]. Additional trials are needed to determine whether newer GLP-1 agonists such as semaglutide are effective for weight management in individuals taking antipsychotic medication.

Due to the increased risk of hyperlipidemia and cardiovascular disease, as well as the shorter life expectancy in this population, some experts have advocated for earlier initiation of statin medications [37]. To determine the risk of atherosclerotic cardiovascular disease (ASCVD) in individuals under the age of 40 with SMI and/or taking a long-term antipsychotic medication, calculations can be made as if the patient were 40 years old. Statin medication can be considered if the calculated 10-year risk is 7.5–10% or greater [37].

Tobacco Use Disorder

A substantial number of individuals with SMI use tobacco products; one meta-analysis found that 30% of adults with major depression, 45% of adults with bipolar disorder, and 55% of adults with schizophrenia are current smokers [38]. The reasons for increased tobacco usage may include high stress levels, self-treatment of clinical symptoms, policies that permit tobacco use in psychiatric and substance use disorder facilities, and culture [39]. Patients, families and caregivers, and clinicians may prioritize other health goals with an assumption that tobacco cessation will not be achievable given comorbid mental illness. However, the standardized mortality ratio for adults with schizophrenia is 9.9 for COPD, 7.0 for influenza and pneumonia (conditions made more lethal by pre-occurring tobacco use), and 2.4 for lung cancer [28].

Most patients with SMI who smoke want to quit and cessation strategies are effective [40]. Nicotine replacement therapy and behavioral counseling carry minimal risk with potentially large benefit. The success rate increases with the addition of varenicline, which has been shown to be effective and to have minimal adverse effects on psychiatric symptoms in this population [41]. Psychiatric consultation should be involved when considering bupropion in patients with SMI, although it has been reported to be safe and effective [42]. Psychiatric and mental health providers can play an important role in encouraging smoking cessation and initiating pharmacotherapy since many patients with SMI see their psychiatric provider more frequently than their primary care provider.

---

[1] Recommendations based on a 2004 consensus statement by the American Diabetes Association, the American Psychiatric Association, the American Association of Clinical Endocrinologists, and the North American Association for the Study of Obesity [36]. It is augmented by more recent European guidelines calling for more frequent glucose and lipid monitoring [26].

Alcohol and Substance Use Disorder

Persons with SMI have increased risks of alcohol use disorder and other substance use disorders when compared to the general population [43]. The risk of substance use disorder is reported to be greater regardless of race, ethnicity, and gender [43]. Medical providers should screen patients with SMI for substance use disorder, and actively engage them in treatment when identified. Individual counseling and peer support groups are effective in supporting sobriety [44]. Medication-assisted treatment, particularly for alcohol use disorder and opioid use disorder, is both effective and underutilized in this population [45, 46].

Intellectual and Developmental Disability

Intellectual disability is defined by significant limitations in intellectual functioning and adaptive behaviors while developmental disability is defined by functional limitations due to a mental or physical impairment, including autism spectrum disorder, and excluding intellectual disability [47]. Impairment in daily functioning is a central characteristic of this class of disorders, and often results in additional challenges to an individual's social, emotional, or occupational activities. Almost one-third of individuals with intellectual and developmental disability (IDD) also experience persistent symptoms of mental illness [48]. Given the cumulative burden of physical and mental health in individuals with co-occurring SMI and IDD, novel approaches are needed to effectively care for these patients. For instance, L'Arche is an organization that facilitates the establishment of peer communities in which individuals with and without developmental disability can live, work, and support each other [49]. Expanding this model to include individuals with SMI could improve the quality of life and health of those living with comorbid IDD and mental illness.

Traumatic Brain Injury

Traumatic brain injury (TBI) is an impact or injury to the head resulting in loss of consciousness, amnesia, confusion, new neurological symptoms, or neuroimaging findings demonstrating injury [50]. Patients who experience TBI can develop new-onset psychotic disorders, including delusions and auditory hallucinations [51]. Individuals with psychotic disorder due to TBI often have other neurological symptoms such as cognitive deficits, memory impairment, and challenges with executive functioning. Brain imaging (MRI or CT) often reveals focal lesions, particularly in the frontal and temporal lobes, which may correlate with electroencephalogram findings showing slowing of brain waves in the affected regions [51].

Despite the difference in pathophysiology between primary psychotic disorder and psychosis due to TBI, pharmacologic treatments are comparable, with antipsychotic medications as a mainstay [51]. Patients with TBI may additionally benefit from anti-epileptic medication, particularly in the case of EEG abnormalities [51]. Because the symptoms and impact on functioning between TBI-associated psychotic disorder and SMI can be similar, patients with these diagnoses respond to many of the same pharmacologic and non-pharmacologic treatment approaches.

Dementia and Cognitive Impairment

Psychotic symptoms can develop in patients with Alzheimer's disease, vascular dementia, Lewy-Body dementia, frontotemporal dementia, or other types of dementia. The initial management of symptoms that do not threaten the safety of the patient, caregivers, or others includes nonpharmacologic interventions such as reorientation, addressing pain and other environmental triggers, as well as pharmacologic treatment of co-occurring depression or anxiety, and consideration for anti-dementia medications such as memantine or donepezil [52]. Antipsychotic medications can be useful if symptoms are severe or progressive, but should be used with caution in these patients. First- and second-generation antipsychotic medications can increase the risk of stroke, hasten cognitive decline, cause sedation, and increase mortality in patients with dementia [53], and should be considered where other interventions have been unsuccessful and the patient is at risk of harming self or others. However, individuals whose psychotic disorder preceded the onset of dementia may require lifelong pharmacotherapy, including antipsychotics. Consultation with a geriatrician, geriatric psychiatrist, or neurologist may be indicated to guide treatment decisions.

Caring for Individuals with Serious Mental Illness

The management of persons with SMI encompasses pharmacological therapy along with intensive multidisciplinary care and support from the community. While pharmacotherapy is often helpful in reducing hospitalizations and improving function and minimizing symptoms, many medications have associated risks of metabolic syndrome, motor disturbances including dystonia and parkinsonism, and cardiac arrhythmias [26]. Care models that co-locate primary care and psychiatric care have been shown to improve identification and management of modifiable risk factors, decrease emergency room visits, and decrease the number of psychiatric relapses [11, 15]. In addition to improving quality of life for persons with SMI, high-quality multidisciplinary treatment and management can mitigate the downstream impact of SMI by improving employment, decreasing crime, and decreasing hospitalizations and length of stay [11].

There are often challenges with medication adherence in patients with SMI. Lack of insight, distrust of the healthcare system and healthcare providers, stigma associated with psychiatric illness, poor access to care, homelessness, concomitant substance use disorders, and other social factors play a role [54]. Patient outreach and education to reduce barriers to medication use are important adjunct interventions. Long-acting injectable medications (LAIs) are often used in patients with schizophrenia to help with medication adherence. In persons with schizophrenia, LAIs decrease rates of hospitalizations compared with oral antipsychotics [55]. LAIs have also been shown to be as effective as oral maintenance therapy in patients with bipolar disorder and schizoaffective disorder. However, LAIs are likely more effective at controlling manic and psychotic symptoms than depressive symptoms in these individuals [56].

Management of Schizophrenia

Psychiatric pharmacotherapy for persons with schizophrenia reduces morbidity and primarily utilizes antipsychotics because of their ability to antagonize dopamine receptors [12, 15]. The mechanism of action of these drugs contributes to adverse side effect profiles and has led to the development of newer "atypical" antipsychotics [15]. These newer drugs modulate serotonin in addition to dopamine which may contribute to their efficacy and decreased side effects. Early treatment with antipsychotic drugs is important and has been shown to decrease the risk of suicide in these individuals [8].

There are multiple antipsychotics available for the treatment of schizophrenia [12, 15]with marked differences in side effect profiles [57]. Antipsychotics take several weeks to demonstrate full clinical effect. Motor side effects such as extrapyramidal symptoms are more common with older antipsychotics, whereas atypical/newer antipsychotics are more likely to cause weight gain, metabolic abnormalities, and sedation [58]. Clozapine is a second-generation antipsychotic used in treatment-resistant schizophrenia or in persons with refractory psychotic symptoms [12]. While clozapine lacks extrapyramidal side effects, it may cause myocarditis and agranulocytosis [12]. Acute dystonia can be managed with anticholinergic therapy, primarily diphenhydramine or benztropine, as well as antipsychotic dosage decreases or medication changes [59].

Management of Schizoaffective Disorder

The lifetime risk for suicide in patients with both schizophrenia and schizoaffective disorder (SAD) is approximately 5% and the presence of depressive symptoms is associated with higher risk [7]. There are limited data on the pharmacologic management of individuals with SAD and most studies have significant overlap with individuals diagnosed with schizophrenia [60]. Individuals with SAD are often treated with antipsychotics but may also require mood stabilizers [12]. Currently, the evidence supports risperidone and paliperidone for the management of both the psychotic and affective components of SAD [61]. In addition, it is unclear if and when antidepressant therapy is a useful adjunct to antipsychotic therapy in these individuals [61].

Management of Bipolar Disorder

The management of bipolar disorder is challenging. Patients with acute mania and unstable mood symptoms require treatment that is focused on both symptom mitigation and safety, and may require inpatient psychiatric admission, either voluntarily or involuntarily. Safety is a key management principle since deliberate self-harm occurs in 30–40% of individuals who are acutely ill, especially in those with either primarily depressive or mixed episodes [17]. Acute management focuses on a combination of pharmacotherapy and cognitive behavioral therapy to address harmful thoughts [17]. The initial pharmacologic selection is dependent on the severity of symptoms. Antipsychotics, lithium, and/or antiepileptics including valproate and carbamazepine are typically used to manage acute mania, occasionally in combination with benzodiazepines [17]. Benzodiazepines should only be used for short period of time to manage symptoms such as agitation and insomnia [17].

Maintenance pharmacotherapy of bipolar disorder often involves combination therapy with both mood stabilizers and antidepressants. Management of depressive symptoms is challenging with few treatment options [62]. Lithium is frequently used to treat bipolar disorder, but necessitates frequent monitoring to avoid toxicity and has a high side effect profile including increased risk of nephrogenic diabetes insipidus and hypothyroidism [63]. However, lithium can prevent manic recurrences [17], and has been demonstrated to lower suicide risk in bipolar disorder by decreasing impulsivity and aggression [18]. Selective serotonin reuptake inhibitors are less likely than serotonin-norepinephrine reuptake inhibitors to induce manic symptoms in those who exhibit primarily depressed mood [17, 62, 64]. Pregnancy and the postpartum period confer an increased risk of relapse in persons with bipolar disorder, and many of the medications used to manage the manic symptoms of bipolar disorder, particularly lithium and valproic acid, are teratogenic and contraindicated in pregnancy [17].

Nonpharmacologic Treatment

Nonpharmacologic management strategies are critical since many patients with SMI still experience symptoms despite appropriate pharmacologic therapy [65]. Cognitive behavioral therapy (CBT) that focuses on coping skills and cognitive restructuring (e.g., cognitive remediation) may help reduce the distress caused by hallucinations and delusions. This approach can be helpful in individuals with bipolar disorder as well as in those with schizophrenia [12, 17] although evidence regarding its effect in bipolar disorder is not definitive [65, 66]. Social and peer support can also be valuable adjuncts to therapy [15]. Social skills training can develop (or re-develop) life skills that may have been diminished during acute psychotic episodes [12]. Vocational training and rehabilitation, along with family-based interventions, can also promote increased function [15].

Psychiatric Emergencies

Emergency departments and primary care clinics are often the first sites where persons with new psychiatric symptoms receive evaluation [67]. The intensity of care for patients with SMI places a high burden on emergency and primary care, and increased access to mental health care would be optimal [68]. Patients who present with acute psychiatric symptoms, such as psychosis, should undergo a directed medical and psychiatric evaluation to rapidly identify potentially life-threatening conditions [67]. Underlying medical conditions, such as severe electrolyte abnormalities, hepatic encephalopathy, thyroid abnormalities, and infection may be contributing factors. Gathering a complete history with collateral information and a physical examination can direct the initial evaluation, including laboratory and imaging studies. It is important to consider acute intoxication with illicit substances or withdrawal, as well as intentional or unintentional overdose or withdrawal of prescription medications.

A safety evaluation is important early in the healthcare encounter since patients may be at risk of suicide and self-harm [58]. Mobile outreach, such as crisis units/teams can also play an important role by offering mental health services to medical providers and enhanced support for patients and families [69]. These teams extend mental healthcare services into the community and can be helpful in engaging with individuals who may be resistant to getting appropriate help by meeting them in a familiar setting. However, mobile crisis may not always be available, particularly in rural communities [69].

Healthcare Models and Programs

The high morbidity and mortality experienced by patients with SMI emphasize the need for whole-person care that integrates both physical and mental health. The Substance Abuse and Mental Health Services Administration (SAMHSA) has delineated six levels of integrated care which range from complete separation of services and processes, to sharing evidence-based screenings and practices at the same location, to creating one treatment plan that includes agreed upon evidence-based practices for all patients with a high functioning team approach that responds to all patient needs as they present [70]. Higher levels of integrated care have been associated with improving preventive services, reducing tobacco and alcohol use, and reductions in emergency room visits [71] and acute hospital days [72].

Assertive Community Treatment Teams

Assertive Community Treatment (ACT) teams are comprised of psychiatrists, social workers, behavioral health specialists, occupational therapists, and peer support specialists. The team is typically compromised of 10–12 members who provide care to up to 100 individuals with SMI [73]. ACT teams provide multidisciplinary outpatient care in the community as opposed to in a traditional office setting, resulting in approximately 80% of the care provided in the community in which the patient lives [73]. Traditionally, ACT teams work with individuals with the most severe forms of mental illness who have the most trouble engaging with traditional medical and psychiatric care [74]. ACT teams work with patients and families to offer wide-ranging support services including medication management, psychotherapy, assistance with accessing social services, life skills training, substance abuse counseling, and home visits [73]. ACT teams work in an integrated manner to promote self-determination and improve integration into the community. They achieve these goals using rapport-building strategies, motivational interviewing, and intensive medical management. An ACT team will typically have a caseload of 10 patients per staff member, with staff including psychiatric providers, nurses, therapists, case managers, and peer support specialists [73].

Ideally, providing care in the community with a constant team of care providers improves the relationship between patients and their care team, which in turn will increase trust in the healthcare system and adherence to treatment regimens. Individuals engaged with ACT teams have reduced psychiatric hospitalizations, improved housing stability, and improved treatment adherence. Unfortunately, ACT teams do not necessarily improve social function or reduce symptoms [74]. The team structure is provided as long as the patient needs this level of service, but is not necessarily indefinite.

Intensive case management (ICM) is another model of SMI care that grew out of the ACT movement. In addition to managing a patient's mental health, ICM teams offer care coordination, rehabilitation, social support, and community-based services such as employment and housing support. The patient-to-staff ratio in this model is no more than 20 to 1. ICM has been shown to increase patient engagement and decrease inpatient hospital days [75].

Community Mental Health Centers

The Community Mental Health Act of 1963 led to the development of community mental health centers around the country, promoting the philosophy that community-based care was a preferable alternative to institutionalization [76]. The network of clinics and outpatient treatment programs that arose subsequently aimed to provide mental health care to individuals with mental illness, with particular energy toward the care of those with SMI. Community mental health centers (CMHCs) are the public or nonprofit entities that were charged with offering psychiatric inpatient, outpatient, partial hospitalization, emergency services, and consultation [76]. In subsequent years, CMHCs faced challenges to their sustainability with inadequate federal or state funding; the limited resources translated into an inability to provide the type of community supports (group homes, family care homes, respite, employment support, etc.) that are required to assist many individuals with SMI to successfully live and integrate into their communities [77].

While many CMHCs were forced to close due to underfunding and lack of resources, those still in operation today provide important services and a safety net for patients with SMI, particularly those who are uninsured or carry public insurance. A typical CMHC is staffed with a psychiatrist, therapists, social workers, and peer support specialists. Funding sources include Medicaid, Medicare, private insurance, grants, and self-payment plans [73, 78]. Most of the care at CMHCs is done in person, but increasingly telehealth is being used to extend the reach of these programs to patients with poor access to transportation, or those living in rural areas.

Psychiatric Residential Treatment Facilities

Psychiatric residential treatment facilities (PRTFs) are specifically designated for persons under the age of 21 who have needs beyond outpatient services and require a safe environment to address these needs [79]. Payment is either through Medicaid, self-pay, or private insurance. These treatment centers house patients in a non-hospital setting where they receive intensive psychiatric and counseling services with the goal of returning them to their families and the community.

Psychiatric Hospitals

Inpatient psychiatric hospitals provide a secure setting to care for patients in acute mental health crisis, most often suicidal ideation, homicidal ideation, mania, or psychosis [80]. Patients can choose to seek care voluntarily, or can be involuntarily committed based on an assessed risk to self or other. The standards for admission to a state or private psychiatric inpatient facility vary slightly by state but usually require that the patient be a danger to themselves or others, or exhibit mental health that has deteriorated to the point where they cannot care for themselves [81]. Commitment procedures can be initiated by family members, law enforcement, health professionals, or court appointed persons [81]. A hearing to adjudicate the commitment is usually with hours to days after a commitment is put in place and patients have a right to protest the commitment. During admission, the treatment team must develop a plan of care that includes both medical management and therapeutic intervention [81]. Discharge is contingent on the medical team's judgment that a patient is safe to return home or to an alternate facility.

Inpatient units are generally locked and the facilities are designed for safety as well as therapeutic activities including medication administration, individual and group counseling, family meetings, and treatment planning. Staffing generally includes mental health technicians, psychiatric nurses, clinician therapists, case managers, and psychiatrists. Some facilities may additionally incorporate recreational therapy, occupational therapy, and pastoral or spiritual care. The use of chemical restraints (using sedative or antipsychotic medication) and physical restraints is rare and limited to instances of acute danger to oneself, other patients, or staff.

While psychiatric hospitalization is a mainstay of the continuum of care for patients with SMI, the goal of inpatient treatment teams is to de-escalate the patient to a lower level of care when able, in order to minimize time in a confined setting and support return to the outpatient setting when it is safe to do so. Community supports such as ACT teams, partial hospitalization, and group homes are designed to make this transition safer and more feasible.

Peer Support Specialists

Peer support specialists (PSS) play an increasing role in supporting persons with mental illness and substance use disorders. PSS are persons with a diagnosis of mental illness or substance use disorder who are stable from a psychiatric standpoint and/or in recovery; and who are trained to provide support to others with similar diagnoses [82]. These specialists offer one-on-one support, group classes on a variety of issues related to healthy living, and home or community visits [83]. Additional research is needed to assess the impact of peer support on mental health outcomes and quality of life for individuals with SMI, but several studies have suggested a potential decrease in mental health symptoms and substance use, and increased time spent in the community [83].

Emerging Service Models

There are innovative models emerging to address the health needs of patients with SMI. The Patient Centered Medical Home [84] and the Collaborative Care (IMPACT) Model [85] are evidence-based foundations that have been useful in guiding healthcare services in the identification and management of mental health disorders. However, these models may still fall short in meeting the complex needs of individuals with SMI. One model of enhanced primary care designed specifically for patients with SMI integrates behavioral health and primary care practice in a medical home that anticipates the medical, mental health, and psychosocial needs of this population [54, 86]. The structural elements of the model include smaller patient panel sizes that facilitate rapport-building and addressing medical complexity; an expanded team of staff and providers cross-trained in both behavioral health and primary care; ancillary services such as case management, financial counseling, and supported employment; and dedicated time for care coordination meetings and collaboration between team members and with community partners [54, 86]. This model has demonstrated improved outcomes in quality of care [86], decreased emergency services utilization [71], and decreased cost of inpatient medical care [72]. Another enhanced primary care model that integrates ACT team services into a medical home demonstrated a significant decrease in inpatient psychiatric utilization, when compared to traditional ACT or primary care settings [54].

Future Directions

The future care of individuals with SMI presents both challenges and opportunities. A significant shortage of behavioral health providers is projected [87]. The need to train, recruit, and retain mental health practitioners—including psychiatrists, psychiatric nurse practitioners, psychologists, clinical social workers, peer support specialists, nurses, and others—is daunting given the disparity in reimbursement for treatment of mental health conditions. Actions required to address the shortage and develop the workforce include public health campaigns to encourage and recruit behavioral health providers; funding for the development of behavioral health education and training programs at the undergraduate and graduate levels; increased loan forgiveness programs for behavioral health specialties; and increased training and reimbursement for peer support services [87]. Training that directly addresses the health needs of patients living with SMI would further bolster efforts to decrease the health disparities experienced by this population. For instance, in 2019 the American Psychological Association approved a new post-doctoral specialty for clinical psychologists in the psychology of serious mental illness [88].

The rapid growth and utilization of telehealth services has provided new opportunities to increase access to psychiatric care for individuals with SMI who reside in rural areas, or those with transportation barriers. Although navigating telehealth platforms can be challenging for individuals with limitations in cognition or inadequate life skills, many patients with SMI are able to connect virtually with their provider, and report a high degree of satisfaction with this mode of service delivery [89, 90]. Incorporating telehealth can further facilitate team-based care by allowing patients, caregivers, and providers in remote locations to meet virtually to coordinate care.

Primary care providers can play an important role in meeting the needs of individuals with SMI. Attention to mental health symptoms, treatments and their associated side effects, and coordination of care with psychiatric providers should be emphasized in primary care training and practice. Integrated models of care can increase access to both behavioral and physical health care, de-stigmatizing psychiatric conditions, minimizing duplication of services, and improving communication and team-based medical decision-making. Integration of peer support specialists into primary care, as well as mental health settings, allows peers to offer both emotional support and targeted interventions that help patients meet their own health goals and improve health outcomes [91].

The United States is transitioning from a fee-for-service to value-based reimbursement model. Value-based reimbursement holds promise for supporting the increased time and services that are needed to support patients with SMI. Enhanced primary care that integrates mental health services requires additional resources, but leads to higher quality of care and significant cost savings to healthcare systems. The extension and further integration of enhanced primary care with community-based programs and organizations are necessary to address the larger social determinants of health that contribute to health disparities. A future healthcare system that provides a continuum of health care and community support will ultimately improve the quality of life and alleviate the barriers to health and health care currently experienced by individuals with serious mental illness.

References

1. National Institutes of Mental Health. NIMH: mental illness. 2019. https://www.nimh.nih.gov/health/statistics/mental-illness. Accessed 16 Nov 2021.
2. SAMHSA National Registry of Evidence-Based Programs and Practices (NREPP). Behind the term: serious mental illness. 2016. https://www.hsdl.org/?view&did=801613. Accessed 14 Nov 2021.
3. Daumit GL, Anthony CB, Ford DE, et al. Pattern of mortality in a sample of Maryland residents with severe mental illness.

Psychiatry Res. 2010;176(2–3):242–5. https://doi.org/10.1016/j.psychres.2009.01.006.
4. de Mooij LD, Kikkert M, Theunissen J, et al. Dying too soon: excess mortality in severe mental illness. Front Psychiatry. 2019;10:855. https://doi.org/10.3389/fpsyt.2019.00855.
5. Druss BG, Zhao L, Von Esenwein S, Morrato EH, Marcus SC. Understanding excess mortality in persons with mental illness: 17-year follow up of a nationally representative US survey. Med Care. 2011;49(6):599–604. https://doi.org/10.1097/MLR.0b013e31820bf86e.
6. Walker ER, Cummings JR, Hockenberry JM, Druss BG. Insurance status, use of mental health services, and unmet need for mental health care in the United States. Psychiatr Serv. 2015;66(6):578–84. https://doi.org/10.1176/appi.ps.201400248.
7. American Psychiatric Association. Diagnostic and statistical manual of mental disorders, 5th edition: DSM-5. 5th ed. American Psychiatric Publishing; 1980. p. 991.
8. Griswold KS, Del Regno PA, Berger RC. Recognition and differential diagnosis of psychosis in primary care. Am Fam Physician. 2015;91(12):856–63.
9. Nevarez-Flores AG, Sanderson K, Breslin M, Carr VJ, Morgan VA, Neil AL. Systematic review of global functioning and quality of life in people with psychotic disorders. Epidemiol Psychiatr Sci. 2019;28(1):31–44. https://doi.org/10.1017/S2045796018000549.
10. Saarni SI, Viertiö S, Perälä J, Koskinen S, Lönnqvist J, Suvisaari J. Quality of life of people with schizophrenia, bipolar disorder and other psychotic disorders. Br J Psychiatry. 2010;197(5):386–94. https://doi.org/10.1192/bjp.bp.109.076489.
11. Jin H, Mosweu I. The societal cost of schizophrenia: A systematic review. Pharmacoeconomics. 2017;35(1):25–42. https://doi.org/10.1007/s40273-016-0444-6.
12. Lieberman JA, First MB. Psychotic disorders. N Engl J Med. 2018;379(3):270–80. https://doi.org/10.1056/NEJMra1801490.
13. Zamanpoor M. Schizophrenia in a genomic era: a review from the pathogenesis, genetic and environmental etiology to diagnosis and treatment insights. Psychiatr Genet. 2020;30(1):1–9. https://doi.org/10.1097/YPG.0000000000000245.
14. van Os J, Kapur S. Schizophrenia. Lancet. 2009;374(9690):635–45. https://doi.org/10.1016/S0140-6736(09)60995-8.
15. Schultz SK, Andreasen NC. Schizophrenia. Lancet. 1999;353(9162):1425–30. https://doi.org/10.1016/s0140-6736(98)07549-7.
16. Miller JN, Black DW. Schizoaffective disorder: a review. Ann Clin Psychiatry. 2019;31(1):47–53.
17. Anderson IM, Haddad PM, Scott J. Bipolar disorder. BMJ. 2012;345:e8508. https://doi.org/10.1136/bmj.e8508.
18. Benard V, Vaiva G, Masson M, Geoffroy PA. Lithium and suicide prevention in bipolar disorder. Encephale. 2016;42(3):234–41. https://doi.org/10.1016/j.encep.2016.02.006.
19. Uher R, Pallaskorpi S, Suominen K, Mantere O, Pavlova B, Isometsä E. Clinical course predicts long-term outcomes in bipolar disorder. Psychol Med. 2019;49(7):1109–17. https://doi.org/10.1017/S0033291718001678.
20. Tondo L, Vázquez GH, Baldessarini RJ. Depression and mania in bipolar disorder. Curr Neuropharmacol. 2017;15(3):353–8. https://doi.org/10.2174/1570159X14666160606210811.
21. National Coalition for the Homeless. Mental illness and homelessness. Jul 2009. https://www.nationalhomeless.org/factsheets/Mental_Illness.pdf. Accessed 15 Nov 2021.
22. Nasrallah HA, Meyer JM, Goff DC, et al. Low rates of treatment for hypertension, dyslipidemia and diabetes in schizophrenia: data from the CATIE schizophrenia trial sample at baseline. Schizophr Res. 2006;86(1-3):15–22. https://doi.org/10.1016/j.schres.2006.06.026.
23. De Hert M, Dekker JM, Wood D, Kahl KG, Holt RIG, Möller HJ. Cardiovascular disease and diabetes in people with severe mental illness position statement from the European Psychiatric Association (EPA), supported by the European Association for the Study of Diabetes (EASD) and the European Society of Cardiology (ESC). Eur Psychiatry. 2009;24(6):412–24. https://doi.org/10.1016/j.eurpsy.2009.01.005.
24. Cobos B, Haskard-Zolnierek K, Howard K. White coat hypertension: improving the patient-health care practitioner relationship. Psychol Res Behav Manag. 2015;8:133–41. https://doi.org/10.2147/PRBM.S61192.
25. Finley PR. Drug interactions with lithium: an update. Clin Pharmacokinet. 2016;55(8):925–41. https://doi.org/10.1007/s40262-016-0370-y.
26. De Hert M, Detraux J, van Winkel R, Yu W, Correll CU. Metabolic and cardiovascular adverse effects associated with antipsychotic drugs. Nat Rev Endocrinol. 2011;8(2):114–26. https://doi.org/10.1038/nrendo.2011.156.
27. Glassman AH, Bigger JT. Antipsychotic drugs: prolonged QTc interval, torsade de pointes, and sudden death. Am J Psychiatry. 2001;158(11):1774–82. https://doi.org/10.1176/appi.ajp.158.11.1774.
28. Olfson M, Gerhard T, Huang C, Crystal S, Stroup TS. Premature mortality among adults with schizophrenia in the United States. JAMA Psychiatry. 2015;72(12):1172–81. https://doi.org/10.1001/jamapsychiatry.2015.1737.
29. Pillinger T, McCutcheon RA, Vano L, et al. Comparative effects of 18 antipsychotics on metabolic function in patients with schizophrenia, predictors of metabolic dysregulation, and association with psychopathology: a systematic review and network meta-analysis. Lancet Psychiatry. 2020;7(1):64–77. https://doi.org/10.1016/S2215-0366(19)30416-X.
30. Vancampfort D, Stubbs B, Mitchell AJ, et al. Risk of metabolic syndrome and its components in people with schizophrenia and related psychotic disorders, bipolar disorder and major depressive disorder: a systematic review and meta-analysis. World Psychiatry. 2015;14(3):339–47. https://doi.org/10.1002/wps.20252.
31. Tiihonen J, Lönnqvist J, Wahlbeck K, et al. 11-year follow-up of mortality in patients with schizophrenia: a population-based cohort study (FIN11 study). Lancet. 2009;374(9690):620–7. https://doi.org/10.1016/S0140-6736(09)60742-X.
32. Allison DB, Newcomer JW, Dunn AL, et al. Obesity among those with mental disorders: a National Institute of Mental Health meeting report. Am J Prev Med. 2009;36(4):341–50. https://doi.org/10.1016/j.amepre.2008.11.020.
33. Cabassa LJ, Ezell JM, Lewis-Fernández R. Lifestyle interventions for adults with serious mental illness: a systematic literature review. Psychiatr Serv. 2010;61(8):774–82. https://doi.org/10.1176/ps.2010.61.8.774.
34. Calkin CV, Gardner DM, Ransom T, Alda M. The relationship between bipolar disorder and type 2 diabetes: more than just co-morbid disorders. Ann Med. 2013;45(2):171–81. https://doi.org/10.3109/07853890.2012.687835.
35. Bellivier F. Schizophrenia, antipsychotics and diabetes: genetic aspects. Eur Psychiatry. 2005;20(Suppl 4):S335–9. https://doi.org/10.1016/s0924-9338(05)80187-7.
36. American Diabetes Association, American Psychiatric Association, American Association of Clinical Endocrinologists, North American Association for the Study of Obesity. Consensus development conference on antipsychotic drugs and obesity and diabetes. Diabetes Care. 2004;27(2):596–601. https://doi.org/10.2337/diacare.27.2.596.
37. Jarskog LF, Yu R. Modifiable risk factors for cardiovascular disease in patients with severe mental illness. UpToDate; 2021.
38. Jackson JG, Diaz FJ, Lopez L, de Leon J. A combined analysis of worldwide studies demonstrates an association between bipolar

39. Lising-Enriquez K, George TP. Treatment of comorbid tobacco use in people with serious mental illness. J Psychiatry Neurosci. 2009;34(3):E1–2.
40. Anthenelli RM, Benowitz NL, West R, et al. Neuropsychiatric safety and efficacy of varenicline, bupropion, and nicotine patch in smokers with and without psychiatric disorders (EAGLES): a double-blind, randomised, placebo-controlled clinical trial. Lancet. 2016;387(10037):2507–20. https://doi.org/10.1016/S0140-6736(16)30272-0.
41. Evins AE, Cather C, Laffer A. Treatment of tobacco use disorders in smokers with serious mental illness: toward clinical best practices. Harv Rev Psychiatry. 2015;23(2):90–8. https://doi.org/10.1097/HRP.0000000000000063.
42. Roberts E, Eden Evins A, McNeill A, Robson D. Efficacy and tolerability of pharmacotherapy for smoking cessation in adults with serious mental illness: a systematic review and network meta-analysis. Addiction. 2016;111(4):599–612. https://doi.org/10.1111/add.13236.
43. Hartz SM, Pato CN, Medeiros H, et al. Comorbidity of severe psychotic disorders with measures of substance use. JAMA Psychiatry. 2014;71(3):248–54. https://doi.org/10.1001/jamapsychiatry.2013.3726.
44. Green AI, Drake RE, Brunette MF, Noordsy DL. Schizophrenia and co-occurring substance use disorder. Am J Psychiatry. 2007;164(3):402–8. https://doi.org/10.1176/ajp.2007.164.3.402.
45. Li KJ, Chen A, DeLisi LE. Opioid use and schizophrenia. Curr Opin Psychiatry. 2020;33(3):219–24. https://doi.org/10.1097/YCO.0000000000000593.
46. Robertson AG, Easter MM, Lin H, Frisman LK, Swanson JW, Swartz MS. Medication-assisted treatment for alcohol-dependent adults with serious mental illness and criminal justice involvement: effects on treatment utilization and outcomes. Am J Psychiatry. 2018;175(7):665–73. https://doi.org/10.1176/appi.ajp.2018.17060688.
47. About Intellectual and Developmental Disabilities (IDDs) | NICHD—Eunice Kennedy Shriver National Institute of Child Health and Human Development. https://www.nichd.nih.gov/health/topics/idds/conditioninfo. Accessed 4 Mar 2022.
48. Munir KM. The co-occurrence of mental disorders in children and adolescents with intellectual disability/intellectual developmental disorder. Curr Opin Psychiatry. 2016;29(2):95–102. https://doi.org/10.1097/YCO.0000000000000236.
49. About L'Arche USA | Communities for Intellectual Disabilities. https://www.larcheusa.org/about/. Accessed 4 Mar 2022.
50. Traumatic Brain Injury Information Page | National Institute of Neurological Disorders and Stroke. https://www.ninds.nih.gov/Disorders/All-Disorders/Traumatic-Brain-Injury-Information-Page. Accessed 4 Mar 2022.
51. Fujii DE, Ahmed I. Psychotic disorder caused by traumatic brain injury. Psychiatr Clin North Am. 2014;37(1):113–24. https://doi.org/10.1016/j.psc.2013.11.006.
52. Press D. Management of neuropsychiatric symptoms of dementia. UpToDate; 2020.
53. American Geriatrics Society. American Geriatrics Society 2019 Updated AGS Beers Criteria® for potentially inappropriate medication use in older adults. J Am Geriatr Soc. 2019;67(4):674–94. https://doi.org/10.1111/jgs.15767.
54. Steiner BD, Wahrenberger JT, Raney L. Providing effective primary care for patients with serious mental illness: additional components to enhance practice. Community Ment Health J. 2020;56(4):592–6. https://doi.org/10.1007/s10597-019-00517-2.
55. Kishimoto T, Hagi K, Kurokawa S, Kane JM, Correll CU. Long-acting injectable versus oral antipsychotics for the maintenance treatment of schizophrenia: a systematic review and comparative meta-analysis of randomised, cohort, and pre-post studies. Lancet Psychiatry. 2021;6 https://doi.org/10.1016/S2215-0366(21)00039-0.
56. Pacchiarotti I, Tiihonen J, Kotzalidis GD, et al. Long-acting injectable antipsychotics (LAIs) for maintenance treatment of bipolar and schizoaffective disorders: a systematic review. Eur Neuropsychopharmacol. 2019;29(4):457–70. https://doi.org/10.1016/j.euroneuro.2019.02.003.
57. Huhn M, Nikolakopoulou A, Schneider-Thoma J, et al. Comparative efficacy and tolerability of 32 oral antipsychotics for the acute treatment of adults with multi-episode schizophrenia: a systematic review and network meta-analysis. Lancet. 2019;394(10202):939–51. https://doi.org/10.1016/S0140-6736(19)31135-3.
58. Keepers GA, Fochtmann LJ, Anzia JM, et al. The American Psychiatric Association practice guideline for the treatment of patients with schizophrenia. Am J Psychiatry. 2020;177(9):868–72. https://doi.org/10.1176/appi.ajp.2020.177901.
59. Stroup TS, Marder S. Schizophrenia in adults: Maintenance therapy and side effect management—UpToDate. https://www.uptodate.com/contents/schizophrenia-in-adults-maintenance-therapy-and-side-effect-management?search=acute%20dystonia&sectionRank=1&usage_type=default&anchor=H2486805191&source=machineLearning&selectedTitle=3~110&display_rank=3#H2486805191. Accessed 4 Mar 2022.
60. Canuso CM, Schooler N, Carothers J, et al. Paliperidone extended-release in schizoaffective disorder: a randomized, controlled study comparing a flexible dose with placebo in patients treated with and without antidepressants and/or mood stabilizers. J Clin Psychopharmacol. 2010;30(5):487–95. https://doi.org/10.1097/JCP.0b013e3181eeb600.
61. Lindenmayer J-P, Kaur A. Antipsychotic management of schizoaffective disorder: a review. Drugs. 2016;76(5):589–604. https://doi.org/10.1007/s40265-016-0551-x.
62. McGirr A, Vöhringer PA, Ghaemi SN, Lam RW, Yatham LN. Safety and efficacy of adjunctive second-generation antidepressant therapy with a mood stabiliser or an atypical antipsychotic in acute bipolar depression: a systematic review and meta-analysis of randomised placebo-controlled trials. Lancet Psychiatry. 2016;3(12):1138–46. https://doi.org/10.1016/S2215-0366(16)30264-4.
63. Dean OM, Gliddon E, Van Rheenen TE, et al. An update on adjunctive treatment options for bipolar disorder. Bipolar Disord. 2018;20(2):87–96. https://doi.org/10.1111/bdi.12601.
64. MacQueen GM, Young LT. Bipolar II disorder: symptoms, course, and response to treatment. Psychiatr Serv. 2001;52(3):358–61. https://doi.org/10.1176/appi.ps.52.3.358.
65. Jones C, Hacker D, Meaden A, et al. Cognitive behavioural therapy plus standard care versus standard care plus other psychosocial treatments for people with schizophrenia. Cochrane Database Syst Rev. 2018;11:CD008712. https://doi.org/10.1002/14651858.CD008712.pub3.
66. Summary E. Treatment for bipolar disorder in adults: a systematic review.
67. Etlouba Y, Laher A, Motara F, Moolla M, Ariefdien N. First presentation with psychotic symptoms to the emergency department. J Emerg Med. 2018;55(1):78–86. https://doi.org/10.1016/j.jemermed.2018.04.014.
68. Bahji A, Altomare J, Sapru A, Haze S, Prasad S, Egan R. Predictors of hospital admission for patients presenting with psychiatric emergencies: a retrospective, cohort study. Psychiatry Res. 2020;290:113149. https://doi.org/10.1016/j.psychres.2020.113149.
69. Murphy SM, Irving CB, Adams CE, Waqar M. Crisis intervention for people with severe mental illnesses. Cochrane Database Syst Rev. 2015;(12):CD001087. https://doi.org/10.1002/14651858.CD001087.pub5.

70. Heath B Jr, Reynolds K, Romero PW. A standard framework for levels of integrated healthcare. SAMSHA-HRSA Center for Integrated Health Solutions; 2013.
71. Belson C, Sheitman B, Steiner B. The effects of an enhanced primary care model for patients with serious mental illness on emergency department utilization. Community Ment Health J. 2020;56(7):1311–7. https://doi.org/10.1007/s10597-020-00645-0.
72. Grove LR, Gertner AK, Swietek KE, et al. Effect of enhanced primary care for people with serious mental illness on service use and screening. J Gen Intern Med. 2021;36(4):970–7. https://doi.org/10.1007/s11606-020-06429-2.
73. U.S. Department of Health and Human Services Substance Abuse and Mental Health Services Administration. Building your program: assertive community treatment. https://store.samhsa.gov/sites/default/files/d7/priv/buildingyourprogram-act_1.pdf. Accessed 2 Mar 2022.
74. Morse G, Monroe-DeVita M, York MM, et al. Implementing illness management and recovery within assertive community treatment teams: a qualitative study. Psychiatr Rehabil J. 2020;43(2):121–31. https://doi.org/10.1037/prj0000387.
75. Dieterich M, Irving CB, Bergman H, Khokhar MA, Park B, Marshall M. Intensive case management for severe mental illness. Cochrane Database Syst Rev. 2017;1:CD007906. https://doi.org/10.1002/14651858.CD007906.pub3.
76. Community Mental Health Act. National Council. https://www.thenationalcouncil.org/about/national-mental-health-association/overview/community-mental-health-act/. Accessed 4 Mar 2022.
77. Erickson B. Deinstitutionalization through optimism: the community mental health act of 1963. Am J Psychiatr Resid J. 2021;16(4):6–7. https://doi.org/10.1176/appi.ajp-rj.2021.160404.
78. Assertive Community Treatment | NCDHHS. https://www.ncdhhs.gov/divisions/mental-health-developmental-disabilities-and-substance-abuse/adult-mental-health-services/assertive-community-treatment. Accessed 4 Mar 2022.
79. Center for Medicare and Medicaid Services. What is a PRTF? http://www.cms.gov/Medicare/Provider-Enrollment-and-Certification/CertificationandComplianc/Downloads/WhatisaPRTF.pdf. Accessed 4 Mar 2022.
80. Psychiatric Hospitals | CMS. https://www.cms.gov/Medicare/Provider-Enrollment-and-Certification/CertificationandComplianc/PsychHospitals. Accessed 4 Mar 2022.
81. Involuntary commitment (assisted treatment) standards (50 states)—treatment advocacy center report. Mental Illness Policy Org. https://mentalillnesspolicy.org/national-studies/state-standards-involuntary-treatment.html. Accessed 4 Mar 2022.
82. Chien WT, Clifton AV, Zhao S, Lui S. Peer support for people with schizophrenia or other serious mental illness. Cochrane Database Syst Rev. 2019;4:CD010880. https://doi.org/10.1002/14651858.CD010880.pub2.
83. An assessment of innovative models of peer support services in behavioral health to reduce preventable acute hospitalization and readmissions. Published online 30 Nov 2015.
84. Bogucki OE, Williams MD, Solberg LI, Rossom RC, Sawchuk CN. The role of the patient-centered medical home in treating depression. Curr Psychiatry Rep. 2020;22(9):47. https://doi.org/10.1007/s11920-020-01167-y.
85. Unützer J, Katon W, Callahan CM, et al. Collaborative care management of late-life depression in the primary care setting: a randomized controlled trial. JAMA. 2002;288(22):2836–45. https://doi.org/10.1001/jama.288.22.2836.
86. Perrin J, Reimann B, Capobianco J, Wahrenberger JT, Sheitman BB, Steiner BD. A model of enhanced primary care for patients with severe mental illness. N C Med J. 2018;79(4):240–4. https://doi.org/10.18043/ncm.79.4.240.
87. Substance Abuse and Mental Health Services Administration. Behavioral health workforce report. Substance Abuse and Mental Health Services Administration; 2021. https://annapoliscoalition.org/wp-content/uploads/2021/03/behavioral-health-workforce-report-SAMHSA-2.pdf. Accessed 4 Mar 2022.
88. Abrams Z. New hope for people with serious mental illness. Monit Psychol. 2019;50(11). https://www.apa.org/monitor/2019/12/new-hope#. Accessed 4 Mar 2022.
89. Santesteban-Echarri O, Piskulic D, Nyman RK, Addington J. Telehealth interventions for schizophrenia-spectrum disorders and clinical high-risk for psychosis individuals: a scoping review. J Telemed Telecare. 2020;26(1–2):14–20. https://doi.org/10.1177/1357633X18794100.
90. Kasckow J, Felmet K, Appelt C, Thompson R, Rotondi A, Haas G. Telepsychiatry in the assessment and treatment of schizophrenia. Clin Schizophr Relat Psychoses. 2014;8(1):21–27A. https://doi.org/10.3371/CSRP.KAFE.021513.
91. Cabassa LJ, Camacho D, Vélez-Grau CM, Stefancic A. Peer-based health interventions for people with serious mental illness: a systematic literature review. J Psychiatr Res. 2017;84:80–9. https://doi.org/10.1016/j.jpsychires.2016.09.021.

Special Population: LGBTQ Community

Julie M. Austen, Rita Lahlou, and Modjulie Moore

Introduction

All people develop a gender identity and sexual orientation via an established developmental trajectory [1]. Some gender identities and sexual orientations have been historically structurally and systematically marginalized, leading to global discrimination, adversity, and stigmatization, all of which affect health outcomes and limit care. The people who experience this marginalization are typically referred to as sexual and gender minority (SGM) populations. The provision of excellent health care to SGM people requires an understanding of the complexity of stigma and its relationship to trauma and subsequent risk behaviors, as well the interaction of biology, social determinants of health, and psychology (the biopsychosocial model). Clinicians who are open, curious, and comfortable with the SGM community (cultural humility) coupled with knowledge of needs, resources, and approaches that are relevant to that community (clinical competence) will provide the best health care. Health systems that reduce stigma within the patient–provider relationship and address systemic inequalities by increasing access and inclusion will further the provision of quality health care.

Definitions and Demographics

Table 26.1 lists common terms that apply to SGM populations. A more exhaustive list of terms is provided by the Human Rights Campaign [2]. Sexual orientation is generally sensed by children between 7 and 14 years of age, and a process of development follows with young people exploring and adopting sexual orientation earlier than in previous generations [3]. Gender identity refers to the persistent and deeply felt psychological sense of being male or female, which is distinct from a person's biological sex, which is the sex assigned at birth based upon initial visualization of genitalia and chromosomes. There is a growing understanding of the complex and dynamic interplay of hormones, genes, and neuroanatomical factors that shape sex characteristics with a resultant paradigm shift away from a binary polarity of sex and gender (male and female) toward a spectrum of developmental trajectories and experiences [4]. People who identify as a gender that is different than their assigned sex at birth may identify as transgender, non-binary, gender non-conforming, gender expansive, genderqueer, or many other identities along the gender spectrum. Gender may be experienced or expressed fluidly at the individual level.

The term queer is a broad category used by individuals or by communities and has been reclaimed as an alternative to sexual orientation and gender labels. Another widely used term is LGBTQIA+, which refers to the community that identifies as lesbian, gay, bisexual, transgender, queer/questioning, intersex, asexual/aromantic/agender, or other identities. Individuals in this community may have other identities, such as those based on race, ethnicity, socioeconomic status, or ability, a phenomenon known as *intersectionality*, the accumulation of which may introduce even more barriers to health and wellness, as well as unique and multiplicative opportunities for resiliency.

Population estimates of SGM people vary widely due to differences in how this data is collected (or not collected) via surveys or medical records. Most large national surveys do not collect sexual orientation and gender identity data (SOGI), and there remains confusion and inconsistency in implementing best practices for collecting this data [5, 6]. Further, SGM people may not feel comfortable sharing SOGI data with providers or organizations they deem to be questionably safe or affirming, and identities may shift overtime. Thus, it is likely that demographic data does not fully

J. M. Austen
Frank Porter Graham Child Development Institute, University of North Carolina at Chapel Hill, Chapel Hill, NC, USA
e-mail: austen@unc.edu

R. Lahlou · M. Moore (✉)
Department of Family Medicine, University of North Carolina at Chapel Hill, Chapel Hill, NC, USA
e-mail: rita_lahlou@med.unc.edu; Modjulie_Moore@med.unc.edu

Table 26.1 Terms used regarding sexual orientation or gender identity

Term	Definition
Sexual orientation	An inherent or immutable enduring emotional, romantic, or sexual attraction to other people; it is independent of gender identity.
Gay	A person who is emotionally, romantically, or sexually attracted to members of the same gender. Men, women, and non-binary people may use this term to describe themselves.
Lesbian	A woman who is emotionally, romantically, or sexually attracted to other women. Women and non-binary people may use this term to describe themselves.
Bisexual	A person whose primary sexual and affectional orientation is toward people of the same and other genders, or toward people regardless of their gender; used interchangeably with pansexual.
Heterosexual	A person whose emotional, romantic, or sexual attraction is toward people of a gender other than their own.
Asexual	Generally characterized by not feeling sexual attraction or a desire for partnered sexuality. Asexuality is distinct from celibacy, which is the deliberate abstention from sexual activity. "Ace" for short.
Gender identity	One's innermost concept of self as male, female, a blend of both or neither—how individuals perceive themselves and what they call themselves; may be the same or different from the sex assigned at birth.
Sex	A categorization based on the appearance of the genitalia at birth.
Sex assigned at birth	The sex (male, female, or intersex) that a medical provider uses to describe a child at birth based on their external anatomy. AMAB = assigned male at birth; AFAB = assigned female at birth. Preferred to "natal sex."
Transgender	An umbrella term for people whose gender identity and/or expression is different from cultural expectations based on the sex they were assigned at birth. This is distinct from sexual orientation.
Cisgender	A term used to describe a person whose gender identity aligns with those typically associated with the sex assigned to them at birth.
Non-binary	A person who does not identify exclusively as a man or a woman; may identify as being both a man and a woman, somewhere in between, or as outside these categories. While many also identify as transgender, not all non-binary people do. Non-binary can also be used as an umbrella term encompassing identities such as agender, bigender, genderqueer, or gender-fluid.
Gender affirmation	An interpersonal, interactive process whereby a person receives social recognition and support for their gender identity and expression.
Queer	A term expressing a spectrum of identities and orientations that are counter to the mainstream; a catch-all term that includes those who do not identify as exclusively straight and/or have non-binary or gender-expansive identities. This term was previously used as a slur but has been reclaimed by many parts of the LGBTQ movement.
Questioning	A term used to describe people who are in the process of exploring their sexual orientation or gender identity; may be testing the waters before coming out.
Two-spirit	A term that honors the inextricable relationship between sexuality and gender in Indigenous cultures [87].
Intersex	People born with a variety of differences in their sex traits and reproductive anatomy, which may include differences in genitalia, chromosomes, gonads, internal sex organs, hormone production, hormone response, and/or secondary sex traits.
Ally	Someone who is actively supportive of LGBTQ people, encompassing straight and cisgender people as well as those within the LGBTQ community who support each other.

represent the population identifying as SGM, and the following statistics may under-represent the population. A 2022 Gallup poll found that 7.1% of respondents identify as lesbian, gay, bisexual, or transgender (LGBT), which is double the percentage from 2012, when Gallup first measured this [7]. One-fifth of people born between 1997 and 2003 (Generation Z) identify as LGBT (mostly bisexual), which is nearly double the proportion of millennials (born between 1981 and 1886) who do so, while the gap widens even further when compared to older generations. Approximately 62% of queer or transgender persons of color (QTPOC) are under 34 years of age, while 45% of White LGBT people are in that age group [8]. Forty percent of QTPOC people are raising children, compared to 22% of LGBT White people. Nearly 13% of US adults 65 years of age and older identify as SGM, an estimate that is expected to grow over the years as young people age [9].

Stigma, Discrimination, and Minority Stress

Both past and present social factors influence risk for health disparities [10]. Examples of past factors include unmet social determinants of health, relative invisibility, historical medical stigma (such as the AIDS epidemic), and the codifying of discrimination into state and federal policies. Present factors include internalized homo- and transphobia and identity masking. These experiences limit access to high-quality health care, reductions in the efficacy of the patient-provider relationship, limited trust of the medical team, and increases in morbidity and mortality. People who identify as SGM are more likely to avoid or delay health care due to fear of discrimination and experience higher rates of stress and adversity [3]. These experiences cause marginalized people to employ high-risk coping strategies, such as substance use, unhealthy eating, and other self-injurious activities in repetitive and unhealthy ways. Suboptimal self-esteem, self-efficacy, and self-worth may exacerbate psychological contexts for interpersonal violence, abuse, and exploitation, all of which contribute to a persistent state of physiological stress, known as minority stress [11]. Minority stress is experienced neurobiologically as activation of the autonomic nervous system via the hypothalamic-pituitary-adrenal axis, known as "fight-or-flight," and is linked to health disparities via excess energy spent in a neurobiologically aroused state [12]. Patients are more likely to delay or disengage from care as a protection strategy to minimize the effects of minority stress. This delay in care may lead to disease progression and sequala in otherwise treatable and preventable diseases, including depression, substance use disorders, diabetes, human immunodeficiency virus (HIV) infection, and cancer. The combined effect of minority stress, reduced access and quality, and risky behaviors contribute to worse health outcomes, known as health disparities.

When SGM people do access to care, they report that providers' lack of knowledge and discrimination within medical settings are barriers to feeling safe enough to participate fully in their medical care [13]. Health care providers who do not identify as SGM report not feeling knowledgeable and untrained about LGBTQ culture (only 9.4% felt very knowledgeable) [14].

Organizing Inclusive Chronic Care

To address the effect of social determinants on a person's health, improve outcomes, and promote well-being, health care systems and individual clinicians must promote trust and patient safety [15, 16]. Clinicians increase the likelihood that SGM patients will receive preventive care and achieve better outcomes when they create inclusive spaces and are trained in culturally relevant models [17]. Health systems must acknowledge that standardized practices often fail to meet the needs of marginalized people and strive to make all patients, regardless of gender and sexual identities, feel safe and comfortable disclosing their SGM identities and health behaviors. The barriers to achieving this are multifaceted and span organizational, clinic, and clinician practices [18].

Health Care System Considerations

The health care system should be inclusive at every level, including the electronic health record (EHR), clinical policies, and medical staff training, with an ongoing accountability for inclusive and equitable treatment, and an understanding of the local, state, and federal contexts that impact the lives of SGM people [19].

The EHR is an important space for sexual orientation and gender identity data entry. Many EHRs include templates for collecting SOGI data in inclusive ways with some especially innovative models including templates for anatomy and body part inventories [20, 21].

System-wide policies should ensure inclusivity, with patients aware of their rights in terms of accessible, inclusive, and equitable care, which can be included in the patient Bill of Rights document that many organizations provide. Organizations should monitor patient satisfaction and outcomes in relation to the service philosophy embedded within a Bill of Rights, and staff should be trained to exemplify this philosophy.

Patients benefit when health care organizations have a sense of the local context of their practices to understand how communities can be supported. For example, practices in communities with a higher prevalence of anal cancer or in a community with a higher number of gender diverse individuals should ensure that they are equipped and skilled to provide relevant services, such as the ability to provide high-resolution anal colposcopy or gender-supportive care. It is also important to understand state laws and policies as some states restrict services to SGM patients, particularly minors, and thereby lead people to black market medications or unsupported approaches to care. Many state and local organizations maintain up-to-date resources for clinicians who must weigh medical ethics against non-evidence-informed policies and law. There are also federal laws on the inclusion of sexual and gender minorities that apply in settings that receive federal funds, such as those that accept Medicare payments or within a federally qualified health center (FQHC).

Clinic and Practice Considerations

Clinics and practices can improve access to services and support patient sense of safety and trust firstly by ensuring low-cost care, such as the access to a FQHC. These low-cost, high-service models improve access and coordination of care for SGM people, who are more likely to be uninsured or underinsured than cisgender/heterosexual peers [22]. Integrated behavioral health models within a primary care practice further enhance access to mental and behavioral health care.

Clinical policies supporting equity and inclusion create an affirming environment in which all staff are trained and held accountable to inclusion principles. Signs, images, health information displays, inclusive bathrooms, and appropriate pronoun use are all ways to communicate safety and welcome to SGM persons. Adequate time and the provision of comprehensive multidisciplinary care, as well as access to urgent care, provide harm reduction strategies and promote connection to primary care and community services. These considerations are best achieved with collaborative models of care, which involve medical, behavioral, social, legal, and financial supports [23].

Youth presenting for chronic disease management require several additional considerations to assure a trusting patient–provider relationship. Like all young people, SGM adolescents need developmentally appropriate privacy with their medical provider to discuss sexual health, mental health, and other general health information [24]. Clinicians should ascertain what experience the young person has had to guide the conversation, such as whether the adolescent has endured sexual trauma or exploitation. The electronic medical record, staff actions, and practice policy must follow state law around youth patient confidentiality. Many youths are developmentally able to provide assent for medical care beginning at age 12 years, though the laws on this vary by state. Familiarity with state laws assures that autonomy is afforded to youth in experientially and developmentally appropriate ways.

Trauma-informed care is defined as an approach to care, on a clinical and organizational level, that recognizes the impact of previous trauma on patients. This model was developed in the 1970s to address the high levels of trauma in US veterans from the Vietnam War and is now used across organizations to provide policies, procedures, and practices that create environments that avoid re-traumatization such as may have been experienced by members of the SGM community.

Cultural Humility and Inclusive Practices

Training clinicians and staff in the provision of care that is respectful and culturally appropriate benefits both patients and providers and is particularly effective in improving the health care experience for SGM people [25]. To carry out medical care ethically, it is helpful for clinicians, nurses, and clerical and administrative staff explore their own beliefs and identity around gender and sexuality, and to be open to providing respectful care to those with different experience. Health care team members can enhance the inclusive care environment by using preferred names and pronouns and inclusive language (Table 26.2). Even providers who identify as members of the SGM community can acknowledge that their experiences differ from some of their patients due to other intersections like race, ethnicity, socioeconomic status, outness, and geography.

Continuity, communication, and coordination of care are enhanced when a patient receives practical knowledge from the clinician, provided in a sensitive manner. Based on negative experiences in the past, SGM identifying patients may be reluctant to trust clinicians, fearing judgment and substan-

Table 26.2 Exclusive and inclusive language

Exclusive language	Inclusive language
Name Ms. Last name or Mr. Last name Ms. First name or Mr. Last name (A not uncommon practice in the southern United States)	Preferred name Mx. Last name or just first name
Male or Female	What is your gender identity? What was your sex assigned at birth? What are your pronouns? (She/her, he/him, they/them, other) Gender _____ (documented)
Marital Status	Relationship Status (single, married, partnered, widowed, separated, divorced, polyamorous)
Mother or Father	Parent or Guardian
Brother or Sister	Sibling, Sibs
Husband or Wife	Partner or Spouse
Pregnant Woman	Pregnant person Birthing person or parent
Breastfeeding	Chestfeeding, Nursing, Lactation
How may I help you, sir (or ma'am)?	How may I help you?

dard care if they reveal aspects of their past medical history or gender and sexual identities. The clinician may unknowingly impair communication during the visit because of lack of training or discomfort with caring for individuals who have different sexual practices and preferences and gender identities than their own [26]. Because most patients may be from non-marginalized groups, many clinicians lack the experience and understanding of SGM patients' health care needs or how to facilitate gender or sexuality affirming care, including the use of "heterosexist concepts" when taking a social or sexual history. Patients can feel more accepted when clinician inquire about family or social history by asking "who are the important people in your life?" rather than asking about marital status or assuming a traditional family structure. Avoiding assumptions and using open-ended questions creates a space for patients to feel comfortable and forthcoming. Patients are generally open to sharing their sexual orientation and history once they feel safe to do so.

Transgender patients report discomfort with unnecessary and invasive questions or examinations in the medical setting [27]. However, the provision of good medical care depends on an understanding of the patient's anatomy, sexual practices, and personal behaviors. Explaining to the patient that an understanding of body parts and sexual practices determines which screening tests for sexually transmitted infections or cancer may be indicated is usually understood by patients and reassures the patient that the clinician is open to hearing non-traditional answers. Awareness that a transgender man who still has a uterus may be having vaginal sex with men leads to a discussion on desire for pregnancy or preference for contraception. It may be useful to explain the rationale for each part of the physical exam—and to ensure there is rationale. With higher rates of trauma in the SGM community, asking for permission to examine the patient, and allowing patient autonomy and involvement (such as offering self-insertion of a speculum), mindful positioning and draping, and professional language create a safe experience that is not re-traumatizing.

Documentation of sexual orientation and gender identity (SOGI) information in the electronic health record (EHR) is recommended by the Institute of Medicine and the Joint Commission, as this helps in population health management, clinical decision support, and the promotion of patient-centered inclusive care at the individual, organizational, and national levels [28, 29]. All EHR systems certified under the federal Meaningful Use Stage 3 Incentive Program are required to record SOGI data, and the US Health Resources and Services Administration's Bureau of Primary Health Care requires all federally qualified health centers (FQHCs) to report patient SOGI data on an annual basis [30, 31].

Patient Care for Chronic Conditions

All patients deserve access to comprehensive primary care including cancer screening, management of chronic conditions, and support for overall wellness. An inclusive approach to health care reduces the isolation felt by many SGM patients and encourages them to engage in their own health care. Common conditions that affect the SGM population are the same as those that affect the adult population including sleep disorders, asthma, high blood pressure, high cholesterol, arthritis, and diabetes [3]. Transgender people are particularly susceptible, with 26% describing their health as poor or fair. Evidence-based guideline driven care is appropriate for these common chronic conditions. Considering psychosocial, mental, and sexual health in the context of physical health, as well as screening for these conditions, builds a trusting relationship with the clinician and improves outcomes for the patient.

Psychosocial Factors

When clinicians address the psychosocial elements of patients' health, including social determinants of health, they build trust by addressing important issues for the individual while demonstrating knowledge of the specific needs of communities [32]. When psychosocial needs are unmet, patients often cope with unhealthy behaviors such as substance use or unhealthy eating practices [33, 34].

The personal relationships of SGM individuals influence psychosocial health. Patients may find their families of origin supportive, or they may have others who they trust and want to include in their health care decisions. Some patients may have more than one partner or family, called polyamorous relationships, and benefit from lack of judgment or marginalization [35].

Clinicians should interview patients both with and without their important people present to ensure privacy and the opportunity to ensure safe relationship dynamics, including the absence of trauma or exploitation. SGM people are more likely to experience intimate violence than their cisgender or heterosexual peers [36]. Trauma-informed care is care that provides the space and time to allow a patient to share life experiences that may affect health. This includes a recognition that past trauma, including abuse, often impacts the psychosocial and physical health of a patient. Patience is required to support the patient while helping find a path to recovery, as well as an understanding that leaving abusive relationships takes time, energy, and planning [37].

Mental Health

People who identify as SGM have higher rates of mental health disorders, including depression, anxiety, unhealthy eating, and substance use, often compounded by the lack of affirming treatment in the community where they grew up or still live [38]. Twenty-eight percent of SGM people report serious mental illness [3]. Validated screening tools for mental health conditions are part of a supportive and comprehensive care plan to identify mental health conditions for all patients, including those in the SGM community. These include the Patient Health Questionnaire 2 and 9 (PHQ-2 and PHQ-9) for depression and the General Anxiety Disorder-7 (GAD-7), among others. Tools that screen for adverse childhood experiences (ACEs) may also be appropriate as 70% of SGM people report bullying and emotional abuse, 41% report physical abuse, and 38% report sexual abuse during childhood [3].

Thirty-six percent of SGM people report having been subjected to conversion therapy by a health care provider [3]. These efforts to change a person's sexual orientation or gender identity have negative effects on the recipients' mental health, including an increased risk of suicide [39]. This practice is misguided, detrimental, and discredited, leading multiple medical, legal, and human rights organizations to formally oppose it [40–45].

Conversion therapy, sexual assault, interpersonal violence, discrimination, minority stress, and other adverse events all contribute to an increased rate of posttraumatic stress disorder (PTSD) in the SGM community or can complicate treatment for PTSD due to other causes. There are evidence-based practices for screening and treatment members of the SGM community [46].

Eating disorders, defined as persistent and extreme disturbance in eating-related behaviors, have a high prevalence rate in the SGM community. Women who identify as lesbian have a higher rate of binge eating and obesity, while men who identify as gay experience anorexia and bulimia at a higher rate [47]. Eating disorders may be coupled with intrusive and distressing preoccupation with the body (body dysmorphic syndrome), and some eating disorder-related behavior overlaps with substance use, which may inhibit or exacerbate appetite, such as stimulant use or marijuana, respectively. Cognitive behavioral therapy, interpersonal therapy, or dialectical behavioral therapy can be helpful in eating and body image disorders.

Though not a mental health issue per se, neurodivergence, specifically autism, is experienced at a higher rate by the transgender and gender diverse community [48]. Affirming and supportive practices benefit autistic people regardless of their sexual or gender identity [49].

It is important to acknowledge the history and harmful effects of pathologizing and criminalizing the behavior of people who identify as sexual and gender minorities, including years of including these characteristics as a psychiatric illness [50]. Patients may fear being labeled with a mental health diagnosis. Implicit bias can be transmitted through electronic health records so clinicians can promote affirming care by discussing and writing about mental health symptoms using descriptive terms such as frequency, intensity, and duration, onset, and effect on life, rather than using diagnostic labels [51].

Suicide

Suicide is a leading cause of death in the United States, especially among men who take their life at nearly four times the rate of females. Men in the SGM community are at even greater risk for suicide or suicide attempts, especially before 25 years of age. Almost a quarter (24%) of high school students identifying as lesbian, gay, or bisexual reported attempting suicide in the prior 12 months [52]. This rate is four times higher than the rate reported among heterosexual students (6.4%). Nearly half of transgender people have thought about or attempted suicide or engaged in non-suicidal self-injury during their lifetime [3, 53].

Universal suicide screening and effective referral and crisis management should be provided in clinical practice. Collaborative Assessment and Management of Suicidality (CAMS) is an evidence-based therapeutic framework that appears promising to reduce suicidal ideation and suicidal cognition [54]. The common practice of "suicide contracting," in which a clinician asks a patient to sign a contract that they will not harm themselves, is considered outdated and harmful with the potential to create division within the patient–provider relationship. The preferred practice is developing and monitoring a safety plan and being aware of SGM specific resources such as The Trevor Project for youth (www.thetrevorproject.org/) and Trans Lifeline (https://translifeline.org/about/), which provides peer-support for trans people in crisis.

Substance Use Disorders

Increased substance use, particularly alcohol, is associated with minority stress in SGM people [55]. Moderate to severe use of alcohol is persistent across the age spectrum, particularly for female SGMs, as is the use of club drugs such as methamphetamine and cocaine by transgender women [12]. Factors associated with substance use include a desire to escape social minority stress, further highlighting the importance of prevention and chronic care management for this population and the need for gender and sexuality affirming mental health support. Screening, Brief Intervention, and Referral to Treatment (SBIRT) is an early intervention model that identifies substance use and encourages intervention including motivational interviewing to raise awareness about risky use and empowering the patient toward behavioral change [56]. SBIRT allows for immediate assessment and intervention without the need for referral, which can be helpful in populations that are historically clinic-averse, or in locations where there is a mismatch between affirming substance abuse practitioners and community need.

Sexual Health and High-Risk Sexual Experiences

Discussions about sexual health in the health care setting should include conversations about which body parts are present and how people prefer to use them (or not) in sexual encounters. Understanding how people use their anatomy can help determine risk, as people may or may not use body parts in ways that increase risk. For example, not all sexual minority men enjoy anal sex, which is a risk factor for anal cancers and sexually transmitted infections, including the human immunodeficiency virus (HIV). Understanding anatomy can promote conversations about safer sex practices and relevant screening tests for specific body parts. In addition, clinicians should ascertain a patient's typical and preferred practices and should offer strategies to support bringing the two closer together and use the opportunity to talk about partners, intimate partner violence, and satisfaction with sexual and romantic relationships.

Men who have sex with men (MSM) accounted for two-thirds of new HIV infections in the United States in 2019, despite representing approximately 2% of the adult population [57]. New infections have decreased significantly among White MSM but not among Black or Latino MSM. White MSM are more likely to be aware of their HIV diagnosis than men from racial minorities. Among MSM with a likely indication for risk-reducing strategies such as pre-exposure prophylaxis (PrEP), minority MSM are less likely to have discussed this with a clinician and have a lower rate of use and adherence. Young MSM aged 18–24 years also have a low rate of adherence (45%). The most common PrEp agents are emtricitabine-tenofovir disoproxil fumarate (Truvada®) and emtricitabine-tenofovir alafenamide (Descovy®) for use in HIV-negative MSM and transwomen. Improving access to and use of HIV health care for MSM, especially those from racial minorities, or younger men, is essential to address health inequity and to end the HIV epidemic.

Clinicians should avoid making assumptions about patient sexual practices and be familiar with potential health issues. For example, people with vaginas experience higher rates of bacterial vaginosis, so education about safe sex toy sharing and cleaning may reduce the transmission of bacterial overgrowth in the vagina [58]. People who identify as asexual or aromantic, meaning that they do not feel a sexual or romantic attraction to anyone, may still be engaging in sexual activity. The SGM community experiences unwanted or undesired experiences, such as sexual exploitation, intimate partner violence, and rape at significantly higher rates than heterosexuals, so clinician should create a safe space where patients can discuss their experiences [59].

Drug use can lower inhibitions, heighten pleasure, and reduce pain, which can lead to risky sexual behavior. Evaluating and supporting patients through a trauma-informed lens can promote the trust necessary to help a patient decrease risky behaviors. Screening for sexually transmitted infections such as HIV, syphilis, chlamydia, and gonorrhea may be indicated.

Cancer Screening

According to the World Health Organization (WHO), breast cancer is the most common cancer diagnosed globally, accounting for 12% of all new cancer diagnoses in women [60]. The US Preventive Services Task Force recommends biennial screening for breast cancer with mammography in women 50–74 years old [61]. Lesbian or bisexual women obtain screening mammograms less often than cisgender women [62]. Consensus groups recommend that female-to-male transmen without bilateral mastectomy follow screening guidelines for cisgender women [63, 64]. Recommendations for male-to-female transwomen are less clear, though the consensus groups recommend that the same guidelines be considered, especially if estrogen or progestin has been used for 5 or more years. Transgender and bisexual patients are less likely than heterosexuals and lesbians to adhere to mammography screening guidelines [65]. Clinicians and radiologists should be familiar with the recommendations for breast cancer screening of transgender people [66]. Table 26.3 lists the recommended guidelines from several professional organizations.

Cervical cancer is the third most common cancer in the world and is almost exclusively caused by infection with one of the high-risk strains of the human papilloma virus [67, 68]. Cervical cancer screening is recommended for all patients with a cervix, including transgender men, who are less likely to be current on cervical cancer screening than non-transgender women, which increases their risk for malignancy, morbidity, and mortality [63, 69, 70]. Oral sex practices can also cause transmission of high-risk HPV. HPV vaccination is routinely recommended for everyone at age 11 or 12 years, and for all persons through age 26 years who have not been previously vaccinated, with the potential to significantly reduce rates of cervical, oral, and anal cancer [71].

Clinicians should use the guidelines for prostate cancer screening in cisgender men in counseling transgender women, even those who have undergone gonadectomy [63]. Colon cancer screening is recommended for all individuals ages 45–75 years old regardless of sexual or gender orientation [72].

Table 26.3 Selected breast cancer screening recommendations for transgender individuals

Patient	UCSF Center of Excellence for Transgender Health [63]	Endocrine Society Clinical Practice Guidelines [64]
Transgender woman with more than 5 years of hormone therapy	Biennial screening mammography beginning at age 50 years	Similar screening to that for cisgender women. Length of hormone exposure not specified
Transgender man without top surgery	Similar screening to that for cisgender women	Similar screening to that for cisgender women
Transgender man who has undergone top surgery	Shared decision making between patient and clinician	Not addressed

Gender Affirming Therapy

Clinicians may wish to support gender diverse patients who are seeking hormone or other affirming care. This can involve initiation of treatment or chronic care with the provision of hormone therapy over many years. Feminizing hormone therapy includes use of estrogen and androgen blockers to achieve feminine embodiment while masculinizing therapy usually involves testosterone. Clinical guidelines for the treatment of gender-dysphoric/gender-incongruent individuals are available from the Endocrine Society [73]. Treatment includes confirmation of symptoms consistent with gender dysphoria, discussion of risks and benefits of medication management, and monitoring and maintenance as appropriate. Patients may benefit from connection to mental health providers, gender affirming surgeons, legal aid resources, and community and peer-support groups. Surgically affirming care might include facial feminization surgery, chondrolaryngoplasty, top surgery, or bottom surgery. Top surgery refers to an elective removal of breast tissue and chest reconstruction for transmasculine patients, and augmentation for transfeminine patients. Bottom surgery or gender affirming genital surgery refers to an array of elective surgery to help align a person's genitals and/or internal reproductive organs with that person's gender identity. For a transfeminine patient, this may include orchiectomy and/or vaginoplasty. For a transmasculine patient, this may include phalloplasty, metoidioplasty (creation of a penis), hysterectomy, bilateral salpingo-oophorectomy, and vaginectomy. Guidelines for transgender health care are available from the World Professional Association for Transgender Health (WPATH) (https://www.wpath.org/), the University of California at San Francisco (UCSF) (https://transcare.ucsf.edu/guidelines), and Fenway Health (https://fenwayhealth.org/care/medical/transgender-health/). Gender Spectrum (www.genderspectrum.com) provides gender affirming resources for young people, caregivers, educators, and medical providers, supporting gender-expansive youth and families with online resources and safe spaces. Better training for clinicians in the health care of trans people can validate the young person's identity and lower the risk of chronic illness [74]. The need for medical care in this vulnerable population with unique needs is increasing, and access to competent and understanding clinicians to provide hormonal treatment that pause or delay puberty may obviate the need for future gender affirmation surgeries [75]. Gender affirming hormone treatment has been found to be safe and improves mental health and other quality of life outcomes.

Youth and Emerging Adults

Youth today live in an environment quite different than that of their parents. They generally spend more time at home, are more likely to live with their family of origin beyond their high school years, have ready access to smart phones and the internet, and live a large portion of their social lives virtually. This developmental environment has fundamentally changed how youth think, communicate, and behave and the timing of developmental milestones. However, today's youth have the same fundamental needs as in the past, such as opportunities to engage in and learn from social relationships, including sexual and romantic relationships if desired; safe environments; and access to safe and supportive relationships with trusted adults including parents. Today's SGM youth tend to come out to their families about 10 years earlier than those in previous generations [3]. Family acceptance and identifying at least one supportive adult are predictive factors of resilience and wellness in SGM youth [76]. Clinicians can identify supportive resources for parents who are struggling to accept their child's gender or sexual orientation identity, as well as those for the young person.

Health care to young people includes the development of healthy coping strategies and lifestyles to prevent later chronic disease, health disparities, and disability. Clinicians should screen for high-risk behaviors and ensure safety within the home, school, and the community, including the virtual world. Practical resources on how to interview and understand adolescents regarding their mental health are available [77].

Young people who identify as SGM are more likely to experience negative social determinants of health than their cisgender and heterosexual peers, including exploitation and homelessness [78, 79]. They also report more psychosocial distress, including suicide attempts and death by suicide, than SGM adults [80, 81]. Transitioning to adulthood is a particularly turbulent time for young adults who experience home ejection or other detachment from their families or communities-of-origin. Young adults presenting for health care may require social support and assistance with medical coordination to achieve or maintain chronic disease management. For young people who are homeless, improvements in health cannot be expected until housing is stabilized. People of color who also identify as SGM experience institutionalization, including incarceration, at higher rates than other groups, with the first experience with the legal system often occurring during transition to adulthood [82]. This trend is the result of centuries of structural and systemic racism coupled with homo- and transphobia.

Older Adults

People over 65 years of age who identify as SGM are thought to comprise approximately 7% of the US population [3]. In SGM adults, loneliness and isolation are more common as people age, and health care providers can provide information on activities and opportunities for community engagement within local inclusive communities [83]. Older SGM adults are more likely to be single and/or living alone and less likely to have children to care for them, compared to non-SGM older adults, relying more on families of choice for support [84]. Many may conceal their sexual and gender identity from health providers and social service professionals for fear of discrimination. Lifetime disparities in employment opportunities and earnings may put SGM older adults at greater financial risk than their non-LGBTQ+ peers.

SGM older adults suffer from chronic disease at higher rates, including mental health issues, depression, smoking, alcohol and substance use, disability, and risky sexual behavior, compared to their non-SGM peers. Many of these problems are associated with a lifetime of victimization and stigma. Dementia may also be of higher prevalence in this population, which may be related to the other chronic problems, low social support, or untreated trauma. Given the aging of the population, including SGM individuals, health care providers will benefit from familiarity with the medical, social, and legal needs of LGBTQ+ individuals living with dementia [85]. It is important to discuss advance directives with all older patients, and perhaps especially so in SGM individuals who may choose a member of their family of choice as their preferred surrogate decision maker (health care power of attorney).

Future Directions

A stated goal in the US Department of Health and Human Services' Healthy People 2030 (https://health.gov/healthypeople) is to *improve the health, safety, and well-being of lesbian, gay, bisexual, and transgender people*. Meeting this goal will require the collection of population-level data, allocation of resources, research, and training, all with the objective of addressing the health disparities experienced by SGM individuals.

Team-based models will promote continuity of care for individuals with chronic conditions, access to urgent care, preventive health, mental health support, and access to reproductive health care. Inclusive care models, such as integrated behavioral health within a patient-centered primary care clinic, can improve care for this population. Culturally sensitive and inclusive training for health care and social service professionals will reduce the fear that many SGM people face when they seek medical care. The growing recognition that social determinants of health must be addressed to improve the overall health of populations is critical. Social factors such as housing, neighborhoods, education, environmental health, and economic stability overlap, with discrimination and minority stress adding to the challenges faced by SGM communities [86]. Policies and practices that address these health disparities will improve health outcomes for many people.

References

1. Hall WJ, Dawes HC, Plocek N. Sexual orientation identity development milestones among Lesbian, Gay, Bisexual, and Queer people: a systematic review and meta-analysis. Front Psychol. 2021;12:753954.
2. Human Rights Campaign. Glossary of terms. https://www.hrc.org/resources/glossary-of-terms.
3. Meyer IH, Wilson BDM, O'Neill K. LGBTQ people in the US: select findings from the generations and TransPop studies. Los Angeles: The Williams Institute; 2021.
4. Fisher AD, Cocchetti C. Biologic basis of gender identity (Chapter 8). In: The plasticity of sex: the molecular biology and clinical features of genomic sex, gender identity and sexual behavior. Academic Press; 2020. p. 89–107.
5. Bates DW. Health inequities and technology. J Health Care Poor Underserved. 2021;32(2):VIII–XIII.
6. Center for Disease Control and Prevention. Collecting sexual orientation and gender identity information. Available at: https://www.cdc.gov/hiv/clinicians/transforming-health/health-care-providers/collecting-sexual-orientation.html.
7. Jones J. LGBT identification in US ticks up to 7.1%. Gallop Poll. Available at: https://news.gallup.com/poll/389792/lgbt-identification-ticks-up.aspx.
8. Wilson BDM, Bouton L, Mallory C. Racial differences among LGBT adults in the U.S. Los Angeles, CA: The Williams Institute, UCLA School of Law; 2021.
9. American Psychological Association. Lesbian, gay, bisexual, and transgender aging. Available at: https://www.apa.org/pi/lgbt/resources/aging.
10. Delozier AM, Kamody RC, Rodgers S, Chen D. Health disparities in transgender and gender expansive adolescents: a topical review from a minority stress framework. J Pediatr Psychol. 2000;45(8):842–7.
11. Meyer IH. Resilience in the study of minority stress and health of sexual and gender minorities. Psychol Sex Orientat Gend Divers. 2015;2(3):209–12.
12. Parent MC, Arriaga AS, Gobble T, Wille L. Stress and substance use among sexual and gender minority individuals across the lifespan. Neurobiol Stress. 2019;10:100146.
13. Ayhan CHB, Bilgin H, Uluman OT, et al. A systematic review of the discrimination against sexual and gender minority in health care settings. Int J Health Serv. 2020;50(1):44–61.
14. Gahagan J, Subirana-Malaret M. Improving pathways to primary health care among LGBTQ populations and health care providers: key findings from Nova Scotia, Canada. Int J Equity Health. 2018;17(1):1–9.
15. Pega F, Veale JF. The case for the World Health Organization's Commission on Social Determinants of Health to address gender identity. Am J Public Health. 2015;105(3):e58–62.
16. Logie C. The case for the World Health Organization's Commission on the Social Determinants of Health to address sexual orientation. Am J Public Health. 2012;102(7):1243–6.
17. McKay T, Tran N, Barbee H, Min JK. Effects of LGBTQ+ affirming care on uptake of preventative care, management of chronic disease, and aging outcomes. MedRxiv. 2022; https://doi.org/10.1101/2022.05.26.22275633.
18. Romanelli M, Hudson KD. Individual and systemic barriers to health care: perspectives of lesbian, gay, bisexual, and transgender adults. Am J Orthopsychiatry. 2017;87(6):714.
19. Hudson KD, Bruce-Miller V. Nonclinical best practices for creating LGBTQ-inclusive care environments: a scoping review of gray literature. J Gay Lesbian Soc Services. 2022; https://doi.org/10.1080/10538720.2022.2057380.

20. Grasso C, Goldhammer H, Brown RJ, Furness BW. Using sexual orientation and gender identity data in electronic health records to assess for disparities in preventive health screening services. Int J Med Inform. 2020;142:104245.
21. Davison K, Queen R, Lau F, Antonio M. Culturally competent gender, sex, and sexual orientation information practices and electronic health records: rapid review. JMIR Med Inform. 2021;9(2):e25467.
22. Furness BW, Goldhammer H, Montalvo W, et al. Transforming primary care for lesbian, gay, bisexual, and transgender people: a collaborative quality improvement initiative. Ann Fam Med. 2020;18(4):292–302.
23. Heredia D, Pankey TL, Gonzalez CA. LGBTQ-affirmative behavioral health services in primary care. Prim Care. 2021;8(2):243–57.
24. Ginsburg KR, Winn RJ, Rudy BJ, et al. How to reach sexual minority youth in the health care setting: the teens offer guidance. J Adolesc Health. 2002;31(5):407–16.
25. Morris M, Cooper RL, Ramesh A, et al. Training to reduce LGBTQ-related bias among medical, nursing, and dental students and providers: a systematic review. BMC Med Educ. 2019;19(1):1–13.
26. Patterson JG, Tree JMY, Kamen C. Cultural competency and microaggressions in the provision of care to LGBT patients in rural and Appalachian Tennessee. Patient Educ Couns. 2019;102(11):2081–90.
27. Romanelli M, Lindsey MA. Patterns of healthcare discrimination among transgender help-seekers. Am J Prev Med. 2020;58(4):e123–31.
28. IOM (Institute of Medicine). Collecting sexual orientation and gender identity data in electronic health records: workshop summary. Washington, DC: The National Academies Press; 2013.
29. The Joint Commission. Advancing effective communication, cultural competence, and patient- and family centered care for the Lesbian, Gay, Bisexual, and Transgender (LGBT) community: a field guide. Oak Brook, IL: The Joint Commission; 2011.
30. Cahill SR, Baker K, Deutsch MB, Keatley J, Makadon HJ. Inclusion of sexual orientation and gender identity in stage 3 meaningful use guidelines: a huge step forward for LGBT health. LGBT Health. 2016;3(2):100–2.
31. Department of Health and Human Services. Program Assistance Letter (PAL 2016-02). Approved uniform data system changes for calendar year 2016. Washington, DC: Bureau of Primary Health Care, Health Resources and Services Administration; 2016.
32. Mink MD, Lindley LL, Weinstein AA. Stress, stigma, and sexual minority status: the intersectional ecology model of LGBTQ health. J Gay Lesbian Soc Services. 2014;26(4):502–21.
33. Brumback T, Thompson W, Cummins K, et al. Psychosocial predictors of substance use in adolescents and young adults: longitudinal risk and protective factors. Addict Behav. 2021;2021(121):106985.
34. Agustina R, Meilianawati F, Atmarita S, et al. Psychosocial, eating behavior, and lifestyle factors influencing overweight and obesity in adolescents. Food Nutr Bull. 2021;42(1_Suppl):S72–91.
35. Sandbakken EM, Skrautvol A, Madsen OJ. 'It's my definition of a relationship, even though it doesn't fit yours': living in polyamorous relationships in a mononormative culture. Psychol Sexual. 2021;13:1–14.
36. Walters ML, Chen J, Breiding MJ. The National Intimate Partner and Sexual Violence Survey (NISVS): 2010 findings on victimization by sexual orientation. Atlanta, GA: National Center for Injury Prevention and Control, Centers for Disease Control and Prevention; 2013.
37. Scheer JR, Poteat VP. Trauma-informed care and health among LGBTQ intimate partner violence survivors. J Interpers Violence. 2021;36(13–14):6670–92.
38. Slemon A, Richardson C, Goodyear T, et al. Widening mental health and substance use inequities among sexual and gender minority populations: findings from a repeated cross-sectional monitoring survey during the COVID-19 pandemic in Canada. Psychiatry Res. 2022;307:114327.
39. Blosnich JR, Henderson ER, Coulter RWS, et al. Sexual orientation change efforts, adverse childhood experiences, and suicide ideation and attempt among sexual minority adults, United States, 2016–2018. Am J Public Health. 2020;10(7):1024–30.
40. American Psychological Association. Report of the American Psychological Association Task Force on appropriate therapeutic responses to sexual orientation. 2009. https://www.apa.org/about/policy/resolution-sexual-orientation-change-efforts.pdf. Accessed 6 Aug 2022,
41. American Academy of Child and Adolescent Psychiatry. Conversion therapy. Posted 2018. https://www.aacap.org/aacap/Policy_Statements/2018/Conversion_Therapy.aspx. Accessed 6 Aug 2022.
42. American Medical Association. Issue brief: LGBTQ change efforts (so-called "conversion therapy"). 2019. https://www.ama-assn.org/system/files/conversion-therapy-issue-brief.pdf. Accessed 6 Aug 2022.
43. American Psychiatric Association. APA reiterates strong opposition to conversion therapy. 2018. https://www.psychiatry.org/getattachment/3d23f2f4-1497-4537-b4de-fe32fe8761bf/Position-Conversion-Therapy.pdf. Accessed 6 Aug 2022.
44. United Nations Human Rights Office of the High Commissioner. Born free and equal: sexual orientation, gender identity and sex characteristics in international human rights law. 2nd ed. 2019. https://www.ohchr.org/sites/default/files/Documents/Publications/Born_Free_and_Equal_WEB.pdf. Accessed 6 Aug 2022.
45. Alempijevic D, Beriashvili R, Beynon J, et al. Statement of the independent forensic expert group on conversion therapy. Torture. 2020;30(1):66–78.
46. Livingston NA, Berke D, Scholl J, et al. Addressing diversity in PTSD treatment: clinical considerations and guidance for the treatment of PTSD in LGBTQ populations. Curr Treat Options psychiatry. 2020;7(2):53–69.
47. National LGBT Health Education Center. Addressing eating disorders, body dissatisfaction, and obesity among sexual and gender minority youth. 2018. https://www.lgbtqiahealtheducation.org/wp-content/uploads/2018/04/EatingDisordersBodyImageBrief.pdf. Accessed 6 Aug 2022.
48. Warrier V, Greenberg DM, Weir E, et al. Elevated rates of autism, other neurodevelopmental and psychiatric diagnoses, and autistic traits in transgender and gender-diverse individuals. Nat Commun. 2020;11:3959. https://doi.org/10.1038/s41467-020-17794-1.
49. Organization for Autism Research. The AASPIRE healthcare toolkit: improving healthcare for autistic adults. Apr 2021. https://researchautism.org/the-aaspire-healthcare-toolkit-improving-healthcare-for-autistic-adults/. Accessed 6 Aug 2022.
50. Haymer M, Buckler-Amabilis S, Lawrence K, Tye M. Language and history of the LGBTQ community. In: The equal curriculum. Springer; 2020. p. 1–12.
51. Dehon E, Weiss N, Jones J, et al. A systematic review of the impact of physician implicit racial bias on clinical decision making. Acad Emerg Med. 2017;24(8):895–904.
52. Ivey-Stephenson AZ, Demissie Z, Crosby AE, et al. Suicidal ideation and behaviors among high school students—youth risk behavior survey, United States, 2019. MMWR Morb Mortal Wkly Rep. 2020;69(Suppl 1):47–55.
53. The Trevor Project. 2022 National survey on LGBTQ youth mental health. 2022. https://www.thetrevorproject.org/survey-2022/assets/static/trevor01_2022survey_final.pdf. Accessed 6 Aug 2022.
54. Ryberg W, Fosse R, Zahl PH, et al. Collaborative assessment and management of suicidality (CAMS) compared to treatment as usual (TAU) for suicidal patients: study protocol for a randomized controlled trial. Trials. 2016;17(1):481.

55. Dyar C, Newcomb ME, Mustanski B. Longitudinal associations between minority stressors and substance use among sexual and gender minority individuals. Drug Alcohol Depend. 2019;201:205–11.
56. Babor T, McRee B, Kassebaum P, Grimaldi P, Ahmed K, Bray J. Screening, brief intervention, and referral to treatment (SBIRT). Subst Abus. 2007;28(3):7–30.
57. Pitasi MA, Beer L, Cha S, et al. Vital signs: HIV infection, diagnosis, treatment, and prevention among gay, bisexual, and other men who have sex with mean—United States, 2010–2019. MMWR Morb Mortal Wkly Rep. 2021;70:1669–75.
58. Berger BJ, Kolton S, Zenilman JM, et al. Bacterial vaginosis in lesbians: a sexually transmitted disease. Clin Infect Dis. 1995;21(6):1402–5.
59. CDC. The national intimate partner and sexual violence survey: an overview of 2010 findings on victimization by sexual orientation. https://www.cdc.gov/violenceprevention/pdf/cdc_nisvs_victimization_final-a.pdf. Accessed 5 Aug 2022.
60. World Health Organization. Breast cancer. 26 Mar 2021. https://www.who.int/nesw-room/fact-sheets/detail/breast-cancer. Accessed 5 Aug 2022.
61. Siu AL. Screening for breast cancer: US preventive services task force recommendation statement. Ann Int Med. 2016;164(4):279–97.
62. Austin SB, Pazaris MJ, Nichols LP, Bowen D, Wei EK, Spiegelman D. An examination of sexual orientation group patterns in mammographic and colorectal screening in a cohort of U.S. women. Cancer Causes Control. 2013;24(3):539–47.
63. UCSF Gender Affirming Health Program, Department of Family and Community Medicine, University of California San Francisco. In: Deutsch MB, editor. Guidelines for the primary and gender-affirming care of transgender and gender nonbinary people. 2nd ed. 2016. Available at: https://transcare.ucsf.edu/guidelines.
64. Hembree WC, Cohen-Kettenis P, Delemarre-van de Wall HA, et al. Endocrine treatment of transsexual persons: an Endocrine Society clinical practice guideline. J Clin Endocrinol Metab. 2009;94(9):3132–54.
65. Bazzi AR, Whorms DS, King D, et al. Adherence to mammography screening guidelines among transgender persons and sexual minority women. Am J Public Health. 2015;105(11):2356–8.
66. Parkh U, Mauser E, Chhor CM, et al. Breast imaging is transgender patients: what the radiologist should know. Radiographics. 2020;40(1):13–27.
67. Jemal A, Bray F, Center MM, Ferlay J, Ward E, Forman D. Global cancer statistics. CA Cancer J Clin. 2011;61(2):69–90.
68. Walboomers JM, Jacobs MV, Manos MM, Bosch FX, Kummer JA, Shah KV, et al. Human papillomavirus is a necessary cause of invasive cervical cancer worldwide. J Pathol. 1999;189(1):12–9.
69. Peitzmeier SM, Khullar K, Reisner SL, Potter J. Pap test use is lower among female-to-male patients than non-transgender women. Am J Prev Med. 2014;47(6):808–12.
70. Sung HY, Kearney KA, Miller M, Kinney W, Sawaya GF, Hiatt RA. Papanicolaou smear history and diagnosis of invasive cervical carcinoma among members of a large prepaid health plan. Cancer. 2000;88(10):2283–9.
71. Meites E, Szilagyi PG, Chesson HW, et al. Human papillomavirus vaccination for adults: updated recommendations of the Advisory Committee on Immunization Practices. MMWR Morb Mortal Wkly Rep. 2019;68(32):698–702.
72. US Preventive Services Task Force. Screening for colorectal cancer. JAMA. 2021;325(19):1965–77.
73. Hembree WC, Cohen-Kettenis PT, Gooren L, et al. Endocrine treatment of gender-dysphoric/gender-incongruent persons: an endocrine society clinical practice guideline. J Clin Endocrinol Metab. 2017;102(11):3869–903. Erratum in: J Clin Endocrinol Metab. 2018 Feb 1;103(2):699. Erratum in: J Clin Endocrinol Metab 2018 Jul 1;103(7):2758–2759.
74. Strauss P, Winter S, Waters Z, et al. Perspectives of trans and gender diverse young people accessing primary care and gender-affirming medical services: findings from trans pathways. Int J Transgend Health. 2022;23(3):295–307.
75. Salas-Humara C, Sequeira GM, Rossi W, Dhar CP. Gender affirming medical care of transgender youth. Curr Probl Pediatr Adolesc Health Care. 2019;49(9):100683.
76. Green AE, Price-Feeney M, Dorison SH. Association of sexual orientation acceptance with reduced suicide attempts among lesbian, gay, bisexual, transgender, queer, and questioning youth. LGBT Health. 2021;8(1):26–31.
77. Melnyk BM, Lusk P. A practical guide to child and adolescent mental health screening, evidence-based assessment, intervention, and health promotion. 3rd ed. Springer; 2022.
78. Bowman E. Chapter on Commercial sexual exploitation of children, special populations and sociological considerations. In: Burke MC, editor. Human trafficking. 3rd ed. Routledge; 2022.
79. Ormiston CK. LGBTQ youth homelessness: why we need to protect our LGBTQ youth. LGBT Health. 2022;9(4):217–21.
80. Hinton JD, De la Piedad GX, Kaufmann LM, et al. A systematic and meta-analytic review of identity centrality among LGBTQ groups: an assessment of psychosocial correlates. J Sex Res. 2022;59(5):568–86.
81. Wang X, Gan Q, Zhou J, et al. A systematic review of the factors associated with suicide attempts among sexual-minority adolescents. MedRxiv. 2022. https://www.medrxiv.org/content/10.1101/2022.01.19.22269164v1.full.
82. Prescott A, Alcala M, Nakamura N. Structural stigma and LGBTQ PoC health. In: Heart, brain and mental health disparities for LGBTQ people of color. Palgrave Macmillan; 2021. p. 149–60.
83. Torres S, Lacy G. Life course transitions, personal networks, and social support for LGBTQ+ elders: implications for physical and mental health. In: Sexual and gender minority health. Emerald Publishing Limited; 2021.
84. Choi SK, Meyer IH. LGBT aging: a review of research findings, needs, and policy implications. Los Angeles: The Williams Institute; 2016.
85. Westwood S, Price E. Lesbian, gay, bisexual and trans individuals living with dementia, concepts, practice and rights. Routledge; 2016.
86. Henderson ER, Goldbach JT, Blosnich JR. Social determinants of sexual and gender minority mental health. Curr Treat Options Psychiatry. 2022;9:1–17.
87. Smithers GD. Reclaiming two-spirits: sexuality, spiritual renewal & sovereignty in native America, vol. 10. Beacon Press; 2022.

Special Population: Care of Incarcerated Persons

27

Rachel Sandler Silva and Evan Ashkin

Introduction

The criminal legal system includes many settings for persons experiencing incarceration. Jails are municipal- and county-administered facilities for individuals who have been detained awaiting charges for a crime, charged with a crime and awaiting trial, or those who have been sentenced to less than 1 year [1]. Prisons are state- and federally administered facilities for persons who are sentenced for greater than 1 year. Community programs include probation and parole and are responsible for persons who have been convicted of a crime but are no longer incarcerated [1]. Probation involves correctional supervision within the community instead of incarceration in a facility after conviction. Parole is a conditional and supervised release from prison [1].

The phenomenon of mass incarceration is unique to the US with historical roots in history and a legacy of national policies. When the Civil War ended, the Thirteenth Amendment preserved involuntary servitude in the event of punishment for a crime [2]. During reconstruction and the subsequent Jim Crow era, new strategies to enslavement involved the passage and enforcement of Black Codes, or laws designed to limit the freedoms of African Americans, which led to an increase of imprisonment and prison farms [3]. Over a century later, the closure of mental health institutions and shift to community-based settings was poorly planned and underfunded [4]. Concomitantly, the federal War on Crime and War on Drugs led to federal policies with strict enforcement for drug possession and created the Drug Enforcement Administration (DEA) [5]. The 1980s expanded enforcement of drug-related law offenses and zero tolerance policies, which included mandatory minimum sentences for drug possession [5], and was followed with three-strike laws, which stipulated life sentences for people with three or more serious or violent offenses [6]. These policy changes dramatically increased the number of persons incarcerated in the US, which now is the leading country for incarceration in the world [7].

Over 2 million people are incarcerated in US jails and prisons and nearly 4.5 million are under community supervision through probation or parole [8]. The prevalence varies by state, with states such as Oklahoma and Louisiana having the highest rates of incarceration, while others like Georgia and Rhode Island focusing on correctional control in the community through probation [9]. Racial disparities are prevalent throughout the criminal legal system. Black (5 times) and Latino populations (1.3 times) are incarcerated at rates greater than White populations [9]. Disparities also vary by state, with Wisconsin having a rate of 2742 per 100,000 Black residents in prison and Arizona having the highest rate of incarceration for Latino residents at 742 per 100,000 [9]. New Jersey has a high ratio of Black to White persons who are incarcerated and Massachusetts has the highest ratio of Latino to White persons incarcerated [9]. American Indian and Alaska Native populations are particularly overrepresented in local jails [10].

Men are overrepresented in the US criminal legal system; however, the rates of women are rising [11, 12]. One in every 15 women in the prison system is serving life-without-parole [13]. Women are more often in the community, but remain in correctional control through probation and parole [14]. In rural areas and smaller counties, the rates of women in jails are growing at a greater rate than urban areas [15]. Compared to men, women who are incarcerated have a higher prevalence of chronic medical illness, mental illness, and substance use disorders [16, 17].

Transgender persons have higher rates of incarceration than the general population [18]. Black, Indigenous, and persons of color who identify as transgender face disproportionate rates of incarceration with 47% of Black, 30% of

R. S. Silva (✉)
Department of Medicine, Hennepin Healthcare, Minneapolis, MN, USA
e-mail: Rachel.Silva@hcmed.org

E. Ashkin
Department of Family Medicine, University of North Carolina at Chapel Hill, Chapel Hill, NC, USA
e-mail: evan_ashkin@med.unc.edu

Indigenous, and 25% of Latino transgender people reporting having been sent to jail or prison for any reason [19]. Gay, Lesbian, and Bisexual persons are three times more likely to be incarcerated than the general population and more likely to face solitary confinement than heterosexual individuals [20, 21]. The average age of the prison population has increased since the 1970s with nearly one-third of people in prison are over age 40 [22]. Older individuals in the criminal legal system suffer from diabetes, cardiovascular conditions, and liver disease in addition to mental health conditions [22, 23].

Chronic illness and conditions have greater prevalence in both adolescents and adults who are involved in the criminal legal system [24, 25]. Diseases such as asthma, hypertension, cardiac disease, cancer, liver disease, HIV/AIDS [16, 26–28], mental health conditions, and substance use disorders are common [24, 29–31]. Social determinants of health (e.g., homelessness and unemployment) create additional barriers to health for people experiencing incarceration [29]. This chapter is a primer to the care of persons who are incarcerated. The first section is an overview of health services that are provided and is followed by clinical care considerations. Next, information about quality of care in carceral settings and post-release care is outlined. The chapter closes with a review of programs that promote reentry as well as future directions.

Health Services During Incarceration

Legal Precedents

Persons who are incarcerated in the US are guaranteed the provision of healthcare under the Eighth Amendment which prohibits cruel and unusual punishment to prisoners [32]. This law was affirmed in Estelle v Gamble in which the US Supreme Court ruled that officials and medical personnel in criminal legal settings cannot deliberately fail to respond to the medical needs of a person who is incarcerated if there is substantial risk of harm to the individual [33]. This standard is known as showing deliberate indifference and has served as precedent in subsequent court cases that protect people who are incarcerated against sexual assault [34], and the provision of dental care [35] and mental healthcare [36]. Deliberate indifference consists in both identifying a serious medical need and demonstrating excessive risk to the health and safety of the individual who is incarcerated [34, 37]. Failing to provide treatment, delaying care, poor medical judgment below professional medical standards, and ignoring obvious conditions are examples of demonstration of deliberate indifference. While individuals who are incarcerated have the constitutional right to healthcare services, multiple cases have upheld the use of co-pays and charging for over-the-counter medications as constitutional [38, 39].

Organization of Care

Health services across the criminal legal system are often interconnected since individuals can be incarcerated in different facilities (e.g., jails to prisons) and the care in each institution is linked to the capacities of the jurisdiction responsible for that facility [40]. In local settings, there are three healthcare delivery models. A partner agency such as the local health department or public hospital may be responsible in the jail setting [41]. Some jails and prisons utilize contractors that are either public or private companies and provide care onsite while others directly employ healthcare personnel [40, 41].

Each state is responsible for administering its prison system and different strategies are used for ambulatory services and hospital-based services [40]. Services can be provided directly through clinicians employed through the department of corrections, through contracts with private companies, through the state's university medical school and affiliated hospital system, or by combinations of these services [40]. Reimbursement in the state prison system varies between a mix of state-allocated funds, capitated contracts, and Medicaid if the state opted for Medicaid expansion under the Affordable Care Act (ACA) [40]. Some states, such as North Carolina, created its own prison hospital which is operated by the Department of Correction [40]. Texas and Georgia also have dedicated hospitals, which are run by university systems that provide healthcare [40].

The federal criminal legal system organizes healthcare services based on location. For individuals who are pre-trial under federal laws, such as those in US Marshalls or Immigration and Customs Enforcement, healthcare is usually provided by a local contracting agency where individuals are detained, which may be the local jail or dedicated detention facility [42, 43]. Native American and Indigenous communities also have tribal jails and prisons. Unlike other federal jurisdictions which fall under the Department of Justice, tribal facilities fall under the Department of the Interior [44].

There are no federal accreditations or regulatory requirements for healthcare services provided in criminal legal settings, in contrast to acute hospitals and long-term care facilities that are accredited by the Joint Commission and have federal regulations under the Center for Medicaid and Medicare [45]. Each state determines rules and regulations that inform care requirements which often fall under the state department of corrections, rather than the department of health. Federal prisons provide care under the standards of the Federal Bureau of Prisons [46]. While accreditation does exist for criminal legal settings through the National Commission on Correctional Healthcare and the American Correctional Association, it is optional [47, 48].

Healthcare financing in criminal legal settings is the responsibility of the jurisdiction. In 1965, the Medicaid Inmate Exclusion Policy (MIEP) prohibited the use of federal Medicaid funding for healthcare for persons who are incarcerated [49]. Because of MIEP, local and state jurisdictions are responsible for the cost of care of individuals who are incarcerated, in contrast to a cost-sharing model between local, state, and federal governments that finances safety-net medical care [41]. MIEP applies whether the individuals who are incarcerated are pre-trial or convicted, both of which disproportionately impact Black, Indigenous, and communities of color [41].

Several payment models have evolved for healthcare services during incarceration. Some facilities may opt to cost share and assume risk in providing care, depending on the health needs of facility population [40, 41]. Facilities that do not risk share may pay healthcare service contractors at an hourly rate or a set fee structure. If financial risk is shared, contractors will use either a flat fee or a capitated payment system. For flat fees, there is a fixed annual amount paid that covers pre-determined costs and can include hospitalization, while capitation involves a set reimbursement per person [40, 41].

Another cost-sharing approach charges patients' co-pays for medications, dental treatment, physician visits, and other health services [50, 51]. The goal is to reimburse states and counties for medical care and reduce unnecessary care. Co-pays, however, create barriers to accessing care and are proportionately more expensive than community rates [50]. People who are incarcerated earn 14–62 cents/h; a $2–$5 for a co-pay is up to 1 month's worth of wages in some facilities [50]. If incarcerated persons cannot afford to pay, some facilities cover the costs with dedicated funds while others create a debt for the patient [51]. Jails typically have fewer resources than prisons given the dependence on funding at the local jurisdiction and greater turn over. Prisons tend to focus on the acute and chronic needs of patients, which do include treatment of chronic diseases like hepatitis C and preventive services [48].

The Health Information Technology for Economic and Clinical Health Act was passed in 2009 which promoted the meaningful use of electronic health records (EHRs) in the US [52]. This legislation did not include healthcare provided in criminal legal settings. In consequence, there is a patchwork system of EHRs across criminal legal institutions; a fully operational EHR; a hybrid electronic and paper system; or a paper system [53]. Most EHRs built for criminal legal care are not integrated with other community health systems, creating barriers in communication and subsequently care. After release, records are not always available to community healthcare providers and may be delayed up to 90 days and have associated fees [54]. The use of aliases in justice-involved populations presents additional challenges in tracking and verifying health records.

Generally, there are dedicated locations in criminal legal settings for healthcare-related activities, including exam rooms, clinical units, and infirmaries with dedicated nursing cares. Although there are standards to promote patient privacy, it is not the same standard as in the community [55, 56]. For example, patients may be evaluated with open doors and security staff nearby in some circumstances. In others, individuals are not allowed out of their housing units as determined by security staff and must be evaluated in their housing unit or even in their cell. The Health Insurance Portability and Accountability Act (HIPAA) stipulates the communication requirements regarding health information that can be shared [57]. HIPAA does allow for sharing protected health information for patients in criminal legal settings [57]. Sharing of protected health information may occur, for example, if an individual is diagnosed with an infectious disease where there is concern that others in the criminal legal facility and staff have been exposed [58]. Information may also be shared for medical conditions that impact housing selection and diet options (e.g., diabetes mellitus).

Dual loyalty arises in criminal legal settings and reflects the duty to treat a patient and to interests of a third party, most notably the jail or prison authority [59]. Dual loyalty is challenging when healthcare professionals are employed by the jail or prison directly, as opposed to separate employment. Healthcare providers should participate in professional relationships with those incarcerated or detained in order to evaluate, protect, or improve their physical and mental health, and avoid participation in activities such as force-feeding during hunger strikes [60]. Providers may be compelled to limit treatment of hepatitis C due to cost, or limit prescriptions for opioid use disorder given security concerns. In these instances, administrative or public health personnel who are independent from direct patient care may provide recommendations [60].

Informed consent is an important principle in carceral settings. The same standards of consent to procedures and treatment that are required in the community apply to carceral settings, including the use of written consent [55, 56]. In some instances, a blanket consent for treatment is signed upon admission. If healthcare is refused, this should be documented and attested by the individual refusing offered care, without repercussions for punishment. In cases where individuals are unable to consent based upon capacity to consent or refuse treatment due to psychiatric illness, there are circumstances in some jurisdictions where medical treatment can be implemented.

Providing Care to Persons Who Are Incarcerated

Clinical Services

An initial medical evaluation consisting of screening, a general health assessment, and clearance is routinely completed when individuals enter a criminal legal facility [55, 56]. Medical clearance includes a documented clinical assessment that is completed prior to entry and may require transfer to a local emergency department if there are acute injuries or conditions, including acute traumatic injury, chest pain, or concern for acute drug ingestion. Screening seeks to identify urgent conditions, such as acute withdrawal syndromes, and potentially contagious conditions like MRSA or influenza (NCCHC J-E-02, J-E-04 [55]). Screening is completed by healthcare staff, if available, but in some facilities is completed by correctional staff. The initial health assessment is a comprehensive review that is required within 14 days of admission to a facility and can be performed by registered nurses or providers [55].

When healthcare providers are not onsite, some facilities designate a healthcare liaison who has special training to address medical conditions (NCCHC J-E-07) [55]. Requests for mental health and substance use disorder care may follow a comparable process; however, facilities may have separate workflows. In general, access to services rely on incarcerated persons to self-advocate for care, and often involve the medicalization of activities of daily living, including dietary modifications, the use of adaptive equipment, and skin care [61]. The use of hardcopy (i.e., written) and electronic systems are challenged due to high rates of limited health literacy [62]. There may be required assessments and exams that are guided by local jurisdiction regulations, such as testing for tuberculosis, HIV, syphilis, and other sexually transmitted diseases.

Healthcare services in carceral facilities depend on the type and size of the facility, the healthcare delivery model, and the local healthcare environment. Detention centers and jails with individuals who are pre-adjudication/pre-trial have greater patient turnover and inconsistent length of stay due to variability in posting bail and changes to court proceedings [55]. Prisons and jails with individuals who are post-adjudication can have a greater predictability [55, 56]. Short-term facilities tend to focus more on urgent medical concerns and may not address non-emergent chronic concerns or preventive services. Prisons generally have resources and protocols that can address chronic conditions and provide preventive screening.

Emergency healthcare and response planning are important components in carceral settings. Facilities routinely have plans for responding to medical emergencies in the facility, depending on resources and the clinical situation. Patients may be treated at the facility or in a contracted emergency department for conditions such as seizures, chest pain, altered mental status, acute opioid overdose, and acute traumatic injury [63]. In many cases, an on-call physician is available to address immediate concerns and to guide care planning.

Non-emergent services are typically considered as acute care and chronic care. This care may be requested through written, electronic, or phone requests in a process described as sick call, which has roots in a US military practice in which personnel would line up for medical attention [64]. Medical requests are triaged by nursing staff, depending on the facility, and may lead to a medical provider visit. Most facilities have nursing protocols for symptoms and conditions that are within a scope of practice. When the acute needs of the patient cannot be addressed in a local setting, several approaches facilitate higher acuity. Some larger facilities have their own urgent care centers, infirmary units, and even hospitals, while others rely on emergency departments and healthcare systems for urgent and emergent health conditions [40]. The logistics for transfer to an outside facility involves coordination with correctional staff and the receiving facility. Depending on patient needs, the correctional facility may transport the patient, or an ambulance service may be utilized. Specialty care referrals or off-site care often involves review by a health authority or health services administrator to determine the need for consultation. In some instances, a formal utilization review process is used.

Chronic disease is often treated using condition-specific protocols that are based on clinical practice guidelines (NCCHC J-F-01) [55]. Conditions such as asthma, diabetes, HIV/AIDS, and hypertension are examples and involve routine monitoring, medication management, lab testing, and providing patient education. Chronic disease management can vary based on the facility. For example, jails that may have short length of stay focus on medication management alone, while prisons with longer sentences can focus on more comprehensive management. Correctional facilities have formularies to help manage healthcare costs, which prioritize generic and less-costly medications [55]. For example, the American Diabetes Association recommends the initial use of metformin and then non-insulin medications prior to beginning insulin [65]. Newer agents, like GLP1 agonists and SGLT2 inhibitors, are infrequently used in criminal legal settings due to cost.

Mental Health

Psychiatric disorders are common in individuals who experience incarceration with prevalence estimates of more 60% of people in jails, and greater than 50% of people in prison [24, 66]. Major psychiatric disorders—including major depressive disorder, bipolar disorder, schizophrenia, and psychotic disorders—are associated with repeat incarceration [67]. Most individuals with mental health conditions are managed with pharmacotherapy while incarcerated, though fewer report adherence at the time of arrest [24].

In pre-trial settings, a psychiatric evaluation may be conducted for individuals who have court cases involving determinations of sanity and competency to stand trial [68]. Typically court-appointed mental health professionals work with legal counsel and hearing judges to inform determinations about the court case. A pre-trial mental health team can develop treatment plans which may include counseling services, group sessions, and pharmacotherapy. When the court issues an order for involuntary medication based upon local case law, the mental health and medical teams are responsible for medication management [69, 70].

Mental health screenings at admission and/or within 14 days of admission are recommended by National Commission of Correctional Healthcare, American Correctional Association, the Bureau of Prisons, and state departments of corrections. Screenings are performed by a member of the patient care team and include psychiatric history including psychiatric hospitalizations, suicide attempts, violent behavior, traumatic brain injury, trauma history, screening for intellectual functioning, and substance use history along with medication history (NCCHC J-E-05) [55, 56]. Although facilities provide access to pharmacotherapy, access to mental health professionals, formulary options, and the use of in-person versus tele-psychiatry vary widely [71, 72]. Mental health teams may contract separately with the criminal legal institution, while other facilities have dedicated mental health units that offer group and individual counseling [73].

Suicide is a particular risk for individuals who are incarcerated since it is the leading cause of death in jails and a significant cause of death in prisons [74]. The most common cause of suicide is by hanging. Institutions use several screening tools for suicide prevention, including the Columbia-Suicide Severity Rating Scale and the Suicide Behaviors Questionnaire-Revised [75, 76]. Policies and protocols to prevent suicide include the use of Kevlar or other resistant clothing, the absence of bedding or other clothing to prevent the use of ligatures, a special diet that limits utensils, and more frequent monitoring by both mental health and security staff [77]. In some settings, individualized care plans can progressively restore incarceration life to the patient [77].

Most US jails and prisons use administrative segregation or solitary confinement, which can involve up to 23 h a day in a cell and meets international definition of torture [78]. Although the psychological consequences of solitary confinement have been well reported, this practice continues in most criminal legal settings despite studies showing that this practice increases the risk for self-harm [79]. New York and other states have limited solitary confinement and have reduced the potential use of solitary confinement for adolescents, those with severe mental illness (SMI), and the elderly [80, 81].

Substance Use Disorders

Substance use disorders are ubiquitous in criminal legal settings, with over half of persons in state prisons and two-thirds of persons sentenced in jails reporting substance use or dependence [82]. Alcohol use has been identified in more than half and illicit substances in three-fourths of all people incarcerated [83]. A history of criminal legal involvement has been associated with more than half of individuals with prescription opioid use disorder or heroin use [31]. Individuals with substance use disorder may have longer jail stays and are more likely to serve time in segregation while incarcerated [84, 85]. Upon release there is a marked increased risk of overdose death within 2 weeks of release [86].

Managing clinical withdrawal syndromes is an important treatment for persons who are incarcerated. Withdrawal is usually managed with clinical protocols, particularly for those substances with known withdrawal syndromes, such as alcohol, benzodiazepines, and opioids (NCCHC J-F-04) [55]. Protocols often utilize validated tools like the Clinical Institute for Withdrawal Assessment for Alcohol (CIWA-Ar) and the Clinical Opioid Withdrawal Scale (COWS) to guide management; however, medically supervised withdrawal can vary. In many settings, clonidine is used for opioid withdrawal rather than an opioid agonist (e.g., methadone) or partial agonist (e.g., buprenorphine) therapy [87]. Scheduled versus as-needed dosing may vary based on the availability of medical personnel for clinical assessment. There is growing evidence about the efficacy of medications for opioid use disorder (MOUD) in carceral settings [31, 86, 88, 89]. Jail and prison systems have adopted different models for prescribing MOUD, which include buprenorphine, methadone, and intramuscular naltrexone [90]. Specific considerations for MOUD administration in criminal legal settings are the potential for diversion and a plan to continue treatment upon release [90, 91].

Special Conditions

Human Immunodeficiency Virus

Human Immunodeficiency Virus (HIV) is prevalent in jails and prisons when compared to the general population given high risk substance use and sexual behaviors in the incarcerated population [92]. Opt-out testing and initiating antiretroviral therapy for HIV have been adopted in many carceral settings [93]. The EnhanceLink Initiative and Transitional Care Coordination Model seeks to connect patients living with HIV to resources and supports in the community in ways that can continue therapy that has been initiated while incarcerated [94].

Hepatitis C

Hepatitis C rates in prison populations is estimated to be as high as 18%; approximately 30% of all individuals living with hepatitis C infection in the US pass through a carceral setting each year [95, 96]. Testing strategies include opt-out testing, risk-based, and mandatory testing with opt-out testing being a recommended strategy to help identify new cases, particularly those who are actively viremic [95–97]. The capacity to treat hepatitis C in carceral settings has greatly expanded with the development of direct-acting antivirals therapies (DAA); however, there are cost and length of stay barriers [97]. Legal action has contributed to improved access to hepatitis C treatment, particularly in state prison systems [98–100]. Jails face challenges with rapid turnover and care linkages to the community [101]. The diagnosis and treatment of hepatitis C in carceral settings remain important for the national strategy to mitigate this disease [102].

Pregnancy

The population of women in prison has increased over 700% in the past 30 years and they are disproportionately from communities of color [103]. Three-quarters of women who are incarcerated are in their childbearing years (ages 18–44) and two-thirds are primary caregivers to young children [104]. Approximately 5% of women entering jails and 4% of women entering state prisons are pregnant upon admission [105]. Prenatal care in carceral settings is variable and dependent on local clinical contracts and resources, though national (e.g., NCCHC) and state policies exist to create standards of care for pregnant women [106, 107].

The use of shackling and restraints during pregnancy varies on the institution and state of incarceration [107]. Only 22 states have legislation prohibiting or limiting the use of shackling of pregnant women, a practice contributing to abdominal trauma and possibly leading to adverse birth outcomes [108–110]. Shackling limits the ability to bond and safely support a newborn in the perinatal period, which is exacerbated by the practice of separating women from their newborns 24 h after birth [110]. Most women deliver alone without social or emotional support, although some doula programs exist [111]. Institutions may adjust the conditions of detention, but in many cases newborn children are placed in the custody of family, friends, or foster care [107].

Women who choose to terminate their pregnancy are legally protected under the law to do so while incarcerated, but the changing landscape around reproductive rights to abortion is threatening access to this care [112]. Transportation to clinic visits for a termination procedure and/or medical treatment can complicate access for incarcerated women seeing care [112]. Often, the incarcerated woman is responsible for costs associated with this care and may be responsible for transportation and security costs despite the legal right to receive this care [113].

Quality of Care

Although no uniform quality of care standards for health services provided in carceral settings exists, several entities provide oversight. For state-operated facilities and many local jurisdictions, the department of corrections or similar agencies have policies and regulations that inform standards, such as minimum standards for healthcare [114]. The first standards for health services in correctional facilities were established by the American Public Health Association in 1976 and the National Commission on Correctional Healthcare (NCCHC) provides dedicated standards regarding healthcare in jails, prisons, and juvenile detention facilities [114]. The American Correctional Association also has a voluntary accreditation process that includes a continuous quality improvement program [47].

Quality improvement (QI) is usually the responsibility of the medical authority, such as the medical director or chief medical officer, who works in collaboration with representatives from service lines including mental health, dentistry, and nursing (NCCHC J-A-06) [55]. QI programs typically involve strategies to improve performance and the collection and analysis of data outcomes (e.g., number of clinic visits) using health records. Because criminal legal settings, particularly jails, involve frequent intakes and a revolving population, the public health needs of the community are reflected in these settings, and quality and novel initiatives may reflect these changing priorities. In Hennepin County Adult Detention Center in Minneapolis, Minnesota, for example, a statewide hepatitis A outbreak led to changes in practice and measuring outcomes metrics regarding the administration of hepatitis A vaccine. The increased prevalence of illicit fentanyl use in the community led to changes in the same facility, including the expansion of prescribing of buprenorphine [115, 116].

Post-Release and Reentry

Persons released from incarceration face enormous challenges for successful reentry, including housing instability, food insecurity, unemployment, lack of transportation, lack of identification cards, compliance with post-release supervision requirements, debt, and reunification with loved ones and family [117]. Over 45,000 US state and local laws create barriers for persons with a criminal record [118], such as criminal background checks for employment. Over 4 million persons were reported in community supervision in 2018, which includes parole and probation [119]. Persons in community supervision are predominantly male (75%) and White (55%), 30% are Black, and 13% are Hispanic. Persons with recidivism report more chronic medical conditions, mental illness, and substance use disorders [120].

For many recently incarcerated persons, the lack of government identification (e.g., driver's license) prevents access to public services and benefits, including healthcare. Obtaining health insurance upon release is highly variable and geographically dependent on states that expanded Medicaid under the Affordable Care Act [121]. In Medicaid expansion states, individuals can often obtain state Medicaid coverage post-release, but may struggle to find providers that accept Medicaid insurance. In non-expansion states, only non-pregnant adults that are aged, blind, or disabled qualify for state Medicaid coverage. Additionally, individuals are often ineligible for ACA insurance subsidies if their incomes are below the qualifying limit of 100% of the federal poverty limit [121].

In the immediate post-release period, there is considerable risk of death for adults and juveniles [122]. The leading cause of post-release death is drug overdose, primarily associated with opioid use [122, 123]. Persons with substance use disorders may receive abstinence-based treatment; however, medication for opioid use disorder (MOUD) has been shown to be effective in reducing post-release overdose death [88]. Unfortunately MOUD is limited in carceral settings, with few people initiating treatment prior to release and connected to care post-release. MOUD is most often discontinued during incarceration for people on treatment for OUD [124]. Another factor associated with post-release death is exposure to solitary confinement from drug overdose, suicide, and homicide [125].

Dedicated transitional care teams and release planners for transition can be effective in reducing morbidity and mortality [117, 126–128]. Medications prescribed during incarceration may be dispensed at release from carceral settings using blister packages or pill bottles. Individuals released to the community can be prescribed medications, except for controlled substances. The practice of prescribing or providing medications at release is not required in all jurisdictions; in some circumstances only 3–7 days are prescribed [128]. Since Medicaid is terminated or suspended when people are incarcerated, even while pre-trial in jails, reobtaining insurance is important in transitioning healthcare services from the carceral setting to the community. Many states have moved toward the suspension of Medicaid, rather than its termination to help facilitate care transitions [129, 130]. There are different models for promoting Medicaid participation. In Massachusetts, individuals can enroll in Medicaid 6 months prior to release [129], a change that was made through Section 1115 waivers [131].

Medical discharge planning from prisons and jails is highly variable. Persons with ongoing medical problems may be given a list of community providers to contact upon release, but effective systems to assure continuity of care are lacking [117]. Post-release referrals for substance use treatment are inconsistent and usually only part of a court order or post-release supervision requirement [140]. Persons with severe mental illness may be given referrals or an appointment with a behavioral health provider in the community, but appointment completion rates are low [140].

Programs to Promote Reentry

Reentry programs, primarily in urban areas, focus on meeting the needs of people returning from incarceration, such as employment readiness, emergency housing, and life skills. Unfortunately, few programs include linkages to essential health services [117]. The Transitions Clinic Network (TCN) is a multistate program that seeks to connect post-release individuals to a primary care medical home [132]. The core of TCN includes community health workers (CHWs) who have lived experience of incarceration and are trained to interface across correctional institutions, reentry service providers, and medical homes. CHWs work to create a comprehensive reentry plan with their clients and are often embedded in primary care practices to facilitate comprehensive services [117]. TCN has been shown to reduce emergency room utilization by 50%, reduce ambulatory care sensitive hospitalizations, and reduce the number of days incarcerated by 25, per client per year [126–128]. There are over 40 TCN clinical sites in 12 states and Puerto Rico and most are in states that expanded Medicaid [132]. However, Texas, Louisiana, and North Carolina have also developed programs. In North Carolina, the North Carolina Formerly Incarcerated Transition Program (NCFIT) has developed eight clinical sites in six counties [133]. Through funding by grants and philanthropy, NCFIT partners with federally qualified health centers and covers costs for chronic medications.

Formerly incarcerated women have a high prevalence of mental health disorders [134, 135], which may be attributed to childhood and intimate partner violence [136]. A Rochester, NY TCN program developed The Women's Initiative Supporting Health and provides screening and vaccinations, mental health treatment, and substance use disorder treatment to recently incarcerated women [137]. In addition, the Women on the Road to Health program, an app-based intervention, focuses on reducing sexually risky behaviors, sexually transmitted infections, and intimate partner violence [138].

Post-release programs and interventions for people afflicted with severe mental illness (SMI) are essential. Without community support after release, people with SMI have high rates of rearrest and reincarceration [139]. Many states have deployed special mental health parole officers to work with individuals upon release, improving linkages to care. Another approach is forensic assertive community treatment, which combines intensive support (e.g., embedded psychiatric services) from justice-informed community treatment teams (e.g., mental health courts and probation and parole) for recently incarcerated person with SMI [140]. Forensic assertive community treatment has been associated with reductions in criminal convictions and increased engagement in outpatient care [141].

One model is transitional healthcare coordination that was started at Riker's Island Jail in New York City. This program involves a multisector transition of care team involving Medicaid, community-based healthcare providers, and departments within the health department and other city agencies [142]. The Transition from Jail to Community model is another approach which incorporates dedicated screening, a care transition plan, and targeted interventions like case management, referrals and education, and additional supports [143].

Although not a specific transitions model, compassionate release allows for changes in sentencing or bail given an individual's life circumstance. For example, a sentence is changed to that of time served while incarcerated and persons can be released to the community. Release may be due to age or declining health status, the incapacitation of a spouse or registered partner, or the incapacitation of the caregiver of the individual's child(ren) [144]. The healthcare team can play a role in advocating for compassionate release for a patient, depending on clinical circumstances and other factors.

Future Directions

The use of telemedicine and electronic consultation has been expanding in carceral settings for primary care, mental health, substance use disorder treatment, and specialty care [145]. Electronic consultation can be used to address a specific clinical question that can then be implemented by a primary provider. This strategy is associated with expedited and efficient care [146]. Telehealth services are an opportunity to expand healthcare resources in carceral facilities, particularly those in resource-constrained settings. Telemedicine has comparable patient satisfaction outcomes compared to in-person visits, but there are many factors in carceral institutions that impact the acceptability of telemedicine for patients and staff [145]. As the electronic and organization infrastructure for telemedicine and electronic consultation expanded during the COVID-19 pandemic, guidelines regarding the use of telemedicine will continue to emerge [147].

References

1. Community Corrections. National Institute of Justice. [cited 2022 Jan 21]. Available from: https://nij.ojp.gov/topics/corrections/community-corrections.
2. U.S. Constitution—Thirteenth Amendment | Resources | Constitution Annotated | Congress.gov | Library of Congress. [cited 2022 Jan 23]. Available from: https://constitution.congress.gov/constitution/amendment-13/.
3. American History, Race, and Prison. Vera Institute of Justice. [cited 2022 Jan 21]. Available from: https://www.vera.org/reimagining-prison-web-report/american-history-race-and-prison.
4. Incarceration Nation. [cited 2022 Jan 23]. Available from: https://www.apa.org/monitor/2014/10/incarceration.
5. A History of the Drug War. Drug Policy Alliance. [cited 2022 Jan 23]. Available from: https://drugpolicy.org/issues/brief-history-drug-war.
6. Sentencing Enhancement—"Three Strikes" Law. 2015 [cited 2022 Jan 23]. Available from: https://www.justice.gov/archives/jm/criminal-resource-manual-1032-sentencing-enhancement-three-strikes-law.
7. Initiative PP. States of incarceration: the global context. 2021 [cited 2022 Jan 23]. Available from: https://www.prisonpolicy.org/global/2021.html.
8. Data toolbox. [cited 2022 Jan 23]. Available from: https://www.prisonpolicy.org/data/.
9. Initiative PP. Correctional control 2018: incarceration and supervision by state. [cited 2022 Jan 23]. Available from: https://www.prisonpolicy.org/reports/correctionalcontrol2018.html.
10. Initiative PP. Visualizing the racial disparities in mass incarceration. [cited 2022 Jan 23]. Available from: https://www.prisonpolicy.org/blog/2020/07/27/disparities/.
11. BOP Statistics: Inmate Gender. [cited 2022 Jan 23]. Available from: https://www.bop.gov/about/statistics/statistics_inmate_gender.jsp.
12. Incarceration of women is growing twice as fast as that of men. Equal Justice Initiative. 2018 [cited 2022 Jan 23]. Available from: https://eji.org/news/female-incarceration-growing-twice-as-fast-as-male-incarceration/.
13. In the extreme: women serving life without parole and death sentences in the United States. The Sentencing Project. [cited 2022 Jan 23]. Available from: https://www.sentencingproject.org/publications/in-the-extreme-women-serving-life-without-parole-and-death-sentences-in-the-united-states/.
14. Initiative PP. Correctional control of women. [cited 2022 Jan 23]. Available from: https://www.prisonpolicy.org/graphs/correctional_control_women.html.
15. Initiative PP. Women's jail incarceration rates are highest in rural and…. [cited 2022 Jan 23]. Available from: https://www.prisonpolicy.org/graphs/women_jail_by_urbanicity.html.
16. Udo T. Chronic medical conditions in U.S. adults with incarceration history. Health Psychol. 2019;38(3):217–25.
17. Binswanger IA, Merrill JO, Krueger PM, White MC, Booth RE, Elmore JG. Gender differences in chronic medical, psychiatric, and substance-dependence disorders among jail inmates. Am J Public Health. 2010;100(3):476–82.
18. National Center for Transgender Equality. LGBTQ people behind bars: a guide to understanding the issues facing transgender prisoners and their legal rights. 2018. Available at: https://transequality.org/transpeoplebehindbars.

19. Initiative PP. BIPOC transgender people have especially high lifetime rates.... [cited 2022 Jan 25]. Available from: https://www.prisonpolicy.org/graphs/bipoc_trans_lifetime_incarc.html.
20. Initiative PP. Visualizing the unequal treatment of LGBTQ people in the criminal justice system. [cited 2022 Jan 25]. Available from: https://www.prisonpolicy.org/blog/2021/03/02/lgbtq/.
21. Meyer IH, Flores AR, Stemple L, Romero AP, Wilson BDM, Herman JL. Incarceration rates and traits of sexual minorities in the United States: National Inmate Survey, 2011–2012. Am J Public Health. 2017;107(2):267–73.
22. Porter LC, Bushway SD, Tsao H-S, Smith HL. How the U.S. prison boom has changed the age distribution of the prison population. Criminology. 2016;54(1):30–55.
23. Skarupski KA, Gross A, Schrack JA, Deal JA, Eber GB. The health of America's aging prison population. Epidemiol Rev. 2018;40(1):157–65.
24. Wilper AP, Woolhandler S, Boyd JW, Lasser KE, McCormick D, Bor DH, et al. The health and health care of US prisoners: results of a nationwide survey. Am J Public Health. 2009;99(4):666–72.
25. Barnert ES, Abrams LS, Tesema L, Dudovitz R, Nelson BB, Coker T, et al. Child incarceration and long-term adult health outcomes: a longitudinal study. Int J Prison Health. 2018;14(1):26–33.
26. Binswanger IA, Krueger PM, Steiner JF. Prevalence of chronic medical conditions among jail and prison inmates in the USA compared with the general population. J Epidemiol Community Health. 2009;63(11):912–9.
27. Wildeman C, Wang EA. Mass incarceration, public health, and widening inequality in the USA. Lancet. 2017;389(10077):1464–74.
28. Wang EA, Green J. Incarceration as a key variable in racial disparities of asthma prevalence. BMC Public Health. 2010;10:290.
29. MacDonald R. The Rikers Island hot spotters: defining the needs of the most frequently incarcerated. Am J Public Health. 2015;105(11):2262–2268 [cited 2022 Jan 25]. Available from: https://ajph.aphapublications.org/doi/10.2105/AJPH.2015.302785.
30. Winkelman TNA, Chang VW, Binswanger IA. Health, polysubstance use, and criminal justice involvement among adults with varying levels of opioid use. JAMA Netw Open. 2018;1(3):e180558.
31. Winkelman TNA, Vickery KD, Busch AM. Tobacco use among non-elderly adults with and without criminal justice involvement in the past year: United States, 2008-2016. Addict Sci Clin Pract. 2019;14(1):2.
32. The Constitution of the United States. Eighth Amendment.
33. Estelle v. Gamble. 429 U.S. 97. 1976.
34. Farmer v Brennan. 511 US 825. 1994.
35. Hoptowit v Ray. 682 F.2d 1337 (9th Cir.). 1982.
36. Bowring V Godwin. 551 F.2d 44 (US Court of Appeals 4th Circuit). 1977.
37. Wilson v Seiter. 501 US 294. 1991.
38. Reynolds v Wagner. 128 F.3d 166 (3d Cir.). 1997.
39. Bihms v. Klevenhagen. 928 F. Supp. 717, 718 (S.D. Tex). 1996.
40. State Prisons and the Delivery of Hospital Care. [cited 2022 Jan 25]. Available from: https://pew.org/2L5PCHm.
41. NACo-NSA Joint Task Force: pre-trial detainee health care and recidivism. [cited 2022 Apr 8]. Available from: https://www.naco.org/resources/featured/healthcareinjails.
42. ICE Health Service Corps. [cited 2022 Apr 8]. Available from: https://www.ice.gov/detain/ice-health-service-corps.
43. Service (USMS) USM. U.S. Marshals Service. [cited 2022 Apr 8]. Available from: https://www.usmarshals.gov/prisoner/healthcare.htm.
44. Hegyi N. Indian affairs promised to reform tribal jails. We found death, neglect and disrepair. NPR. 2021 Jun 10 [cited 2022 Jan 25]; Available from: https://www.npr.org/2021/06/10/1002451637/bureau-of-indian-affairs-tribal-detention-centers-deaths-neglect.
45. Regulations & Guidance | CMS. [cited 2022 Apr 8]. Available from: https://www.cms.gov/Regulations-and-Guidance/Regulations-and-Guidance.
46. BOP: Inmate Medical Care. [cited 2022 Apr 8]. Available from: https://www.bop.gov/inmates/custody_and_care/medical_care.jsp.
47. About Health Care. [cited 2022 Apr 8]. Available from: https://aca.org/ACA_Member/Healthcare/About_Us/ACA/ACA_Member/Healthcare_Professional_Interest_Section/HC_About.aspx?hkey=e9d55fc8-f10b-4222-ad99-f994031d2bec.
48. NCCHC leads in correctional health care accreditation and certification. [cited 2022 Apr 8]. Available from: https://www.ncchc.org/.
49. Social Security Act Amendments of 1965, Pub L No. 97, 42 USC §1396d. 9 Apr 1965.
50. Initiative PP. The steep cost of medical co-pays in prison puts health at risk. [cited 2022 Jan 25]. Available from: https://www.prisonpolicy.org/blog/2017/04/19/copays/.
51. Initiative PP. Prison co-pays: Appendix. [cited 2022 Jan 25]. Available from: https://www.prisonpolicy.org/reports/copay_policies.html.
52. National Commission on Correctional Healthcare Standards Health IT Legislation. HealthIT.gov. [cited 2022 Jan 31]. Available from: https://www.healthit.gov/topic/laws-regulation-and-policy/health-it-legislation.
53. Goldstein MM. Health information privacy and health information technology in the US correctional setting. Am J Public Health. 2014;104(5):803–9.
54. Woods GT, Cross K, Williams BC, Winkelman TNA. Accessing prison medical records in the United States: a national analysis, 2018. J Gen Intern Med. 2019;34(11):2331–2.
55. Standards for Health Services in Jails. National Commission on Correctional Healthcare. 2018.
56. Standards for Health Services in Prisons. National Commission on Correctional Healthcare. 2018.
57. Rights (OCR) O for C. When does the privacy rule allow covered entities to disclose protected health information to law enforcement officials? HHS.gov. 2007 [cited 2022 Jan 31]. Available from: https://www.hhs.gov/hipaa/for-professionals/faq/505/what-does-the-privacy-rule-allow-covered-entities-to-disclose-to-law-enforcement-officials/index.html.
58. Information sharing in criminal justice-mental health collaborations: working with HIPAA and other privacy laws. CSG Justice Center. [cited 2022 Jan 31]. Available from: https://csgjusticecenter.org/publications/information-sharing-in-criminal-justice-mental-health-collaborations/.
59. Physicians for Human Rights. Dual loyalty & human rights in health professional practice: proposed guidelines & institutional mechanisms. Boston, MA: Physicians for Human Rights; 2002. 145 p.
60. Pont J, Stöver H, Wolff H. Dual loyalty in prison health care. Am J Public Health. 2012;102(3):475–80.
61. Friedman E, Burr E, Sufrin C. Seeking recognition through carceral health care bureaucracy: analysis of medical care request forms in a county jail. Soc Sci Med. 2021;291:114485.
62. Hadden KB, Puglisi L, Prince L, Aminawung JA, Shavit S, Pflaum D, et al. Health literacy among a formerly incarcerated population using data from the transitions clinic network. J Urban Health. 2018;95(4):547–55.
63. Koester L, Brenner JM, Goulette A, Wojcik SM, Grant W. Inmate health care provided in an emergency department. J Correct Health Care. 2017;23(2):157–61.
64. Schroeder-Lein GR. The encyclopedia of civil war medicine. M.E. Sharpe; 2008. 458 p.
65. Volume 44 Issue Supplement_1 | Diabetes Care | American Diabetes Association. [cited 2022 Jan 28]. Available from: https://diabetesjournals.org/care/issue/44/Supplement_1.

66. Growth of incarceration in the United States: exploring causes and consequences. Office of Justice Programs. [cited 2022 Jan 28]. Available from: https://www.ojp.gov/library/publications/growth-incarceration-united-states-exploring-causes-and-consequences.
67. Baillargeon J, Binswanger IA, Penn JV, Williams BA, Murray OJ. Psychiatric disorders and repeat incarcerations: the revolving prison door. Am J Psychiatry. 2009;166(1):103–9.
68. Roesch R, Zapf PA, Golding SL, Skeem JL. Defining and assessing competency to stand trial. p. 24.
69. Jarvis v. Levine. 418 N.W.2d 139. 1988.
70. Sell v. United States. 539 U.S. 166. 2003.
71. Police Executive Research Forum. Managing mental illness in jails: sheriffs are finding promising new approaches. 2018.
72. Reingle Gonzalez JM, Connell NM. Mental health of prisoners: identifying barriers to mental health treatment and medication continuity. Am J Public Health. 2014;104(12):2328–33.
73. Cohen TR, Mujica CA, Gardner ME, Hwang M, Karmacharya R. Mental health units in correctional facilities in the United States. Harv Rev Psychiatry. 2020;28(4):255–70.
74. Mortality in local jails and state prisons, 2000–2013. The Marshall Project. [cited 2022 Jan 31]. Available from: https://www.themarshallproject.org/documents/2191181-mortality-in-local-jails-and-state-prisons.
75. The Lighthouse Project. The Columbia Lighthouse Project. [cited 2022 Jan 31]. Available from: https://cssrs.columbia.edu/.
76. Osman A, Bagge CL, Guittierez PM, Konick LC, Kooper BA, Barrios FX. The suicidal behaviors questionnaire-revised (SBQ-R): validation with clinical and nonclinical samples. Assessment. 2001;5:443–54.
77. Boring A. Suicide prevention in correctional facilities: reflections and next steps. NCIA. 2013 [cited 2022 Jan 31]. Available from: http://www.ncianet.org/suicide-prevention-in-correctional-facilities-reflections-and-next-steps/.
78. UN Nelson Mandela Rules | SolitaryConfinemen.org. Solitary Confinement. [cited 2022 Apr 8]. Available from: https://www.solitaryconfinement.org/un-nelson-mandela-rules.
79. Kaba F, Lewis A, Glowa-Kollisch S, Hadler J, Lee D, Alper H, et al. Solitary confinement and risk of self-harm among jail inmates. Am J Public Health. 2014;104(3):442–7.
80. Closson T. New York will end long-term solitary confinement in prisons and jails. The New York Times. 1 Apr 2021 [cited 2022 Jan 31]. Available from: https://www.nytimes.com/2021/04/01/nyregion/solitary-confinement-restricted.html.
81. Senate Passes the 'HALT' Solitary Confinement Act. NY State Senate. 2021 [cited 2022 Jan 31]. Available from: https://www.nysenate.gov/newsroom/press-releases/senate-passes-halt-solitary-confinement-act.
82. Bronson J. Drug use, dependence, and abuse among state prisoners and jail inmates, 2007–2009. 2017. p. 27.
83. Substance abuse and America's prison population 2010. Partnership to End Addiction. [cited 2022 Jan 31]. Available from: https://drugfree.org/reports/behind-bars-ii-substance-abuse-and-americas-prison-population/.
84. Improving outcomes for people with mental illnesses involved with New York City's criminal court and correction systems. CSG Justice Center. [cited 2022 Jan 31]. Available from: https://csgjusticecenter.org/publications/improving-outcomes-for-people-with-mental-illnesses-involved-with-new-york-citys-criminal-court-and-correction-systems/.
85. Metzner JL, Fellner J. Solitary confinement and mental illness in U.S. prisons: a challenge for medical ethics. J Am Acad Psychiatry Law. 2010;38(1):104–8.
86. Binswanger IA, Stern MF, Deyo RA, Heagerty PJ, Cheadle A, Elmore JG, et al. Release from prison—a high risk of death for former inmates. N Engl J Med. 2007;356(2):157–65.
87. Lewis DD. Detoxification of chemically dependent inmates. Federal Bureau of Prisons; 2014. p. 34.
88. Green TC, Clarke J, Brinkley-Rubinstein L, Marshall BDL, Alexander-Scott N, Boss R, et al. Postincarceration fatal overdoses after implementing medications for addiction treatment in a statewide correctional system. JAMA Psychiat. 2018;75(4):405–7.
89. Lee JD, Malone M, McDonald R, Cheng A, Vasudevan K, Tofighi B, et al. Comparison of treatment retention of adults with opioid addiction managed with extended-release buprenorphine vs daily sublingual buprenorphine-naloxone at time of release from jail. JAMA Netw Open. 2021;4(9):e2123032.
90. Opioid use disorder treatment in jails and prisons. [cited 2022 Jan 31]. Available from: https://pew.org/2VJkT5F.
91. Medication-assisted treatment (MAT) for opioid use disorder in jails and prisons. National Council. [cited 2022 Jan 31]. Available from: https://www.thenationalcouncil.org/medication-assisted-treatment-for-opioid-use-disorder-in-jails-and-prisons/.
92. Spaulding AC, Anderson EJ, Khan MA, Taborda-Vidarte CA, Phillips JA. HIV and HCV in U.S. prisons and jails: the correctional facility as a bellwether over time for the community's infections. AIDS Rev. 2017;19(3):134–47.
93. Flanigan TP. Jails: the new frontier. HIV testing, treatment, and linkage to care after release. AIDS Behav. 2013;17(2) https://doi.org/10.1007/s10461-013-0552-7.
94. Spaulding AC, Booker CA, Freeman SH, Ball SW, Stein MS, Jordan AO, et al. Jails, HIV testing, and linkage to care services: an overview of the EnhanceLink initiative. AIDS Behav. 2013;17(Suppl 2):S100–7.
95. Varan AK, Mercer DW, Stein MS, Spaulding AC. Hepatitis C seroprevalence among prison inmates since 2001: still high but declining. Public Health Rep. 2014;129(2):187–95.
96. Spaulding AC, Adee MG, Lawrence RT, Chhatwal J, von Oehsen W. Five questions concerning managing hepatitis C in the justice system: finding practical solutions for hepatitis C virus elimination. Infect Dis Clin N Am. 2018;32(2):323–45.
97. Core concepts—treatment of HCV in a correctional setting—treatment of key populations and unique situations—hepatitis C online. [cited 2022 Jan 31]. Available from: https://www.hepatitisc.uw.edu/go/key-populations-situations/treatment-corrections/core-concept/all.
98. Maru DS-R, Bruce RD, Basu S, Altice FL. Clinical outcomes of hepatitis C treatment in a prison setting: feasibility and effectiveness for challenging treatment populations. Clin Infect Dis. 2008;47(7):952–61.
99. NC DPS: N.C. Department of Public Safety Settles Hepatitis C Lawsuit. [cited 2022 Jan 31]. Available from: https://www.ncdps.gov/news/press-releases/2021/03/08/nc-department-public-safety-settles-hepatitis-c-lawsuit.
100. Hepatitis C fight hinges on prisons. US News & World Report. [cited 2022 Jan 31]. Available from: //www.usnews.com/news/healthiest-communities/articles/2019-02-05/hepatitis-c-fight-hinges-on-prisons-inmate-care.
101. Chan J, Schwartz J, Kaba F, Bocour A, Akiyama MJ, Hobstetter L, et al. Outcomes of hepatitis C virus treatment in the New York City jail population: successes and challenges facing scale up of care. Open Forum Infect Dis. 2020;7(7):ofaa263.
102. Ocal S, Muir AJ. Addressing hepatitis C in the American incarcerated population: strategies for nationwide elimination. Curr HIV/AIDS Rep. 2020;17(1):18–25.
103. Glaze L, Bonczar T. Probation and parole in the United States, 2007—statistical tables. New York. p. 32.
104. Sufrin C, Beal L, Clarke J, Jones R, Mosher WD. Pregnancy outcomes in US Prisons, 2016–2017. Am J Public Health. 2019;109(5):799–805.
105. Maruschak LM. Medical problems of prisoners: (448112008-001). American Psychological Association; 2008 [cited 2022 Jan 31].

Available from: http://doi.apa.org/get-pe-doi.cfm?doi=10.1037/e448112008-001.
106. ACOG Committee Opinion No. 511: Health care for pregnant and postpartum incarcerated women and adolescent females. Obstet Gynecol. 2011;118(5):1198–202.
107. State standards for pregnancy-related health care and abortion for women in prison. American Civil Liberties Union. [cited 2022 Jan 31]. Available from: https://www.aclu.org/state-standards-pregnancy-related-health-care-and-abortion-women-prison-0.
108. Ferszt GG, Palmer M, McGrane C. Where does your state stand on shackling of pregnant incarcerated women? Nurs Womens Health. 2018;22(1):17–23.
109. Sufrin C. Pregnancy and postpartum care in correctional settings. 2014;9.
110. Clarke JG, Simon RE. Shackling and separation: motherhood in prison. AMA J Ethics. 2013;15(9):779–85.
111. Home. mnprisondoulaproject. [cited 2022 Jan 31]. Available from: https://www.mnprisondoulaproject.org.
112. Sufrin CB, Creinin MD, Chang JC. Incarcerated women and abortion provision: a survey of correctional health providers. Perspect Sex Reprod Health. 2009;41(1):6–11.
113. Kasdan D. Abortion access for incarcerated women: are correctional health practices in conflict with constitutional standards. Perspect Sex Reprod Health. 2009;41(1):59–62.
114. Correctional Health Care Standards and Accreditation. [cited 2022 Jan 31]. Available from: https://www.apha.org/policies-and-advocacy/public-health-policy-statements/policy-database/2014/07/02/12/07/correctional-health-care-standards-and-accreditation.
115. Zellmer L, Peters L, Silva RS. Hennepin county adult detention center's response to a 2019 hepatitis A outbreak in Minnesota. Am J Public Health. 2021;111(5):839–841 [cited 2022 Jan 31]. Available from: https://ajph.aphapublications.org/doi/abs/10.2105/AJPH.2021.306159.
116. Duncan A, Sanders N, Schiff M, Winkelman TNA. Adaptations to jail-based buprenorphine treatment during the COVID-19 pandemic. J Subst Abus Treat. 2021;121:108161.
117. Shavit S, Aminawung JA, Birnbaum N, Greenberg S, Berthold T, Fishman A, Busch SH, Wang EA. Transitions clinic network: challenges and lessons in primary care for people released from prison. Health Aff (Millwood). 2017;36(6):1006–15. https://doi.org/10.1377/hlthaff.2017.0089.
118. Brennan Center for Justice. Collateral consequences and the enduring nature of punishment. Jun 2021 [cited 2022 Jan 12]. Available from: https://www.brennancenter.org/our-work/analysis-opinion/collateral-consequences-and-enduring-nature-punishment.
119. Office of Justice Programs. Probation and parole in the United States, 2017–2018. US Dept of Justice. Aug 2020 [cited 2022 Jan 12]. Available from: https://www.ojp.gov/library/publications/probation-and-parole-united-states-2017-2018.
120. Bureau of Justice Statistics. Drug use, dependence, and abuse among state prisoners and jail inmates, 2007–2009. US Dept of Justice. Jun 2017 (updated 2020 Aug 10, cited 2022 Jan 12). Available from: https://www.bjs.gov/content/pub/pdf/dudaspji0709.pdf.
121. Market Place Eligibility. U.S. Centers for Medicare and Medicaid Services. HealthCare.gov. [cited 2022 April 18]. Available from: https://www.healthcare.gov/quick-guide/eligibility/.
122. Binswanger IA, Blatchford PJ, Mueller SR, Stern MF. Mortality after prison release: opioid overdose and other causes of death, risk factors, and time trends from 1999 to 2009. Ann Intern Med. 2013;159(9):592–600.
123. Ranapurwala SI, Shanahan ME, Alexandridis AA, Proescholdbell SK, Naumann RB, Edwards D Jr, Marshall SW. Opioid overdose mortality among former North Carolina inmates: 2000-2015. Am J Public Health. 2018;108(9):1207–13. https://doi.org/10.2105/AJPH.2018.304514. Epub 2018 Jul 19.
124. Moore KE, Roberts W, Reid HH, Smith KMZ, Oberleitner LMS, McKee SA. Effectiveness of medication assisted treatment for opioid use in prison and jail settings: a meta-analysis and systematic review. J Subst Abus Treat. 2019;99:32–43. https://doi.org/10.1016/j.jsat.2018.12.003. Epub 2018 Dec 15.
125. Brinkley-Rubinstein L, Sivaraman J, Rosen DL, Cloud DH, Junker G, Proescholdbell S, Shanahan ME, Ranapurwala SI. Association of restrictive housing during incarceration with mortality after release. JAMA Netw Open. 2019;2(10):e1912516. https://doi.org/10.1001/jamanetworkopen.2019.12516.
126. Wang EA, Wang Y, Krumholz HM. A high risk of hospitalization following release from correctional facilities in Medicare beneficiaries: a retrospective matched cohort study, 2002 to 2010. JAMA Intern Med. 2013;173(17):1621–8.
127. Wang EA, Lin HJ, Aminawung JA, Busch SH, Gallagher C, Maurer K, Puglisi L, Shavit S, Frisman L. Propensity-matched study of enhanced primary care on contact with the criminal justice system among individuals recently released from prison to New Haven. BMJ Open. 2019;9(5):e028097. https://doi.org/10.1136/bmjopen-2018-028097.
128. Wang EA, Hong CS, Shavit S, Sanders R, Kessell E, Kushel MB. Engaging individuals recently released from prison into primary care: a randomized trial. Am J Public Health. 2012;102(9):e22–9. https://doi.org/10.2105/AJPH.2012.300894. Epub 2012 Jul 19.
129. How Medicaid enrollment of inmates facilitates health coverage after release. [cited 2022 Jan 31]. Available from: http://pew.org/1XSt64R.
130. Feb. 20 BB, 2019. Termination of Medicaid coverage during incarceration: set-up for failure? NACo. [cited 2022 Jan 31]. Available from: https://www.naco.org/articles/termination-medicaid-coverage-during-incarceration-set-failure.
131. 1115 Application Process | Medicaid. [cited 2022 Jan 31]. Available from: https://www.medicaid.gov/medicaid/section-1115-demonstrations/1115-application-process/index.html.
132. Transitions Clinic Network. [cited 2022 April 18]. Available from: https://transitionsclinic.org/.
133. Waters R. After prison, healthy lives built on access to care and community. Health Aff (Millwood). 2019;38(10):1616–21. https://doi.org/10.1377/hlthaff.2019.01163.
134. Visher CA, Bakken NW. Reentry challenges facing women with mental health problems. Women Health. 2014;54(8):768–80. https://doi.org/10.1080/03630242.2014.932889.
135. Green BL, Dass-Brailsford P, Hurtado de Mendoza A, Mete M, Lynch SM, DeHart DD, Belknap J. Trauma experiences and mental health among incarcerated women. Psychol Trauma Theory Res Pract Policy. 2016;8(4):455–63. https://doi.org/10.1037/tra0000113.
136. Finney C, Oliver H, Oliver W. Domestic violence and prisoner reentry: experiences of African American women and men. New York: Vera Institute of Justice; 2006. Available at: http://www.vera.org/publications.
137. Morse DS, Wilson JL, McMahon JM, Dozier AM, Quiroz A, Cerulli C. Does a primary health clinic for formerly incarcerated women increase linkage to care? Womens Health Issues. 2017;27(4):499–508. https://doi.org/10.1016/j.whi.2017.02.003. Epub 2017 Mar 13.
138. El-Bassel N, Gilbert L, Goddard-Eckrich D, Chang M, Wu E, Hunt T, Epperson M, Shaw SA, Rowe J, Almonte M, Witte S. Efficacy of a group-based multimedia HIV prevention intervention for drug-involved women under community supervision: project WORTH. PLoS One. 2014;9(11):e111528. https://doi.org/10.1371/journal.pone.0111528.

139. Substance Abuse and Mental Health Services Administration. Forensic assertive community treatment action brief. SAMHSA. [cited 2022 Jan 12]. Available from: https://store.samhsa.gov/product/Forensic-Assertive-Community-Treatment-FACT-A-Service-Delivery-Model-for-Individuals-With-Serious-Mental-Illness-Involved-With-the-Criminal-Justice-System/PEP19-FACT-BR.
140. Bryson WC, Cotton BP, Barry LC, Bruce ML, Piel J, Thielke SM, Williams BA. Mental health treatment among older adults with mental illness on parole or probation. Health Justice. 2019;7(1):4. https://doi.org/10.1186/s40352-019-0084-y.
141. Lamberti JS, Weisman RL, Cerulli C, Williams GC, Jacobowitz DB, Mueser KT, Marks PD, Strawderman RL, Harrington D, Lamberti TA, Caine ED. A randomized controlled trial of the Rochester forensic assertive community treatment model. Psychiatr Serv. 2017;68(10):1016–24. https://doi.org/10.1176/appi.ps.201600329. Epub 2017 Jun 1.
142. Transitional Healthcare Coordination—NYC Health. [cited 2022 Jan 31]. Available from: https://www1.nyc.gov/site/doh/health/health-topics/transitional-healthcare-coordination.page.
143. Transition from Jail to Community. [cited 2022 Jan 31]. Available from: https://info.nicic.gov/tjc/.
144. Compassionate release/reduction of sentence: procedures for implementation of 18 U.S.C. 3582(c)(A) and 4205(g). National Institute of Corrections. 2013 [cited 2022 Jan 31]. Available from: https://nicic.gov/compassionate-releasereduction-sentence-procedures-implementation-18-usc-3582ca-and-4205g.
145. Tian EJ, Venugopalan S, Kumar S, Beard M. The impacts of and outcomes from telehealth delivered in prisons: a systematic review. PLoS One. 2021;16(5):e0251840.
146. Frencher S, Steinberg K, Aubry L, Sanchez D, Kwong A, Baqai W, et al. A tale of two jails: leveraging electronic consultation to address the specialty care needs of the vulnerable county jail population. NEJM Catal. 2(3) [cited 2022 Jan 31]. Available from: https://catalyst.nejm.org/doi/full/10.1056/CAT.20.0472.
147. Prescribing controlled substances via telehealth | Telehealth.HHS.gov. [cited 2022 Jan 31]. Available from: https://telehealth.hhs.gov/providers/policy-changes-during-the-covid-19-public-health-emergency/prescribing-controlled-substances-via-telehealth/.

Special Population: Care of Immigrants and Refugees

Martha C. Carlough and Rana Alkhaldi

Introduction

As a result of political conflict, ethnic or religious persecution, violence, poverty, or climate change, people have been forced to flee their homes throughout the course of history. After World War II, the office of the United Nations High Commissioner for Refugees (UNHCR) was established in order to assist the millions of Europeans who had been forced from their homes. Since its foundation, the UNHCR has assisted over 50 million individuals across the globe [1]. As of 2020, an estimated 82 million people were displaced from their homes, 20 million of whom were classified under international law as refugees. While refugees are resettled in a number of countries around the world, the US has taken in close to one million since 2003 alone [2]. In this chapter, we will provide an overview of the care of refugees and asylum seekers in the US. We will describe the process of immigration and resettlement to the US, review common health issues facing this population, and discuss behavioral and lifestyle factors, as well as social and community issues, to consider while caring for refugees. Finally, we propose a framework for primary care of the refugee population.

Populations and Terminology

The term *refugee* was defined under international law during the 1951 Refugee Convention, commonly referred to as the Geneva Convention. According to the UNHCR, an individual is eligible for refugee status if they have been forced to flee their country due to war, violence, or religious or ethnic persecution, often without warning. These individuals receive special protection under international law, as they typically lack the protection of their native country [3]. The term *asylum seeker* refers to an individual who flees their home country before their refugee status has been determined legally, and who subsequently applies for protection in their country of destination [4]. Table 28.1 provides definitions of terms used in describing various types of displaced persons. In this chapter, we will primarily focus on refugees and asylum seekers.

There exists a number of reasons why people are forcibly displaced, including human trafficking, economic crises, and natural disasters. While an in-depth discussion of each of these types of migrants is beyond the scope of this chapter, the chronic illnesses all subtypes of forced migrants face are not dissimilar, as the experience of forced displacement itself is a source of toxic stress and, by extension, a risk factor for disease.

M. C. Carlough (✉) · R. Alkhaldi
Department of Family Medicine, University of North Carolina at Chapel Hill, Chapel Hill, NC, USA
e-mail: martha_carlough@med.unc.edu; ranaunc@email.unc.edu

Table 28.1 Terms and definitions

Term	Description
Refugee	• A legal term under international law referring to someone who has been forced to flee their country because of war, violence, or persecution, often without warning • Designated by the United Nations High Commission on Refugees (UNHCR)
Asylum seeker	• Someone seeking international protection from dangers in their home country, but whose claim for refugee status has not been determined legally • Must apply for protection in the country of destination, meaning they must arrive at or cross a border in order to apply
Migrant	• Someone moving from place to place • Can include moving within a country or crossing borders • Usually migrate for economic reasons such as seasonal work
Internally displaced person	• Someone forced to move from their home because of conflict, persecution, or natural disaster • These individuals remain in their home country

Processes of Immigration and Resettlement

International Policies and Governing Bodies

The international body overseeing international refugee assistance and resettlement or repatriation is the United Nations High Commission on Refugees (UNHCR). UNHCR is responsible for upholding fundamental principles of human rights and solidarity to protect and assist refugees by enhancing self-reliance, supporting countries of origin for their safe return, and/or expanding access to third-country resettlement as detailed in the Global Compact on Refugees [5]. UNHCR works in tandem with countries willing to accept refugees, including the opportunity to become naturalized citizens of the resettlement country. Usually, individual countries will establish annual limits on the number of incoming refugees they are able to accept based on their internal regulations.

Refugees for whom resettlement is deemed the most appropriate or only durable solution go through a lengthy process of screening and assessment by UNHCR in the country to which they fled, often through urban resettlement centers, as well as refugee camp administration. An initial resettlement interview usually includes all family members available, and questions are addressed to verify family composition, refugee claim, and resettlement needs, including particular medical needs or other vulnerabilities. Following this, a Refugee Registration Form (RRF) is used by UNHCR to identify a suitable resettlement situation in a third country.

US Refugee Resettlement Processes

Refugees matched to the US for resettlement then are screened and assisted by the International Organization of Migration (IOM), refugee officers from the Department of Homeland Security's US Citizenship and Immigration Services (USCIS), and non-profit sector staff (e.g., International Red Cross) and prepared for resettlement. Each resettlement country may set their own protocols for medical screening. Travel is organized and financed by the country of resettlement, and often the cost of this "travel loan" is subsequently paid back to the host country by the refugee [6]. This process can easily take up to 2 years and as long as 20 years in protracted refugee crisis situations.

Once refugees are selected for US resettlement, they undergo a pre-departure medical evaluation conducted according to the Centers for Disease Control (CDC) guidelines by an approved physician, also known as a *panel physician* who has been appointed by a local US embassy or consulate [7]. The primary purpose of this overseas medical examination is to ensure incoming refugees do not have any inadmissible or acute conditions that would worsen or be transmissible during travel and in the immediate resettlement period. The depth of this screening varies depending on the local resources available but is intended to include a medical and psychological evaluation; screening for tuberculosis, leprosy, gonorrhea, syphilis; and a review of vaccine records [8]. For more details, see the referenced information on the CDC website listed in resources.

US-based voluntary resettlement agencies (e.g., World Relief, Church World Service) coordinate incoming refugee placement and assist with initial needs including housing, transportation, school enrollment, and employment services, all within the first 30–90 days after arrival. This is often an intense period of adjustment and support for refugees but quickly subsides as most refugee resettlement agencies only receive federal support for newly arrived refugees for a short time.

Domestic Medical Examination

The initial domestic medical examination (DME) is generally completed within the first 90 days and typically occurs at local health departments. In certain situations, community health centers or other sites of primary care able to bill Medicaid can also provide this service, in cooperation with state refugee health programs. The DME includes a detailed history and physical, administration of vaccines necessary for school enrollment or employment in the US, and a nutrition assessment including screening for lead and anemia [9]. It is not intended to provide ongoing care for chronic illness, but rather is an opportunity to connect with the healthcare system and make plans and connections for ongoing primary and specialty care. Individuals approved for asylum and certified victims of human trafficking are also eligible for this refugee benefit. Although some refugees and asylees may continue to receive primary care services at the site of their DME, they can also choose to go elsewhere and use their Medicaid benefits for health care as long as they are covered.

The US refugee resettlement processes are designed to encourage self-sufficiency. Governmental cash assistance and refugee medical assistance (RMA), which includes full Medicaid benefits, are usually discontinued after 8 months. Though many refugee children qualify for Medicaid, adult refugees must identify their own source of health insurance, either through an employer or marketplace insurance program similar to other legal residents of the US. It is critical that refugees and others in similar categories, including asylum seekers and victims of human trafficking, understand options for healthcare coverage, including local, low-cost, and accessible care.

Adjustment of Status and Citizenship Trajectory

After 1 year in the US, refugees are expected to adjust their legal status by applying for a green card for lawful permanent residency, and after 5 years, refugees may apply to become US citizens. Refugees and asylees who do not seek citizenship remain legal residents of the US; however, without citizenship, they will eventually not be able to receive benefits including Social Security, Medicaid, and Medicare. Individuals who have a physical or developmental disability or mental impairment that impacts their ability to complete the English and civics testing requirements may apply for an exception using the N-648 form [10]. This form must be completed by a physician or, in some situations, a psychologist. In addition, most immigration attorneys encourage individuals seeking asylum in the US to undergo a medical examination to document any physical evidence or sequelae of torture or ill-treatment to support their application for asylum and improve the likelihood of asylum status being granted [11]. Training to complete these forensic medical evaluations is available through several organizations including Physicians for Human Rights and the Society of Refugee Health Care Providers. For more information, refer to the list of resources at the end of the chapter.

It is important that healthcare providers caring for refugees and other forced migrants be aware of these processes and support refugees and other newly arrived immigrants in the complexities of healthcare benefits and access and realize that, ultimately, US citizenship is also a social determinant of health. The path to US citizenship is illustrated in Fig. 28.1.

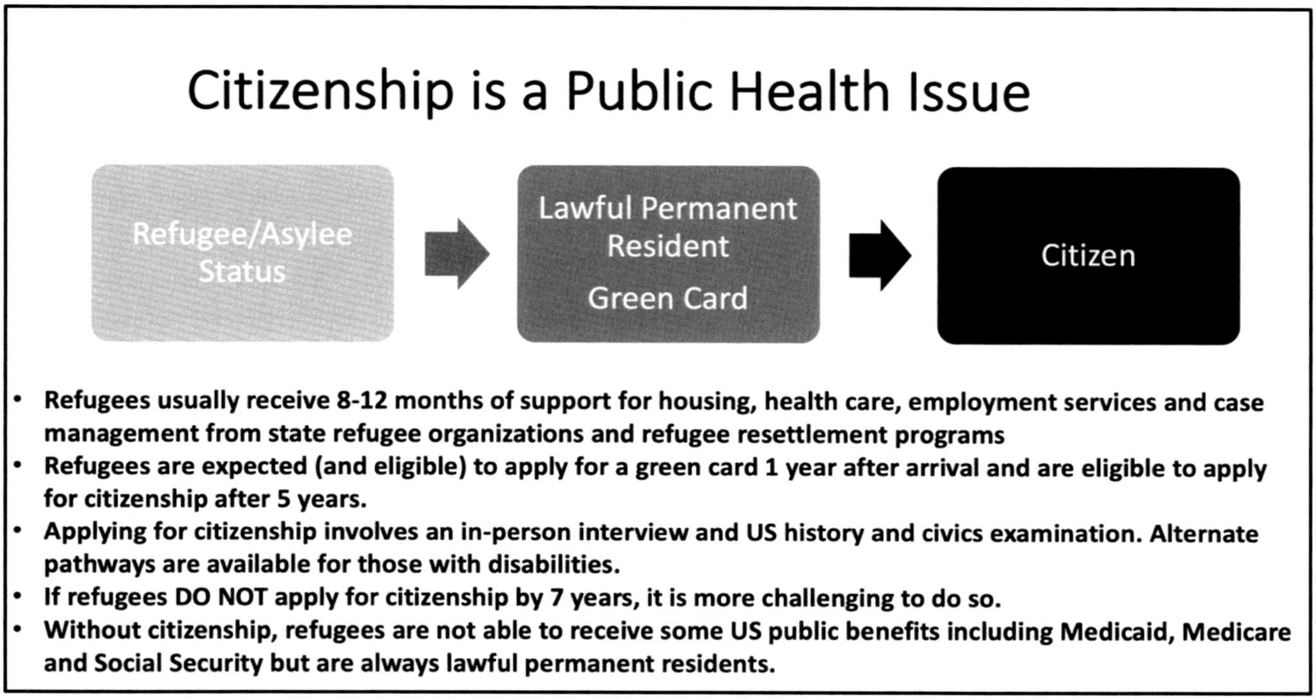

Citizenship is a Public Health Issue

Refugee/Asylee Status → Lawful Permanent Resident Green Card → Citizen

- Refugees usually receive 8-12 months of support for housing, health care, employment services and case management from state refugee organizations and refugee resettlement programs
- Refugees are expected (and eligible) to apply for a green card 1 year after arrival and are eligible to apply for citizenship after 5 years.
- Applying for citizenship involves an in-person interview and US history and civics examination. Alternate pathways are available for those with disabilities.
- If refugees DO NOT apply for citizenship by 7 years, it is more challenging to do so.
- Without citizenship, refugees are not able to receive some US public benefits including Medicaid, Medicare and Social Security but are always lawful permanent residents.

Fig. 28.1 The path to citizenship. (Figure developed by Martha Carlough)

Social and Community Issues

Stages of Migration

Migration as a refugee or other forced migrant broadly has been described in three stages [12]. During *pre-migration*, or all that precipitates the need and decision to move, individuals and families have usually experienced and witnessed significant civil unrest, trauma, and deprivation on many levels. Families are often separated, with many more women and children ending up in refugee situations. The second stage, termed *migration*, involves physical relocation by organizations overseeing the refugee crisis, such as the UNHCR and International Red Cross. Traditionally, refugees and other displaced persons were temporarily relocated in refugee camps. Increasingly, as the need for havens of safety has outpaced available space and situations, refugees are temporarily located in urban resettlement areas in adjacent countries willing to receive them. The third stage, or *post-migration*, may last a lifetime as individuals are assimilated to varying degrees within a new country and society willing to accept them as refugees. This three-step process has also been referred to as the *triple trauma paradigm*, as forced migrants repeatedly experience trauma and adjustment at each stage as described in Fig. 28.2 [13]. Those working with refugees need to understand these stages and utilize a trauma-informed approach to care recognizing the complexities involved [14].

PRE-FLIGHT *(Note: Symptoms often develop as adaptations that promote survival under life-threatening circumstances.)*	FLIGHT	POST-FLIGHT *(Note: Symptoms often develop as adaptations that promote survival under life-threatening circumstances.)*
- Harassmnt, intimidation, threats. - Fear of unexpected arrest. - Loss of job/livelihood. - Loss of home and possessions. - Disruption of studies, life dreams. - Repeated relocation. - Living in hiding/underground. - Societal chaos/breakdown. - Prohibition of traditional practices. - Lack of medical care. - Separation, isolation of family. - Malnutrition. - Need for secrecy, silence, distrust. - Brief arrests. - Being followed or monitored. - Imprisonment. - Torture. - Other forms of violence. - Witnessing violence. - Disappearances/ deaths.	- Fear of being caught or returned. - Living in hiding/underground. - Detention at checkpoints/borders. - Loss of home/possessions. - Loss of job/schooling. - Illness. - Robbery. - Exploitation: bribes, falsification. - Physical assault, rape, or injury. - Witnessing violence. - Lack of medical care. - Separation, isolation of family. - Malnutrition - Crowded, unsanitary conditions. - Long waits in refugee camps. - Great uncertainty about future.	- Low social and economic status. - Lack of legal status. - Language barriers. - Transportation, service barriers. - Loss of identity, roles. - Bad news from home. - Unmet expectations. - Unemployment/underemployment. - Racial/ethnic discrimination. - Inadequate, dangerous housing. - Repeated relocation/migration. - Social and cultural isolation. - Family separation/reunification. - Unresolved losses/disappearances. - Conflict: internal, marital, generational, community. - Unrealistic expectations from home. - Shock of new climate, geography.

Fig. 28.2 The triple trauma paradigm. (Source: Center for Victims of Human Torture. Improving Well-Being for Refugees in Primary Care. A Toolkit for Providers. 2019. Pg. 16 [13])

Changes in Family Structure

There are many and varied circumstances precipitating a refugee situation, but most have a slow onset of civil unrest and breakdown of societal structures. In these situations, family dynamics often change even before migration, with women and children more often staying put while men are working away from homes or involved in fighting or fleeing conflict situations. This may lead to situations where older children become caretakers for younger children or cultural brokers for the extended family. The risk of older children becoming unaccompanied and fleeing alone or being caught in human trafficking is significant. By the time individuals and families arrive in the US, they may have functioned for many years in family structures that look very different than would be typical in their countries of origin. This may be exacerbated as refugee children are exposed to American culture and forced to quickly adapt in US schools, while their parents or other elders lag behind learning English and struggle to find employment, widening a generational gap as well as acculturation gap. While refugee resettlement agencies work to place refugees in geographic proximity to others going through similar resettlement processes from their home countries, this is challenging. Even within a given nationality, different ethnic groups, languages, or other issues including class and caste structures may impact their ability to form a cohesive community in their new home country. Refugees are also faced with the challenges of a largely individualistic American culture, whereas many other cultures are community-based, with multiple family units living together or in proximity supporting one another.

While refugees and other forced migrants may be some of the most resilient people anywhere, the trauma, loss, and stress they experience also may have an enormous impact on their ability to care for themselves and their families and to seek healthcare when needed. It is important for healthcare workers to recognize the impact of refugee resettlement on family structure and to use best practices in clinical care. This includes planning for extra time and complexities of health education and decision-making and not using family members as interpreters. Providers should recognize and respect culture-specific familial and communal relationships, while also being aware of unhealthy relationships, including situations of unsupervised minors, intimate partner violence, or child or elder abuse.

Impact of Poverty and Limited Resources

In addition to the enormous social and physical consequences of leaving one's home country during a humanitarian crisis, refugees and forced migrant populations are at risk of long-term limited resources of food, housing, health care, employment, and other public benefits. Some evidence suggests that refugees are more likely to be employed than equally educated US citizens and less likely to be on other public benefits after establishing residence in the US; however, there is still significant public discrimination against refugees in many places, impacting employment and housing opportunities [15]. There is also confusion and concern about how receiving public benefits including federally funded Supplemental Nutritional Assistance Program (SNAP), subsidized housing assistance under Section 8, and Temporary Assistance for Needy Families (TANF) could impact the approval of permanent immigration processes which impacts many families, including refugee families, and limits their seeking of and receiving available resources [16]. These issues only exacerbate the fear and mistrust of authorities that many refugees and forced migrants already have as a result of previous experiences in their countries of origin. This may extend to healthcare-seeking behavior and trust in healthcare providers, who need to understand how power and experience of limited human rights and freedom may impact the experience of health care and healthcare-seeking behaviors.

Differences in Understanding of Health and Health Literacy

Personal health literacy is defined as *the degree to which individuals have the ability to find, understand, and use information and services to inform health-related decisions and actions for themselves and others* [17]. While refugees and other forced migrants obviously may have no or limited English language proficiency, necessitating the use of trained medical interpreters, health literacy is a more complex issue and is impacted by cultural models of health that may be significantly different than the predominantly bio-medical model common in the US. These beliefs and models may be unspoken but can impact care-seeking behavior, experience, or denial of specific symptoms, and ability to follow through with offered advice and treatment plans. Access to understandable, actionable information offered with sensitivity to different perspectives and understanding of health and well-being is essential for refugees to thrive.

Refugees and Chronic Disease

Infectious diseases and mental illnesses both contribute significantly to the morbidity and mortality of refugee and migrant populations. As a result of the migratory experience, communicable diseases rank higher as causes of death within these communities than chronic conditions such as cardiovascular disease [18]. Additionally, trauma before or during migration, as well as stressors after settling in their host countries, results in higher rates of mental illness among these individuals [19]. While non-communicable diseases are certainly prevalent in these populations and should not be neglected, this section will focus primarily on common infectious diseases and mental illnesses that disproportionately affect refugee and migrant populations.

Infectious Disease

The process of forced migration carries with it an increased risk for transmission of communicable disease, whether due to crowding, poor sanitation in refugee camps, subpar living conditions, or limited healthcare in transit or in the country of resettlement [20–22]. For refugees resettling in the US, the CDC requires pre-entry screening for tuberculosis (TB), gonorrhea, and syphilis; provides recommendations for vaccinations; and presumptively treats parasitic infections [8]. However, many communicable diseases evade these medical screening exams, and asylum seekers and other migrant populations do not undergo the same pre-screening process as refugees. As such, clinicians caring for refugee and migrant populations should have an understanding of infectious diseases that may impact these individuals. This section will review the most common transmissible illnesses prevalent in these communities after settling in the US.

Tuberculosis

In 2020, the US had an incidence rate of tuberculosis (TB) of 2.2 per 100,000 individuals with 7174 cases that year [23]. Origin of birth remains the greatest risk factor for contracting TB, with 72% of domestic cases occurring in persons born outside of the US [24]. Consequently, TB screening is a prerequisite for entry to the US for refugees. As of 2007, all refugees and immigrants bound for the US aged 15 years and older receive a chest radiograph to screen for TB. Individuals with positive chest radiographs, HIV positivity, or symptoms suggestive of active TB are tested additionally with sputum smears, cultures, and drug susceptibility testing. Children ages 2–14 years who come from TB-endemic areas also receive a tuberculin skin test or an interferon-gamma release assay, with a follow-up chest radiograph if positive. Anyone with active TB is required to complete treatment with directly observed therapy prior to being granted permission to travel to the US [8]. Despite this, latent TB continues to contribute to a significant burden of disease. In some refugee populations, the prevalence of latent TB exceeds 40%. Furthermore, chronic stress from migration and resettlement is thought to be a contributor to increased reactivation rates in these individuals [22]. Multidrug resistance is also more common in migrants, thought to be a result of the acquisition of multidrug-resistant pathogens during the process of migration [25].

Due to its prevalence in these communities, TB should be a consideration when clinicians are evaluating undifferentiated symptoms in refugee or migrant patients. In addition to pulmonary involvement, extrapulmonary tuberculosis (e.g., miliary TB, lymphadenitis, otitis media, or cutaneous infections) may also manifest [18, 22]. Once diagnosed, treatment adherence for these individuals can be a challenge, given barriers to healthcare access and the risk of being lost to follow-up [21].

Chronic Hepatitis and HIV

Chronic viral diseases such as chronic hepatitis B and C or human immunodeficiency virus (HIV) have a prevalence in some migrant populations up to 14%, 1.3%, and 2.3%, respectively, depending on country of origin, and can lead to significant morbidity and mortality [20]. Chronic hepatitis B and C are leading causes of cirrhosis and hepatocellular carcinoma globally [26, 27], and HIV/AIDS continues to have a dramatic impact on the health of millions of individuals worldwide [28].

According to estimates by the World Health Organization (WHO), 296 million people had a diagnosis of chronic hepatitis B in 2019, with the highest burden of disease in the WHO Western Pacific (i.e., East Asia, Southeast Asia, and Pacific Islands) and African regions [29]. Due to a large efflux of migration coming from these regions, the burden of chronic hepatitis B in the US falls primarily on foreign-born individuals. An estimated 60–90% of domestic cases of chronic hepatitis B are found in persons born outside of the US [30, 31]. Screening guidelines for hepatitis B specific for refugee or migrant populations do not exist at present; the risk within this population is dependent on their country of origin, and often their ethnicity, as certain ethnic groups may have a higher prevalence of infection within a country or region [32]. Hepatitis B vaccination is not readily available to individuals in all parts of the world, and although it is a recommended vaccination prior to entry to the US, no vaccinations are mandatory for immigration or resettlement [8]. As such, primary prevention is of utmost importance by ensuring vaccination against hepatitis B for all migrants and refugees, regardless of country of origin.

Chronic hepatitis C also presents a public health risk to refugee and migrant populations. In 2019, the WHO estimated that 58 million people were living with chronic hepatitis C around the world. Hepatitis C is endemic to the entire globe; however, it is most prevalent in the Eastern Mediterranean and in Europe, as well as Southeast Asia and the Western Pacific. Despite improved access to hepatitis C treatment due to generic forms of medications, treatment rates continue to be low globally. According to data from the WHO, only 21% of the 58 million people infected with chronic hepatitis C were aware of their diagnosis, and of those, only an estimated 62% completed treatment by the end of 2019 [33]. As a result, following established CDC recommendations for all refugees and migrants (i.e., one-time screening for all adults and for pregnant women in every pregnancy) regardless of country of origin is advised [34].

Within high-income countries including the US, migrants are disproportionately affected by infection with HIV [35, 36]. Globally, about 38 million individuals are living with HIV as of late 2020, with greater than two-thirds being from African nations [28]. Migration itself, particularly if forced or under duress, is thought to place individuals at higher risk of HIV, due to overcrowding, limited access to healthcare, psychological and physical trauma, sexual violence, and malnutrition [37]. As such, the CDC requires HIV testing as part of routine pre-entry screening for refugees and immigrants to the US [8]. Screening for HIV should be offered again to all settling domestically to allow the initiation of early treatment when indicated [38]. After resettlement, outcomes for migrants and refugees tend to be worse than those for patients native to the US [36, 37]. This is partly due to late entry to care, which may be a result of lack of awareness of their diagnosis, lack of education about their disease, or lack of health insurance [36]. Long-term adherence to treatment has similarly been documented as an issue with refugee and migrant populations, likely as a result of the same factors [37]. HIV-related stigma in migrant communities may be another contributor as to why these patients are late to seeking care or to follow up with treatment. As such, interventions that aim to increase access to treatment and reduce stigma may work to reduce disparities in these populations [36].

Vaccine-Preventable Diseases

As a consequence of displacement and migration, refugees often miss doses of vaccines prior to departure or are left out of vaccination programs in countries providing them asylum. While immigrants moving voluntarily to the US are required by law to be vaccinated against certain diseases prior to entry, refugees are not subject to this statute. However, the CDC does highly recommend routine vaccination for incoming refugees prior to arrival and has developed an immunization schedule that includes 11 vaccines listed in Table 28.2. Refugees may receive up to two doses of each, depending on vaccine availability and the individual's age. Patients with certain medical conditions may have additional recommended vaccines or doses [8].

As outbreaks of vaccine-preventable diseases in resettled refugee populations have been documented throughout the years, confirming immunity against these diseases among newly arriving refugees can have a significant impact on preserving the health of a local community [38]. Deciding to perform serology testing to confirm immunity can be made on a case-by-case basis, depending on cost and likelihood of exposure [39]. It is not necessary to screen for immunity if an individual provides documentation of vaccination; otherwise, refugees should be vaccinated according to the official CDC immunization schedule for the US. If documentation is sparse or of questionable reliability, or if children were severely malnourished at the time of vaccination, revaccination is indicated [38].

Table 28.2 Recommended immunizations

Diphtheria, tetanus, and pertussis (DTP or DTaP)
Hepatitis B
H. influenzae type b (Hib)
Measles, mumps, and rubella (MMR)
Oral polio vaccine (OPV) or inactivated polio vaccine (IPV)
Pneumococcal
Rotavirus
Tetanus and diphtheria (Td)
Meningococcal ACWY
Varicella
Influenza

Intestinal Parasites

Around the globe, intestinal parasites can contribute to significant morbidity and mortality [18, 22]. Perhaps the most serious and potentially deadly infections are schistosomiasis and *Strongyloides*, both of which are easily detected and treatable and are highly prevalent in migrant populations [18, 20, 38, 40]. Based on data from newly arrived refugees, the CDC requires presumptive treatment for parasitic infections for individuals settling in the US, specifically targeting schistosomiasis and *Strongyloides* infections (in addition to malaria and soil-transmitted intestinal helminths) based on country of origin. This intervention has proven to be quite successful, with one study demonstrating a decline in *Strongyloides* prevalence by serologic assays and stool polymerase chain reaction (PCR) after treatment with ivermectin prior to departure among refugees bound to the US between 2012 and 2015 [8]. However, these parasites continue to be present in recently settled migrant populations and should be suspected in patients with persistent eosinophilia since schistosomiasis and *Strongyloides* together account for about 20–50% of elevated eosinophil counts in these patients. Serology testing is the most reliable method for diagnosing infections caused by both of these organisms [22].

Mental Health Issues

Refugees, asylum seekers, and other migrants have proportionally higher rates of depression, generalized anxiety disorder, and posttraumatic stress disorder (PTSD) as compared to age-matched individuals in the population of the host countries in which they settle [19, 39, 41–43]. Estimations of the prevalence of these disorders vary widely from study to study, with higher quality data indicating slightly lower rates [42, 43]. Among adults and children within these communities, depression occurs at an estimated rate between 4% and 62%, generalized anxiety disorder between 4% and 40%, and PTSD between 8% and 49%. Refugee and asylum seeker women tend to have higher rates of postpartum depression, as compared to women native to the host country. Individuals who identify as lesbian, gay, bisexual, transgender, or queer or questioning (LGBTQ) experience depression and PTSD at higher numbers than members of the LGBTQ community who are native-born. Rates of psychotic disorders, such as schizophrenia, schizoaffective disorder, delusional disorder, and bipolar disorder, are about 2%, which is equivalent to other populations. Substance use disorders tend to be lower initially upon migration, which is thought to be connected to the "healthy immigrant effect"—the phenomenon that migrants undergo extensive screening and medical examinations prior to arrival; however, over time, rates of substance use among these populations trend up to match the rates of the host country [19].

Causes and Social Determinants of Mental Disorders

Experiences of trauma in all phases of migration contribute to the higher prevalence of depression, generalized anxiety disorder, and PTSD in refugee and migrant communities. Prior to migration, individuals may undergo religious, ethnic, political, or gender-based persecution or violence that leads them to flee their homes for their and their family's safety. Additionally, they may have witnessed violence firsthand, lost family members to violence prior to departure, or been forcefully conscripted as child soldiers in their home country [19, 39, 44]. During migration, individuals continue to be at risk of violence, food insecurity, and housing insecurity. Refugee camps are known to have high rates of violence, overcrowding, and disease, often worsening or adding to the trauma experienced during their migration journey, and putting them at higher risk of chronic depression and anxiety [19, 43, 44].

Perhaps the factors that contribute most significantly to risk for chronic mental illness are the conditions in the host country post-migration [41, 43]. Once they have resettled, they are often subject to much of the same social determinants of health that impact other vulnerable populations: poverty, housing insecurity, food insecurity, access to health care, and discrimination [41, 43, 45]. Unstable housing, inconsistent income, and increased xenophobic sentiments and discrimination have impacts on chronic stress, resulting in chronic mental disorders [41, 43]. As a result of loss of social networks, women and older adults, in particular, tend to become socially isolated after resettlement, and social isolation is another risk factor known to lead to or worsen anxiety and depression [43, 45].

Mental Health Screening

With higher rates of chronic depression, PTSD, and anxiety disorders, screening can be an important tool to identify and treat individuals within these communities. Refugees and migrants access mental health care less frequently than other populations, and as a result, these disorders will often manifest as somatization [19]. As such, the CDC recommends screening for depression and PTSD in all refugees and migrants over the age of 16. For depression screening, the Patient Health Questionnaire-9 (PHQ-9) is the recommended tool and has been studied in various communities of refugees and different cultural groups. PTSD screening can be accomplished with the Posttraumatic Stress Disorder (PTSD) Checklist—Civilian version. The Harvard Trauma Questionnaire includes a PTSD portion, which can also be used [19, 39]. The Generalized Anxiety Disorder-7 item scale (GAD-7) is the recommended tool for screening for anxiety and can be used for adults and adolescents as young as age 13. The Refugee Health Screener-15 (RHS-15) is a questionnaire that is specifically validated for newly arrived refugees to screen for common mental disorders, including depression, anxiety, and PTSD [19]. As an aid to frame questions in a culturally sensitive way that can help patients understand them better, the *Diagnostic and Statistical Manual of Mental Disorders* (Fifth Edition) (DSM-5) includes a resource entitled the Cultural Formulation Interview (CFI). This evidence-based tool can assist clinicians in making assessments and treatment plans that are patient-centered and culturally specific [19, 41, 42].

Cultural Factors

Screening for mental health disorders is of utmost importance in these communities since refugees and migrants seek care for mental illness less frequently than other populations [19, 41, 44]. In discussing refugees and migrants broadly, it is important to remember that cultural beliefs about mental health vary widely among groups, and generalization should be avoided. Differing cultural norms and conceptions of mental health can affect individuals' willingness to agree to or engage in the treatment, and language barriers and difficulty navigating the healthcare system are significant obstacles to presenting for care or following through with treatment. Perceived stigmatization or lack of sensitivity of healthcare providers are other factors that limit individuals' willingness to seek care [19, 41, 44]. When refugees and migrants do access mental health services, additional barriers such as limited or inappropriate use of interpreters can affect the quality of care they receive [44].

Treatment Considerations

Several strategies can be implemented to improve the quality of care for refugees and migrants being treated for mental health disorders. Increasing accessibility through the use of interpreters and cultural brokers, using culturally sensitive services, and understanding familial and social structures can all positively impact care.

The use of professional interpreters is of utmost importance in the treatment of psychiatric illnesses. Out of convenience, providers may attempt to use family members or community members as interpreters. While family or community members can act as cultural brokers to help with explaining cultural differences or contexts, it is inappropriate to use them as interpreters due to potential breaches in confidentiality and possible limitations in the disclosure of information as a result. Professional interpreters are often more accurately able to convey and describe diagnoses and treatment options to the patients, which ultimately leads to improved quality of care [41, 42].

Considering cultural traditions and taking them into account when constructing a treatment plan can improve outcomes as well. The CFI mentioned above that is featured in the DSM-5 can assist with this [19, 41, 42]. While this is not always possible, constructing a practice in a way that is openly welcoming to refugees and migrants (e.g., by providing signage in the clinic that is translated into their native languages, hiring staff that is representative of the migrant community, partnering with local refugee resettlement organizations, etc.) can foster trust and improve care [19]. Collaborative care models featuring integrated behavioral health within primary care clinics are effective in improving patient outcomes, as well as provider resilience [19, 44]. Incorporating the family and community into the assessment and plan of care may be appropriate and beneficial in certain circumstances, particularly since the same trauma may have impacted multiple members of the family [42].

Framework for Refugee Primary Care

While refugees and other forced migrants come to the US from a vast array of experiences and different geographic regions, there are common conditions that may present in these populations in primary care offices [46, 47]. Many of these conditions will only become clear after initial resettlement health screenings are completed and acute needs are attended to. These may include mental health issues, such as PTSD, depression, and anxiety, developmental disabilities, as well as undiagnosed chronic conditions including chronic pelvic or musculoskeletal pain, headaches, and impaired nutrition due to poor oral health and other issues. A slow and staged approach to building rapport, team-based care using trained medical interpreters and other specifically skilled providers who may have additional time for health education, mental health services, and connecting refugees to local community and social services resources is essential.

Including the care of refugees and other forced migrant and immigrant patients in a primary care practice requires particular attention to specific issues that should be common for all sites of health care—a welcoming, respectful, and safe environment and adequate time and resources to provide comprehensible and appropriate care to any at-risk population. There are many resources to support and connect healthcare providers interested in providing excellent care for refugees and immigrants, a number of which are listed in the resources. Despite the numerous challenges, caring for refugees, asylum seekers, and other migrant populations can be highly rewarding.

References

1. UNHC for Refugees. History of UNHCR. UNHCR. https://www.unhcr.org/history-of-unhcr.html. Accessed 4 Oct 2021.
2. UNHC for Refugees. Figures at a Glance. UNHCR. https://www.unhcr.org/figures-at-a-glance.html. Accessed 4 Oct 2021.
3. UNHC for Refugees. Refworld | "Refugees" and "Migrants"—Frequently Asked Questions (FAQs). Refworld. https://www.refworld.org/docid/56e81c0d4.html. Accessed 4 Oct 2021.
4. UNHCR—Asylum-Seekers. https://www.unhcr.org/en-us/asylum-seekers.html. Accessed 21 Oct 2021.
5. UNHC for Refugees. The Global Compact on Refugees. UNHCR. https://www.unhcr.org/the-global-compact-on-refugees.html. Accessed 30 Nov 2021.
6. Refugee Council USA. Resettlement Process. https://rcusa.org/resettlement/resettlement-process/. Accessed 26 Nov 2021.
7. Centers for Disease Control. Technical Instruction for Panel Physicians. https://www-cdc-gov.libproxy.lib.unc.edu/immigrantrefugeehealth/panel-physicians.html. Accessed 26 Nov 2021.
8. Mitchell T, Weinberg M, Posey DL, Cetron M. Immigrant, and refugee health. Pediatr Clin N Am. 2019;66(3):549–60. https://doi.org/10.1016/j.pcl.2019.02.004.
9. Centers for Disease Control. Guidance for the US Domestic Refugee Examination for Newly Arriving Refugees. https://www-cdc-gov.libproxy.lib.unc.edu/immigrantrefugeehealth/guidelines/domestic-guidelines.html. Accessed 26 Nov 2021.
10. Medical Certification for Disability Exceptions | USCIS. Published 30 Oct 2020. https://www.uscis.gov/n-648. Accessed 30 Nov 2021.
11. Lustig SL, Kureshi S, Delucchi KL, Iacopino V, Morse SC. Asylum grant rates following medical evaluations of maltreatment among political asylum applicants in the United States. J Immigr Minor Health. 2008;10(1):7–15. https://doi.org/10.1007/s10903-007-9056-8.
12. Bhugra D, Becker MA. Migration, cultural bereavement and cultural identity. World Psychiatry. 2005;4(1):18–24.
13. Improving well-being for refugees in primary care: toolkit for providers. The Center for Victims of Torture; 2019. https://www.cvt.org/resources/publications. Accessed 26 Nov 2021
14. The Triple Trauma of Refugees. UNC Global. https://global.unc.edu/news-story/the-triple-trauma-of-refugees/. Accessed 30 Nov 2021.
15. Evans WN, Fitzgerald D. The economic and social outcomes of refugees in the United States: evidence from the ACS. National Bureau of Economic Research; 2017. https://doi.org/10.3386/w23498.
16. Haq C, Hostetter I, Zavala L, Mayorga J. Immigrant health and changes to the public-charge rule: family physicians' response. Ann Fam Med. 2020;18(5):458–60. https://doi.org/10.1370/afm.2572.
17. Health Literacy in Healthy People 2030 | health.gov. https://health.gov/our-work/national-health-initiatives/healthy-people/healthy-

people-2030/health-literacy-healthy-people-2030. Accessed 30 Nov 2021.
18. Castelli F, Sulis G. Migration and infectious diseases. Clin Microbiol Infect. 2017;23(5):283–9. https://doi.org/10.1016/j.cmi.2017.03.012.
19. Griswold KS, Loomis DM, Pastore PA. Mental health and illness. Prim Care. 2021;48(1):131–45. https://doi.org/10.1016/j.pop.2020.09.009.
20. Abbas M, Aloudat T, Bartolomei J, et al. Migrant and refugee populations: a public health and policy perspective on a continuing global crisis. Antimicrob Resist Infect Control. 2018:7. http://dx.doi.org.libproxy.lib.unc.edu/10.1186/s13756-018-0403-4.
21. Seedat F, Hargreaves S, Nellums LB, Ouyang J, Brown M, Friedland JS. How effective are approaches to migrant screening for infectious diseases in Europe? A systematic review. Lancet Infect Dis. 2018;18(9):e259–71. https://doi.org/10.1016/S1473-3099(18)30117-8.
22. Stauffer WM, Weinberg M. Emerging clinical issues in refugees. Curr Opin Infect Dis. 2009;22(5):436–42. https://doi.org/10.1097/QCO.0b013e32832f14a4.
23. CDCTB. Reported TB in the U.S., 2020—National Data. Centers for Disease Control and Prevention. Published 25 Oct 2021. https://www.cdc.gov/tb/statistics/reports/2020/national_data.htm. Accessed 20 Nov 2021.
24. CDCTB. Reported TB in the U.S., 2020—Demographics. Centers for Disease Control and Prevention. Published 25 Oct 2021. https://www.cdc.gov/tb/statistics/reports/2020/demographics.htm. Accessed 20 Nov 2021.
25. Hargreaves S, Lönnroth K, Nellums LB, et al. Multidrug-resistant tuberculosis and migration to Europe. Clin Microbiol Infect. 2017;23(3):141–6. https://doi.org/10.1016/j.cmi.2016.09.009.
26. Te HS, Jensen DM. Epidemiology of hepatitis B and C viruses: a global overview. Clin Liver Dis. 2010;14(1):1–21. https://doi.org/10.1016/j.cld.2009.11.009.
27. Averhoff FM, Glass N, Holtzman D. Global burden of hepatitis C: considerations for healthcare providers in the United States. Clin Infect Dis. 2012;55:S10–5.
28. HIV/AIDS. https://www.who.int/news-room/fact-sheets/detail/hiv-aids. Accessed 21 Nov 2021.
29. Hepatitis B. https://www.who.int/news-room/fact-sheets/detail/hepatitis-b. Accessed 21 Nov 2021.
30. Wong RJ, Brosgart CL, Welch S, et al. An updated assessment of chronic hepatitis B prevalence among foreign-born persons living in the United States. Hepatology (Baltimore, MD). 2021;74(2):607–26. https://doi.org/10.1002/hep.31782.
31. People Born Outside of the United States and Viral Hepatitis | CDC. Published 24 Sept 2020. https://www.cdc.gov/hepatitis/populations/Born-Outside-United-States.htm. Accessed 20 Nov 2021.
32. Mixson-Hayden T, Lee D, Ganova-Raeva L, et al. Hepatitis B virus and hepatitis C virus infections in United States-bound refugees from Asia and Africa. Am J Trop Med Hyg. 2014;90(6):1014–20. https://doi.org/10.4269/ajtmh.14-0068.
33. Hepatitis C. https://www.who.int/news-room/fact-sheets/detail/hepatitis-c. Accessed 21 Nov 2021.
34. CDC. Hepatitis C | CDC. Centers for Disease Control and Prevention. Published 14 Jun 2021. https://www.cdc.gov/hepatitis/hcv/index.htm. Accessed 21 Nov 2021.
35. Valverde E, DiNenno E, Oraka E, Bautista G, Chavez P. HIV testing among foreign-born men and women in the United States: results from a nationally representative cross-sectional survey. J Immigr Minor Health. 2018;20(5):1118–27. https://doi.org/10.1007/s10903-017-0655-8.
36. Ross J, Cunningham CO, Hanna DB. HIV outcomes among migrants from low- and middle-income countries living in high-income countries: a review of recent evidence. Curr Opin Infect Dis. 2018;31(1):25–32. https://doi.org/10.1097/QCO.0000000000000415.
37. Winston SE, Montague BT, Lopez MJ, et al. Evaluation of longitudinal clinical outcomes and adherence to care among HIV-infected refugees. J Int Assoc Provid AIDS Care. 2013;12(3):202–7. https://doi.org/10.1177/1545109712459680.
38. Pottie K, Girard V. Common infectious diseases. Prim Care. 2021;48(1):45–55. https://doi.org/10.1016/j.pop.2020.11.002.
39. Reese K, Moyer B. Refugee medical screening. Prim Care. 2021;48(1):9–21. https://doi.org/10.1016/j.pop.2020.09.003.
40. Janda A, Eder K, Fressle R, et al. Comprehensive infectious disease screening in a cohort of unaccompanied refugee minors in Germany from 2016 to 2017: a cross-sectional study. PLoS Med. 2020;17(3):e1003076. https://doi.org/10.1371/journal.pmed.1003076.
41. Rousseau C, Frounfelker RL. Mental health needs and services for migrants: an overview for primary care providers. J Travel Med. 2019;26(2). http://dx.doi.org.libproxy.lib.unc.edu/10.1093/jtm/tay150.
42. Kronick R. Mental health of Refugees and asylum seekers: assessment and intervention. Can J Psychiatry Rev Can Psychiatr. 2018;63(5):290–6. https://doi.org/10.1177/0706743717746665.
43. Hynie M. The social determinants of refugee mental health in the post-migration context: a critical review. Can J Psychiatr. 2018;63(5):297–303. https://doi.org/10.1177/0706743717746666.
44. Lu J, Jamani S, Benjamen J, Agbata E, Magwood O, Pottie K. Global mental health and services for migrants in primary care settings in high-income countries: a scoping review. Int J Environ Res Public Health. 2020;17(22):8627. https://doi.org/10.3390/ijerph17228627.
45. Johnson K, Carpenter E, Walters T. Special issues in immigrant medicine. Prim Care. 2021;48(1):147–61. https://doi.org/10.1016/j.pop.2020.09.010.
46. Mishori R, Aleinikoff S, Davis D. Primary care for refugees: challenges and opportunities. Am Fam Physician. 2017;96(2):112–20.
47. Eckstein B. Primary care for refugees. Am Fam Physician. 2011;83(4):9.

Resources/Websites

Centers for Disease Control—Immigrant, Refugee and Migrant Health. https://www.cdc.gov/immigrantrefugeehealth/.
Church World Service. http://cwsglobal.org/.
EthnoMed. https://ethnomed.org/.
North America Society of Refugee Health Providers. https://refugee-society.org/.
Office of Refugee Resettlement. https://acf.hhs.gov/orr/programs/refugee-health.
Physicians for Human Rights. https://phr.org/.
Refugee Health Technical Assistance Center. https://refugeehealthta.org/.
The Center for Victims of Torture. https://www.cvt.org/.
World Relief. http://www.worldelief.org/.

Special Population: COVID-Associated Chronic Conditions

John M. Baratta and Louise King

Introduction

Severe Acute Respiratory Syndrome Coronavirus-2 (SARS-CoV-2) is a highly infectious, single-stranded RNA coronavirus that was first detected as a cause of mysterious pneumonia-like illnesses in a Wuhan Province, China, seafood market in December 2019 [1]. SARS-CoV-2 is principally a respiratory virus and transmission is primarily by exposure to respiratory fluids carrying the infectious virus. Exposure may occur through inhalation of respiratory droplets and aerosolized particles; deposition of respiratory droplets on exposed mucous membranes (e.g., mouth, nose, or eyes); or by touching mucous membranes with soiled hands [2].

Persons infected with SARS-CoV-2 can have a wide spectrum of illness severity, from critical illness and death to asymptomatic illness. Illness caused by SARS-CoV-2 was termed COVID-19 by the World Health Organization, the acronym derived from "coronavirus disease 2019" [3]. For many affected by COVID-19, the presentation is similar to that of other viral illnesses and includes symptoms such as fever, shortness of breath, fatigue, cough, nausea, diarrhea, myalgias, and arthralgias. It is theorized that the virus may exert pathophysiologic effects through numerous processes, including direct viral toxicity, endothelial damage and microvascular injury, immune system dysregulation, stimulation of a hyperinflammatory state, hypercoagulability with resultant micro- and macro-clotting, and maladaptation of the angiotensin-converting enzyme 2 (ACE2) pathway [4].

In the beginning months of the pandemic, early COVID-19 survivors began to report lingering symptoms after resolution of the acute illness. In the setting of widespread closures and social distancing, these affected persons frequently took their concerns to online platforms such as social media. Their anecdotes of persistent symptoms led to the formation of patient support and advocacy groups which have worked tirelessly to strive for recognition of the lingering effects, colloquially termed "Long COVID," and to develop patient-led research [5].

Emerging research has demonstrated a high prevalence of patients with persistent symptoms after acute infection, most commonly seen in patients who had been hospitalized for the acute illness [6]. Findings of a delayed return to usual health have also been noted in people with more mild initial illness who did not require hospitalization [7]. A cohort of hospitalized and non-hospitalized patients from Washington State, the site of the first outbreak in the United States, reported a greater than 30% prevalence of persistent symptoms between 3 and 9 months after the initial illness [8]. A subsequent larger-scale study has demonstrated similar incidence of persons affected by post-COVID conditions (PCC) [9].

The COVID-19 pandemic has led to unprecedented global medical, economic, and social challenges. While healthcare advances have helped save the lives of many COVID-19 patients, countless survivors of this disease have struggled with its aftereffects. Post-COVID Condition (PCC) is a broad term which can be used to describe persistent symptoms or health effects after resolution of the acute illness. PCCs are strikingly common, estimated to affect 1 in 5 COVID-19 survivors, suggesting that tens of millions in the United States may have been affected by this syndrome [9, 10]. This chapter will offer a discussion on PCC, with an emphasis on evaluation and management of major symptoms.

J. M. Baratta (✉)
Department of Physical Medicine and Rehabilitation, University of North Carolina at Chapel Hill, Chapel Hill, NC, USA
e-mail: john_baratta@med.unc.edu

L. King
Department of Medicine, University of North Carolina, Chapel Hill, NC, USA
e-mail: louise_king@med.unc.edu

Defining Post-COVID Conditions

Post-COVID Conditions (PCCs) can broadly be described as "lack of return to a usual state of health following COVID-19 illness" [11]. The two key criteria for diagnosis of a PCC include (1) prior confirmed or presumed COVID illness and (2) persisting symptoms or health effects which are attributable to a post-infectious process. Given the emerging nature of PCCs, there is a lack of universal agreement on more specific terminology and case definitions. The Centers for Disease Control (CDC) describes PCCs as "the wide range of health consequences that are present more than four weeks after infection with SARS-CoV-2" [12]. The United Kingdom's National Institute for Health and Care Excellence describes three phases: "acute COVID-19" up to 4 weeks; "ongoing symptomatic COVID-19" from 4 to 12 weeks; and "post-COVID-19 syndrome" in those who have symptoms for more than 12 weeks without explanation by an alternative diagnosis [13]. The WHO definition describes that PCC "occurs in individuals with a history of probable or confirmed SARS-CoV-2 infection, usually 3 months from the onset of COVID-19 with symptoms and that last for at least 2 months and cannot be explained by an alternative diagnosis" [3].

It is important to note that a variety of terminology has been used to describe PCC. Other terms that are used synonymously with PCC include but are not limited to long COVID, long haul COVID, post-acute sequelae of SARS-CoV-2 infection, late sequelae of COVID, long-term effects of COVID, and chronic COVID. As of October 2021, a specific ICD-10 Code, U09.9, has been implemented to denote "Post COVID Condition." The code should be used for patients with a probable or confirmed history of SARS-CoV-2 infection who are diagnosed with a PCC [14].

Symptoms, Natural History, and Risk Factors

The effects of PCC can be wide-ranging and heterogeneous. Symptom constellations can vary by type, severity, and time course but often have an impact on everyday functioning [15]. The most prominent symptoms associated with PCC include fatigue, respiratory complaints (e.g., dyspnea, cough, chest pain), and cognitive impairments (e.g., memory loss, inattention). Patients can present with one primary symptom, although upon review of systems there are often multiple active concerns attributable to the PCC. Table 29.1 lists common symptoms by organ system.

The severity of symptoms may range from a mild to severe and debilitating. The trajectory of symptoms can also be variable with patients experiencing: (1) persisting symptoms from time of acute COVID; (2) new onset of symptoms after initial symptom relief; (3) crescendo symptoms; or (4) a combination of symptoms [5]. Figure 29.1 illustrates the varying patterns of symptom burden which might occur in patients.

Table 29.1 Common post-COVID condition symptoms

Constitutional	Musculoskeletal	Psychiatric
Fatigue	Joint pain	Anxiety
Decreased endurance	Muscle pain	Depression
Sleep disturbance	Muscle weakness	Post-traumatic stress disorder
Respiratory	*Neurological*	*Immunologic*
Cough	Memory and attention impairment	Skin rashes
Dyspnea	Dizziness	Hypersensitivity
Hypoxia	Headaches	
	Peripheral neuropathy	
Cardiovascular	*Gastrointestinal*	
Chest tightness and pain	Abdominal pain	
Arrhythmias	Diarrhea	
Hypercoagulability	Nausea	

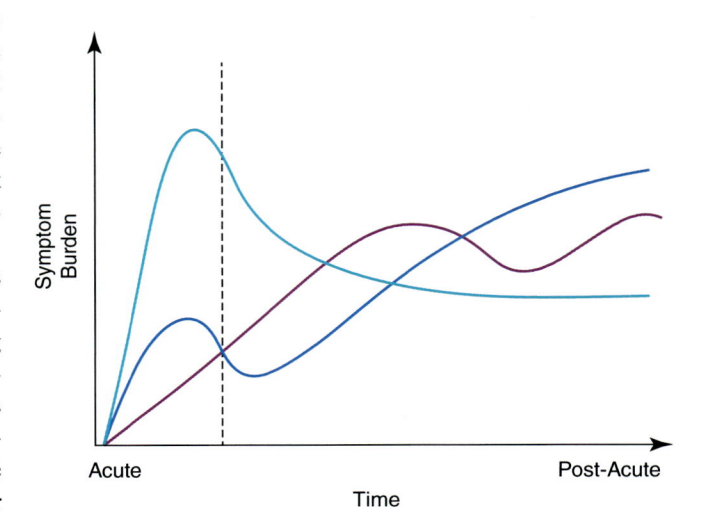

Fig. 29.1 Post-COVID condition (PCC) symptom trajectories. The burden of PCC symptoms can be variable and fluctuating. Patients may experience symptom worsening (dark blue line), symptom lessening (light blue line), episodic symptom flares (purple line), or a combination thereof during the post-acute period

The time course of PCC can be varied, affecting COVID survivors from weeks to months to years [5, 6, 16]. Persistent health effects have been shown to correspond with higher rates of medical and psychiatric diagnoses, use of healthcare resources, and risk of death beyond 30 days after illness onset [17, 18]. Future, longer-term cohort analyses will provide further insight on expectations and prognosis.

Emerging data have identified several key risk factors for developing PCC, including severity of acute COVID illness, older age, and the presence of medical comorbidities such as diabetes and obesity [4, 19, 20]. Females are more commonly affected by persistent symptoms, constituting a majority of PCC cases [20, 21]. It has furthermore been shown that persons with lower socioeconomic status and tobacco use are at higher risk [19]. Risk factors for development of PCCs continue to be investigated and will be further elucidated with time.

Pathophysiology

Persons with PCCs may or may not have demonstrable organ damage as a cause for their persistent health impairments. Organ damage, such as lung fibrosis or myocarditis, is more likely to occur in COVID survivors who experienced a severe acute illness [17]. Health consequences for these patients overlap significantly with other known conditions that affect people recovering from severe illness. For example, post-intensive care syndrome (PICS) is a constellation of physical, mental, and emotional health effects known to complicate recovery of persons after critical illness [22].

More challenging are cases in which COVID survivors experience persistent symptoms in the absence of identified organ damage or diagnostic testing abnormalities. In these patients, the mechanisms underlying the development of PCC are thought to be multiple and linked to several factors. Key processes may include excessive inflammation or an autoimmune phenomenon secondary to a dysregulated immune response, remnants of whole SARS-CoV-2 virus or viral fragments causing organ dysfunction, microclot formation, endothelial injury, excessive histamine release, mitochondrial dysfunction, Epstein-Barr Virus (EBV) reactivation, and an altered microbiome, among other potential causes [15, 23–26].

PCC is not the first recognized, post-infectious syndrome. Chronic fatiguing illnesses after acute viral and bacterial infections have been described since the 1700s and are comparable to PCC in historical descriptions. For example, *febricula*, meaning "little fever," was first recognized in the 1750s and consisted of low-grade temperature elevation, lassitude, and cognitive dysfunction [27]. Other similar conditions have included neurocirculatory asthenia, Akureyri disease, Royal Free disease, Tapanui flu, and chronic Epstein-Barr virus [28].

Some post-infectious fatiguing illnesses fall under the umbrella of Myalgic Encephalomyelitis/Chronic Fatigue Syndrome (ME/CFS). ME/CFS is a complex and underdiagnosed illness which has been estimated to affect up to 2.5 million Americans [29]. While the cause of this condition is not fully understood, the syndrome is often thought to be triggered by an infection and numerous outbreaks have been reported [29, 30]. It is characterized by at least 6 months of incapacitating fatigue, post-exertional malaise, unrefreshing sleep, memory and attention impairments, and orthostatic intolerance. In 2015, the Institute of Medicine (IOM), now the National Academy of Medicine (NAM), published updated diagnostic criteria for ME/CFS (Fig. 29.2) [31]. Of people who continue to remain ill 6 months after mild or moderate acute COVID-19, it has been shown that about half met criteria for ME/CFS [29].

Fig. 29.2 Proposed diagnostic criteria for ME/CFS [31]

> **The 2015 IOM diagnostic criteria for ME/CFS state that three symptoms and at least one of two additional manifestations are required for diagnosis.**
>
> The three required symptoms are:
>
> 1. *A substantial reduction or impairment in the ability to engage in pre-illness levels of activity* (occupational, educational, social, or personal life) that:
>   a. lasts for more than 6 months
>   b. is accompanied by fatigue that is:
>   i. often profound
>   ii. of new onset (not life-long)
>   iii. not the result of ongoing or unusual excessive exertion
>   iv. not substantially alleviated by rest
> 2. *Post-exertional malaise (PEM)**
> 3. *Unrefreshing sleep**
>
> At least one of the following two additional manifestations must be present:
>
> 1. *Cognitive impairment**
> 2. *Orthostatic intolerance*
>
> * The IOM committee specified that "The diagnosis of ME/CFS should be questioned if patients do not have these symptoms at least half of the time with moderate, substantial, or severe intensity."

Management Principles

Persons with PCCs benefit from comprehensive, knowledgeable, and timely care and there are several evaluation and treatment approaches that can promote recovery. This care may be offered by primary care providers, medical specialists, or specialty post-COVID centers.

History and Symptom Review

Given the complex nature of PCCs, careful history-taking by the provider is critical to understand a patient's syndrome. The history of present illness is a chronological description which traditionally includes elements such as location of concern, quality, severity, duration, timing, context, modifying factors, and associated signs or symptoms. PCCs often include vague, constitutional symptoms and may require targeted questions. In addition, a focused review of systems is important to understand the larger picture of symptom burden, particularly as many PCC patients are overwhelmed and have cognitive symptoms which limit their ability to recall. Table 29.2 lists key items to consider.

Standardized questionnaires can screen for comorbid conditions: Patient Health Questionnaire (PHQ) for depression; General Anxiety Disorder-7 for anxiety; STOP-BANG for sleep apnea; and DePaul Symptom Questionnaire (DSQ) for post-exertional malaise [32]. Persons with PCCs often struggle with substantial challenges in adjusting to the syndrome and associated health effects [33]. Compassion and empathy in the care of this population are critical since patients report frustration with providers and the healthcare community for being terse or dismissive [34]. Dedicated time to PCC patient encounters can be challenging from an organizational perspective, but can yield later rewards by allowing the patient to feel heard and validated.

Table 29.2 Symptom questions and review of systems

Interview questions	Review of systems
What symptoms after COVID have been the most troubling?	Fatigue, weakness, numbness, paresthesias, headaches, tinnitus, anosmia, ageusia, sleep impairment
Did symptoms start during the initial illness or come on later?	Dyspnea, cough, or excessive sputum
Are symptoms constant or do they come in episodes?	Chest pain, pressure, or palpitations
Have symptoms been worsening, improving, or stable recently?	Nausea, vomiting, diarrhea, constipation
Are there any factors that worsen or improve the symptoms?	Joint or muscle pains, rash
	Anxiety, depression, stress

Manage Comorbid Conditions

The presence of comorbid medical conditions is a risk factor for the development of PCCs [4, 19, 20] and it is important to evaluate and treat comorbidities to optimize recovery. Common medical comorbidities such as asthma, chronic obstructive pulmonary disease, sleep apnea, coronary artery disease, chronic kidney disease, hypertension, hyperlipidemia, and diabetes mellitus can be managed according to their respective standards of care. Less common comorbid conditions which can potentiate fatiguing illness include fibromyalgia, dysautonomia, mast cell activation disorder, connective tissue disease, and ME/CFS. Management of these conditions should be considered in the patient's ongoing treatment plan.

Evaluate Impact on Functioning and Activities

There is a spectrum of impairments associated with PCCs and persons are often limited in their abilities to perform regular activities, including home and work responsibilities, schooling, hobbies, and exercise. Some may require compensatory or adaptive techniques to activities of daily living (ADLs), mobility, and cognitive tasks. In such cases, it is prudent to incorporate a multidisciplinary approach including physical therapists to improve endurance and mobility; occupational therapists to provide training on activities of daily living and energy conservation techniques; and speech language pathologists to provide cognitive rehabilitation. A patient's vocational and avocational goals should be considered as part of a treatment plan, as returning to prior activities will aid in satisfaction with recovery and quality of life.

Consider Psychosocial Stressors

The COVID-19 pandemic has been a time of new and unprecedented stressors for most persons, and life challenges are intensified for those living with PCCs. COVID-19 survivors are at a higher risk for developing new anxiety and mood disorders, sleep impairments, and substance use disorders [18]. Additionally, there are often financial, relationship, caregiving, and transportation challenges to consider for a newly disabled person. When feasible, the provider should consider involving a social worker to evaluate and coordinate care. Psychotherapy counseling services should be considered for those who are in need.

Utilize a Focused Medical Evaluation

Currently there is no diagnostic testing that can definitively distinguish PCC from other etiologies, in part due to the heterogeneous and multifactorial nature of the condition. A targeted medical workup to evaluate and exclude other causes of persistent symptoms is critical. For example, persons with symptoms longer than 4 weeks may benefit from laboratory testing, including complete blood counts, metabolic panel, inflammatory markers, thyroid function, and Vitamin D and B12 levels. Testing may be broadened if symptoms persist for 12 weeks or longer and should be guided by the patient's primary symptoms and clinical findings. Patients with myalgias and arthralgias may benefit from testing for antinuclear antibody, rheumatoid factor, anti-cyclic citrullinated peptide, anti-cardiolipin, and creatine phosphokinase. Clinical guidelines exist from the CDC and specialty medical organizations [11, 32, 35–38]. Many laboratory and imaging studies of persons with PCC are nonrevealing, emphasizing the importance of the judicious testing selection. It is also important to note that the absence of laboratory-confirmed abnormalities should not lead to dismissal of the patient's symptoms or the impact on their functioning [34].

Care of Symptoms Associated with Post-COVID Conditions

Patients with PCCs can experience a constellation of symptoms with varying severity and impact on daily life. Fatigue tends to be the most common persisting symptom with other frequent symptoms and syndromes including respiratory, cardiovascular, and cognitive sequelae [39].

Fatigue

Persistent fatigue is the most common PCC complaint, occurring in both hospitalized and non-hospitalized individuals [8, 16, 40]. While fatigue often improves over time, in many cases it can persist for more than 6 months. PCC-related fatigue can be multidimensional, often being described as physical, cognitive, emotional, or a combination thereof. Those who experience mild fatigue may be able to continue most daily activities without interruption, but those who are moderately or severely impacted can be limited in the ability to perform a variety of activities in home or work settings. Those with profound fatigue may require homebound or bedbound accommodations.

The evaluation of patients with PCC-related fatigue should include assessment of the characteristics and patterns of fatigue, pre-existing or new medical conditions, and medications and supplements. First, patients should be evaluated for fatigue patterns throughout the normal day with several questions: *Is fatigue a daily issue? Are there times of the day when fatigue is less prominent? Do changes in physical or cognitive activities affect the degree of fatigue?* This line of questioning is useful to determine an "energy window," a daily timeframe during which patients may experience a lessening of symptoms. Next, attention should be paid to comorbid conditions which may contribute to fatigue, such as diabetes, heart failure, and anemia.

Optimal recovery from PCC-related fatigue will be dependent on adequate management of comorbid conditions. Finally, there should be a review of the patient's medicines and supplements which may contribute to fatigue. Antihistamine, anticholinergic, and anxiolytic medications are frequently used to manage PCC-related symptoms and can contribute to fatigue. Laboratory testing may be considered, including a complete blood count, chemistries including renal and hepatic function tests, thyroid-stimulating hormone, C-reactive protein or erythrocyte sedimentation rate, and creatinine kinase [11, 32].

Treatment of PCC-associated fatigue utilizes a multi-pronged approach which is tailored to the patient's situation and includes: (1) an individualized return to activity program; (2) implementation of energy conservation techniques; (3) use of a healthy dietary pattern and hydration; and (4) management of other medical conditions which may contribute to fatigue. Return to activity programs should be structured and adapted based on the degree of the individual's fatigue. The following consensus recommendations from The American Academy of Physical Medicine and Rehabilitation's Multi-Disciplinary PASC (Post-Acute Sequelae of SARS-CoV-2 Infection) Collaborative can inform treatment [32].

Return to Activity Program

A person with *mild fatigue* can perform ADLs, work, and school activities but may require modifications to their schedule and cessation of other, non-essential activities. Individuals should be encouraged to continue household and community activities which have been tolerated and initiate a slow progression of return to higher intensity activity. One such approach is the *Rule of Tens*, which consists of increasing duration, intensity, and frequency of activity by 10% every 10 days. Patients can report their level of activity fatigue using the Borg Rate of Perceived Exertion (RPE) scale, starting at RPE 10–11/Light (Table 29.3).

A person with *moderate fatigue* has decreased community mobility and is limited in performing instrumental activities of daily living, such as meal preparation, shopping, and housework. They may require frequent rest breaks and may have stopped work or school. Individuals should be encouraged to continue household and limited community activities which have been tolerated. Individuals should begin an activity or aerobic exercise program with exertion at sub-maximal levels, starting at RPE 9–11/Very Light-Light.

A person with *severe fatigue* is mostly confined to the home and may have difficulty with basic activities of daily

Table 29.3 Borg Rate of Perceived Exertion (RPE) scale

6	No exertion at all	No muscle fatigue, breathlessnes or difficulty in breathing.
7	Extremely light	Very, very light.
8		
9	Very light	Like walking slowly for a short while. Very easy to talk.
10		
11	Light	Like a light exercise at your own pace.
12	Moderate	
13	Somewhat hard	Fairly strenuous and breathless. Not so easy to talk.
14		
15	Hard	Heavy and strenuous. An upper limit for fitness training, as when running or walking fast.
16		
17	Very hard	Very strenuous. You are very tired and breathless. Very difficult to talk.
18		
19	Extremely hard	The most strenuous effort you have ever experienced.
20	Maximal exertion	Maximal heaviness.

The Borg RPE scale (© Gunnar Borg, 1970, 1998, 2017). Scale printed with permission. The scale and full instruction can be obtained through BorgPerception. www.borgperception.se

living, such as eating, bathing, dressing, and toileting. They require frequent, extended rest periods and have generally stopped work or school. Individuals should be encouraged to continue the limited household and community activities that can be performed without symptom exacerbation. Individuals should be encouraged to start a physical activity program which should initially consist of upper and lower extremity stretching and light muscle strengthening before any targeting aerobic activity. Once tolerated, patients can begin an activity or exercise program at sub-maximal levels (i.e., RPE 7–9/Extremely Light-Very Light).

Across all levels, patients should be encouraged to gradually advance activity as long as it does not cause worsening of symptoms, which may be delayed in onset for several days after the activity. If symptoms worsen, activity should be returned to the previously tolerated level. Referral to a rehabilitation therapist with knowledge of post-COVID care may be considered to further guide the treatment program.

Energy Conservation Techniques

Strategies that conserve energy has been shown to improve fatigue [41]. One approach is termed the "Four P's": Planning, Prioritizing, Pacing, and Positioning. *Planning* encourages the patient to consider the day or week ahead, scheduling activities in the energy windows to minimize overexertion. *Prioritizing* suggests that patients consider which activities must get done and which can be postponed to a later time or delegated to someone else. *Pacing* is the concept of staggering activities throughout a day or week to reduce development of excessive fatigue. *Positioning* involves modifying activities to reduce energy expenditure, such as sitting instead of standing.

Accommodations can also be useful to help patients remain in the workplace or return to work. Providers may consider offering written documentation to support work accommodations, including limiting hours, providing rest breaks, modifying work activities, allowing seated work, permitting work from home, and permitting assistive devices or durable medical equipment.

Healthy Dietary Approaches

Although data are limited to support specific diets for PCC-associated fatigue, a balanced selection of whole grains, vegetables, fruits, and healthy proteins is ideal [42]. Patients with PCC may experience new food intolerances and should be encouraged to eat sensibly while being mindful of their body's reaction. They should also be encouraged to remain well-hydrated, primarily consuming water and minimizing sugary drinks. Fatigue related to autonomic dysfunction, specifically postural orthostatic tachycardia syndrome, can be mitigated with adequate water and salt intake [43]. Fatigue due to muscle atrophy in the context of weight loss can be improved with adequate caloric and protein intake. Additionally, anti-inflammatory nutritional supplements have been proposed to help management of fatigue, including Vitamin B12, Vitamin C, Vitamin D, branched-chain amino acids, and omega-3 fatty acids [44].

Management of Comorbid Conditions

Treatment of PCC-associated fatigue can be compromised if co-existing conditions are not addressed. People with PCC also may experience comorbid conditions such as anemia, fibromyalgia, chronic fatigue syndrome, thyroid dysfunction, sleep disorders, autoimmune disorders, diabetes, heart failure, and respiratory sequelae which could contribute to the overall presentation. Providers are encouraged to treat such conditions in collaboration with appropriate specialists. Finally, in some cases, there may be a role for pharmacologic therapy for management of PCC-related fatigue. Medications which are commonly used for fatigue in other populations and have shown promise in those with PCC-related fatigue include methylphenidate, modafinil, and amantadine [45].

Respiratory Symptoms

Dyspnea is the second most common symptom in patients with PCC [46, 47]. Breathing difficulties can lead to reduced function at home and work, in addition to negatively impacting quality of life [48]. Persistent respiratory symptoms (e.g., dyspnea) are a contributing factor to increased healthcare utilization after acute COVID, as noted by an increase in the prescription of respiratory medicines, including inhalers, antitussives, and expectorants [17].

The assessment of PCC-associated respiratory symptoms begins with the patient's history. Persons with a history of severe COVID illness, marked by hospitalization, ventilation, or admission to the ICU, are more likely to develop persistent respiratory symptoms [36]. However, patients with mild symptoms during the acute infection can develop persistent PCC-associated respiratory symptoms [49, 50]. The review of systems should cover related symptoms, including chest pain, cough, palpitations, orthopnea, and anxiety. The single-item Modified Medical Research Council (mMRC) scale or the modified Borg dyspnea scale can be used to document dyspnea symptoms [48].

Evaluation of patients with PCC-associated respiratory symptoms should include a comprehensive physical examination, an oxygen saturation at rest and with exercise, and a chest X-ray [51]. If possible, it can be helpful to perform a Six Minute Walk Test (6MWT) since patients often report symptoms that occur or are worsened with exertion [52]. If the 6MWT is not available, ambulating with a patient in the office with an oxygen saturation meter can be informative. Patients with persistent dyspnea on exertion should also undergo pulmonary function tests (PFTs), which include spirometry, diffusion capacity, and lung volumes [48]. Repeating testing pre- and post-bronchodilation is useful to detect reactive airways disease. The most common finding on PFTs in patients with PCC-associated respiratory symptoms is a reduced diffusing capacity of lung for carbon monoxide (DLCO), which reflects decreased function of the alveolar tissue to transfer gas from inspired air into the bloodstream. Lower DLCO measures have been associated with more severe initial disease [51, 53]. In patients with more significant respiratory complaints, reductions in total lung capacity (TLC) and residual volumes have been reported [54]. Many patients with pre-existing asthma report a worsening of their symptoms and some may interpret increased PCC-related breathlessness with worsening of their asthma. Providers should be mindful of this possibility to identify patients that may be self-treating their asthma inappropriately [55].

Further diagnostic workup with chest computed tomography (CT) is indicated in patients with diminished DLCO, abnormal lung volumes, oxygen desaturation, or significant respiratory symptoms. Patients who are found to have fibrotic lung disease on the chest CT can benefit from a referral to a pulmonologist and intensive pulmonary rehabilitation [56]. Cardiopulmonary exercise testing (CPET) can be a valuable tool to assess the cause of persistent dyspnea, particularly in patients with higher activity and exercise tolerance [57].

Patients who have had COVID have a two-fold increase in risk for pulmonary embolism in the year after their acute illness [9]. Clinicians should have a low threshold for suspecting pulmonary embolism, especially those who had more severe COVID. The standard of care for diagnosis and treatment of pulmonary embolism is the same as in any other patient, often beginning with the measurement of a d-dimer and proceeding to a chest CT with contrast if the d-dimer is elevated. If chronic venous thromboembolism is suspected, a ventilation/perfusion scan (V/Q scan) should be ordered, as chronic pulmonary emboli may not be detected in a CT scan [51].

In the absence of pulmonary testing abnormalities, an exercise program for pulmonary rehabilitation is frequently helpful [36] although energy conservation techniques should be considered due to fatigue. The benefits of breathing exercises that emphasize controlled, diaphragmatic breathing have been supported by evidence which demonstrates that people with PCC-associated respiratory issues often have disordered, shallow breathing which can be exacerbated by activity [57, 58]. Videos and internet-derived programs can provide training for improving breathing techniques [59, 60]. Respiratory therapists and speech language pathologists also provide directive instruction for breathing techniques. The use of vocal techniques from opera has furthermore been demonstrated as a method to retrain breathing [60, 61]. The course of dyspnea is variable and has been described as increasing over time, decreasing, or staying stable [16, 51,

62]. The myriad of diagnostic testing may be normal, even for patients with significant symptom burden. It is important to acknowledge and validate the patient's symptoms and to offer close follow-up [63].

Cough is a common PCC-associated respiratory complaint [51]. A chest x-ray, PFTs, and a search for other etiologies of chronic cough, such as GERD or the use of ACE inhibitor, should be considered. Underlying, predisposing conditions should be identified and symptomatic treatment of cough can be provided. Some guidelines allow for the use of empiric treatment with a steroid inhaler, especially in patients who have a history of asthma [53]. Fortunately the symptom of cough usually dissipates with time [16, 51, 62].

Cardiovascular Symptoms

Long-term cardiovascular symptoms and sequelae, such as chest pain, palpitations, and dyspnea, are common after COVID [64]. A diagnostic evaluation may include electrocardiogram (EKG), ambulatory cardiac rhythm monitoring, echocardiogram, cardiac stress test, serum markers of myocardial stress such as pro-brain natriuretic peptide (pro-BNP), and consultation with a cardiologist. Treatment should be guided from diagnostic findings and established guidelines. In addition to the evaluation of cardiovascular symptoms, there are several principles to consider when caring for a person with PCC-related issues. First, persons recovering from COVID have an increased risk of cardiovascular disease in the year following their diagnosis, including myocardial infarction, angina, and ischemic cardiomyopathy [16, 17, 64]. Chest pain in patients with PCC should be thoroughly evaluated, taking into account a patient's risk factors for coronary artery disease, the nature and quality of the chest pain, and associated signs and symptoms. Laboratory and other studies should include a serum troponin level, EKG, and echocardiogram and persistent chest pain suggestive of angina pectoris should be further evaluated with an exercise stress test [37]. Consultation with a cardiologist is recommended in patients with a high probability of coronary artery disease, or patients with atypical chest pain.

A second principle is that etiologies other than coronary artery disease should be considered in PCC patients with chest pain. Pericarditis and myocarditis are more prevalent in patients who are recovering from COVID, although the absolute increase in disease burden is less than what is reported in coronary artery disease [16, 65, 66]. Pericarditis may show EKG changes and the diagnosis can be confirmed by an echocardiogram. Cardiac magnetic resonance imaging (MRI) is helpful in the diagnosis of myocarditis. As noted earlier, the risk of pulmonary embolism is also increased in people recovering from COVID-19 and should also be considered.

Next, COVID survivors are at increased risk for arrhythmias, particularly atrial fibrillation [64]. Palpitations, which are reported in as many as 20% of patients with recovering from COVID, should be thoroughly evaluated with an EKG and ambulatory cardiac monitoring [65, 67]. An evaluation of chest pain in patients with PCC may be unrevealing, but this should not result in dismissal of the patient's symptoms. If there are no clear etiologies after a comprehensive workup, symptomatic care is appropriate. Musculoskeletal inflammation or neuropathic pain may be contributors and should be considered when developing a plan for symptom management.

Special Consideration: Postural Orthostatic Tachycardia Syndrome (POTS) Dysautonomia

Patients with PCCs may experience dysregulation of the autonomic nervous system [68, 69]. Dysautonomia is used to describe the wide-ranging effects of this syndrome, which frequently include cardiovascular, gastrointestinal, and secretomotor issues [70]. Manifestations of dysautonomia include postural orthostatic tachycardia syndrome (POTS), neurocardiogenic syncope, inappropriate sinus tachycardia, and orthostatic intolerance [68]. Key symptoms for POTS include orthostatic symptoms of dizziness, fatigue, and palpitations. POTS is defined by the Heart Rhythm Society as an increase in heart rate of ≥30 beats/min when going from supine to standing position, with orthostatic symptoms such as lightheadedness, palpitations, tremor, weakness, and fatigue [71].

POTS symptoms may be episodic and, in clinical scenarios with a high clinical suspicion and normal bedside orthostatic measurements, a tilt table test which measures blood pressure and heart rate with increasing positional gradations can be used to make the diagnosis [69]. Treatment of POTS consists of non-pharmacologic and pharmacologic measures. Non-pharmacologic treatments include: (1) volume repletion with adequate hydration of at least 3 L/day [72]; (2) increased salt consumption up to 8–10 g/day or the addition of 1–2 teaspoons of salt/day [73]; (3) use of compression stockings, preferably thigh-high stocking with at least medium compression [72]; (4) avoidance of potentially exacerbating factors such as alcohol and anticholinergic medications [72]; and the use of recumbent exercise, such as swimming, rowing, or recumbent bicycling [73].

Pharmacotherapy is indicated when POTS symptoms are severe or poorly responsive to non-pharmacologic interventions. Beta blockers are a first-line therapy and propranolol is often used as an initial choice [72] since it has the advantage of mitigating common PCC-associated symptoms, including headache, anxiety, and tremor. However, as a non-selective beta blocker, care must be taken not to use propranolol in patients with known or suspected asthma. Metoprolol, bisoprolol, and atenolol are other beta blockers that have been used with success in POTS [74].

Persons with PCC-associated POTS who have low-normal to normal blood pressure limit the utility of a beta blocker. Fludrocortisone is an alternate therapy and can be started at a low dose and increased gradually [72]. The patient should be monitored for electrolyte disturbances, leg swelling, and secondary hypertension. Other pharmacologic treatments include pyridostigmine, clonidine, and ivabradine. Pyridostigmine is effective and also useful for patients without hypertension but many patients cannot tolerate it due to frequent side effects of diarrhea [75]. Clonidine can be used in patients with POTS with hypertension and is effective in treating excessive sweating related to dysautonomia, but has a narrow therapeutic window [73]. Ivabradine specifically targets heart rate and is well-tolerated; however, its cost in the United States makes it less practical for many patients [72].

Cognitive Symptoms

Cognitive symptoms, often termed *brain fog*, include impairments of attention, short-term memory, word finding, processing speed, and executive function, and can be major sequelae of PCC [38, 76, 77]. Contributing etiologies for PCC-associated cognitive symptoms include direct infection of the central nervous system, coagulopathy causing microclots and stroke, immune response with cytokine production, autonomic dysfunction, physical symptoms such as fatigue, and the emotional impact of being ill [4, 38]. Cognitive effects can range in severity and have variable impact on functioning. Mild symptoms might be a nuisance, such as briefly forgetting a name or set of keys. Moderate symptoms can result in difficulty with complex tasks such as sequencing steps of a recipe or managing one's medications. Severe symptoms can impact the performance of basic activities of daily living and may impede a person's ability to hold competitive employment.

The evaluation of cognitive symptoms begins with a clinical interview and physical examination and is inclusive of developmental and educational histories, screening for medical risk factors for cognitive impairment, and assessing current sleep, mood, and substance use. Screening can include validated tools such the MoCA© (Montreal Cognitive Assessment) or PROMIS© (Patient-Reported Outcomes Measurement Information System) Cognitive Function scales. A thorough neurologic examination should be performed, with a focus on new or worsening focal neurological deficits. Abnormal findings would warrant further urgent evaluation with neuroimaging [38, 76]. Initial laboratory testing includes complete blood count, Vitamin B12, thiamine, folate, homocysteine, Vitamin D, comprehensive metabolic panel, and thyroid function tests [38].

Neuropsychology testing can be useful to interpret a variety of cognitive dimensions with demographically adjusted norms. Testing may include objective estimation of baseline functioning; tests of attention, processing speed, executive functioning, visuospatial ability, and memory; standardized questionnaires about depression, anxiety, cognitive function, and fatigue; and a formal assessment of adequacy of effort. Results are interpreted within the context of medical and psychiatric histories and current symptoms with the goal of providing patients and providers information about current function and recommendations to support future recovery.

Several approaches support cognitive recovery in persons with PCCs. First, comorbid conditions such as sleep impairment, mood disorders, substance use, and sedating medications should be identified and treated. Next, cognitive rehabilitation with a speech language pathologist should be considered. This is a cornerstone approach for many people with cognitive symptoms, such as stroke and traumatic brain injury, and has been successfully adapted to assist those with PCCs [78]. Treatment techniques utilized during cognitive rehabilitation sessions can improve attention, memory, problem solving, and reasoning skills. Home cognitive exercises are often provided to patients to continue their training. Additionally, physical activity has been demonstrated to have positive effects in cognitive impairment related to other conditions, and should be encouraged when safe [79, 80]. Furthermore, anti-inflammatory diets and mind-body medicine—such as mindfulness meditation, yoga, and tai chi—should be considered [81–83]. Off-label use of medications for symptom management may also be considered on a case-by-case basis. Promise has been shown with some stimulants, such as methylphenidate, and activating antidepressants, such as bupropion.

There are other persisting symptoms in patients with PCCs and Table 29.4 presents these by category with an evaluation summary and initial management strategies.

Table 29.4 Evaluation and management of additional common PCC symptoms

Category	Symptom	Summary of evaluation	Initial management strategies
Neurologic	Headaches	• Assess location, frequency, pain characteristics, and aggravating/alleviating factors. • Perform complete neurological examination including evaluation for red flag symptoms including focal neurologic deficits, meningismus, temporal artery tenderness, and papilledema.	• Non-pharmacologic approaches include avoidance of triggers; resting in a quiet, dark room; and hot or cold compresses to the head or neck. • Attempt acute treatment with oral analgesics such as acetaminophen, NSAIDS, metoclopramide, triptans, ergots, and butalbital compounds. • For frequent headache sufferers, prophylaxis with certain beta blockers, calcium channel blockers, antidepressants, and anti-seizure medications can be recommended. • Consider referral to a neurologist.
Neurologic	Neuropathy	• Assess distribution and characteristics such as sensory loss, numbness, pain, or burning sensations. • Perform complete musculoskeletal and neurological examinations. • Initial laboratory testing includes a complete blood count; a comprehensive metabolic profile; fasting blood glucose, vitamin B12, and thyroid-stimulating hormone levels; and serum protein electrophoresis with immunofixation. • Consider electrodiagnostic studies.	• Treatment of neuropathy focuses on managing the underlying etiology, such as improving blood sugar control, correcting thyroid dysfunction, or repleting vitamin levels. Appropriate treatment should slow progression of neuropathy but may not reverse existing effects. • Non-pharmacologic approaches include light yoga, massage, acupuncture, and TENS (transcutaneous electrical nerve stimulation). • Attempt trial of gabapentin, pregabalin, or serotonin and norepinephrine reuptake inhibitors (SNRIs). Topical agents such as lidocaine or capsaicin gel could also be considered. • Referral to physical therapy is indicated if there is an associated balance impairment. • Consider referral to a neurologist.
Neurologic	Sleep disturbance	• Collect a history of sleep patterns, including the time it typically takes to fall asleep; the number and duration of nighttime awakenings; the final morning awakening; and day-to-day variability of the schedule. • Assess for anxiety or worries which could contribute to poor rest; daytime sleepiness; and mental and physical fatigue. • Review medications and substance use to determine whether any might contribute to a CNS-simulating effect. • Screen for sleep apnea, such as with the STOP-BANG assessment.	• Counsel on sleep hygiene techniques, including regular exercise; a consistent sleep pattern; a cool, dark, and quiet bedroom; and avoidance of electronic devices for approximately 1 h before bed. • Address psychosocial stressors as needed with empathy, counseling services, and medication. • Offer cognitive behavioral therapy for insomnia (CBT-I). • Minimize CNS-stimulating medicines when possible. If necessary, encourage morning administration. • Consider a sleep study or a referral to a sleep specialist.
Neurologic	Changes to smell	• Concerns may include anosmia (inability to smell), hyposmia (decreased ability to smell), phantosmia (perception of odor without stimulus present), and parosmia (altered perception of an odor in the presence of an odorant stimulus). • Assess the characteristics of symptoms, timing, progression, and impact on lifestyle. Patient examples can be helpful. Inquire about nasal congestion and drainage. • Review patient's history with special attention to sinus problems, allergies, and nasal obstruction. • Perform a complete ears, nose, and throat examination with emphasis on the nasal airways.	• Smell training, or olfactory training, has shown promise in helping recover lost sense of smell. While protocols can vary, the most common involves smelling four scents for approximately 20 s each on a twice daily basis. Recommended scents include four essential oils: lavender, lemon, clove, and eucalyptus. During the smelling process, the patient should practice guided imagery by viewing a picture or attempting to visualize the scent they are smelling. Olfactory training kits can be purchased or assembled at home. • Offer patient resources on loss of smell, such as are available at as https://www.fifthsense.org.uk/ or https://abscent.org/. • Consider referral to an otolaryngologist for further evaluation including possible nasal endoscopy.

Psychiatric	Mood, anxiety, and stress disorders	• Assess presence of depression, anxiety, PTSD, and suicidal ideation. Consider potential co-existence of delirium or substance use. • Perform validated symptom screening, such as PHQ-9 and GAD-7, being mindful that traditional measures have limitations including overlap with other frequent PCC symptoms (e.g., fatigue, inattention). • Evaluate for reversible causes including nutritional deficiencies (B12, folate, vitamin D), endocrinopathies (TSH, free T4), and sleep disorders. • Brain imaging such as MRI is frequently unrevealing but can be considered in select cases.	• Provide reassurance to patients that psychiatric symptoms after COVID are common. Medical attention and provider acknowledgment can be a source of hope to patients. Psychiatric issues should be addressed as part of the overall recovery plan. • Psychotherapy services and post-COVID support groups can be particularly useful to assist with symptom management and adjustment to a new disability. • Traditional pharmacotherapy—including selective serotonin reuptake inhibitors (SSRIs), serotonin and norepinephrine reuptake inhibitors (SNRIs), tricyclic antidepressants (TCAs), and stimulants—can play an important role. Particular considerations may also include bupropion (can improve cognitive impairments), mirtazapine (can reduce nausea and assist sleep), and propranolol (can lower heart rate and reduce tremor). • Consider referral to a psychiatrist.
Dermatologic	Rash	• Assess for pruritus and the time course of lesions. • Perform a full skin examination with particular attention to fingers and toes. • Obtain lab work for inflammatory markers (ESR, CRP). • Consider a skin biopsy.	• Provide reassurance that most PCC-related skin manifestations are self-limiting. • If needed, initiate symptomatic treatment such as with steroid creams, hydroxyzine, or diphenhydramine. • Consider referral to a dermatologist.
Dermatologic	Hair loss	• Assess the degree of hair loss and time course. • Inquire about other life stressors which could contribute to sudden hair loss, such as pregnancy, rapid weight loss, nutritional deficiency, and chemotherapy. • Perform a thorough scalp examination.	• Provide education on telogen effluvium, the most common hair disorder associated with COVID-19, which is characterized by diffuse generalized shedding. Hair loss is expected to be self-limiting and correct after 3–6 months. • Encourage consumption of a healthy, varied diet and use of multivitamin and biotin supplements.
Gastrointestinal	Nausea	• Assess for medication adverse effects. • Assess for dysautonomia with orthostatic blood pressure and heart rate. • Consider a GI motility study or endoscopy.	• Encourage small, frequent meals. Some patients do better with lower-carbohydrate diets. • Initiate regular probiotics. • Attempt a trial of ondansetron. • Treat anxiety and depression when present.
Rheumatologic	Myalgias, arthralgias	• Perform careful physical exam, looking for arthritis or skin changes. • Check CBC, renal function, inflammatory markers, ANA, rheumatoid factor, creatine kinase, and thyroid studies. • Consider checking other autoantibodies, such as antinuclear antibody and anti-cyclic citrullinated peptide, depending on specific symptoms.	• Treat any underlying pathologies if identified. • Use NSAIDS if there are no contraindications. • Consider agents to treat chronic pain, such as gabapentin or similar agents. • Consider referral to a rheumatologist.

Health Care Service Models

The high prevalence of COVID-19 during the pandemic and sequelae of persistent health effects will result in substantial and sustained health care utilization. Much of the care for patients with PCCs will be provided in primary care settings with consultations and referrals based on individual patient situations [35]. However, due to the nuances and complexities associated with this syndrome, outpatient centers for post-COVID care have emerged throughout the United States. Many of these programs have been centered at large medical centers, with varied structures depending on the services available at a particular institution. For example, the spectrum of programs can range from solely therapy-based treatments to single- or multi-specialty evaluation. The majority of programs are led by providers specializing in physical medicine & rehabilitation (PM&R), pulmonology, and general internal medicine [84].

There are numerous benefits to multidisciplinary models of care for patients with complex conditions, as has been evidenced in the care of people with a disorders such as Parkinson's Disease, amyotrophic lateral sclerosis, and post-ICU syndrome [85–87]. Multidisciplinary centers for patients with PCCs may include primary care providers; medical specialists in PM&R, pulmonology, cardiology, neurology, and psychiatry; physical, occupational, and speech therapists; neuropsychologists; nutrition specialists; social workers; and care coordinators [88–90]. By integrating a team of medical providers, therapists, and other health professionals, this model provides more comprehensive services than those in traditional, outpatient settings. This approach can increase patient-centered care by facilitating provider collaboration and minimizing patient travel.

Future Directions

The evidence base of the pathophysiology, diagnostic approaches, and treatment strategies of PCCs will continue to substantially evolve in the coming years. This information will be critical in providing clinical care to persons with PCCs, since this syndrome may represent the largest disabling event in the United States since post-polio syndrome [49, 91]. Given the limited understanding of the multifactorial mechanisms contributing to PCCs, current care approaches remain primarily symptomatic. However, major research is underway to further understand the epidemiology and risk factors of PCCs, as well as to develop evaluation and treatment approaches. For example, the US Congress provided $1.15 billion in funding over 4 years for the National Institutes of Health to support research into PCCs, the centerpiece of which has been the Researching COVID to Enhance Recovery (RECOVER) national study [92]. This initiative and related investigations are shedding light on post-infectious chronic illnesses and will hopefully lead to new understanding and syndrome management for related conditions, such as ME/CFS. Finally, ongoing provider and community outreach and advocacy efforts remain critical to continued awareness of persistent PCC-related health effects and disability.

References

1. Holmes EC, Goldstein SA, Rasmussen AL, Robertson DL, Crits-Christoph A, Wertheim JO, et al. The origins of SARS-CoV-2: a critical review. Cell. 2021;184(19):4848–56.
2. Harrison AG, Lin T, Wang P. Mechanisms of SARS-CoV-2 transmission and pathogenesis. Trends Immunol. 2020;41(12):1100–15.
3. Coronavirus. [cited 2022 Jun 23]. Available from: https://www.who.int/health-topics/coronavirus.
4. Crook H, Raza S, Nowell J, Young M, Edison P. Long covid-mechanisms, risk factors, and management. BMJ. 2021;374:n1648.
5. Davis HE, Assaf GS, McCorkell L, Wei H, Low RJ, Re'em Y, et al. Characterizing long COVID in an international cohort: 7 months of symptoms and their impact. EClinicalMedicine. 2021;38:101019.
6. Carfì A, Bernabei R, Landi F, Gemelli Against COVID-19 Post-Acute Care Study Group. Persistent symptoms in patients after acute COVID-19. JAMA. 2020;324(6):603–5.
7. Tenforde MW, Kim SS, Lindsell CJ, Billig Rose E, Shapiro NI, Files DC, et al. Symptom duration and risk factors for delayed return to usual health among outpatients with COVID-19 in a multistate health care systems network—United States, March-June 2020. MMWR Morb Mortal Wkly Rep. 2020;69(30):993–8.
8. Logue JK, Franko NM, McCulloch DJ, McDonald D, Magedson A, Wolf CR, et al. Sequelae in adults at 6 months after COVID-19 infection. JAMA Netw Open. 2021;4(2):e210830.
9. Bull-Otterson L. Post–COVID conditions among adult COVID-19 survivors aged 18–64 and ≥65 years—United States, March 2020–November 2021. MMWR Morb Mortal Wkly Rep. 2022;71 [cited 2022 Jun 21]. Available from: https://www.cdc.gov/mmwr/volumes/71/wr/mm7121e1.htm.
10. PASC Dashboard. [cited 2022 Jun 23]. Available from: https://pascdashboard.aapmr.org/.
11. CDC. Healthcare workers. Centers for Disease Control and Prevention. 2020 [cited 2022 Jun 23]. Available from: https://www.cdc.gov/coronavirus/2019-ncov/hcp/clinical-care/post-covid-conditions.html.
12. Datta SD, Talwar A, Lee JT. A proposed framework and timeline of the Spectrum of disease due to SARS-CoV-2 infection: illness beyond acute infection and public health implications. JAMA. 2020;324(22):2251–2.
13. Shah W, Hillman T, Playford ED, Hishmeh L. Managing the long term effects of covid-19: summary of NICE, SIGN, and RCGP rapid guideline. BMJ. 2021;372:n136.
14. Centers for Disease Control and Prevention. [cited 2022 Jun 23]. Available from: https://www.cdc.gov/nchs/data/icd/announcement-new-icd-code-for-post-covid-condition-april-2022-final.pdf.
15. Nalbandian A, Sehgal K, Gupta A, Madhavan MV, McGroder C, Stevens JS, et al. Post-acute COVID-19 syndrome. Nat Med. 2021;27(4):601–15.
16. Huang L, Yao Q, Gu X, Wang Q, Ren L, Wang Y, et al. 1-year outcomes in hospital survivors with COVID-19: a longitudinal cohort study. Lancet. 2021;398(10302):747–58.

17. Al-Aly Z, Xie Y, Bowe B. High-dimensional characterization of post-acute sequelae of COVID-19. Nature. 2021;594(7862):259–64.
18. Taquet M, Geddes JR, Husain M, Luciano S, Harrison PJ. 6-month neurological and psychiatric outcomes in 236 379 survivors of COVID-19: a retrospective cohort study using electronic health records. Lancet Psychiatry. 2021;8(5):416–27.
19. Whitaker M, Elliott J, Chadeau-Hyam M, Riley S, Darzi A, Cooke G, et al. Persistent COVID-19 symptoms in a community study of 606,434 people in England. Nat Commun. 2022;13(1):1957.
20. Yong SJ. Long COVID or post-COVID-19 syndrome: putative pathophysiology, risk factors, and treatments. Infect Dis. 2021;53(10):737–54.
21. Sykes DL, Holdsworth L, Jawad N, Gunasekera P, Morice AH, Crooks MG. Post-COVID-19 symptom burden: what is long-COVID and how should we manage it? Lung. 2021;199(2):113–9.
22. Yong SJ, Liu S. Proposed subtypes of post-COVID-19 syndrome (or long-COVID) and their respective potential therapies. Rev Med Virol. 2021;9:e2315.
23. Kell DB, Laubscher GJ, Pretorius E. A central role for amyloid fibrin microclots in long COVID/PASC: origins and therapeutic implications. Biochem J. 2022;479(4):537–59.
24. Meringer H, Mehandru S. Gastrointestinal post-acute COVID-19 syndrome. Nat Rev Gastroenterol Hepatol. 2022;19(6):345–6.
25. Weinstock LB, Brook JB, Walters AS, Goris A, Afrin LB, Molderings GJ. Mast cell activation symptoms are prevalent in long-COVID. Int J Infect Dis. 2021;112:217–26.
26. Gold JE, Okyay RA, Licht WE, Hurley DJ. Investigation of long COVID prevalence and its relationship to Epstein-Barr virus reactivation. Pathogens (Basel, Switzerland). 2021;10(6):763.
27. The symptoms, nature, causes, and cure of the febricula, or little fever: commonly called the nervous or hysteric fever: the fever on the spirits: vapours, hypo, or spleen/By Sir Richard Manningham. Wellcome Collection. [cited 2022 Jun 26]. Available from: https://wellcomecollection.org/works/tt26ftah.
28. Sharif K, Watad A, Bragazzi NL, Lichtbroun M, Martini M, Perricone C, et al. On chronic fatigue syndrome and nosological categories. Clin Rheumatol. 2018;37(5):1161–70.
29. Bateman L, Bested AC, Bonilla HF, Chheda BV, Chu L, Curtin JM, et al. Myalgic encephalomyelitis/chronic fatigue syndrome: essentials of diagnosis and management. Mayo Clin Proc. 2021;96(11):2861–78.
30. Chronic Fatigue Syndrome. 11 Nov 1990. Available from: http://www.newsweek.com/chronic-fatigue-syndrome-205712.
31. IOM 2015 Diagnostic Criteria | Diagnosis | Healthcare Providers | Myalgic encephalomyelitis/chronic fatigue syndrome (ME/CFS) | CDC. 2021 [cited 2022 Jun 26]. Available from: https://www.cdc.gov/me-cfs/healthcare-providers/diagnosis/iom-2015-diagnostic-criteria.html.
32. Herrera JE, Niehaus WN, Whiteson J, Azola A, Baratta JM, Fleming TK, et al. Multidisciplinary collaborative consensus guidance statement on the assessment and treatment of fatigue in post-acute sequelae of SARS-CoV-2 infection (PASC) patients. PM R. 2021;13(9):1027–43.
33. Lamontagne SJ, Winters MF, Pizzagalli DA, Olmstead MC. Post-acute sequelae of COVID-19: evidence of mood & cognitive impairment. Brain Behav Immun Health. 2021;17:100347.
34. Rushforth A, Ladds E, Wieringa S, Taylor S, Husain L, Greenhalgh T. Long Covid—the illness narratives. Soc Sci Med. 2021;286:114326.
35. Vance H, Maslach A, Stoneman E, Harmes K, Ransom A, Seagly K, et al. Addressing post-COVID symptoms: a guide for primary care physicians. J Am Board Fam Med. 2021;34(6):1229–42.
36. Maley JH, Alba GA, Barry JT, Bartels MN, Fleming TK, Oleson CV, et al. Multi-disciplinary collaborative consensus guidance statement on the assessment and treatment of breathing discomfort and respiratory sequelae in patients with post-acute sequelae of SARS-CoV-2 infection (PASC). PM R. 2022;14(1):77–95.
37. Whiteson J, Azola A, Barry JT, Bartels MN, Blitshteyn S, Fleming TK, et al. Multi-disciplinary collaborative consensus guidance statement on the assessment and treatment of cardiovascular complications in patients with post-acute sequelae of SARS-CoV-2 infection (PASC). PM R. 2022;14:855.
38. Fine JS, Ambrose AF, Didehbani N, Fleming TK, Glashan L, Longo M, et al. Multi-disciplinary collaborative consensus guidance statement on the assessment and treatment of cognitive symptoms in patients with post-acute sequelae of SARS-CoV-2 infection (PASC). PM R. 2022;14(1):96–111.
39. Lopez-Leon S, Wegman-Ostrosky T, Perelman C, Sepulveda R, Rebolledo PA, Cuapio A, et al. More than 50 long-term effects of COVID-19: a systematic review and meta-analysis. Sci Rep. 2021;11(1):16144.
40. Michelen M, Manoharan L, Elkheir N, Cheng V, Dagens A, Hastie C, et al. Characterising long COVID: a living systematic review. BMJ Glob Health. 2021;6(9):e005427.
41. Jason LA, Brown M, Brown A, Evans M, Flores S, Grant-Holler E, et al. Energy conservation/envelope theory interventions to help patients with myalgic encephalomyelitis/chronic fatigue syndrome. Fatigue Biomed Health Behav. 2013;1(1–2):27–42.
42. Barrea L, Grant WB, Frias-Toral E, Vetrani C, Verde L, de Alteriis G, et al. Dietary recommendations for post-COVID-19 syndrome. Nutrients. 2022;14(6):1305.
43. Abed H, Ball PA, Wang LX. Diagnosis and management of postural orthostatic tachycardia syndrome: a brief review. J Geriatr Cardiol. 2012;9(1):61–7.
44. Haß U, Herpich C, Norman K. Anti-inflammatory diets and fatigue. Nutrients. 2019;11(10):2315.
45. Farooqi M, Khan A, Jacobs A, D'Souza V, Consiglio F, Karmen CL, et al. Examining the long-term sequelae of SARS-CoV2 infection in patients seen in an outpatient psychiatric department. Neuropsychiatr Dis Treat. 2022;18:1259–68.
46. Aiyegbusi OL, Hughes SE, Turner G, Rivera SC, McMullan C, Chandan JS, et al. Symptoms, complications and management of long COVID: a review. J R Soc Med. 2021;114(9):428–42.
47. Nasserie T, Hittle M, Goodman SN. Assessment of the frequency and variety of persistent symptoms among patients with COVID-19: a systematic review. JAMA Netw Open. 2021;4(5):e2111417.
48. Antoniou KM, Vasarmidi E, Russell AM, Andrejak C, Crestani B, Delcroix M, et al. European Respiratory Society statement on long COVID-19 follow-up. Eur Respir J. 2022;60:2102174.
49. Groff D, Sun A, Ssentongo AE, Ba DM, Parsons N, Poudel GR, et al. Short-term and long-term rates of postacute sequelae of SARS-CoV-2 infection: a systematic review. JAMA Netw Open. 2021;4(10):e2128568.
50. Bell ML, Catalfamo CJ, Farland LV, Ernst KC, Jacobs ET, Klimentidis YC, et al. Post-acute sequelae of COVID-19 in a non-hospitalized cohort: results from the Arizona CoVHORT. PLoS One. 2021;16(8):e0254347.
51. Daines L, Zheng B, Pfeffer P, Hurst JR, Sheikh A. A clinical review of long-COVID with a focus on the respiratory system. Curr Opin Pulm Med. 2022;28(3):174–9.
52. Thomas M, Price OJ, Hull JH. Pulmonary function and COVID-19. Curr Opin Physiol. 2021;21:29–35.
53. Funke-Chambour M, Bridevaux PO, Clarenbach CF, Soccal PM, Nicod LP, von Garnier C, et al. Swiss recommendations for the follow-up and treatment of pulmonary long COVID. Respiration. 2021;100(8):826–41.
54. Boutou A, Asimakos A, Kortianou E, Vogiatzis I, Tzouvelekis A. Long COVID-19 pulmonary sequelae and management considerations. J Pers Med. 2021;11(9):838.
55. Philip KEJ, Buttery S, Williams P, Vijayakumar B, Tonkin J, Cumella A, et al. Impact of COVID-19 on people with asthma: a

56. Yan Z, Yang M, Lai CL. Long COVID-19 syndrome: a comprehensive review of its effect on various organ systems and recommendation on rehabilitation plans. Biomedicine. 2021;9(8):966.
57. Mancini DM, Brunjes DL, Lala A, Trivieri MG, Contreras JP, Natelson BH. Use of cardiopulmonary stress testing for patients with unexplained dyspnea post–coronavirus disease. JACC Heart Fail. 2021;9(12):927–37.
58. Singh I, Joseph P, Heerdt PM, Cullinan M, Lutchmansingh DD, Gulati M, et al. Persistent exertional intolerance after COVID-19. Chest. 2022;161(1):54–63.
59. Coronavirus recovery: breathing exercises. 2022 [cited 2022 Jul 5]. Available from: https://www.hopkinsmedicine.org/health/conditions-and-diseases/coronavirus/coronavirus-recovery-breathing-exercises.
60. Philip KEJ, Owles H, McVey S, Pagnuco T, Bruce K, Brunjes H, et al. An online breathing and wellbeing programme (ENO breathe) for people with persistent symptoms following COVID-19: a parallel-group, single-blind, randomised controlled trial. Lancet Respir Med. 2022 [cited 2022 Jul 6]. Available from: https://www.thelancet.com/journals/lanres/article/PIIS2213-2600(22)00125-4/fulltext.
61. Cahalan R, Meade C, Mockler S. SingStrong—a singing and breathing retraining intervention for respiratory and other common symptoms of long COVID: a pilot study. Can J Respir Ther. 2022;58:20–7.
62. Tran VT, Porcher R, Pane I, Ravaud P. Course of post COVID-19 disease symptoms over time in the ComPaRe long COVID prospective e-cohort. Nat Commun. 2022;13(1):1812.
63. CDC. Healthcare workers. Centers for Disease Control and Prevention. 2020 [cited 2022 Jun 27]. Available from: https://www.cdc.gov/coronavirus/2019-ncov/hcp/clinical-care/post-covid-index.html.
64. Xie Y, Xu E, Bowe B, Al-Aly Z. Long-term cardiovascular outcomes of COVID-19. Nat Med. 2022;28(3):583–90.
65. Dixit NM, Churchill A, Nsair A, Hsu JJ. Post-acute COVID-19 syndrome and the cardiovascular system: what is known? Am Heart J Plus Cardiol Res Pract. 2021;5:100025.
66. Jiang DH, Roy DJ, Gu BJ, Hassett LC, McCoy RG. Postacute sequelae of severe acute respiratory syndrome coronavirus 2 infection. JACC Basic Transl Sci. 2021;6(9–10):796–811.
67. Ashton R, Ansdell P, Hume E, Maden-Wilkinson T, Ryan D, Tuttiett E, et al. COVID-19 and the long-term cardio-respiratory and metabolic health complications. Rev Cardiovasc Med. 2022;23(2):053.
68. Blitshteyn S, Whitelaw S. Postural orthostatic tachycardia syndrome (POTS) and other autonomic disorders after COVID-19 infection: a case series of 20 patients. Immunol Res. 2021;69(2):205–11.
69. Bisaccia G, Ricci F, Recce V, Serio A, Iannetti G, Chahal AA, et al. Post-acute sequelae of COVID-19 and cardiovascular autonomic dysfunction: what do we know? J Cardiovasc Dev Dis. 2021;8(11):156.
70. Eldokla AM, Mohamed-Hussein AA, Fouad AM, Abdelnaser MG, Ali ST, Makhlouf NA, et al. Prevalence and patterns of symptoms of dysautonomia in patients with long-COVID syndrome: a cross-sectional study. Ann Clin Transl Neurol. 2022;9(6):778–85.
71. Sheldon RS, Grubb BP, Olshansky B, Shen WK, Calkins H, Brignole M, et al. 2015 Heart Rhythm Society expert consensus statement on the diagnosis and treatment of postural tachycardia syndrome, inappropriate sinus tachycardia, and vasovagal syncope. Heart Rhythm. 2015;12(6):e41–63.
72. Raj SR, Fedorowski A, Sheldon RS. Diagnosis and management of postural orthostatic tachycardia syndrome. Can Med Assoc J. 2022;194(10):E378–85.
73. Dani M, Dirksen A, Taraborrelli P, Torocastro M, Panagopoulos D, Sutton R, et al. Autonomic dysfunction in 'long COVID': rationale, physiology and management strategies. Clin Med. 2021;21(1):e63–7.
74. Goodman BP. Treatment updates in postural tachycardia syndrome. Curr Treat Options Neurol. 2020;22(10):35.
75. Kanjwal K, Karabin B, Sheikh M, Elmer L, Kanjwal Y, Saeed B, et al. Pyridostigmine in the treatment of postural orthostatic tachycardia: a single-center experience: pyridostigmine in the treatment of pots. Pacing Clin Electrophysiol. 2011;34(6):750–5.
76. Graham EL, Clark JR, Orban ZS, Lim PH, Szymanski AL, Taylor C, et al. Persistent neurologic symptoms and cognitive dysfunction in non-hospitalized Covid-19 "long haulers". Ann Clin Transl Neurol. 2021;8(5):1073–85.
77. Ceban F, Ling S, Lui LMW, Lee Y, Gill H, Teopiz KM, et al. Fatigue and cognitive impairment in post-COVID-19 syndrome: a systematic review and meta-analysis. Brain Behav Immun. 2022;101:93–135.
78. Mathern R, Senthil P, Vu N, Thiyagarajan T. Neurocognitive rehabilitation in COVID-19 patients: a clinical review. South Med J. 2022;115(3):227–31.
79. Nuzum H, Stickel A, Corona M, Zeller M, Melrose RJ, Wilkins SS. Potential benefits of physical activity in MCI and dementia. Behav Neurol. 2020;2020:7807856.
80. Hötting K, Röder B. Beneficial effects of physical exercise on neuroplasticity and cognition. Neurosci Biobehav Rev. 2013;37(9 Pt B):2243–57.
81. McGrattan AM, McGuinness B, McKinley MC, Kee F, Passmore P, Woodside JV, et al. Diet and inflammation in cognitive ageing and Alzheimer's disease. Curr Nutr Rep. 2019;8(2):53–65.
82. Huston P, McFarlane B. Health benefits of tai chi: what is the evidence? Can Fam Physician. 2016;62(11):881–90.
83. Panjwani U, Dudani S, Wadhwa M. Sleep, cognition, and yoga. Int J Yoga. 2021;14(2):100–8.
84. Dundumalla S, Barshikar S, Niehaus WN, Ambrose AF, Kim SY, Abramoff BA. A survey of dedicated PASC clinics: characteristics, barriers and spirit of collaboration. PM R. 2022;14(3):348–56.
85. Fereshtehnejad SM, Rodríguez-Violante M, Martinez-Ramirez D, Ramirez-Zamora A. Editorial: managing Parkinson's disease with a multidisciplinary perspective. Front Neurol. 2021;12:799017.
86. Hogden A, Foley G, Henderson RD, James N, Aoun SM. Amyotrophic lateral sclerosis: improving care with a multidisciplinary approach. J Multidiscip Healthc. 2017;10:205–15.
87. Svenningsen H, Langhorn L, Ågård AS, Dreyer P. Post-ICU symptoms, consequences, and follow-up: an integrative review. Nurs Crit Care. 2017;22(4):212–20.
88. Puchner B, Sahanic S, Kirchmair R, Pizzini A, Sonnweber B, Wöll E, et al. Beneficial effects of multi-disciplinary rehabilitation in postacute COVID-19: an observational cohort study. Eur J Phys Rehabil Med. 2021;57(2):189–98.
89. Baratta JM, Tompary A, Siano S, Floris-Moore M, Weber DJ. Postacute sequelae of COVID-19 infection and development of a physiatry-led recovery clinic. Am J Phys Med Rehabil. 2021;100(7):633–4.
90. Sivan M, Halpin S, Hollingworth L, Snook N, Hickman K, Clifton IJ. Development of an integrated rehabilitation pathway for individuals recovering from COVID-19 in the community. J Rehabil Med. 2020;52(8):jrm00089.
91. Jubelt B. Post-polio syndrome. Curr Treat Options Neurol. 2004;6(2):87–93.
92. RECOVER: Researching COVID to Enhance Recovery. [cited 2022 Jun 23]. Available from: https://recovercovid.org.

Special Population: Care of Cancer Survivors

Bogda Koczwara

Introduction

With advances in screening, early detection, and treatment, many cancers diagnosed today will either be cured or lead to a long-term control of cancer, with patients experiencing extended life expectancy but some requiring ongoing or intermittent treatment for cancer [1]. This evolution of the trajectory from a disease that was rapidly fatal less than a century ago has led to a recognition of cancer as a chronic illness and to the growing number of cancer survivors [2]. As of today, more than 50 million worldwide, or approximately 1.3% of world population are alive within 5 years of the cancer diagnosis with many more living beyond this 5 year cut off, although the detailed estimates for the long-term survivors are harder to obtain [3].

The effectiveness of cancer treatments and resulting survival rates differ between cancers with broadly three disease trajectories: for those whose cancers are highly curable (e.g., testicular cancer) with resulting high proportion of cancer survivors; for those whose cancers that have poor outcomes (e.g., pancreatic cancer); and for those with cancers that have intermediate survival rates, such as colorectal cancer or bladder cancer [4]. For cancers with short life expectancy, the disease trajectory does not follow that of a chronic illness with the term more applicable to the other two groups. Furthermore, the expected trajectories continue to change with the continuing advancements in anticancer treatment. For example, metastatic melanoma was almost uniformly associated with a very short life expectancy less than 10 years ago. Today, with the introduction of immunotherapy, there are many long-term survivors of this disease [5].

Background

The evolution of cancer disease trajectories has led to the emergence of unique cohorts of individuals commonly described as cancer survivors, and the establishment of a clinical and research field of cancer survivorship that is focused on the care of cancer survivors. There have been many definitions of cancer survivor [6, 7]. The definition of a cancer survivor developed by the National Coalition for Cancer Survivorship notes that a survivor is a person diagnosed with cancer from the time of diagnosis for the remainder of their life [8]. Recently, four distinct phases of survivorship have been proposed including acute, chronic, long-term, and cured survivors, which reflects the phase of their illness and their anticipated care needs [9]. Chronic survivorship recognizes the experience of individuals living with incurable and progressive cancer who until recently were not considered as cancer survivors despite facing similar, and often greater, challenges [10]. Chronicity applies to the cancer itself, rather than the symptoms and associated conditions that are the result of being a cancer survivor (i.e., late effects), which may manifest months or years after cancer treatment is completed. Within the scope of these definitions every person diagnosed with cancer is a cancer survivor, although the focus of their cancer care may be more on the antitumor therapy in the acute phase of their illness and on survivorship challenges in the post-treatment phase.

Survivorship care is generally viewed in the timeframe that commences once the acute anticancer treatment has been completed. This care focuses on recovery from acute treatment and ongoing follow-up; the foundations of this approach are laid at the time of diagnosis. For example, prevention of long-term treatment toxicities such as cardiac disease requires recognition and management of risk factors at the time of treatment selection. Many cancer survivors fully recover, with no identifiable sequelae and excellent long-term quality of life and survival. For other survivors, the cancer may no longer be detectable but the long-term effects of the disease and its treatment can lead

B. Koczwara (✉)
Flinders University and Flinders Medical Centre,
Adelaide, SA, Australia
e-mail: bogda.koczwara@flinders.edu.au

to the development of other chronic conditions. It is important to consider cancer survivorship as not a disease but rather a risk factor for disease. Cancer survivors are at increased risk of late effects, premature death from cancer and non-cancer causes, increased disability, and inferior quality of life, resulting in greater health service utilization and personal financial burden [11]. This chapter will provide an overview to the care of cancer survivors. The first section will review the current knowledge regarding the burden of disease experienced by cancer survivors. Next, the principles of survivorship care, with particular focus on the management of cancer survivors through the lens of chronic disease management, will be outlined. The chapter will close with future opportunities in clinical care, research, and policy in this field.

Epidemiology of Cancer Survivorship

To understand the disease burden in cancer survivorship at the individual and societal levels, one must consider the prevalence of the specific cancer, the risk of adverse outcomes caused by disease process itself, and the sequelae of cancer treatment, relative to general population. Furthermore, the burden of disease should be viewed in terms of multiple health and health care outcomes including mortality, morbidity, service utilization, and cost.

Prevalence

It is estimated that there are approximately 50 million individuals alive within 5 years of a cancer diagnosis in the world today, with the rates higher in developed countries [12]. The most prevalent cancers include breast, prostate, and colorectal cancer, reflecting both high incidence and high cure rates (Fig. 30.1). To illustrate the relationship between incidence and prevalence, representative data from Australia shows that for every case of breast cancer diagnosed in Australia in 2019, there were 10 cancer survivors living with the history of breast cancer, four of them diagnosed within past 5 years [13].

The proportion of individuals with history of cancer varies by nation, ranging from 5.5% in the United States to

Share of population with cancer, World, 2019

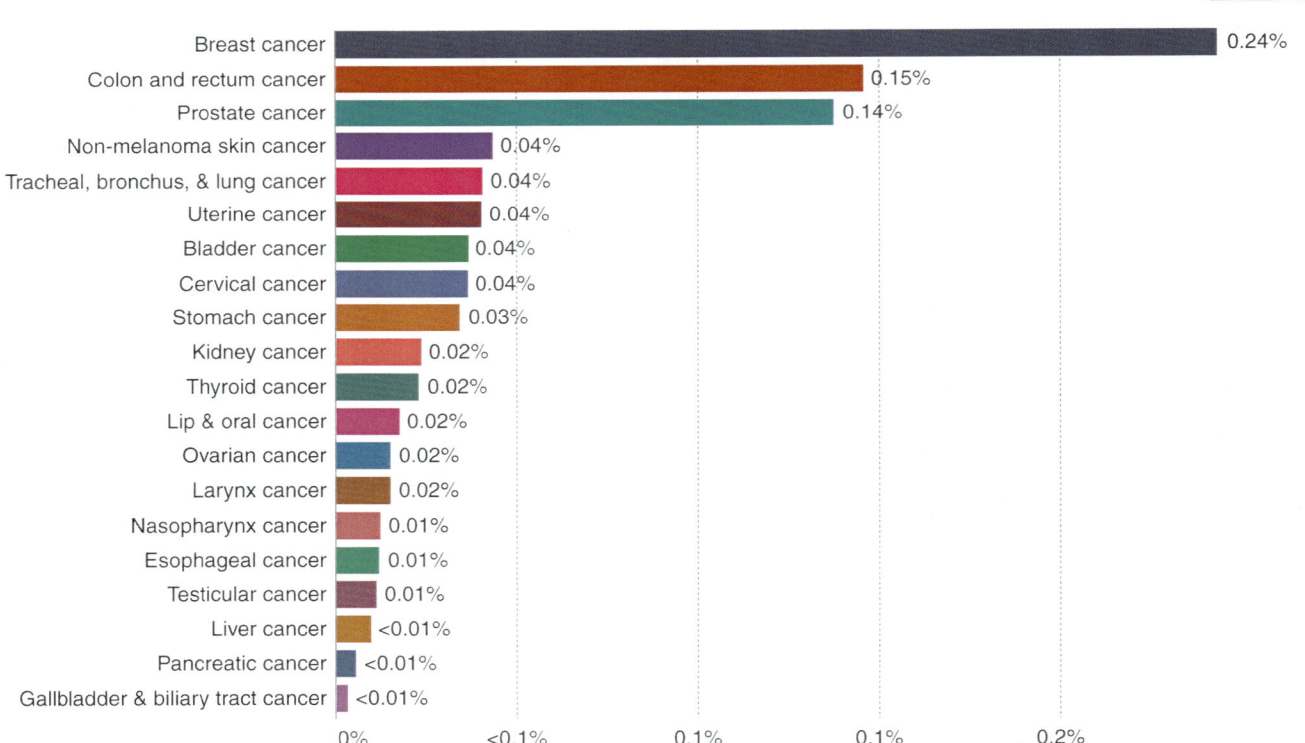

Cancer type	Share
Breast cancer	0.24%
Colon and rectum cancer	0.15%
Prostate cancer	0.14%
Non-melanoma skin cancer	0.04%
Tracheal, bronchus, & lung cancer	0.04%
Uterine cancer	0.04%
Bladder cancer	0.04%
Cervical cancer	0.04%
Stomach cancer	0.03%
Kidney cancer	0.02%
Thyroid cancer	0.02%
Lip & oral cancer	0.02%
Ovarian cancer	0.02%
Larynx cancer	0.02%
Nasopharynx cancer	0.01%
Esophageal cancer	0.01%
Testicular cancer	0.01%
Liver cancer	<0.01%
Pancreatic cancer	<0.01%
Gallbladder & biliary tract cancer	<0.01%

Source: IHME, Global Burden of Disease
Note: To allow comparisons between countries and over time this metric is age-standardized
OurWorldData.org/cancer • CC BY

Fig. 30.1 Distribution of cancer types worldwide. (Reproduced with permission [12])

0.4 in Central Africa [12]. The variation reflects better treatment outcomes as well as the demographics of the population, with greater proportions of older adults and concomitantly higher cancer incidence rates reported in Western countries. These changes are reflected in the demographic characteristics of people affected by cancer, with 70% occurring in people older than 50 and approximately 5% in those 15 years and younger [12]. While the absolute numbers of survivors of childhood cancers are small, this group represents some of the longest survivors of cancer and reflects the successful treatment of early childhood cancers. Data on survivorship health in this population provides important insights into the long-term consequences of cancer treatment for older adults with cancer. As the global population ages and the advances in cancer treatment expand beyond developed countries, there will be more cancer survivors in lower- and middle-income countries and need for innovative care models.

There are significant numbers of older adults with multiple chronic conditions, including cancer, who need to manage not only the chronic disease, such as hypertension and osteoarthritis, but also the active treatment and sequelae of cancer. Data from Medicare beneficiaries in the United States reports that only 10% had no other conditions independent of cancer, but approximately one-third had five or more conditions [14]. For these cancer survivors, cancer treatment and care management need to be provided in the context of pre-existing multimorbidity.

Mortality

Cancer survivors are at increased risk of premature death due to a recurrence of the primary cancer, development of the second cancer, or death from co-existing conditions that might have been precipitated or made more severe due to cancer and/or its treatment [15]. While the risk of cancer recurrence, and to a lesser degree risk of a second cancer, can be monitored and mitigated by treatment, the risk associated with comorbid non-cancer diseases and conditions is less well known. For example, a 2016 study from the United States Surveillance, Epidemiology and End Results (SEER) database noted that the comparative risks of cancer and non-cancer death differed markedly by cancer type, and that more than 40% of non-cancer deaths were from cardiovascular disease [16]. Cardiovascular disease is the most common competing cause of premature death in cancer survivors, with increased risk reflecting the cardiotoxicity of many treatment regimens either early after cancer diagnosis or [17] in long-term cancer survivors [18, 19]. A large analysis of individuals with cancer from South Australia who survived at least 5 years of survivorship has reported that 45% of deaths were attributed to cancer and the remainder to non-cancer causes at a median follow-up of 17 years. Cardiovascular disease was the most common cause of death with increased risk of premature death across all cancer types and all age groups, except in ages 80 years or older [19].

Such increased risk may be due to cancer treatment that adversely impacts cardiac and/or vascular function, or a cumulative and combined risk of both cancer and cardiovascular disease due to primary risk factors such as smoking. There is evidence that patients and health care providers prioritize cancer care over the management of comorbid chronic disease [20] such as diabetes [21] and the mitigation of modifiable risk factors (e.g., physical inactivity) [22]. Further research is needed to understand the mechanisms behind this increased risk to develop effective interventions for risk reduction.

There is increased risk of suicide after cancer diagnosis and treatment. The risk varies according to cancer type and world region; higher rates are reported in Asia, lowest in Oceania, and sparse data from low- and middle-income countries [23]. The risk of premature death from suicide after cancer is approximately four times that of a cancer-free controls with older, white, unmarried men at highest risk [24].

Functional Status and Quality of Life

Cancer survivorship is associated with development and progression of preexisting physical and psychosocial conditions that impact quality of life and functional status [25]. Although long-term survival is important, quality of life, functional status, mental health, and social and economic participation are also important outcomes for survivors [26]. There are limited data documenting these and other person-centered outcomes. For example, an Australian population-based cohort study of 22,505 survivors and 244,000 individuals without cancer demonstrated greater disability and poor quality of life in individuals with cancer; however, the outcomes varied significantly by cancer type and were worse with recent diagnosis, treatment, and advanced cancer stage [27]. Physical disability was a major contributor to adverse distress and quality of life outcomes.

The disability and functional limitations in cancer survivors negatively impacts the capacity to maintain employment with downstream effects on social function and financial status. Approximately 40–50% of survivors are younger than 65 and in an age of employment [28]. Cancer survivors who remain working are more likely to experience inferior work performance and absenteeism when compared to persons without cancer [29, 30]. Survivors are also at higher risk of job loss or inability to return to employment after cancer treatment [31]. The inability to work or reduced work capacity is an important driver of financial toxicity, defined as financial consequences of cancer and its treatment and the resulting distress [32]. The financial toxicity and limited financial reserves of cancer survivors with poor functional status are particularly salient since survivors will likely require health services to manage their disability. A survey data from National Health Services in Australia reported that cancer survivors were more likely to consult their primary care providers and other health care providers with the presence of comorbid conditions associated with greater health service utilization [33].

Multimorbidity

Most cancer survivors experience multiple health conditions and comorbidities [34]. Cancer shares risk factors with other chronic conditions and cancer treatment predisposes patients to developing new conditions as well [35]. Multimorbidity is common in the general population, particularly in older adults [36]; however, there are limited data reporting the prevalence of multimorbidity in cancer patients. A study of Medicare beneficiaries noted that 90% had more than one health condition, and approximately a third had five or more [1]. Multimorbidity is the major driver of health care utilization and associated cost in cancer survivors [33], creating challenges in the prioritization and management of cancer and other co-existing chronic conditions. Patients and their health care providers tend to focus on cancer care, and there is a lack of point-of-care tools to assist in clinical decision making [37]. Prioritization and management challenges can be exacerbated in patients who are socioeconomically disadvantaged and where access to specialized care may be more limited [38]. The complexity of multimorbidity impacts both disease management and symptom management. In cancer survivors, symptoms tend to cluster [39]. A study of cancer survivors from the Netherlands identified fatigue as a primary symptom [40].

Cancer Survivor Syndromes

Cancer survivors experience several clusters of symptoms and clinical entities. Fear of cancer recurrence/progression is a commonly reported syndrome in cancer survivors [41]. Fear of cancer recurrence was more common in patients who were younger, had physical symptoms and/or distress, and poorer quality of life [41]. Cancer-related cognitive impairment is another condition experienced by approximately 30% of patients [42]. While initially attributed to cancer treatment, and labeled "chemobrain", its etiology is poorly understood; the etiologies include cancer treatment and the underlying cancer. Premature aging and associated frailty are observed in cancer survivors of any age, including survivors of childhood cancer [43]. A cohort of 1922 adult childhood cancer survivors found that the prevalence of frailty was comparable to adults who were 65 years old without cancer. Frailty is associated with the presence of chronic conditions and a higher risk of death [44]. Frailty and pre-frailty in young adult survivors of childhood cancer provide insight into the biology of chronic diseases that are associated with cancer survivorship, with the main contributing factor considered to be cancer and its treatment.

Cancer Survivorship Care

Survivorship care involves the prevention, surveillance, and management of the physical and psychosocial adverse consequences of cancer (i.e., "late effects"); cancer recurrence and development of secondary cancers; and preexisting and new chronic conditions [45]. In addition to disease and symptom management, survivorship care incorporates health promotion strategies and secondary prevention to mitigate future risks of new conditions. Effective cancer survivorship care needs to be multidisciplinary in scope and integrated across multiple health care settings and providers, due to the diversity of adverse health care outcomes and the variability of risk factors. Figure 30.2 depicts a conceptual framework that incorporates the many domains and outcomes of optimal survivorship care [46].

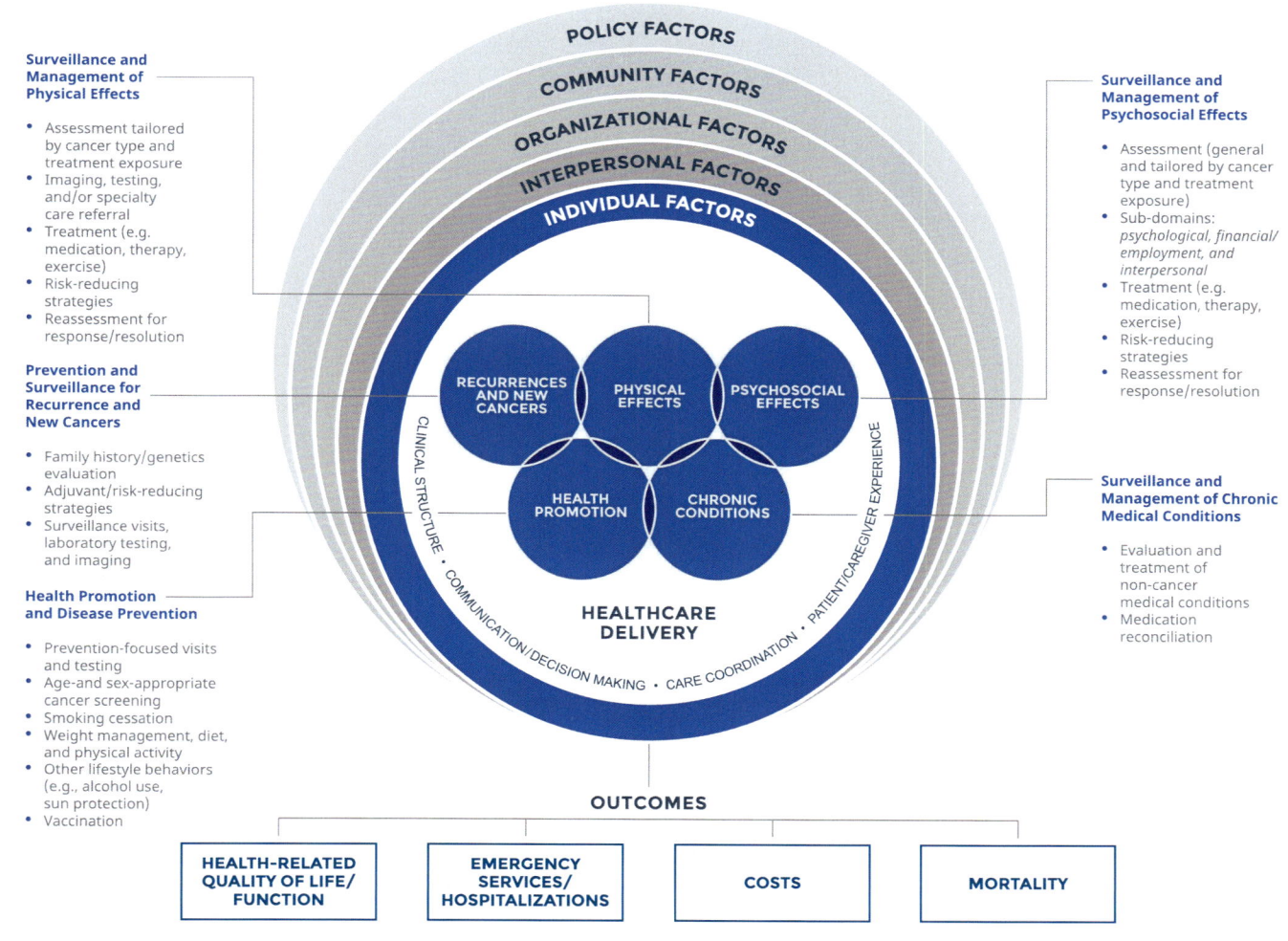

Fig. 30.2 Conceptual framework of survivorship care [46]

Models and Guidelines

There are several models and guidelines that have been developed to promote the implementation of survivorship care in clinical settings. Some are applicable across all cancer types (e.g., Clinical Oncology Society of Australia Model [47] or Livestrong Essential Elements [48]), while others are specific to a cancer type (e.g., Prostate Cancer Framework [49]), and some are specific to designated subpopulations (e.g., Aboriginal Optimal Care Pathway [50]). Each can be considered with several health service approaches, including specialist led, specialist consultative survivorship care, nurse led care, primary care, shared care between primary and specialist and self-management. Unfortunately, there is a limited evidence base and no consensus regarding the effectiveness of each respective model, and it appears that different models are best suited to different survivor subgroups [51, 52].

Many cancer organizations have developed specific guidelines and clinical pathways to guide cancer survivorship care (Table 30.1). Some focus on a specific population group, while others focus on a symptom or clinical condition. Most guidelines are developed to inform health care providers, but a few are directed to patients or have a patient-focused application. The key component of survivorship care common to guidelines and frameworks has been the development of a treatment summary and a survivorship care plan to ensure understanding of what is required and appropriate in planning and providing care. Despite the original enthusiasm of guidelines, there are very few studies that demonstrate benefits of survivorship care plan for health care outcomes of cancer survivors [53].

Table 30.1 Cancer organization guidelines

Organization (country)	Available survivorship care guidelines including a web link
American Cancer Society	Breast cancer Colorectal cancer Head and neck cancer Prostate cancer https://www.cancer.org/health-care-professionals/american-cancer-society-survivorship-guidelines.html
American Society of Clinical Oncology	Breast cancer Fatigue management Sexual function Fertility preservation Anxiety and depression Peripheral neuropathy https://www.asco.org/news-initiatives/current-initiatives/cancer-care-initiatives/prevention-survivorship/survivorship-4
Cancer Australia	Principles of Cancer Survivorship https://www.canceraustralia.gov.au/publications-and-resources/cancer-australia-publications/principles-cancer-survivorship
Children Oncology Group (USA)	Long-Term Follow-Up Guidelines for Survivors of Childhood, Adolescent, and Young Adult Cancers http://www.survivorshipguidelines.org/
Clinical Oncology Society of Australia	Position Statement on Exercise https://www.cosa.org.au/media/332488/cosa-position-statement-v4-web-final.pdf
European Society of Medical Oncology	Patient Guide on Survivorship https://www.esmo.org/for-patients/patient-guides/survivorship
eviQ (Australia)	Cancer survivorship education module https://education.eviq.org.au/courses/supportive-care/cancer-survivorship
International	Exercise guidelines for cancer survivors https://www.ncbi.nlm.nih.gov/pmc/articles/PMC8576825/
The National Comprehensive Cancer Network (USA)	General survivorship guidelines https://jnccn.org/view/journals/jnccn/18/8/article-p1016.xml
McMillan Cancer Support (UK)	Assessment and care planning for cancer survivors. A concise evidence review https://www.macmillan.org.uk/_images/assessment-and-care-planning-for-cancer-survivors_tcm9-297790.pdf

Gaps in Clinical Practice

Despite the many guidelines and frameworks, dedicated survivorship care programs are not widespread. The associated evidence on survivorship care interventions is inconsistent and siloed, with limited data on health services and economic outcomes that would inform the adoption and implementation into clinical practice [54]. Most notably, cancer survivorship care is not considered and integrated into existing operational and funding models for chronic disease management in the general population. With the significant global growth of cancer survivors with associated complex health care conditions, there is a heightened need for survivorship care that leverages longstanding and novel approaches to address patients' needs within health care systems [11].

Advancing Survivorship Care

Promoting improvements in cancer survivorship care at the health system level must reflect the best evidence, contribute to demonstrated outcomes that are cost-effective, be acceptable to patients and health care providers, and be organizationally feasible within existing and emerging health care environments. Some of the best improvement opportunities in survivorship care are approaches and strategies that have been successfully demonstrated in the general population and have potential to be applied in the context of cancer.

Chronic Illness Care Models

There is substantial evidence of improved health care outcomes with chronic illness care models that have be developed in the general population, but the translation to cancer survivorship care remains understudied [55]. These models of care emphasize the sharing of information between the patient, their informal supports, and service providers, emphasizing care integration and timely communication. This approach is particularly applicable to cancer survivorship, given the complexity of cancer treatment and the complexity of patients' needs. It also aligns well with the existing funding models for chronic disease management in most health care systems, and many elements have already been established in primary care settings, which can facilitate the integration of survivorship care.

Self-Management, Peer, and Family Support

Patient self-management and support are important components of chronic illness care models, emphasizing the role and capacities of patients and their informal support networks (e.g., family, friends, and other informal caregivers) in addressing the day-to-day health care needs [56]. These resources are particularly relevant to care of cancer survivors since engagement with health care providers and resources may be limited and often diminishes after time of diagnosis and initial treatment. Furthermore, lifestyle management, including healthy eating and physical activity, is an important component of survivorship care. Cancer survivors need to employ a range of core skills to manage their health care needs relating to cancer (see Fig. 30.3).

The COVID19 pandemic has further emphasized the critical importance of self-management support for cancer survivors [57].

A review of the potential benefits of self-management and self-management support in cancer contributed to six priorities for action including: (1) preparing patients for active involvement in care, (2) shifting the care culture to embed self-management support in daily operations, (3) preparing the workforce, (4) developing consensus on patient reported outcomes, (5) advancing the evidence base, and (6) expanding reach and access [58]. The experience of self-management in cancer survivorship does not occur in isolation but relies on effective social support from family and peers. Patients who report their social wellbeing more positively are more likely to accept aggressive treatment [59]. Conversely, loneliness has been reported to be associated with increased cancer mortality [60]. For cancer survivors, effective social networks, both family and peer support, provide a buffer from stress and assist in navigating complex health care challenges [61, 62].

Health Care System Considerations

Effective cancer survivorship care is provided to patients in the broader context of health care systems. Specifically, health care systems should be responsive to care needs at both the individual and population levels. The structures and processes of the respective health care system need to adapt as care needs evolve and change. Many require information technology (IT) platforms and applications that can provide data to inform care requirements, drive change when needed, and evaluate its impact. These IT platforms and applications should also support the communication modalities that are foundational to continuity of care and information exchange. For many survivors, care will continue over many years and involve multiple health care providers across a variety of health care settings, including acute cancer services and community-based facilities [63]. Finally, as health care systems are becoming increasingly complex with a multitude of providers, they should seek to increase efficiencies of care, minimizing unnecessary duplication of services, with horizontal and vertical integration across different levels of care [64]. A number of potential strategies have been shown to be effective in overcoming the challenge of complexity and improving patient outcomes.

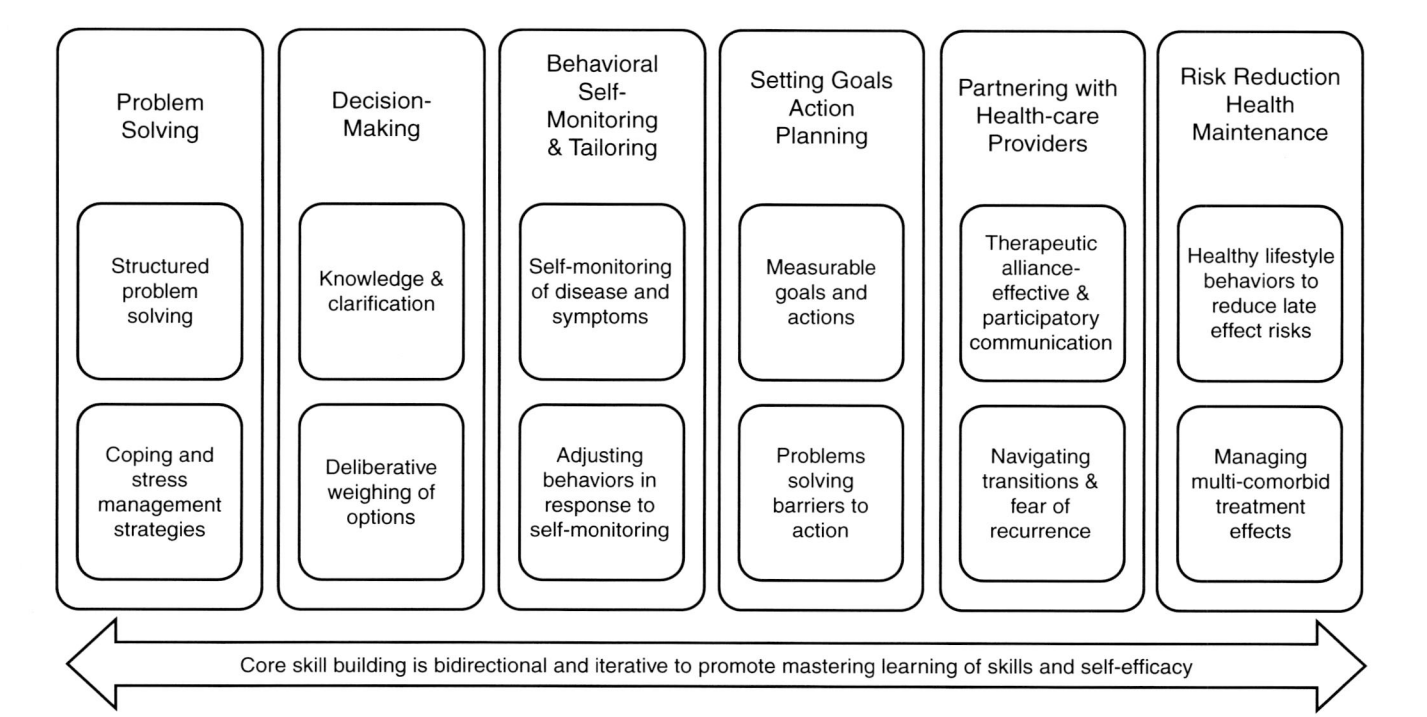

Problem Solving	Decision-Making	Behavioral Self-Monitoring & Tailoring	Setting Goals Action Planning	Partnering with Health-care Providers	Risk Reduction Health Maintenance
Structured problem solving	Knowledge & clarification	Self-monitoring of disease and symptoms	Measurable goals and actions	Therapeutic alliance-effective & participatory communication	Healthy lifestyle behaviors to reduce late effect risks
Coping and stress management strategies	Deliberative weighing of options	Adjusting behaviors in response to self-monitoring	Problems solving barriers to action	Navigating transitions & fear of recurrence	Managing multi-comorbid treatment effects

Core skill building is bidirectional and iterative to promote mastering learning of skills and self-efficacy

Fig. 30.3 Core self-management skills [58]

Care Coordination and Navigation

Effective care coordination, defined as deliberate organization of patient care activities, to facilitate the appropriate delivery of health care services, is particularly important in cancer care because of its complexity [65]. Poor care coordination is associated with poor symptom control, medical errors, and increased cost of care [66]. A recent systematic review and meta-analysis of over 30 years of empirical studies of care coordination showed that patient navigation was the most common form of coordination reported followed by home telehealth and nurse case management [67]. Collectively, cancer care coordination was associated with improvements across many outcomes including patient experience with care and appropriate health care utilization and reduced cost. Despite these positive findings, measurement of cancer care coordination varies across studies, access to coordination varies across populations, and most studies focus on patient-level interventions with little impact on the health care system, highlighting many areas for future research [67]

Patient Reported Outcomes

Patient reported outcomes (PROs) are defined as any report which documents the status of patients' health condition and comes directly from the patient [68]. PROs that are collected and analyzed in a systematic way can promote care that is responsive to patient needs [69]. Some symptoms, such as anxiety and depression, are not readily apparent and often require specific screening to identify an underlying mental health disorder [70]. A systematic approach to PRO collection using validated questionnaires can assist in identifying symptoms and needs and has been shown to improve satisfaction with care, reduce health care cost, and improve survival [71–73]. PROs can also serve as adjuncts and proxies to other biomarker that identify patients who are at risk for specific conditions and where interventions may be indicated [74, 75]. Lastly, PROs can be a useful tool to monitor health system performance and identify gaps and areas of system-level improvement [76].

Digital Health

Digital health technology, such as electronic health (eHealth), wearables, telehealth, and health information technology, offers a promise of health care that is accessible, user friendly, and efficient. These digital technologies can enable a systematic approach to communication and data collection, such as routine PRO collection, or remote monitoring [77]. As with other health care technologies, the effectiveness of digital approaches is user-dependent, and uptake is dependent on patients who may have different levels of comfort and skill with usability. In consequence, the benefits of digital technology need to recognize the limitations of access to technology, e-health literacy, digital inclusion [78], and the usability of the technology itself.

One area where digital health can have potential benefit is through the integration and communication of multiple health providers—both synchronously and asynchronously—for cancer survivors. It also offers an opportunity to address challenges to health care access due to geographical barriers, mitigating distance, and reducing language barriers of care that have potential for creating a system of survivorship care that is globally connected [79, 80]. This promise is tempered by the reality that a globally connected world is dependent on the access to technologies that are limited in many low- and middle-income countries.

Future Directions

As the number of cancer survivors continues to increase, health care systems will need to develop innovative and effective approaches to implementing best practice models of care that can address the unique needs of cancer survivors. The challenge and the opportunity for advancement revolve around the same issue: the tension between focusing on the unique needs of cancer survivors, as distinct from other populations of people with chronic disease, and the integration of their care within the principles of chronic disease management and the larger health care system. Reconciling this tension calls for innovative research that overcomes silos and improves research translation [81]. One specific area is the opportunity for learning from different health care settings and different models of survivorship care delivery across the globe with health system–level data. To do so, a global collaborative effort is needed that not only facilitates research collaborations but embeds it with the broader health care policy [82]. Only through global collaborative effort can we improve outcomes for cancer survivors, irrespective of where they live and what cancer they may be diagnosed with.

References

1. Siegel RL, Miller KD, Fuchs HE, Jemal A. Cancer statistics, 2021. CA Cancer J Clin. 2021;71(1):7–33. https://doi.org/10.3322/caac.21654. Epub 2021 Jan 12. Erratum in: CA Cancer J Clin. 2021;71(4):359.
2. Boele F, Harley C, Pini S, Kenyon L, Daffu-O'Reilly A, Velikova G. Cancer as a chronic illness: support needs and experiences. BMJ Support Palliat Care. 2019; https://doi.org/10.1136/bmjspcare-2019-001882. Epub ahead of print.
3. Global Burden of Disease 2019 Cancer Collaboration. Cancer incidence, mortality, years of life lost, years lived with disability, and

disability-adjusted life years for 29 cancer groups from 2010 to 2019: a systematic analysis for the Global Burden of Disease Study 2019. JAMA Oncol. 2021;8:e216987. https://doi.org/10.1001/jamaoncol.2021.6987. Epub ahead of print.
4. McConnell H, White R, Maher J. Categorising cancers to enable tailored care planning through a secondary analysis of cancer registration data in the UK. BMJ Open. 2017;7(11):e016797. https://doi.org/10.1136/bmjopen-2017-016797.
5. Michielin O, Atkins MB, Koon HB, Dummer R, Ascierto PA. Evolving impact of long-term survival results on metastatic melanoma treatment. J Immunother Cancer. 2020;8(2):e000948. https://doi.org/10.1136/jitc-2020-000948.
6. Twombly R. What's in a name: who is a cancer survivor? J Natl Cancer Inst. 2004;96(19):1414–5. https://doi.org/10.1093/jnci/96.19.1414.
7. Marzorati C, Riva S, Pravettoni G. Who is a cancer survivor? A systematic review of published definitions. J Cancer Educ. 2017;32(2):228–37. https://doi.org/10.1007/s13187-016-0997-2.
8. National Coalition for Cancer Survivorship. https://canceradvocacy.org/about/our-mission/. Accessed 14 Jan 2022.
9. Surbone A, Tralongo P. Categorization of cancer survivors: why we need it. J Clin Oncol. 2016;34(28):3372–4. https://doi.org/10.1200/JCO.2016.68.3870. Epub 2016 Jul 25.
10. Langbaum T, Smith TJ. Time to study metastatic-cancer survivorship. N Engl J Med. 2019;380(14):1300–2. https://doi.org/10.1056/NEJMp1901103.
11. Alfano CM, Leach CR, Smith TG, Miller KD, Alcaraz KI, Cannady RS, Wender RC, Brawley OW. Equitably improving outcomes for cancer survivors and supporting caregivers: a blueprint for care delivery, research, education, and policy. CA Cancer J Clin. 2019;69:35–49. https://doi.org/10.3322/caac.21548.
12. Roser M, Ritchie H. Cancer. 2015. Published online at OurWorldInData.org. Retrieved from: https://ourworldindata.org/cancer. Accessed 4 Apr 2022.
13. Australian Institute of Health and Welfare. Cancer in Australia 2019. Cat. no. CAN 123. Canberra: AIHW; 2019.
14. Ward BW, Schiller JS, Goodman RA. Multiple chronic conditions among US adults: a 2012 update. Prev Chronic Dis. 2014;11:E62. https://doi.org/10.5888/pcd11.130389.
15. Corner J. Addressing the needs of cancer survivors: issues and challenges. Expert Rev Pharmacoecon Outcomes Res. 2008;8(5):443–51. https://doi.org/10.1586/14737167.8.5.443.
16. Zaorsky NG, Churilla TM, Egleston BL, Fisher SG, Ridge JA, Horwitz EM, Meyer JE. Causes of death among cancer patients. Ann Oncol. 2017;28(2):400–7. https://doi.org/10.1093/annonc/mdw604.
17. Ye Y, Otahal P, Marwick TH, Wills KE, Neil AL, Venn AJ. Cardiovascular and other competing causes of death among patients with cancer from 2006 to 2015: an Australian population-based study. Cancer. 2019;125(3):442–52. https://doi.org/10.1002/cncr.31806. Epub 2018 Oct 12.
18. Shin DW, Ahn E, Kim H, Park S, Kim YA, Yun YH. Non-cancer mortality among long-term survivors of adult cancer in Korea: national cancer registry study. Cancer Causes Control. 2010;21(6):919–29. https://doi.org/10.1007/s10552-010-9521-x. Epub 2010 Feb 19.
19. Koczwara B, Meng R, Miller MD, Clark RA, Kaambwa B, Marin T, Damarell RA, Roder DM. Late mortality in people with cancer: a population-based Australian study. Med J Aust. 2021;214(7):318–23. https://doi.org/10.5694/mja2.50879. Epub 2020 Dec 9.
20. Clark RA, Marin TS, Berry NM, Atherton JJ, Foote JW, Koczwara B. Cardiotoxicity and cardiovascular disease risk assessment for patients receiving breast cancer treatment. Cardiooncology. 2017;3:6. https://doi.org/10.1186/s40959-017-0025-7.
21. Harding JL, Andes LJ, Gregg EW, Cheng YJ, Weir HK, Bullard KM, Burrows NR, Imperatore G. Trends in cancer mortality among people with vs without diabetes in the USA, 1988-2015. Diabetologia. 2020;63(1):75–84. https://doi.org/10.1007/s00125-019-04991-x. Epub 2019 Sep 12.
22. Zhang YB, Pan XF, Chen J, Cao A, Zhang YG, Xia L, Wang J, Li H, Liu G, Pan A. Combined lifestyle factors, incident cancer, and cancer mortality: a systematic review and meta-analysis of prospective cohort studies. Br J Cancer. 2020;122(7):1085–93. https://doi.org/10.1038/s41416-020-0741-x. Epub 2020 Feb 10.
23. Du L, Shi HY, Yu HR, Liu XM, Jin XH, Yan-Qian FXL, Song YP, Cai JY, Chen HL. Incidence of suicide death in patients with cancer: a systematic review and meta-analysis. J Affect Disord. 2020;276:711–9. https://doi.org/10.1016/j.jad.2020.07.082. Epub 2020 Jul 20.
24. Zaorsky NG, Zhang Y, Tuanquin L, Bluethmann SM, Park HS, Chinchilli VM. Suicide among cancer patients. Nat Commun. 2019;10(1):207. https://doi.org/10.1038/s41467-018-08170-1. Erratum in: Nat Commun. 2020 Jan 31;11(1):718.
25. Treanor CJ, Donnelly M. The late effects of cancer and cancer treatment: a rapid review. J Commun Support Oncol. 2014;12(4):137–48. https://doi.org/10.12788/jcso.0035.
26. Laidsaar-Powell R, Konings S, Rankin N, Koczwara B, Kemp E, Mazariego C, Butow P. A meta-review of qualitative research on adult cancer survivors: current strengths and evidence gaps. J Cancer Surviv. 2019;13(6):852–89. https://doi.org/10.1007/s11764-019-00803-8. Epub 2019 Nov 19.
27. Joshy G, Thandrayen J, Koczwara B, Butow P, Laidsaar-Powell R, Rankin N, Canfell K, Stubbs J, Grogan P, Bailey L, Yazidjoglou A, Banks E. Disability, psychological distress and quality of life in relation to cancer diagnosis and cancer type: population-based Australian study of 22,505 cancer survivors and 244,000 people without cancer. BMC Med. 2020;18(1):372. https://doi.org/10.1186/s12916-020-01830-4.
28. de Boer AG. The European cancer and work network: CANWON. J Occup Rehabil. 2014;24(3):393–8. https://doi.org/10.1007/s10926-013-9474-5.
29. Mehnert A, de Boer A, Feuerstein M. Employment challenges for cancer survivors. Cancer. 2013;119(Suppl 11):2151–9. https://doi.org/10.1002/cncr.28067.
30. Thandrayen J, Joshy G, Stubbs J, Bailey L, Butow P, Koczwara B, Laidsaar-Powell R, Rankin NM, Beckwith K, Soga K, Yazidjoglou A, Bin Sayeed MS, Canfell K, Banks E. Workforce participation in relation to cancer diagnosis, type and stage: Australian population-based study of 163,556 middle-aged people. J Cancer Surviv. 2021;16:461. https://doi.org/10.1007/s11764-021-01041-7. Epub ahead of print.
31. Islam T, Dahlui M, Majid HA, Nahar AM, Mohd Taib NA, Su TT, MyBCC Study Group. Factors associated with return to work of breast cancer survivors: a systematic review. BMC Public Health. 2014;14(Suppl 3):S8. https://doi.org/10.1186/1471-2458-14-S3-S8. Epub 2014 Nov 24.
32. Pearce A, Tomalin B, Kaambwa B, Horevoorts N, Duijts S, Mols F, van de Poll-Franse L, Koczwara B. Financial toxicity is more than costs of care: the relationship between employment and financial toxicity in long-term cancer survivors. J Cancer Surviv. 2019;13(1):10–20. https://doi.org/10.1007/s11764-018-0723-7. Epub 2018 Oct 24.
33. Ng HS, Koczwara B, Roder D, Chan RJ, Vitry A. Patterns of health service utilisation among the Australian population with cancer compared with the general population. Aust Health Rev. 2020;44(3):470–9. https://doi.org/10.1071/AH18184.
34. Ritchie CS, Zhao F, Patel K, Manola J, Kvale EA, Snyder CF, Fisch MJ. Association between patients' perception of the comorbidity burden and symptoms in outpatients with common solid tumors. Cancer. 2017;123(19):3835–42. https://doi.org/10.1002/cncr.30801. Epub 2017 Jun 13.
35. Ng HS, Koczwara B, Roder D, Vitry A. Changes in the prevalence of comorbidity in the Australian population with cancer, 2007-

36. Fortin M, Hudon C, Haggerty J, Akker MV, Almirall J. Prevalence estimates of multimorbidity: a comparative study of two sources. BMC Health Serv Res. 2010;10:111. https://doi.org/10.1186/1472-6963-10-111.
37. Lawn S, Fallon-Ferguson J, Koczwara B. Shared care involving cancer specialists and primary care providers—what do cancer survivors want? Health Expect. 2017;20(5):1081–7. https://doi.org/10.1111/hex.12551. Epub 2017 May 3.
38. Pathirana TI, Jackson CA. Socioeconomic status and multimorbidity: a systematic review and meta-analysis. Aust N Z J Public Health. 2018;42(2):186–94. https://doi.org/10.1111/1753-6405.12762. Epub 2018 Feb 14.
39. Molassiotis A, Wengström Y, Kearney N. Symptom cluster patterns during the first year after diagnosis with cancer. J Pain Symptom Manag. 2010;39(5):847–58. https://doi.org/10.1016/j.jpainsymman.2009.09.012. Epub 2010 Mar 11.
40. de Rooij BH, Oerlemans S, van Deun K, Mols F, de Ligt KM, Husson O, Ezendam NPM, Hoedjes M, van de Poll-Franse LV, Schoormans D. Symptom clusters in 1330 survivors of 7 cancer types from the PROFILES registry: a network analysis. Cancer. 2021;127(24):4665–74. https://doi.org/10.1002/cncr.33852. Epub 2021 Aug 13.
41. Simard S, Thewes B, Humphris G, Dixon M, Hayden C, Mireskandari S, Ozakinci G. Fear of cancer recurrence in adult cancer survivors: a systematic review of quantitative studies. J Cancer Surviv. 2013;7(3):300–22. https://doi.org/10.1007/s11764-013-0272-z. Epub 2013 Mar 10.
42. Janelsins MC, Kesler SR, Ahles TA, Morrow GR. Prevalence, mechanisms, and management of cancer-related cognitive impairment. Int Rev Psychiatry. 2014;26(1):102–13. https://doi.org/10.3109/09540261.2013.864260.
43. Cupit-Link MC, Kirkland JL, Ness KK, Armstrong GT, Tchkonia T, LeBrasseur NK, Armenian SH, Ruddy KJ, Hashmi SK. Biology of premature ageing in survivors of cancer. ESMO Open. 2017;2(5):e000250. https://doi.org/10.1136/esmoopen-2017-000250.
44. Ness KK, Krull KR, Jones KE, Mulrooney DA, Armstrong GT, Green DM, Chemaitilly W, Smith WA, Wilson CL, Sklar CA, Shelton K, Srivastava DK, Ali S, Robison LL, Hudson MM. Physiologic frailty as a sign of accelerated aging among adult survivors of childhood cancer: a report from the St Jude Lifetime cohort study. J Clin Oncol. 2013;31(36):4496–503. https://doi.org/10.1200/JCO.2013.52.2268. Epub 2013 Nov 18.
45. Institute of Medicine and National Research Council. From cancer patient to cancer survivor: lost in transition. Washington, DC: The National Academies Press; 2006. https://doi.org/10.17226/11468.
46. Nekhlyudov L, Mollica MA, Jacobsen PB, Mayer DK, Shulman LN, Geiger AM. Developing a quality of cancer survivorship care framework: implications for clinical care, research, and policy. J Natl Cancer Inst. 2019;111(11):1120–30. https://doi.org/10.1093/jnci/djz089. Erratum in: J Natl Cancer Inst. 2021;113(2):217.
47. Vardy JL, Chan RJ, Koczwara B, Lisy K, Cohn RJ, Joske D, Dhillon HM, Jefford M. Clinical Oncology Society of Australia position statement on cancer survivorship care. Aust J Gen Pract. 2019;48(12):833–6. https://doi.org/10.31128/AJGP-07-19-4999.
48. The essential elements of survivorship care: a livestrong brief. https://www.livestrong.org/sites/default/files/what-we-do/reports/essentialelementsbrief.pdf. Accessed 14 Jan 2022.
49. Dunn J, Green A, Ralph N, Newton RU, Kneebone A, Frydenberg M, Chambers SK. Prostate cancer survivorship essentials framework: guidelines for practitioners. BJU Int. 2021;128(Suppl 3):18–29. https://doi.org/10.1111/bju.15159. Epub 2020 Aug 18.
50. Optimal Care Pathway for Aboriginal and Torres Strait Islander people with cancer. https://www.canceraustralia.gov.au/sites/default/files/publications/optimal-care-pathway-aboriginal-and-torres-strait-islander-people-cancer/pdf/optimal-care-pathway-for-aboriginal-and-torres-strait-islander-people-with-cancer.pdf. Accessed 14 Jan 2022.
51. Chan RJ, Crawford-Williams F, Crichton M, Joseph R, Hart NH, Milley K, Druce P, Zhang J, Jefford M, Lisy K, Emery J, Nekhlyudov L. Effectiveness and implementation of models of cancer survivorship care: an overview of systematic reviews. J Cancer Surviv. 2021;17:1–25. https://doi.org/10.1007/s11764-021-01128-1. Epub ahead of print.
52. Høeg BL, Bidstrup PE, Karlsen RV, Friberg AS, Albieri V, Dalton SO, Saltbæk L, Andersen KK, Horsboel TA, Johansen C. Follow-up strategies following completion of primary cancer treatment in adult cancer survivors. Cochrane Database Syst Rev. 2019;2019(11):CD012425. https://doi.org/10.1002/14651858.CD012425.pub2.
53. Hill RE, Wakefield CE, Cohn RJ, Fardell JE, Brierley ME, Kothe E, Jacobsen PB, Hetherington K, Mercieca-Bebber R. Survivorship care plans in cancer: a meta-analysis and systematic review of care plan outcomes. Oncologist. 2020;25(2):e351–72. https://doi.org/10.1634/theoncologist.2019-0184. Epub 2019 Oct 25.
54. Kemp E, Geerse O, Knowles R, Woodman R, Mohammadi L, Nekhlyudov L, Koczwara B. Mapping systematic reviews of breast cancer survivorship interventions: a network analysis. J Clin Oncol. 2022;40:2083–93.
55. Lawn S, Battersby M. Chronic condition management models for cancer care and survivorship. In: Cancer and chronic conditions. Addressing the problem of multimorbidity in cancer patients and survivors. Springer; 2016.
56. Grady PA, Gough LL. Self-management: a comprehensive approach to management of chronic conditions. Am J Public Health. 2014;104(8):e25–31. https://doi.org/10.2105/AJPH.2014.302041. Epub 2014 Jun 12.
57. Koczwara B. Cancer survivorship care at the time of the COVID-19 pandemic. Med J Aust. 2020;213(3):107–108.e1. https://doi.org/10.5694/mja2.50684. Epub 2020 Jun 28.
58. Howell D, Mayer DK, Fielding R, Eicher M, Verdonck-de Leeuw IM, Johansen C, Soto-Perez-de-Celis E, Foster C, Chan R, Alfano CM, Hudson SV, Jefford M, Lam WWT, Loerzel V, Pravettoni G, Rammant E, Schapira L, Stein KD, Koczwara B, Global Partners for Self-Management in Cancer. Management of cancer and health after the clinic visit: a call to action for self-management in cancer care. J Natl Cancer Inst. 2021;113(5):523–31. https://doi.org/10.1093/jnci/djaa083.
59. Yellen SB, Cella DF. Someone to live for: social well-being, parenthood status, and decision-making in oncology. J Clin Oncol. 1995;13(5):1255–64. https://doi.org/10.1200/JCO.1995.13.5.1255.
60. Kraav SL, Awoyemi O, Junttila N, Vornanen R, Kauhanen J, Toikko T, Lehto SM, Hantunen S, Tolmunen T. The effects of loneliness and social isolation on all-cause, injury, cancer, and CVD mortality in a cohort of middle-aged Finnish men. A prospective study. Aging Ment Health. 2021;25(12):2219–28. https://doi.org/10.1080/13607863.2020.1830945. Epub 2020 Oct 14.
61. Schroevers MJ, Helgeson VS, Sanderman R, Ranchor AV. Type of social support matters for prediction of posttraumatic growth among cancer survivors. Psychooncology. 2010;19(1):46–53. https://doi.org/10.1002/pon.1501.
62. Ussher J, Kirsten L, Butow P, Sandoval M. What do cancer support groups provide which other supportive relationships do not? The experience of peer support groups for people with cancer. Soc Sci Med. 2006;62(10):2565–76. https://doi.org/10.1016/j.socscimed.2005.10.034. Epub 2005 Nov 21.
63. Nekhlyudov L, O'Malley DM, Hudson SV. Integrating primary care providers in the care of cancer survivors: gaps in evidence and future opportunities. Lancet Oncol. 2017;18(1):e30–8. https://doi.org/10.1016/S1470-2045(16)30570-8.

64. Cortis LJ, Ward PR, McKinnon RA, Koczwara B. Integrated care in cancer: what is it, how is it used and where are the gaps? A textual narrative literature synthesis. Eur J Cancer Care (Engl). 2017;26(4) https://doi.org/10.1111/ecc.12689. Epub 2017 Apr 20.
65. McDonald K, Schultz E, Albin L, et al. Care coordination atlas version 3. Rockville, MD: Agency for Healthcare Research and Quality; 2010.
66. National Cancer Policy Board. Ensuring quality cancer care. Washington, DC: National Academies Press; 1999.
67. Gorin SS, Haggstrom D, Han PKJ, Fairfield KM, Krebs P, Clauser SB. Cancer care coordination: a systematic review and meta-analysis of over 30 years of empirical studies. Ann Behav Med. 2017;51(4):532–46. https://doi.org/10.1007/s12160-017-9876-2.
68. Weldring T, Smith SM. Patient-reported outcomes (PROs) and patient-reported outcome measures (PROMs). Health Serv Insights. 2013;6:61–8. https://doi.org/10.4137/HSI.S11093.
69. Clinical Oncology Society of Australia (COSA) Patient Reported Outcomes Working Group, Koczwara B, Bonnamy J, Briggs P, Brown B, Butow PN, Chan RJ, Cohn RJ, Girgis A, Jefford M, Joske DJ, Licqurish S, Mackay G, Saunders CM, Webber K. Patient-reported outcomes and personalised cancer care. Med J Aust. 2021;214(9):406–408.e1. https://doi.org/10.5694/mja2.50893. Epub 2020 Dec 13.
70. Butow P, Price MA, Shaw JM, Turner J, Clayton JM, Grimison P, Rankin N, Kirsten L. Clinical pathway for the screening, assessment and management of anxiety and depression in adult cancer patients: Australian guidelines. Psychooncology. 2015;24(9):987–1001. https://doi.org/10.1002/pon.3920. Epub 2015 Aug 13.
71. Basch E, Deal AM, Dueck AC, Scher HI, Kris MG, Hudis C, Schrag D. Overall survival results of a trial assessing patient-reported outcomes for symptom monitoring during routine cancer treatment. JAMA. 2017;318(2):197–8. https://doi.org/10.1001/jama.2017.7156.
72. Girgis A, Durcinoska I, Arnold A, Descallar J, Kaadan N, Koh ES, Miller A, Ng W, Carolan M, Della-Fiorentina SA, Avery S, Delaney GP. Web-based patient-reported outcome measures for personalized treatment and care (PROMPT-care): multicenter pragmatic nonrandomized trial. J Med Internet Res. 2020;22(10):e19685. https://doi.org/10.2196/19685.
73. Kotronoulas G, Kearney N, Maguire R, Harrow A, Di Domenico D, Croy S, MacGillivray S. What is the value of the routine use of patient-reported outcome measures toward improvement of patient outcomes, processes of care, and health service outcomes in cancer care? A systematic review of controlled trials. J Clin Oncol. 2014;32(14):1480–501. https://doi.org/10.1200/JCO.2013.53.5948. Epub 2014 Apr 7.
74. Subbiah IM, Charone MM, Roszik J, Haider A, Vidal M, Wong A, Bruera E. Association of Edmonton symptom assessment system global distress score with overall survival in patients with advanced cancer. JAMA Netw Open. 2021;4(7):e2117295. https://doi.org/10.1001/jamanetworkopen.2021.17295.
75. Hershman DL, Neugut AI, Moseley A, Arnold KB, Gralow JR, Henry NL, Hillyer GC, Ramsey SD, Unger JM. Patient-reported outcomes and long-term nonadherence to aromatase inhibitors. J Natl Cancer Inst. 2021;113(8):989–96. https://doi.org/10.1093/jnci/djab022.
76. Ramsey I, Corsini N, Hutchinson AD, Marker J, Eckert M. A core set of patient-reported outcomes for population-based cancer survivorship research: a consensus study. J Cancer Surviv. 2021;15(2):201–12. https://doi.org/10.1007/s11764-020-00924-5. Epub 2020 Aug 31.
77. Kreps GL. Achieving the promise of digital health information systems. J Public Health Res. 2014;3(3):471. https://doi.org/10.4081/jphr.2014.471.
78. Kemp E, Trigg J, Beatty L, Christensen C, Dhillon HM, Maeder A, Williams PAH, Koczwara B. Health literacy, digital health literacy and the implementation of digital health technologies in cancer care: the need for a strategic approach. Health Promot J Austr. 2021;32(Suppl 1):104–14. https://doi.org/10.1002/hpja.387. Epub 2020 Sep 21.
79. Morris BB, Rossi B, Fuemmeler B. The role of digital health technology in rural cancer care delivery: a systematic review. J Rural Health. 2021; https://doi.org/10.1111/jrh.12619. Epub ahead of print.
80. Bhatt S, Evans J, Gupta S. Barriers to scale of digital health Systems for Cancer Care and Control in last-mile settings. J Glob Oncol. 2018;4:1–3. https://doi.org/10.1200/JGO.2016.007179. Epub 2017 Mar 21.
81. Chan RJ, Hollingdrake O, Bui U, Nekhlyudov L, Hart NH, Lui CW, Feuerstein M. Evolving landscape of cancer survivorship research: an analysis of the Journal of Cancer Survivorship, 2007-2020. J Cancer Surviv. 2021;15(4):651–8. https://doi.org/10.1007/s11764-021-01042-6. Epub 2021 May 4.
82. Lawler M, De Lorenzo F, Lagergren P, Mennini FS, Narbutas S, Scocca G, Meunier F. Challenges and solutions to embed cancer survivorship research and innovation within the EU Cancer Mission. Mol Oncol. 2021;15:1750–8. https://doi.org/10.1002/1878-0261.13022.

Special Populations: Care of Military Veterans

Shawn Kane

"The willingness with which our young people are likely to serve in any war, no matter how justified, shall be directly proportional to how they perceive the veterans of earlier wars were treated and appreciated by their nation."
George Washington

Introduction

A veteran is defined as someone who has served but is not currently serving on active duty in the US Army, Navy, Air Force, Marine Corps, Space Force, or Coast Guard and those who served in the US Merchant Marine during World War II. Those who served in the National Guard, or the Reserves, are only classified as veterans if they were called to active duty [1]. Over the course of our nation's history, more than 41 million Americans have served in the military and the US Census Bureau in 2018 reported the veteran population as 18 million, or 7% of the adult population. This decrease in the veteran population is due to the smaller sized standing military population and the loss of older veterans from World War II and the Korean War. It is estimated there will be 200,000 new veterans annually, with projections of 12.9 million veterans living in the United States in 2040 [2, 3]. Despite the definition of who is a veteran, many veterans deny their status based on their own definition, such as serving in peacetime or serving only in the continental United States.

The veteran population have physical, mental, and psychosocial health needs unique to their service. Currently, less than half of veterans receive care from the Veterans Health Administration or the Defense Health Agency, leaving many to receive health care from community-based clinicians [4, 5]. It is vital that primary care physicians recognize and understand this unique patient population.

S. Kane (✉)
Department of Family Medicine, University of North Carolina at Chapel Hill, Chapel Hill, NC, USA
e-mail: shkane@email.unc.edu

Veteran Population

Though veterans come from different cultures and subcultures, they share values and customs including respect for hierarchy and etiquette, loyalty, teamwork, and selfless service. The traditions are further characterized by both the branch of the military and the era in which the veteran served. Different wartime eras have varying and specific health-related issues. Younger veterans from more recent conflicts have different health issues compared to veterans from World War II, the Korean and Vietnam wars, and the first Persian Gulf War [6].

The post-9/11 veteran population is more racially diverse than in any prior service era, with more non-white and Latinos and fewer African Americans. More than 30% of post-9/11 veterans are women and they are even more ethnically diverse than the men. When compared to prior eras, the post-9/11 veteran is more likely to be non-white, single, younger, and uninsured and have less income [4, 6].

Better protective gear, better health care, and advances in battlefield medicine have resulted in survival rates of 90–93% for those wounded in combat, compared to survival rates of 70% in World War II to 76% in the Vietnam War and the first Persian Gulf War [7, 8]. These medical advances create unique challenges in the care of younger veterans, who are more likely to have survived horrific, life-changing injuries, returned to combat after being severely wounded, and served in combat longer, resulting in complex health care needs. It is natural, based on proximity to the conflict, to assume that the current era of veterans is the worse off and the most negatively affected by service. Caring for the post-9/11 veteran population is indeed challenging; however, compared to veterans of the Persian Gulf and Vietnam conflicts, they tend to be more socially integrated, have fewer issues with substance abuse, and require less disability compensation for post-traumatic stress disorder (PTSD) [9].

Veteran Care

History

The city-states of ancient Greece were the first governments to take some responsibility in caring for wounded soldiers, their families, and the families of soldiers killed in combat. Since then, nations have implemented and evolved ways to care for casualties of war [10]. The United States has the most robust veteran care system of any nation in the world. In 1776, to boost enlistments the Continental Congress provided pensions to disabled soldiers and, until 1811, individual states and communities provided medical care to veterans. Since 1811 the federal government has assumed the responsibility for veteran care. The world wars saw massive increases in the veteran population and services provided, leading to the establishment of a federal Veterans Administration (VA). The passing of the GI Bill in June 1944 placed the VA second only to the Departments of War and Navy in funding and personnel. The VA department of medicine and surgery was established in 1946. In 1989, the VA was elevated to a cabinet-level position and renamed the Department of Veterans Affairs (VA). In 1991, the health care arm of the VA became known as the Veterans Health Administration [11].

Veterans Health Administration

The Veterans Health Administration (VHA) traces its roots back to the US Civil War and legislation signed into law by Abraham Lincoln. In 1873 the first government-sponsored veteran's home opened in Augusta, Maine, and served soldiers from the Union Army, including US Colored Troops. This campus and the others that followed set the template for succeeding generations of VA hospitals [11].

The VHA is the largest of the three administrations in the VA, the Veteran Benefits Administration and the National Cemetery Administration being the other two. The current VHA is America's largest integrated health care system and consists of approximately 1600 facilities that range from large medical centers to small outpatient community clinics [12]. In addition to the provision of medical care to veterans, the VHA provides training to health professionals and conducts medical research that benefits society at large.

Eligibility and Cost

Determining eligibility for VA health care can be complicated and confusing. The basic requirements are successful completion of 24 months of active military service and not receiving a dishonorable discharge (there are some individual circumstances that may allow for eligibility without serving for 24 months). Those serving in the National Guard and the Reserves must have been called to active duty and completed that service period to be eligible for VHS care [13].

The amount an individual pays for health care in the VHA is determined by a combination of their VA disability rating, ability to hold gainful employment, Medicaid eligibility, and military service record. The VA classifies veterans into one of eight priority groups which determines the veteran's co-payment for all health care services, including pharmacy services. The acquisition of VA eligibility can significantly impact the life and health of a veteran and can be facilitated by contacting a local Veteran Service Organization, the local VA health care facility, or using the VA website (www.va.gov) [13].

Veteran-Specific Chronic Health Issues

While health-related conditions are treated similarly whether the patient is a veteran or not, recognizing the common comorbidities seen in veterans optimizes the patient-physician relationship. Some comorbidities are easily identified and diagnosed, while others are not obvious and require a high index of suspicion and good clinical acumen. Understanding any symptom overlap may identify undiagnosed comorbidities earlier and lead to better treatment outcomes. Some of these topics are emotionally charged and sensitive and require compassion and the establishment of a confident veteran–health care provider relationship. There are three key concepts to caring for veterans: (1) identifying veterans in your patient population, (2) appropriate screening, and (3) understanding available resources. Asking a simple question, "Have you or a loved one ever served in the military?" is a great way to start. Screening for multiple conditions can identify undisclosed issues and the presence of chronic pain, emotional distress, or brain injury should increase concern for other disorders.

Musculoskeletal

Musculoskeletal injuries are a leading cause of lost duty time and separation for active-duty members and the sequelae of osteoarthritis (OA) and chronic pain are common morbidities in veterans. OA affects 30 million Americans, with a prevalence of 14% in those aged 25 years and older and up to 34% in those aged 65 years or older [14]. As daunting as those statistics are they underestimate the prevalence of this condition in the veteran population where the rate is twice that of age matched nonveterans. Female veterans have an adjusted incidence rate that is nearly 20% higher than males and African Americans have a higher incidence than other populations [5, 15]. Osteoarthritis and chronic pain from musculoskeletal injuries are not unique to American veterans with other militaries reporting similar incidence and prevalence and negative impact on individuals and societies [16].

The impact of chronic pain, from OA and other musculoskeletal injuries, on the overall health, well-being, and quality of life of veterans cannot be overestimated. Veterans with chronic musculoskeletal pain have a higher incidence of mood disorders, post-traumatic stress disorder, substance abuse disorders, and traumatic brain injury [17]. Veterans who suffer from OA, specifically in the hip or the knee, have an increased prevalence of insomnia and obstructive sleep apnea compared to veterans without those diagnoses. Though challenging to establish causality, the association between pain, mood, and sleep on an individual's overall health is well established [18]. As a result of these interactions the treatment of OA needs to focus on more than just the joints, rather should be an integrated, patient-centered biopsychosocial model that addresses the whole person. In 2020, the Department of Veterans Affairs and the Department of Defense published a clinical practice guideline on the nonsurgical management of hip and knee osteoarthritis which emphasizes the importance of whole-person care [14, 19, 20].

Traumatic Brain Injury

A traumatic brain injury (TBI) is temporary or permanent physiological disruption or structural injury from a traumatic force [6, 21]. TBIs are a result of direct impacts, rapid accelerations/decelerations, or blast exposure. TBI is classified as mild, moderate, or severe based on clinical symptoms such as loss or alteration of the level of consciousness and post-traumatic amnesia. The clinical evaluation is enhanced by validated tools such as the Glasgow Coma Scale and by brain imaging. The Brain Injury Screening Questionnaire (BISQ) screens for lifetime history of TBI with the intention of reducing the consequences of undiagnosed. This and other useful screening tools for veterans are listed in Table 31.1.

A mild traumatic brain injury (mTBI, also known as concussion) is a clinical diagnosis and the absence of obvious physical injuries, situational chaos, and motivated service members can result in missed or delayed diagnosis. At the peak of the conflicts in Iraq and Afghanistan, it was estimated that 28–60% of service members evacuated from the theater of war had a TBI, with 77% of those being mTBI [22, 23]. Overall, 20–30% of veterans of the conflicts in Iraq and Afghanistan sustained a TBI. Blast injuries are the primary cause of TBIs sustained in these more recent conflicts [24].

Table 31.1 Validated screening tools beneficial in the care of veterans

Traumatic brain injury
Defense Veteran Brain Injury Center (DVBIC) 3 Question TBI Screen [75]
Traumatic Brain Injury-4 (TBI-4) [76]
Brain Injury Screening Tool (BIST) [77]
Veteran Traumatic Brain Injury Screening Tool (VATBIST) [78]
Post-traumatic stress disorder
Clinician-Administered PTSD Scale (CAPS-5)
Post-traumatic Check List 5 (PCL-5)
Mood disorders
Patient Health Questionnaire 2 and 9 (PHQ-2 and PHQ-9)
General Anxiety Disorder-7 (GAD-7)
Substance use disorders
Alcohol Use Disorders Identification Tool (AUDIT)
Opioid Risk Tool (ORT)
CAGE (Cut down, Annoyance, Guilt, and Eye-opener) questions
Drug Abuse Screening Test (DAST)
Suicide
Columbia Suicide Severity Rating Scale (C-SSRS)
Ask Suicide Screening Questions (ASQ) [79]
Pain
Defense and Veterans Pain Rating Scale (DVPRS) [80, 81]
Health status
Short Form Health Survey (SF-36)

Early recognition and diagnosis of mTBI is essential. The 3 Question DVBIC TBI Screening Tool was designed to evaluate US military veterans and identify those who may need further evaluation for mTBI (Table 31.1). If diagnosed and treated appropriately, most mTBI patients will recover within 30 days. Despite the best treatment, an estimated 10–35% of patients who sustained a combat-related mTBI will suffer from prolonged symptoms [25]. The symptoms associated with the sequelae of mTBI are broad and vague and overlap with many of the other comorbidities seen in veterans, such as chronic pain, poor sleep, mood disturbances, and substance abuse. Up to 90% of veterans with persistent TBI symptoms suffer from chronic pain and approximately 35% suffer from PTSD [17, 25].

TBI is referred to as one of the "signature wounds" of the recent American conflicts. The condition is more common due to the type of warfare, the protracted nature of the conflict, and the initially unappreciated differences between civilian and combat-related trauma. When compared to civilian cohorts with similar brain trauma, post-9/11 veterans are 30% more likely to suffer from persistent symptoms [26]. Risk factors for protracted TBI symptomatology include older age, female sex, lower education levels, reduced resiliency, lack of support system, chronic pain, premorbid or reoccurrence of mental health problems, substance abuse, and severity of injury [27, 28]. The symptom overlap and the known high prevalence of comorbidities should drive screening of all veterans for possible persistent TBI symptoms.

Post-traumatic Stress Disorder

Post-traumatic stress disorder (PTSD) is classified by the *Diagnostics and Statistical Manual of Mental Disorders, fifth edition*, as a trauma or stress-related disorder that is characterized by four symptom clusters: reexperiencing symptoms, avoidance symptoms, negative alternations in cognition and mood, and alterations in arousal or reactivity [29]. Six to seven percent of the US population will experience PTSD in their lifetime, with 10.6% of veterans receiving care at the VA having a PTSD diagnosis. Nearly one in four (23–26%) of veterans of the most recent conflicts suffer from PTSD [30–32].

The diagnosis of PTSD requires the presence of symptoms that lead to distress and functional impairment, with no substance or comorbid condition as an explanation of symptoms, for 1 month after exposure to an actual or perceived traumatic event. Without early diagnosis, the patient may develop negative coping strategies. Recognition and treatment may be delayed because the patient is reluctant to seek treatment due to perceived weakness, stigma surrounding mental health issues, and unfamiliarity with treatment effectiveness.

The negative and magnifying impact of PTSD on other comorbidities common to veterans cannot be overstated. The symptom overlaps between PTSD, chronic pain, TBI, and other conditions make dual diagnoses highly probable, and 50–60% of veterans will have two or more of these conditions [16, 33, 34]. Understanding this complicated association and screening for these overlapping conditions is vital for health care providers caring for veterans. Common tools used for PTSD screening are listed in Table 31.1.

Moral Injury

A moral injury is defined as persistent symptoms resulting from perpetuating, failing to prevent, bearing witness to, or learning about acts that transgress deeply held moral beliefs and expectations. This term or situation has historically been absent in the mental health literature but more recently has garnered more attention and research. Veterans who have sustained a moral injury suffer intense feelings of guilt, shame, sadness, and anger. PTSD and a moral injury can result from the same event and co-occur in a veteran, though may occur separately. Understanding the existence of this condition is important as treatment is unique and requires referral to a specialist skilled in this area [35].

Depression

Depression and major depressive disorder are major causes of morbidity and disability worldwide, with an estimated annual prevalence of 7% in the US population [36]. Historically, veterans of World War II and the Korean War had a lower lifetime prevalence of depression than nonveterans. However, this changed during the Vietnam conflict and has persisted to this day [37]. Despite the fact that depression is more prevalent in the veteran population, with upwards of 40% of veterans of recent conflicts receiving care at the VA meeting diagnostic criteria, PTSD tends to be more researched and thought about as the mental health condition affecting veterans [38]. PTSD and depression are not mutually exclusive and their coexistence can be a challenging dual diagnosis with one condition impacting the other. The comorbid combination of PTSD and depression in the veteran population results in more severe symptoms and is associated with an increased risk of significant, life-threatening conditions such as suicide, substance abuse disorder, and homelessness [39]. While PTSD garners significant attention in the veteran community, depression is highly prevalent and warrants appropriate screening using standardized measures such as the Patient Health Questionnaire-9 (PHQ-9).

Substance Abuse Disorder

Substance use and abuse is unfortunately common in the veteran population with cigarette smoking and alcohol consumption rates that are higher than those of nonveterans [40]. There is an estimated 32% and 20% prevalence of alcohol use disorder and drug use disorder (both illicit and inappropriate use of prescription medications) respectively in veterans [41]. Comorbidities such as TBI, PTSD, and chronic pain put male veterans at twice the risk of a substance abuse disorder than female veterans with a corresponding increase in adverse clinical outcomes [42, 43]. Screening for substance abuse disorders in veterans is essential as the high prevalence can complicate other comorbidities and lead to negative outcomes. Commonly used screening tools such as the Alcohol Use Disorders Identification Test (AUDIT), CAGE (Cut down, Annoyance, Guilt, and Eye-opener) questions, and Drug Abuse Screening Test (DAST) are appropriate for screening veterans for substance use concerns (Table 31.1).

Suicide

Suicide is an epidemic that continues to worsen and take a toll on the veteran population. Male and female veterans have a 1.4- and 1.8-time higher risk of suicide than nonveterans [44]. In the post-9/11 veteran population, men aged 18–34 years have the highest suicide rate which is highest in the first 3 years after leaving the military. Though the rate lowers with age, veterans aged 50 years and older are still twice as likely to commit suicide compared to nonveterans [44]. Risk factors for suicide include PTSD, depression, chronic pain, substance use and abuse, and other comorbid mental health conditions. Veterans who have attempted suicide are at least 11% more likely to try again. Veterans should be screened for suicide risk (Table 31.1). Veterans should be asked about their access to firearms, given their frequent use when committing suicide compared to nonveterans [45].

Chronic Pain

Chronic pain is defined as pain that persists past the expected healing time, lacks the normal warning function of acute pain, and persists beyond 3–6 months. Chronic pain affects up to 20% of the world's population and accounts for 15–50% of physician visits [46]. In the veteran population the challenge of managing chronic pain is magnified by the presence of multiple comorbidities including PTSD, TBI, substance abuse disorder, and depression. An active-duty service member who is suffering from and has been treated for chronic or persistent pain while serving has a high likelihood of seeking care for those conditions from the VA [47].

Since the Vietnam conflict, the presence of comorbid PTSD and chronic pain has continued to increase, and veterans of the more recent conflicts have the highest co-occurrence rate for these conditions [48]. Almost 50% of veterans treated for chronic pain have PTSD and 66% of veterans treated for PTSD have chronic pain [49]. The etiology of the increase in prevalence in veterans of more recent wars is thought due to the extended and repeated deployments, resulting in higher injury rates and trauma exposures. The complex entanglement of these comorbidities is now better understood. Veterans with comorbid PTSD often feel as if they have less control over their pain, believe that their emotions affect their pain, and catastrophize more about their pain. Comorbid PTSD results in increased pain severity, disability, and pain-related interference. Appreciating this complex relationship will allow clinicians to better diagnose and treat these comorbidities [49, 50].

All veterans should be screened for both chronic pain and PTSD to identify these comorbid conditions early on to maximize treatment outcomes [48]. Patients with chronic pain and other mental health comorbidities will likely require interdisciplinary collaboration including the orchestration and coordination of care. Establishing a therapeutic primary care relationship is critical and facilitates nonconfrontational discussions that will help in working through mental health comorbidities [51].

Women's Health Care

As of 2015 there were 1.6 million women veterans of the US Armed Forces, accounting for 8.4% of the total veteran population [52]. Along with a total increase in the number of women in the Armed Forces, there have been drastic changes in the opportunities available to women including due in part to the repeal of the combat exclusion policy that previously restricted many roles to men. The increase in female veterans has increased the number of female patients seeking care at the VA with an associated increase in women's health services provided at the VA. As of 2016, 6.5% of VA users were women, a doubling since 2000 and a rate that outpaces the increase in male patients [53]. Women veterans develop the same medical conditions and comorbidities as male veterans with the same potential for complications and merit the same screening [54].

Military Sexual Trauma

Military sexual trauma (MST) is sexual assault or harassment that is experienced during military service. Although not limited to women, the prevalence rate in female veterans is significantly higher than that of men. Due to underreporting, the prevalence of MST is unclear but estimated to be 15–38% for women and 1–4% for men. The negative health consequences and outcomes related to MST are significant and include multiple comorbidities that have the potential for life-altering or lifelong consequences. Depression, anxiety, PTSD, suicidal ideation, and suicide attempts are all higher in victims of MST as is substance abuse, poorer physical well-being, and negative economic impact [55, 56].

Occupational Exposures

Hearing and Tinnitus

Hearing loss and tinnitus are two of the most prevalent service-connected disabilities in veterans and the leading causes of auditory dysfunction [57, 58]. Hearing loss results from the loss of function of the outer hair cells in the cochlea and as the condition progresses there is also dysfunction in the inner hair cells. Audiology testing can objectively document the degree of hearing loss across the frequency ranges of the human ear. Tinnitus, the subjective experience of sound within the ear commonly referred to as ringing in the ears, is harder to assess and the exact etiology is unclear [57, 59]. These conditions can occur in isolation or together with a wide range of overlap. Auditory dysfunction typically results from either increasing age or exposures to loud noises [60]. In the United States, the prevalence of hearing loss and tinnitus in the general population is 20% and 15–25%

respectively [58, 61]. The prevalence of hearing loss and tinnitus in the veteran population is as high as 58% and 75%, respectively [62]. This significant increase is likely the result of the increased exposures to blasts and blast-related trauma.

The negative impact of auditory dysfunction on a veteran's quality of life cannot be overestimated. The presence of these conditions negatively impacts sleep quality, reduces independence, and increases frustration, stress, depression, and anxiety. Hearing loss can have a major impact on a veteran, but there are multiple options available to ameliorate and treat this condition, such as hearing aids or hearing assistive listening devices. Tinnitus is a challenging condition due to limited treatment options. Tinnitus is associated with depression and anxiety and possibly an increased risk of suicide. The presence of multiple comorbidities such as blast-related TBI, PTSD, and depression makes the direct establishment of causality a challenge. Understanding and appreciating the complex interactions of these conditions can improve identification and treatment for the veteran [57, 58].

Airborne Hazards

Any contaminant or potentially toxic substance that is inhaled is referred to as an airborne hazard. Veterans are exposed to multiple airborne hazards from a combination of environmental (sand and dust), occupational (fuel and aircraft exhaust), and pollutant (smoke from oil wells and burn pits) sources [63, 64]. The potential for these inhalation exposures to cause post-deployment respiratory conditions led the VA to create the Airborne Hazards and Open Burn Pit Registry, which allows for research into the long-term effects of these environmental exposures. The data from this registry has allowed for new diagnosis of asthma, rhinitis, and sinusitis to be service connected based on presumptive exposure in Southwest Asia and elsewhere [65].

Agent Orange

The conflict in Vietnam brought about the widespread use of tactical herbicides to defoliate the jungle with the intent of minimizing the enemy's freedom to maneuver. Between 1962 and 1971, the US military sprayed an estimated 19 million gallons of herbicide across Vietnam and other Southeast Asian nations. Agent Orange, the most used herbicide in Vietnam, was made from mixing equal parts of two potent herbicides. The combination of these herbicides results in the production of 2,3,7,8-tetrachlorodibenzo-p-dioxin (TCDD), the most potent dioxin. The contemporary commercial standard for TCDD concentration at the time was less than 0.05 parts per million (ppm). The concentration of Agent Orange used in Vietnam ranged from 2 to 50 ppm with an average of 13 ppm [66, 67].

Up to 4.3 million Americans served in Vietnam with a substantial number still living. A growing list of medical conditions including malignancies and neurologic conditions have been presumptively linked to herbicide exposure in Vietnam. This list is continuously updated as sound medical and scientific evidence continues to link illnesses with herbicide exposure [65].

Social Issues

Health Disparities Among Veterans

An increasing number of women and ethnic minorities seek health care from the VA. The current generation of veterans is more diverse than in the past with 11% being women and 30% being ethnic minorities [68]. Forty percent of female veterans are from a racial or ethnic minority compared to 23% of male veterans. The growth of female veterans is outpacing their male counterparts leading to a higher proportion of veterans identifying as women, though overall most veterans are male. Female VA patients are a medically complex subpopulation, and compared to civilian women and their male VA counterparts they have a higher prevalence of mental illness and medical comorbidities [53]. Even in a system with minimal financial barriers, such as the VA, there are documented health care disparities that affect women and racial and ethnic minorities across a range of clinical areas. The reasons behind these disparities are complex and multifactorial, but with data collection and quality improvement the VA is well positioned to impact these disparities [69].

Homelessness

Veteran homelessness has been an issue since the US Civil War and continues to be a contemporary public health problem in the United States [70]. Twelve percent of the homeless adult population are veterans, while less than 8% of the total population are veterans, leading the VA to aspire to address and end homelessness among veterans. Homeless veterans tend to be older and better educated and more likely to have married, been employed, and have health coverage, compared to the overall homeless population [71, 72]. These characteristics should be advantages and lower the risk of homelessness in veterans; however, that is not the case. Substance abuse, severe mental illness, and low income are common risk factors for homelessness and veterans have a higher rate of these conditions, along with unique risks of problematic military discharges, low military pay grade, and social isolation. The VA programs have been successful as by 2017 there was a 47% drop in veteran homelessness. There is a large overlap in the risk factors for homelessness and suicide in the veteran population and those who are or have been homeless are five times more likely to attempt suicide.

The VA has made great strides in decreasing homelessness, but continued attention is needed to control this public health crisis [71].

Non-health Care Benefits to Veterans

The VA provides veterans with multiple benefits beyond health care with some of these benefits available to their family members. The list of benefits includes but is not limited to disability compensation, vocational rehabilitation, housing loans, life insurance, and even burial assistance. The entire list of VA benefits and how to apply can be accessed at www.va.gov; individual states also have a wide range of veteran benefits that can be accessed through the states' departments of veteran affairs.

Future Directions

Timely access to health care is a challenge everywhere, and as the largest integrated health system in the country, the VA is no different. Due to highly publicized concerns with veterans' access to timely health care, the US Congress passed the Veterans Access, Choice, and Accountability Act of 2014 (Veterans Choice Program) with the intent of improving access. This was followed by the Department of Veteran Affairs Maintaining Internal Systems and Strengthening Integrated Outside Networks (MISSION) Act of 2018 [73]. Prior to passage of these two acts, almost all veteran care was delivered within the VA. Allowing veterans to be seen in a civilian health care network may address the issue of access, but it may sacrifice quality and cost more. The quality of general and preventative medical care delivered at the VA typically exceeds the community when measured by national quality measures. The VA cares for veterans on a fixed budget and there is concern that the use of non-VA care may deplete this budget. It is imperative that the ease of access is balanced with quality and cost as the United States strives to provide ongoing excellent health care to the men and women who have served in the US Military [74].

References

1. Bureau, U.C. https://www.census.gov/topics/population/veterans/about/glossary.html.
2. Vespa JE. Those Who Served: America's Veterans from World War II to the War on Terror, A.C.S.R. ACS-32, Editor. Washington DC: US Census Bureau; 2020.
3. Oster C, et al. The health and wellbeing needs of veterans: a rapid review. BMC Psychiatry. 2017;17(1):414.
4. Waszak DL, Holmes AM. The Unique Health Needs of Post-9/11 U.S. Veterans. Workplace Health Saf. 2017;65(9):430–44.
5. Yedlinsky NT, Neff LA, Jordan KM. Care of the military veteran: selected health issues. Am Fam Physician. 2019;100(9):544–51.
6. Olenick M, Flowers M, Diaz VJ. US veterans and their unique issues: enhancing health care professional awareness. Adv Med Educ Pract. 2015;6:635–9.
7. Howard JT, et al. Use of combat casualty care data to assess the US military trauma system during the Afghanistan and Iraq Conflicts, 2001-2017. JAMA Surg. 2019;154(7):600–8.
8. Gawande A. Casualties of war—military care for the wounded from Iraq and Afghanistan. N Engl J Med. 2004;351(24):2471–5.
9. Fontana A, Rosenheck R. Treatment-seeking veterans of Iraq and Afghanistan: comparison with veterans of previous wars. J Nerv Ment Dis. 2008;196(7):513–21.
10. Rostker BD. Providing for the casualties of war: the American Experience Through World War II. Santa Monica, CA: RAND Corporation; 2013.
11. VA History. 2021. http://www.va.gov/history.
12. Veterans Health Administration https://www.va.gov/health/ originally accessed 13 Nov 21 and reaccessed 2 Apr 23.
13. Eligibility for VA Health Care https://www.va.gov/health-care/eligibility/ originally accessed 13 Nov 21 and reaccessed 2 Apr 23.
14. Krishnamurthy A, et al. Synopsis of the 2020 US Department of Veterans Affairs/US Department of Defense Clinical Practice Guideline: the non-surgical management of hip and knee osteoarthritis. Mayo Clin Proc. 2021;96(9):2435–47.
15. Stanishewski M, Zimmermann B. Osteoarthritis treatment in the veteran population. Fed Pract. 2015;32(Suppl 12):21S–5S.
16. Gauntlett-Gilbert J, Wilson S. Veterans and chronic pain. Br J Pain. 2013;7(2):79–84.
17. Higgins DM, et al. Persistent pain and comorbidity among Operation Enduring Freedom/Operation Iraqi Freedom/operation New Dawn veterans. Pain Med. 2014;15(5):782–90.
18. Taylor SS, et al. Prevalence of and characteristics associated with insomnia and obstructive sleep apnea among veterans with knee and hip osteoarthritis. BMC Musculoskelet Disord. 2018;19(1):79.
19. Department of Veterans Affairs, D.o.D., VA/DoD Clinical Practice Guideline for the Non-surgical management of hip and knee osteoarthritis. 2020.
20. Allen KD, et al. A combined patient and provider intervention for management of osteoarthritis in veterans: a randomized clinical trial. Ann Intern Med. 2016;164(2):73–83.
21. Kane SF, et al. When war follows combat veterans home. J Fam Pract. 2013;62(8):399–407.
22. Lew HL, et al. Soldiers with occult traumatic brain injury. Am J Phys Med Rehabil. 2005;84(6):393–8.
23. Marshall KR, et al. Mild traumatic brain injury screening, diagnosis, and treatment. Mil Med. 2012;177(8 Suppl):67–75.
24. Daggett VS, et al. Needs and concerns of male combat Veterans with mild traumatic brain injury. J Rehabil Res Dev. 2013;50(3):327–40.
25. Schneiderman AI, Braver ER, Kang HK. Understanding sequelae of injury mechanisms and mild traumatic brain injury incurred during the conflicts in Iraq and Afghanistan: persistent postconcussive symptoms and posttraumatic stress disorder. Am J Epidemiol. 2008;167(12):1446–52.
26. Hoge CW, Goldberg HM, Castro CA. Care of war veterans with mild traumatic brain injury—flawed perspectives. N Engl J Med. 2009;360(16):1588–91.
27. Tsai J, et al. Examining the relation between combat-related concussion, a novel 5-factor model of posttraumatic stress symptoms, and health-related quality of life in Iraq and Afghanistan veterans. J Clin Psychiatry. 2012;73(8):1110–8.
28. Wall PL. Posttraumatic stress disorder and traumatic brain injury in current military populations: a critical analysis. J Am Psychiatr Nurses Assoc. 2012;18(5):278–98.

29. APA. Diagnostic and statistical manual of mental disorders (DSM-5). 5th ed. 2013.
30. Fulton JJ, et al. The prevalence of posttraumatic stress disorder in Operation Enduring Freedom/Operation Iraqi Freedom (OEF/OIF) Veterans: a meta-analysis. J Anxiety Disord. 2015;31:98–107.
31. Ostacher MJ, Cifu AS. Management of posttraumatic stress disorder. JAMA. 2019;321(2):200–1.
32. VA/DoD Clinical Practice Guideline for the Management of Posttraumatic Stress Disorder and Acute Stress Disorder. 2017.
33. Aase DM, et al. Impact of PTSD on post-concussive symptoms, neuropsychological functioning, and pain in post-9/11 veterans with mild traumatic brain injury. Psychiatry Res. 2018;268:460–6.
34. Tanev KS, et al. PTSD and TBI co-morbidity: scope, clinical presentation and treatment options. Brain Inj. 2014;28(3):261–70.
35. Griffin BJ, et al. Moral injury: an integrative review. J Trauma Stress. 2019;32(3):350–62.
36. Burnett-Zeigler I, et al. Depression treatment in older adult veterans. Am J Geriatr Psychiatry. 2012;20(3):228–38.
37. Boakye EA, et al. Self-reported lifetime depression and current mental distress among veterans across service eras. Mil Med. 2017;182(3):e1691–6.
38. Blore JD, et al. Depression in Gulf War veterans: a systematic review and meta-analysis. Psychol Med. 2015;45(8):1565–80.
39. Arenson MB, et al. Posttraumatic stress disorder, depression, and suicidal ideation in veterans: results from the mind your heart study. Psychiatry Res. 2018;265:224–30.
40. Johnson BS, et al. Enhancing veteran-centered care: a guide for nurses in non-VA settings. Am J Nurs. 2013;113(7):24–39; quiz 54, 40.
41. Lan CW, et al. The epidemiology of substance use disorders in US Veterans: a systematic review and analysis of assessment methods. Am J Addict. 2016;25(1):7–24.
42. Seal KH, et al. Trends and risk factors for mental health diagnoses among Iraq and Afghanistan veterans using Department of Veterans Affairs health care, 2002-2008. Am J Public Health. 2009;99(9):1651–8.
43. Seal KH, et al. Association of mental health disorders with prescription opioids and high-risk opioid use in US veterans of Iraq and Afghanistan. JAMA. 2012;307(9):940–7.
44. Kang HK, et al. Suicide risk among 1.3 million veterans who were on active duty during the Iraq and Afghanistan wars. Ann Epidemiol. 2015;25(2):96–100.
45. Department of Veterans Affairs, D.o.D. VA/DoD clinical practice guideline for the assessment and management of patients at risk for suicide. 2013.
46. Treede RD, et al. A classification of chronic pain for ICD-11. Pain. 2015;156(6):1003–7.
47. Adams RS, et al. Predictors of Veterans Health Administration utilization and pain persistence among soldiers treated for postdeployment chronic pain in the Military Health System. BMC Health Serv Res. 2021;21(1):494.
48. Outcalt SD, et al. Does comorbid chronic pain affect posttraumatic stress disorder diagnosis and treatment? Outcomes of posttraumatic stress disorder screening in Department of Veterans Affairs primary care. J Rehabil Res Dev. 2016;53(1):37–44.
49. Outcalt SD, et al. Pain experience of Iraq and Afghanistan Veterans with comorbid chronic pain and posttraumatic stress. J Rehabil Res Dev. 2014;51(4):559–70.
50. Alschuler KN, Otis JD. Coping strategies and beliefs about pain in veterans with comorbid chronic pain and significant levels of posttraumatic stress disorder symptoms. Eur J Pain. 2012;16(2):312–9.
51. Thompson JM, et al. A sailor's pain: Veterans' musculoskeletal disorders, chronic pain, and disability. Can Fam Physician. 2009;55(11):1085–8.
52. Lofquist DA. Characteristics of female veterans—an analytic view across age-cohorts: 2015. 2017.
53. Carter A, et al. Racial and ethnic health care disparities among women in the veterans affairs healthcare system: a systematic review. Womens Health Issues. 2016;26(4):401–9.
54. Asmundson GJ, Wright KD, Stein MB. Pain and PTSD symptoms in female veterans. Eur J Pain. 2004;8(4):345–50.
55. Johnson NL, et al. Establishing a new military sexual trauma treatment program: issues and recommendations for design and implementation. Psychol Serv. 2015;12(4):435–42.
56. Stahlman S, et al. Mental health and substance use factors associated with unwanted sexual contact among U.S. Active Duty Service Women. J Trauma Stress. 2015;28(3):167–73.
57. Martz E, et al. Tinnitus, depression, anxiety, and suicide in recent veterans: a retrospective analysis. Ear Hear. 2018;39(6):1046–56.
58. Swan AA, et al. Prevalence of hearing loss and tinnitus in Iraq and Afghanistan Veterans: a chronic effects of neurotrauma consortium study. Hear Res. 2017;349:4–12.
59. Burns-O'Connell G, Stockdale D, Hoare DJ. Soldiering on: a survey on the lived experience of tinnitus in aged military veterans in the UK. Med Humanit. 2019;45(4):408–15.
60. Moore BCJ. The effect of exposure to noise during military service on the subsequent progression of hearing loss. Int J Environ Res Public Health. 2021;18(5):2436.
61. Henry JA, et al. Tinnitus: an epidemiologic perspective. Otolaryngol Clin N Am. 2020;53(4):481–99.
62. Theodoroff SM, et al. Hearing impairment and tinnitus: prevalence, risk factors, and outcomes in US service members and veterans deployed to the Iraq and Afghanistan wars. Epidemiol Rev. 2015;37:71–85.
63. Falvo MJ, et al. Airborne hazards exposure and respiratory health of Iraq and Afghanistan veterans. Epidemiol Rev. 2015;37:116–30.
64. Thatcher TH, et al. Analysis of Postdeployment Serum Samples Identifies Potential Biomarkers of Exposure to Burn Pits and Other Environmental Hazards. J Occup Environ Med. 2019;61(Suppl 12):S45–54.
65. VA, Service Connection for Respiratory Condition Due to Exposure to Particulate Matter. 2021.
66. National Academies of Sciences, E.g., and Medicine, et al. Veterans and agent orange: update 11 (2018). 2018.
67. Public Health Agent Orange. https://www.publichealth.va.gov/exposures/agentorange.
68. Davis TD, et al. Utilization of VA mental health and primary care services among Iraq and Afghanistan veterans with depression: the influence of gender and ethnicity status. Mil Med. 2014;179(5):515–20.
69. Saha S, et al. Racial and ethnic disparities in the VA health care system: a systematic review. J Gen Intern Med. 2008;23(5):654–71.
70. Tsai J, Rosenheck RA. Risk factors for homelessness among US veterans. Epidemiol Rev. 2015;37:177–95.
71. Tsai J, et al. Addressing veteran homelessness to prevent veteran suicides. Psychiatr Serv. 2018;69(8):935–7.
72. Tsai J, Pietrzak RH, Szymkowiak D. The problem of veteran homelessness: an update for the new decade. Am J Prev Med. 2021;60(6):774–80.
73. Mattocks KM, et al. Understanding VA's use of and relationships with community care providers under the MISSION act. Med Care. 2021;59(Suppl 3):S252–8.
74. Massarweh NN, Itani KMF, Morris MS. The VA MISSION act and the future of Veterans' access to quality health care. JAMA. 2020;324(4):343–4.
75. Schwab KA, et al. Screening for traumatic brain injury in troops returning from deployment in Afghanistan and Iraq: initial investigation of the usefulness of a short screening tool for traumatic brain injury. J Head Trauma Rehabil. 2007;22(6):377–89.

76. Olson-Madden JH, et al. Validating the traumatic brain injury-4 screening measure for veterans seeking mental health treatment with psychiatric inpatient and outpatient service utilization data. Arch Phys Med Rehabil. 2014;95(5):925–9.
77. Theadom A, et al. The Brain Injury Screening Tool (BIST): tool development, factor structure and validity. PLoS One. 2021;16(2):e0246512.
78. Donnelly KT, et al. Reliability, sensitivity, and specificity of the VA traumatic brain injury screening tool. J Head Trauma Rehabil. 2011;26(6):439–53.
79. NIMH. Ask Suicide Screening Questions Tool Kit. https://www.nimh.nih.gov/research/research-conducted-at-nimh/asq-toolkit-materials.
80. Defense and Veterans Pain Rating Scale. 2022. https://www.dvcipm.org/clinical-resources/defense-veterans-pain-rating-scale-dvprs/.
81. Polomano RC, et al. Psychometric testing of the defense and veterans pain rating scale (DVPRS): a new pain scale for military population. Pain Med. 2016;17(8):1505–19.

Special Populations: Care of Persons Experiencing Homelessness

Richard Moore II and Timothy P. Daaleman

Introduction

Individuals experiencing homelessness are pushed to the margins of society and health care. The number of persons experiencing homelessness (PEH) and who are vulnerably housed continues to increase in both rural and urban areas of the United States (US) [1]. These individuals have increased risk of unsafe living conditions, and a higher likelihood of infectious and non-infectious medical and psychological conditions that impact their short- and long-term health [2–4]. PEH and vulnerably housed individuals include those who have an absence of stable, permanent housing and who have limited means of obtaining housing [1]. A multitude of factors contribute to the prevalence of experiencing homelessness including: historical factors such as the de-institutionalization of mental health treatment, urbanization, and gentrification [5]; policies that inform variable access and strategies to housing resources at the municipal level, and; individual circumstances such as severe, persistent mental illness and substance use disorders [6].

There are a limited number of healthcare clinics, programs, and initiatives that are primarily designed to provide care for PEH which promote access and are responsive to their needs [7]. As a result, many PEH seek health care through emergency departments and hospital settings, limiting the capacity to form continuity relationships with providers that could mitigate future morbidity and mortality [3]. Evidence-based practices can inform healthcare providers in their care of PEH that promotes health and quality of life [8]. Healthcare systems, in turn, can develop initiatives that are responsive to the diverse health needs of PEH by fostering an environment in which individuals feel understood, and that their needs are addressed.

This chapter will provide an overview to the care of persons experiencing homelessness (PEH) and draws upon consensus guidelines developed in Canada [8], a review of interventions that have been found to be effective in marginalized populations [9], and recommendations from subject matter experts [10]. It will first describe the characteristics and medical comorbidities that are associated with the experience of homelessness. The chapter will then outline strategies that can be used to screen for persons who are vulnerably housed and experiencing homelessness. The final section will provide information regarding the integrated care of PEH, including evidence-based strategies and programs that can mitigate the adverse impacts of homelessness on health and health care.

Characteristics of Persons Experiencing Homelessness

In the US, an estimated 1.5% of individuals experience homelessness per year, and 4.5% experience homelessness in their lifetime [11]. Table 32.1 provides the US Department of Housing and Urban Development's definition of homelessness [12]. Recent point-in-time counts note that approximately 580,000 people are facing homelessness on a given day [1]. Sixty percent are staying in sheltered environments, while four in ten are in unsheltered locations, such as abandoned buildings or on the street [1]. The prevalence of people experiencing homelessness has increased consecutively over 4 years, beginning in 2016, and rising 2% from 2019 to 2020 [1]. The number of people experiencing chronic homelessness, including individuals who have either been homeless for one consecutive year, or experienced homelessness for a cumulative 12 months in a 3-year period, has also grown with time [1].

The majority of homeless populations are located in urban environments (58%), however a significant number of individuals are found in suburban (22%) and rural (20%) settings [1]. Nearly 172,000 individuals are in families in both sheltered and, as of 2020, increasingly unsheltered environments [1]. Individual risk for homelessness in youth and young

R. Moore II · T. P. Daaleman (✉)
Department of Family Medicine, University of North Carolina at Chapel Hill, School of Medicine, Chapel Hill, NC, USA
e-mail: rick_moore@med.unc.edu; tim_daaleman@med.unc.edu

Table 32.1 Homelessness definitions. (Adapted from reference [12])

Category	Definition
Literally homeless	1. Individual or family who lacks a fixed, regular, and adequate nighttime residence, as typified by: (a) Has a primary nighttime residence that is a public or private place not meant for human habitation; (b) Is living in a publicly or privately operated shelter designated to provide temporary living arrangements (c) Is exiting an institution where (s)he has resided for 90 days or less and who resided in an emergency shelter or place not meant for human habitation immediately before entry into that institution
Imminent risk of homelessness	2. Individual or family who will imminently lose their primary nighttime residence, such that: (a) Residence will be lost within 14 days of the date of application for homeless assistance; (b) No subsequent residence has been identified; and (c) The individual or family lacks the resources or support networks needed to obtain other permanent housing
Homeless under other federal statutes	3. Unaccompanied youth under 25 years of age, or families with children and youth, who do not otherwise qualify as homeless, but who: (a) Are defined as homeless under the other listed federal statutes; (b) Have not had a lease, ownership interest, or occupancy agreement in permanent housing during the 60 days prior to the homeless assistance application; (c) Have experienced persistent instability as measured by two moves or more during the preceding 60 days; and (d) Can be expected to continue in such status for an extended period of time due to special needs or barriers
Fleeing/Attempting to flee DV	4. Any individual or family who: (a) Is fleeing, or is attempting to flee, domestic violence; (b) Has no other residence; and (c) Lacks the resources or support networks to obtain other permanent housing

adults increases with an experience of family conflict and history of abuse [13], in LGBTQ youth [14], and in those who have been part of the foster system [15]. Military veterans are at higher risk of homelessness, with a lifetime prevalence rate of 10.2% that is greater (19.9%) in veterans who are between 30 and 44 years of age [16]. African Americans bear a disproportionate impact, comprising 39% of all individuals and 53% of families with children experiencing homelessness [1]. Comparable rates are reported in people identifying as Hispanic or Latino, who make up 16% of the general population but 23% of the homeless population [1].

The Mental and Physical Health Hazards of Experiencing Homelessness

Persons experiencing homelessness are disproportionately impacted by both communicable and non-communicable disease, which contributes to lower life expectancy in both men and women [3]. Despite lower life expectancy, the majority of PEH are over 55 years of age and are at increased risk of cardiovascular and other chronic diseases associated with older age [17].

Mental Illness and Substance Use Disorders

Serious and persistent mental illness (SMI), such as schizophrenia, bipolar disorder, and major depression, are associated with higher rates of experiencing homelessness [18]. A mental health diagnosis is associated with greater risk of becoming homeless and a reduced likelihood of exiting homelessness [19]. Prior suicide attempts and a history of behavioral health conditions are independently associated with homelessness over 1 year and lifetime periods [11]. The deinstitutionalization of patients with SMI began in the 1950s and did not take into account the social and housing support needs of those released into the community [20]. The result of this policy was a progressive increase in homelessness and higher rates of SMI in those experiencing homelessness [20]. The provision of safe, secure housing can facilitate mental health services and reduce emergency service and hospital utilization, while promoting the coordination of outpatient mental health follow-up at the time of discharge [21].

Psychiatric conditions and substance use disorders have a significant impact on homeless youth and adults [22, 23]. Substance use disorders are prevalent among homeless and vulnerably housed populations, who experience higher rates of adverse childhood experiences, trauma, and toxic stress that contribute to use of substance-related coping strategies in an effort to mitigate symptoms [24, 25]. PEH are subject to higher rates of trauma and adverse life experiences and, during periods of homelessness, encounter further psychologic distress through economic insecurity, unsafe living conditions, diminished access to basic needs, and re-exposure to trauma [26]. Physical and sexual assault, neglect, and domestic violence contribute to the heightened rates of anxiety, depression, and post-traumatic stress disorder seen in homeless children and adults [26, 27]. In addition to the increased prevalence of trauma, there is reduced access to medical and behavioral health services for PEH, which further exacerbates mental health comorbidities [7, 21].

The exposure to trauma and higher rates of adverse childhood experiences that are common in the context of homelessness also contribute to the higher rates of substance use disorders [24]. Many PEH may seek to self-treat their trauma and other life stressors through alcohol and substance use [25]. Among PEH, death due to overdose can be responsible for a third of total deaths in adults younger than 45 years of age, offsetting reduced mortality related to human immunodeficiency virus (HIV) that contributes to a stable mortality rate in homeless populations [28]. Screening for substance use disorders using tools such as the Drug Abuse Screening Test (DAST-10) and Alcohol Use Disorders Identification Test (AUDIT-C) may facilitate the identification of at-risk individuals and linkages to resources, including harm reduction services, opioid substitution therapy, and enhanced case management [29].

Case management and access to primary care can reduce the likelihood of PEH having unmet mental health needs [23]. The integration of mental health services into a medical home can also enhance the quality of care for PEH, with behavioral health providers delivering on-site care and serving as liaisons that can link individuals to community-based services [30]. The integration of substance use treatment in primary care can benefit PEH who may have significant barriers to care [31]. Medication assisted treatment is often a core treatment modality that can promote recovery.

Opioid agonist therapy has demonstrated efficacy, including reductions in opioid-related death, risk of suicide, and cardiovascular mortality [31]. These outcomes are irrespective of the type of opioid agonist therapy (e.g., buprenorphine-based treatment or methadone) that is employed. A systematic review of harm reduction interventions reported that supervised consumption facilities were linked to a 35% reduction in opioid overdose death within 500 m of the facility, as well as higher likelihood of reversal of opioid toxicity, reductions in syringe sharing and reuse, and reduction of injection in public spaces [8]. Managed alcohol programs have reported mixed hepatic-related outcomes but with stabilization of consumption and enhanced linkage to medical and social services [8].

Infectious Disease

Persons experiencing homelessness (PEH) have a higher risk of viral hepatitis infections, including Hepatitis A and B, due to injection and non-injection drug use, higher risk sexual encounters, reduced access to sanitary living conditions, and impaired access to clean food and water [2, 4, 32, 33]. HIV and viral hepatitis are major causes of mortality [34, 35] and disproportionally impact individuals who are homeless or unstably housed, as well as people who inject drugs (PWID) [2]. For example, a pooled analysis from 16 countries reported an increased risk of infection with HIV and Hepatitis C for PWID experiencing recent unstable housing or homelessness [2]. In the US, approximately 1.2 million people are living with HIV and approximately 34,800 were newly diagnosed in 2019 [36]. PEH with HIV are less likely to achieve virologic suppression [4] and, by extension, greater viral transmission rates are reported [37]. Differences in suppression rates are due to the absence of a stable address and the lack of transportation, which contributes to barriers to antiretroviral therapy (ART). Substantial numbers of patients with PWID do not begin treatment and have higher rates of re-infection [38]. If treatment is initiated, they have a greater likelihood of treatment completion and cure [38].

Access to recommended screening and follow-up care for PEH with HIV and viral hepatitis, as well as linkage to vaccination and harm reduction services, are important parts in comprehensive treatment. Hepatitis C treatment is feasible in primary care settings, with direct acting antiviral medication regimens that are efficacious, and safety and tolerability profiles that are less likely to interact with other drugs [39, 40]. Primary care homeless models for Hepatitis C may promote access by taking into account financial barriers, (e.g., co-pays), access to public transportation, and other challenges in navigating healthcare systems. Similarly, HIV treatment models for PEH that co-locate with patient centered medical homes can leverage the resources of the clinical environment to improve health outcomes for people with HIV [30].

Promoting access to vaccinations is important in chronic disease management. The Centers for Disease Control (CDC) and Advisory Committee on Immunization Practices (ACIP) recommend routine vaccination against Hepatitis A for PEH due to increased risk [32]. The CDC and ACIP do not have specific recommendations for Hepatitis B vaccination, however many PEH have associated factors such as chronic liver disease, injection drug use, HIV, and Hepatitis C infection in which vaccination is recommended. Recent guidelines have been expanded to include eligibility for all adults [41]. Pneumococcal vaccination can also be considered for PEH with health conditions such as chronic heart and lung disease, alcoholism, liver disease, diabetes, tobacco use, and HIV infection[42].

Chronic Medical Conditions

The majority of individuals experiencing chronic homelessness are 50 years of age and older [1]. The medical conditions that older PEH experience are comparable to the general population, but factors such as environmental exposure, barriers to healthcare access, chronic stress, lack of adequate nutrition, and substance use, contribute to more advanced stages of disease [43, 44]. Cardiovascular disease is a major cause of morbidity and mortality, due to a combination of increased exposure to both non-traditional (e.g., cocaine use, heavy alcohol use, HIV infection) as well as traditional risk factors (e.g., smoking, hypertension) risk factors [43]. Diabetes mellitus, hypertension, and hyperlipidemia are not more common in PEH but are often not well controlled, leading to poorer cardiovascular outcomes [44].

Since cardiovascular disease is more prevalent in homeless populations and present at more advanced stages [43–45], early screening and treatment for traditional (e.g., tobacco use, uncontrolled hypertension) and non-traditional (e.g., cocaine use, heavy alcohol use) risk factors should be considered for primary and secondary prevention. Assessing for behavior change and working with patients in prioritizing their health goals—with an understanding that housing and other social determinants (e.g., food insecurity, intimate partner violence)—may reprioritize medical conditions, such as treatment for substance use disorders or hypertension.

Cognitive impairment is also disproportionately experienced in PEH when compared to the general population [45, 46]. The lifetime risk of traumatic brain injury is approximately five times greater and contributes to greater prevalence [47]. Screening for cognitive impairment using tools such as the Mini-Mental State Examination can help identify at-risk patients as well as treatment response [6].

Exposure-related injuries, such as frostbite and hypothermia, are common in PEH due to contact with temperature extremes without adequate protection, as well as predisposing factors such as alcohol use, neuropathy, and peripheral vascular disease [48, 49]. Other factors such as poor-fitting shoes, wet socks, prolonged standing, and lack of adequate housing can lead to fungal and bacterial skin infections, immersion foot conditions, and skin ulceration [50, 51]. Proper foot care, the prompt identification of these underlying conditions, and the initiation of treatment can mitigate the risk of amputation associated with more profound tissue injury, as well as promoting follow-up care [52].

Screening for Vulnerably Housed and Persons Experiencing Homelessness

Systematically addressing social determinants of health (SDOH), such has housing instability, is an important part of ongoing US health policy reforms that incentivize healthcare systems to identify and mitigate SDOH as strategies for improving population health [53, 54]. Reliably identifying persons experiencing housing instability is an ongoing challenge to healthcare systems and many are exploring workflows to screen patients during clinical encounters [55]. Since homelessness is experienced at a significant rate among US military veterans, the US Department of Veterans Affairs (VA) introduced universal screening for homelessness in 2012 using the Homelessness Screening Clinical Reminder (HSCR) [56, 57].

The HSCR is administered at least annually during VA outpatient visits and includes the following questions: (1) "In the past 60 days, have you been living in stable housing that you own, rent, or stay in as part of a household?" and; (2) "Are you worried or concerned that in the next 60 days you may not have stable housing that you own, rent, or stay in as part of a household?" [55] With this approach, the VA improved the identification of veterans who were homeless or at risk for homelessness, and linked them to services which led to an 85% resolution of housing instability on re-screening [57].

SDOH screening approaches for housing can also begin with informal questions, such as "How is your living situation?" that are integrated into clinical encounters and allow patients to voice their current life circumstance in their own words [7, 58]. This approach can be inclusive of a broader screening context for SDOH, including food insecurity and transportation limitations, and are important steps in identifying needs and linkage to additional services [58].

Providing Integrated Care to Persons Experiencing Homelessness

The experience of homelessness is stigmatizing, and the adverse effects extend to the healthcare settings. A trauma-informed care perspective is vital since individuals experiencing homelessness have a higher prevalence of adverse childhood experiences, as well as ongoing experiences of trauma and toxic stress [26]. Developing and implementing a trauma-informed care organizational framework involves an appreciation of the pervasive impact of trauma in the lives of individuals experiencing homelessness, and an understanding by the care team of how current and prior trauma can trigger physical and behavioral symptoms [59, 60]. Healthcare settings can be adapted to create environments that promote emotional safety, where trauma and the downstream effects of traumatic experiences (e.g., substance use, psychiatric disorders) can be identified and managed. The incorporation of screening and assessment tools for traumatic events (e.g., adverse childhood experiences) [61], the creation of outreach protocols to engage individuals who may be lost to care, and the coordination and co-location of care management, substance use treatment, and mental health services, are important structural elements in providing clinical care [62]. Table 32.2 presents a summary of the reported evidence-base for effective interventions to address the health and social needs of PEH by structure, process, and outcome components.

The integration of social and behavioral services is a key element in the organization of care for persons experiencing

Table 32.2 Effective interventions for people experiencing homelessness. (Adapted from references [8–10])

Structure
• The following values should guide the delivery of services: ample time and patience for communication; promoting trust and acceptance; providing supportive, unbiased, open, honest, and transparent services in inclusive spaces; encouraging clients to accept personal responsibility for health; allowing clients to take ownership and participate in decisions, and; promoting accessibility, fairness, and equality
• Multicomponent interventions with coordinated care are most effective and should include both health and social services. Whole person care designs and service partnerships are keys to successful interventions
• Primary care programs specifically tailored to homeless individuals are more likely to achieve higher patient-reported quality of care
• Healthcare service providers should collaborate with organizations that have active outreach to homeless people who are difficult to engage. Team-based care can provide general medical and mental health care as well as linkages to housing services
• Interventions that provide case management and supportive housing have the greatest effect when they target individuals who are the highest utilizers of services
Process
• Providers should be mindful and understanding of the lived experience of people who are marginalized. Efforts should focus on the delivery of high-quality comprehensive services in the community and on the streets
• Staff training, technical assistance, and fidelity to protocols help mitigate communication, bureaucracy, or stigma barriers to accessing services
• Standard case management with coordination of services improves housing outcomes
• A positive interpersonal relationship with individuals who are homeless is essential; the key ingredients for a positive patient–provider relationship include respect for the individual, upholding the person's dignity, building mutual trust, and showing warmth and care
• Healthcare providers need to be familiar with, or work closely with staff who have, expertise in the full range of programs and services that are available in their community for persons who are homeless
• Adapted clinical guidelines are available to help healthcare providers tailor their practice to better meet the physical and mental health needs of persons who are homeless
Outcome
• When assessing health, well-being, and other outcomes, use tools and measures that provide objective data but are also meaningful to the client group. The collection and sharing of data are required to support service planning, policy, and research

homelessness (PEH). After social needs and priorities are identified, a team approach can facilitate linkages to community-based service providers and government agencies [7, 30]. Services may include referrals to resources that coordinate housing assistance and food banks, connect individuals to sheltered environments as an interim solution, and provide vouchers for transportation and prescription medicines. This approach can also facilitate and coordinate medical and surgical subspecialty care, including treatment of mental health conditions, substance use disorders, viral hepatitis, and HIV.

Well-integrated healthcare teams have the capacity to improve outcomes by promoting coordination and continuity of care [8]. Some models include integrated programs for women that incorporate on-site pregnancy or child services alongside substance use treatment [63]. Care teams that are embedded in larger systems of care should be mindful of barriers, such as access to transportation and working telecommunications [7]. The administrative practice of updating contact information (e.g., addresses, phone numbers), collecting preferred and alternate modes of communication, avoiding punitive policies for missed or canceled appointments, and partnering with patients to address transportation needs can promote entry and continuity of care. Providing coordinated care often requires high-level partnership across settings [64] and a non-judgmental approach that provides safe communal space [65].

Collaboration between healthcare providers, government agencies, and community-based services can promote care that is accessible and responsive to the needs of PEH [8]. Effective collaboration involves case managment and has several models: traditional case management; assertive community treatment (ACT) teams, and; critical time intervention (CTI)s which takes a briefer interventional approach during times of transition to enhance emotional support and linkage to necessary services [8]. A systematic review reported a variable impact of standard case management on exiting homelessness and reducing depressive symptoms [8]. The effectiveness of ACT teams is mixed, with some studies showing fewer days homeless but no significant differences in mental health outcomes [8]. Intensive case management has been demonstrated to reduce the number of days homeless, however no major reduction in psychological symptoms [8]. Critical time intervention strategies have been demonstrated to reduce the number of homeless nights, but no significant effects on substance use or quality of life [8].

Housing First and Associated Strategies

The provision of housing improves a range of health and social outcomes for PEH, especially among those experiencing mental illness and substance use disorders [9].

Housing First is an established intervention for PEH with mental health and substance use disorders [66]. This approach provides individuals with housing and subsequently attempts engagement in mental health and other services [66]. A series of randomized controlled trials using a Housing First strategy improved stable housing status and quality of life, reduced contacts with the criminal justice system, however evidence was mixed for improving mental health, substance use, and community functioning outcomes compared with usual treatment [66]. A review of housing interventions, including Housing First, found that the provision of housing improved sustained housing after hospital discharge, reduced substance use and relapses, decreased health services use, and improved health outcomes of PEH with HIV [67].

The Continuum of Care (CoC) program is administered by the US Department of Housing and Urban Development (HUD), and is designed to assist sheltered and unsheltered homeless persons by providing the housing and/or services that are needed to help individuals move into transitional and permanent housing, with the goal of long-term stability [68]. The CoC Program broadly promotes community-wide planning, the coordinated use of resources to address homelessness, and utilizes integrated data systems and information technology. HUD awards CoC funding to nonprofit organizations and/or units of local governments [68]. Coordinated Entry, also known as coordinated assessment or coordinated intake, is a process that is frequently used by CoC programs to identify, assess, and connect PEH to housing assistance and other services [68]. The Homeless Management Information System (HMIS) is an information technology system that collects client, program, and system-level data related to the provision of housing services. Each CoC is responsible for operating an HMIS system according to HUD data standards [69].

Income assistance interventions have been developed and tested, including financial empowerment, rental assistance, compensated work therapy, and social enterprise strategies. Financial empowerment approaches build upon traditional policies for income assistance, such as Temporary Assistance for Needy Families (TANF), which may be insufficient in building self-sufficiency and independence over time [70]. A study that compared standard TANF to either financial education, or financial education with integrated trauma-informed peer support, found that the full intervention showed enhanced self-efficacy, reduction in symptoms of depression, and reduced financial hardship [70]. Rental assistance has resulted in reduction of homelessness rates, increases in the number of individuals living above the poverty line, reduced healthcare expenditures, and global improvement in outcomes (educational, developmental, health) for children [71, 72].

Compensated work therapy has been coordinated with substance use treatment and supervised, performance-based engagement that required regular toxicology screening and addiction treatment [73]. Some studies have reported higher rates of engagement in substance use treatment, fewer physical symptoms and problems associated with substance use, reduction in incarceration rates, and decreased episodes of homelessness compared to controls over a 1-year period [73]. Among homeless youth, employment-based interventions are targeted at skill development and engagement and retention in the workforce [74]. A train and place approach, in which skills are taught in advance of seeking employment, includes workshops, apprenticeships, and internships, focusing on building specific and generally applicable work skills such as interpersonal communication and professionalism [75]. A place and train strategy involves securing competitive employment and then offering ongoing, individualized support in maintaining work over time [75, 76]. Social Enterprise Interventions (SEI) involve skills development specific to supporting and maintaining a business, so that learning and application phases are integrated and skills are acquired and developed with increasing levels of experience [77, 78].

Medical Respite and Recuperative Care

Medical respite and recuperative care programs (MRPs) characterize a care model that has been developed to address the specific health care and social needs of PEH [79]. MRPs provide acute and post-acute care for PEH who do not require hospitalization, but are too medically vulnerable to recover from a physical illness or injury on the streets [79].

A randomized trial reported that an MRP paired with permanent supportive housing reduced hospitalizations by 29%, and ED visits by 24% for PEH [80]. However MRPs vary in their organizational models, as well as in the services provided and patient populations that they serve [81]. A 2013 systematic review concluded that MRPs can promote health outcomes and facilitate access to health services for PEH, but demonstrating the value of this care model and identifying best practices are limited by the heterogeneity and quality of existing research [82]. In 2000, the Health Resources and Services Administration (HRSA) conducted a descriptive evaluation that reported variation in MRP settings (e.g., shelters, apartments, stand-alone facilities) and highlighted the complex care needs of the PEH population, but it did not examine MRP-level factors that impacted care provision and PEH outcomes [83]. Another VA-based study focused on the primary care experience of PEH [84], however the generalizability of these findings to MRP and other care settings is uncertain.

Outreach and Engagement

PEH who have the greatest need often live nomadically or in hard-to-find locations and report mistrust of established institutions such as clinics or hospitals. The **US Interagency Council on Homelessness** has identified four elements of effective street outreach [85].

1. Street Outreach Efforts are Systematic, Coordinated, and Comprehensive. Collaboration is required among multiple stakeholders and a broad network of programs and services, such as law enforcement, healthcare providers, and community-based homeless service providers. Data systems are critical to document contact with PEH and to access information on available resources [85].
2. Street Outreach Efforts Are Housing Focused. A Housing First approach is utilized, with the goal of connecting PEH to stable housing with tailored services and supports of their choice [85].
3. Street Outreach Efforts Are Person-Centered, Trauma-Informed, and Culturally Responsive. A person-centered approach focuses on the individual's strengths and resources, without assumptions about what a person might need [85].
4. Street Efforts Emphasize Safety and Reduce Harm. Strategies ensure the safety of all individuals seeking assistance and employ harm reduction principles, recognizing that some PEH may not initially accept offers of emergency shelter or housing assistance [85].

Drop-In Centers

For PEH who may be hard to reach, engaged outreach workers and initiatives are an integral part of engagement [86]. Co-locating clinical and ancillary services in homeless drop-in sites have been reported to reduce barriers to accessing care and enable healthcare providers to engage with vulnerable patients and build trust [87]. The drop-in center is a service model where PEH receive an array of self-directed health care and social services as a first step of engagement and gateway to greater services [88]. This model has been found to offer a more acceptable and effective alternative to shelter-based care by increasing engagement with housing services, medical and mental health treatment, and other social supports [88]. Although these programs have primarily focused on younger persons experiencing homelessness [88–90], drop-in centers that have provided collaborative mental health and primary care have been developed in Canada [91].

COVID Mitigation Strategies

Persons experiencing homelessness (PEH) are at increased risk of COVID-19 infection due to the lack of safe housing and shelter environment conditions that are conducive to a disease epidemic [92, 93]. Congregate living settings in shelters, encampments, or abandoned buildings, as well as barriers to basic hygiene supplies and showering facilities, can potentiate virus transmission [92, 93]. The chronic mental and physical conditions and reduced access to health care also limit screening, quarantining, and treatment of PEH who have been exposed to, or are actively infected with COVID-19 [92, 93]. Homeless populations may be transient and geographically mobile, creating challenges in the tracking, prevention, and treatment of those who need care [92, 93].

The Centers for Disease Control and Prevention (CDC) provided guidance for homeless service providers to plan and respond to COVID-19 [94]. The CDC promoted a "whole community" approach, which involved connecting with key partners and identifying additional sites and resources for PEH [94]. This approach includes a community coalition that should include: local and state health departments, homeless service providers and Continuum of Care leadership, emergency management services, law enforcement, healthcare providers, and other support services like outreach, case management, and behavioral health support [94]. The CDC noted the need to maintain homeless services during community spread of COVID-19, and that homeless shelters should not exclude people who are having symptoms or test positive for COVID-19 without a plan for where these clients can safely access services and stay [94].

The guidelines emphasized that community coalitions should identify additional temporary housing and shelter sites that are able to provide appropriate services, supplies, and staffing with the capacity: to decompress shelter beds to reduce crowding; to provide isolation and quarantine sites for people who are at-risk, have been exposed, tested positive, or have symptoms of COVID-19 [94]. Non-group housing options, such as hotels/motels, that have individual rooms should be considered for the overflow, quarantine, and protective housing sites for isolation [94].

In the US, passage of the CARES Act and approval of other funding sources, such as FEMA Public Assistance, have made it possible for communities to conduct emergency protective measures and to plan for recovery [95].

PEH have difficulty accessing health services settings, such as a clinics, and state and local vaccine distribution plans should have strategies to provide vaccines at homeless service sites like shelters, day programs, or food service locations [96]. Implementation plans should include

Table 32.3 COVID-19 vaccination implementation strategies. (Adapted from reference [96])

Reinforce partnerships
• Strengthen and leverage partnerships that were established in community-based COVID-19 mitigation responses to develop vaccine distribution pathways
• Consider prior vaccination plans (e.g., hepatitis A outbreak) for reaching people experiencing homelessness
Estimate the population size
• Use the Department of Housing and Urban Development's point-in-time count to estimate the number of people experiencing homelessness by region
• Consider geographic information systems to map the population distribution and facilities that are accessed
Develop a communication strategy
• Enlist trusted communicators, such as people with lived experience of homelessness, in planning and implementation of vaccination events
• Advertise vaccination events using multiple communication strategies
Identify vaccine policies and establish protocols and logistics
• Review state and local vaccination plans to identify when homeless service staff and people experiencing homelessness are prioritized for COVID-19 vaccination
• Work with case managers, healthcare agencies, and community organizations to identify people experiencing homelessness who might be eligible for vaccination in earlier phases
• Identify responsible entities (e.g., health department), providers, and staff who are known and trusted and that will be responsible for ordering, storing, distributing, administering, and documenting data pertaining to vaccines
• Involve people experiencing homelessness and homeless service provider staff in the decision-making process for vaccination planning
• Ensure that vaccines can be offered on a recurring basis and plan to offer repeat events and multiple, focused strategies:
– Points of Dispensing are convenient locations that people experiencing homelessness can easily access
– On-site clinics are temporary locations where homeless services are offered, such as meal service sites, homeless shelters
– Outreach teams or mobile vans can include from public health and community outreach organizations
• Consider complementary strategies to reach people experiencing homelessness through other venues
• Review existing vaccine checklists and ensure adequate supplies, including epinephrine
• Reinforce to staff and vaccination recipients the core COVID-19 prevention measures (masks, physical distancing, avoiding crowds, handwashing) and provide masks as needed during vaccination events and post-vaccination observation periods
Provide post-vaccination observation and care
• Ensure adequate space and staff for potential adverse reactions
• Use multiple second-dose reminder methods simultaneously to improve completion of each vaccinee's two-dose series. Record complete contact information at the time of vaccination to improve follow-up. Consider innovative strategies for second-dose reminders such as providing prepaid phone cards, prepaid cell phones with programmed reminders, or second-dose incentives
• Review strategies for vaccine documentation and reporting and ensure that vaccination teams have sufficient vaccination record cards

strategies to offer vaccination in areas frequented by people experiencing unsheltered homelessness, such as encampments [96]. A communication plan to reach PEH is also critical and should include strategies such as: flyers at encampments, shelters, and on public transportation; announcements at healthcare programs, and email, text messages, social media, television, and radio [96]. Working with people with lived experience of homelessness can provide insight and advice regarding vaccination education [96]. Table 32.3 summarizes general principles provided by the CDC regarding COVID-19 vaccine implementation [96].

In response to the COVID-19 pandemic, Continuums of Care, Emergency Solutions Grant recipients, health care for homeless programs, public health departments, hospital systems, and community-based organizations have come together to design new solutions and approaches to care for people experiencing homelessness (PEH) [97]. The creation or adaptation of partnerships with these stakeholders, often involving a rapid assessment of gaps specific to PEH, has led to the development of strategies to address these gaps, and facilitated cross-sector coordination [97]. COVID-19 has driven a system-level response—government agencies, community-service providers, and healthcare systems working collaboratively—in addressing the health and social needs of PEH across the US [97].

The Framework for an Equitable COVID-19 Homelessness Response project has been designed to help communities and homelessness assistance programs respond to COVID-19 with a racial justice and equity approach [95]. Through a partnership of national organizations and leaders, the framework provides guidance to communities on a range of key public health and economic recovery strategies that can meet public health goals, increase housing stability, and prevent future increases in homelessness that result from an economic downturn [95]. The framework is organized into five Action Areas.

- *Action Area A: Unsheltered People*—Activities that connect people experiencing unsheltered homelessness to

non-congregate shelter to promote social distancing or quarantine and facilitate access to healthcare services and resources to permanent housing. This action area calls upon communities to reduce unsheltered homelessness through housing and public health strategies [95].
- *Action Area B: Shelters*—Activities that establish non-congregate emergency shelter to promote social distancing or quarantine and that can keep people safer within decompressed congregate shelter settings. This action area encourages communities to sustain and expand to transform their sheltering system to focus on non-congregate environments and other safer models of sheltering people [95].
- *Action Area C: Housing*—Activities that promote access to diverse housing models and an array of services. This action area calls upon communities to broaden housing resources, strengthen landlord engagement, and ensure an equitable access to resources [95].
- *Action Area D: Diversion and Prevention*—Activities that reduce new entries into shelter or unsheltered homelessness through diversion prevention strategies, targeting individuals with the greatest risk, such as those who have been previously homeless, those impacted by COVID-19, those at the lowest income levels, and those who have resource limited support networks [95].
- *Action Area E: Strengthening Systems for the Future*—Activities that strengthen a systematic homelessness response systems and rehousing operations by promoting stronger partnerships across systems and sectors, and better preparedness for future health crises [95].

These actions will need to be coordinated across many stakeholders, partners and systems, as well as across levels of government, including emergency management offices and emergency operations; public health, and healthcare systems; and homelessness and housing services [95].

Final Comments

Although homelessness remains an ongoing challenge that adversely impacts the health of individuals, there is an evidence-base of effective strategies and a framework for the effective implementation of these interventions. Homeless services are predominantly offered through a network of programs and providers, which requires an implementation framework that can ensure fidelity to the effective components, and flexibility to adapt and innovate at the local environment. In addition, frameworks need to incorporate program operating principles, the intended population, intervention protocols, defined outcomes, and service utilization [98].

The Interactive Systems Framework for Dissemination and Implementation is an enhanced framework that incorporates these components and involves the capacity to synthesize best practices, translate this information to practical application, analyze the intervention model, and provide ongoing support to ensure adoption and fidelity [98]. Several homeless service intervention models under the US Department of Veterans Affairs and the National Center on Homelessness Among Veterans use an enhanced implementation framework, providing the flexibility to allow change "from" and "across" the sites as well as "up" to program managers. The model promotes feedback from service providers that can inform modifications and adaptations [98]. In addition, program components that have been found to be effective at respective sites can be disseminated through information technology platforms and adopted by other sites [98].

The establishment of a homelessness-focused special needs plan may be a fiscal model that can sustainably finance healthcare delivery for homeless individuals [99]. Traditional fee-for-service Medicare and Medicaid is not designed to be responsive to persons experiencing homelessness (PEH), who have a wide range of complex social and behavioral needs. PEH receive care by clinicians in non-traditional settings (e.g., shelters, medical respite program) and require intensive case management and care coordination with homeless service providers and government agencies [99]. The creation of a homeless special needs plan that would fully capitate monthly payments to organizations, who would assume full financial risk for the care of PEH, may be an effective strategy in achieving better outcomes and higher degrees of care coordination [99]. These plans would need to receive adequate risk-adjust payments per member per month that reflect the total true cost of caring for PEH. The care model requirements might include medical respite, street-outreach, intensive behavioral health and substance use treatment services, case management in collaboration with local housing agencies, work and job training to secure permanent housing [99].

In summary, COVID-19 has led to an unprecedented level of collaboration between homeless service providers, local government entities, and healthcare providers. Improving care of homeless populations is a necessary step toward health equity and can serve to enhance both patient and provider outcomes and satisfaction [100]. The transformation of health care in the US provides an optimal environment for initiating and sustaining change and the time is right for investments in system-level change that has the potential to solve the problem of homelessness.

References

1. US Department of Housing and Urban Development. Annual homelessness assessment report. Washington, DC; 2021. https://www.huduser.gov/portal/sites/default/files/pdf/2020-AHAR-Part-1.pdf.
2. Arum C, Fraser H, Artenie AA, et al. Homelessness, unstable housing, and risk of HIV and hepatitis C virus acquisition among people who inject drugs: a systematic review and meta-analysis. Lancet Public Health. 2021;6(5):e309–e23.
3. Hwang SW, Wilkins R, Tjepkema M, et al. Mortality among residents of shelters, rooming houses, and hotels in Canada: 11 year follow-up study. BMJ. 2009;339:b4036.
4. Thakarar K, Morgan JR, Gaeta JM, Hohl C, Drainoni ML. Homelessness, HIV, and incomplete viral suppression. J Health Care Poor Underserved. 2016;27(1):145–56.
5. Winkler P, Barrett B, McCrone P, Csémy L, Janouskova M, Höschl C. Deinstitutionalised patients, homelessness and imprisonment: systematic review. Br J Psychiatry. 2016;208(5):421–8.
6. Maness DL, Khan M. Care of the homeless: an overview. Am Fam Physician. 2014;89(8):634–40.
7. Andermann A, Bloch G, Goel R, et al. Caring for patients with lived experience of homelessness. Can Fam Physician. 2020;66(8):563–70.
8. Pottie K, Kendall CE, Aubry TM, et al. Clinical guideline for homeless and vulnerably housed people, and people with lived homelessness experience. CMAJ. 2020;192(10):E240–E54.
9. Luchenski S, Maguire N, Aldridge RW, Hayward A, et al. What works in inclusion health: overview of effective interventions for marginalised and excluded populations. Lancet. 2014;391:266–80.
10. National Health Care for the Homeless Council. Who we are. Nashville, TN; 2019. https://nhchc.org/who-we-are/.
11. Tsai J. Lifetime and 1-year prevalence of homelessness in the US population: results from the National Epidemiologic Survey on Alcohol and Related Conditions-III. J Public Health. 2018;40(1):65–74.
12. US Department of Housing and Urban Development. Criteria and Recordkeeping Requirements for Definition of Homelessness HUD Exchange: US Department of Housing and Urban Development; 2012. https://files.hudexchange.info/resources/documents/HomelessDefinition_RecordkeepingRequirementsandCriteria.pdf.
13. Van den Bree MB, Shelton K, Bonner A, Moss S, Thomas H, Taylor PJ. A longitudinal population-based study of factors in adolescence predicting homelessness in young adulthood. J Adolesc Health. 2009;45(6):571–8.
14. Corliss HL, Goodenow CS, Nichols L, Austin SB. High burden of homelessness among sexual-minority adolescents: findings from a representative Massachusetts high school sample. AJPH. 2011;101(9):1683–9.
15. Kelly P. Risk and protective factors contributing to homelessness among foster care youth: an analysis of the National Youth in Transition Database. Child Youth Serv Rev. 2020;108:104589.
16. Tsai J, Pietrzak RH, Szymkowiak D. The problem of veteran homelessness: an update for the new decade. Am J Prev Med. 2021;60(6):774–80.
17. Lee CT, Guzman D, Ponath C, Tieu L, Riley E, Kushel M. Residential patterns in older homeless adults: results of a cluster analysis. Soc Sci Med. 2016;153:131–40.
18. Greenberg GA, Rosenheck RA. Mental health correlates of past homelessness in the National Comorbidity Study Replication. J Health Care Poor Underserved. 2010;21(4):1234–49.
19. Nilsson SF, Nordentoft M, Hjorthøj C. Individual-level predictors for becoming homeless and exiting homelessness: a systematic review and meta-analysis. J Urban Health. 2019;96(5):741–50.
20. Hamden A, Newton R, McCauley-Elsom K, Cross W. Is deinstitutionalization working in our community? Int J Men Hlth Nurs. 2011;20(4):274–83.
21. Sawyer AM. From therapy to administration: deinstitutionalisation and the ascendancy of psychiatric 'risk thinking'. Health Sociol Rev. 2005;14(3):283–96.
22. Winiarski DA, Rufa AK, Bounds DT, et al. Assessing and treating complex mental health needs among homeless youth in a shelter-based clinic. BMC Health Serv Res. 2020;20(1):1–10.
23. Kaplan LM, Vella L, Cabral E, et al. Unmet mental health and substance use treatment needs among older homeless adults: results from the HOPE HOME Study. J Community Psychol. 2019;47(8):1893–908.
24. Brown DW, Anda RF, Tiemeier H, Felitti VJ, Edwards VJ, Croft JB, et al. Adverse childhood experiences and the risk of premature mortality. AJPM. 2009;37(5):289–396.
25. Palepu A, Gadermann A, Hubley AM, Farrell S, Gogosis E, Aubry T, et al. Substance use and access to health care and addiction treatment among homeless and vulnerably housed persons in three Canadian cities. PLoS One. 2013;8(10):e75133.
26. Bransford C, Cole M. Trauma-informed care in homelessness service settings: challenges and opportunities. In: Larkin H, Aykanian A, Streeter CL, editors. Homelessness prevention and intervention in social work: policies, programs, and practices. Switzerland: Springer; 2019.
27. The National Center on Family Homelessness. The characteristics and needs of families experiencing homelessness. Needham, MA; 2011. https://files.eric.ed.gov/fulltext/ED535499.pdf.
28. Baggett TP, Hwang SW, O'Connell JJ, Porneala BC, Stringfellow EJ, Orav EJ, et al. Mortality among homeless adults in Boston: shifts in causes of death over a 15-year period. JAMA Intern Med. 2013;173(3):189–95.
29. Maisto SA, Carey MP, Carey KB, Gordon CM, Gleason JR. Use of the AUDIT and the DAST-10 to identify alcohol and drug use disorders among adults with a severe and persistent mental illness. Psychol Assess. 2000;12(2):186.
30. Sarango M, Hohl C, Gonzalez N, et al. Strategies to build a patient-centered medical home for multiply diagnosed people living with HIV who are experiencing homelessness or unstable housing. Am J Public Health. 2018;108:S519–S21.
31. Santo T, Clark B, Hickman M. Association of opioid agonist treatment with all-cause mortality and specific causes of death among people with opioid dependence: a systematic review and meta-analysis. JAMA Psych. 2021;78(9):979–93.
32. Doshani M, Weng M, Moore KL, et al. Recommendations of the Advisory Committee on Immunization Practices for use of hepatitis A vaccine for persons experiencing homelessness. Morb Mortal Wkly Rep. 2019;68(6):153.
33. Noska AJ, Belperio PS, Loomis TP, et al. Prevalence of human immunodeficiency virus, hepatitis C virus, and hepatitis B virus among homeless and nonhomeless United States veterans. Clin Infect Dis. 2017;65(2):252–8.
34. Roth GA, Abate D, Abate KH, et al. Global, regional, and national age-sex-specific mortality for 282 causes of death in 195 countries and territories, 1980–2017: a systematic analysis for the Global Burden of Disease Study 2017. Lancet. 2017;392:1736–88.
35. Stanaway JD, Flaxman AD, Naghavi M, et al. The global burden of viral hepatitis from 1990 to 2013: findings from the Global Burden of Disease Study 2013. Lancet. 2016;388:1081–8.
36. US Department of Health and Human Services. US Statistics. 2021. https://www.hiv.gov/hiv-basics/overview/data-and-trends/statistics.
37. Cohen MS, Chen YQ, McCauley M, et al. Prevention of HIV-1 infection with early antiretroviral therapy. N Engl J Med. 2011;365(6):493–505.

38. Beiser ME, Smith K, Ingemi M, Mulligan E, Baggett TP. Hepatitis C treatment outcomes among homeless-experienced individuals at a community health centre in Boston. Int J Drug Policy. 2019;72:129–37.
39. Wade AJ, Doyle JS, Gane E, et al. Outcomes of treatment for hepatitis C in primary care, compared to hospital-based care: a randomized, controlled trial in people who inject drugs. Clin Infect Dis. 2020;70(9):1900–6.
40. Moore RA, Fried MW, Wright B. Primary care providers in federally qualified health centers can treat hepatitis C effectively without ongoing consultative support from specialists. Med Care. 2021;59(8):699–703.
41. Mast EE, Weinbaum CM, Fiore AE, et al. A comprehensive immunization strategy to eliminate transmission of hepatitis B virus infection in the United States: recommendations of the Advisory Committee on Immunization Practices (ACIP) Part II: immunization of adults. MMWR Recomm Rep. 2006;55:1–33.
42. Tomczyk S, Bennett NM, Stoecker C. Use of 13-valent pneumococcal conjugate vaccine and 23-valent pneumococcal polysaccharide vaccine among adults aged ≥65 years: recommendations of the Advisory Committee on Immunization Practices (ACIP). MMWR Morb Mortal Wkly Rep. 2014;19(63):822–5.
43. Baggett TP, Liauw SS, Hwang SW. Cardiovascular disease and homelessness. J Am Coll Cardiol. 2018;71(22):2585–97.
44. Lee TC, Hanlon JG, Ben-David J, et al. Risk factors for cardiovascular disease in homeless adults. Circulation. 2005;111(20):2629–35.
45. Stone B, Dowling S, Cameron A. Cognitive impairment and homelessness: a scoping review. Health Soc Care Community. 2019;27(4):e125–e42.
46. Hurstak E, Johnson JK, Tieu L, et al. Factors associated with cognitive impairment in a cohort of older homeless adults: results from the HOPE HOME study. Drug Alcohol Depend. 2017;178:562–70.
47. Hwang SW, Colantonio A, Chiu S, et al. The effect of traumatic brain injury on the health of homeless people. CMAJ. 2008;179(8):779–84.
48. Nygaard RM, Endorf FW. Frostbite vs burns: increased cost of care and use of hospital resources. J Burn Care Res. 2018;39(5):676–9.
49. O'Connell JJ, Petrella DA, Regan RF. Accidental hypothermia & frostbite: cold-related conditions. Boston, MA: Boston Healthcare for Homeless Program; 2004. https://www.bhchp.org/sites/default/files/BHCHPManual/pdf_files/Part2_PDF/Hypothermia.pdf.
50. Brooks LK, Kalyanaraman N, Malek R. Diabetes care for patients experiencing homelessness: beyond metformin and sulfonylureas. Am J Med. 2019;132(4):408–12.
51. Moes J. Proper fitting shoes: reducing pain, increasing activity, and improving foot health among adults experiencing homelessness. Public Health Nurs. 2019;36(3):321–9.
52. Endorf FW, Nygaard RM. Social determinants of poor outcomes following frostbite injury: a study of the national inpatient sample. J Burn Care Res. 2021;
53. de la Vega PB, Losi S, Martinez LS, et al. Implementing an EHR-based screening and referral system to address social determinants of health in primary care. Med Care. 2019;57:S133–S9.
54. Alley DE, Asomugha CN, Conway PH, al. e. Accountable health communities—addressing social needs through Medicare and Medicaid. New Engl J Med. 2016;374:8–11.
55. Montgomery AE, Byrne T, Cusack MC, et al. Patients' perspectives on elements of stable housing and threats to housing stability. J Society Soc Work Res. 2020;11(4)
56. Fargo JD, Montgomery AE, Byrne TB, et al. Needles in a haystack: screening and healthcare system evidence for homelessness. Stud Health Technol Inform. 2017;235:574–8.
57. Byrne T, Fargo JD, Montgomery AE, et al. Screening for homelessness in the Veterans Health Administration: monitoring housing stability through repeat screening. Public Health Rep. 2015;130(6):684–92.
58. Brcic V, Eberdt C, Kaczorowski J. Development of a tool to identify poverty in a family practice setting: a pilot study. Int J Family Med. 2011;2011:812182.
59. Dinnen S, Kane V, Cook JM. Trauma-informed care: a paradigm shift needed for services with homeless veterans. Prof Case Mgmt. 2014;19(4):161–70.
60. Milaney K, Williams N, Lockerbie SL. Recognizing and responding to women experiencing homelessness with gendered and trauma-informed care. BMC Pub Hlth. 2020;20(1):1–6.
61. Glowa PT, Olson AL, Johnson DJ. Screening for adverse childhood experiences in a family medicine setting: a feasibility study. J Am Board Fam Med. 2016;29(3):30–307.
62. Elliott DE, Bjelajac P, Fallot RD, et al. Trauma-informed or trauma-denied: principles and implementation of trauma-informed services for women. J Community Psychol. 2005;33(4):461–77.
63. Niccols A, Milligan K, Sword W, et al. Maternal mental health and integrated programs for mothers with substance abuse issues. Psychol Addict Behav. 2010;24:466–74.
64. Bartlett A, Jhanji E, White S, et al. Interventions with women offenders: a systematic review and meta-analysis of mental health gain. J Forens Psychiatry Psychol. 2015;26:133–65.
65. Kerrigan D, Kennedy CE, Morgan-Thomas R, et al. A community empowerment approach to the HIV response among sex workers: effectiveness, challenges, and considerations for implementation and scale-up. Lancet. 2015;385:172–85.
66. Woodhall-Melnik JR, Dunn JR. A systematic review of outcomes associated with participation in Housing First programs. Hous Stud. 2016;31:287–304.
67. Fitzpatrick-Lewis D, Ganann R, Krishnaratne S, et al. Effectiveness of interventions to improve the health and housing status of homeless people: a rapid systematic review. BMC Public Health. 2011;11:638.
68. United States Department of Housing and Urban Development. Introductory Guide to the Continuum of Care (CoC) Program Washington DC: US Department of Housing and Urban Development; 2012. https://files.hudexchange.info/resources/documents/CoCProgramIntroductoryGuide.pdf.
69. US Department of Housing and Urban Development. Homeless management information system. Washington, DC: US Department of Housing and Urban Development; 2012. https://www.hudexchange.info/programs/hmis/.
70. Booshehri LG, Dugan J, Patel F, et al. Trauma-informed Temporary Assistance for Needy Families (TANF): a randomized controlled trial with a two-generation impact. J Child Fam Stud. 2018;27(5):1594–604.
71. Fischer W, Rice D, Mazzara A. Research shows rental assistance reduces hardship and provides platform to expand opportunity for low-income families. Washington, DC; 2019.
72. Gubits D, Shinn M, Wood M, et al. What interventions work best for families who experience homelessness? Impact estimates from the family options study. J Policy Anal Manage. 2018;37(4):835–66.
73. Kashner TM, Rosenheck R, Campinell AB, et al. Impact of work therapy on health status among homeless, substance-dependent veterans: a randomized controlled trial. Arch Gen Psych. 2002;59(10):938–44.
74. Ferguson KM. Employment outcomes from a randomized controlled trial of two employment interventions with homeless youth. J Soc Soc Work Res. 2018;9(1):1–21.
75. Burns T, Catty J, Becker T, et al. The effectiveness of supported employment for people with severe mental illness: a randomised controlled trial. Lancet. 2007;370:1146–52.

76. Drake RE, Bond GR, Becker DR. Individual placement and support. An evidence-based approach to supported employment. Oxford University Press; 2012.
77. Ferguson KM. Implementing a social enterprise intervention with homeless, street-living youth in Los Angeles. Soc Work. 2007;52:103–12.
78. Ash SL, Clayton PH. Generating, deepening, and documenting learning: the power of critical reflection in applied learning. J Appl Learn High Educ. 2009;1:25–48.
79. United States Interagency Council on Homelessness. Opening doors: federal strategic plan to prevent and end homelessness. Washington, DC: United States Interagency Council on Homelessness; 2015. https://www.usich.gov/resources/uploads/asset_library/USICH_OpeningDoors_Amendment2015_FINAL.pdf.
80. Sadowski LS, Kee RA, VanderWeele TJ, et al. Effect of a housing and case management program on emergency department visits and hospitalizations among chronically ill homeless adults: a randomized trial. JAMA. 2009;301:1771–8.
81. Zerger S, Doblin B, Thompson L. Medical respite care for homeless people: a growing national phenomenon. J Health Care Poor Underserved. 2009;20:36–41.
82. Doran KM, Ragins KT, Gross CP, Zerger S. Medial respite programs for homeless patients: a systematic review. J Health Care Poor Underserved. 2013;24:499–524.
83. Zerger S. An evaluation of the respite pilot initiative: final report Washington, DC; 2006. https://nhchc.org/wp-content/uploads/2019/08/RespiteRpt0306-1.pdf.
84. Kertesz SG, Pollio DE, Jones RN, et al. Development of the primary care quality-homeless (PCQ-H) instrument: a practical survey of homeless patients' experiences in primary care. Med Care. 2014;52(8):734–42.
85. United States Interagency Council on Homelessness. Core elements of effective street outreach to people experiencing homelessness. Washington DC; 2019. https://www.usich.gov/resources/uploads/asset_library/Core-Components-of-Outreach-2019.pdf.
86. Blankertz LE, Cnaan RA, White K, Fox J, Messinger K. Outreach efforts with dually diagnosed homeless persons. Fam Soc. 1990;71:387–97.
87. Zlotnick C, Zerger S, Wolfe PB. Health care for the homeless: what we have learned in the past 30 years and what's next. Am J Public Health. 2013;103(S2):S199–205.
88. Slesnick N, Feng X, Guo X, Brakenhoff B, et al. A test of outreach and drop-in linkage versus shelter linkage for connecting homeless youth to services. Prev Sci. 2016;17:450–60.
89. Pederson ER, Tucker JS, Kovalchik SA. Facilitators and barriers of drop-in center use among homeless youth. J Adol Hlth. 2016;59:144–53.
90. Slesnick N, Kang MJ, Bonomi AE, Prestopnik JL. Six and twelve month outcomes among homeless youth accessing therapy and case management services through an urban drop-in center. Health Serv Res. 2008;43:211–29.
91. Tam C. Developing collaborative mental health care for homeless persons at a drop-in center. Psychiatr Serv. 2010;61:549–51.
92. Tsai J, Wilson M. COVID-19: a potential public health problem for homeless populations. Lancet Public Health. 2020;5(4):e186–e7.
93. Perri M, Dosani N, Hwang SW. COVID-19 and people experiencing homelessness: challenges and mitigation strategies. CMAJ. 2020;192(26):E716–e9.
94. US Department of Health and Human Services. Interim Guidance for Homeless Service Providers to Plan and Respond to Coronavirus Disease 2019 (COVID-19): CDC; 2021. https://www.cdc.gov/coronavirus/2019-ncov/community/homeless-shelters/plan-prepare-respond.html.
95. National Alliance to End Homelessness. The Framework for an Equitable COVID-19 Homelessness Response. 2021. https://endhomelessness.org/wp-content/uploads/2020/04/COVID-Framework-4.29.2020-1.pdf.
96. US Department of Health and Human Services. Interim Guidance for Health Departments: COVID-19 Vaccination Implementation for People Experiencing Homelessness: CDC; 2021. https://www.cdc.gov/coronavirus/2019-ncov/community/homeless-shelters/vaccination-guidance.html.
97. United States Department of Housing and Urban Development. Homeless system response: operational healthcare partnerships. Washington, DC: United States Department of Housing and Urban Development; 2020. https://files.hudexchange.info/resources/documents/COVID-19-Homeless-System-Response-Operational-Healthcare-Partnerships.pdf.
98. Casey R, Clark C, Smits P, Peters R. Application of implementation science for homeless interventions. Am J Public Health. 2013;103:S183–S5.
99. Jain SH, Baackes J, O'Connell JJ. Homeless special needs plans for people experiencing homelessness. JAMA. 2020;323(10):927–38.
100. Kung A, Cheung T, Knox M. Capacity to address social needs affects primary care clinician burnout. Ann Fam Med. 2019;17(6):487–94.

Part IV
Organizational Frameworks for Chronic Illness Care

Integrated Behavioral Health Care

Linda Myerholtz, Nathaniel A. Sowa, and Brianna Lombardi

Introduction

Many terms are used to describe the incorporation of mental health care in primary care settings including collaborative care, primary care behavioral health, embedded care, and co-located care. Peek and colleagues developed a lexicon that defines integrated behavioral health (IBH) as "the care that results from a practice team of primary care and behavioral health clinicians, working together with patients and families, using a systematic and cost-effective approach to provide patient-centered care for a defined population" [1]. In addition to treating mental health needs of patients in primary care, especially those with chronic conditions, IBH addresses stress-related physical illness, behaviors contributing to unhealthy lifestyles, adherence issues, coordination of care, and ineffective use of emergency and hospital-based health care services. The authors of the lexicon created a "family tree" of interrelated terms that describe the integration of behavioral health and primary care (Fig. 33.1).

The IBH movement gained momentum in the late 1980s due to growing recognition that a fragmented, siloed system of care, where the care of the body and the mind are artificially separated, was not meeting the needs of patients, especially those with chronic conditions. Almost half of adults and more than a quarter of adolescents experience a mental illness or substance use concern at some point in their lifetime [2–4]. The COVID-19 pandemic has intensified psychological distress with 30–50% of the general population experiencing anxiety and 34–48% experiencing depression, a more than threefold increase compared to prior to the outbreak [5–7]. Chronic stress related to fear, social isolation, and losses (i.e., jobs, social activities, meaningful life events, and deaths) has likely contributed to the increase in the number of people experiencing mental health distress during the pandemic.

L. Myerholtz (✉) · B. Lombardi
Department of Family Medicine, University of North Carolina at Chapel Hill, Chapel Hill, NC, USA
e-mail: linda_myerholtz@med.unc.edu; brianna_lombardi@med.unc.edu

N. A. Sowa
Department of Psychiatry, University of North Carolina at Chapel Hill, Chapel Hill, NC, USA
e-mail: nate_sowa@med.unc.edu

Illustration: A family tree of related terms used in behavioral health and primary care integration
See glossary for details and additional definitions

Integrated Care
Tightly integrated, on-site teamwork with unified care plan as a standard approach to care for designated populations. Connotes organizational integration involving social & other services. "Altitudes" of integration: 1) Integrated treatments, 2) integrated program structure; 3) integrated system of programs, and 4) integrated payments. (Based on SAMHSA)

Patient-Centered Care
"The experience (to the extent the informed, individual patient desires it) of transparency, individualization, recognition, respect, dignity, and choice in all matters, without exception, related to one's person, circumstances, and relationships in health care"—or "nothing about me without me" (Berwick, 2011).

Coordinated Care
The organization of patient care activities between two or more participants (including the patient) involved in care, to facilitate appropriate delivery of healthcare services. Organizing care involves the marshaling of personnel and other resources needed to carry out required care activities, and often managed by the exchange of information among participants responsible for different aspects of care" (AHRQ, 2007).

Shared Care
Predominately Canadian usage—PC & MH professionals (typically psychiatrists) working together in shared system and record, maintaining 1 treatment plan addressing all patient health needs. (Kates et al, 1996; Kelly et al, 2011)

Collaborative Care
A general term for ongoing working relationships between clinicians, rather than a specific product or service (Doherty, McDaniel & Baird, 1996). Providers combine perspectives and skills to understand and identify problems and treatments, continually revising as needed to hit goals, e.g. in collaborative care of depression (Unützer et al, 2002)

Co-located Care
BH and PC providers (i.e. physicians, NP's) delivering care in same practice. This denotes shared space to one extent or another, not a specific service or kind of collaboration. (adapted from Blount, 2003)

Integrated Primary Care or Primary Care Behavioral Health
Combines medical & BH services for problems patients bring to primary care, including stress-linked physical symptoms, health behaviors, MH or SA disorders. For any problem, they have come to the right place—"no wrong door" (Blount). BH professional used as a consultant to PC colleagues (Sabin & Borus, 2009; Haas & deGruy, 2004; Robinson & Reiter, 2007; Hunter et al, 2009).

Behavioral Health Care
An umbrella term for care that addresses any behavioral problems bearing on health, including MH and SA conditions, stress-linked physical symptoms, patient activation and health behaviors. The job of all kinds of care settings, and done by clinicians and health coaches of various disciplines or training.

Patient-Centered Medical Home
An approach to comprehensive primary care for children, youth and adults—a setting that facilitates partnerships between patients and their personal physicians, and when appropriate, the patient's family. Emphasizes care of populations, team care, whole person care—including behavioral health, care coordination, information tools and business models needed to sustain the work. The goal is health, patient experience, and reduced cost. (Joint Principles of PCMH, 2007).

Mental Health Care
Care to help people with mental illnesses (or at risk)—to suffer less emotional pain and disability—and live healthier, longer, more productive lives. Done by a variety of caregivers in diverse public and private settings such as specialty MH, general medical, human services, and voluntary support networks. (Adapted from SAMHSA)

Substance Abuse Care
Services, treatments, and supports to help people with addictions and substance abuse problems suffer less emotional pain, family and vocational disturbance, physical risks—and live healthier, longer, more productive lives. Done in specialty SA, general medical, human services, voluntary support networks, e.g. 12-step programs and peer counselors. (Adapted from SAMHSA)

Primary Care
Primary care is the provision of integrated, accessible health care services by clinicians who are accountable for addressing a large majority of personal health care needs, developing a sustained partnership with patients, and practicing in the context of family and community. (Institute of Medicine, 1994)

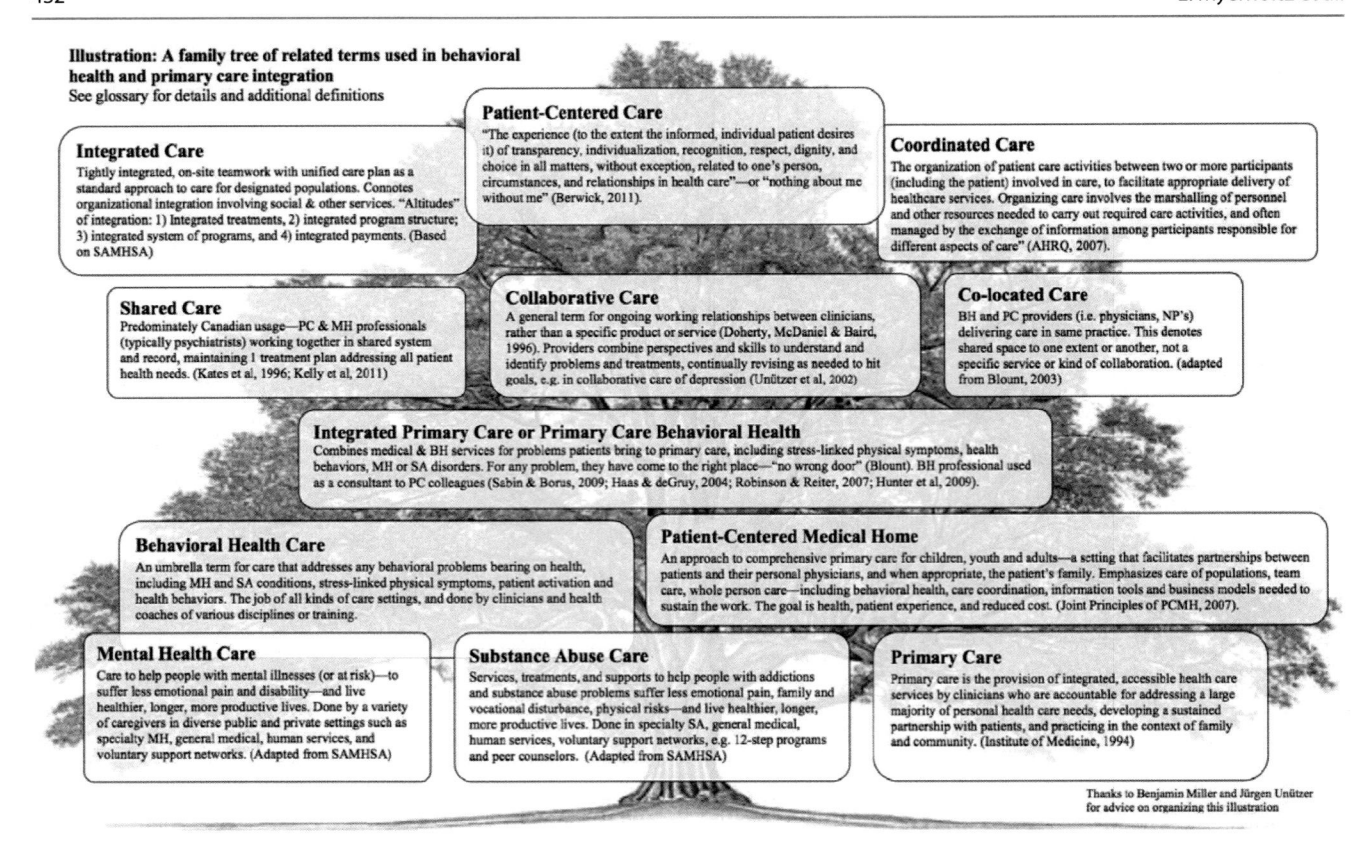

Thanks to Benjamin Miller and Jürgen Unützer for advice on organizing this illustration

Fig. 33.1 Family tree of related terms used in behavioral health and primary care integration [1]. From: Peek CJ and the National Integration Academy Council. *Lexicon for Behavioral Health and Primary Care Integration:* AHRQ Publication No. 13-IPOO1-EF. Rockville, MD: Agency for Healthcare Research and Quality. 2013. Available at http://integrationacademy.ahrq.gov/sites/default/files/Lexicon.pdf

Meeting the Need in Primary Care

Despite growing behavioral health problems, the majority of individuals with behavioral health disorders do not receive treatment [4, 8, 9]. The reasons for this are complex and include underdiagnosis, stigma about receiving mental health treatment, perceived and real cost barriers, lack of knowledge on how to access care, and a shortage of behavioral health providers [10]. Many individuals may not seek treatment from a behavioral health professional (BHP) but are comfortable visiting their medical provider, making primary care practices well poised to identify behavioral health treatment needs. Twenty percent of primary care visits are behavioral health related [11–13], 59% of psychotropic medications are prescribed by primary care clinicians [14], and many patients with depression who do seek treatment reach out to their primary care provider first. As a result, primary care is the de facto mental health system [15]. This is widely recognized and the American Academy of Family Physicians recommends co-location of behavioral health services in primary care settings and has issued principles for integrating behavioral health into Patient-Centered Medical Homes (PCMH) [16, 17]. The Institute of Medicine (IOM), Agency for Health Care Research and Quality (AHRQ), Patient-Centered Primary Care Collaborative [18], and the 2021 National Academies of Sciences, Engineering, and Medicine report *Implementing High-Quality Primary Care: Rebuilding the Foundation of Health Care* [19] have endorsed IBH as a critical element in the transformation of our current health care system.

Interplay of Emotional and Physical Health

Behavioral health disorders, especially depression and anxiety, are among the top five chronic conditions contributing to overall health care costs in the United States [20], and mental illness ranks first in global disease burden in terms of years lived with a disability [21]. Individuals with mental illness have higher rates of chronic disease including cardiovascular disease, asthma, diabetes, and cancer, resulting in a life expectancy up to 30 years less than adults without serious mental illness [22] and a mortality rate that is 2.2 times higher than the general population [23]. Many chronic conditions, such as diabetes, pain, headache, cardiac conditions, and gastrointestinal problems, are impacted directly and indirectly by emotional well-being and behavioral issues. Integrating behavioral health care into a primary care setting increases the opportunity for patient engagement in his or her own health care and skill building focused on health behavior change.

Reducing Stigma in Mental Health

The stigma around mental health is a significant barrier to care as people fear being labeled and judged [10]. Only 57% of adults without behavioral health concerns and 25% of adults who have behavioral health symptoms believe that people are sympathetic toward individuals who have mental illness [24]. Stigma toward individuals with mental illness is prevalent among medical students and other health care providers [25]. Seventy percent of individuals with behavioral health concerns would not access services in a behavioral health treatment organization that is separate from their primary source of medical care [26]. When behavioral health treatment is integrated into primary care, the stigma of receiving mental health care may be reduced.

Health Care Disparities and Access

IBH is particularly salient in meeting the needs of racial and ethnic minority groups, including Black and African American, Latinx, Asian, and indigenous populations, as significant behavioral health disparities for minoritized populations persist [27–29]. Rates of behavioral health diagnoses vary among racial and ethnic groups, but overall, the need is high and worsened by the COVID-19 pandemic [30]. Disparities in access to and treatment of behavioral health conditions in people living in marginalized communities lead to fewer referrals to appropriate behavioral health services [31, 32], and those services are less likely to be located in the communities or delivered by providers from diverse backgrounds [33, 34]. Disparities reflect the deeply imbedded societal inequities in the United States including factors such as underinsurance, underemployment, housing and school segregation, and discrimination. Behavioral concerns among minority youth often result in disciplinary action from schools or incarceration rather than treatment [35].

IBH can address many of the barriers to care that people in marginalized communities experience. Standardized screening in IBH clinics may identify behavioral health needs of racial and ethnic minorities that were previously missed or ignored by health providers. Co-locating physical and behavioral providers in the same space may reduce the burden placed on patients to find transportation and time to attend multiple visits at separate clinics. IBH delivered in primary care can be an entry point to behavioral health intervention and may destigmatize treatment when delivered as part of a total plan of health care.

Disparities also exist in access to behavioral health care in rural communities [36]. The lack of trained behavioral health clinicians, in particular providers that prescribe and manage psychotropic medication, is significant. In rural US counties, 47% of people do not have access to a psychologist and 65% do not have access to a psychiatrist [37]. IBH can increase access to mental health treatment in rural communities through telepsychiatry and collaborative care [38, 39].

Across the United States, patients often struggle to access behavioral health treatment due to a lack of awareness or unavailability of resources within their community and payment barriers. A common access point to the complicated US health care system is via primary care, making it strategically poised to facilitate both medical and behavioral health care. Individuals needing behavioral health care may be more likely to consider behavioral health services when provided in the context of a primary care practice where the setting and providers are familiar.

Improving Continuity of Care

In traditional care settings, primary care clinicians and behavioral health providers may have different treatment goals for the same patient and may have limited communication with each other due to logistical issues and strict state confidentiality laws governing behavioral health care. Integrated care allows for continuity and collaboration on treatment plans for patients since communication within a team is not limited by state confidentiality laws in the same manner as between practitioners who are not in the same practice.

Improving Outcomes at Reduced Cost

A significant proportion of patients have chronic comorbid behavioral and physical health conditions resulting in 60–75% higher total medical health care costs than the general population [40, 41]. Integrating care reduces total health care costs and improves outcomes for patients and providers, which will be discussed later in this chapter.

Models of Integrated Behavioral Health Care

There are a multitude of ways that practices integrate behavioral health care including co-located care, consultation models involving telepsychiatry or web-based services, the primary care behavioral health model, and team-based col-

COORDINATED — KEY ELEMENT: COMMUNICATION		CO-LOCATED — KEY ELEMENT: PHYSICAL PROXIMITY		INTEGRATED — KEY ELEMENT: PRACTICE CHANGE	
LEVEL 1 Minimal Collaboration	LEVEL 2 Basic Collaboration at a Distance	LEVEL 3 Basic Collaboration Onsite	LEVEL 4 Close Collaboration Onsite with Some System Integration	LEVEL 5 Close Collaboration Approaching an Integrated Practice	LEVEL 6 Full Collaboration in a Transformed/Merged Integrated Practice
Behavioral health, primary care and other healthcare providers work:					
In separate facilities, where they:	In separate facilities, where they:	In same facility not necessarily same offices, where they:	In same space within the same facility, where they:	In same space within the same facility (some shared space), where they:	In same space within the same facility, sharing all practice space, where they:
• Have separate systems • Communicate about cases only rarely and under compelling circumstances • Communicate, driven by provider need • May never meet in person • Have limited understanding of each other's roles	• Have separate systems • Communicate periodically about shared patients • Communicate, driven by specific patient issues • May meet as part of larger community • Appreciate each other's roles as resources	• Have separate systems • Communicate regularly about shared patients, by phone or e-mail • Collaborate, driven by need for each other's services and more reliable referral • Meet occasionally to discuss cases due to close proximity • Feel part of a larger yet non-formal team	• Share some systems, like scheduling or medical records • Communicate in person as needed • Collaborate, driven by need for consultation and coordinated plans for difficult patients • Have regular face-to-face interactions about some patients • Have a basic understanding of roles and culture	• Actively seek system solutions together or develop work-a-rounds • Communicate frequently in person • Collaborate, driven by desire to be a member of the care team • Have regular team meetings to discuss overall patient care and specific patient issues • Have an in-depth understanding of roles and culture	• Have resolved most or all system issues, functioning as one integrated system • Communicate consistently at the system, team and individual levels • Collaborate, driven by shared concept of team care • Have formal and informal meetings to support integrated model of care • Have roles and cultures that blur or blend

Fig. 33.2 A standard framework for levels of integrated health care: six levels of collaboration/integration. (Reprinted with permission from the SAMHSA-HRSA Center for Integrated Health Solutions)

laborative care management. The different models fall on a spectrum of integration (from co-location of care to fully integrated engagement of a team of providers), program structure (from very loose to highly structured using treatment protocols and clinical measures to evaluate clinical effectiveness), and intensity of behavioral health services offered (from screening and brief intervention to ongoing therapy and psychiatry services). The Substance Abuse and Mental Health Services Administration (SAMSHA) provides a useful framework of six levels of integration to facilitate meaningful dialogue about service design and research (Fig. 33.2) [42]. Popular behavioral health integration models are described below.

Co-located Behavioral Health

On the most basic level, integrated care may involve physically co-locating a behavioral health professional (BHP) in a primary care setting. These models may embed different types of BHPs (e.g., licensed therapists, psychologists, social workers, psychiatrists, and psychiatric nurses) and may utilize a variety of practice patterns, including long-term psychotherapy, short-course psychotherapy, targeted interventions (i.e., weight management, diabetes management, tobacco cessation, etc.), consultation or diagnostic services, or psychopharmacology management. The level of integration can vary greatly from practice to practice, but there is likely at least some degree of regular communication and collaboration between BHPs and medical team members. Co-location allows for shared services essential to care, such as scheduling, staff, and medical records, with ample opportunity to consult and coordinate care for difficult-to-treat patients [42].

Co-location of a BHP results in higher patient-reported quality of life scores [43–45], reduced treatment costs to patients [44, 46], increased patient and provider satisfaction [44, 47, 48], decreased appointment wait time [44, 49, 50], and reduction in referral rate to specialty behavioral health care [51]. Co-located behavioral health contributes to a reduction in depression severity in an integrated care setting [45]. Available evidence suggests there are no effects on patient physical functioning, patient social functioning, or hospital admission rates [45].

Co-located behavioral health is popular, due to the relative ease of implementation, low overhead costs, low financial risk, and success in meeting behavioral health needs of patients. However, providers and administrators should not overlook the limitations of co-located models, including varying degrees of integration, other unaddressed barriers to access, the limited evidence base, and the lack of a population health approach, which may limit the impact to the overall patient panel.

Primary Care Behavioral Health

Primary Care Behavioral Health (PCBH) is a team-based primary care approach to behavioral health problems and health conditions that are influenced by biopsychosocial factors [52]. A behavioral health consultant (BHC) is incorporated into the primary care team and works with patients of all ages with mild to severe health conditions. The BHC meets patients in a timely manner, often on the day of referral, is fully integrated into the biopsychosocial care provided by the entire primary care team, works with a large proportion of the clinic patients, and provides education and consultation to the primary care clinicians [52, 53]. BHCs typically provide short (15–30 min), focused interactions with patients and utilize techniques aimed at improving specific symptoms and/or functional limitations. To maintain accessibility while serving a high proportion of a practice population, follow-up interactions are limited, with a primary care provider (PCP) resuming sole care of a patient as soon as possible with re-engagement as indicated or if needed higher levels of behavioral health services are unavailable or declined by the patient [52].

The PCBH model has been implemented in a variety of primary care settings, including large systems, such as the US Veterans Health Administration [54] and the US Department of Defense [55], as well as in systems that serve economically disadvantaged populations, such as Federally Qualified Health Centers, community health organizations, primary care training clinics, and homeless clinics [52, 56–58]. The PCBH model has high rates of patient satisfaction and leads to improvement in Global Behavioral Health assessment of function at work or school [53]. Six studies using pre- to post-treatment designs (including one randomized control trial (RCT)) have examined specific symptom outcome measures using validated tools and have shown improvement in anxiety, depression, PTSD, sleep, tobacco use, and weight loss [59–64]. Other data suggest that the model may reduce referrals to specialty behavioral health [51, 65] and change antidepressant prescribing patterns by the team PCPs [51, 65, 66]. Patients who received care through PCBH had fewer preventable inpatient hospitalizations compared to those receiving medical treatment only [67].

The PCBH model depends on the integration of well-trained behavioral health professionals into the BHC role, which can be challenging for many nonphysician behavioral health professionals and may require "retraining" in certain aspects of the work [68]. The generalist approach of primary care that treats patients across the lifespan may be uncomfortable for many BHCs, whose training may be limited to pediatrics, adult, or geriatric care. Further, the role of consultant may be unfamiliar for professionals who lack training or exposure to such a model or have never worked or trained in a medical setting [69]. Hence, the BHC role requires the adoption of a unique professional identity [68, 70]. Tools that teach the core competencies necessary for BHCs can be useful in retraining [69]. Other training initiatives for the BHC role include academic programs (graduate and certificate programs), community-based training, and self-study resources.

Financial challenges can limit implementation of the PCBH model. Specifically, the lack of reimbursement for same-day visits is a barrier that is especially relevant to this model. Some payers do not reimburse for behavioral health visits conducted on the same day as primary care visits, limiting the ability to generate revenue in a model that emphasizes immediate availability [71]. Further, given the relatively brief nature of individual visits, reimbursement for such visits is typically lower, if there is any reimbursement available at all [72]. Thus, in fee-for-service models, the PCBH model may not be directly self-sufficient. However, there is some evidence that incorporation of a BHC into a primary care practice can actually increase overall revenue through increased PCP efficiency [73]. Further, some financial risk can be mitigated through utilization of value-based or accountable care payment models that recognize the return on investment that can be achieved through behavioral health integration.

The PCBH model depends on the efficient utilization of the skills of the BHC. Barriers to this include hesitation to interrupt patient visits to involve BHCs and low productivity due to limited consultation, which limits the impact on the patient population [74]. This could be due to inadequate BHC training or cultural challenges that prevent adequate integration of the BHC into the clinic workflow and treatment team [69].

Screening, Brief Intervention, and Referral to Treatment

Screening, Brief Intervention, and Referral to Treatment (SBIRT) is a comprehensive, integrated public health approach to early intervention and treatment for people at risk for or currently afflicted with substance use disorders [75]. The components of the intervention include (1) universal **Screening** for substance use, (2) delivery of **Brief Interventions** to those individuals with low to moderate risk of harm, and (3) **Referral** to treatment services for individuals with more serious signs of substance use and resultant serious harms. The basis of the intervention comes from the trans-theoretical change model [76] and motivational interviewing [77] which work together to identify an individual's readiness to change and assist them in making movement toward healthy, adaptive responses related to substance use. The model aligns with the *5 A's* approach to behavioral counseling adopted by the US Preventative Services Task Force (Ask, Advise, Assess, Assist, and Arrange) [78].

Universal screening is typically accomplished using evidence-based tools to detect risky alcohol and other substance misuse. These tools include the Alcohol Use Disorders Identification Test-Consumption (AUDIT-C) [79] and the Drug Abuse Screening Test (DAST), which screens for any substance use other than alcohol [80]. Additional tools are available for specific populations, as well as for children and adolescents. After screening, those determined to be at risk of harm from substance use are provided brief intervention and/or are referred to treatment. Interventions are short (5–30 min in duration), semi-structured discussions to raise awareness of substance use and increase motivation to avoid, reduce, or discontinue harmful use of substances [75, 81, 82]. There are variations in the duration, the number of conversations or meetings, and the structure and nature of the interventions. Successful brief interventions incorporate six elements captured in the acronym FRAMES: **F**eedback on behavior and consequences, **R**esponsibility to change placed on the patient, **A**dvice to change from the provider, **M**enu of options to bring about change, **E**mpathy from the provider, and **S**elf-efficacy for change engendered in the patient [81, 83].

The SBIRT model in primary care prevents or reduces the serious long-term harms associated with heavy alcohol use, including automobile accidents, arrests, incarcerations, work absences, and other societal costs [82]. The efficacy of SBIRT targeting use of other substances is suggestive of benefit, but less clear [81].

Despite the potential benefits of SBIRT in primary care settings, the intervention is underutilized [84]. Barriers to use include challenges with implementation of screening, inadequate reimbursement for the service, limited education on substance use disorders among health care professionals, and inconsistent use of the tools necessary for the intervention [75, 84]. Successful implementation of SBIRT into primary care must include training and education of key stakeholders, utilization of strategies to support clinicians (such as reminders in electronic health records and task shifting), and regular reporting to summarize program data [84]. Strategies that address patients, professionals, and organizations are more effective than strategies that only address individual health care professionals [85]. More intensive implementation strategies are associated with greater efficacy in primary care [86]. There should be fidelity to the core features of the SBIRT model, but flexibility in the peripheral components of the intervention (who performs the screen, whether it is done in person or electronically, duration of the intervention, etc.) may lead to greater success.

The Collaborative Care Management Model

The collaborative care management model (CoCM) is one of the most widely studied integrated care models and is based on the principles of Wagner and colleagues' chronic care model [87]. Developed at the University of Washington, CoCM involves caseload-focused psychiatry consultation supported by a behavioral health care manager. It is a dynamic model of care that improves access to behavioral health care, enhances communication between team members, and provides consultation with psychiatrists.

Expert consensus has identified four essential elements of CoCM including care that is (1) patient-centered, (2) population-focused, (3) measurement-guided, and (4) evidence-based [88]. The model is team-based and includes the patient, the primary care provider (PCP), a behavioral health care manager, and a consulting psychiatrist (Fig. 33.3). The care manager role may be fulfilled by a social worker, nurse, psychologist, or other mental health professional. The PCP identifies patients for treatment, retains the primary treatment relationship with the patient, prescribes medications, collaborates with the care manager, and is ultimately responsible for treatment decisions. The care manager conducts comprehensive behavioral health assessments; creates a patient-centric treatment plan; provides brief, evidence-based behavioral interventions (motivational interviewing, problem-solving therapy, brief cognitive behavioral therapy, behavioral activation, etc.); actively engages the patient through frequent outreach; and coordinates care among team members. The care manager meets regularly (typically weekly) with the psychiatric consultant to review challenging cases and systematically monitors patient progress using evidence-based tools and a patient registry. The psychiatric consultant documents treatment recommendations, provides education to the care manager and PCP, and is available to consult as needed with team members. Generally, the psychiatric consultant does not examine the patient directly, but rather develops treatment recommendations based on information documented in the medical record and verbal and written communication from team members. This indirect method allows the psychiatric consultant to be involved in a larger number of cases than they would be able to see in traditional face-to-face visits. Some CoCM models add additional team members, including psychologists, clinical pharmacists, or specialty care physicians.

As a population health model, registries are used in CoCM to track patient progress and outreach efforts to ensure that no one "falls through the cracks." Treatment progress and

Fig. 33.3 Collaborative care model. (Reprinted with permission from the University of Washington)

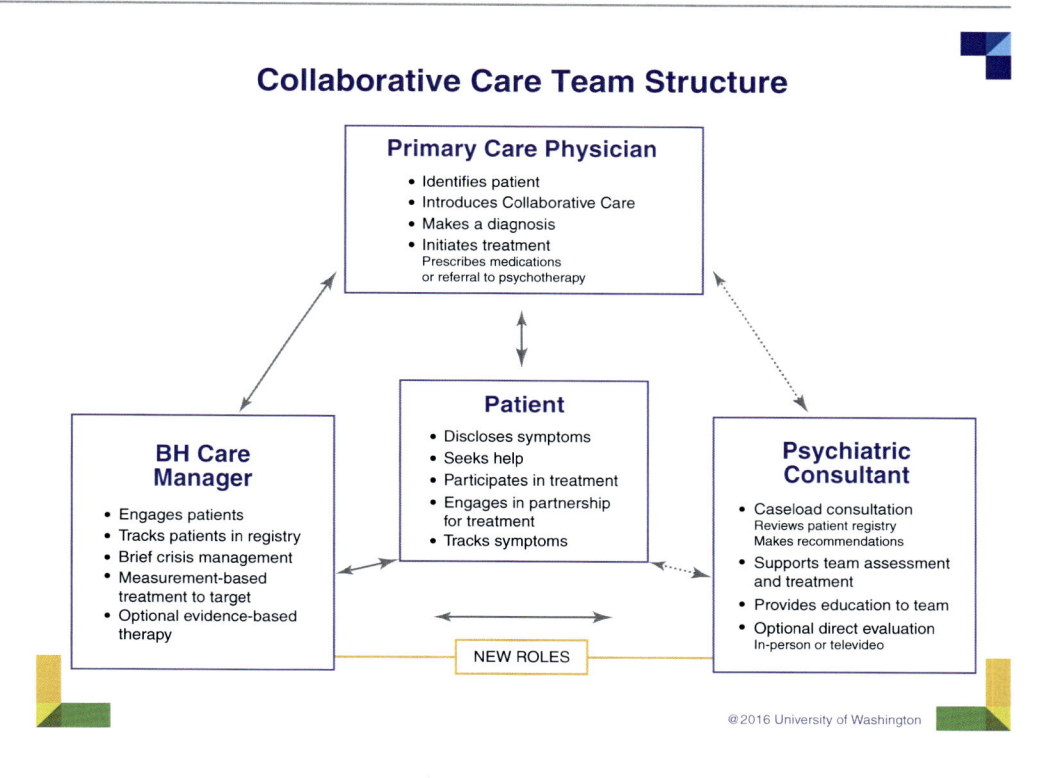

response is closely followed using standardized illness-specific measures such as the Patient Health Questionnaire-9 (PHQ-9) for depression and the Generalized Anxiety Disorder-7 (GAD-7). Regular review of the registry by the care manager and the psychiatrist allows for dynamic treatment recommendations, with timely adjustments to treatment plans [89]. The goal in CoCM is to *treat-to-target*, meaning that treatment is continuously modified until specific outcome measures are achieved [90]. The DIAMOND CoCM program, for example, considers a depression response as a 50% or greater decrease in PHQ-9 score from baseline at 6 months, and remission is defined as a PHQ-9 score of less than 5 at 6 months [91]. Typically, if the patient has not had at least a 50% improvement in symptoms using a validated measure, the treatment plan is modified every 10–12 weeks [92]. When patients do not respond to treatment, the care manager facilitates any needed referrals and treatment with other resources, such as community mental health centers and substance use treatment centers. In addition to treatment response, other metrics are monitored in collaborative care models including process measures such as access times, cost savings, resource utilization (e.g. emergency room visits and hospitalizations), and caregiver and patient satisfaction [92].

Historically, CoCM models were disease-specific, focusing commonly on depression and anxiety. For example, the initial randomized controlled trial (RCT) of CoCM, the Improving Mood-Promoting Access to Collaborative Treatment (IMPACT) trial, targeted treatment of depression in older adults and demonstrated up to three times higher rates of depression response and remission with CoCM compared to usual primary care treatment [92]. In addition, CoCM resulted in greater patient and provider satisfaction, higher rates of antidepressant and psychotherapy use, greater patient-reported quality of life, and lower rates of health-related functional impairment, with a reduced total cost of care and a return on investment of $6.5 for every $1 spent, predominantly through reductions in utilization of emergency and inpatient medical care [93]. Subsequently, over 90 RCTs have confirmed the effectiveness of CoCM for depression [94], as well as other behavioral health conditions including anxiety [95, 96], post-traumatic stress disorder [97], substance use disorders [98, 99], ADHD [100], and bipolar disorder [101, 102]. In addition, CoCM improves comorbid chronic physical health conditions in individuals with concurrent disease including diabetes [103], hypertension [103], cancer [104], obesity [105], and HIV [106]. CoCM is also effective in treatment of socioeconomically disadvantaged populations [107, 108], rural populations [38, 109], and racial and ethnic minorities [110]. Finally, while the initial CoCM model emphasized physically embedding care managers within primary care clinics, fully remote, virtual care management and psychiatric consultation models are as effective as physically co-located CoCM programs [109, 111].

Despite its well-established evidence base, implementation of CoCM is not widespread. Several barriers to implementation exist, largely due to cultural, structural, and financial challenges. Cultural barriers include acceptance of the model by leadership and clinical staff, as CoCM may represent a paradigm shift in a primary care practice's approach to behavioral health treatment. Structural challenges include appropriately trained staff to serve as care managers, contracting with a psychiatrist who is comfortable and familiar with the model, incorporation of a patient registry, and clinic workflow changes that facilitate CoCM. The largest barriers are financial, as care management programs often are not cost-neutral in traditional fee-for-service billing. Despite studies that show the cost-effectiveness of CoCM to health systems [93, 112–114], some systems are reluctant to take on the additional expense of care managers and psychiatric consultants whose work is not directly compensated. Despite the introduction of billing codes by the Centers for Medicare and Medicaid Services (CMS), utilization remains limited [115, 116] due to a variety of factors including spotty payment of these billing codes by private and public payers, workflow changes, documentation, and monitoring burden required to utilize the codes [117]. Substantial effort is necessary to make CoCM a cost-neutral model in a fee-for-service payment paradigm [117]. Ongoing refinement of the model is underway with several resources available through the University of Washington Advancing Integrated Mental Health Solutions (AIMS) Center [118], the Safety Net Medical Home Initiative [119], the Substance Abuse and Mental Health Services Administration [120], and the American Psychiatric Association [121].

Implementation Strategies and Considerations

Several resources can help facilitate the development and implementation of an IBH program within a primary care setting:

- The *Integration Playbook*, an online, interactive guide for integrating behavioral health in ambulatory care developed by the Academy for Integrating Behavioral Health and Primary Care (part of the Agency for Healthcare Research and Quality (AHRQ): https://integrationacademy.ahrq.gov/playbook/about-playbook).
- *The Organized, Evidence-Based Care: Behavioral Health Integration Guide* and the *GROW Pathway Planning Worksheet* [122] developed by the Safety Net Medical Home Initiative are available online at http://www.safetynetmedicalhome.org/change-concepts/organized-evidence-based-care/behavioral-health
- *Quick Start Guide to Behavioral Health Integration* developed by SAMHSA-HRSA Center for Integrated Health Solutions: https://www.thinglink.com/channel/622854013355819009/slideshow
- SAMHSA also has a general listing of other integration tools available on their integrated behavioral health care website: http://www.samhsa.gov/children/behavioral-health-care-integration-resources
- The Advancing Integrated Mental Health Solutions (AIMS) Center through the University of Washington focuses on the Collaborative Care Model and has trainings, online resources, and virtual "office hours" providing consultation for organizations: https://aims.uw.edu/

Translating and introducing IBH models, developed and evaluated as part of RCTs, to community primary care practices can be challenging. The Advancing Care Together (ACT) program and the Integration Workforce Study (IWS) examined methods for integrating care within "real-world" primary care settings [123–130]. By longitudinally studying the implementation approaches within primary care practices and behavioral health agencies over several years, ACT and IWS showed that successful integration must include changes in organizational processes and interprofessional relationships. Challenges common among the practices were categorized into four themes—(1) engaging leadership and culture change, (2) workflow, (3) access, and (4) tracking and using data in meaningful ways. Common key characteristics of successful integration include support and vision from influential leadership, a focus on vulnerable populations, community-wide collaborations, team-based care including the patient and family, data-driven decisions, and diverse funding streams [131]. The following sections outline the considerations for an IBH program.

Mission and Vision

To guide the transformation process, practices must commit to a shared mission and clear vision for the integration of care. The population to be served should be clarified such as whether all adult patients are screened for depression versus only screening and treating high-risk/high-utilizing patients. The scope of care the practice is prepared to offer should also be clarified.

Staffing and Training

Strong interdisciplinary teams committed to mutual respect, collaboration, and a shift from the traditional hierarchy of medical practice is necessary for the success of IBH. Primary care clinicians and behavioral health professionals benefit from understanding each other's different training and perspectives which can synergize to create an integrated team that provides excellent patient care.

Behavioral health professionals must learn to adapt traditional assessment and therapy models to brief, solution-focused interventions with limited time spent on assessment. BHPs also need to function outside of the traditional 50-min hour and consider intervention strategies that work within the busy pace and workflow of a medical practice. This can be a substantial cultural shift for behavioral health providers. A foundation in the interplay of physical illness and emotional well-being, knowledge of common chronic health care conditions, and knowledge of medical culture is also essential for BHPs to be successful in primary care settings [132]. The American Psychological Association Interorganizational Work Group on Competencies for Primary Care Psychology Practice has delineated six competency domains with associated essential components for behavioral scientists practicing in primary care [133]. These include competency in science related to the biopsychosocial approach, research and evaluation, leadership and administration, interdisciplinary systems, advocacy, and practice management. Additional clinical skills in assessment, intervention, clinical consultation, and supervision and teaching are also essential. Although more training is now available for BHPs in integrated care models, finding providers able and eager to work in primary care settings continues to be a challenge [126].

Primary care clinicians need to be able to screen patients for common behavioral health concerns (i.e., depression, anxiety, substance use issues) and recognize variations in signs and symptoms of behavioral health concerns across the life spectrum. Without standardized screening processes, depression, for example, goes undetected in greater than 50% of primary care patients [134]. Also, PCPs need to consider when and how best to involve a BHP in a patient's care. This includes developing strategies for effectively introducing the BHP to the patient and communicating needs efficiently to the BHP [135].

As new staff join the team, orientation and training should help them understand the goals, processes, and cultural expectations involved in integrated care. This can involve shadowing different members of the team, reviewing training manuals that describe the mission and vision, and reviewing the standardized protocols and workflows that support IBH. These efforts solidify an organization's conceptualization and commitment to IBH. Ongoing education and mentoring further facilitates the maturation of a truly integrated care system [126].

Workflow

As practices develop their model for IBH, attention needs to be paid to workflow. Developing standardized practice protocols facilitate clarity and process consistency. These protocols should cover screening, team communication expectations, treatment guidelines, and referral considerations. Practices need to consider what behavioral health screening to use, the frequency of use, who will be screened, and which staff will administer and score the screening tools. Having a systematic approach to screening helps to identify patients needing service as well as inform the practice on population-based behavioral health needs. Practices will need to decide on the behavioral health needs that are feasible to address, however. Full population-based screening for many behavioral health problems could easily overwhelm the resources available to respond to the identified needs.

Commonly used screening tools in primary care settings include the PHQ-2, PHQ-9, and Edinburgh Postnatal Depression Scale to screen for depression. The GAD-7 scale is often used to screen for anxiety disorders and the post-traumatic stress disorder (PTSD) checklist for the Diagnostic and Statistical Manual of Mental Disorders, 5th edition (DSM-V, PCL-5), screens for trauma impact. The Alcohol Use Disorders Identification Test (AUDIT), CAGE (Cut down, Annoyance, Guilt, and Eye-opener) questions, and Drug Abuse Screening Test (DAST) are used to screen for substance use concerns. Many of these tools have modified versions appropriate for use with adolescents. The Modified Checklist for Autism in Toddlers-Revised (M-CHAT-R) is used for screening for autism spectrum disorders. Tools such as the Ages and Stages Questionnaire and Parents' Evaluation of Developmental Status (PEDS) milestone questionnaires are used to assess achievement of expected developmental milestones. These tools are designed for the patient or a parent to complete rather than the provider. This is an important consideration, given that provider ratings can be biased and may miss the worsening of symptoms [136]. Tools need to be reliable and sensitive for the population, easy for patients to complete, and simple for staff to score and interpret. These tools must be available in the moment and useful in clinical decision making. Protocols should be developed regarding how often the measure is administered and what results indicate that treatment is effective versus needing to be modified.

Workspace Design

Practices need to consider the logistics of workflow and usage of space. Having workspace for behavioral health team members centralized so that the BHP is visible and easily accessed by all practice members facilitates real-time communication and the integration of behavioral health care. Shared or centralized workspace also increases the likelihood of "curbside" consultations and the development of robust interpersonal working relationships.

Schedules

The design of the schedule for the BHP will influence his or her availability and flexibility regarding patient needs. The ability to quickly access the BHP at the time of need greatly impacts the success and level of integration. In some models, the BHP has no scheduled follow-up visits outside of a return visit with the PCP. In other models, the schedule has a mix of available consultation times interspersed with brief scheduled follow-up appointments, usually 20–30 min, which are aligned with the clinic schedule. Time for making follow-up phone calls for outreach and treatment monitoring is needed for practices that implement a population management approach.

Communication

Clear communication processes are essential for the success of IBH. Communicating impressions and treatment plans through the shared electronic health record (EHR) has the advantage of being easy, reducing duplication of documentation, and data consolidation. It should be clear where within the EHR the BHP will document, such as within the same note as the physician or a separate note. There should be strategies on how to communicate and collaborate on shared treatment plans. Standardized templates for documenting care can facilitate communication among team members. There are some challenges with shared EHRs and most EHR systems are not designed with behavioral health care documentation standards and regulations in mind. Practices may need to create processes that ensure clear communication within the EHR that is accessible, meaningfully enhances patient care, and meets regulatory and billing requirements for medical and behavioral health care. An additional consideration for documentation of behavioral health care within an integrated and shared EHR is how to maintain standards of confidentiality and privacy that in some states are stricter than federal Health Insurance Portability and Accountability Act (HIPAA) privacy rules.

To facilitate integrated team care it is helpful to have a standard process that defines what should trigger a provider to provider "warm handoff" and what should be communicated during the handoff. Interdisciplinary pre-clinic huddles where the team meets to review the clinic schedule and identify possible patient care needs in advance help organize the day. Complex care team meetings also improve care for the patient and foster collaboration and ongoing training for team members. Finally, it helps to have an understanding among team members regarding the practice of care professionals interrupting each other, particularly when care team members are providing service to other patients.

Practice Improvement

Registries to track patients and monitor program metrics are critical elements in IBH models. Successful programs use data and quality metrics to respond to patient needs and enhance the overall program. As practices systematically collect patient-level data tied to behavioral health and other outcomes, they must consider how to use and manage the information. Some EHR systems have the ability to access data over time (i.e., PHQ-9 scores, GAD-7, HbA1c, blood pressure, etc.) and can collate this into reports that measure and track patient-specific health targets. This data can be used to monitor individual treatment response, identify patients who have not been engaged in care for a specified period of time, and inform and evaluate practice change efforts. Data is powerful and it is important to have adequate infrastructure to use the data. The practice must decide what data to track, at both individual and population levels, what information should be aggregated, and who will run, interpret, and act on the reports. In practices without EHR systems that can access and report data, tracking patient data is challenging.

An important step in designing an IBH program is the determination of metrics that show whether the program is effective and valuable. These measures should include patient-oriented outcomes, patient and staff satisfaction scales, and costs. While definitions of effectiveness and value may vary from practice to practice, standardized measures allow comparisons across practices which facilitate the process of continuous quality improvement. Practices or programs that perform well on outcome measures can inform other practices. In addition, having a structured continuous quality improvement plan protects against the natural process whereby systems slowly revert to old patterns of care.

Future Directions and Trends

No one IBH model is likely to address every local population's needs and ongoing innovation and creativity is needed. While the data supporting the effectiveness of IBH continue to grow, one of the limitations with much of the literature is that the outcome studies have focused on specific diseases (depression and anxiety) in specific populations (e.g., older adult populations). Future research must examine IBH models that address multiple comorbidities, behavioral health concerns that occur across the life spectrum (children, adolescents, perinatal, etc.), and diagnoses that fall on the more debilitating end of the spectrum such as schizophrenia and bipolar disorders. In addition, we need to expand our understanding of how IBH models can be adapted to engage and meet the needs of culturally diverse populations and how these models can complement other population health models of care (i.e., chronic care management and programs to address social determinants of health). The development of flexible, stepped care approaches that address changing mental health treatment needs of individuals and access to diverse resources in the practice and community are essential for successful integration of behavioral health.

The future of integrated care depends on adaptability and innovation in terms of implementation. The COVID pandemic, for example, accelerated the adoption of virtual care via telecommunications via video and phone. Research is showing that patients value this form of care [137] and that treatment outcomes are comparable to in-person care [110, 138, 139]. The federal government, state Medicaid programs, and private insurers have all expanded coverage for telehealth during the COVID-19 public health emergency. Most insurance companies also cover telehealth services, often including behavioral telemedicine. Advocacy is needed to continue reimbursement for tele-behavioral health beyond the public health emergency and to ensure that virtual behavioral health care is treated with fiscal parity with in-person care and parity with virtual medical care. Hybrid models that include in-person, phone/video-based, and asynchronous interventions will help address the diversity of behavioral health needs based on the population, community, and resources.

IBH can be a mechanism to address long-standing health and behavioral health disparities among individuals from marginalized racial and ethnic groups if delivered using culturally informed methods [140, 141]. Unfortunately, training providers in culturally appropriate techniques and adapting IBH interventions to the needs of diverse communities has lagged. IBH teams of the future need to be trained to practice as culturally competent providers of care.

Family consultations, family therapy, and parenting training are rarely described in studies on integrated primary care programs [142]. Given that the discipline of family medicine represents a substantial portion of primary care practices, future IBH models should consider how to keep the "family" in IBH.

Future studies should also examine how enhanced resiliency and self-engagement in chronic disease management may improve outcomes and satisfaction while reducing overall health care costs. Most IBH models focus on moderating the impact of emotional distress that is already present. Integrating resiliency models such as mindfulness-based stress reduction, peer support, and chronic disease self-management may help to improve outcomes for an even broader array of patients.

Finally, integrated care must be financially sustainable. Value-based payment models may address the financial limitations of IBH delivered in clinics with fee-for-service visits in which only the PCP receives a billable encounter and other team members are paid for as overhead. Bundled payment mechanisms, like those developed for CoCM, demonstrate the importance of incentivizing team-based care models. Focusing on payment for teams rather than providers may be a pathway for sustainability [19]. CMS encourages innovation and integration of behavioral health as a means of providing whole-person care, which will improve outcomes while reducing overall costs [143].

Summary

The integration of behavioral health and primary care is transformative and can help achieve the quadruple aim of better health, better patient experience, lower costs, and improved physician experience [144, 145]. It is especially important for patients with chronic diseases and can complement the management and treatment of often complex and serious medical conditions. The growing recognition of the biopsychosocial interplay in chronic disease ensures that behavioral health will remain critical in the care of patients and there is no more apt place to reach them than in the primary care setting.

References

1. Peek CJ. Lexicon for behavioral health and primary care integration: concepts and definitions developed by expert consensus. Rockville, MD: Agency for Healthcare Research and Quality; 2013.
2. Kessler RC, Wang PS. The descriptive epidemiology of commonly occurring mental disorders in the United States. Annu Rev Public Health. 2008;29:115–29.
3. Merikangas KR, He J-P, Burstein M, Swanson SA, Avenevoli S, Cui L, et al. Lifetime prevalence of mental disorders in U.S. adolescents: results from the National Comorbidity Survey Replication—Adolescent Supplement (NCS-A). J Am Acad Child Adolesc Psychiatry. 2010;49(10):980–9.
4. Substance Abuse and Mental Health Services Administration. Key substance use and mental health indicators in the United States: results from the 2019 National Survey on Drug Use and Health. Department of Health and Human Services; 2020.
5. Salari N, Hosseinian-Far A, Jalali R, Vaisi-Raygani A, Rasoulpoor S, Mohammadi M, et al. Prevalence of stress, anxiety, depression among the general population during the COVID-19 pandemic: a systematic review and meta-analysis. Glob Health. 2020;16(1):57.
6. Xiong J, Lipsitz O, Nasri F, Lui LMW, Gill H, Phan L, et al. Impact of COVID-19 pandemic on mental health in the general population: a systematic review. J Affect Disord. 2020;277:55–64.
7. Ettman CK, Abdalla SM, Cohen GH, Sampson L, Vivier PM, Galea S. Prevalence of depression symptoms in US adults before and during the COVID-19 pandemic. JAMA Netw Open. 2020;3(9):e2019686.
8. Park-Lee E, Lipari RN, Hedden SL, Kroutil LA, Porter JD. Receipt of Services for Substance Use and Mental Health Issues Among Adults: results from the 2016 National Survey on Drug Use and Health. CBHSQ Data Review. Rockville (MD): Substance Abuse and Mental Health Services Administration (US); 2017.

9. Walker ER, Cummings JR, Hockenberry JM, Druss BG. Insurance status, use of mental health services, and unmet need for mental health care in the United States. Psychiatr Serv. 2015;66(6):578–84.
10. Mochari-Greenberger, H, Pande, RL. Barriers to Behavioral Health Care: Consumer Insights Reveal Low Engagement and Unmet Needs Persist. 2018. https://www.ableto.com/wp-content/uploads/2018/10/AbleTo_Barriers-to-Behavioral-Health-Care_WhitePaper.pdf.
11. Center for Disease Control and Prevention. Percentage of Mental Health-Related Primary Care Office Visits, by Age Group—National Ambulatory Medical Care Survey, United States, 2010. 2014. p. 1118.
12. Olfson M, Kroenke K, Wang S, Blanco C. Trends in office-based mental health care provided by psychiatrists and primary care physicians. J Clin Psychiatry. 2014;75(3):247–53.
13. Olfson M, Blanco C, Wang S, Laje G, Correll CU. National trends in the mental health care of children, adolescents, and adults by office-based physicians. JAMA Psychiatry. 2014;71(1):81–90.
14. Mark TL, Levit KR, Buck JA. Datapoints: psychotropic drug prescriptions by medical specialty. Psychiatr Serv. 2009;60(9):1167.
15. Kessler R, Stafford D. Primary care is the de facto mental health system. In: Kessler R, Stafford D, editors. Collaborative medicine case studies. New York, NY: Springer; 2008. p. 9–21.
16. American Academy of Family Physicians. Mental health care services by family physicians (position paper). 2011. http://www.aafp.org/about/policies/all/mental-services.html.
17. Working Party Group on Integrated Behavioral Healthcare, Baird M, Blount A, Brungardt S, Dickinson P, Dietrich A, et al. Joint principles: integrating behavioral health care into the patient-centered medical home. Ann Fam Med. 2014;12(2):183–5.
18. Nielsen M. Behavioral health integration: a critical component of primary care and the patient-centered medical home. Fam Syst Health. 2014;32(2):149–50.
19. National Academies of Sciences, Engineering, and Medicine; Health and Medicine Division; Board on Health Care Services; Committee on Implementing High-Quality Primary Care. Implementing high-quality primary care: rebuilding the foundation of health care. Robinson SK, Meisnere M, Phillips RL, McCauley L, editors. Washington, DC: National Academies Press (US); 2021.
20. Loeppke R, Taitel M, Haufle V, Parry T, Kessler RC, Jinnett K. Health and productivity as a business strategy: a multiemployer study. J Occup Environ Med. 2009;51(4):411–28.
21. Vigo D, Thornicroft G, Atun R. Estimating the true global burden of mental illness. Lancet Psychiatry. 2016;3(2):171–8.
22. Hert DE, Correll CU, Bobes J, Cetkovich-Bakmas M, Cohen D, Asai I, et al. Physical illness in patients with severe mental disorders. I. Prevalence, impact of medications and disparities in health care. World Psychiatry. 2011;10(1):52–77.
23. Walker ER, McGee RE, Druss BG. Mortality in mental disorders and global disease burden implications: a systematic review and meta-analysis. JAMA Psychiatry. 2015;72(4):334–41.
24. Centers for Disease Control and Prevention (CDC). Attitudes toward mental illness—35 states, District of Columbia, and Puerto Rico, 2007. MMWR Morb Mortal Wkly Rep. 2010;59(20):619–25.
25. Chiles C, Stefanovics E, Rosenheck R. Attitudes of students at a US medical school toward mental illness and its causes. Acad Psychiatry. 2017;41(3):320–5.
26. Kessler RC, Demler O, Frank RG, Olfson M, Pincus HA, Walters EE, et al. Prevalence and treatment of mental disorders, 1990 to 2003. N Engl J Med. 2005;352(24):2515–23.
27. Sanchez K, Chapa T, Ybarra R, Martinez ON. Eliminating health disparities through culturally and linguistically centered integrated health care: consensus statements, recommendations, and key strategies from the field. J Health Care Poor Underserved. 2014;25(2):469–77.
28. Ida DJ, SooHoo J, Chapa T. Integrated Care for Asian American, Native Hawaiian and Pacific Islander Communities: a blueprint for action: Consensus Statement and Recommendations. Department of Health and Human Services, Office of Minority Health. 2012. p. 43.
29. Huang H-C, Liu S-I, Hwang L-C, Sun F-J, Tjung J-J, Huang C-R, et al. The effectiveness of Culturally Sensitive Collaborative Treatment of depressed Chinese in family medicine clinics: a randomized controlled trial. Gen Hosp Psychiatry. 2018;50:96–103.
30. McKnight-Eily LR, Okoro CA, Strine TW, Verlenden J, Hollis ND, Njai R, et al. Racial and Ethnic Disparities in the Prevalence of Stress and Worry, Mental Health Conditions, and Increased Substance Use Among Adults During the COVID-19 Pandemic—United States, April and May 2020. MMWR Morb Mortal Wkly Rep. 2021;70(5):162–6.
31. Kugelmass H. "Sorry, I'm not accepting new patients": an audit study of access to mental health care. J Health Soc Behav. 2016;57(2):168–83.
32. Garb HN. Race bias and gender bias in the diagnosis of psychological disorders. Clin Psychol Rev. 2021;90:102087.
33. Lasser KE, Himmelstein DU, Woolhandler S. Access to care, health status, and health disparities in the United States and Canada: results of a cross-national population-based survey. Am J Public Health. 2006;96(7):1300–7.
34. Santiago CD, Miranda J. Progress in improving mental health services for racial-ethnic minority groups: a ten-year perspective. Psychiatr Serv. 2014;65(2):180–5.
35. Marrast L, Himmelstein DU, Woolhandler S. Racial and ethnic disparities in mental health care for children and young adults: a national study. Int J Health Serv. 2016;46(4):810–24.
36. Kirby JB, Zuvekas SH, Borsky AE, Ngo-Metzger Q. Rural residents with mental health needs have fewer care visits than urban counterparts. Health Aff (Millwood). 2019;38(12):2057–60.
37. Andrilla CHA, Patterson DG, Garberson LA, Coulthard C, Larson EH. Geographic variation in the supply of selected behavioral health providers. Am J Prev Med. 2018;54(6 Suppl 3):S199–207.
38. Powers DM, Bowen DJ, Arao RF, Vredevoogd M, Russo J, Grover T, et al. Rural clinics implementing collaborative care for low-income patients can achieve comparable or better depression outcomes. Fam Syst Health. 2020;38(3):242–54.
39. Renn BN, Johnson M, Powers DM, Vredevoogd M, Unützer J. Collaborative care for depression yields similar improvement among older and younger rural adults. J Am Geriatr Soc. 2021;70(1):110–8.
40. Kathol RG, McAlpine D, Kishi Y, Spies R, Meller W, Bernhardt T, et al. General medical and pharmacy claims expenditures in users of behavioral health services. J Gen Intern Med. 2005;20(2):160–7.
41. Shen C, Sambamoorthi U, Rust G. Co-occurring mental illness and health care utilization and expenditures in adults with obesity and chronic physical illness. Dis Manag. 2008;11(3):153–60.
42. Heath B Jr, Reynolds K, Romero PW. A standard framework for levels of integrated healthcare. Washington, DC: SAMSHA-HRSA Center for Integrated Health Solutions; 2013.
43. Callahan CM, Kroenke K, Counsell SR, Hendrie HC, Perkins AJ, Katon W, et al. Treatment of depression improves physical functioning in older adults. J Am Geriatr Soc. 2005;53(3):367–73.
44. van Orden M, Hoffman T, Haffmans J, Spinhoven P, Hoencamp E. Collaborative mental health care versus care as usual in a primary care setting: a randomized controlled trial. Psychiatr Serv. 2009;60(1):74–9.
45. Elrashidi MY, Mohammed K, Bora PR, Haydour Q, Farah W, DeJesus R, et al. Co-located specialty care within primary care practice settings: a systematic review and meta-analysis. Healthc (Amst). 2018;6(1):52–66.

46. Wiley-Exley E, Domino ME, Maxwell J, Levkoff SE. Cost-effectiveness of integrated care for elderly depressed patients in the PRISM-E study. J Ment Health Policy Econ. 2009;12(4):205–13.
47. Chen H, Coakley EH, Cheal K, Maxwell J, Costantino G, Krahn DD, et al. Satisfaction with mental health services in older primary care patients. Am J Geriatr Psychiatry. 2006;14(4):371–9.
48. Hedrick SC, Chaney EF, Felker B, Liu C-F, Hasenberg N, Heagerty P, et al. Effectiveness of collaborative care depression treatment in Veterans' Affairs primary care. J Gen Intern Med. 2003;18(1):9–16.
49. Ayalon L, Areán PA, Linkins K, Lynch M, Estes CL. Integration of mental health services into primary care overcomes ethnic disparities in access to mental health services between black and white elderly. Am J Geriatr Psychiatry. 2007;15(10):906–12.
50. Haggarty JM, Jarva JA, Cernovsky Z, Karioja K, Martin L. Wait time impact of co-located primary care mental health services: the effect of adding collaborative care in northern Ontario. Can J Psychiatr. 2012;57(1):29–33.
51. Felker BL, Barnes RF, Greenberg DM, Chaney EF, Shores MM, Gillespie-Gateley L, et al. Preliminary outcomes from an integrated mental health primary care team. Psychiatr Serv. 2004;55(4):442–4.
52. Reiter JT, Dobmeyer AC, Hunter CL. The primary care behavioral health (PCBH) model: an overview and operational definition. J Clin Psychol Med Settings. 2018;25(2):109–26.
53. Hunter CL, Funderburk JS, Polaha J, Bauman D, Goodie JL, Hunter CM. Primary care behavioral health (PCBH) model research: current state of the science and a call to action. J Clin Psychol Med Settings. 2018;25(2):127–56.
54. Kearney LK, Post EP, Pomerantz AS, Zeiss AM. Applying the interprofessional patient aligned care team in the Department of Veterans Affairs: transforming primary care. Am Psychol. 2014;69(4):399–408.
55. Hunter CL, Goodie JL, Dobmeyer AC, Dorrance KA. Tipping points in the Department of Defense's experience with psychologists in primary care. Am Psychol. 2014;69(4):388–98.
56. Kanapaux W. The road to integrated care: commitment is the key. Tennessee CMHC demonstrates promise of co-located behavioral and primary care. Behav Healthc Tomorrow. 2004;13(2):15.
57. Hill JM. Behavioral health integration: transforming patient care, medical resident education, and physician effectiveness. Int J Psychiatry Med. 2015;50(1):36–49.
58. Funderburk JS, Fielder RL, DeMartini KS, Flynn CA. Integrating behavioral health services into a university health center: patient and provider satisfaction. Fam Syst Health. 2012;30(2):130–40.
59. Angantyr K, Rimner A, Nordén T, Norlander T. Primary care behavioral health model: perspectives of outcome, client satisfaction, and gender. Soc Behav Personal. 2015;43(2):287–301.
60. Katon W, Robinson P, Von Korff M, Lin E, Bush T, Ludman E, et al. A multifaceted intervention to improve treatment of depression in primary care. Arch Gen Psychiatry. 1996;53(10):924–32.
61. Cigrang JA, Rauch SAM, Mintz J, Brundige A, Avila LL, Bryan CJ, et al. Treatment of active duty military with PTSD in primary care: a follow-up report. J Anxiety Disord. 2015;36:110–4.
62. Goodie JL, Isler WC, Hunter C, Peterson AL. Using behavioral health consultants to treat insomnia in primary care: a clinical case series. J Clin Psychol. 2009;65(3):294–304.
63. Sadock E, Auerbach SM, Rybarczyk B, Aggarwal A. Evaluation of integrated psychological services in a university-based primary care clinic. J Clin Psychol Med Settings. 2014;21(1):19–32.
64. McFeature B, Pierce T. Primary care behavioral health consultation reduces depression levels among mood-disordered patients. J Health Dispar Res Pract. 2012;5(2):4.
65. Brawer PA, Martielli R, Pye PL, Manwaring J, Tierney A. St. Louis Initiative for Integrated Care Excellence (SLI(2)CE): integrated-collaborative care on a large scale model. Fam Syst Health. 2010;28(2):175–87.
66. Serrano N, Monden K. The effect of behavioral health consultation on the care of depression by primary care clinicians. WMJ. 2011;110(3):113–8.
67. Lanoye A, Stewart KE, Rybarczyk BD, Auerbach SM, Sadock E, Aggarwal A, et al. The impact of integrated psychological services in a safety net primary care clinic on medical utilization. J Clin Psychol. 2017;73(6):681–92.
68. Serrano N, Cordes C, Cubic B, Daub S. The state and future of the primary care behavioral health model of service delivery workforce. J Clin Psychol Med Settings. 2018;25(2):157–68.
69. Robinson PJ, Reiter JT. Behavioral consultation and primary care: a guide to integrative services. Cham: Springer International Publishing; 2016.
70. Robinson PJ, Strosahl KD. Behavioral health consultation and primary care: lessons learned. J Clin Psychol Med Settings. 2009;16(1):58–71.
71. Freeman DS, Manson L, Howard J, Hornberger J. Financing the primary care behavioral health model. J Clin Psychol Med Settings. 2018;25(2):197–209.
72. Freeman D. The behavioral health medical home. In: Cummings NA, O'Donohue WT, editors. Understanding the behavioral healthcare crisis: the promise of integrated care and diagnostic reform. Routledge; 2011. p. 250–65.
73. Gouge N, Polaha J, Rogers R, Harden A. Integrating behavioral health into pediatric primary care: implications for provider time and cost. South Med J. 2016;109(12):774–8.
74. Miller BF, Brown Levey SM, Payne-Murphy JC, Kwan BM. Outlining the scope of behavioral health practice in integrated primary care: dispelling the myth of the one-trick mental health pony. Fam Syst Health. 2014;32(3):338–43.
75. Strobbe S. Prevention and screening, brief intervention, and referral to treatment for substance use in primary care. Prim Care. 2014;41(2):185–213.
76. Prochaska JO, DiClemente CC, Norcross JC. In search of how people change. Applications to addictive behaviors. Am Psychol. 1992;47(9):1102–14.
77. Miller WR, Rollnick S. Motivational interviewing: helping people change. Illustrated. Guilford Press; 2012.
78. Centers for Medicare and Medicaid Services. Screening and behavioral counseling interventions in primary care to reduce alcohol misuse. 2021. https://www.cms.gov/medicare-coverage-database/view/ncacal-decision-memo.aspx?proposed=N&NCAId=249.
79. Saunders JB, Aasland OG, Babor TF, de la Fuente JR, Grant M. Development of the Alcohol Use Disorders Identification Test (AUDIT): WHO Collaborative Project on Early Detection of Persons with Harmful Alcohol Consumption—II. Addiction. 1993;88(6):791–804.
80. Gavin DR, Ross HE, Skinner HA. Diagnostic validity of the drug abuse screening test in the assessment of DSM-III drug disorders. Br J Addict. 1989;84(3):301–7.
81. Young MM, Stevens A, Galipeau J, Pirie T, Garritty C, Singh K, et al. Effectiveness of brief interventions as part of the Screening, Brief Intervention and Referral to Treatment (SBIRT) model for reducing the nonmedical use of psychoactive substances: a systematic review. Syst Rev. 2014;3:50.
82. Kaner EF, Beyer FR, Muirhead C, Campbell F, Pienaar ED, Bertholet N, et al. Effectiveness of brief alcohol interventions in primary care populations. Cochrane Database Syst Rev. 2018;2:CD004148.
83. Bien TH, Miller WR, Tonigan JS. Brief interventions for alcohol problems: a review. Addiction. 1993;88(3):315–35.
84. Thoele K, Moffat L, Konicek S, Lam-Chi M, Newkirk E, Fulton J, et al. Strategies to promote the implementation of Screening,

85. Keurhorst M, van de Glind I, Bitarello do Amaral-Sabadini M, Anderson P, Kaner E, Newbury-Birch D, et al. Implementation strategies to enhance management of heavy alcohol consumption in primary health care: a meta-analysis. Addiction. 2015;110(12):1877–900.
86. Nilsen P, Aalto M, Bendtsen P, Seppä K. Effectiveness of strategies to implement brief alcohol intervention in primary healthcare. A systematic review. Scand J Prim Health Care. 2006;24(1):5–15.
87. Wagner EH, Glasgow RE, Davis C, Bonomi AE, Provost L, McCulloch D, et al. Quality improvement in chronic illness care: a collaborative approach. Jt Comm J Qual Improv. 2001;27(2):63–80.
88. Dissemination of integrated care within adult primary care settings: the collaborative care model. American Psychiatric Association & Academy of Psychosomatic Medicine; 2016. https://psychiatry.org/psychiatrists/practice/professional-interests/integrated-care/collaborative-care-model.
89. Garrison GM, Angstman KB, O'Connor SS, Williams MD, Lineberry TW. Time to Remission for Depression with Collaborative Care Management (CCM) in Primary Care. J Am Board Fam Med. 2016;29(1):10–7.
90. McGough PM, Bauer AM, Collins L, Dugdale DC. Integrating Behavioral Health into Primary Care. Popul Health Manag. 2016;19(2):81–7.
91. Solberg LI, Crain AL, Jaeckels N, Ohnsorg KA, Margolis KL, Beck A, et al. The DIAMOND initiative: implementing collaborative care for depression in 75 primary care clinics. Implement Sci. 2013;8:135.
92. Unützer J, Katon W, Callahan CM, Williams JW, Hunkeler E, Harpole L, et al. Collaborative care management of late-life depression in the primary care setting: a randomized controlled trial. JAMA. 2002;288(22):2836–45.
93. Unutzer J, Katon WJ, Fan M-Y, Schoenbaum MC, Lin EHB, Della Penna RD, et al. Long-term cost effects of collaborative care for late-life depression. Am J Manag Care. 2008;14(2):95–100.
94. Archer J, Bower P, Gilbody S, Lovell K, Richards D, Gask L, et al. Collaborative care for depression and anxiety problems. Cochrane Database Syst Rev. 2012;10:CD006525.
95. Roy-Byrne PP, Craske MG, Stein MB, Sullivan G, Bystritsky A, Katon W, et al. A randomized effectiveness trial of cognitive-behavioral therapy and medication for primary care panic disorder. Arch Gen Psychiatry. 2005;62(3):290–8.
96. Roy-Byrne P, Craske MG, Sullivan G, Rose RD, Edlund MJ, Lang AJ, et al. Delivery of evidence-based treatment for multiple anxiety disorders in primary care: a randomized controlled trial. JAMA. 2010;303(19):1921–8.
97. Fortney JC, Pyne JM, Kimbrell TA, Hudson TJ, Robinson DE, Schneider R, et al. Telemedicine-based collaborative care for posttraumatic stress disorder: a randomized clinical trial. JAMA Psychiatry. 2015;72(1):58–67.
98. Suzuki J, Matthews ML, Brick D, Nguyen M-T, Wasan AD, Jamison RN, et al. Implementation of a collaborative care management program with buprenorphine in primary care: a comparison between opioid-dependent patients and patients with chronic pain using opioids nonmedically. J Opioid Manag. 2014;10(3):159–68.
99. Watkins KE, Ober AJ, Lamp K, Lind M, Setodji C, Osilla KC, et al. Collaborative care for opioid and alcohol use disorders in primary care: the SUMMIT randomized clinical trial. JAMA Intern Med. 2017;177(10):1480–8.
100. Silverstein M, Hironaka LK, Walter HJ, Feinberg E, Sandler J, Pellicer M, et al. Collaborative care for children with ADHD symptoms: a randomized comparative effectiveness trial. Pediatrics. 2015;135(4):e858–67.
101. Fortney JC, Bauer AM, Cerimele JM, Pyne JM, Pfeiffer P, Heagerty PJ, et al. Comparison of teleintegrated care and telereferral care for treating complex psychiatric disorders in primary care: a pragmatic randomized comparative effectiveness trial. JAMA Psychiatry. 2021;78(11):1189–99.
102. Kruzer K, Avery A, Lavakumar M. Collaborative care for bipolar disorder in people living with HIV. Gen Hosp Psychiatry. 2020;64:117–8.
103. Katon WJ, Lin EHB, Von Korff M, Ciechanowski P, Ludman EJ, Young B, et al. Collaborative care for patients with depression and chronic illnesses. N Engl J Med. 2010;363(27):2611–20.
104. Sharpe M, Walker J, Holm Hansen C, Martin P, Symeonides S, Gourley C, et al. Integrated collaborative care for comorbid major depression in patients with cancer (SMaRT Oncology-2): a multicentre randomised controlled effectiveness trial. Lancet. 2014;384(9948):1099–108.
105. Ma J, Rosas LG, Lv N, Xiao L, Snowden MB, Venditti EM, et al. Effect of integrated behavioral weight loss treatment and problem-solving therapy on body mass index and depressive symptoms among patients with obesity and depression: the RAINBOW randomized clinical trial. JAMA. 2019;321(9):869–79.
106. Pyne JM, Fortney JC, Curran GM, Tripathi S, Atkinson JH, Kilbourne AM, et al. Effectiveness of collaborative care for depression in human immunodeficiency virus clinics. Arch Intern Med. 2011;171(1):23–31.
107. Grote NK, Katon WJ, Russo JE, Lohr MJ, Curran M, Galvin E, et al. Collaborative care for perinatal depression in socioeconomically disadvantaged women: a randomized trial. Depress Anxiety. 2015;32(11):821–34.
108. Katon W, Russo J, Reed SD, Croicu CA, Ludman E, LaRocco A, et al. A randomized trial of collaborative depression care in obstetrics and gynecology clinics: socioeconomic disadvantage and treatment response. Am J Psychiatry. 2015;172(1):32–40.
109. Fortney JC, Pyne JM, Mouden SB, Mittal D, Hudson TJ, Schroeder GW, et al. Practice-based versus telemedicine-based collaborative care for depression in rural federally qualified health centers: a pragmatic randomized comparative effectiveness trial. Am J Psychiatry. 2013;170(4):414–25.
110. Hu J, Wu T, Damodaran S, Tabb KM, Bauer A, Huang H. The effectiveness of collaborative care on depression outcomes for racial/ethnic minority populations in primary care: a systematic review. Psychosomatics. 2020;61(6):632–44.
111. Whitfield J, Lepoire E, Stanczyk B, Ratzliff A, Cerimele JM. Remote collaborative care with off-site behavioral health care managers: a systematic review of clinical trials. J Acad Consult Liaison Psychiatry. 2021;63(1):71–8.
112. Katon W, Russo J, Lin EHB, Schmittdiel J, Ciechanowski P, Ludman E, et al. Cost-effectiveness of a multicondition collaborative care intervention: a randomized controlled trial. Arch Gen Psychiatry. 2012;69(5):506–14.
113. Simon GE, Katon WJ, Lin EHB, Rutter C, Manning WG, Von Korff M, et al. Cost-effectiveness of systematic depression treatment among people with diabetes mellitus. Arch Gen Psychiatry. 2007;64(1):65–72.
114. Jacob V, Chattopadhyay SK, Sipe TA, Thota AB, Byard GJ, Chapman DP, et al. Economics of collaborative care for management of depressive disorders: a community guide systematic review. Am J Prev Med. 2012;42(5):539–49.
115. Cross DA, Qin X, Huckfeldt P, Jarosek S, Parsons H, Golberstein E. Use of medicare's behavioral health integration service codes in the first two years: an observational study. J Gen Intern Med. 2020;35(12):3745–6.
116. Brown JD, Urato C, Ogbuefi P. Uptake of Medicare behavioral health integration billing codes in 2017 and 2018. J Gen Intern Med. 2021;36(2):564–6.

117. Carlo AD, Corage Baden A, McCarty RL, Ratzliff ADH. Early Health System Experiences with Collaborative Care (CoCM) billing codes: a qualitative study of leadership and support staff. J Gen Intern Med. 2019;34(10):2150–8.
118. Advancing Integrated Mental Health Solutions (AIMS) Center. 2021. http://aims.uw.edu/.
119. The Organized. Evidence-based care: behavioral health integration guide. 2021. http://www.safetynetmedicalhome.org/change-concepts/organized-evidence-based-care/behavioral-health.
120. Substance Abuse and Mental Health Services Administration Integration tools. 2021. http://www.samhsa.gov/children/behavioral-health-care-integration-resources.
121. Integrated Care. 2021. https://www.psychiatry.org/psychiatrists/practice/professional-interests/integrated-care.
122. Ratzliff A, Phillips KE, Sugarman JR, Unützer J, Wagner EH. Practical approaches for achieving integrated behavioral health care in primary care settings. Am J Med Qual. 2017;32(2):117–21.
123. Davis M, Balasubramanian BA, Waller E, Miller BF, Green LA, Cohen DJ. Integrating behavioral and physical health care in the real world: early lessons from advancing care together. J Am Board Fam Med. 2013;26(5):588–602.
124. Cohen DJ, Balasubramanian BA, Davis M, Hall J, Gunn R, Stange KC, et al. Understanding care integration from the ground up: five organizing constructs that shape integrated practices. J Am Board Fam Med. 2015;28(Suppl 1):S7–20.
125. Cohen DJ, Davis M, Balasubramanian BA, Gunn R, Hall J, deGruy FV, et al. Integrating behavioral health and primary care: consulting, coordinating and collaborating among professionals. J Am Board Fam Med. 2015;28(Suppl 1):S21–31.
126. Hall J, Cohen DJ, Davis M, Gunn R, Blount A, Pollack DA, et al. Preparing the workforce for behavioral health and primary care integration. J Am Board Fam Med. 2015;28(Suppl 1):S41–51.
127. Gunn R, Davis MM, Hall J, Heintzman J, Muench J, Smeds B, et al. Designing clinical space for the delivery of integrated behavioral health and primary care. J Am Board Fam Med. 2015;28(Suppl 1):S52–62.
128. Cifuentes M, Davis M, Fernald D, Gunn R, Dickinson P, Cohen DJ. Electronic health record challenges, workarounds, and solutions observed in practices integrating behavioral health and primary care. J Am Board Fam Med. 2015;28(Suppl 1):S63–72.
129. Balasubramanian BA, Fernald D, Dickinson LM, Davis M, Gunn R, Crabtree BF, et al. REACH of interventions integrating primary care and behavioral health. J Am Board Fam Med. 2015;28(Suppl 1):S73–85.
130. Wallace NT, Cohen DJ, Gunn R, Beck A, Melek S, Bechtold D, et al. Start-up and ongoing practice expenses of behavioral health and primary care integration interventions in the advancing care together (ACT) program. J Am Board Fam Med. 2015;28(Suppl 1):S86–97.
131. Grazier KL, Smiley ML, Bondalapati KS. Overcoming barriers to integrating behavioral health and primary care services. J Prim Care Community Health. 2016;7(4):242–8.
132. Fisher L, Dickinson WP. Psychology and primary care: new collaborations for providing effective care for adults with chronic health conditions. Am Psychol. 2014;69(4):355–63.
133. McDaniel SH, Grus CL, Cubic BA, Hunter CL, Kearney LK, Schuman CC, et al. Competencies for psychology practice in primary care. Am Psychol. 2014;69(4):409–29.
134. Mitchell AJ, Vaze A, Rao S. Clinical diagnosis of depression in primary care: a meta-analysis. Lancet. 2009;374(9690):609–19.
135. Martin M, Allison L, Banks E, Bauman D, Harsh J, Cahill A, et al. Essential skills for family medicine residents practicing integrated behavioral health A Delphi study. Fam Med. 2019;51(3):227–33.
136. Hatfield D, McCullough L, Frantz SHB, Krieger K. Do we know when our clients get worse? an investigation of therapists' ability to detect negative client change. Clin Psychol Psychother. 2010;17(1):25–32.
137. Bleyel C, Hoffmann M, Wensing M, Hartmann M, Friederich H-C, Haun MW. Patients' perspective on mental health specialist video consultations in primary care: qualitative preimplementation study of anticipated benefits and barriers. J Med Internet Res. 2020;22(4):e17330.
138. Tully PJ, Baumeister H. Collaborative care for comorbid depression and coronary heart disease: a systematic review and meta-analysis of randomised controlled trials. BMJ Open. 2015;5(12):e009128.
139. Woltmann E, Grogan-Kaylor A, Perron B, Georges H, Kilbourne AM, Bauer MS. Comparative effectiveness of collaborative chronic care models for mental health conditions across primary, specialty, and behavioral health care settings: systematic review and meta-analysis. Am J Psychiatry. 2012;169(8):790–804.
140. McGregor B, Belton A, Henry TL, Wrenn G, Holden KB. Improving behavioral health equity through cultural competence training of health care providers. Ethn Dis. 2019;29(Suppl 2):359–64.
141. O'Loughlin K, Donovan EK, Radcliff Z, Ryan M, Rybarczyk B. Using integrated behavioral healthcare to address behavioral health disparities in underserved populations. Trans Issues Psychol Sci. 2019;5(4):374–89.
142. Martin MP, White MB, Hodgson JL, Lamson AL, Irons TG. Integrated primary care: a systematic review of program characteristics. Fam Syst Health. 2014;32(1):101–15.
143. CMS white paper on CMS Innovation Center's strategy: driving health system transformation—a strategy for the CMS Innovation Center's second decade. 2021. https://innovation.cms.gov/strategic-direction-whitepaper.
144. Bodenheimer T, Sinsky C. From triple to quadruple aim: care of the patient requires care of the provider. Ann Fam Med. 2014;12(6):573–6.
145. Berwick DM, Nolan TW, Whittington J. The triple aim: care, health, and cost. Health Aff (Millwood). 2008;27(3):759–69.

Transitions of Care

Catherine L. Coe, Mallory McClester Brown, and Christine E. Kistler

Introduction

With an aging population and advances in medical science, people with serious illness are living longer and chronic disease management for these patients now dominates the healthcare system. Approximately half of all adults in the United States (US) have a chronic disease [1]. Effective management for patients with chronic disease requires robust and ongoing coordination across various care settings from outpatient primary care to the hospital and skilled nursing facility. Fragmentation and discoordination of health care increase the risks to patient safety and are significant causes of inappropriate care and increased healthcare costs.

Due to their serious illnesses, patients with chronic disease are often hospitalized. "Readmission" is defined by the Centers for Medicare & Medicaid Services (CMS) as hospitalization within 30 days of discharge from a prior acute care admission to a hospital [2]. In 2018, the Healthcare Cost and Utilization Project reported a 30-day readmission rate of 14% for all payers. Patients with Medicare account for 60% of the reported readmissions costing approximately $35 billion for Medicare alone [3]. Poorly executed transitions of care negatively affect patients' health, well-being, and family resources, unnecessarily increase healthcare system costs [4], and raise the probability of readmission [5–7]. Medicare reimbursement penalties were instituted by the federal Patient Protection and Affordable Care Act for hospitals with high rates of readmissions, focusing attention on ways to reduce the risk of patients returning to the hospital soon after discharge [8]. Policymakers and providers recognize that avoiding rehospitalizations improves quality of care and reduces healthcare costs. Readmissions may be reduced by developing a system that is anticipatory and supportive across care settings, rather than reactionary.

Definition and History of Transitions of Care

Transitions of care is defined as the set of actions taken to ensure coordination and continuity of health care as patients are transferred across various care settings (Fig. 34.1) [9]. Transitions of care, when done well, considers the patient's safety, goals, and well-being, and reduces the use of resources by decreasing emergency room utilization and the need for rehospitalization, decreasing cost to the healthcare system and increasing patient, family, and provider satisfaction. As an example, consider a frail 70-year-old woman with heart failure who is admitted to the hospital for a hip fracture. If she tolerates the procedure, does not have post-operative complications, and stabilizes medically, her care will likely be transitioned to a skilled nursing facility (SNF) for rehabilitation. Once at the SNF, if she decompensates medically and becomes delirious, or has an exacerbation of her heart failure, she will likely be sent back to the emergency room and readmitted to the hospital. However, if her rehabilitation at the SNF progresses well without medical complications, she will successfully transition from the SNF to home with home health care and follow up with her primary care clinician and the orthopedic surgeon who performed the hip repair. This example shows the possible outcomes of a patient with chronic disease moving through the healthcare system, which involves multiple medical providers, various physical locations, and changing care settings. To ensure patients receive the best quality of care, each team of nurses, therapists, physicians, and social workers must work together to successfully transition patients from one care setting to the next which includes moving among healthcare venues as varied as hospitals, acute rehabilitation centers, skilled and subacute nursing facilities, long-term care facilities, assisted living homes, home with home health care, and hospice facilities.

C. L. Coe · M. M. Brown
Department of Family Medicine, University of North Carolina at Chapel Hill, Chapel Hill, NC, USA
e-mail: catherine_coe@med.unc.edu; mallory_mcclester@med.unc.edu

C. E. Kistler (✉)
Department of Family Medicine, University of North Carolina at Chapel Hill, Chapel Hill, NC, USA
e-mail: Christine_Kistler@med.unc.edu

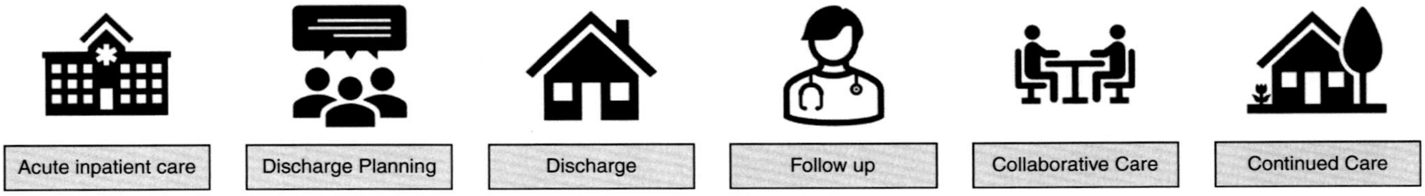

Fig. 34.1 Transitions of Care ensures coordination and continuity of health care as patients transfer across care settings

Table 34.1 Components of effective discharge planning, from the Project Reengineering Discharge program [12]

Components of patient and system navigation
1. Educate the patient about his or her diagnosis throughout the hospital stay
2. Make appointments for clinician follow-up and post-discharge testing
3. Discuss with the patient any tests or studies completed in the hospital and clarify who is responsible for following up the results
4. Organize post-discharge services
5. Confirm the medication plan
6. Reconcile the discharge plan with national guidelines and critical pathways
7. Review the appropriate steps to take if a problem arises
8. Expedite transmission of the discharge summary to the physicians (and other services such as home health nurses) responsible for the patient's care after discharge
9. Assess the degree of understanding by asking patient to explain the details of the plan
10. Give the patient a written plan at the time of discharge
11. Provide telephone reinforcement of the discharge plan and problem-solving 2–3 days after discharge

Table 34.2 Effective transitional care management after discharge [17]

Patient questions and care manager assessment during post-hospitalization phone call
1. Which healthcare facility were you discharged from?
2. How have you been feeling since your discharge from the hospital?
3. Do you have any questions about your discharge instructions?
4. Do you have any unanswered questions from your hospitalization?
5. What changes were made to your medications now that you are home?
6. In the judgment of the care manager, is a clinical pharmacist needed for this patient?
7. Do you have a primary care physician? (name and location)
8. Do you have a follow-up appointment with your primary care provider?
9. Do you have a follow-up appointment with another healthcare provider? (name and specialty)
10. Do you know the danger signs that would indicate that you need to call a healthcare provider?
11. Who is helping you now that you are out of the hospital?

Programs in Transitions of Care

Several landmark programs have demonstrated effective practices in transitions of care. The Care Transitions Intervention (CTI) utilizes a nurse transition coach who educates and empowers patients to better navigate their own care. The CTI emphasizes four "pillars": medication self-management, a patient-owned health record, follow-up with a primary care clinician or specialist, and awareness of "red flags." The intervention lowered 30- and 90-day readmission rates and reduced readmissions [10, 11].

Project Reengineering Discharge (RED), developed at Boston University, addresses both the system and patients' navigation of the discharge process through 11 mutually reinforcing components (Table 34.1) [12, 13]. When implemented in an urban university hospital, participants randomized to the intervention group had a lower rate of 30-day hospital utilization (emergency department visits and rehospitalizations) [11, 12, 14].

Project BOOST (Better Outcomes by Optimizing Safe Transitions) identifies high-risk older adult patients early in the admission process [15]. This program provides resources to optimize the hospital discharge process and minimize issues older patients face after leaving the hospital. There are five key elements: (1) a comprehensive intervention, (2) a comprehensive implementation guide, (3) longitudinal technical assistance (provides face-to-face training and a year of expert mentoring and coaching), (4) the BOOST collaborative, and (5) the BOOST data center. Incorporating health coaching into the patient teaching component of hospitalization allows patients to take an active role in self-care, allowing them to determine goals and readiness to make lifestyle changes.

Post-discharge multidisciplinary clinics reduce 30-day rehospitalization rates [16]. When staffed by a primary care clinician (physician or advanced practice provider), social worker, pharmacist, and nurse, these clinics provide significant cost savings in addition to the reduction in readmissions. A multicomponent Transitional Care Management (TCM) service from the University of Utah implemented by care managers (either nurses or social workers) included phone calls within 72 hours of discharge and primary care appointments within 1 week [17]. The TCM care manager asked 11 questions during the post-hospitalization phone call, which effectively reduced rehospitalization up to 180 days (Table 34.2).

In 2015, the Patient-Centered Outcomes Research Institute (PCORI) sponsored Project ACHIEVE (Achieving patient-centered Care and optimized Health In care transitions by

Fig. 34.2 Transitional care core components of the ACHIEVE project (Achieving patient-centered Care and optimized Health In care transitions by Evaluating the Value of Evidence) [18]

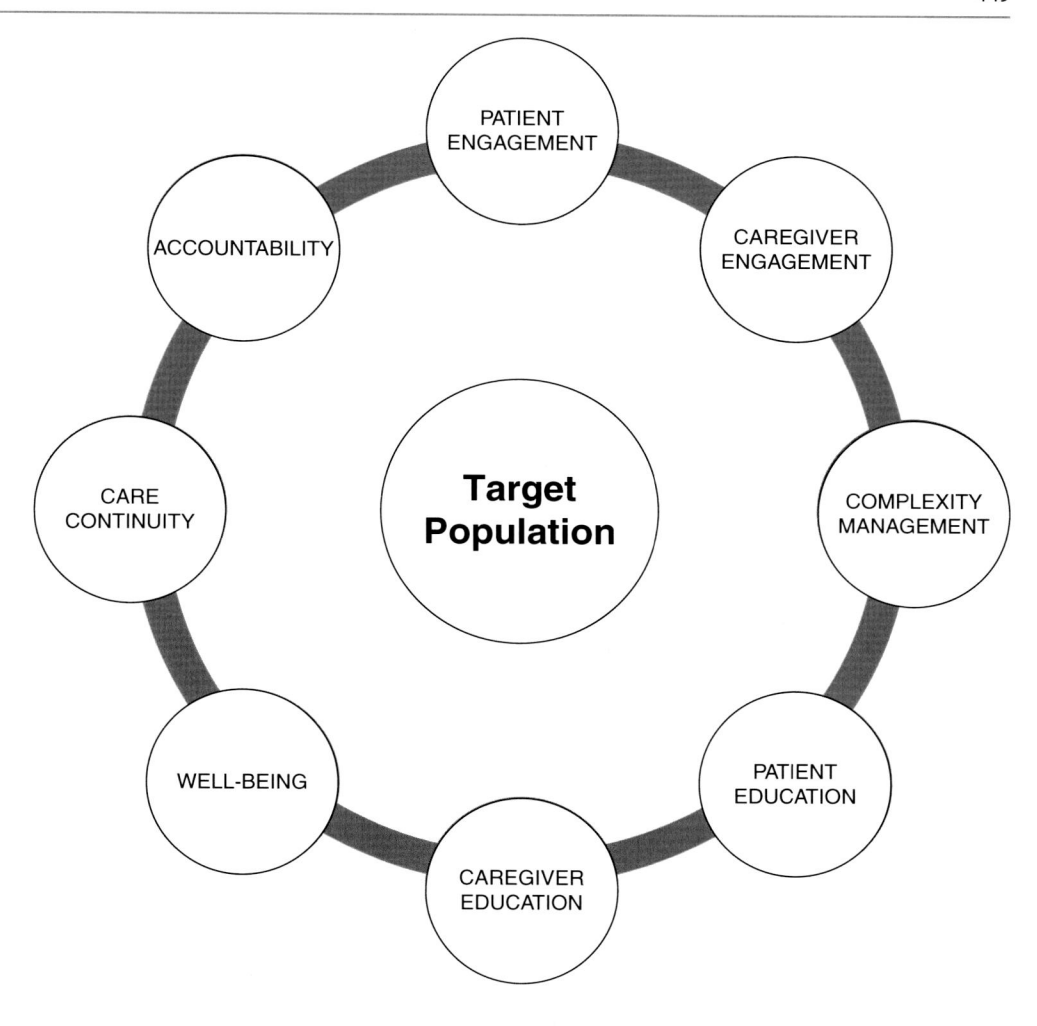

Evaluating the Value of Evidence) to evaluate key components of transitional care that support desired patient and caregiver outcomes (Fig. 34.2) [18]. The project concluded that each of the components should be considered when planning a transition of care to support patients and caregivers.

Finance and Transitions of Care

Transitional Care Management (TCM) payment codes were implemented by CMS in 2013 to encourage primary care clinics to provide transitions care services to patients leaving inpatient care and returning to their primary care providers, including Current Procedural Terminology (CPT) codes for billing (Table 34.3). Medicare beneficiaries who receive TCM from their primary care providers have lower mortality rates than those who do not [19, 20]. Despite evidence of reduced mortality and healthcare costs among TCM recipients, initial implementation was slow [19]. The federal Affordable Care Act initiated a Hospital Readmissions Reduction Program (HRRP) which went into effect on October 1, 2012, and applies financial penalties to hospitals with higher-than-expected readmission rates for targeted conditions [21]. This program was initially met with criticism given concerns that larger hospitals caring for disadvantaged and therefore sicker patients might shoulder more penalties, thereby decreasing resources available to improve quality. However, a large retrospective cohort study of 2823 US hospitals participating in HRRP found that penalty incentives associated with HRRP were associated with fewer readmissions [22].

Table 34.3 Current Procedural Terminology (CPT) Codes for Transitional Care Management

CPT Code 99495	Transitional Care Management services with the required elements: Medical decision making of at least moderate complexity during the service period; face-to-face visit within 14 calendar days of discharge
CPT Code 99496	Transitional Care Management services with the required elements: Medical decision making of high complexity during the service period; Face-to-face visit within 7 calendar days of discharge

CMS TCM payment codes provide coverage for services rendered during the 30-day period following discharge from an inpatient acute care, psychiatric, or long-term care hospital, or an inpatient rehabilitation or skilled nursing facility [23]. It can also include discharge from hospital outpatient observation units or partial hospitalization, including at a community mental health center. It does not include discharge from the emergency department. Patients must be discharged to a community setting, either home, group home, long-term care nursing home, or assisted living facility. Dialysis codes, anticoagulant codes, and chronic care management codes can be billed in addition to the TCM codes.

There are several requirements for TCM payment. First, within two business days of discharge, a medical provider or clinical staff member must contact the discharged patient or their caregiver via phone, email, or face-to-face encounter. If two or more attempts occur in a timely manner and are documented in the medical record, even if unsuccessful, these attempts will count toward this contact requirement. Certain non-face-to-face services must also be rendered which include review of discharge information, need for follow-up tests/treatments, education of the patient/caregiver, execution of referrals, and community provider follow-up. To complete the process, a face-to-face visit is required within 7 or 14 days depending on the complexity of the medical decision making. Decision making is considered more complex if the patient has multiple comorbidities and diagnoses, with extensive data and testing to review. This visit may be conducted in a video format but cannot be a telephone encounter. At a minimum, the encounter must document the dates of discharge, first contact after discharge, and the face-to-face visit, and describe the complexity of medical decision making (moderate or high).

Effective Transitions of Care

Planning for a TCM visit begins while a patient is in the hospital. As part of the Medicare conditions of participation, hospitals are required to employ and document a discharge planning process for all patients and must identify those who are likely to suffer adverse health consequences after discharge in the absence of adequate discharge planning. Due to increasing pressure to shorten the length of a hospital stay, patients are less likely to stay hospitalized until they feel "better," as was the case in the past. Decreasing length of stays leave limited time for educating patients and families in the hospital [24].

Anticipating and Preventing Reasons for Readmission

The success or failure of transitions of care management in preventing rehospitalizations depends on the nature of the intervention, the setting of implementation, and the population of patients [25]. Many tools exist to predict hospital readmission but inconsistencies in the data prevent the understanding of which risk factors are most predictive [4]. Older age, prior hospitalization, poor family or social support, low health literacy, high medication burden, and numerous specific medical conditions increase the likelihood of readmission (Table 34.4) [9, 26].

In addition to these risk factors, readmissions have other causes that are harder to measure and ameliorate including poor communication, misunderstandings of instructions during hospitalization or at discharge, lack of transportation to access medicines or post-discharge health care, inadequate patient comprehension of diagnoses and follow-up needs, and failure to complete planned outpatient diagnostic or treatment plans [27]. The risk of readmission is highest in the transition of care period shortly after discharge. This period is when medication errors are most likely to occur and intended or pending tests are not followed up (outpatient test recommended but did not take place). Avoidable rehospitalizations are often due to poor communication between hospital physicians and the clinician seeing the patient after discharge or between the discharge team and the patient. Patients often do not understand risks and benefits of medication changes, when they can resume normal activity, what questions they should ask, and warning signs for which they should watch. Discharging patients from the hospital with

Table 34.4 Risk factors for readmission

Category	Examples
Medical history	Prior hospital stays Extensive medication list Poor compliance
Medical condition	Heart disease History of stroke Diabetes Cancer Depression Multimorbidity
Physical function	Requires caregiver for assistance with activities of daily living (ADLs)
Mental health function	Cognitive impairment
Social determinants of health	Inadequate social support Inadequate preparation from caregivers Poor health literacy Medicare/Medicaid ineligible

intravenous access lines, complex wound care, enteral feeding devices, urinary catheters, surgical drains, or other invasive devices is complicated and can lead to readmission if the patient is not prepared or managed appropriately [24].

Interventions to reduce readmissions are classified by timing (pre-discharge, post-discharge, or bridging interventions that start before discharge and continue afterwards) and use several methods such as discharge planning protocols, comprehensive assessments, discharge support arrangements, and educational interventions [8]. Single discharge planning components do not decrease hospital readmissions, rather multicomponent, comprehensive interventions and wholistic approaches yield the highest and most durable degree of reduction [11].

Table 34.5 Key components of the discharge summary for a patient with risk factors for readmission

Risk factors for readmission	Discharge summary component
History of hospitalization	Chief complaint, reasons for admission Medical hospital course
Medical condition	Medication list, including changes
Physical functional impairment	Functional status (ADLs, IADLs) Therapy needs Durable medical equipment
Mental health functional impairment	Advance directives Overall goals of care
Social determinants of health	Typical residence Primary caregiver, support at home Transportation needs

Pre-discharge Transitional Care Management

Pre-discharge transitional care management begins during hospitalization and includes patient education and other efforts. It starts with the work involved in the discharge summary and medication reconciliation. It also ensures appropriate care such as durable medical equipment (DME), infusions, and transportation are available at discharge [9, 28]. Collaborating with the outpatient provider during hospitalization and asking the patient and caregiver's preference for appointment scheduling after discharge helps optimize outpatient follow-up care [29, 30].

Patient Education
In the State Action on Avoidable Rehospitalizations (STAAR) trial, a hospital discharge nurse, pharmacist, or social worker identified patients at high risk for readmission and ensured thorough discharge planning including educating the patient prior to discharge [31]. Nurses developed a systematic way of providing discharge information to the patient, with a folder that included information about the patient's care team, follow-up appointments, and treatment plan, with educational materials specifically tailored for the patient. Patients were also encouraged to write down their questions, to be answered by the nurse prior to discharge. The discharge nurse also led discussions at multidisciplinary rounds including reaching consensus on the estimated day of discharge for the patient.

Discharge Summary
As a key mode of communication bridging care from the hospital to the next setting, the discharge summary can provide a clear, organized, and complete story of the hospitalization, functional limitations, medications, and patient education (Table 34.5) [30]. Medication reconciliation including any discontinued medications, new medications, or changes in medication dosing or frequency is an important part of this process, as medication errors or effects are a leading cause of readmission [32]. Education at discharge helps the patient and caregiver understand the relevant disease process, the events during the hospitalization, medication changes, expected follow-up, and who to contact if concerns arise. For higher-risk patients, a "coach" improves self-management skills [10, 30].

Some practices will send a liaison from the practice to the hospital to help coordinate care by sharing information about the patient with the hospital team, alerting the practice of the admission along with the anticipated date of discharge, and ensuring that the practice anticipates post-discharge issues and provides timely follow-up [4].

Medications
A thorough assessment of the patient's discharge medications and potential barriers promotes safety and is often performed by the team pharmacist. Compounded or special medications needed for post-discharge use my require special effort to ensure the medications are ready at discharge, such as running test claims to see if insurance prior-authorization is needed. Other helpful efforts include sending medication refills to a home-delivery pharmacy, training on the use of complicated medications such as insulin, inhalers, or intravenous infusions, and education on side effects or adverse reactions. Addressing each of these potential barriers helps avoid medication non-adherence or incorrect dosing following discharge [33].

Durable Medical Equipment
If consulted during hospitalization, the physical, occupational, and respiratory therapy teams will provide an

assessment of the patient's ability to care for themselves at home and recommend durable medical equipment (DME), including oxygen. If the patient requires skilled nursing facility care or home health therapy services, this should be identified prior to discharge. If homebound, assessment for needed DME ensures that the patient and caregivers keep the patient safe while facilitating continued recovery. Obtaining DME requires orders, documentation of necessity, and coordination with insurance companies, and streamlining this process while the patient is in the hospital will improve the transition process and prevent readmissions [34].

Some patients have chronic, serious illnesses that require additional care following discharge such as heart failure, wounds, or conditions requiring intravenous medications. Prior to discharge, the transition team should make arrangements for any needed supplies, remote monitoring equipment, or licensed professionals to help with the care or administration of medications. Sometimes a patient's family or caregiver can render the needed services once trained by either the pre-discharge or post-discharge nurses. In most cases, a small quantity of supplies should be provided pre-discharge and arrangements made for timely post-discharge provision of all necessary equipment.

Transportation

Transportation needs should be assessed prior to discharge, including the immediate transport to the next level of care as well as transportation to needed follow-up appointments. For hospital discharge, care managers can arrange either basic or advanced life support ambulance services depending on the patient's care needs. A wheelchair van is another option if family or friends are unable to provide transportation. Patients may qualify for assistance with transportation that the inpatient care managers or post-discharge TCM team members can facilitate.

Post-discharge Transitional Care Management

Post-discharge components of TCM interventions include telephone calls, hotlines, home visits, and timely outpatient follow-up, all of which further reduce the likelihood of rehospitalization than inpatient interventions alone [25].

Phone Calls

Follow-up telephone calls have been studied with and without a script. A script may include plans for follow-up, discussion of new symptoms, and review of medication availability [9]. In addition to the pre-discharge components in the STAAR trial, post-discharge phone calls from a STAAR pharmacist found that 52% of patients deviated from medication instructions after leaving the hospital which included patients continuing on medications that had been discontinued during the hospitalization, using over-the-counter medications that were not mentioned during the hospitalization, and confusion regarding proper dosing instructions for medications that were initiated or changed at discharge [31]. The highest risk patients benefit from close follow-up which can include a phone call, a home health visit, or an office visit within 48 h, all of which can reduce the risk of rehospitalization. Post-hospitalization phone calls are a cost-effective readmission prevention strategy [4, 7]. These phone calls should include asking the patient if they have filled their prescriptions, ensuring the patient knows how and when to take the medications, discussing the patient's understanding of critical elements of self-care, reviewing why, when, and how to recognize worsening symptoms, when and whom to call for help, and confirming the date and time of the follow-up physician appointment as well as ensuring adequate transportation [4].

Follow-Up Visits

Outpatient follow-up is best if provided with the patient's primary care clinician as the risk of readmission is higher when patients see an unfamiliar provider [27]. Follow-up appointments with the primary care clinician are especially effective in decreasing readmissions if scheduled within 1–2 weeks of discharge. Timely appointments require good communication between the inpatient team and the outpatient clinician's office. In one study, only 44% of Medicare beneficiaries had a follow-up visit within 7 days of discharge [35]. In addition to timeliness, other key components of a successful hospital follow-up office visit include preparing the patient and the office clinical team before the visit, assessing the patient and initiating a new care plan or revising the existing care plan during the visit, reviewing the patient's health-related goals, and communicating and coordinating the ongoing care plan at the conclusion of the visit with the patient and the care team [4]. The patient should be asked about factors that contributed to the hospitalization or emergency department visit and correct modifiable factors that might reduce the likelihood of a future admission. The medications should be reviewed again to reduce medication errors and increase compliance with an updated medication list printed for them. Follow-up labs, tests, and discussion of the need for additional work-up should also be addressed. The patient's understanding of the plan is assessed and reviewed in language they can understand along with the opportunity to ask questions. The visit should end with agreed-upon goals of self-management, a scheduled follow-up visit, and instructions on reasons to return earlier. Checklists can help with post-hospital follow-up visits [4]. Note templates can also be created in the electronic medical record to standardize the visit and ensure consistent high-quality TCM care.

Primary care TCM programs are beneficial even for patients with serious illness. Cancer patients did not have more recurrence or death when seen in follow-up by their primary care clinicians versus their oncologist and had higher patient satisfaction [36, 37]. Heart failure patients have similar rates of readmissions or deaths whether seen by a primary care clinician versus a specialist in heart failure [38]. Populations that likely benefit from specialty care TCM include seriously ill pediatric patients or those with severe persistent mental illness, though definitive research on this is lacking.

Bridging Components of Transitional Care Management

Bridging TCM interventions are provided during a vulnerable time and educate, empower, and activate the patient regarding self-care. Useful strategies include coaches, and provider continuity across the inpatient to outpatient transition. One of the oldest bridging programs was developed in the 1990s and utilizes an advanced practice provider (APP) who conducts an in-hospital assessment and a home visit within 24 h of discharge, followed by weekly visits, including one primary care visit [39]. For higher-risk patients, a "coach" is helpful in improving the patient's self-management skills [10, 30]. A transition coach bridges between the inpatient setting where efforts focus on disease-specific education and assessment of social needs to the outpatient setting where the coach focuses on medication adherence, ambulatory follow-up, and symptom monitoring.

Another approach involves home-based medical programs devoted to transitions of care. The Mayo clinic's program identifies and meets with high-risk patients prior to discharge and continues to follow them for 180 days post-hospitalization with a multidisciplinary team including an APP providing direct in-home care and pharmacy, nursing, specialty geriatrics, and palliative medicine support remotely [40]. All three of these programs show improvements in rehospitalization, cost-savings, and patient-centered outcomes. A similar program for homebound older adults that included an APP who conducted in hospital and post-discharge visits improved communication but did not change length of stay or rehospitalization rates [41].

Evidence is scarce to support any one strategy over another for reducing the likelihood of readmissions [8]. Single interventions, when evaluated in isolation, have not consistently demonstrated statistically significant changes in readmission rates. Even when interventions are bundled, there is no consistent solution to decreasing readmissions. Still, there is agreement that a multidisciplinary approach to care coordination must be a part of ongoing efforts to reduce avoidable readmissions [25, 42].

Advance Care Planning

Hospitalized patients with serious illness may benefit from advance care planning. A change in condition requiring hospitalization provides an opportunity to discuss goals of care and personal priorities. The inpatient team should elicit patient and family values and goals, understand their fears and worries, explore trade-offs in quantity and quality of life, determine a healthcare proxy, and discuss prognosis [43]. Sometimes patients need time to process their hospitalization in the context of their serious illness, making the post-discharge TCM visit an ideal time to discuss the experience and their wishes for repeat hospitalization. Hospice should be discussed if prognostically appropriate and congruent with patient's values [44].

Paperwork can be completed during hospitalizations or post-discharge, including forms that designate the healthcare power of attorney. Living wills and documents such as the Physician Orders for Life-Sustaining Treatment (POLST) provide a framework for medical preferences for patients with serious illness [45]. Clinicians should sign *Do Not Resuscitate* (DNR) forms for those patients who express this preference. These forms should be readily available and, in the case of a DNR form, travel with the patient upon discharge.

Interprofessional Approach to Transitions of Care

In 2013, almost 42% of Medicare patients were discharged from a hospital stay to a nursing home or rehabilitation facility [46]. Transitioning from one place of care to the next increases the likelihood that vital information will be lost, and care plans will be fragmented [9]. To address this, many healthcare systems have instituted TCM programs that recognize that discharges from the hospital are most successful when a team-based approach is taken, including the physician/APP, nurse, pharmacist, case manager, patient, and family/caregiver.

While many hospitals have a discharge planning team to facilitate the transitions from the hospital, not all primary care settings have a dedicated TCM program. However, a primary care nested interprofessional transition-of-care clinic is associated with reduced hospital readmissions [47]. Clear communication is essential for effective interprofessional teams [48]. Several standardized communication tools exist and many utilize the TeamSTEPPS approach (Team Strategies and Tools to Enhance Performance and Patient Safety) [49]. Supported by the Agency for Healthcare Research and Quality (AHRQ), TeamSTEPPS is an evidence-based system to improve communication and teamwork skills among healthcare professionals [50].

Physician and Advance Practice Provider Role

Physicians and APPs play an important role on the discharge planning team, informing the team on the timing and needs of discharge. The hospital physician is often the one who contacts the patient's primary care physician for input on medical history as well as updating them on the patient's progress. A complete discharge summary available in a timely manner is an important role of the physician and includes several key pieces of information that can reduce the risk of readmission. At the time of discharge a "warm-handoff" to the receiving outpatient provider (clinic or SNF) improves clear communication of the admission and discharge planning and shares items for follow-up [51].

Nurse Role

During a patient's hospitalization, the nursing staff is most often present at the bedside and providing integral insight into the patient's hospitalization. The discharging team should incorporate the nursing assessment and evaluation of trajectory during discharge planning including any nursing needs when the patient transitions to next level of care, or to home, such as assistance with wound management, intravenous antibiotic administration, daily weights, blood pressure monitoring, and medication management [52]. Nurses can answer patients' medical questions and serve as a liaison between the patient and the primary care clinic.

Pharmacist Role

In most inpatient settings, a pharmacist works with the providers throughout care, and in planning for discharge. The pharmacist anticipates medication issues and changes, educates the patient on the recommended medication regimen prior to discharge, reconciles the medications on the day of discharge, and provides counseling and a discussion about barriers to adherence [53]. Many healthcare systems have developed and implemented a medication delivery program where discharge medications are delivered to the patient's bedside prior to discharge [54]. When paired with a pharmacist, these programs reduce readmission rates [55]. Once discharged, community pharmacists and embedded clinical pharmacists evaluate adherence and access to medications, and make adjustments as needed. These actions are both feasible and beneficial [56]. Visits with the pharmacist can continue after the TCM visit to provide ongoing management of chronic conditions, such as diabetes or anticoagulation.

Social Worker Role

Hospital-based case managers, most of whom are social workers, have an important role in the discharge process. Case managers can uncover psychosocial issues or other causes that likely contributed to an admission or readmission. These members of the team are often best equipped to determine the level of care the patient entered the hospital with and to advise on the appropriate services needed at discharge [57]. Once identified, the case manager can coordinate delivery of durable medical equipment (DME) and medications, and arrange home-based services or transportation. In the outpatient setting, the post-discharge TCM case manager can ensure delivery of the intended services and assess for new needs. Although many needs can be anticipated prior to discharge, there often arise unexpected challenges with access to medications, nutrition, transportation, or assistance with activities of daily living that patients and caregivers need assistance navigating [58]. They can assist in the completion of forms for CMS-qualifying home aids and schedule follow-up as needed.

Medical Assistant Role

For patients who desire to remain at home despite needing additional care and support, certified nursing assistants are a helpful resource. Many times, however, insurance limits the number of hours that a patient may receive this service, limiting the availability as patients transition out of the hospital. Local health departments may provide home aids, but these services have specific regulations and are often limited in availability and coverage.

Physical and Occupational Therapist Roles

Hospitalizations can promote debility, particularly in chronically ill and older populations [59]. The transition out of the hospital might find them weaker and more dependent on others than when they entered. A thorough assessment of their physical strength and ability to complete ADLs should occur as a part of the discharge planning process. The physical and occupational therapy teams can assess what additional therapy resources and DME a patient might need when transitioning out of the hospital. After discharge, the patients will transition to outpatient therapists who will continue the plan of care and rehabilitation. They can also provide recommendations for DME best suited to the home and ask for other types of therapy such as speech therapy, when indicated.

Family and Patient Role

The patient and the family also play an important role in the discharge process. They help in deciding the next location of the patient's care, when follow-up will occur, and who to contact if a problem arises. They must also understand the updated medication list, when and how to take the medications, and potential side effects. Ideally, they can describe a system for taking their medication prior to discharge. It is also important to ensure that the patient and family have some understanding of the reason for admission and the diagnosis [9].

Disparities in Transitions of Care

Racial and Ethnic Disparities

Several studies have demonstrated disparities in care among non-White hospitalized patients. When patients are discharged and require post-discharge analgesia, African American patients are less likely to receive opioid medication and for shorter durations than White patients and Asian patients were more likely to receive opioid pain medication than White patients [60]. After a total knee replacement, African American patients had a higher likelihood of discharge to a SNF and were more likely to be readmitted within 90 days [61]. In a study of Medicare fee-for-service beneficiaries, post-discharge follow-up within 7 days lowered risk for readmission, however, Non-Hispanic Black beneficiaries had a higher risk for readmission [35]. A national study also identified a higher likelihood for readmission among African American and Hispanic patients, compared to White patients, even within the same SNF facility [62]. Racial/ethnic disparities exist in transitions of care patterns and hospice use during the last 6 months of life for Medicare beneficiaries, with African American patients more likely to have multiple transitions of care during this time compared to White patients while Hispanic and Asian American patients were more likely to die without any transitions [63]. Efforts to ensure seamless transitions of care for African American patients and timely education and promotion of end-of-life options for Hispanic and Asian American patients are urgently needed.

Language Barriers

Patients who speak little or no English have additional barriers to a safe and comprehensive transition of care following discharge. Patients with limited English proficiency are more likely to report a problem with post-discharge issues compared to English proficient patients [64]. Post-discharge issues included difficulty obtaining prescriptions, medication concerns, questions about follow-up care, and new or worsening symptoms. To decrease or minimize the barriers related to limited English proficiency, a trained medical interpreter (in-person, video, or telephone) should be made available to the patient to review the discharge plan. Family or friends should not be relied upon as interpreters, rather medically trained language professionals should be available in a timely fashion. A post-discharge outreach program using an interpreter can help identify and remedy post-discharge issues [64].

Future Directions

Future efforts to improve TCM should include a patient-centered and patient-desired approach to improve outcomes [65]. The future of TCM will need to be flexible to address all spheres of care including transitions to home, nursing facilities, and assisted living facilities, with palliative care options available. Novel integration of the use of telehealth, mobile apps, or remote monitoring to reduce rehospitalizations shows promise, though their feasibility and improvement of outcomes such as readmission or death have yet to be determined [66–68]. As payment for healthcare transitions to a value-based model, even greater attention will need to be paid to the transition points to ensure optimal, cost-effective, and safe patient care.

References

1. Buttorff C, Ruder T, Bauman M. Multiple Chronic Conditions in the United States. RAND Corporation. https://www.rand.org/content/dam/rand/pubs/tools/TL200/TL221/RAND_TL221.pdf. Accessed 19 Jan 2022.
2. Adams CJ, Stephens K, Whiteman K, Kersteen H, Katruska J. Implementation of the Re-Engineered Discharge (RED) toolkit to decrease all-cause readmission rates at a rural community hospital. Qual Manag Health Care. 2014;23(3):169–77. https://doi.org/10.1097/QMH.0000000000000032.
3. Weiss AJ, Jiang HJ. Overview of clinical conditions with frequent and costly hospital readmissions by payer, 2018: statistical brief #278. In: Healthcare cost and utilization project (HCUP) statistical briefs. Rockville (MD): Agency for Healthcare Research and Quality (US); 2006.
4. Schall M, Coleman E, Rutherford P, Taylor J. How-to guide: improving transitions from the hospital to the clinical office practice to reduce avoidable rehospitalizations. Cambridge: Institute for Healthcare Improvement; 2011.
5. Peter D, Robinson P, Jordan M, Lawrence S, Casey K, Salas-Lopez D. Reducing readmissions using teach-back: enhancing patient and family education. J Nurs Adm. 2015;45(1):35–42. https://doi.org/10.1097/NNA.0000000000000155.
6. Peikes D, Chen A, Schore J, Brown R. Effects of care coordination on hospitalization, quality of care, and health care expenditures among Medicare beneficiaries: 15 randomized trials. JAMA. 2009;301(6):603–18. https://doi.org/10.1001/jama.2009.126.

7. Jencks SF, Williams MV, Coleman EA. Rehospitalizations among patients in the Medicare fee-for-service program. N Engl J Med. 2009;360(14):1418–28. https://doi.org/10.1056/NEJMsa0803563.
8. McCoy KA, Bear-Pfaffendof K, Foreman JK, et al. Reducing avoidable hospital readmissions effectively: a statewide campaign. Jt Comm J Qual Patient Saf. 2014;40(5):198–204. https://doi.org/10.1016/s1553-7250(14)40026-6.
9. Halter JB, Ouslander JG, Tinetti ME, Studenski S, High KP. Hazzard's geriatric medicine and gerontology. 6th ed. McGraw Hill; 2009.
10. Coleman EA, Smith JD, Frank JC, Min S-J, Parry C, Kramer AM. Preparing patients and caregivers to participate in care delivered across settings: the Care Transitions Intervention. J Am Geriatr Soc. 2004;52(11):1817–25. https://doi.org/10.1111/j.1532-5415.2004.52504.x.
11. Kripalani S, Theobald CN, Anctil B, Vasilevskis EE. Reducing hospital readmission rates: current strategies and future directions. Annu Rev Med. 2014;65:471–85. https://doi.org/10.1146/annurev-med-022613-090415.
12. Jack BW, Chetty VK, Anthony D, et al. A reengineered hospital discharge program to decrease rehospitalization: a randomized trial. Ann Intern Med. 2009;150(3):178–87. https://doi.org/10.7326/0003-4819-150-3-200902030-00007.
13. Jack BW, Paasche-Orlow MK, Mitchell SM, Forsythe S. An overview of the Re-Engineered Discharge (RED) toolkit. Prepared by Boston University under Contract No HHSA290200600012i. Agency for Healthcare Research and Quality: Rockville, MD; 2013.
14. Greenwald JL, Denham CR, Jack BW. The hospital discharge. J Patient Saf. 2007;3(2):97–106. https://doi.org/10.1097/01.jps.0000236916.94696.12.
15. Enderlin CA, McLeskey N, Rooker JL, et al. Review of current conceptual models and frameworks to guide transitions of care in older adults. Geriatr Nurs. 2013;34(1):47–52. https://doi.org/10.1016/j.gerinurse.2012.08.003.
16. Baldwin SM, Zook S, Sanford J. Implementing posthospital interprofessional care team visits to improve care transitions and decrease hospital readmission rates. Prof Case Manag. 2018;23(5):264–71. https://doi.org/10.1097/NCM.0000000000000284.
17. Farrell TW, Tomoaia-Cotisel A, Scammon DL, et al. Impact of an integrated transition management program in primary care on hospital readmissions. J Healthc Qual. 2015;37(1):81–92. https://doi.org/10.1097/01.JHQ.0000460119.68190.98.
18. Naylor MD, Shaid EC, Carpenter D, et al. Components of comprehensive and effective transitional care. J Am Geriatr Soc. 2017;65(6):1119–25. https://doi.org/10.1111/jgs.14782.
19. Bindman AB, Cox DF. Changes in health care costs and mortality associated with transitional care management services after a discharge among Medicare beneficiaries. JAMA Intern Med. 2018;178(9):1165–71. https://doi.org/10.1001/jamainternmed.2018.2572.
20. Agarwal SD, Barnett ML, Souza J, Landon BE. Adoption of Medicare's transitional care management and chronic care management codes in primary care. JAMA. 2018;320(24):2596–7. https://doi.org/10.1001/jama.2018.16116.
21. Zuckerman RB, Sheingold SH, Orav EJ, Ruhter J, Epstein AM. Readmissions, observation, and the hospital readmissions reduction program. N Engl J Med. 2016;374(16):1543–51. https://doi.org/10.1056/NEJMsa1513024.
22. Hoffman GJ, Yakusheva O. Association between financial incentives in Medicare's hospital readmissions reduction program and hospital readmission performance. JAMA Netw Open. 2020;3(4):e202044. https://doi.org/10.1001/jamanetworkopen.2020.2044.
23. Transitional Care Management Services. Centers for Medicare and Medicaid Services. 2021. https://www.cms.gov/Outreach-and-Education/Medicare-Learning-Network-MLN/MLNProducts/Downloads/Transitional-Care-Management-Services-Fact-Sheet-ICN908628.pdf. Accessed 13 Jan 2022.
24. Stevens S. Preventing 30-day readmissions. Nurs Clin North Am. 2015;50(1):123–37. https://doi.org/10.1016/j.cnur.2014.10.010.
25. Hansen LO, Young RS, Hinami K, Leung A, Williams MV. Interventions to reduce 30-day rehospitalization: a systematic review. Ann Intern Med. 2011;155(8):520–8. https://doi.org/10.7326/0003-4819-155-8-201110180-00008.
26. Kansagara D, Chiovaro JC, Kagen D, et al. So many options, where do we start? An overview of the care transitions literature. J Hosp Med. 2016;11(3):221–30. https://doi.org/10.1002/jhm.2502.
27. Weinberger M, Oddone EZ, Henderson WG. Does increased access to primary care reduce hospital readmissions? Veterans Affairs Cooperative Study Group on Primary Care and Hospital Readmission. N Engl J Med. 1996;334(22):1441–7. https://doi.org/10.1056/NEJM199605303342206.
28. Davidson GH, Austin E, Thornblade L, et al. Improving transitions of care across the spectrum of healthcare delivery: a multidisciplinary approach to understanding variability in outcomes across hospitals and skilled nursing facilities. Am J Surg. 2017;213(5):910–4. https://doi.org/10.1016/j.amjsurg.2017.04.002.
29. Naylor M, Brooten D, Jones R, Lavizzo-Mourey R, Mezey M, Pauly M. Comprehensive discharge planning for the hospitalized elderly. A randomized clinical trial. Ann Intern Med. 1994;120(12):999–1006. https://doi.org/10.7326/0003-4819-120-12-199406150-00005.
30. Burke RE, Kripalani S, Vasilevskis EE, Schnipper JL. Moving beyond readmission penalties: creating an ideal process to improve transitional care. J Hosp Med. 2013;8(2):102–9. https://doi.org/10.1002/jhm.1990.
31. Carter JA, Carr LS, Collins J, et al. STAAR: improving the reliability of care coordination and reducing hospital readmissions in an academic medical centre. BMJ Innov. 2015;1(3):75–80. https://doi.org/10.1136/bmjinnov-2015-000048.
32. Forster AJ, Murff HJ, Peterson JF, Gandhi TK, Bates DW. The incidence and severity of adverse events affecting patients after discharge from the hospital. Ann Intern Med. 2003;138(3):161–7. https://doi.org/10.7326/0003-4819-138-3-200302040-00007.
33. Redmond P, Grimes TC, McDonnell R, Boland F, Hughes C, Fahey T. Impact of medication reconciliation for improving transitions of care. Cochrane Database Syst Rev. 2018;8:CD010791. https://doi.org/10.1002/14651858.CD010791.pub2.
34. Teel J, Wang JY, Loschiavo M. Durable medical equipment: a streamlined approach. Fam Pract Manag. 2021;28(2):15–20.
35. Anderson A, Mills CW, Willits J, et al. Follow-up post-discharge and readmission disparities among Medicare fee-for-service beneficiaries, 2018. J Gen Intern Med. 2022;37(12):3020–8. https://doi.org/10.1007/s11606-022-07488-3.
36. Grunfeld E, Levine MN, Julian JA, et al. Randomized trial of long-term follow-up for early-stage breast cancer: a comparison of family physician versus specialist care. J Clin Oncol. 2006;24(6):848–55. https://doi.org/10.1200/JCO.2005.03.2235.
37. Grunfeld E, Fitzpatrick R, Mant D, et al. Comparison of breast cancer patient satisfaction with follow-up in primary care versus specialist care: results from a randomized controlled trial. Br J Gen Pract. 1999;49(446):705–10.
38. Luttik MLA, Jaarsma T, van Geel PP, et al. Long-term follow-up in optimally treated and stable heart failure patients: primary care vs. heart failure clinic. Results of the COACH-2 study. Eur J Heart Fail. 2014;16(11):1241–8. https://doi.org/10.1002/ejhf.173.
39. Naylor MD, Brooten D, Campbell R, et al. Comprehensive discharge planning and home follow-up of hospitalized elders: a randomized clinical trial. JAMA. 1999;281(7):613–20. https://doi.org/10.1001/jama.281.7.613.

40. Takahashi PY, Leppin AL, Hanson GJ. Hospital to community transitions for older adults: an update for the practicing clinician. Mayo Clin Proc. 2020;95(10):2253–62. https://doi.org/10.1016/j.mayocp.2020.02.001.
41. Ornstein K, Smith KL, Foer DH, Lopez-Cantor MT, Soriano T. To the hospital and back home again: a nurse practitioner-based transitional care program for hospitalized homebound people. J Am Geriatr Soc. 2011;59(3):544–51. https://doi.org/10.1111/j.1532-5415.2010.03308.x.
42. Leppin AL, Gionfriddo MR, Kessler M, et al. Preventing 30-day hospital readmissions: a systematic review and meta-analysis of randomized trials. JAMA Intern Med. 2014;174(7):1095–107. https://doi.org/10.1001/jamainternmed.2014.1608.
43. Bernacki RE, Block SD. American College of Physicians High Value Care Task Force. Communication about serious illness care goals: a review and synthesis of best practices. JAMA Intern Med. 2014;174(12):1994–2003. https://doi.org/10.1001/jamainternmed.2014.5271.
44. Electronic Code of Federal Regulations. Title 42, Chapter IV, Subchapter B, Part 418. Hospice Care. 2017. https://www.ecfr.gov/current/title-42/chapter-IV/subchapter-B/part-418. Accessed 25 Jan 2022.
45. Hickman SE, Keevern E, Hammes BJ. Use of the physician orders for life-sustaining treatment program in the clinical setting: a systematic review of the literature. J Am Geriatr Soc. 2015;63(2):341–50. https://doi.org/10.1111/jgs.13248.
46. Tian W. An All-Payer View of Hospital Discharge to Postacute Care, 2013: Statistical Brief #205. In: Healthcare Cost and Utilization Project (HCUP) Statistical Briefs. Rockville, MD: Agency for Healthcare Research and Quality (US); 2006.
47. Nall RW, Herndon BB, Mramba LK, Vogel-Anderson K, Hagen MG. An interprofessional primary care-based transition of care clinic to reduce hospital readmission. Am J Med. 2020;133(6):e260–8. https://doi.org/10.1016/j.amjmed.2019.10.040.
48. Scotten M, Manos EL, Malicoat A, Paolo AM. Minding the gap: interprofessional communication during inpatient and post discharge chasm care. Patient Educ Couns. 2015;98(7):895–900. https://doi.org/10.1016/j.pec.2015.03.009.
49. Chen AS, Yau B, Revere L, Swails J. Implementation, evaluation, and outcome of TeamSTEPPS in interprofessional education: a scoping review. J Interprof Care. 2019;33(6):795–804. https://doi.org/10.1080/13561820.2019.1594729.
50. About TeamSTEPPS | Agency for Healthcare Research and Quality. https://www.ahrq.gov/teamstepps/about-teamstepps/index.html. Accessed 17 Jan 2022.
51. Campbell Britton M, Hodshon B, Chaudhry SI. Implementing a warm handoff between hospital and skilled nursing facility clinicians. J Patient Saf. 2019;15(3):198–204. https://doi.org/10.1097/PTS.0000000000000529.
52. Davisson E, Swanson E. Nurses' heart failure discharge planning part I: the impact of interdisciplinary relationships and patient behaviors. Appl Nurs Res. 2020;56:151337. https://doi.org/10.1016/j.apnr.2020.151337.
53. Lech LVJ, Husted GR, Almarsdottír AB, Andersen TRH, Rossing C, Nørgaard LS. Hospital and community pharmacists' views of and perspectives on the establishment of an intraprofessional collaboration in the transition of care for newly discharged patients. Inov Pharm. 2020;11(3). https://doi.org/10.24926/iip.v11i3.2440.
54. Agarwal P, Poeran J, Meyer J, Rogers L, Reich DL, Mazumdar M. Bedside medication delivery programs: suggestions for systematic evaluation and reporting. Int J Qual Health Care. 2019;31(8):G53–9. https://doi.org/10.1093/intqhc/mzz014.
55. Lash DB, Mack A, Jolliff J, Plunkett J, Joson JL. Meds-to-Beds: the impact of a bedside medication delivery program on 30-day readmissions. J Am Coll Clin Pharm. 2019;2(6):674–80. https://doi.org/10.1002/jac5.1108.
56. Cossette B, Ricard G, Poirier R, et al. Pharmacist-led transitions of care between hospitals, primary care clinics, and community pharmacies. J Am Geriatr Soc. 2021;70(3):766–76. https://doi.org/10.1111/jgs.17575.
57. Hunter T, Nelson JR, Birmingham J. Preventing readmissions through comprehensive discharge planning. Prof Case Manag. 2013;18(2):56–63; quiz 64. https://doi.org/10.1097/NCM.0b013e31827de1ce.
58. Fabbre VD, Buffington AS, Altfeld SJ, Shier GE, Golden RL. Social work and transitions of care: observations from an intervention for older adults. J Gerontol Soc Work. 2011;54(6):615–26. https://doi.org/10.1080/01634372.2011.589100.
59. Surkan MJ, Gibson W. Interventions to mobilize elderly patients and reduce length of hospital stay. Can J Cardiol. 2018;34(7):881–8. https://doi.org/10.1016/j.cjca.2018.04.033.
60. Rambachan A, Fang MC, Prasad P, Iverson N. Racial and ethnic disparities in discharge opioid prescribing from a hospital medicine service. J Hosp Med. 2021;16(10):589–95. https://doi.org/10.12788/jhm.3667.
61. Singh JA, Kallan MJ, Chen Y, Parks ML, Ibrahim SA. Association of race/ethnicity with hospital discharge disposition after elective total knee arthroplasty. JAMA Netw Open. 2019;2(10):e1914259. https://doi.org/10.1001/jamanetworkopen.2019.14259.
62. Rivera-Hernandez M, Rahman M, Mor V, Trivedi AN. Racial disparities in readmission rates among patients discharged to skilled nursing facilities. J Am Geriatr Soc. 2019;67(8):1672–9. https://doi.org/10.1111/jgs.15960.
63. Wang S-Y, Hsu SH, Aldridge MD, Cherlin E, Bradley E. Racial differences in health care transitions and hospice use at the end of life. J Palliat Med. 2019;22(6):619–27. https://doi.org/10.1089/jpm.2018.0436.
64. Malevanchik L, Wheeler M, Gagliardi K, Karliner L, Shah SJ. Disparities after discharge: the association of limited English proficiency and postdischarge patient-reported issues. Jt Comm J Qual Patient Saf. 2021;47(12):775–82. https://doi.org/10.1016/j.jcjq.2021.08.013.
65. Brock J, Jencks SF, Hayes RK. Future directions in research to improve care transitions from hospital discharge. Med Care. 2021;59(Suppl 4):S401–4. https://doi.org/10.1097/MLR.0000000000001590.
66. Diehl TM, Barrett JR, Abbott DE, et al. Protocol for the MobiMD trial: a randomized controlled trial to evaluate the effect of a self-monitoring mobile app on hospital readmissions for complex surgical patients. Contemp Clin Trials. 2021;113:106658. https://doi.org/10.1016/j.cct.2021.106658.
67. Moitra E, Park HS, Gaudiano BA. Development and initial testing of an mhealth transitions of care intervention for adults with schizophrenia-spectrum disorders immediately following a psychiatric hospitalization. Psychiatry Q. 2021;92(1):259–72. https://doi.org/10.1007/s11126-020-09792-9.
68. Ben-Zeev D, Scherer EA, Gottlieb JD, et al. mHealth for schizophrenia: patient engagement with a mobile phone intervention following hospital discharge. JMIR Ment Health. 2016;3(3):e34. https://doi.org/10.2196/mental.6348.

Population Health

Amy N. Prentice, Rayhaan Adams, Deborah S. Porterfield, and Timothy P. Daaleman

Introduction

Population health examines the health outcomes of a group of individuals and the distribution of defined outcomes within the group [1]. Measuring, and ideally improving, the health of a population is especially relevant to chronic illness care. The core principles of population health include care management, data measurement, and analytics, all of which have the potential for improving health outcomes and cost savings in chronically ill patients. This chapter provides an overview to population health and care management. The first section introduces the principles of population health, and the historical development of these ideas. The following section grounds an understanding of care management in health care settings by defining important concepts and by operationalizing key workflows. The chapter closes with strategies for implementing population health strategies, including as care management, and future directions in the field.

Defining Population Health

Population health is best understood as an outcome, rather than in terms of structure or process, which distinguishes it from other related concepts [1]. In this way of thinking, population health can be conceptualized of as the sum of specific health outcomes, in domains such as mortality rates, disease burden, and health behaviors, that collectively provide a measure of the health of a defined group of individuals. A more refined understanding of population health would examine the health outcomes of a group of individuals and the distribution of such outcomes within that group [2]. Specific measures of population health include infant mortality rates, the prevalence of diabetes, and the prevalence of smoking in a population such as adolescents.

A related concept is population health management, which is the collective systems and policies that seek to impact health care quality, access, and outcomes for a defined population, with an ultimate goal of improving the health of that group [3]. Population health management focuses on the strategies that promote population health. When the defined population is a clinical or health-associated population rather than a general population, the concept of population medicine may be used. This associated term is sometimes synonymous with population health management and has been defined by the Institute of Healthcare Improvement as the design, delivery, coordination, and payment of high-quality health care services to manage the Triple Aim for a population, using the resources available within a health care system [4].

There are several strategies that may be designed and implemented in a population management or population medicine approach, such as the use of data registries to identify persons in need of specific clinical preventive service and the use of care managers. For clarity, the term population medicine may be used when clinical populations are being considered, and population health for more geographically based populations [5]. However, the term population health can be applied in both situations. One additional clarification is needed to distinguish between public health and population health. These two concepts have sometimes been used interchangeably, for example, to describe the impact of an intervention (e.g., smoking cessation) for a specific population's health (e.g., smokers with emphysema), as well as the public's health (e.g., nonsmokers who benefit from reduction in second-hand smoke). In addition, the term public health is most often used to describe an approach to protecting and improving the health of a geographic population, such as a city, county, or state, which is often tied to government or other regulatory agencies (e.g., health departments) with jurisdiction over that population [6].

A. N. Prentice (✉) · R. Adams · T. P. Daaleman
Department of Family Medicine, University of North Carolina at Chapel Hill, Chapel Hill, NC, USA
e-mail: amy_prentice@med.unc.edu; Rayhaan.adams@unchealth.unc.edu; tim_daaleman@med.unc.edu

D. S. Porterfield
Gillings School of Global Public Health, University of North Carolina at Chapel Hill, Chapel Hill, NC, USA

Population Health Conceptual Models

It is important to have a conceptual framework, theory, or an evidence-base to guide the selection of measures and interventions when considering approaches to measuring, and ultimately improving, the health of populations. A model provides an organizing framework in terms of plausible interventions to improve health outcomes. Specificity is required when applying a model in order to gauge fidelity to the intervention, and in development of measurement and analytic approaches to determine the effect of the intervention. This is important when working with health care systems and/or health insurance plans that may be underdeveloped with methods to identify and address more "upstream" factors, such as social determinants of health. A well-informed theory, which elucidates important drivers of population health, can map out pathways to determine how health system-level factors influence drivers of population health. A theoretical or empirically based model can also identify potential levers to upstream drivers, identifying strategies to synergistically work with clinical care services in improving health.

There have been several models of population health; two are particularly applicable to chronic illness care [7, 8]. The Chronic Care Model (CCM) is a foundational framework for improving chronic disease population health [9] (Fig. 35.1).

The CCM focuses on clinical service delivery and is comprised of several domains; organization of health care, decision support, delivery system design, clinical information systems, and self-management support. The sixth domain in the model—community resources and policies—is the most underdeveloped of the domains. The CCM has been widely evaluated, most recently in a review that included 77 original studies of CCM implementation for patients with chronic disease [10]. All but two studies reported improvements in healthcare practice or health outcomes and the review described specific elements of the CCM that were included in the interventions. Self-management support and delivery system design were the most common approaches; however, it was unclear which combinations of interventions were most effective.

The CCM has had broad influence in clinical practice and policy [11]. An "Expanded Chronic Care Model" of the CCM includes elements of chronic disease prevention, social determinants of health, and the role of community supports to positively impact population health for patients with chronic disease [12]. These targeted areas enrich the original CCM, which had a primary focus on care delivery for chronic disease, by expanding the scope beyond clinical settings and by highlighting the importance of primary and secondary prevention. An "eHealth Enhanced Chronic Care Model" potentiated each of the CCM elements by applying health

Fig. 35.1 Chronic Care Model

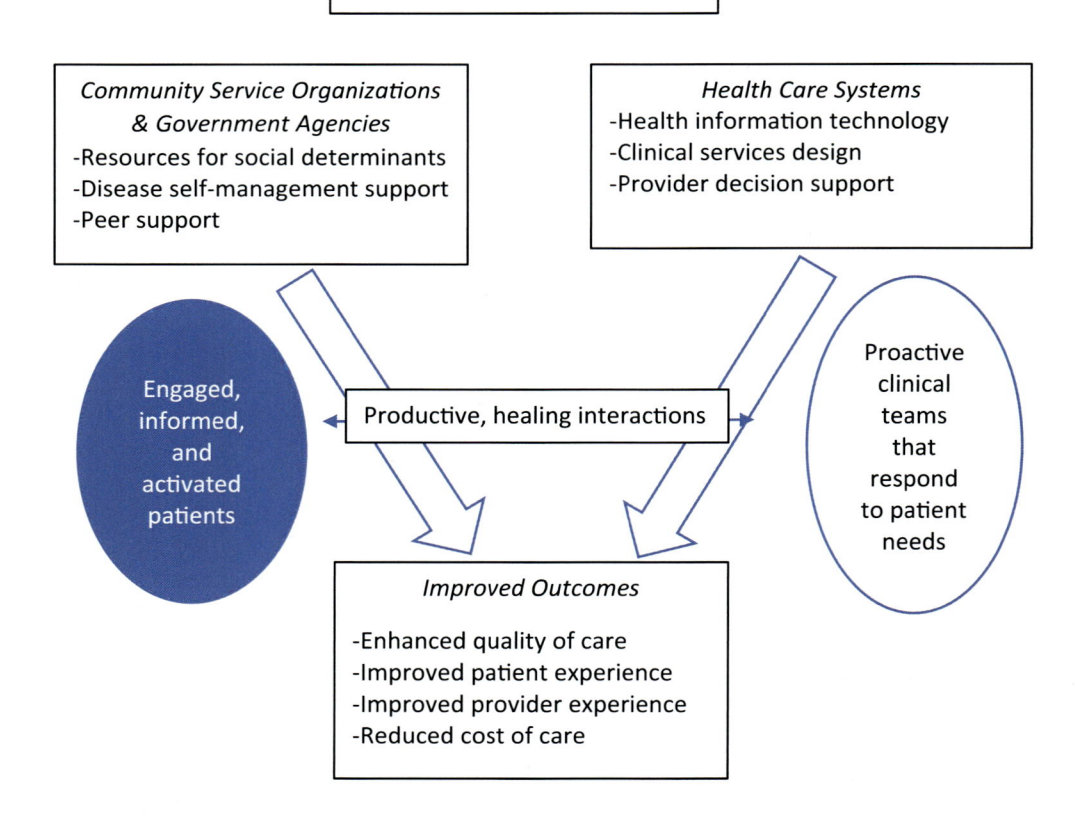

Table 35.1 Population health management and Chronic Care Model

• Population identification	• Clinical knowledge of determinants of health
• **Registry/data warehouse**	
• Risk stratification modeling	• **Integration with public health/community systems**
• *Use of registry/electronic medical record for: identification of subpopulations for tailored interventions; tracking of referrals to specialists and other providers in the medical neighborhood*	
	• Utilization of evidence-based guidelines *and embedded decision support*
• Personalized patient-centered care that includes: **self-management,** health promotion, disease management, case management	• Providing of culturally and linguistically appropriate care
	• Ongoing evaluation of outcomes with feedback loops
• Medical home	• Interoperable cross sector health information technology
• Interdisciplinary health care team	
	• *Ongoing quality improvement efforts addressing prioritized health and health care areas*

Adapted from Siderov and Romney [14]
Bold = also named in the Chronic Care Model; *italicized* = added by the authors

and communication technologies, as well as adding a new element of "eHealth Education," or the promotion of skills for persons with chronic disease in areas such as texting, websites, and mobile phone applications [13]. Table 35.1 compares a set of population health management elements to the Chronic Care Model [14].

The Institute of Healthcare Improvement's guide to measurement of the Triple Aim A is a second model of population health that is applicable to chronic disease care [7]. This framework organizes a menu of measures for the Triple Aim components, and is comparable to the Expanded Chronic Care Model in its depiction of how health care delivery systems can work with preventive services to promote population health [7]. In the model, prevention and health promotion efforts influence upstream factors, such as the social determinants of health, and individual factors, such as health behaviors. In contrast, health care is depicted as influencing disease burden, health and function, and mortality.

Defining Care Management

Care management is an important component of population health and was a term that was initially adopted by British social service agencies in 1993 to describe their approach to case management [15]. Although this understanding differentiated care managers from other related workers by their long-term involvement with clients and by their work with multiple teams and services, there was no common understanding operationalizing care management or the recipients of these services. As a result, there was confusion as to whether care management described an approach to working with patients, or the actual tasks and functions that were required [18]. Clinical case management, a related concept, stressed the importance of small, manageable caseloads that had a wide, inclusive scope, including individualized treatments, programmatic flexibility, outreach, care of patients with serious mental illness, interagency cooperation, and continuity of care [17]. This concept was developed in response to the increased need for a direct patient interface, a focus on small caseloads, and interagency care coordination [15]. The role and responsibilities of a clinical case manager have been adopted and its central components are comparable to the traditional case manager, since there is a focus on needs assessments, coordination of care, linkage to community resources, and ongoing follow-up, largely in practice-based settings [15].

There are several interpretations of what constitutes care management; however, at its core, care management seeks to improve the coordination and effectiveness of health care services. Care management can be more formally defined as a collaborative process of assessment, planning, facilitation, and advocacy for options and services to meet a patient's health needs through communication and available resources that promote high quality, cost-effective care [19]. The overall goal of care management is to optimize wellness and improve the coordination of health care services while providing cost-effective, evidence-based services [20]). Care management programs apply systems-level strategies, such as practice incentives and access to collateral information, as ways to improve health care settings and encourage patients and their support system to engage in a collaborative process that manages social and behavioral factors [20]. Care managers, in turn, are responsible for identifying, coordinating, and monitoring patients' psychosocial needs over a longitudinal timeframe, which is guided by the patient and health care team [16].

The responsibilities of care managers may include assisting patients to access needed preventive services, such as breast and colorectal cancer screening. Another task might involve reaching out to patients after emergency room visits or hospitalizations to ensure timely access to primary care and appropriate transitional care. Care managers can also follow up on needs that are identified during outpatient visits, and connect patients with other allied health care resources, such as health educators, nutritionists, social workers, and community-based resources [21–29].

Care Management Functions

The scope of work for care management has evolved over the past two decades. The Bureau of Primary Health Care (BPHC), for example, identified five major functions: developing and maintaining rapport with patients and providers; patient and family education; symptom surveillance; developing and maintaining self-care action plans, and; promoting treatment adherence through problem solving of treatment-emergent problems [16]. With the rise of patient-centered medical homes, care managers have assumed additional responsibilities in these settings, including assistance in coordinating care, providing one-on-one personalized self-management education, and facilitating focused care and attention for patients with complex needs [17]. Care managers often serve as liaisons between multiple patient care stakeholders, such as specialists and allied health professionals, health insurance companies, community-based services, and hospital-based services. They often conduct in-depth patient assessments and spend time discussing, locating, and coordinating patient resources and services [30]. As a result of the diverse skill set that is required, care managers are usually nurses, social workers, or other allied health professionals who have the training and expertise to work alongside health care providers, patients, and ancillary care services [16, 22, 23, 30, 31].

When embedded in health care settings, care managers can be a readily available resource for patients with chronic health conditions and psychosocial barriers, often through in-person and telephonic interactions. The continuity and quality of the relationship between patient and care manager often leads to a level of trust and rapport, empowering patients to self-managers their health care [32]. The scope of responsibilities for embedded care managers (ECM) include many of the previously noted functions—comprehensive patient assessments, patient education, development of individualized care plans, facilitation of care across different care settings—in addition to data gathering for ongoing quality improvement and evidence-based practice [33].

One evolving care management model focuses on identifying and improving the psychosocial factors that contribute to helplessness and hopelessness in chronically ill patients to facilitate health behavior change [34]. This approach leverages the relationship between patient and care manager and is designed to guide patients to be co-producers of their own health [34]. The model seeks to increase patient capacity by developing consistent, validating relationships that are focused on promoting patient agency. This occurs through dialogue with patients about their self-defined medical concerns, which are then co-constructed into patient-centered plans for health [34].

Another approach incorporates principles from the Patient Centered Medical Home and Accountable Care Organization frameworks to promote population health management. Here the focus of care management is on proactive outreach to medically vulnerable patients, who may be high utilizers of healthcare resources. Care management services are provided on a continuous basis, rather than a reactive, episodic approach, and include patient assessments, resource planning, and facilitation of patient-centered services. This strategy is supported by data that prospectively identifies and stratifies different patient populations to tailor intervention to specific subgroups. Many healthcare organizations have opted to embed population-based care managers within targeted practices that have a high concentration of at-risk patients to promote greater patient engagement. The use of predictive analytics and the case reviews of patients who are high utilizers of health care services aids in the identification of prospective patients. In this approach, the care manager would either receive point of care referrals from physicians and other care providers, or use an information technology tool that would identify patients who have screened positive, using specific criteria [21].

Transitional Care Management (TCM) is an interdisciplinary service model that provides coordination and continuity of care as patients navigate across care settings [18]. The service aims to minimize gaps or delays in care through care management and care coordination, with the goal of reducing potentially avoidable utilization (e.g., Emergency Department visits, Admissions, Readmissions). Patients are seen within their primary care medical home in 7–14 days after discharge, and they receive support from care managers, population health specialists, social workers, pharmacists, and nurses for a 30-day period [18]. Management strategies include identifying and mitigating non-clinical barriers to care/social determinants of health, discussion of medication access and self-management, assessment of behavioral health needs, review of advanced directives, and the development of care plans that promote access to health care services [18].

Implementing Care Management

The effectiveness of any innovation, such as care management, is dependent on the effective implementation of that intervention [35]. Health care organizations often quickly adopt complex innovations and subsequently find that sustained implementation proves challenging, time consuming, and costly [36]. This is an evolving area of research and three theory-based studies have examined care management implementation strategies, as well as factors that may influence the successful adoption of the intervention. A care management trial for depression was implemented through a strategy that supported practice change [37]. The implementation strategy relied on established quality improvement programs and was informed by diffusion of innovations theory [37].

The implementation strategy was grounded in the Three Component Model (TCM), a practice change process model that is derived from diffusion of innovations. There were several "readiness" principles for identifying candidate practices and clinicians who would be participants in the study; (1) an interest in the innovation (i.e., enhancing depression care); (2) viewing the innovation as aligned with their needs, values, and resources; (3) have capacity to pilot the innovation with minimal competing resources, and; (4) can assess the impact of the innovation [37].

Engagement was the first step and involved getting buy-in from health care organization (HCO) leadership before tasking the clinical staff. The team generally included the HCO medical director, a representative from the quality improvement program, and a representative from the care management [37]. This group was responsible for identifying and recruiting practices that are ready to participate in the project phase. Step 2 involved building HCO capacity for the care management model. The organizational and study teams needed to develop a capacity within the HCO to support the clinical model and practice change strategy, and subsequently capacity within the practices to adopt the program. The existing HCO quality improvement program provided practice support in implementing and sustaining the depression care management model [37].

The study team led capacity building efforts in pilot practices while each respective HCO quality improvement program became the central and sustaining source of ongoing practice support as the care management program was adopted. For example, capacity was developed within the HCO for telephone care management of depressed patients; a psychiatrist provided weekly supervision for care managers, as well as needed or requested consultation with primary care clinicians [37]. Care managers and the psychiatrist received standardized training, including a suicide risk assessment protocol and protocols for follow-up interventions for patients at risk. A patient registry was developed to track patients receiving care management and their progress [37].

Step 3 of the implementation strategy involved building primary care capacity for the care management model. Through participation in the "prepared practice" component of the TCM model, clinicians were provided with a 2-h interactive skills training program, including the diagnostic assessment of depressive disorders, the role of care management, and use of decision support to modify management and achieve remission [37]. Care managers and psychiatrists were introduced to primary care clinicians at these sessions and office staff receive a one-hour inservice session about the clinical model. The fourth and final step of the model involved ongoing support for maintaining the practice-level change, which targeted supervision of care management and providing feedback on the patient's clinical response [37]. The supervising psychiatrist working with the HCO quality improvement program and study staff monitored referral rates to care management and the appropriateness of referrals. This mechanism provided formative feedback to clinicians who were having difficulty implementing the care management model [37].

The project used process and outcome measures to provide an assessment of implementation. Clinician surveys and care manager logs were used to describe the process of care. The overall outcome of the intervention was assessed using the PHQ-9 with measurements at baseline, three months, and six months post intervention through telephone interviews with independent evaluators [37]. Care manager logs and HCO administrative data were used to assess cooperation with implementation and changes in the process of care in each practice [37].

A second study described and evaluated an implementation strategy for embedding a generalist care management program in a patient-centered medical home [21]. Here, implementation was considered as the period during which the intended users of an innovation (i.e., physicians and clinical staff) became skillful in adopting a new program; evaluating the implementation process required determining how well the innovation was consistently used. An organizational model of innovation implementation was used to guide the parameters of implementation and evaluation. This framework looks to determine how courses of action taken to execute a program or innovation result in observed patterns of initial use by examining an organization's readiness for change, the quality of the implementation policies and practices, and the climate for implementation.

There were three phases to the implementation strategy for embedding the care manager. The first phase engaged clinical leadership and identified champions around the concept and evidence-base of care management [21]. Although initial funding for the care manager position was provided through state agency grants for defined populations, such as Medicaid and uninsured patients, an operational decision was made for care management services to be made accessible for all clinic patients. A job description was developed for the care manager position with a requirement of clinical licensure (e.g., RN or MSW), excellent communication and problem-solving skills, and a minimum of three years of experience in health care [21].

Phase II began post-hiring and included several promotional strategies to raise the visibility of the care manager, such as screen-savers at computer workstations, bookmarks for providers and patients, and attendance and announcements at practice meetings and other clinical venues [21]. The information technology unit created a care management template in the electronic health record during this phase. Phase III of implementation focused on effectively integrating the care manager within the clinic operational structure and workflow [21]. Strategies included locating the care manager workplace centrally within the practice site, securing access to the appointment scheduling and health care system care management informatics system, embedding the position into ongoing practice quality initiatives, and establishing a plan for reporting interventions and utilization, such as point-of-care contacts and referrals [21].

Physicians and support staff were surveyed and most physicians (75%) and support staff (82%) reported interactions with the care manager, primarily via face-to-face, telephone, or electronic means [21]. Nearly 70% of the contacts were for facilitating referrals for behavioral health services; however, assistance with financial, social, and community-based resources was also prevalent (60–70%) [21]. Satisfaction with care management services was very high (98% of respondents reporting satisfied or very satisfied), and 79% of the clinician and care staff reported that the care manager was frequently or always accessible when needed [21].

Regarding the implementation strategy, clinicians and care staff noted that the most effective strategy was the outreach and direct contact that the care manager made with stakeholders (80%) [21]. In addition, personal introductions and an ongoing presence at practice meetings were also cited (63%), but other strategies such as handout cards and screen-savers on clinic laptops were reported as less effective. Regarding outcomes, over a 24-month implementation period, there was a trend of an absolute decrease of eight emergency department visits per month and an absolute decrease in inpatient admissions of 7.5 admissions per month [21].

The third and most recent study used normalization process theory (NPT) as a grounding to understand the organization of care management implementation in practice [38]. Semi-structured interviews and observations were conducted at 25 practices in five physician organizations. There were two key organizational structures for care management; practice-based care management (i.e., care managers were embedded in the practice as part of the practice team), and centralized care management (i.e., care managers worked independently of the practice workflow and were located outside the practice) [38].

Information Technology

Information technology (IT) is a central component in population health management. The federal Office of the National Coordinator defines health information technology as the "array of technologies to store, share, and analyze health information," [39] including EHRs, personal health records (PHRs), and e-prescribing. Well-integrated and high functioning IT systems can potentially facilitate population health management in multiple ways: through the identification of a population at risk, either by health outcomes or lack of preventive or clinical services; by tailoring clinical services to subpopulation identified through queries or risk modeling, and by ongoing evaluation of outcomes and quality improvement efforts. One framework of health IT describes a set of tools needed to accomplish the functions of IT and population health management: electronic health records, clinical data warehouses, registries, predictive modeling/risk stratification abilities, decision support tools, patient portals, and data analytics tools [40]. An Agency for Healthcare Research and Quality report specified requirements and functions for IT systems in order to support population health management [41]. These requirements include technical functionalities to identify subpopulations of patients, examine detailed characteristics of identified subpopulations, create reminders for patients and providers, track performance measures, and make data available in multiple forms [41].

IT applications are being adopted across organizational levels, particularly Accountable Care Organizations (ACOs) and other initiatives such as recognition of clinical practices as Patient Centered Medical Homes (PCMH) and the spread of Meaningful Use. The PCMH Recognition Program of the NCQA [42] includes a specific standard of "Population Health Management" with elements such as clinical data and use of data for population management. Meaningful Use of certified electronic health record technology, a term developed and promoted by the federal government, promotes the use of EHRs to improve care delivery, population health, and health data security [43]. The sustained adoption of the meaningful use of EHRs will be incentivized through payment programs of Medicare and Medicaid.

Table 35.2 displays the domains and features of IT systems that are required to support respective functions. Of note, the second and third domains support population health management [44].

A survey of early ACOs found that about half reported complete or near complete capability for the most common IT functions [40]. Only 36% of ACOs were able to integrate outpatient and inpatient data from providers within the organization, and only 34% had the IT capability for primary care physicians to bi-directionally share referral information with specialists.

Table 35.2 Domains of information technology systems for provider organizations [44]

Domain	System features	Purpose
Transaction systems	Patient registration and scheduling Electronic health record, including orders, e-prescribing, and patient portal Patient billing and collection General financial systems	Care of the individual patient
Population management	Patient registries; care coordination and case management Risk stratification: predictive analytics, protocols for intervention Task tracking and documentation	Population level view
Data warehouse and analytics	Analytical models Cost accounting Comparative data, benchmarking Exploratory analyses Practice profiles for clinicians External reporting	To develop knowledge

Future Directions

There is increased awareness by individual health care providers and organizations to address the social determinants of health (SDOH), which are key drivers of population health [45]. The World Health Organization defines SDOH as "conditions in which people are born, grow, work, live, and age, and the wider set of forces and systems shaping the conditions of daily life" [46]. Some proponents of population health improvement have advocated for measurement of SDOH indices (e.g., unstable housing, food insecurity), as part of the medical record, a first step to identify and address these factors [47]. In addition, the Centers for Medicare and Medicaid Services has promoted the Accountable Health Communities initiative, a program to promote screening approaches for adverse SDOH in clinical care settings as a central part of in managing of the health of the populations [30]. This initiative has drawn some criticism since criteria for an effective SDOH screening is underdeveloped [23].

Independent of the Accountable Health Communities program, there has been interest in promoting collaborations between health care systems and public health or community-based organizations, in order to address behavioral and social determinants of health [23]. Early work in this area was led by the Agency for Healthcare Research and Quality (AHRQ), specifically for the delivery of preventive services [31], but other sources of resources to promote these collaborations, in addition to AHRQ, are now available, such as the Practical Playbook [24]. However, evidence for these collaborations is early and emerging research will need to elucidate efficacy for chronic disease states and effectiveness in health care organizational contexts [25, 26].

As population management continues as a focal point for health care transformation, the need for services such as care coordination and care management will continue to grow [48]. Payment reform, and ultimately, investment in non-physician resources and staffing models will be essential to managing indirect care in a cost efficient and effective manner [49]. Reimbursement and investment in care management staffing and infrastructure have not been historically supported by the fee-for-service model and subsequently, is not responsive to an aging population with advanced and complex medical and psychosocial needs [50]. Primary care and other health services will need to determine how to balance business models that have typically been linked to in-person physician visits, with the need to build capacity to address the indirect care, which is non-revenue generating work that is required to treat patients and account for their resource and community needs [50].

Identifying barriers to care and engaging in health promotion and prevention yield long-term patient benefits, such as improved patient engagement, increased care team wellbeing and productivity, and decreased total cost of care, payors have explored upfront per member per month payments to support practices in achieving those outcomes [51]. A capitated and/or value-based reimbursement model provides incentives for time-intensive indirect care work (e.g., health coaching, case management, referral coordination, etc.). These financial models allow capacity for additional staff to proactively manage care needs that would otherwise require a visit with a physician, therefore providing a lower-cost, more convenient care platform, while also allowing practices to grow their populations and maintain access for the acute care needs of the most complex patients [51].

The COVID-19 pandemic disrupted traditional health care delivery models and spurred the adoption of virtual and telephonic care delivery models, the same approaches that have historically been utilized by care managers to identify, engage, and track patients and their health outcomes [52]. Care management during this time provided strategies to mitigate the risks of in-person care that was not available, by maintaining patient connection to the medical home [53]. The rise in virtual care has also exposed the vulnerabilities in the US healthcare system, particularly SDOHs determinants, by highlighting the systemic non-clinical barriers to care within vulnerable populations and communities [54]. The marked gap of SDOH contributed to the onset or worsening of chronic health conditions, like asthma, diabetes, heart disease, and hypertension—all conditions that contribute to increased total cost of care, disability and mortality [54]. The acknowledgment and inclusion of these social care needs in healthcare data has strengthened the need for investment in care management to not only address acute gaps in care but also to focus on upstream issues that impede patients from improving their health.

References

1. Donabedian A. The quality of care. How can it be assessed? JAMA. 1988;260(12):1743–8.
2. Kindig D, Stoddart G. What is population health? Am J Public Health. 2003;93(3):380–3.
3. Meiris DC, Nash DB. More than just a name. Popul Health Manag. 2008;11(4):181.
4. Lewis N. Institute for Healthcare Improvement Leadership Blog. 2014. http://www.ihi.org/communities/blogs/_layouts/ihi/community/blog/itemview.aspx?List=81ca4a47-4ccd-4e9e-89d9-14d88ec59e8d&ID=50.
5. Kindig D. Health Affairs Blog. 2015. http://healthaffairs.org/blog/2015/04/06/what-are-we-talking-about-when-we-talk-about-population-health/.
6. What is Public Health?: CDC Foundation. https://www.cdcfoundation.org/content/what-public-health.
7. Stiefel M, Nolan K. A guide to measuring the triple aim: population health, experience of care, and per capita cost 2012. 2016. http://www.jvei.nl/wp-content/uploads/A-Guide-to-Measuring-the-Triple-Aim.pdf.
8. Wagner EH, Austin BT, Von Korff M. Organizing care for patients with chronic illness. Milbank Q. 1996;74(4):511–44.
9. Wagner E. Chronic disease management: what will it take to improve care for chronic illness? Eff Clin Pract. 1998;1(1):2–4.
10. Davy C, Bleasel J, Liu H, Tchan M, Ponniah S, Brown A. Effectiveness of Chronic Care Models: opportunities for improving healthcare practice and health outcomes: a systematic review. BMC Health Serv Res. 2015;15:194.
11. Improving Chronic Illness Care: About ICI and Our Work: The Robert Wood Johnson Foundation. http://www.improvingchroniccare.org/index.php?p=About_US&s=6.
12. Barr VJ, Robinson S, Marin-Link B, Underhill L, Dotts A, Ravensdale D, et al. The expanded Chronic Care Model: an integration of concepts and strategies from population health promotion and the Chronic Care Model. Hosp Q. 2003;7(1):73–82.
13. Gee PM, Greenwood DA, Paterniti D, Ward D, Miller LS. The eHealth Enhanced Chronic Care Model: a theory derivation approach. J Med Internet Res. 2015;17(4):e86.
14. Sidorov J, Romney M. The spectrum of care. In: Nash DB, Reifsnyder J, Fabius RJ, Pracilio VP, editors. Population health: creating a culture of wellness. 1st ed. Burlington, MA: Jones & Bartlett Learning; 2016. p. 3–22.
15. Burns T. Case management, care management and care programming. Br J Psychiatry. 1997;170(5):393–5.
16. Lewis J, Bernstock P, Bovell V, Wookey F. Implementing care management: issues in relation to the new community care. Br J Soc Work. 1997;27(1):5–24.
17. Patchner LS. In the belly of the beast: a case study of social work in a managed care organization. Adv Soc Work. 2002;3(1):16–32.
18. Rachman R. Community care: changing the role of hospital social work. Health Soc Care Community. 1995;3(3):163–72.
19. Case Management Society of America. Standards of Practice for Case Management. 2010. http://www.cmsa.org/portals/0/pdf/memberonly/StandardsOfPractice.pdf.
20. Center for Health Care Strategies I. Care Management Definition and Framework. 2007 https://www.chcs.org/media/Care_Management_Framework.pdf.
21. Daaleman TP, Hay, Prentice A, Gwynne M. Embedding care management in the medical home: a case study. J Prim Care Community Health. 2014;5:97–100.
22. S Findley et al. ugly construction to get trailing dot after citation, or after journals slug if citation is not defined J Ambul Care Manage 37 (1), 82–91. Jan-Mar 2014.
23. Haas SA, Swan BA. Developing the value proposition for the role of the registered nurse in care coordination and transition management in ambulatory care settings. Nurs Econ. 2014;32(2):70–9.
24. Hall AG, Webb FJ, Scuderi CB, Tamayo-Friedel C, Harman JS. Differences in patient ratings of medical home domains among adults with diabetes: comparisons across primary care sites. J Prim Care Community Health. 2014;5(4):247–52. https://doi.org/10.1177/2150131914538455. Epub 2014 Jun 13
25. Hiss RG, Armbruster BA, Gillard ML, McClure LA. Nurse care manager collaboration with community-based physicians providing diabetes care: a randomized controlled trial. Diabetes Educ. 2007;33(3):493–502.
26. Sepers CE Jr, Fawcett SB, Lipman R, Schultz J, Colie-Akers V, Perez A. Measuring the implementation and effects of a coordinated care model featuring diabetes self-management education within four patient-centered medical homes. Diabetes Educ. 2015;41(3):328–42.
27. Taliani CA, Bricker PL, Adelman AM, Cronholm PF, Gabbay RA. Implementing effective care management in the patient-centered medical home. Am J Manag Care. 2013;19(12):957–64.
28. Wang QC, Chawla R, Colombo CM, Snyder RL, Nigam S. Patient-centered medical home impact on health plan members with diabetes. J Public Health Manage Pract. 2014;20(5):E12–20.
29. Howard H, Malouin R, Callow-Rucker M. Care managers and knowledge shift in primary care patient-centered medical home transformation. Human Organization, Vol. 75. the Society for Applied Anthropology. 2016. 0018–7259/16/010010–11$1.60/1.
30. Ackroyd SA, Wexler DJ. Effectiveness of diabetes interventions in the patient-centered medical home. Curr Diab Rep. 2014;14:471. https://doi.org/10.1007/s11892-013-0471-z.
31. Thom DH, Hessler D, Willard-Grace R, Bodenheimer T, Najmabadi A, Araujo C, Chen EH. Does health coaching change patients' trust in their primary care provider? Patient Educ Couns. 2014;96(1):135–8. https://doi.org/10.1016/j.pec.2014.03.018. Epub 2014 Apr 2
32. Howard HA, Malouin R, Callow-Rucker M. Care managers and knowledge shift in primary care patient-centered medical home transformation. Hum Organ. 2016;75(1):10–20.
33. Hines P, Mercury M. Designing the role of the embedded care manager. Prof Case Manag. 2013;18(4):182–7.
34. Rose SM, Hatzenbuehler S, Gilbert E, Bouchard MP, McGill D. A population health approach to clinical social work with complex patients in primary care. Health Soc Work. 2016;41(2):93–100.
35. Beresford P, Croft S, Adshead L. 'We don't see her as a social worker': a service user case study of the importance of the social worker's relationship and humanity. Br J Soc Work. 2008;38(7):1388–407.
36. Davis TS, Guada J, Reno R, Peck A, Evans S, Sigal LM, et al. Integrated and culturally relevant care: a model to prepare social workers for primary care behavioral health practice. Soc Work Health Care. 2015;54(10):909–38.
37. Dietrich AJ, Oxman TE, Williams JW Jr, et al. Going to scale: re-engineering systems for primary care treatment of depression. Ann Fam Med. 2004;2(4):301–4.
38. Holtrop JS, Potworowski G, Fitzpatrick L, Kowalk A, Green LA. Effect of care management program structure on implementation: a normalization process theory analysis. BMC Health Serv Res. 2016;16(a):386. https://doi.org/10.1186/s12913-016-1613-1.

39. Basics of Health IT: HeatlhIT.gov. https://www.healthit.gov/patients-families/basics-health-it.
40. Wu FM, Rundall TG, Shortell SM, Bloom JR. Using health information technology to manage a patient population in accountable care organizations. J Health Organ Manag. 2016;30(4):581–96.
41. Cusack CM, Knudson AD, Kronstadt JL, Singer RF, Brown AL. Practice-based population health: information technology to support transformation to proactive primary care. AHRQ Publication; 2010. https://pcmh.ahrq.gov/sites/default/files/attachments/Information%20Technology%20to%20Support%20Transformation%20to%20Proactive%20Primary%20Care.pdf.
42. Assurance NCQA. Patient-Centered Medical Home (PCMH) Recognition. http://www.ncqa.org/programs/recognition/practices/patient-centered-medical-home-pcmh.
43. HeatlhIT.gov. Meaningful Use Objectives and Definitions. https://www.healthit.gov/providers-professionals/meaningful-use-definition-objectives.
44. Cuddeback JK, Fisher DW. Information technology. In: Nash DB, Reifsnyder J, editors. Population health: creating a culture of wellness. 1st ed. Burlington, MA: Jones & Bartlett Learning; 2016. p. 153–80.
45. Designing a High-Performing Health Care System for Patients with Complex Needs, The Commonwealth Fund and the London School of Economics and Political Science. 2017.
46. Steiner BD, Denham AC, Ashkin E, et al. Community Care of North Carolina: improving care through community health networks. Ann Fam Med. 2008;6:361–7.
47. Luo Z, Chen Q, Annis AM, Piatt G, Green LA, Tao M, Holtrop JS. Comparison of health plan- and provider-delivered chronic care management models on patient clinical outcomes. J Gen Intern Med. 2016;31(7):762–70. https://doi.org/10.1007/s11606-016-3617-2. Epub 2016 Mar 7
48. Population Health Management: Meeting the Demand for Value Based Care. https://www.ncqa.org/wp-content/uploads/2021/02/20210202_PHM_White_Paper.pdf.
49. Fraher E, Brandt B. Toward a system where workforce planning and interprofessional practice and education are designed around patients and populations not professions. J Interprof Care. 2019;33(4):389–97. https://doi.org/10.1080/13561820.2018.1564252. Epub 2019 Jan 23
50. Park B, Gold SB, Bazemore A, Liaw W. How evolving United States payment models influence primary care and its impact on the quadruple aim. J Am Board Fam Med. 2018;31(4):588–604. https://doi.org/10.3122/jabfm.2018.04.170388.
51. Miller BF, Ross KM, Davis MM, Melek SP, Kathol R, Gordon P. Payment reform in the patient-centered medical home: enabling and sustaining integrated behavioral health care. Am Psychol. 2017;72(1):55–68. https://doi.org/10.1037/a0040448.
52. Dupraz J, Le Pogam M-A, Peytremann-Bridevaux I. Early impact of the COVID-19 pandemic on in-person outpatient care utilisation: a rapid review. BMJ Open. 2022;12(3):e056086.
53. Amon C, King J, Colclasure J, Hodge K, DuBard CA. Leveraging Accountable Care Organization infrastructure for rapid pandemic response in independent primary care practices. Healthc (Amst). 2022;10(2):100623.
54. Flor LS, Friedman J, Spencer CN, Cagney J, Arrieta A, Herbert ME, et al. Quantifying the effects of the COVID-19 pandemic on gender equality on health, social, and economic indicators: a comprehensive review of data from March, 2020, to September, 2021. Lancet. 2022;399(10344):2381–97.

Artificial Intelligence, Machine Learning, and Natural Language Processing

Kimberly A. Shoenbill, Suranga N. Kasturi, and Eneida A. Mendonca

Introduction

Artificial intelligence has become a popular "buzz word" in the medical and lay literature that elicits both high hopes and bitter disillusionment. The applications, promise, and shortcomings of this emerging science are relevant to the field of medicine and chronic illness care.

Definitions

The relationship between artificial intelligence and two related terms that are often confused or merged is illustrated in Fig. 36.1 [1–3]. *Artificial intelligence* (AI) is the branch of computer science that centers on computer simulation of human intelligence and includes the study and application of machine learning, logic, problem-solving, and decision science. *Machine learning* (ML) is a subdomain of AI in which computers (machines) identify patterns in data that identify similar or increasingly complex patterns in new data. The computer "learns" from the original data to make more accurate classifications or predictions on subsequent data inputs. *Natural language processing* (NLP) is a subdomain of AI that converts written or spoken words into computer-interpretable datasets to be analyzed with statistical and machine learning methods. NLP is used in speech recognition (i.e., dictations, virtual assistant, and chatbot tools) and free-text medical record analysis to identify care details or discourse characteristics as recorded by the provider. NLP is used with medical record discrete (structured text) analysis to provide a more complete assessment of care delivery. NLP can also be used for information retrieval to assist with literature searches on topics of interest.

K. A. Shoenbill (✉)
Department of Family Medicine, Program on Health and Clinical Informatics, University of North Carolina at Chapel Hill, Chapel Hill, NC, USA

Lineberger Comprehensive Cancer Center, University of North Carolina at Chapel Hill, Chapel Hill, NC, USA
e-mail: kimberly_shoenbill@med.unc.edu

S. N. Kasturi
Black Dog Institute, University of New South Wales, Sydney, NSW, Australia

Center for Biomedical Informatics, Regenstrief Institute, Indianapolis, IN, USA
e-mail: s.kasturi@unsw.edu.au

E. A. Mendonca
Division of Biomedical Informatics, Department of Pediatrics, Cincinnati Children's Hospital and University of Cincinnati, Cincinnati, OH, USA
e-mail: eneida.mendonca@cchmc.org

Fig. 36.1 The relationship between artificial intelligence and the subdomains of machine learning and natural language processing

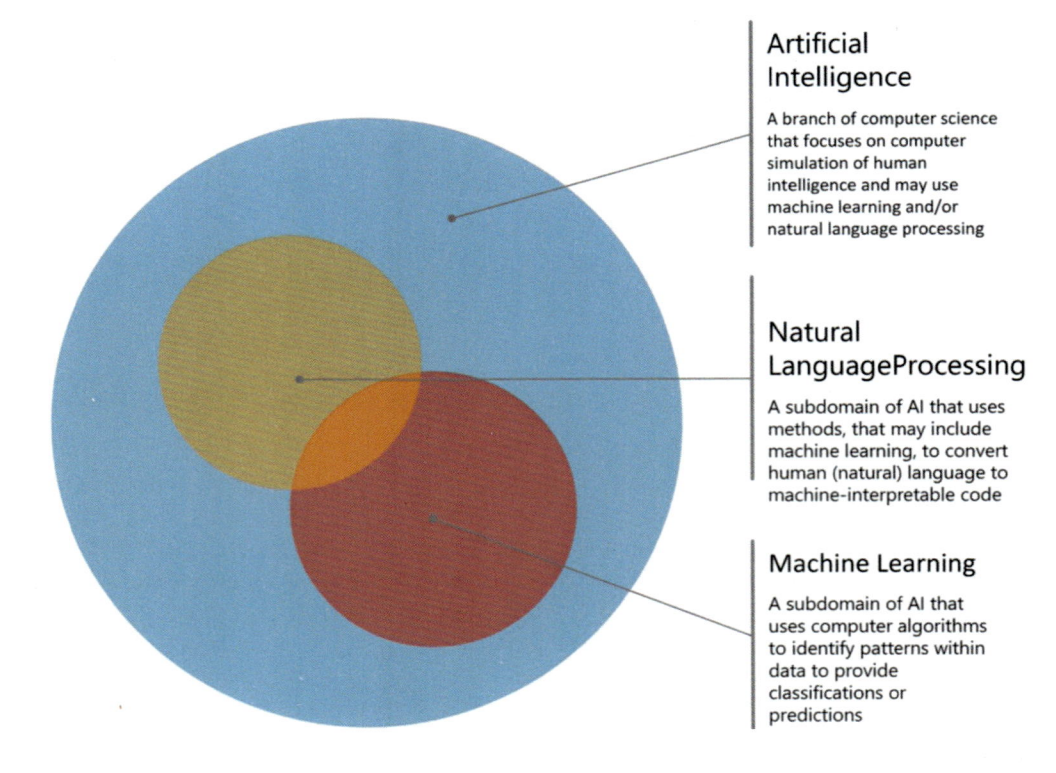

Artificial Intelligence

A branch of computer science that focuses on computer simulation of human intelligence and may use machine learning and/or natural language processing

Natural LanguageProcessing

A subdomain of AI that uses methods, that may include machine learning, to convert human (natural) language to machine-interpretable code

Machine Learning

A subdomain of AI that uses computer algorithms to identify patterns within data to provide classifications or predictions

Differences from Statistics

A common question from clinicians and researchers new to machine learning is how it differs from statistical analysis. Although there are overlaps, in statistical methods the analytical goal is to make an *inference*, specifically to uncover relationships between variables from a sample population and extrapolate that information to the whole population. Although some statistical methods can make predictions about new data (e.g., logistic and linear regression), these methods focus on the relationships between variables. In contrast, machine learning methods focus on *prediction* of an outcome from input variables. In machine learning, the relationships between large numbers of variables can be complex and non-linear with each variable making a small contribution to the final prediction. These variable relationships may not be easily understood by humans, but it is the "what" of the machine learning model (i.e., the prediction) that is the investigative goal more than the "how" of the model (i.e., the inter-variable relationships) [4].

Another difference between machine learning and statistics is the meaning of the term *regression*. In statistics, *regression is an analytic method to identify relationships* between one or more independent input variables and a dependent outcome variable that is either categorical or continuous. In machine learning, *regression refers to prediction of only continuous outcome variables* from one or more continuous or categorical input variables. Machine learning models are based on mathematical models (algorithms) and make predictions by completing a *classification task*, with a discrete outcome variable predicted (e.g., a diagnosis) or a *regression task* with a continuous variable predicted (e.g., time to disease recurrence).

Machine learning is broadly divided into supervised and unsupervised models. Supervised models are created from input data and known (labeled) output data. Unsupervised models are created from input data, without labeled output data, and the computer finds associations to identify potential prevalent or recurrent connections between the input data and the output data. Unsupervised machine learning is often used in exploratory analysis to begin to identify patterns and connections in the data. A conceptual model of a machine learning process is provided in Fig. 36.2.

To enhance understanding of the literature surrounding research and applications of AI, ML, and NLP, a table of key concepts is provided in Table 36.1 [3, 5, 6].

Fig. 36.2 Conceptual model of a machine learning process

Conceptual Model of Machine Learning Process

Input Data (Instances)
Input data (often called "instances" in ML) can be patient-level data with each patient represented as a collection of features (i.e., variables such as diagnoses, lab values etc.). Each patient (instance) may have a known class (known outcome variable = supervised ML) or unknown class (unknown outcome variable = unsupervised ML). The input data will be mixed in respect to final outcome variables.

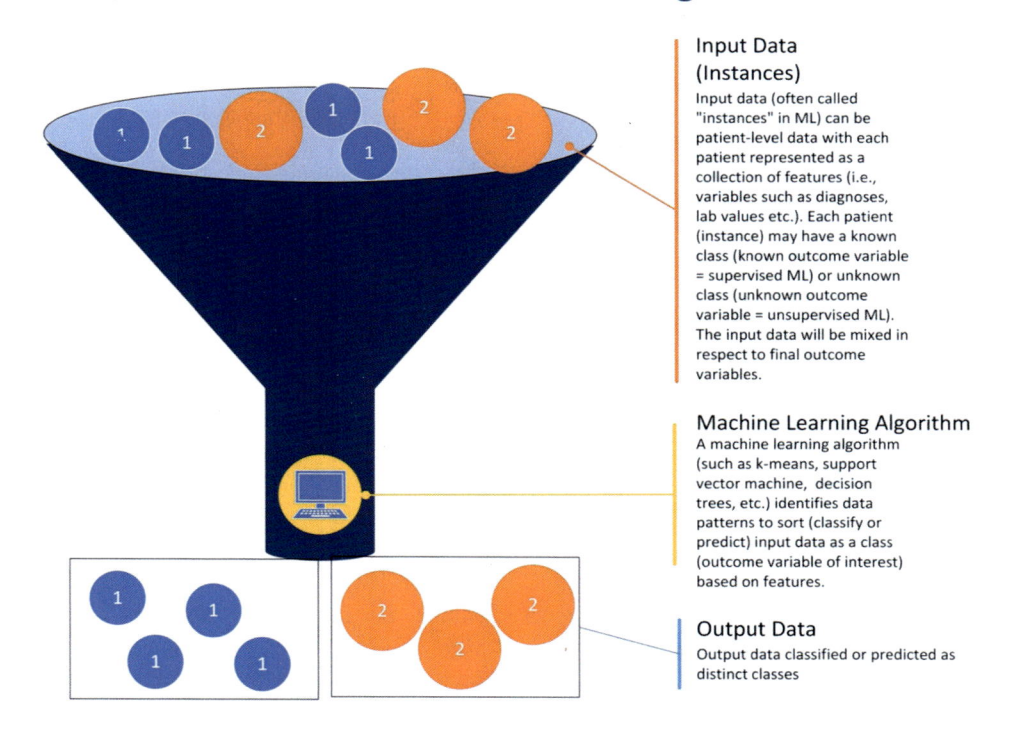

Machine Learning Algorithm
A machine learning algorithm (such as k-means, support vector machine, decision trees, etc.) identifies data patterns to sort (classify or predict) input data as a class (outcome variable of interest) based on features.

Output Data
Output data classified or predicted as distinct classes

Table 36.1 Key concepts in artificial intelligence (AI), machine learning (ML), and natural language processing (NLP) [3, 5, 6]

Concepts	Descriptions
Black box	Machine learning or artificial intelligence algorithm is not understood by humans due to: (1) complexity (often with multiple variables each with a small contribution to the result) and/or (2) the algorithm is proprietary
Corpus	A collection of textual documents used in NLP
Explainability (auditability)	A desirable feature of AI and ML algorithms that allows the mathematical functions and code to be understood by humans and investigated, if needed, to ensure equity and accuracy
Deep learning	A type of AI employing neural networks or similar methods requiring big data inputs to learn prediction models. Deep learning often employs black box algorithms
Dimensionality reduction	ML techniques that reduce the number of variables used in a model while retaining critical data points within the dataset
Ensemble learning	ML methods using multiple algorithms to construct a more predictive model than could be achieved with a single algorithm
Feature selection	Choosing of variables that will be used in a ML model
Overfitting	A problem in ML where the model learns the training data set (and its idiosyncrasies) too well, producing near 100% accuracy in predictions using the training data, but poor prediction accuracy in new data
Metrics	**Measures of model success**
Accuracy	Proportion of correctly identified cases among all cases examined
F-measure	An assessment of the overall accuracy of precision and recall (i.e., the harmonic mean)
Precision	In information retrieval and NLP, a measure of a system's ability to retrieve relevant information. This measure is calculated as relevant terms retrieved divided by the total number of terms retrieved. Precision is also called positive predictive value in a diagnostic test evaluation
Receiver operator curve	A graph with false positive rate plotted on the x axis and the true positive rate plotted on the y axis providing a measure (area under the receiver operator curve [AUROC]) of how well a model can distinguish between two groups

(continued)

Table 36.1 (continued)

Concepts	Descriptions
Sensitivity (recall)	Proportion of true positives that are correctly identified by a model (also called the true positive rate and recall). In information retrieval and NLP, a second measure of the ability of a system to retrieve relevant information. This measure is calculated as relevant terms retrieved divided by all relevant terms in the data set
Specificity	Proportion of true negatives that are correctly identified by a model (also called the true negative rate)
Types of ML models	**Descriptions**
Supervised	Model training method using input (independent) variables (also called features) and labeled dependent variables
Unsupervised	Model training method using input (independent) variables (also called features) and unlabeled/unknown dependent variables
Reinforcement learning	Model training method that rewards correct prediction of desired outcome variables and punishing incorrect predictions. This method continually "learns" from its actions based on its input and mistakes

Historical Highlights

Artificial intelligence is a term attributed to John McCarthy during a Dartmouth Conference in 1956. Machine learning started in 1959 with Arthur Samuel demonstrating that a computer could "learn" to play checkers. Over the next 60+ year trajectory, early artificial intelligence applications in medicine included Internist I (an internal medicine consultant on diagnosis), Cas-Net (a causal association network), and the Mycin system (antibiotic selection based on clinical presentation prior to culture results being available). Early systems were novel, but not well-accepted due to their cumbersome data entry requirements (pre-auto-population from electronic health records).

The *Black Box* Problem

Pervasive uptake of AI was hindered by the *black box* computational approaches underlying early AI systems. These systems required the user to enter data into the system, but the methods and calculations that resulted in the recommended diagnosis or course of treatment were unknown (a "black box") to the end-user. Understandably, many providers were not comfortable trusting the results of an AI recommendation or diagnosis unless they understood the data and decisions used to produce the result. As methods and algorithms evolved, more transparent processes were employed for many AI applications to medicine. Such methods included decision trees or Bayes net algorithms, but what was gained in transparency often required a compromise on model prediction accuracy. For example, a decision tree small enough to be comprehensible on human review usually contains few splits of the data, meaning few variables were assessed to determine which variables were informative in arriving at a prediction. With larger trees having more variables or with the assessment of multiple decision trees at once (called random forest models using ensemble methods), accuracy of prediction often increases, but at the expense of easy comprehension by the end-user.

The late 2000s showed a resurgence of interest in AI with the emergence of electronic health records (EHRs) and potential for improved care using clinical decision support tools. This interest led to more investigations into "deep learning" and explorations of multi-layered neural networks. These models were again viewed suspiciously by many providers as these *black box* recommendations were presented, but the data and calculations leading to the recommendation were not explained or discoverable. Today, attraction to and rejection of AI and Clinical Decision Support (CDS) tools continue in medical applications with ongoing concerns about "explainability" (or auditability) of the algorithm specifics and appropriate application to specific populations.

Health Inequity

There is increased interest in identifying and critically evaluating existing AI models and CDS tools to determine if the data used in model building was representative of the general population and specifically inclusive of historically marginalized people. Without data from these significant populations, the models can provide biased recommendations that can exacerbate disparities in care with inequitable recommendations for or against treatment based on race, gender, and ethnicity. The need to ensure that data used to build machine learning models are unbiased and representative of all populations on which the model or CDS will be used cannot be overstated or overlooked in predictive model design, application, and life-cycle review. Concerns and hope for AI applications in health care are discussed in detail in the recent National Academy of Medicine Report on AI and will be reviewed throughout this chapter [7].

Applications to Chronic Illness Care

Chronic disease (illness) is broadly defined as an adverse medical condition that is present for at least 1 year and requires either ongoing medical management, limitations of activities of daily living (ADLs), or both. Six in ten US adults have one chronic disease and four in ten live with two or more chronic diseases [8].

The most prevalent chronic diseases in US adults are heart disease, cancer, chronic lung disease, stroke, Alzheimer's disease, diabetes, chronic kidney disease, and arthritis. Advancing research and treatment options in chronic disease management have made longer-term survival possible for many patients living with these diseases. This can present unique challenges and opportunities for healthcare providers to use the large amounts of data, generated in the care of these patients, to better identify evidence-based best practices in chronic disease care for current and future patients. This is an area poised for automation and use of artificial intelligence [9, 10]. NLP and ML algorithms can be employed to analyze clinical notes, including free-text and discrete data, to identify patient characteristics and patterns of care that can assist with detection of patient cohorts having a disease (phenotyping), prediction of disease development or progression, or guide important interventions for disease treatment. Examples of some of these areas of investigation in the NLP and/or ML literature include polypharmacy reduction [11], cancer regression [12], optimizing geriatric care [13, 14], and addressing mental health diagnosis and treatment issues [15]. Studies of NLP and/or ML have looked at specific chronic disease detection, stabilization, or regression in multiple chronic illnesses including COPD [16–19], cardiovascular disease and heart failure [20–23], liver disease [24], and diabetes mellitus [25–29]. An excellent overview of medical AI applications presented by stakeholder groups, application types, and methods used can be found in Chapter 3 of the National Academy of Medicine's special publication on AI in Health Care [7].

Individual Patient Applications

Evidence-based medicine is informed from research and quality improvement (QI) studies. AI and machine learning provide an important service in collating and analyzing large amounts of data to discover connections, correlations, and outcomes that may not be evident in smaller trials or studies with fewer patients or less diverse populations. AI, ML, and NLP can be the key methods to uncover "hidden information" that is present in medical records or clinical trial data [30–32]. With these discoveries of data correlation, new areas of investigation are uncovered to inform future studies and randomized clinical trials that can identify stronger associations or causalities. This evidence can be applied to individual patients in the form of chronic disease prediction and risk mitigation [33]. These findings can also inform optimal disease monitoring methods or schedules, disease prognosis, genomic data applications for precision medicine, and selecting personalized summary information, at the point of care, for patients to take home [34–37].

Home Applications

As medicine moves from siloed care in clinics and hospitals to comprehensive whole-person care in varied settings, there is an increasing need for in-home resources and caregiver support tools. Identifying home-care needs, tool efficacy, support/tool effectiveness, and valuable information and community resources are areas of ongoing investigation. AI, ML, and NLP can assist with these research and QI endeavors by collating and analyzing large amounts of data from patients and their caregivers to identify best practices and methods for primary care providers to support patient goals and needs as they receive more care at home. Some of the tools to assist in home care and monitoring include wearable devices to detect falls and "living laboratories" set up in research centers that simulate home environments to identify how to set up home supports to maximize patient comfort, safety, and ability to manage chronic diseases at home [38–40]. With the design and expansion of "in-home hospitals," increasingly sophisticated data collection, monitoring, and data-interoperability models are needed for seamless integration with clinical care [41]. AI, ML, and NLP can also assist caregivers in locating more information on their own regarding their loved-ones' disease, community resources, or medication side-effects. This empowers patients and their caregivers to fully partner with providers, retain agency over their healthcare goals, and inform future questions to pose to the primary care provider.

Healthcare Provider Applications

Whole-person care across healthcare sites can also be supported by AI, ML, and NLP to ensure accurate patient data matching and data interoperability from specialist, primary, and community care facilities [42]. Although a seemingly simple task, without a national patient identifier in the US, this basic patient identification task is a challenging problem with fragmented care across multiple sites, specialties, and payor systems for patients with chronic illnesses.

Machine learning is routinely used in electronic health records to use patients' data to provide clinical decision support (CDS) as prompts for providers at the point of care (e.g., Best Practice Advisories [BPAs]). The suggestions can range from alerts about potential drug interactions to suggestions about recommended preventive screenings for cancer. CDS prompts have the potential to improve and streamline providers' work and cognitive load during a patient encounter, but can also have the unintended consequence of recurrent distractions and impedance to efficient care delivery. This intrusion to the workflow often results from the CDS prompt not adhering to the 5 "Rights" of CDS design and implementation. These "Rights" include delivering:

1. The right **information** (i.e., evidence-based, actionable information appropriate to the patient based on EHR data and visit goal).
2. To the right **person** (e.g., physician, nurse, or physical therapist).
3. Using the right intervention **format** (e.g., alerts, order sets, or protocols).
4. Through the right **channel** (e.g., EHR, Patient Health Record (PHR), or computerized provider order entry [CPOE] tool).
5. At the right time in the **workflow** (e.g., alerting a provider of a drug interaction when the provider begins to write a prescription instead of after the prescription is entered and ready to send to the pharmacy).

Alert fatigue is an unintended consequence of CDS and more prevalent when the above "rights" are not considered in CDS design and deployment. As described by the Agency for Healthcare Research and Quality (AHRQ) Patient Safety Network, alert fatigue occurs when healthcare clinicians become desensitized to safety alerts and ignore them, increasing the risk of missing clinically important alerts in the barrage of unimportant or inappropriate alerts [43].

To mitigate alert fatigue risks, CDS designers and implementers must remain cognizant of the potential intrusive power of the CDS tool. A prompt can be designed as *interruptive* (popping up on the user's screen regardless of what the user is doing) or *non-interruptive* (available to click on in the background if the user requests more information). Additionally, the prompt can be offered with a "hard stop," requiring some action/input from the user before the user can proceed with other EHR activities, or as a fleeting reminder that can disappear after a specified time limit is reached or the user clicks off the region of interest. Judicious design, deployment, and ongoing evaluation of CDS tools are essential components of these AI applications in support of safe, efficient, and effective medical care delivery. To this end, many healthcare systems have appointed CDS (e.g., BPA) committees that collect and review data on numbers and types of alerts that fire and are ignored versus those with which users actively engage. In so doing, unhelpful CDS prompts are identified and voted on as potential alerts to be removed from the system to decrease alert fatigue.

Practice Applications

The healthcare domain continues to advance at a rapid pace with ever increasing discoveries in medical sciences, widespread uptake of health information systems, and the development and adoption of AI in response to a variety of healthcare needs. Despite the diffusion of knowledge enabled by these advances, they have not led to transformative impacts seen in other industries that have embraced similar knowledge-driven ecosystems [44]. This is attributed to:

(a) challenges caused by the exponential increase in health data generation and curation [45];
(b) significant time lag of up to 17 years between the discovery of knowledge and its application at clinical settings [46]; and
(c) the lack of system-level innovation driven by a diverse, interdisciplinary community to share ideas and learn from these evolving scientific endeavors [47].

Learning Health Systems (LHS) are an emerging approach that addresses these challenges. They are defined as a sociotechnical system in which science, informatics, incentives, and culture are aligned for continuous improvement and innovation, with best practices seamlessly embedded in the delivery process and new knowledge captured as an integral by-product of the delivery experience [44]. The LHS concept was first proposed during a 2007 workshop organized by the US National Academy of Medicine [48]. Since then, LHSs have gained widespread interest and adoption globally. Examples of LHS global adoption include the TRANSFoRm project [49] and the Swiss Learning Health System [50].

The fundamental operational process of a LHS is a learning cycle. A LHS can consist of multiple learning cycles, each seeking to address a specific health problem or challenge. Each learning cycle consists of converting data to knowledge (D2K), applying this knowledge to drive performance (K2P), and measuring changes in performance to generate new data that seeds the next iteration of the cycle (P2D) [45]. Each of these phases is driven by communities of interest composed of key actors and stakeholders who have come together to challenge a collective healthcare problem [51].

LHSs can be implemented at varying levels of scale across a single organization, by networks of organizations, or by specialties that span organizational boundaries. They may occur across geographic regions from counties to states or entire countries. Further, different LHS cycles may progress at different speeds based on the health problem that is being addressed.

Community Applications

Healthcare delivery and associated decision-making activities are driven by a variety of patient-level demographics, diagnoses, medications, past encounter data, and other clinical information collected by providers or self-reported by patients during routine medical care. Increased awareness of precision health and US reimbursement policies that favor value-based care have promoted interest in leveraging social, economic, and environmental factors to address upstream risks that impact patient health and wellbeing. These concerns have led to the concept of Social Determinants of Health (SDoH), which are defined as conditions in the environment where people are born, live, work and age that have a major impact on people's health, wellbeing, and quality of life [52]. It is increasingly recognized that these factors play a major role in addressing health disparities. The Kaiser Family Foundation [53] has categorized key SDoH factors (Table 36.2).

SDoH factors may be measured at a patient or population level. To date, patient-level SDoH elements are under-documented and underutilized in clinical practice [54]. Although SDoH data collection efforts are improving at many health systems, historically SDoH variables have not been systematically collected by providers as part of structured health data or reported by patients as part of survey instruments. The quality of self-reported SDoH data is also suspect [55, 56]. In contrast, a variety of SDoH-related elements that describe an individual's financial wellbeing (debt, unemployment, homelessness, need of public assistance) as well as negative behaviors or risks (feelings of safety, lack of healthcare access, limited education) are often present in unstructured free-text notes collected by other providers, particularly nurses, social workers, and mental health specialists. Unfortunately, extracting viable SDoH elements from large repositories of free-text data is challenging and time-consuming, and may still lead to an incomplete picture of individual health. In contrast, population-level SDoH measured at geographic levels such as census tract, zip code, or county levels are more widely available and are of higher quality and completeness [57]. They are collected by a variety of government and community organizations involved in environmental justice and public welfare. These elements have also been used to create composite indices such as the Social Vulnerability Index (SVI) [58] and the Area Deprivation Index (ADI) [59], which are used to inform population-level social risk factors.

Routine collection of patient-level SDoH elements in the form of structured data has grown due to increased awareness of their value [60, 61]. They have also been integrated into existing medical terminologies such as the Logical Observation Identifiers Names and Codes (LOINC) [62] and the International Classification of Diseases (ICD). While their utilization to date has been limited, their adoption within the healthcare domain is on the uptake [63] and is increasingly collected as part of routine patient screening practices [64].

Due to limited availability of SDoH elements, their use in patient care delivery, particularly for AI and decision-making tools, is limited. Use of SDoH in analytical modeling is also challenging given that SDoH elements are likely to be associated with each other, thereby resulting in issues of multi-collinearity and presenting challenges in interpretation [65]. To date, only a limited number of efforts have been made to incorporate SDoH factors for AI [66]. There is significant potential to include SDoH for AI-driven efforts to predict patient-level need of services, particularly as their availability, completeness, and quality increase over time. Effective mechanisms to generate population-wide SDoH-related phenotypes using unstructured and structured data also offer much potential to inform patient care delivery and better outcomes.

Health Policy Applications

Identifying and implementing effective and equitable health care practices relies heavily on analysis of large amounts of data, an area of strength for ML and NLP models. One example is the Medicaid expansion initiatives that are informed by vast quantities of claims data to identify healthcare use, underuse, and requested (or denied) use. Only through thorough evaluation of what is being done can we correlate care (or lack thereof) with improved or worsened outcomes. This information can inform policy on coverage, including to whom and for what services, to provide the greatest number of patients the most improved health outcomes for a given amount of resource investment.

Similar use of ML and NLP to identify correlates of chronic disease development and progression can inform public policies to protect large numbers of patients. Policy implications of AI and ML in specific chronic illnesses and

Table 36.2 Important social determinants of health, as defined by the Kaiser Family Foundation [53]

Determinant	Factors
Economic stability	Employment, income, expenses, debt, medical bills, other financial support
Neighborhood and physical environment	Housing, transportation, access to safe walking areas
Education	Literacy, early childhood, vocational or higher education
Food	Hunger, access to healthy food options
Community and social context	Social integration, discrimination, support systems, community engagement
Healthcare system	Health coverage, provider availability, quality of care, and providers' linguistic and cultural competency

in health care in general have been proposed in the literature and provide insights on prudent future paths to safe and effective application of these technologies to improve patient care [7, 25–27]. Additionally, in evaluating large amounts of data using ML and NLP methods, beyond single trial analyses, researchers can identify environmental, lifestyle and behavior factors, and product-use risks that can then inform policies and guidelines to protect patients from newly understood harms.

Health Equity Concerns

Increasing attention is given to the diversity of communities in terms of individual demographics such as race, ethnicity, gender, and age; socio-economic factors such as income-level, residence (urban or rural), education levels, and literacy; and health status factors such as chronic disease burden and special healthcare needs. The principle of health equity states that everyone has a fair and just opportunity to be as healthy as possible irrespective of these differences [67]. Unfortunately, different patient populations are often not treated equally or equitably. A large body of research highlights significant disparities in access to health care, as well as provider and health system-level biases that impact patient care and outcomes.

Historical disparities and biases are reflected in datasets collected across health systems. If used for analytics, such datasets may lead to the "garbage in—garbage out" problem [68], resulting in biased models that are harmful to vulnerable, underserved, and minority populations [69–71]. Given evidence of harm caused by biased models [72], there is significant interest in improving model behaviors to mitigate biases. Efforts include ensuring proper representation in data used for modeling [73], investigation of causality in model predictions [74], as well as explainability and interpretability of model predictions to assess fairness.

Given the multi-faceted nature of fairness [75], what constitutes bias may vary based on the use case under test. A variety of metrics can be used to investigate models for each of these biases. However, the decision on which metric to apply must be made based on the clinical use case and application of a model. As an example, a model that is intended to deliver an assistive treatment may be assessed using false negative rate or false omission rate parity, while a model which delivers a harmful outcome may be assessed using false discovery rate or false positive rate parity. Once biases are identified, they may be rectified by a variety of mitigation methods such as reweighing and optimizing pre-processing, which are applied to model training, adversarial debiasing, and prejudice removal, which are applied during model training, and equalized odds post-processing, which is applied to model outputs. In addition to such static metrics which consider a snapshot of analytical fairness at a specific time, it is also important to consider health equity as an ongoing process. This process has been named *algorithmovigilance* and defined as the scientific methods and activities relating to the evaluation, monitoring, understanding, and prevention of adverse effects of algorithms in health care [76]. These processes should occur prior to, during, and after implementation of algorithms to ensure their safe and appropriate use in the populations where they will be employed [77].

Future Directions

Artificial intelligence has the potential to revolutionize health care with improved diagnostic and predictive capabilities over prior rule-based, solely human-dependent methods of care delivery and surveillance. However, current challenges must be addressed to optimize this largely untested potential and support care delivery in real-world environments. The US presidential mandate of 2019 directed federal agencies to develop a plan to ensure AI and ML standards [78]. As evidenced by IBM Watson Health's inability to tackle large treatment prediction problems requiring use of voluminous and disparate cancer and genomic data, many challenges still impede widespread AI and ML adoption and use at the point of care [79]. Some of these challenges include [2, 78, 80]:

1. Regulatory challenges—lack of AI standards and easy methods of *algorithmovigilance* to ensure equity, validity, and population applicability.
2. Data governance challenges—lack of standardized data governance policies.
3. Data-interoperability challenges—lack of an integrated global healthcare database.
4. Data accessibility—lack of large, freely available (open-source), labeled data sets for machine learning and NLP model training and testing.
5. Method adoption and implementation challenges—lack of easy integration into workflows.
6. Method development for automatic term relationship identification in textual data analysis.
7. Method development for automatic temporal extraction to facilitate identification of disease progression and outcome onset.
8. Workforce development to ensure clinicians, informaticians, clinical data scientists, and computer science specialists can work together to create, validate, apply, interpret, and monitor these methods in the service of better patient care.

Artificial intelligence, including ML and NLP methods, holds tremendous potential for both advancing healthcare delivery and unintended consequences of worsening health equity disparities or advising providers to follow inaccurate treatment pathways based on incomplete, inaccurate, or out-of-date data [81–83]. As in medicine in general, the first rule of AI in health care is, *Do no harm* [84]. Increasing government oversight along with professional guidance documents are providing guardrails to inform future AI development and implementation [85–90].

The recent Agency for Healthcare Research and Quality (AHRQ) research agenda emphasized improving chronic care and learning with some emphasis on the use of health information technology supporting these goals [91]. Guidance on prudent and realistic paths forward to using these technologies has been offered by the recent National Academy of Medicine report with a key insight recognizing that the next best step in greater AI use and adoption requires AI tools to focus on *augmentation* of provider cognition and care of patients instead of *autonomous* AI methods without human oversight [92]. Provider commitment to patient-centered care requires patient-provider relationships, continuity of care, and holistic approaches in chronic illness management. Machines can help collate and present voluminous data, and provide new insights on correlations within these data, but machines are not able to replace the human touch and knowing that comes from seeing and understanding the whole patient. Our path forward as tech-savvy providers is *partnering* with AI tools to deliver the most effective, efficient, and patient-centered care possible.

References

1. Panch T, Szolovits P, Atun R. Artificial intelligence, machine learning and health systems. J Glob Health. 2018;8(2):020303. https://doi.org/10.7189/jogh.08.020303.
2. Sheikhalishahi S, Miotto R, Dudley JT, Lavelli A, Rinaldi F, Osmani V. Natural language processing of clinical notes on chronic diseases: systematic review. JMIR Med Inform. 2019;7(2):e12239. https://doi.org/10.2196/12239.
3. Shortliffe EH, Cimino J. Biomedical informatics: computer applications in health care and biomedicine. 5th ed. Cham: Springer; 2021.
4. Sidey-Gibbons JAM, Sidey-Gibbons CJ. Machine learning in medicine: a practical introduction. BMC Med Res Methodol. 2019;19(1):64. https://doi.org/10.1186/s12874-019-0681-4.
5. Mitchell TM. Machine learning. THe McGraw-Hill Companies, Inc.; 1997. p. 400.
6. Rudin C. Stop explaining black box machine learning models for high stakes decisions and use interpretable models instead. Nature. Machine Intelligence. 2019;1(5):206–15. https://doi.org/10.1038/s42256-019-0048-x.
7. Matheny ME, Whicher D, Thadaney IS. Artificial intelligence in health care: a report from the National Academy of Medicine. JAMA. 2020;323(6):509–10. https://doi.org/10.1001/jama.2019.21579.
8. CDC: National Center for Chronic Disease Prevention and Health Promotion. About Chronic Diseases. US Department of Health and Human. Services. https://www.cdc.gov/chronicdisease/about/index.htm. Accessed 10 July 2021.
9. Souza-Pereira L, Pombo N, Ouhbi S, Felizardo V, Garcia N. Clinical decision support systems for chronic diseases: a systematic literature review. Comput Methods Prog Biomed. 2020;195:105565. https://doi.org/10.1016/j.cmpb.2020.105565.
10. Yin J, Ngiam KY, Teo HH. Role of artificial intelligence applications in real-life clinical practice: systematic review. J Med Internet Res. 2021;23(4):e25759.
11. Sönnichsen A, Trampisch US, Rieckert A, et al. Polypharmacy in chronic diseases-Reduction of Inappropriate Medication and Adverse drug events in older populations by electronic Decision Support (PRIMA-eDS): study protocol for a randomized controlled trial. Trials. 2016;17:57. https://doi.org/10.1186/s13063-016-1177-8.
12. Sasaki K, Jabbour EJ, Ravandi F, et al. The LEukemia Artificial Intelligence Program (LEAP) in chronic myeloid leukemia in chronic phase: a model to improve patient outcomes. Am J Hematol. 2021;96(2):241–50. https://doi.org/10.1002/ajh.26047.
13. Boekhout JM, Berendsen BAJ, Peels DA, Bolman CAW, Lechner L. Evaluation of a computer-tailored healthy ageing intervention to promote physical activity among single older adults with a chronic disease. Int J Environ Res Public Health. 2018;15(2):346. https://doi.org/10.3390/ijerph15020346.
14. Boekhout JM, Volders E, Bolman CAW, de Groot RHM, Lechner L. Long-term effects on loneliness of a computer-tailored intervention for older adults with chronic diseases: a randomized controlled trial. J Aging Health. 2021;33:865–76. https://doi.org/10.1177/08982643211015027.
15. Le Glaz A, Haralambous Y, Kim-Dufor DH, et al. Machine learning and natural language processing in mental health: systematic review. J Med Internet Res. 2021;23(5):e15708. https://doi.org/10.2196/15708.
16. Bibault JE, Xing L. Screening for chronic obstructive pulmonary disease with artificial intelligence. Lancet Digit Health. 2020;2(5):e216–7. https://doi.org/10.1016/s2589-7500(20)30076-5.
17. Feng Y, Wang Y, Zeng C, Mao H. Artificial intelligence and machine learning in chronic airway diseases: focus on asthma and chronic obstructive pulmonary disease. Int J Med Sci. 2021;18(13):2871–89. https://doi.org/10.7150/ijms.58191.
18. Fischer AM, Varga-Szemes A, Martin SS, et al. Artificial Intelligence-based fully automated per lobe segmentation and emphysema-quantification based on chest computed tomography compared with global initiative for chronic obstructive lung disease severity of smokers. J Thorac Imaging. 2020;35(Suppl 1):S28–s34. https://doi.org/10.1097/rti.0000000000000500.
19. Li X, Zhou HP, Zhou ZJ, et al. Artificial intelligence-powered remote monitoring of patients with chronic obstructive pulmonary disease. Chin Med J. 2021;134(13):1546–8. https://doi.org/10.1097/cm9.0000000000001529.
20. Romiti S, Vinciguerra M, Saade W, Anso Cortajarena I, Greco E. Artificial Intelligence (AI) and cardiovascular diseases: an unexpected alliance. Cardiol Res Pract. 2020;2020:4972346.
21. Mathur P, Srivastava S, Xu X, Mehta JL. Artificial intelligence, machine learning, and cardiovascular disease. Clin Med Insights Cardiol. 2020;14:1–9. https://doi.org/10.1177/1179546820927404.
22. Barrett M, Boyne J, Brandts J, et al. Artificial intelligence supported patient self-care in chronic heart failure: a paradigm shift from reactive to predictive, preventive and personalised care. EPMA J. 2019;10(4):445–64. https://doi.org/10.1007/s13167-019-00188-9.
23. Wan TT, Gurupur V, Wang BL, Matthews S. A patient-centric care approach to facilitate the design of an artificial intelligence application in geriatric care management of heart failure readmissions. Biomed Res Clin Rev. 2021;3(5).
24. Decharatanachart P, Chaiteerakij R, Tiyarattanachai T, Treeprasertsuk S. Application of artificial intelligence in

25. Broome DT, Hilton CB, Mehta N. Policy implications of artificial intelligence and machine learning in diabetes management. Curr Diab Rep. 2020;20(2):1–5.
26. Dankwa-Mullan I, Rivo M, Sepulveda M, Park Y, Snowdon J, Rhee K. Transforming diabetes care through artificial intelligence: the future is here. Popul Health Manag. 2019;22(3):229–42.
27. Ellahham S. Artificial intelligence: the future for diabetes care. Am J Med. 2020;133(8):895–900.
28. Tarumi S, Takeuchi W, Chalkidis G, et al. Leveraging artificial intelligence to improve chronic disease care: methods and application to pharmacotherapy decision support for type-2 diabetes mellitus. Methods Inf Med. 2021;60(S 01):e32–43. https://doi.org/10.1055/s-0041-1728757.
29. Zhu T, Li K, Herrero P, Georgiou P. Deep learning for diabetes: a systematic review. IEEE J Biomed Health Inform. 2021;25(7):2744–57.
30. Aldhyani THH, Alshebami AS, Alzahrani MY. Soft clustering for enhancing the diagnosis of chronic diseases over machine learning algorithms. J Healthc Eng. 2020;2020:4984967. https://doi.org/10.1155/2020/4984967.
31. Battineni G, Sagaro GG, Chinatalapudi N, Amenta F. Applications of machine learning predictive models in the chronic disease diagnosis. Journal of personalized medicine. 2020;10(2):21.
32. Soni VD. Chronic disease detection model using machine learning techniques. Int J Sci Technol Res. 2020;9(9):262–6.
33. Daowd A, Faizan S, Abidi S, Abusharekh A, Shehzad A, Abidi SSR. Towards personalized lifetime health: a platform for early multimorbid chronic disease risk assessment and mitigation. Stud Health Technol Inform. 2019;264:935–9. https://doi.org/10.3233/shti190361.
34. Ahmed Z, Mohamed K, Zeeshan S, Dong X. Artificial intelligence with multi-functional machine learning platform development for better healthcare and precision medicine. Database (Oxford). 2020;2020:baaa010. https://doi.org/10.1093/database/baaa010.
35. Ng K, Kartoun U, Stavropoulos H, Zambrano JA, Tang PC. Personalized treatment options for chronic diseases using precision cohort analytics. Sci Rep. 2021;11(1):1139. https://doi.org/10.1038/s41598-021-80967-5.
36. Silva P, Jacobs D, Kriak J, et al. Implementation of pharmacogenomics and artificial intelligence tools for chronic disease management in primary care setting. J Pers Med. 2021;11(6):443. https://doi.org/10.3390/jpm11060443.
37. Subramanian M, Wojtusciszyn A, Favre L, et al. Precision medicine in the era of artificial intelligence: implications in chronic disease management. J Transl Med. 2020;18(1):472. https://doi.org/10.1186/s12967-020-02658-5.
38. Chae SH, Kim Y, Lee KS, Park HS. Development and clinical evaluation of a web-based upper limb home rehabilitation system using a smartwatch and machine learning model for chronic stroke survivors: prospective comparative study. JMIR Mhealth Uhealth. 2020;8(7):e17216. https://doi.org/10.2196/17216.
39. Griffin AC, Xing Z, Khairat S, et al. Conversational agents for chronic disease self-management: a systematic review. AMIA Annu Symp Proc. 2020;2020:504–13.
40. Schachner T, Keller R, Wangenheim FV. Artificial intelligence-based conversational agents for chronic conditions: systematic literature review. J Med Internet Res. 2020;22(9):e20701. https://doi.org/10.2196/20701.
41. Castelyn G, Laranjo L, Schreier G, Gallego B. Predictive performance and impact of algorithms in remote monitoring of chronic conditions: a systematic review and meta-analysis. Int J Med Inform. 2021;156:104620. https://doi.org/10.1016/j.ijmedinf.2021.104620.
42. Kooij L, Groen WG, van Harten WH. The effectiveness of information technology-supported shared care for patients with chronic disease: a systematic review. J Med Internet Res. 2017;19(6):e221. https://doi.org/10.2196/jmir.7405.
43. Network PS. Alert Fatigue. AHRQ. US Department of Health & Human Services. https://psnet.ahrq.gov/primer/alert-fatigue. Accessed 20 July 2021.
44. Friedman C, Rubin J, Brown J, et al. Toward a science of learning systems: a research agenda for the high-functioning Learning Health System. J Am Med Inform Assoc. 2015;22(1):43–50.
45. Friedman C, Rubin J, Sullivan K. Toward an information infrastructure for global health improvement. Yearb Med Inform. 2017;26(01):16–23.
46. Morris ZS, Wooding S, Grant J. The answer is 17 years, what is the question: understanding time lags in translational research. J R Soc Med. 2011;104(12):510–20.
47. University of Michigan Medical School. Learning Health Systems. https://medicine.umich.edu/dept/lhs/service-outreach/learning-health-systems.
48. Olsen L, Aisner D, McGinnis JM. The learning healthcare system: workshop summary. Washington, DC: National Academies Press (US); 2007.
49. Delaney BC, Curcin V, Andreasson A, et al. Translational medicine and patient safety in Europe: TRANSFoRm—architecture for the learning health system in Europe. Biomed Res Int. 2015;2015:961526.
50. Boes S, Mantwill S, Kaufmann C, et al. Swiss learning health system: a national initiative to establish learning cycles for continuous health system improvement. Learning health systems. 2018;2(3):e10059.
51. Menear M, Blanchette M-A, Demers-Payette O, Roy D. A framework for value-creating learning health systems. Health research policy and systems. 2019;17(1):1–13.
52. Marmot M, Bell R. Fair society, healthy lives. Public Health. 2012;126(Suppl 1):S4–S10. https://doi.org/10.1016/j.puhe.2012.05.014.
53. Artiga S, Hinton, E. Beyond health care: the role of social determinants in promoting health and health equity. 2018. http://www.ccapcomcare.org/Newsletters/2018-05%20INSIGHT%20KFF%20Brief.pdf. Accessed 20 Nov 2021.
54. McCormack LA, McCormack M-B. Social determinant of health documentation trends and their association with emergency department admissions. AMIA Ann Symp Proc. 2020;2020:823–32.
55. Cook LA, Sachs J, Weiskopf NG. The quality of social determinants data in the electronic health record: a systematic review. J Am Med Inform Assoc. 2021;29(1):187–96. https://doi.org/10.1093/jamia/ocab199.
56. Kasthurirathne SN. The use of clinical, behavioral, and social determinants of health to improve identification of patients in need of advanced care for depression. Indiana University-Purdue University; 2018. https://scholarworks.iupui.edu/handle/1805/17765
57. Kolak M, Bhatt J, Park YH, Padron NA, Molefe A. Quantification of Neighborhood-Level Social Determinants of Health in the Continental United States. JAMA Netw Open. 2020;3(1):e1919928. https://doi.org/10.1001/jamanetworkopen.2019.19928.
58. Flanagan BE, Gregory EW, Hallisey EJ, Heitgerd JL, Lewis B. A social vulnerability index for disaster management Journal of Homeland Security and Emergency Management. 2011;8(1):3. https://doi.org/10.2202/1547-7355.1792.
59. Knighton AJ, Savitz L, Belnap T, Stephenson B, VanDerslice J. Introduction of an area deprivation index measuring patient socioeconomic status in an integrated health system: implications for population health. EGEMS (Wash DC). 2016;4(3):1238. https://doi.org/10.13063/2327-9214.1238.

60. Bako AT, Walter-McCabe H, Kasthurirathne SN, Halverson PK, Vest JR. Reasons for social work referrals in an urban safety-net population: a natural language processing and market basket analysis approach. J Soc Serv Res. 2020;47(3):414–25. https://doi.org/10.1080/01488376.2020.1817834.
61. Feller D, Zucker J, Bear Don't Walk O, Yin M, Gordon P, Elhadad N. Longitudinal analysis of social and behavioral determinants of health in the EHR: exploring the impact of patient trajectories and documentation practices. AMIA Annu Symp Proc. 2019;2019:399–407.
62. Inc. RI. LOINC from Regenstrief: Social Determinants of Health. https://loinc.org/sdh/. Accessed 20 Nov 2021.
63. Truong HP, Luke AA, Hammond G, Wadhera RK, Reidhead M, Joynt Maddox KE. Utilization of social determinants of health ICD-10 Z-codes among hospitalized patients in the United States, 2016–2017. Med Care. 2020;58(12):1037–43. https://doi.org/10.1097/MLR.0000000000001418.
64. Buitron de la Vega P, Losi S, Sprague Martinez L, et al. Implementing an EHR-based screening and referral system to address social determinants of health in primary care. Med Care. 2019;57(Suppl 6 Suppl 2):S133–9. https://doi.org/10.1097/MLR.0000000000001029.
65. Fuchs VR. Social determinants of health: caveats and nuances. JAMA. 2017;317(1):25–6. https://doi.org/10.1001/jama.2016.17335.
66. Kasthurirathne SN, Grannis S, Halverson PK, Morea J, Menachemi N, Vest JR. Precision health-enabled machine learning to identify need for wraparound social services using patient- and population-level data sets: algorithm development and validation. JMIR Med Inform. 2020;8(7):e16129. https://doi.org/10.2196/16129.
67. Braveman P, Arkin E, Orleans T, Proctor D, Acker J, Plough P. What is health equity? Behav Sci Policy. 2018;4(1):1–14.
68. Kim Y, Huang J, Emery S. Garbage in, garbage out: data collection, quality assessment and reporting standards for social media data use in health research, infodemiology and digital disease detection. J Med Internet Res. 2016;18(2):e41. https://doi.org/10.2196/jmir.4738.
69. Buolamwini J, Gebru T. Gender shades: intersectional accuracy disparities in commercial gender classification. ML Research Press; 2018. p. 77–91.
70. Shankar S, Halpern Y, Breck E, Atwood J, Wilson J, Sculley D. No classification without representation: assessing geodiversity issues in open data sets for the developing world. 2017.
71. Tommasi T, Patricia N, Caputo B, Tuytelaars T. Chapter 2. Advances in computer vision and pattern recognition. In: A deeper look at dataset bias. Domain adaptation in computer vision applications. 2017. p. 37–55.
72. Obermeyer Z, Powers B, Vogeli C, Mullainathan S. Dissecting racial bias in an algorithm used to manage the health of populations. Science. 2019;2019(366):477–53.
73. Kay M, Matuszek C, Munson SA. Unequal representation and gender stereotypes in image search results for occupations. Paper Presented at Proceedings of the 33rd Annual ACM Conference on Human Factors in Computing Systems; 2015.
74. Sharma S, Henderson H, Ghosh J. CERTIFAI: Counterfactual Explanations for Robustness, Transparency, Interpretability, and Fairness of Artificial Intelligence models. TBD. 2019.
75. Bellamy RK, Dey K, Hind M, Hoffman SC, Houde S, Kannan K, et al. AI fairness 360: an extensible toolkit for detecting, understanding, and mitigating unwanted algorithmic bias. TBD. 2018.
76. Embi PJ. Algorithmovigilance-advancing methods to analyze and monitor artificial intelligence-driven health care for effectiveness and equity. JAMA Netw Open. 2021;4(4):e214622. https://doi.org/10.1001/jamanetworkopen.2021.4622.
77. Kun-Hsing YKIS. Artificial intelligence, bias and clinical safety. BMJ Qual Saf. 2019;28(3):231–7. https://doi.org/10.1136/bmjqs-2018-008370.
78. Choudhury A, Renjilian E, Asan O. Use of machine learning in geriatric clinical care for chronic diseases: a systematic literature review. JAMIA Open. 2020;3(3):459–71. https://doi.org/10.1093/jamiaopen/ooaa034.
79. Lohr S. What ever happened to IBM's Watson? New York Times. 2021.
80. Meskó B, Hetényi G, Győrffy Z. Will artificial intelligence solve the human resource crisis in healthcare? BMC Health Serv Res. 2018;18(1):1–4.
81. Kueper JK, Terry AL, Zwarenstein M, Lizotte DJ. Artificial intelligence and primary care research: a scoping review. Ann Fam Med. 2020;18(3):250–8. https://doi.org/10.1370/afm.2518.
82. Liyanage H, Liaw ST, Jonnagaddala J, et al. Artificial intelligence in primary health care: perceptions, issues, and challenges. Yearb Med Inform. 2019;28(1):41–6. https://doi.org/10.1055/s-0039-1677901.
83. Yang Z, Silcox C, Sendak M, et al. Advancing primary care with Artificial Intelligence and Machine Learning. Healthc (Amst). 2022;10(1):100594. https://doi.org/10.1016/j.hjdsi.2021.100594.
84. Wiens J, Saria S, Sendak M, et al. Do no harm: a roadmap for responsible machine learning for health care. Nat Med. 2019;25(9):1337–40. https://doi.org/10.1038/s41591-019-0548-6.
85. Bender E, Friedman B. Data statements for natural language processing: toward mitigating system bias and enabling better science. Transactions of the Association for Computational Linguistics. 2018;6:587–604.
86. Gebru T, Morgenstern J, Vecchione B, et al. Datasheets for datasets. Commun ACM. 2021;64(12):86–92. https://doi.org/10.1145/3458723.
87. Mitchell M, Wu S, Zaldivar A, et al. Model cards for model reporting. Paper presented at Proceedings of the Conference on Fairness, Accountability, and Transparency. 2019.
88. Munoz C, Smith M, Patil DJ. Big data: a report on algorithmic systems, opportunity, and civil rights. 2016.
89. Saria S, Subbaswamy A. Tutorial: safe and reliable machine learning. In: ACM Conference on Fairness, Accountability, and Transparency (FAT* 2019). 2019.
90. Taber P, Radloff C, Del Fiol G, Staes C, Kawamoto K. New standards for clinical decision support: a survey of the state of implementation. Yearb Med Inform. 2021;30(1):159–71. https://doi.org/10.1055/s-0041-1726502.
91. Bierman AS, Wang J, O'Malley PG, Moss DK. Transforming care for people with multiple chronic conditions: Agency for Healthcare Research and Quality's research agenda. Health Serv Res. 2021;56(Suppl 1):973–9. https://doi.org/10.1111/1475-6773.13863.
92. National Academy of Medicine. Artificial intelligence in health care: the hope, the hype, the promise, the peril. National Academy of Medicine Special Publication; 2019. Accessed 10 Sept 2021.

Health Information Technology

Carlton Moore

Introduction

Health information technology (IT) is a broad concept that encompasses an array of technologies that collect, store, share, and analyze electronic healthcare information [1]. Health IT includes a range of functionality from medical billing systems to electronic health records (EHRs). EHRs are repositories of electronically maintained longitudinal records of patients' health status and health care. Many EHR systems have additional information management tools that facilitate computerized order-entry, clinical reminders and alerts, and linkages to knowledge sources for clinical decision support. In 2004, less than 25% of ambulatory practices were using electronic health records (EHRs); however, over a decade later the number of practices using EHRs increased to more than 86% (Fig. 37.1) [2].

This chapter will provide an overview of health IT, particularly as it applies to chronic illness care. The first section will give an historical perspective on the development of health IT, as well as an operational understanding of its many elements. Next, the expansion of health IT into applications of chronic disease management will be discussed. The subsequent section will outline the policy and operational components of Meaningful Use (MU) and be followed by an assessment of the effectiveness of health IT in chronic disease management. The chapter will close with an appraisal of the state of the science and future trends in health IT.

From Paper to Electrons: An Historical Perspective of Health IT

"You have to know the past to understand the present" [attributed to Carl Sagan] [3].

C. Moore (✉)
Department of Medicine, University of North Carolina at Chapel Hill, Chapel Hill, NC, USA
e-mail: crmoore@med.unc.edu; carlton_moore@med.unc.edu

Many factors have led to a dramatic increase in the use of health IT and away from paper-based medical records in clinical care. The modern paper chart arose in the nineteenth century as clinical casebooks, daybooks, and diaries commonly used by physicians to record observations and treatment plans for their patients [4]. They served as longitudinal medical records that were updated on a regular basis as patients' medical conditions and treatment plans changed. Early on, clinical notes in paper charts were handwritten with few formatting requirements or standards which specified the necessary information that should be included in the notes. This led to communication and other challenges related to the legibility of handwritten notes, as well as significant variability in completeness and accuracy of information that was documented in medical records. Additionally, a single patient that was cared for by multiple physicians would have multiple paper charts distributed across various hospitals and/or physician offices. This partitioning of paper records contributed to poor coordination of care.

Most early advances in paper-based medical records were developed in academic teaching hospitals and then slowly disseminated to ambulatory care settings and private physician practices. For example, a major innovation to improve patient care, based on models from industry, was introduced in 1907 at St. Mary's Hospital and the Mayo Clinic in order to address the problem of scattered, disorganized patient information. In this setting, new patients were assigned a unique clinic number and all data for that patient were combined into a single paper medical chart, designated by the assignment number. An early study found that the charts consistently listed chief complaint, objective and subjective symptoms, and diagnosis [4].

From these early days, as practices and hospitals grew, laboratory and other diagnostic study results were added to the paper chart. Typically, blood specimens were sent to outside labs and the results were facsimiled (faxed) back to the office, and results were placed in the corresponding patient chart; there was a similar workflow for radiology and pathology studies. Additionally, notes from nurses and other

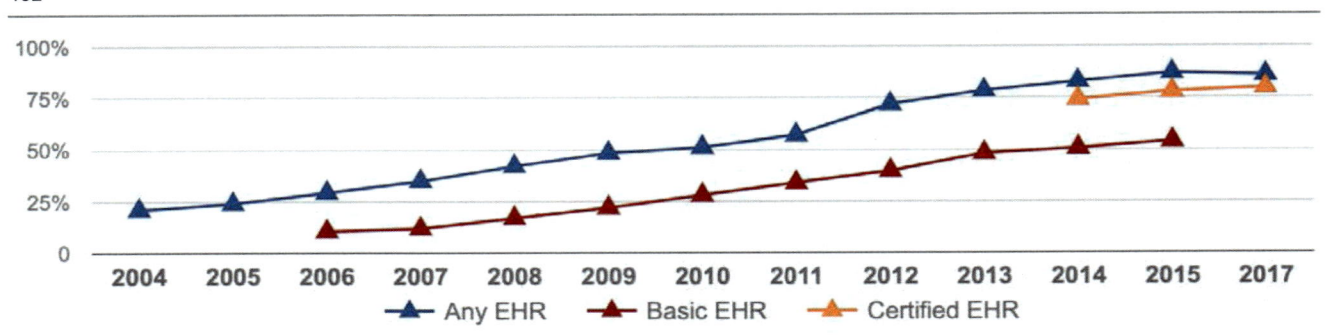

Fig. 37.1 Percentage of office-based physicians with electronic health records

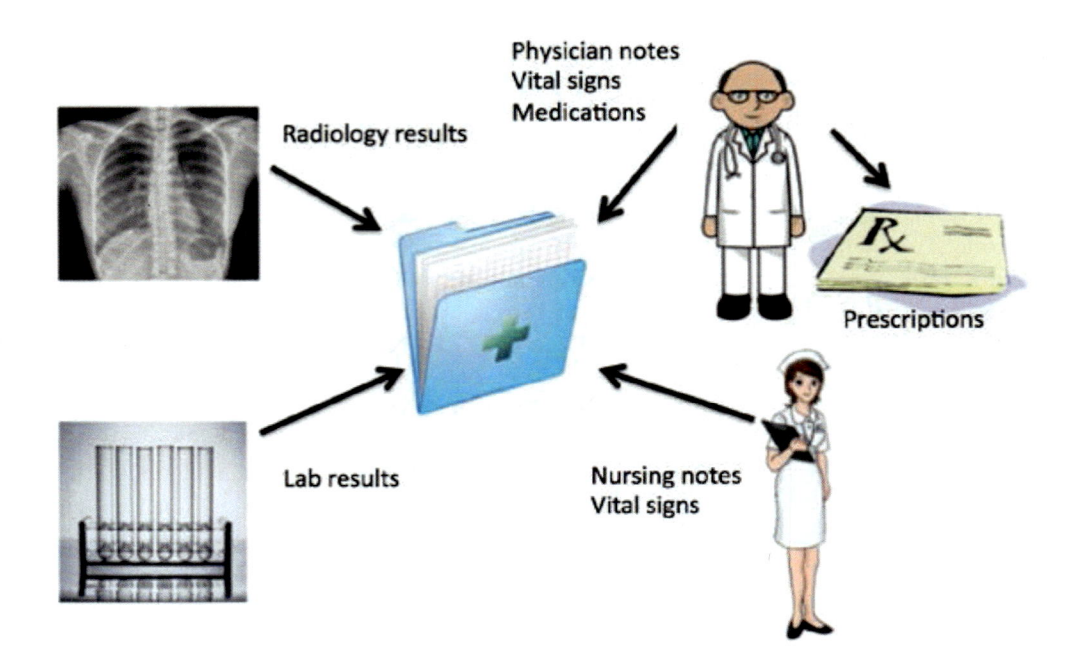

Fig. 37.2 Inputs to the medical record

healthcare professionals involved in patient care were added to charts (Fig. 37.2). For office practices with many patients, medical records were filed away in a medical records room where they were stored until needed for subsequent patient encounters.

This system was prevalent in ambulatory practices throughout the U.S. prior to the expansion of EHR use. The advantage of the paper chart was that it provided a relatively quick and easy way of documenting and viewing a patient's medical information, once a chart was obtained from the medical records location. However, for patients with chronic disease, there were several disadvantages of the paper system [5]. The first was difficulty in determining the quality of care provided to chronically ill patients. Due to the unstructured manner in which information was stored in paper charts, it became both time and resource intensive for individual physicians and practices to identify specific subsets of chronic disease patient populations, in order to assess the quality of care being provided.

The paper-based system also did not facilitate identifying high-risk patients for improving the quality of their care. For example, a primary care physician who wanted to find and aggregate patients with poorly controlled diabetes (i.e., hemoglobin A1c $\geq$ 9.0%) would have to manually review paper charts to create a list, and then proactively schedule these high-risk patients for appointments to optimize medication regimens. Often, paper-based rosters utilized software programs to create spreadsheets in which data was manually entered as each individual chart was reviewed. This process would need to be repeated for other chronic diseases or conditions, and the information would need to be updated over time. For physicians and physician practices with large patient panels and limited support staff, this was an impracticable process.

A second challenge was having a single user of the information at one time, which limited accessibility for any other user. Inaccessibility of the paper chart, especially in large organizations, is a major limitation of paper records. For example, a patient's chart may be unavailable to other providers for days while the physician completes documentation of his clinical note from the patient visit. Also, researchers may borrow paper charts for data abstraction in clinical studies, during which time the charts may not be available for patient care.

The lack of remote access to paper charts can also compromise patient care, particularly in situations when physicians do not have access to patients' clinical information. For example, an after-hours call to a physician about a patient complaining of chest pain is problematic, since the provider cannot view the patient's chart to determine if this is a new or longstanding complaint, or if there are pertinent diagnostic test results (e.g., a recently performed cardiac stress test) that would inform appropriate triage for the patient. Documentation clarity was another limitation of the paper record. Since physician notes and medication prescriptions were handwritten, legibility was frequently a problem. This resulted in substantial rates of adverse drug events, due to incorrectly prescribed or administered medications.

One study that reviewed 1411 handwritten prescriptions from an internal medicine clinic in a large health system found that approximately 28% of the prescriptions contained one or more errors or potential errors [6]. Another study of 4 adult primary care practices found that prescribing errors occurred in 7.6% of outpatient prescriptions and many could have caused patient harm [7]. One example of a prescription error described [8] involved an elderly nursing home resident who was prescribed oral hydroxyzine, 10 mg every 6 h, to alleviate itching. The pharmacist misread the physician's handwriting and dispensed oral hydralazine (a blood pressure medication), 10 mg every 6 h instead.

The inability to support clinical decision making is another limitation with paper-based medical records. As a passive recording tool that documents clinical information about patients, it requires that clinicians manually search for key information needed to make evidence-based clinical decisions during patient encounters. For example, if a physician wants to make an informed decision about which antihypertensive to prescribe a patient, she must know about relevant medication allergies, potential drug-drug-interactions, relevant laboratory results (e.g., creatinine and potassium), as well as disease-specific recommendations. This patient-specific information is either hidden and difficult to access in the paper chart (e.g., relevant laboratory results and allergies), or the disease-specific guideline and recommendations reside outside of the paper chart. As a result, a physician must actively search for, acquire, and then process this information prior to prescribing. The process must be repeated for multiple medications and for multiple patients with multiple chronic medical conditions.

This process not only applies to medications, but also to other chronic disease management interventions such as diagnostic screening. Physicians must be cognizant of preventive service and care guidelines which is daunting. A primary care physician, for example, is estimated to require over 7 h per working day in order to counsel and provide preventive services based on U.S. Preventive Services Task Force recommendations [9]. This workflow is in the context of an environment in which there are competing demands during patient encounters, such as troubleshooting acute medical issues and addressing psychosocial barriers to care [10]. Unsurprisingly, patients only received approximately 50% of recommended services in the era of paper charts [11].

Genesis and Evolution of Health IT for Chronic Disease Management

"If you want to make an apple pie from scratch, you must first create the universe" [attributed to Carl Sagan] [3].

The intersection of two events spurred expansion of EHRs from large healthcare systems and academic medical centers and into small medical groups and community practices; publication of the Institute of Medicine's (IOM) 2001 report *Crossing the Quality Chasm: A New Health System for the 21st Century* [12] and the 2008 great recession.

Crossing the Quality Chasm: Putting a Spotlight on the Healthcare System's Failures

The IOM report, *Crossing the Quality Chasm*, admonished that the U.S. healthcare delivery system did not provide consistent, high-quality medical care to all people, that patients were harmed too frequently, and that health care failed to deliver its potential benefit [12]. The report highlighted that Americans were living longer, due in part to advances in medical science and technology, however the aging population was associated with an increase in the incidence and prevalence of chronic conditions. Although these conditions, including heart disease, diabetes, and asthma, are now the leading cause of illness, disability, and death, the contemporary health system remained overly focused on acute, episodic care [12].

The failures described in the IOM report were corroborated in a study that reviewed medical records from adult patients living in 12 U.S. metropolitan areas to determine if they received evidence-based recommended care for several chronic medicine conditions [11]. The study concluded that patients received less than half of the recommended care for their chronic medical conditions. For example, only about 24% of participants in the study who had diabetes received three or more glycosylated hemoglobin tests over a 2-year period [11]. The gaps in quality of care highlighted here and by other researchers led the IOM to conclude that the current healthcare system required major redesign in order to effectively improve outcomes for patients with chronic diseases.

A major redesign proposed by IOM was effective use of health IT and EHRs in patient care [12]. There was a strong belief that IT must play a central role in the redesign of the healthcare system if a substantial improvement in healthcare quality is to be achieved. A final recommendation was for a national commitment to building an information infrastructure to support healthcare delivery, consumer health, quality measurement and improvement, public accountability, clinical and health services research, and clinical education. A goal of this commitment was the elimination of handwritten clinical data by the end of the decade [12].

An Opportunity Through the 2008 Great Recession

The American Recovery and Reinvestment Act (ARRA) of 2009 [13], commonly referred to as "The Stimulus," was a financial incentives package enacted by the U.S. Congress in February 2009 and signed into law on February 17, 2009, by President Barack Obama. It was a response to the 2008 Great Recession and its primary objective was to quickly promote jobs in an economy in which the unemployment rate was increasing. A secondary objective was to invest in infrastructure, education, and health care, most notably the development of the health IT infrastructure described in the IOM report. As a consequence, a key component of ARRA was the Health Information Technology for Economic and Clinical Health Act (HITECH Act) [14] that was designed to stimulate the adoption of EHRs and support health IT. HITECH sought to provide incentive payments to individual physicians (and hospitals) if they achieved "meaningful use" of "certified" EHR technology. The rule also established payment penalties in future years for healthcare providers who did not meet the requirements for the "meaningful use" of EHRs, thus using a carrot and stick approach for implementing health IT functionality.

The HITECH Act included funding of approximately $22 billion, with the majority of funding allocated as follows: (1) $18 billion allocated to Center for Medicare and Medicaid Services (CMS) for Medicare and Medicaid reimbursements to incentivize hospitals and physicians to adopt and "meaningfully use" EHR systems; (2) $2 billion to the Office of the National Coordinator (ONC) for health IT to develop regulations for the certification of EHRs and for advising CMS on defining EHR "meaningful use" criteria, and; (3) $677 million to establish Health Information Technology Regional Extension Centers (RECs) to provide technical assistance, guidance and information on best practices to support and accelerate healthcare providers efforts to "meaningfully use" EHRs (Fig. 37.3).

Fig. 37.3 ARRA support for EHR adoption

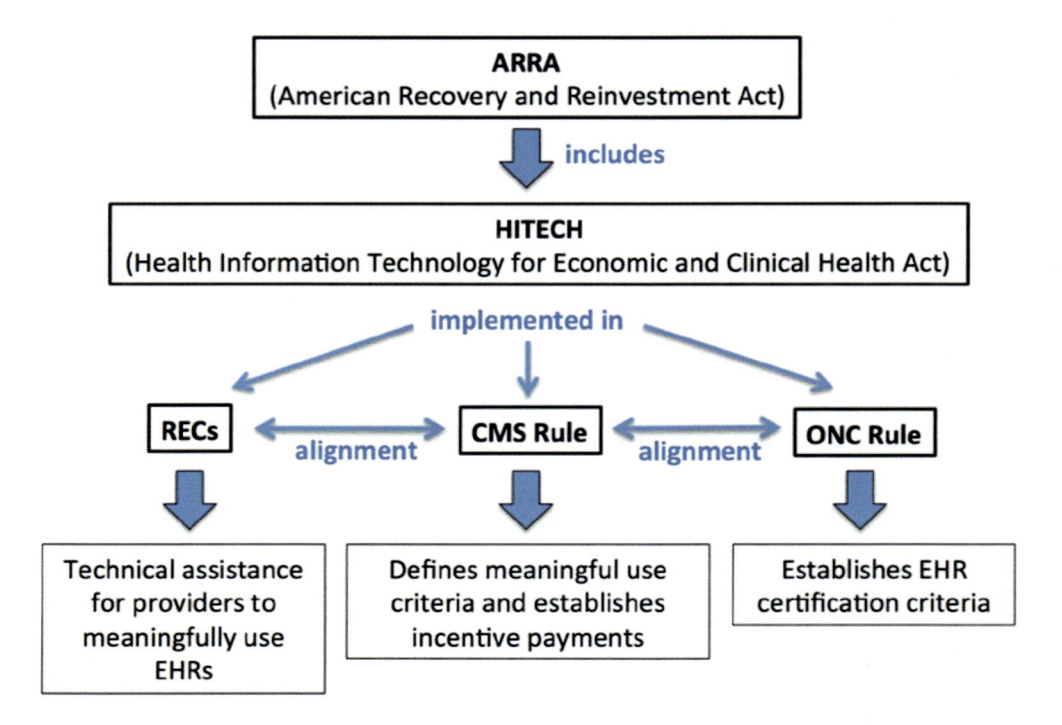

Electronic Health Records (EHRs)

Although the historical development of the paper-based medical record parallels advances in clinical care, the advancement of health IT and EHRs was more closely associated with changes in reimbursement models. Starting in the early 1980s with the advent of managed health care, reimbursement started to shift from a fee-for-service model (i.e., providers are paid based on the quantity of services provided) to a capitation or fixed fee model (i.e., providers are paid a fixed amount per patient). As a result, there began a transition to environments in which the adoption of health IT tools that facilitate cost-effective and efficient care outside of hospital settings held a competitive advantage. Additionally, the ambulatory environment was changing from a model in which a single physician was responsible for all or a majority of chronically ill patient's care, to a model in which teams of healthcare providers, often from multiple medical specialties, provide care to a single patient. As a consequence, ambulatory medical records started to become complex information sources, containing large amounts of data, such as comprehensive clinical notes written by different healthcare providers from multiple specialties, laboratory and pathology results, and radiology images and reports.

The contemporary EHR goes beyond a simple computerized version of the paper record and can be characterized by the following functional components: consolidated view of patient data; clinical decision support; computerized physician order entry (CPOE); access to medical knowledge resources, and integrated communication support for clinicians [5]. A key function of an EHR is its capability to provide a single portal of access to, and visualization of, all patient data. Before the advent of comprehensive EHRs, patient data resided in independent databases and clinicians had to access one computer system to view lab results, another system to view radiology images, and still another to view pathology reports (Fig. 37.4). EHRs moved to consolidate patient data from disparate clinical data systems—often manufactured by different vendors—by connecting to each individual system, thus providing clinicians with the ability to view all patient data (e.g., labs, radiology, etc.) via a single EHR interface (Fig. 37.5) [5].

To enable this functionality, EHR administrators (i.e., IT specialists responsible for maintaining EHR systems) are required to revise the coding format of each clinical data system to match the coding format of the EHR, a task that is accomplished by the Interface Engine (Fig. 37.5). An Interface Engine is a translational buffer that allows clinical data systems manufactured by different vendors to communicate with one another [5]. Most clinical data systems and

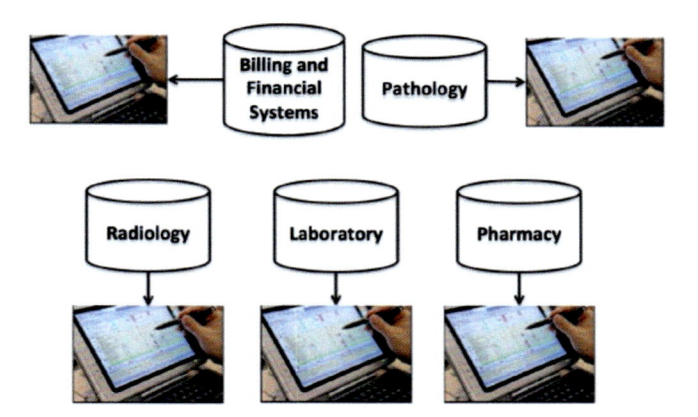

Fig. 37.4 Separate logon required for each clinical data system

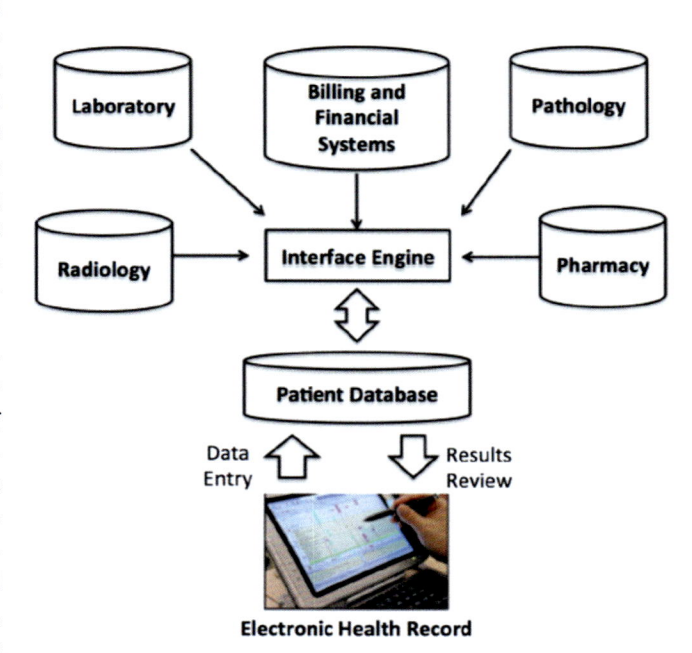

Fig. 37.5 Single EHR logon to access all clinical data systems

EHRs use a standardized format called health level 7 (HL 7) to transfer data, but clinical data systems occasionally deviate from this common format, and EHR administrators have to modify the formatting via an Interface Engine for compatibility with the EHR. As a result, hospitals and ambulatory practices can connect to different vendor clinical data systems and achieve consolidated access to all clinical data via the single EHR interface.

The consolidated access to patient data provided by EHRs thus enables robust capacities for clinicians to access and review data. EHRs can provide summary views of patient data on a single screen that shows the active problem list, medications, allergies, health maintenance reminders, and other summary information relevant to chronic disease management. Lab results can be trended over time in a flowsheet format or as graphs and chest x-ray images can be annotated by clinicians to measure the size of pulmonary nodules.

Clinical Decision Support (CDS) is a key feature of EHRs that is relevant to improving chronic disease management. CDS is defined as the use of computers to bring relevant knowledge to bear on the health care and well-being of patients [15]. Decision support is most effective at the point of patient care, when the clinician is processing clinical information and starting to make decisions regarding diagnostic testing and treatment plans. This may take the form of a health maintenance reminder, or an alert that a diabetic patient has not had a hemoglobin A1C checked in over 6 months. There are several key elements that contribute to successful implementation of CDS [16, 17]. The first is that decision support should be provided automatically as part of provider workflow at the time and location of decision making. CDS should provide actionable recommendations with the philosophy that "the user is alright right" and that users should have the ability to override nearly any CDS recommendation. Next, CDS systems often lack sufficient detail to accurately anticipate every patient's unique clinical situation and CDS recommendations may need accommodation.

To avoid "alert fatigue" (i.e., prompting providers with numerous clinically insignificant or inappropriate alerts), providers should have some control over the alerts they receive by giving them the electronic capacity to modify or turn off certain alerts. An important activity is seeking user feedback with regularly scheduled meetings in order to develop user-friendly systems, and to troubleshoot problems. Finally, system downtime needs to be minimized and quickly resolved since providers have limited tolerance for systems that are slow or behaving erratically.

Clinical Physician Order Entry (CPOE) is an electronic functionality allowing clinicians to order lab and other diagnostic tests, as well as prescribing medications. Before the advent of modern EHRs, these were stand-alone computer systems that clinicians had to access separately. Most advanced CPOE systems are integrated with CDS so that alerts are generated if, for example, clinicians are ordering a drug that the patient has a known allergy, or if there is a potential drug-drug interaction. Also, many systems generate alerts if the dose of an ordered drug is adjusted, based for example, on the patient's most recent glomerular filtration rate. Another EHR functionality is real-time access to medical information sources. This may range from links to publicly available or proprietary sources such as PubMed or Up-To-Date® or "Infobuttons" that link information sources to "home-grown" or institutionally specific resources [18]. Finally, most EHRs have robust systems to facilitate communication between providers. This may take the form of communication that is "pushed" from one provider to another via email or pager services, or "pulled" in by a provider during a patient encounter while using the EHR.

The Meaningful Use (MU) of EHRs

As noted earlier, the HITECH Act included funding to incentivize hospitals and physicians to adopt and "meaningfully use" EHR systems and empowered the Office of the National Coordinator (ONC) for health IT to develop regulations to certify EHRs and to define EHR "meaningful use" criteria. The overall objectives for meaningful use (MU) are to: electronically capture key patient health information in an accurate and comprehensive manner; use electronic patient information to facilitate clinical decision support (CDS) that informs evidence-based decision making by providers; facilitate quality reporting of care processes and patient outcomes in order to inform quality improvement efforts and to facilitate pay-for-performance reimbursement structures; engage patients (and families) in their care and encourage patient self-management, and; facilitate sharing of patient information among treating providers in order to improve transitions of care [14]. The ONC defined the EHR certification criteria and specified "what" an EHR system must be able to do, while meaningful use criteria (defined by CMS) specified "how" a certified EHR system must be used by providers for patient care. Table 37.1 provides an overview of the various objectives of Stage 1 (i.e., the first phase of implementation) MU with the corresponding components.

As originally conceived by ONC, MU would be rolled out in three distinct stages. Stage 1 would focus on electronically capturing health information in a standardized format as well as reporting quality measures. Part of the data capture involved transitioning from paper prescription and test ordering to electronic prescribing and computerized physician order entry (CPOE). Stage 2 focused on using structured data for clinical decision support in order to improve processes of care. Additionally, during the transitioning from stage 1 to stage 2, there would be a greater requirement to provide patients with on-line access to their health information along with patient-specific educational material to promote patient self-management. Finally, stage 3 of meaningful use would focus on enhancing and further utilizing EHR tools developed in the first 2 MU stages to improve patient outcomes.

37 Health Information Technology

Table 37.1 Stage 1 meaningful use objectives [14]

Objectives	Components	Details
1. Electronically capture health information in a standardized format	Record demographics	Gender, age, race, ethnicity, date of birth, and preferred language
	Record vitals	Document changes in: heart rate, blood pressure, height, weight, calculate and display BMI
	Medication and medication allergy list	Maintain active medication and active medication allergy list
	Problem list	Maintain an up-to-date problem list of current and active diagnoses
	Lab/test results	Incorporate clinical lab test results into EHR technology as structured data
	Smoking status	Record smoking status
2. Use electronic patient information to facilitate clinical decision support (CDS) that informs evidence-based decision making	Drug formulary	Implement drug-formulary checks
	Drug-drug/drug-allergy check	Implement drug-drug and drug-allergy interaction checks
	Computerized physician order entry (CPOE)	Use CPOE for medication orders directly entered by any licensed healthcare professional who can enter orders into the medical record
	e-Prescribing	Generate and transmit permissible prescriptions to pharmacies electronically
	Decision support rules	Implement one clinical decision support rule relevant to specialty or high clinical priority along with the ability to track compliance with that rule
	Create reports by condition	Generate lists of patients by specific conditions to use for quality improvement, reduction of disparities, research, or outreach
3. Facilitate quality reporting of care processes and patient outcomes	Quality reporting	Report ambulatory quality measures to Center for Medicare and Medicaid Services or the state-level agencies
	e-Report registry	Capability to submit electronic data to immunization registries or immunization information systems and actual submission in accordance with applicable law and practice
	e-Report public health	Capability to provide electronic syndromic surveillance data to public health agencies and actual transmission in accordance with applicable law and practice
4. Engage patients in their care and encourage patient self-management	Patient clinical summary	Provide clinical summaries for patients for each office visit
	Patient e-health information	Provide patients with an electronic copy of their health information (including diagnostic test results, problem list, medication list, medication allergies), upon request
	Prevention and follow-up reminders	Send reminders to patients per patient preference for preventive and follow-up care
	Patient education	Use certified EHR technology to identify patient-specific education resources and provide those resources to the patient if appropriate
5. Facilitate sharing of patient information among treating providers in order to improve transitions of care	Electronic information exchange	Capability to exchange key clinical information (e.g., diagnostic test results, problem list, medication list, medication allergies), among providers of care and patient authorized entities electronically
	Transition summary	The eligible provider who transitions their patient to another setting of care or refers their patient to another provider of care should provide summary care record for each transition of care referral
	Medication reconciliation	Physicians who receive patients from other settings of care for providers of care should perform medication reconciliation

MU Objective #1: Electronic Capture of Health Information in a Standardized Format

Electronically capturing clinical data in a standardized format, and subsequently using the data for patient care, is the foundation for all other MU objectives and it is the primary advantage EHRs have over paper-based records. There are tradeoffs between coded or structured data, and narrative or unstructured data. The major advantage of coded data entry into an EHR is that information is standardized and can easily be used in clinical decision support (CDS), quality improvement (QI), billing, and research. Standardized codes allow computers to "understand" and "interpret" clinical information and therefore process it to help inform clinical decision making. For example, if the diagnosis of diabetes is entered into the EHR as coded data, the EHR's CDS system will "understand" the diagnosis and can send reminders to the treating clinician about evidence-based health maintenance recommendations. However, if the diabetes diagnosis is entered into the EHR as free-text, the computer cannot "understand" the data and therefore, cannot use it for CDS. Another important example is coded medication lists. If medications are not entered into EHRs as structured or coded data, CDS systems that support drug-allergy and drug-drug interaction alerts would not be possible.

The major disadvantage of coded data is that it often does not provide the detailed and nuanced description of patients' symptomatology when compared with narrative free-text. For example, the coded patient symptom "chest pain" is much less informative than a free-text clinical narrative describing the patient's symptoms (e.g., "the patient presents with burning epigastric chest pain that worsens when he eats fatty foods and improves when he takes antacid medication"). Because of the trade-offs between structure and narrative data, MU does not completely prohibit free-text unstructured data entry, it simply mandates that specific clinical variables (described in Table 37.1) that are key for implementation of the remaining MU objectives be collected and maintained as structured data.

EHR vendors and end-users determine the balance of how other clinical information is entered and stored in determining the balance between structured and narrative data entry, which is the art of EHR interface design and implementation. The optimal balance is determined by several factors (Fig. 37.6) including medical specialty (e.g., PCPs may be more likely to prefer narrative data entry vs. ophthalmologists who may prefer a more structured or templated format), personal clinician preference, and end-user data needs (QI, billing, reporting, etc.).

MU Objective #2: Clinical Decision Support (CDS) Systems

Clinical decision support can be defined as the use of health IT to bring relevant knowledge to the management of health care for an individual patient [15]. A key point is that support means the facilitation of clinician decision making, rather than computer-generated recommendations about patient care. Relevant means the selection of information that is pertinent to patient care [15]. For a CDS system to optimally function it must have the following features: access to structured or coded data in the EHR relevant to the patient (e.g., age, gender, diagnoses, lab results, medications, and allergies); a high-quality, evidence-based medical knowledge source; a software program or algorithm (e.g., rules engine) for processing the medical knowledge and patient-specific data to generate an output (e.g., patient-specific treatment recommendations), and; a mechanism for presenting the prompt or recommendation to the clinician (information automatically presented to clinician vs. information only presented at request of clinician—"on demand"). Figure 37.7 shows a diagram of the typical architecture of a CDS system [19].

The data accessed by the CDS system is usually processed via a rules engine that can range in complexity from simple if …, then … logic to an artificial neural network. The outputs of CDS systems are reminders, alerts, and/or diagnostic and therapeutic recommendations. CDS systems can range in

Fig. 37.6 Trade-offs between structured and unstructured data entry

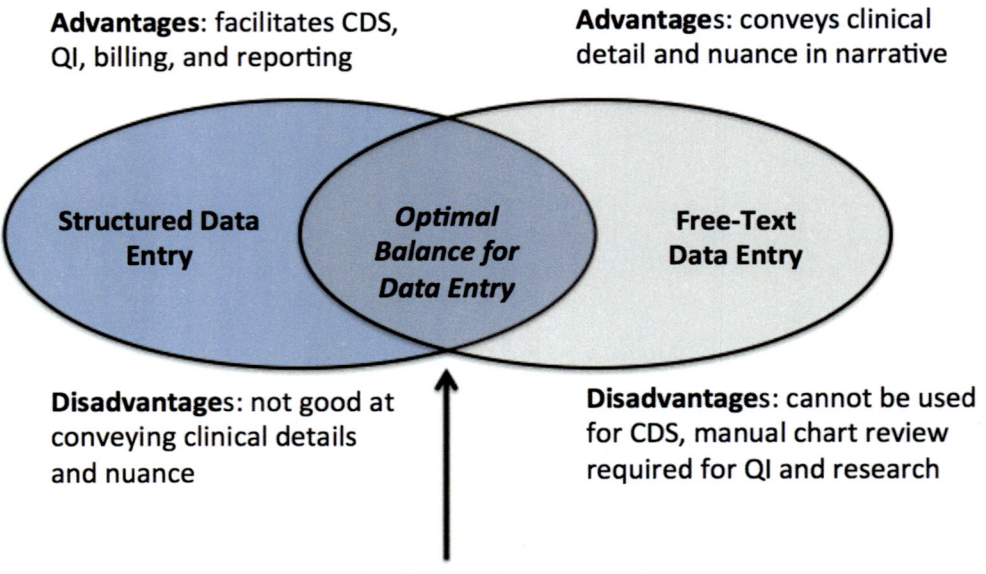

Fig. 37.7 Architecture of clinical decision support systems [19]

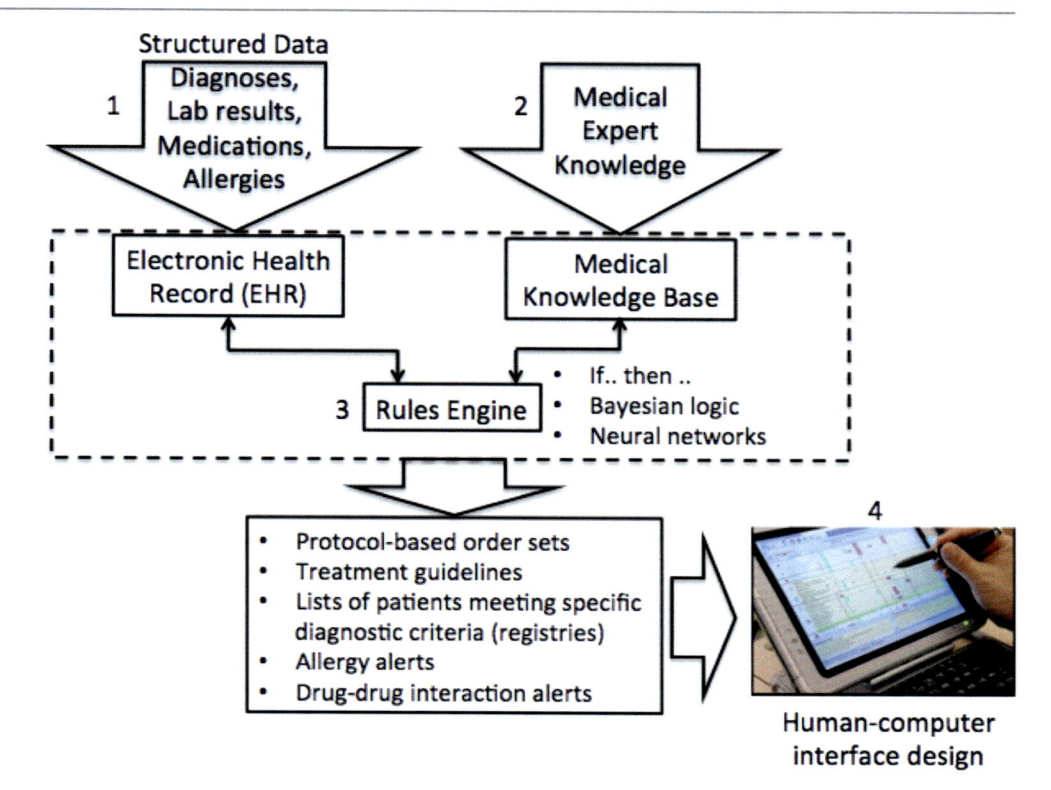

complexity from simple systems that generate alerts and reminders that a diabetic patient is due for screening for diabetic retinopathy, to a more complex system that recommends starting a patient on a statin medication because her 10-year risk of atherosclerotic cardiovascular disease is ≥7.5% [20].

At first glance, implementation of CDS systems may appear to be straightforward. For example, from a programming viewpoint, creation of an if … then … rule for checking that a patient's age is ≥50 years AND there is no procedure code in the EHR database indicating the patient has ever had a colonoscopy appear to be fairly simple. The larger problem with successful implementation of CDS systems has less to do with technology and more to do with human-computer interaction, clinical workflow, and organizational commitment. For example, a CDS rules engine needs to be optimized to avoid false-positives (minimizing alert fatigue), or the CDS system should complement existing provider workflow rather than disrupting it (e.g., generating reminders not relevant to the current patient encounter). In addition, the information sources grounding the CDS system rule needs to be updated over time, as evidence-based guidelines change [21].

CDS-generated alerts, reminders, and recommendations can be designed to: remind clinicians of things they intend to do but should not have to remember; provide information when clinicians are unsure what to do and, identify potential errors clinicians have made in prescribing medications. A key factor in CDS effectiveness in improving care processes and patient outcomes is the way in which CDS output is rolled out to clinicians. The Institute of Medicine has emphasized that health IT and CDS systems should be optimally designed to make it "easy (for clinicians) to do the right thing" [22].

CDS systems differ in how much control users have over decisions to use CDS-generated alerts, reminders, and recommendations. These decisions involve not only whether information generated by CDS systems is displayed on demand, so that users have full control over whether information is displayed, but also the circumstances under which users can, after viewing CDS recommendations, choose to accept them. A key issue involved in CDS implementation is the balance between clinician autonomy with their workflows and adherence to guideline-based care. Table 37.2 outlines several key implementation areas.

Some of these implementation issues have been addressed by research studies [15, 17, 23–27], however there are few accepted guidelines regarding standardization, in part because clinicians often differ in their preferences and approaches to care. However, one consensus opinion highlights that, CDS systems need to be minimally disruptive to "cognitive workflow" to be successful. For example, clinicians receiving multiple inappropriate alerts can start exhibiting "alert fatigue" which results in ignoring alerts and/or overriding alerts and reminders. There is a risk that the few clinically significant alerts will be buried in the numerous alerts [28]. For CDS to be integrated and consistently used in clinician workflow, unique customization to local processes and adaptations to previous clinical workflows may be required [17].

Table 37.2 Clinical decision support (CDS) intent and key issues with implementation

CDS intent	Delivered	Potential for workflow disruption	Key issues for success	Example
Reminder of actions user intends to do, but should not have to remember	Automatic	Low	Timing	Reminder for influenza vaccination
Provide information when user is unsure what to do	On demand	Low	Speed Ease of access	Link to clinical knowledge-database (e.g., UpToDate®)
Correct user's errors and/or recommend user change plans	Automatics vs. on demand	High	Timing Ability to override alert Minimize false-positives Minimize alert fatigue	Alert about a potential drug-drug interaction

Table 37.3 Advancing personal health record functionality [31]

Level	Functionality
1	Collect patient information, such as self-reported demographic and risk factor information (e.g., health behaviors, symptoms, diagnoses, and medications)
2	Integrate patient information with clinical information through links to the EHR and/or claims data
3	Interpret clinical information for the patient by translating clinical findings into lay language and delivering health information via a user-friendly interface
4	Provide individualized clinical recommendations to the patient, such as screening and on evidence-based guidelines

MU Objective #3: Facilitate Quality Reporting of Care Processes and Patient Outcomes

This MU objective seeks to facilitate tracking and reporting of clinical quality measures (CQMs) to payers (e.g., CMS) and for public reporting. As discussed earlier, about half of patients with chronic illness receive recommended care, and low value care is provided to patients from 20% to 30% of the time [11, 29]. In this context, a primary goal of CMS in implementing MU is promoting the transition of the U.S. healthcare system from a free-for-service model to a value-based model. A prerequisite for a functioning value-based system is the capacity to capture and report CQM to payers. Over the past several years CQMs have become an integral part of CMS and commercial payor strategies to improve quality of care and reduce costs for their beneficiaries. Meaningful use of EHRs assists in the collection and reporting of this data, which may be increasingly tied to future reimbursement schedules for healthcare providers.

MU Objective #4: Engage Patients in Their Care and Encourage Patient Self-Management

This MU objective focuses on using EHR technology to engage patients in their care by providing electronic access to personal health information (e.g., lab results, radiology reports, etc.), as well as evidence-based information sources to promote patient informed decision making and self-management. The EHR systems that facilitate this process are personal health records (PHRs) and patient web portals [30]. A PHR is a comprehensive health record where data is housed within (e.g., imported from EHRs, pharmacies, patient-entered data, etc.) and where patients have access and input to the data.

There are three types of PHRs. Free standing PHRs are completely controlled by the patient and usually hosted by an internet-based platform (e.g., Microsoft Health Vault). The PHR is not usually associated with any other record or healthcare providers. The second type is called a tethered PHR, which is hosted by the patient's healthcare provider and linked to the EHR. In a tethered PHR, patients can view a subset of the personal health information contained in the EHR and, for example, trend their lab results over the last year or view their immunization history. Finally, a sponsored PHR is provided by a patient's employer or health insurance plan and generally contains information based on insurance claims data.

A model for advancing PHR functionality to enable patient-centered care and self-management is displayed in Table 37.3.

First-generation PHRs function at Level 1 and are simply electronic replacements for the home medical file; data is manually entered by patients and stored on a secure website. The amount of medical detail entered is patient-dependent and the information may be inaccurate or inconsistent. More advanced PHRs (Level 2 and above) address this problem by linking electronically to clinical information in EHRs (i.e., tethered PHR). At the next level, PHRs have functional capacity that can translate technical medical information in ways that are understandable to patients (Level 3). Finally, at Level 4, the PHR can make patient-specific recommendations on issues such as preventive services and screening tests that are indicated or health behavior prompts that are based on an individual patient's specific risk factors.

A patient web portal is a secure website for patients that is usually maintained by a patient's healthcare provider and offers access to functions and services linked to an EHR [30]. This functionality can include secure messaging, protected health information (e.g., lab results, medication lists, diagnoses), appointment scheduling, a tethered PHR, and patient self-management programs. Patient web portals can provide functionality that allows communication between patients and providers (i.e., secure messaging), chronic disease self-management tools, and administrative tools (e.g., appointment scheduling).

MU Objective #5: Facilitate Sharing of Patient Information Among Treating Providers

The full potential of health IT system integration into health care cannot be realized if EHR information is housed in data silos and impedes the ability of EHRs to exchange patient data. The compartmentalization of patient information by EHRs does not support high-quality transitions of patient care across different healthcare providers and organizations. For example, if a patient with several chronic illnesses changes primary care providers, it is important for the new provider to have complete information regarding the patient's medication regimen, previous lab results, diagnoses, preventive screening history, previous diagnostic testing (e.g., cardiac stress test), etc. Historically, this transfer of information occurred by the patient requesting paper records from the previous provider and transferring documents to the new provider who then reviewed the information and incorporated it into the new record.

The promise of the health information exchange (HIE) (Fig. 37.8) is that an information-transfer process occurs seamlessly, and that relevant clinical data is automatically transferred from previous provider(s) to current provider(s) via their respective EHRs, even if the EHRs are from different vendors. By facilitating the sharing of information between providers, health care will plausibly become more efficient by reducing the redundancy of healthcare services (e.g., repeating a cardiac stress test performed by previous provider).

A focus of MU, especially stage 2, is that healthcare systems and providers demonstrate that their certified EHR can exchange clinical data among providers outside of their respective systems. Nearly $600 million in federal funding

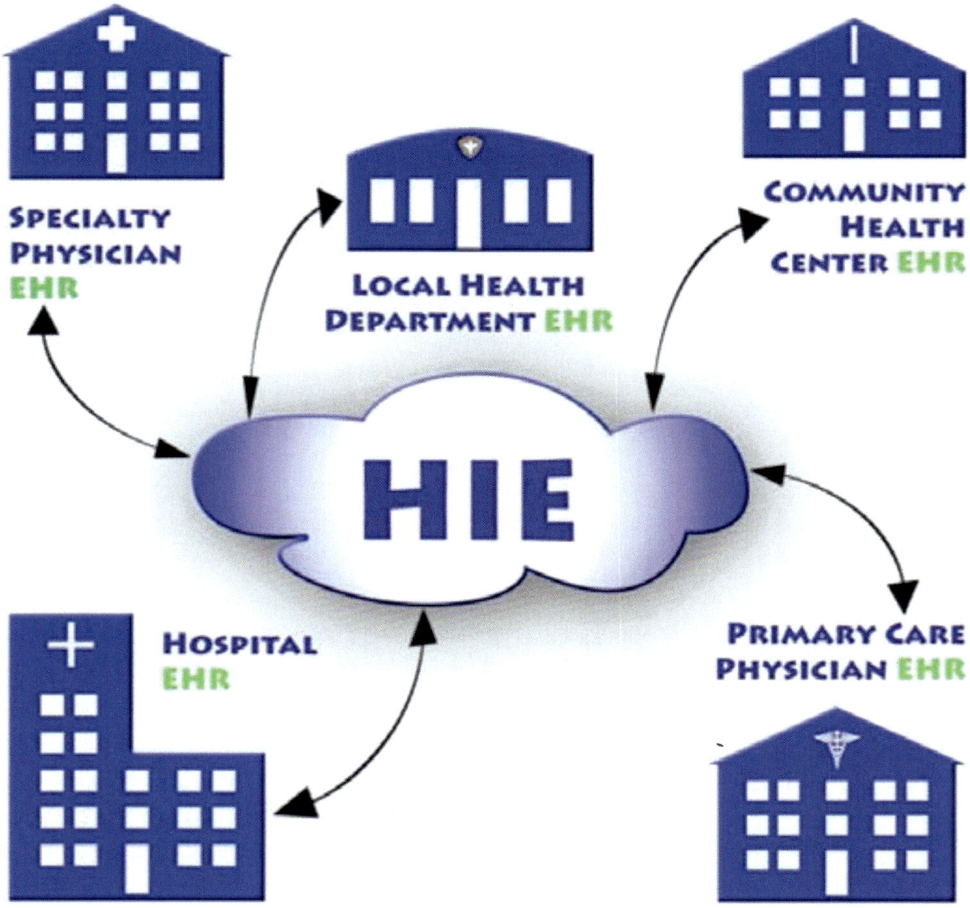

Fig. 37.8 Health information exchange (HIE)

was designated to support statewide HIE organizations and a few states have invested additional funding [32]. Currently, more than 100 organizations facilitate HIE among healthcare providers, and 30% of hospitals and 10% of ambulatory practices participate [33]. The key issues to facilitate HIE and EHR interoperability include: establishing standards for clinical data exchange between EHR systems; the need to identify and consistently use unique patient identifiers or establishing patient identity using demographic data across different providers; a framework for assuring patient privacy, and; a model for the financial sustainability of the HIE infrastructure.

A systematic review [34] concluded that use of HIE likely reduces emergency department usage and costs via reductions in repeat imaging studies. However, the impact on other health outcomes is unknown and further study is needed to identify and understand the role of HIE in chronic disease management, as well as factors for successful HIE implementation [32].

Effectiveness of Health IT in Chronic Disease Management

A systematic review was performed to better understand the effects that various components of health IT have on chronic disease processes of care and health outcomes [35]. The review included 109 articles involving 112 health IT systems and the index chronic diseases included: diabetes (42.9% of articles), heart disease (36.6%), and mental health (23.2%). About one-third of studies addressed multiple chronic disorders. Most of the studies (60%) used health IT systems implemented in the outpatient setting, including 59% in primary care and 28% in specialty care. Physicians were most frequently the intended users of the systems (39%), with nurses and patients being the intended users, 39% and 17% respectively. The impact on processes of care and health outcomes (positive, neutral, or negative) that were associated with implementation of health IT is shown in Table 37.4.

Most studies showed some improvements in chronic disease processes of care or outcomes, with the most impressive gains in screening (100% of studies positive), cost (91% positive), documentation (83% positive), guideline adherence (79% positive), and treatment adherence (67% positive). Referral rates and scores on standardized instruments (e.g., depression) showed least improvement (0% and 30% positive, respectively).

When reviewers looked at sociotechnical determinants for successful implementation of health IT systems, they found that involving end-users in the development process, responsiveness to end-user feedback, and adequate training were important factors [35]. A major barrier to success was failure to consider increased time for clinicians to use the system (i.e., performance usability) and/or significant alterations in clinical workflow resulting in health IT implementation.

Population Health and Chronic Disease Management

"Absence of evidence is not evidence of absence" [attributed to Carl Sagan] [3].

Prior to implementation of health IT systems with the functionality to summarize health outcomes in patient populations, there was scant data on the performance of healthcare providers to deliver quality of care. As noted previously, the evolution of health IT functionality was driven, in large part, by unsustainable increases in healthcare costs. The HITECH act that catalyzed adoption of the "meaningful use" of EHRs help build the foundations for the major reforms that were to come just over the horizon; transitioning the U.S. healthcare system from primarily a "fee-for-service" model to models focused on reimbursement based on population health.

Table 37.4 Impact of health IT on processes of care and health outcomes [35]

Processes of care and outcomes	Examples	Intervention effect		
		Positive	Neutral	Negative
Guideline adherence	Screening for target disorders, conducting lab tests on recommended schedule	79%	21%	0%
Visit frequency	Decrease in emergency visits	50%	50%	0%
Documentation	Provider documentation of diagnostic criteria for specified disorder	83%	17%	0%
Treatment adherence	Adherence to medication regimens	67%	33%	0%
Referral rate	Referrals to specialist or nurse care manager	0%	100%	0%
Screening and testing	Mood disorders, Papanicolaou tests, and mammography	100%	0%	0%
Cost	Typically involving analysis of health IT system cost and savings to the organization	91%	9%	0%
Changes in lab values	Glycosylated hemoglobin	50%	50%	0%
Scores on standardized instruments	Depression	30%	60%	10%
Hospitalizations	Number of hospitalizations	43%	57%	0%

A major delivery system reform built on the foundation created by HITECH was the Affordable Care Act (ACA) enacted in 2010 [36]. The ACA set in motion the changes in healthcare delivery that lead to the growth of Accountable Care Organizations (ACOs). An ACO is a network of ambulatory practices and hospitals that share financial and medical responsibility for providing coordinated care to patient populations for the purpose of reducing cost and improving quality of care [37]. One might argue that the ultimate goal of "meaningful use" of EHRs was to facilitate tracking the health of patient populations and provide feedback to both provider and payors on the quality of care delivered in order to make population-based healthcare delivery and reimbursement systems feasible [38]. The carrot for healthcare organizations to form ACOs is that they get to share in savings gained by integrating and coordinating care, and successfully achieving quality measure goals for the patient populations they care for.

Currently there are more than 900 ACOs in the U.S., covering over 32 million patients [39]. A recent systematic review [40] investigated the association between health IT as determinant of ACO participation and performance. The review found that hospitals and physicians participating in an ACO are more likely to have more advanced health IT infrastructure. For example, ACO-affiliated providers are more likely to perform population management, patient engagement, and quality improvement activities electronically than those not affiliated with an ACO. Additionally, there is a positive association between increased EHR capabilities and disease prevention, information exchange and care management processes. However, the study described some troubling barriers to organizations forming ACOs. For example, 43% of rural health clinics reported that lack of capitol for health IT improvements impeded their ability to track care provided to their patient populations, thus limiting their participation in ACOs.

Another key health IT functionality that supports population health is the ability to create disease registries. Registries allow healthcare organizations to identify patient cohorts within a population with specific diagnoses. This allows healthcare organizations to pro-actively target high-risk populations for evidence-based interventions shown to improve health outcomes. For example, identifying all patients with diabetes in order to assess optimization of glycemic control. In an ideal health IT system, these patients would be accurately identified using structured data stored in the EHR (e.g., diagnosis codes). However, the performance of diagnosis codes (e.g., ICD codes) in identifying patient populations with specific chronic diseases is often suboptimal. For example, ICD-9 codes lack the sensitivity (31%) to effectively identify and manage asthmatic children in real-time [41]. Therefore, the future of population-based management of patients is linked to developing technologies and processes that accurately capture chronic disease diagnoses using both structured and unstructured data (e.g., free-text).

Future Directions

"Somewhere, something incredible is waiting to be known" [attributed to Carl Sagan] [3].

Natural Language Processing, Machine Learning, and Genomic Medicine are promising developments in health information technology. Since passage of the HITECH act in 2009 and the ACA in 2010, the use of EHR data to identify and target specific patient populations (e.g., diabetes and heart failure) for evidence-based interventions has become a necessary condition for many healthcare systems to survive in the current reimbursement environment. However, structured data (e.g., diagnostic codes) perform poorly when compared to manual chart review, because much of the information stored in EHRs is free-text or narrative information in clinical notes. Natural language processing (NLP) and machine learning (ML) have the potential of utilizing unstructured data in EHRs to accurately identify and target patient cohorts for evidence-based interventions that improve health outcomes. For example, a study comparing identification of patient satisfying Framingham heart failure phenotype at four geographically dispersed hospitals using different EHRs found good performance characteristics (sensitivity = 79%, specificity = 82%, positive-predictive value = 85%) using NLP, with manual chart abstraction as the reference standard [42].

We are entering a new age of genomics in chronic disease management. It is now possible to develop genetic prediction models to assess patients at high risk for developing certain medical conditions, as well a prediction models for treatment response to medications (pharmacogenetics). Organizations, such as the Electronic Medical Records and Genomics (eMERGE) network [43] and Implementing Genomics in Practice (IGNITE) network [44] are working to develop genomic prediction models that can be used in EHR clinical decision support (CDS) systems for use by clinicians to identify patients at high risk for developing certain medical conditions and/or are likely to have an adverse reaction to certain medications. Each participating site in the network provides extensive genomic (genotype) and clinical data (phenotype) derived from their EHRs. The sites are geographically dispersed and have diverse patient populations.

One clear challenge is creating accurate phenotypes (e.g., the patient population with type-2 diabetes) from a large network of institutions with different EHRs. This is achieved by using both structured data (e.g., billing codes, lab results, medications) and unstructured data (e.g., clinical notes) from EHRs to identify the valid phenotype cohort of interest [45].

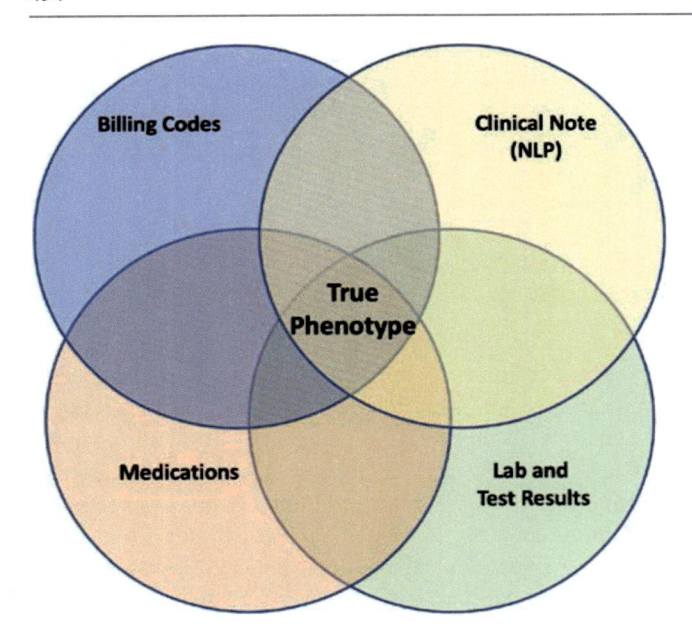

Fig. 37.9 EHR data structure and phenotyping

Figure 37.9 shows a graphical display of the data types used to identify phenotypes. An example of an algorithms used to calculate various phenotypes can be found on the eMERGE website [43].

Participating institutions provide patient's genotype information, and the data is examined for specific traits and alleles. At this point monogenic determinant (involving a single gene) and polygenic determinants (involving multiple genes) associated with specific disease entities (phenotypes) are assessed. Several healthcare organizations, such as Mayo Clinic, have modified their EHRs to incorporate genomic data into their CDS systems to alert prescribers of significant drug-gene interactions, such as warfarin sensitivity [46]. A Mayo study highlights that using genetic information for CDS has a promising future and may revolutionize chronic disease management; however, EHRs need to be adapted to handle new and large classes of information, new standards must be created and adopted, and CDS should be refined to ensure that validated genetic findings are seamlessly integrated into clinical workflow [45].

References

1. HealthIT.gov. Basics of Health IT. 2013. https://www.healthit.gov/patients-families/basics-health-it.
2. ONC. Office-based Physician Electronic Health Record Adoption: 2004–2014 Washington, DC: The Office of the National Coordinator (ONC) for Health Information Technology; 2015. http://dashboard.healthit.gov/quickstats/pages/physician-ehr-adoption-trends.php.
3. BrainyQutes. Carl Sagan Quotes: BrainyQuotes. 1996. https://www.brainyquote.com/quotes/carl_sagan_589698.
4. Gillum RF. From papyrus to the electronic tablet: a brief history of the clinical medical record with lessons for the digital age. Am J Med. 2013;126(10):853–7.
5. Tang PC, McDonald CJ. Electronic health record systems. In: Shortliffe EH, Cimino JJ, editors. Biomedical informatics: computer applications in health care and biomedicine. 3rd ed. Springer Science; 2006.
6. Devine EB, Wilson-Norton JL, Lawless NM, Hansen RN, Hazlet TK, Kelly K, et al. Characterization of prescribing errors in an internal medicine clinic. Am J Health Syst Pharm. 2007;64(10):1062–70.
7. Gandhi TK, Weingart SN, Seger AC, Borus J, Burdick E, Poon EG, et al. Outpatient prescribing errors and the impact of computerized prescribing. J Gen Intern Med. 2005;20(9):837–41.
8. Brodell RT, Helms SE, KrishnaRao I, Bredle DL, Prescription errors. Legibility and drug name confusion. Arch Fam Med. 1997;6(3):296–8.
9. Yarnall KS, Pollak KI, Ostbye T, Krause KM, Michener JL. Primary care: is there enough time for prevention? Am J Public Health. 2003;93(4):635–41.
10. Jaen CR, Stange KC, Nutting PA. Competing demands of primary care: a model for the delivery of clinical preventive services. J Fam Pract. 1994;38(2):166–71.
11. McGlynn EA, Asch SM, Adams J, Keesey J, Hicks J, DeCristofaro A, et al. The quality of health care delivered to adults in the United States. N Engl J Med. 2003;348(26):2635–45.
12. IOM. Crossing the quality chasm: a new health system for the 21st century. Washington, DC: National Academy Press; 2001.
13. Congress.gov. American Recovery and Reinvestment Act of 2009 Washington, DC: Library of Congress; 2009. https://www.congress.gov/bill/111th-congress/house-bill/1.
14. HealthIT.gov. Health IT Legislation and Regulations. 2016. https://www.healthit.gov/policy-researchers-implementers/health-it-legislation.
15. Greenes RG. Clinical decision support: the road ahead. 1st ed. Academic Press; 2011.
16. Friedlin J, Dexter PR, Overhage JM. Details of a successful clinical decision support system. AMIA Annu Symp Proc. 2007;254-8
17. Kawamoto K, Houlihan CA, Balas EA, Lobach DF. Improving clinical practice using clinical decision support systems: a systematic review of trials to identify features critical to success. BMJ. 2005;330(7494):765.
18. Cimino JJ, Li J. Sharing infobuttons to resolve clinicians' information needs. AMIA Annu Symp Proc. 2003;815
19. El-Sappagh S, El-Masri S. A distributed clinical decision support system architecture. J King Saud Univ - Comput Inf Sci. 2013;26(1):69–78.
20. ACC. 2013 Prevention guidelines ASCVD risk estimator. American College of Cardiology; 2013. http://www.acc.org/tools-and-practice-support/mobile-resources/features/2013-prevention-guidelines-ascvd-risk-estimator.
21. Sittig DF, Singh H. A new sociotechnical model for studying health information technology in complex adaptive healthcare systems. Qual Saf Health Care. 2010;19(Suppl 3):i68–74.
22. IOM. To err is human: building a safer health system. Washington, DC: Institute of Medicine (IOM), National Academy Press; 1999.
23. Fathima M, Peiris D, Naik-Panvelkar P, Saini B, Armour CL. Effectiveness of computerized clinical decision support systems for asthma and chronic obstructive pulmonary disease in primary care: a systematic review. BMC Pulm Med. 2014;14:189.
24. Jeffery R, Iserman E, Haynes RB, Team CSR. Can computerized clinical decision support systems improve diabetes management? A systematic review and meta-analysis. Diabet Med. 2013;30(6):739–45.
25. Nies J, Colombet I, Degoulet P, Durieux P. Determinants of success for computerized clinical decision support systems integrated

25. in CPOE systems: a systematic review. AMIA Annu Symp Proc. 2006;2006:594–8.
26. Roshanov PS, Misra S, Gerstein HC, Garg AX, Sebaldt RJ, Mackay JA, et al. Computerized clinical decision support systems for chronic disease management: a decision-maker-researcher partnership systematic review. Implement Sci. 2011;6:92.
27. Souza NM, Sebaldt RJ, Mackay JA, Prorok JC, Weise-Kelly L, Navarro T, et al. Computerized clinical decision support systems for primary preventive care: a decision-maker-researcher partnership systematic review of effects on process of care and patient outcomes. Implement Sci. 2011;6:87.
28. Nanji KC, Slight SP, Seger DL, Cho I, Fiskio JM, Redden LM, et al. Overrides of medication-related clinical decision support alerts in outpatients. J Am Med Inform Assoc. 2014;21(3):487–91.
29. Wennberg JE. Practice variation: implications for our health care system. Manag Care. 2004;13(9 Suppl):3–7.
30. RWJF. The value of personal health records and web portals to engage consumers and improve quality. Robert Wood Johnson Foundation; 2012. http://www.rwjf.org/en/library/research/2012/07/the-value-of-personal-health-records-and-web-portals-to-engage-c.html.
31. Krist AH, Woolf SH. A vision for patient-centered health information systems. JAMA. 2011;305(3):300–1.
32. Kern LM, Barron Y, Abramson EL, Patel V, Kaushal R. HEAL NY: promoting interoperable health information technology in New York State. Health Aff (Millwood). 2009;28(2):493–504.
33. Adler-Milstein J, Bates DW, Jha AK. Operational health information exchanges show substantial growth, but long-term funding remains a concern. Health Aff (Millwood). 2013;32(8):1486–92.
34. Rudin RS, Motala A, Goldzweig CL, Shekelle PG. Usage and effect of health information exchange: a systematic review. Ann Intern Med. 2014;161(11):803–11.
35. Dorr D, Bonner LM, Cohen AN, Shoai RS, Perrin R, Chaney E, et al. Informatics systems to promote improved care for chronic illness: a literature review. J Am Med Inform Assoc. 2007;14(2):156–63.
36. HHS. What is the Affordable Care Act? Washington, DC: US Department of Health and Human Services; 2017. https://www.hhs.gov/answers/health-insurance-reform/what-is-the-affordable-care-act/index.html.
37. Burke T. Accountable care organizations. Public Health Rep. 2011;126(6):875–8.
38. Bitton A, Flier LA, Jha AK. Health information technology in the era of care delivery reform: to what end? JAMA. 2012;307(24):2593–4.
39. Muhlestein D, Saunders RS, McClellan MB. Growth of ACOs and alternative payment models in 2017. Health Aff. 2017;
40. Balio CP, Apathy NC, Danek RL. Health information technology and accountable care organizations: a systematic review and future directions. EGEMS (Wash DC). 2019;7(1):24.
41. Wu ST, Sohn S, Ravikumar KE, Wagholikar K, Jonnalagadda SR, Liu H, et al. Automated chart review for asthma cohort identification using natural language processing: an exploratory study. Ann Allergy Asthma Immunol. 2013;111(5):364–9.
42. Moore CR, Jain S, Haas S, Yadav H, Whitsel E, Rosamand W, et al. Ascertaining Framingham heart failure phenotype from inpatient electronic health record data using natural language processing: a multicentre Atherosclerosis Risk in Communities (ARIC) validation study. BMJ Open. 2021;11(6):e047356.
43. eMERGE. Electronic Medical Records and Genomics (eMERGE) Network. 2021. https://emerge-network.org/.
44. IGNITE. Implementing GeNomics In praTicE (IGNITE). 2019. https://gmkb.org/.
45. Wei WQ, Denny JC. Extracting research-quality phenotypes from electronic health records to support precision medicine. Genome Med. 2015;7(1):41.
46. Caraballo PJ, Sutton JA, Giri J, Wright JA, Nicholson WT, Kullo IJ, et al. Integrating pharmacogenomics into the electronic health record by implementing genomic indicators. J Am Med Inform Assoc. 2020;27(1):154–8.

Quality Improvement

38

Dana Neutze and Brian Wiggs

Introduction

Health care systems across the United States have an interest in improving the quality of care, reducing care costs, and improving patient satisfaction [1]. The transition from a production-based to value-based paradigm for reimbursement has further heightened these efforts across a wide range of health care settings, especially in patients with chronic health conditions [2]. Consequently, there has been ongoing development and implementation of health information technology, and the adoption of quality improvement strategies and tools in hospitals and clinics [3].

Fundamentally, quality improvement (QI) is the process by which providers and organizations strive to improve outcomes, decrease cost, improve accessibility, and improve the care experience for providers and staff. This chapter provides an overview of quality improvement in the health care setting. The first section surveys the roots of quality improvement in other industries and looks at the genesis of the movement in health care. Next, basic QI principles are introduced and described in relation to health services. The subsequent section outlines several QI models and approaches and is accompanied by key areas of change management and managing data. The chapter closes with some future directions for quality improvement.

Movements and Initiatives Promoting Quality Improvement

The roots of quality improvement in health care are found in other industries, particularly manufacturing. Walter Shewhart, regarded as the father of quality control, integrated the subjects of engineering, economics, and statistics [4, 5].

In his 1931 book *Economic Control of Quality of Manufactured Product,* Shewhart theorized that there are two sources of variation within a given process: assignable and chance causes, and then emphasized the importance of identifying and removing assignable causes to improve quality. W. Edwards Deming espoused continuous improvement in the Japanese manufacturing industry. Deming believed quality was a key driver of success, requiring a cultural transformation in how individuals manage and lead and that if an organization prioritizes quality, costs will decrease through improved productivity and resource utilization. Joseph Juran emphasized the importance and role of management in quality, known as the *Juran Trilogy*. The trilogy includes three distinct processes: quality planning (customer-focused quality products and services), quality control (addressing gaps in performance), and quality improvement (correct gaps in customer needs). Stakeholder teams execute improvement projects to eliminate root causes of process performance or create new processes to meet customer requirements and needs with the goal of achieving self-control by engaging individuals at every level within the organization [4, 5]. Henry Ford revolutionized the car industry with flow production of the Model-T in 1908. Before this time, cars were custom-made, resulting in the production of only a few expensive cars. Ford developed the assembly line, producing cars for the masses. However, Ford's Model-T cars were only available in one color. Customer choice was advanced when Taiichi Ohno and Eiji Toyoda created the Toyota Production System, which decreased waste while improving production, creating better customer service and greater profits [6]. The manufacturing industry realized that quality control and serving the customer were essential for business.

Quality Enters Health Care

It was not until the turn of the twenty-first century that the ideas born in industry crossed over into health care, driven

D. Neutze (✉) · B. Wiggs
Department of Family Medicine, University of North Carolina at Chapel Hill, Chapel Hill, NC, USA
e-mail: Dana_neutze@med.unc.edu; brian.wiggs@unchealth.unc.edu

Table 38.1 The six aims for better health care. (Source: *Crossing the Quality Chasm*)

Aim	Purpose	Example
Safe	Health care should cause no harm to individuals	Electronic health records automatically check for drug interactions
Effective	Should be based on the latest scientific evidence without doing unnecessary interventions	Cervical cancer screening for women limited to ages 21–65
Patient-Centered	Providing care based on the values of the patient and respect for the patient	Shared decision making
Timely	Reducing waits and delays	Same-day appointments
Efficient	Reducing waste of supplies and equipment	Stocking only necessary supplies so that they do not expire
Equitable	Providing care to everyone that is the same irrespective of race, gender, and socioeconomic status	Free prevention screenings that can be accessed by all individuals

by the transition of health care from predominantly acute episodic care to the management of chronic illness. In 1999, the Institute of Medicine's (IOM) Committee on the Quality of Health Care in America released the groundbreaking report *To Err is Human: Building a Safer Health System* [7], citing the 44,000 deaths a year in US hospitals caused by medical errors. The report was a wakeup call in health care. A second report, *Crossing the Quality Chasm: A New Health System for the 21st Century* [8] was published by the IOM in 2001 and proposed how the health care system should change to make it "safe, effective, patient-centered, timely, efficient, and equitable." Table 38.1 displays their six aims for high quality patient care. The report challenged health care providers, patients, administrators, and lawmakers to rethink the ways in which care was delivered and to restructure the system to support new models of care. These two landmark reports set the stage for innovation and launched federal initiatives to test and implement new approaches. *Crossing the Quality Chasm* identified both the need and the framework to redesign America's health care system and promoted an impetus to move from pay for performance to pay for value.

Patient-Centered Medical Home

An early driver of QI was the National Committee for Quality Assurance (NCQA), which is a private, not-for-profit organization established in 1990, that provides consulting, data analytic, and accreditation services to clinics, hospitals, and other health care entities that meet specified organizational and performance standards [9]. Certification programs like this are voluntary, but some insurance payers link their contracting with participation in various programs. One such program is the Patient-Centered Medical Home (PCMH), which has three levels of accreditation that are indexed by patient-centered access, team-based care, population health management, care management, care coordination, care transitions, and performance measurement and quality improvement [10]. The PCMH is a refinement of the concept of Advanced Medical Homes, proposed by the American College of Physicians (ACP) in 2006 and intended to promote a patient-centered, physician-guided model of health care [11]. The PCMH was soon endorsed by the American Academy of Pediatrics, the American Academy of Family Physicians, and the American Osteopathic Association [12]. The key elements of the PCMH include: (1) a personal physician responsible for all of a patient's care; (2) an emphasis on quality and safety; (3) enhanced access to care for patients. Since existing payment models were fee-for-service based, the PCMH model called for reimbursing physicians differently with enhanced payments based on quality and safety of care. As value-based care has evolved, fewer insurance payers require specific NCQA certification, though they do still rely on the Healthcare Effectiveness Data and Information Set (HEDIS) metrics, for which healthcare systems are held accountable.

Institute for Healthcare Improvement

The Institute for Healthcare Improvement (IHI) was founded in 1991 as an independent not-for-profit organization based on the work of the Committee on the Quality of Health Care in America and the National Demonstration Project on Quality Improvement in Health Care [13]. The mission of the organization is to revolutionize health care along the six aims set out in *Crossing the Quality Chasm* (Table 38.1). In 2007, IHI introduced the *Triple Aim* with the goal of "improving the individual experience of care; improving the health of populations; and reducing the per capita costs of care for populations" [14]. This has been expanded to the *Quadruple Aim*, which includes improving the experience of clinicians and staff [15]. This approach led to new initiatives by national organizations such as Family Medicine for America's Health [16] and new approaches to healthcare, including telemedicine [17]. IHI develops and spreads best practices through strategic initiatives such as the campaign to decrease the mortality of hospitalized patients by avoiding medical errors and improving efficiency [18]. Other campaigns focus on maternal health, aging, and joy in practice. Organizations can get involved in active initiatives through the IHI website.

Federal Government Enters Quality Improvement

The federal government is the single largest payer of healthcare in the US through the Centers for Medicare and Medicaid Services (CMS), and joined the QI initiative in 2006 with the Physician Quality Reporting System (PQRS) which was established to align payment with the reporting of quality data [19]. Initially there were incentive payments up to 2% for data provided, but these ended in 2014. In 2010, penalties for non-reporting data were introduced and providers were incented to submit data on a subset of over 200 different metrics. These metrics included preventive measures such as vaccine and cancer screening rates and chronic disease targets such as hemoglobin A1c control.

PQRS was reconstituted under the Medicare and CHIPS Reauthorization Act (MACRA) of 2015 and expanded the push to value-based payments by focusing not just on quality, but also on total costs of care [19]. Part of the reimbursement is for demonstrated quality, such as decreasing readmission rates and providing preventative care. Most of these models share risk with the health care organizations to incentivize good health outcomes at a lower cost. As a result of these programs and initiatives, the ongoing transition from a production-based to value-based reimbursement model has focused QI efforts across a wide range of health care settings [2].

Quality Improvement Principles

Four key principles are essential for any QI project, irrespective of the models or methodology used [20]. The first is that QI work should be viewed systematically as health care is complex with many inputs, processes, and outputs. Processes can be further divided into what care is provided and how it is delivered, and altering one factor within the system can have positive and negative effects. QI work looks not only at the individual outcome metric or behavior change but at the underlying system. One useful tool is a process map, which provides a visual overview of the different steps in workflows and stakeholders that may be contributing to them. A process map allows team members to understand workflows on a more global scale—from start to finish—since most members typically think and work in a limited part of the organization.

The second principle is a focus on patients. Improvements in health care should center on patient wellness and experience. QI initiatives can get sidetracked by paying more attention to process measures than to the patients who are receiving care. Teamwork is the third principle, highlighting that different members of a health care team understand different aspects of clinical processes and contribute distinctive skills. A diverse but cohesive team is necessary for a QI intervention to be successful in both the short and long term. A team approach creates buy-in, which is critical to the success of a program.

The fourth principle is the use of data, which ensures that an intervention is necessary and impactful. Data allows a team to learn from an intervention rather than taking a trial-and-error approach [21]. Both quantitative and qualitative data are important to gauging progress. Qualitative data, including surveys and interviews, are often overlooked but provide crucial information, such as calibrating organizational culture, which cannot be determined from quantitative data alone.

Quality Improvement Models and Frameworks

Deming Cycle/PDSA

W. Edwards Deming is often incorrectly credited with developing the Plan-Do-Study-Act (PDSA) model, otherwise known as the Deming Cycle (Fig. 38.1) [5, 21]. In fact, Deming adapted the Plan-Do-Check-Act (PDCA) model from his men-

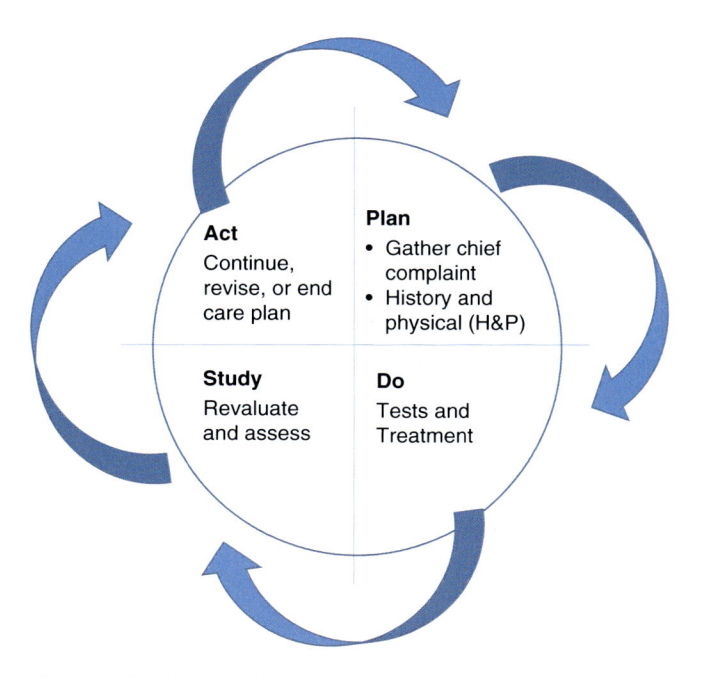

Fig. 38.1 PDSA cycle with clinical example [22]

Fig. 38.2 The Model for Improvement

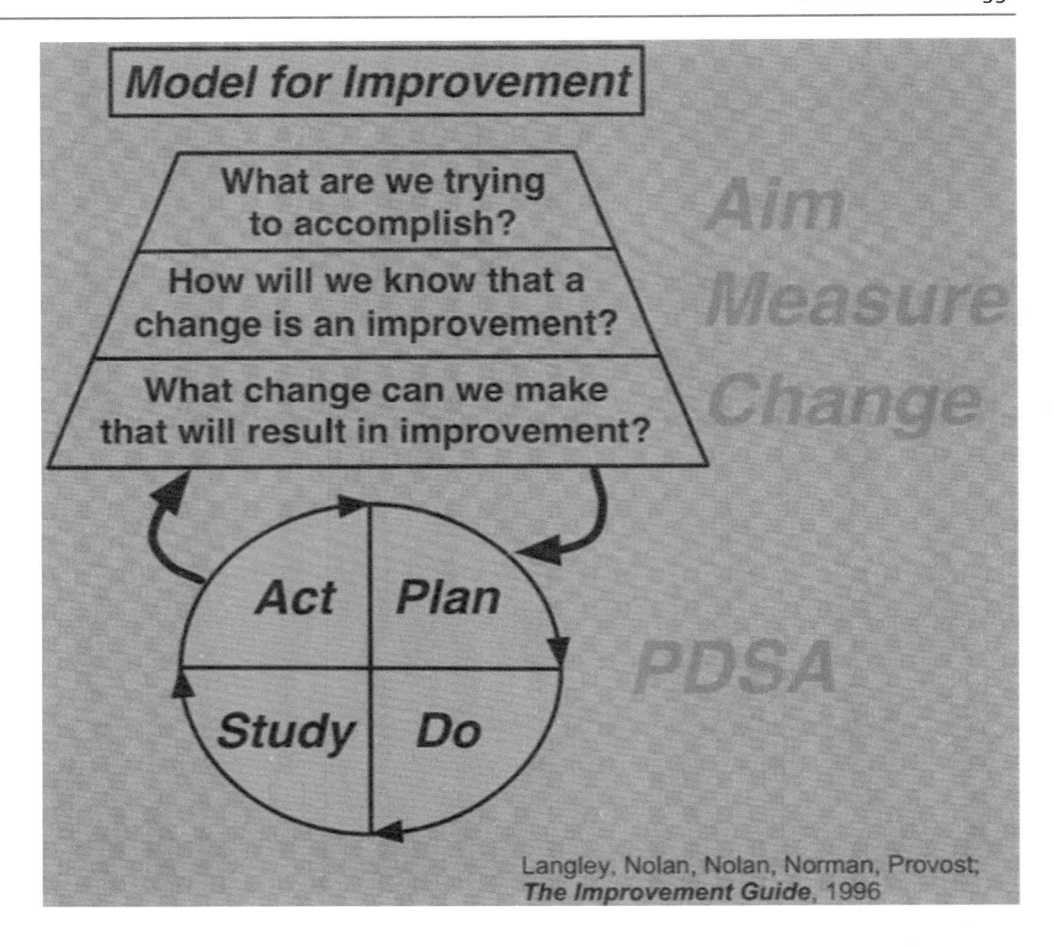

tor, Walter Shewhart, to better reflect the actions required to test change [5, 21]. An initial plan determines the experiment and outlines the proposed metrics (Plan). The experiment is carried out (Do), and the lessons learned from it are evaluated (Study/Check). The success and failures of the experiment are used to inform the next set of experiments (Act). In this way, the cycle is continuous as one trial informs the next, leading to ongoing and iterative gains in knowledge and advancement.

The PDSA improvement cycle is similar to the "SOAP" model whereby clinicians seek to understand the **S**ubjective complaint and symptoms, evaluate **O**bjective data through a physical exam, labs, and so on, develop an **A**ssessment to determine diagnosis, and enact and re-evaluate care **P**lan over the appropriate course of time [22].

IHI proposed The Model for Improvement, which places the PDSA cycle within a larger framework (Fig. 38.2) [21, 23]. Prior to initiating the PDSA cycle, the model asks three key questions that determine the aim, measurement strategies, and interventions of a project: *What are we trying to accomplish?* (Aim); *How will we know that a change is an improvement?* (Measure); and *What change can we make that will result in improvement?* (Selecting changes).

Forming the Team

Teamwork is critical for a successful QI project, and there are three key players who have different roles [21]. The *clinical leader* ensures that changes can be made within the organization and understands how changes will affect the system as a whole. The *technical expert* knows the process being improved, has increased knowledge of QI methodologies, and makes recommendations. The *day-to-day leader* implements the proposed innovation and oversees the collection of data. Effective teams should have all three types of members.

Teams naturally go through a development process known as *forming, storming, norming, and performing* [24]. In the *forming* stage, the team comes together with members who may or may not know each other and learns the task before them. Sometimes there is a *storming* stage with conflict between members as individuals voice opposing opinions and varying working styles become evident. During the *norming* stage, the group accepts one another and works together despite differences. Eventually, the team enters the *performing* stage and operates at full potential to reach goals. Changes in team membership may cause a regression to earlier stages.

Setting Aims

Once the team is formed, the aim of the improvement project is clarified. Aim statements should be specific, measurable, attainable, relevant, and time-bound (SMART). A clinical example of a SMART aim statement would be to increase cervical cancer screening rates by 5% in the next 3 months:

- Specific: Cervical cancer screening in women ages 21–65
- Measurable: The change in the percent of women getting screened
- Attainable: A 5% change is a realistic goal for the time frame
- Relevant: Screening detects cancers early and impacts the lives of patients.
- Time-bound: 3 months.

Selecting Measures

There are three types of measures collected during PDSA cycles; *outcome, process, and balancing* [21]. *Outcome* metrics measure the ultimate desired effect of the change, and can include biometric measures such as hemoglobin A1c, or rates such as screenings, morbidity, and mortality. *Process* measures look at the protocols and procedures that are used during PDSA cycles and are important if there is a time dependency to demonstrate change. Some process measures gauge participation rates among health care staff, or adherence to the standard work of the improvement. These metrics could include rates of referral for screening tests, even if the screening has not been completed. Process measures can be useful to identify and remediate improvements to the QI process itself. *Balancing* measures ascertain how QI interventions in one area positively or negatively impact other areas of clinical operations. For example, visit cycle time—the total time that a patient spends during a clinical encounter—may be lengthened when changing workflow patterns around preventive screening services in a clinic.

Selecting, Testing, Implementing and Spreading Change

Change can be sought for a variety of reasons, and typically involves thinking about the current process and using logic to come up with opportunities to make it work better. Even without major changes, novel approaches can modify workflows and improve results. Not all change initiatives result in the desired outcome, so it is critical to evaluate and test any adopted changes. After a process has gone through PDSA cycles to ensure it is effectively adopted on a small scale, the change is implemented into standard work, becoming the new way the process is carried out. Once a change has been successfully implemented, it can be disseminated across the organization to other clinical teams.

Six Sigma

Six Sigma is a process improvement strategy developed by Motorola in 1986 that focuses on eliminating defects and decreasing variability [25]. Six Sigma's roots go back to the early days of manufacturing, and build on the work of quality control pioneers Walter Shewhart and W. Edwards Deming. The term Six Sigma derives from the manufacturing industry's desire to reduce variability in products or processes to within six standard deviations of the mean (represented by σ), ensuring that their products are statistically 99.9997% free of defects. Six Sigma projects use the DMAIC methodology: Define the system, Measure the process, Analyze the data, Improve the process, Control the future state [26]. DMAIC identifies defects in the system and uses analytics and statistics to identify why they are occurring. Once defects are identified, the process is redesigned to prevent them in the future. The control stage is essential for maintaining a zero-defect process through continuous monitoring.

Six Sigma creates a hierarchal structure that is dependent upon training and certification and is often designated by the colored belts used in martial arts. Black belts and green belts, trained in statistical analysis and Six Sigma, manage projects throughout the organization. There are differences in Lean (see below) and Six Sigma approaches and methodologies, but their principles and tools can be combined to reduce both waste and defects [27]. Six Sigma principles and methods have been applied to health care, including improving the delivery of preventive services and diabetes care [28, 29].

Lean

Since the implementation of the Affordable Care Act, organizations across the health care industry have launched initiatives to improve quality and cost. However, health care in the US is still delivered mainly through fragmented, siloed, and uncoordinated care models funded by misaligned payment models [30]. Lean has emerged as one of the leading strategies to address the many challenges facing the health care industry as it transitions from fee-for-service to value-based reimbursement models [31, 32].

Lean is the practice of increasing value for patients by continuously eliminating waste from patient care pathways to improve quality, safety, and efficiency of care [33, 34]. Lean is a structured organizational approach for prioritizing and aligning strategic and process improvements to achieve transformative change in patient care, operational efficiency, and human development [30, 34]. Lean philosophy centers around two pillars: continuous improvement and respect for people. Lean seeks to reduce waste and bring value to the customer through continual improvement. An integral component of Lean is going to *gemba*, the "place of truth," to see what is really happening rather than what is believed to be happening, such as observing the operations floor or the clinic to truly understand the process and culture [35].

The core principle in Lean is that value is based on the customer or patient's perspective, and then specific actions identify and eliminate steps that do not create value. Another principle empowers customers/patients to determine value by customer demand. Throughout the process, there is an aim for perfection ("zero harm") by continuously removing wasteful steps and using flow and pull to create value [36]. All types of waste are identified and eliminated (Table 38.2).

Another guiding principle of Lean is to embrace the scientific method for problem-solving (i.e., PDSA or PDCA) at all levels of an organization [22]. Many Lean organizations have adopted A3 thinking from the Toyota Production System as a problem-solving framework. The term A3 refers to a standard paper size—11 by 17 inches—and connotes a standard consensus-building and communication tool that is used to study and solve a problem and then to communicate that change. A3 thinking is a transparent, logical, and structured process to drive change [35].

While A3 processes and reports can take on varying recording and reporting formats, the concept remains unchanged. One example is the 9-box A3 Report (Table 38.3). The reason for action (Box 1) lays out the problem and associated importance statements and answers the "burning platform" question of what problem we are trying to solve, why it is important to solve the problem, and what is involved [37, 38]. The current state (Box 2) and target state (Box 3) help individuals depict the existing workspace, both subjectively and objectively, as well as an ideal, future state. Box 4 identifies gaps that exist between the current and target state and uses a root cause analysis for a deeper dive into why these gaps exist. There are different tools that can be used at this stage of the project, such as the 5 Whys and a Fishbone Diagram, which determine what countermeasures or solutions presented in Box 5, would help solve the problem. Some solutions are straightforward and readily implemented, such as purchasing new ergonomically correct supply carts to decrease physical strain to staff.

Several PDSA cycles are often contained within experiments, as these cycles are the heart of A3 thinking [39]. Box 6 outlines the experiment plan(s), which includes metrics, process owners, and timelines. Box 7 delineates a completion plan with attention to remaining issues and unintended consequences. Box 8 examines what was achieved through the experiments and relies on the regular collection and reporting of data to verify change. In Box 9, lessons and insights are documented from reflection sessions held throughout the project to communicate with stakeholders and apply in future improvement work [38].

A3 thinking, and indeed all Lean tools, can be applied at any level of the organization and can promote a learning environment. Projects can be contained in one clinic or integrated into the entire healthcare system. Ideally, an organization commits to Lean and uses its philosophies and tools to transform the entire enterprise, known as Lean transformation. Lean goes beyond an improvement model since it requires a culture change in an organization, with support and buy-in from all stakeholders [35].

Most of the published literature on Lean implementation in health care has been siloed or project-based, focused on short-term results of continuous improvement efforts [40, 41]. Few studies have evaluated Lean's contributions to system-wide change, including the long-term effects of embedding a culture of continuous improvement rooted in Lean principles and behaviors [31, 41–43]. The limited literature on system-wide implementation of Lean in health care may reflect the shared misunderstanding of Lean among health care stakeholders. All too often, Lean is viewed as a set of tools or an improvement program sepa-

Table 38.2 Types of waste in health care [37, 38]

Muda	Description	Health care example
Waiting	Waiting for information, people, or materials	Patients waiting for discharge clearance
Overproduction	Doing more work than is absolutely required, over-processing	Ordering more lab work than is necessary to treat a patient
Rework (or defect)	Having to undertake remedial work of any kind because it was done incorrectly the first time	Medication sent to the wrong pharmacy
Motion	The movement of human beings, when not necessary	Nurses walking five miles in a single shift
Transportation	The movement of information, materials, and equipment	A form moving from person to person or department to department
Inventory	Any unnecessary materials, unnecessary queuing of people, tasks, or forms	More medication on hand than is necessary
Non-utilized talent	The waste of expertise of human beings by asking them to do something better undertaken by someone else	Staff not being given the opportunity to improve a process. Staff not using the full scope of their licensure.
Over-processing	Extra steps that do not provide value	Having to fill out multiple copies of the same paperwork

Table 38.3 A3 nine-box A3 report template [37, 38]

Box 1 Reasons for Action *Why is this problem important and why are you talking about it now?* Business Case	Box 4 Gap Analysis *Why are we experiencing the problems and what constraints prevent us from the goal?* Root cause analysis Possible tools: – 5 Whys – Fishbone – Pareto Analysis	Box 7 Completion Plan *What is the specific work plan for testing various solutions?* Who will do what and when? Ensure ongoing PDSA
Box 2 Current State *What is the condition that the business or operation feels?* Metrics, description, visual displays	Box 5 Solution Approach *What alternatives and options will be considered to solve the problem?* Ideas to remedy root causes discovered in Box 4	Box 8 Confirmed State *What was achieved related to the current state?* Metrics gathered and reported at regular intervals
Box 3 Target State *What is the specific change that you want to accomplish and how will you measure success?* Target metrics, description of target state, visual displays	Box 6 Experiments *What will you do to test the alternatives and options?* Gantt Chart or other project plan Indicators of performance	Box 9 Insights *What did we learn from this experience and where are the opportunities for improvement?* Plus (+)/deltas Aha moments

rate from the organization's business system, with tools and thinking limited to project-based work and short-term results which does not enable an organization to embed the culture necessary to make breakthrough strategic improvement and innovation [44]. The incorrect use of Lean in health care has resulted in it being viewed as "Medical Taylorism" by certain segments of the provider community who see Lean as a threat to autonomy and patient-centered care [45].

Lean is not just a technical methodology focused solely on process improvement tools. Lean is a socio-technical system that incorporates the social, behavioral, and other contextual factors within an organization to empower people and enable change [41, 46]. The core work of any Lean transformation is to change the culture, which involves changing how all stakeholders in the organization respond to problems, think about patients, and work with each other [47–49]. Health care leaders should view Lean transformation as a different approach to managing an organization and a continuous journey in developing a learning organization focused on delivering high-quality care to its patients [44].

Practice Level Quality Improvement

There are several quality improvement strategies, such as PDSA cycles, that can be used at the practice level. For example, a primary care clinic found that only 55% of their patients had lipid surveillance for cardiovascular disease prevention and only 68% of those patients were prescribed statins. An improvement team was assembled, agreed that this performance could be improved, and used an IHI framework to guide their quality improvement project. First, the team defined their problem (Aim) and chose a process measure (i.e., percentage of patients that received yearly lipid panels) as well as an outcome measure (e.g., triglycerides, total cholesterol). They identified the data management approach that would track their initiative. A first test of change within the PDSA cycle was to create and implement an automated system to remind clinical support staff that a patient was due for yearly cholesterol screening (Plan-Do). After implementation, screening rates improved from 55 to 64%.

While this was a significant improvement, the team built on their intervention by reviewing their experience, using this information to inform and refine their activity (Study-Act). For the next PDSA cycle, the team generated a list of patients with diabetes mellitus who were due for cholesterol screening and involved front desk administrative staff. At patient check-in, administrative staffs were asked to direct the patient to the laboratory, where there was a standing order for drawing a lipid panel. After implementing this change in the workflow, the screening rate went from 64 to 75%.

For the third PDSA cycle, the team provided ongoing data to administrative staff regarding their performance in directing eligible patients to the lab. The team set a process measure of greater than 90% fidelity for directing patients to the lab and provided incentives, such as individual recognition and social events, such as a pizza party. Initially there was 94% fidelity to the process and, remarkably, fidelity was sustained at nearly 90% for over 2 years after the incentives were discontinued. Screening patients at the start of the visit and having the result readily available, allowed physicians to use that information to make decisions at the point of care regarding statins and other interventions. Over the same period, average total cholesterol fell from 185 mg/dL to 170 mg/dL. LDL fell from 99 mg/dL to 81 mg/dL (Fig. 38.3).

Fig. 38.3 Run charts of total cholesterol and lipids for a patient population

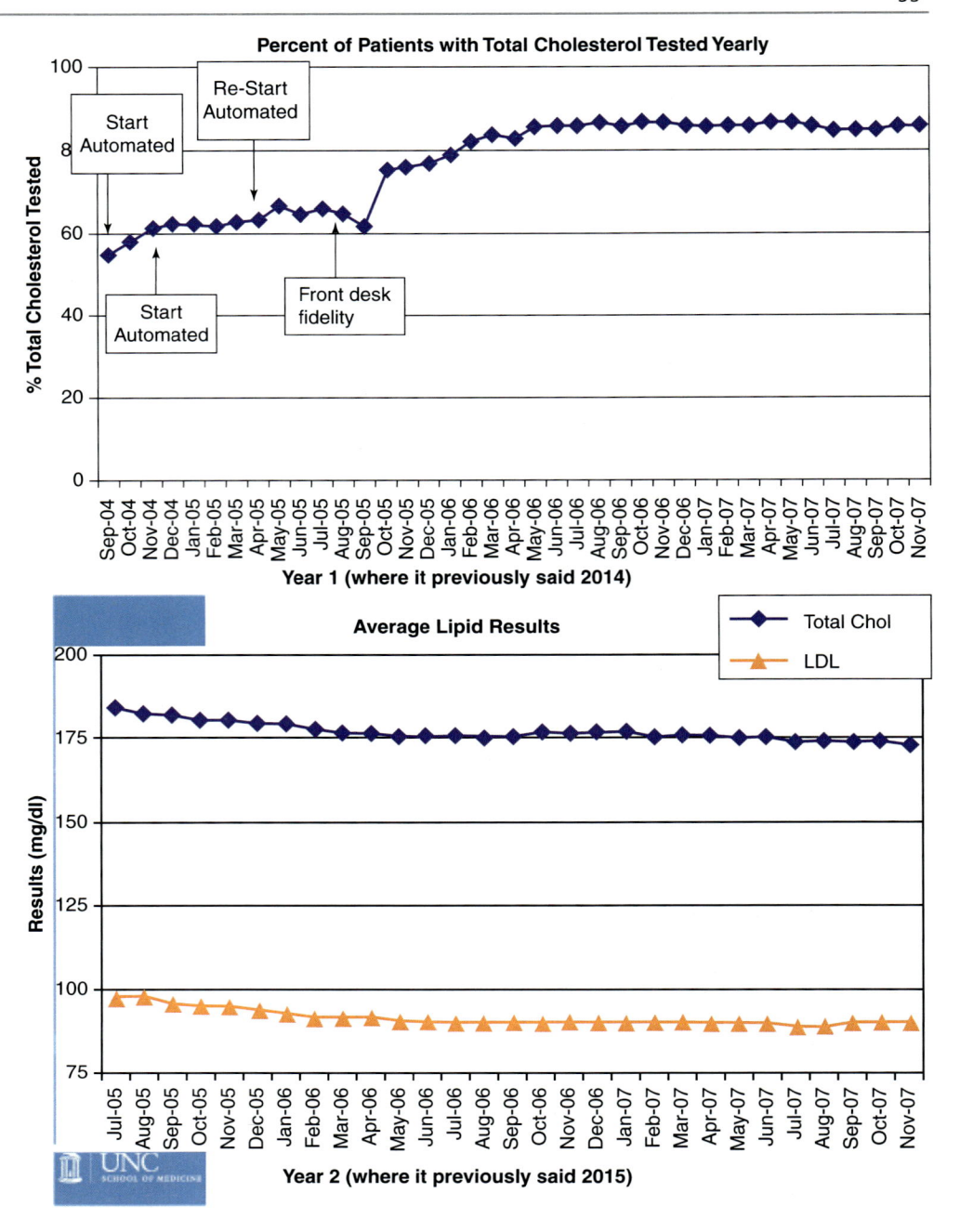

System Level Quality Improvement and Transformation

Some hospitals and health care systems have embarked on a process to transform their entire organizations in a way that is guided by quality and value across every aspect of the enterprise. Virginia Mason Medical Center, Thedacare, and Sutter Health have all successfully lowered cost and improved the quality of care by changing how they approach quality improvement, putting quality at the center of all of their planning and operations, and creating central support and directives for quality [50, 51]. Using different approaches, all have demonstrated strong evidence for organizational level transformation.

Approximately 20 years ago, Virginia Mason Medical Center (VM) was a 336-bed acute care hospital, with multiple outpatient clinics around Seattle, that was losing money. It was clear that VM needed to transform as an organization if they were going to survive. In a drive to patient-centeredness, the organization investigated different management frameworks that would help the organization transform into a patient-centered, high-quality organization. VM decided on Lean as embodied in the Toyota Production

System and sent leaders and staff to manufacturing plants in Japan and the United States to learn how to create value for the patient by eliminating waste [50–52].

Virginia Mason credits Lean with their ongoing success. For example, improvements that targeted reducing wasted, non-patient focused activity of nursing staff decreased wasted motion so that now 90% of a nurse's shift is focused on patient care [50]. Using Lean methods, the VM Kirkland clinic created a standardized diabetes care plan that resulted in 82% of diabetic patients having hemoglobin A1c levels of less than 8. VM not only improved care but also achieved positive margins every year since beginning their Lean journey. Professional liability decreased 27% from 2007 to 2008 and then dropped an additional 12%. Leadership and staff now teach their management and improvement methods via the Virginia Mason Institute.

ThedaCare is a health care system in northeast Wisconsin made up of five hospitals and associated outpatient clinics that began their "Lean journey" in 2003. From 2004 to 2009, their operating income doubled, and as of 2013, it has remained at or above 4% of revenue [54]. In addition to ongoing QI projects, ThedaCare has changed the way they lead by implementing a Lean Management system, which they refer to as a Business Performance System, or BPS [53]. Although there are limited evaluation studies of the ThedaCare experience, prior CEO John Toussaint points to Lean as the method by which the organization decreased inpatient costs by 25%, improved patient satisfaction to 100%, and committed zero medication errors when a pharmacist was involved in medication reconciliation [51]. He also cites one area surgery center that improved its non-operative time by 50%.

Sutter Health includes a large, not-for-profit ambulatory care delivery system that serves over one million patients and includes 17 full-service primary care facilities, housing 40 family medicine, internal medicine, and pediatric clinics [31, 40, 48]. In response to external market forces such as changing health policy, growing patient population, and pressure to contain costs, Sutter Health established a proactive strategic initiative to improve efficiency and cost across the system. To achieve the strategic goal, senior leaders launched a system-wide Lean transformation starting in primary care. In addition to improving quality and cost, implementing Lean in primary care was seen as a viable way to reduce provider burnout, workplace stress, and improve patient experience [31]. Primary care Lean redesigns were conducted in three implementation phases, with each phase lasting 4–6 months. Phase one included a single pilot clinic, phase two comprised of three additional pilot clinics, and phase three added all remaining primary care clinics. Redesigns within the clinics in all phases followed the same Lean implementation approach: (1) reorganization of supplies, equipment, and education material in patient exam rooms, (2) optimization of call center functions, (3) co-location of provider and care teams to facilitate collaboration and communication, and (4) redesign of care team workflows to promote a higher level of service quality by optimizing care team collaboration. Redesigned care team workflows included pre-session huddles between providers and certified medical assistants (CMAs), CMAs and patients setting the agenda to be covered with the provider, and expansion of CMA's role to co-manage the provider's in-basket messages [31, 53]. Sutter Health's lean transformation in primary care has improved provider workflow efficiency, provider productivity, patient satisfaction, clinic cycle times, staff satisfaction, and collaboration among care teams [32, 48, 53].

Change Management

Change comes with quality improvement, which can be challenging for stakeholders in an organization. Change management is the process of creating change and sustaining it within an organization [37]. Each improvement model is a socio-technical system that incorporates the social, behavioral, and other relevant contextual factors within an organization to empower people and enable change [41, 46]. All too often, health care stakeholders lose sight of quality improvement's social aspect involving leadership, behavior, and other elements of an organization's underlying culture, which can produce challenges with engagement, sustainment, and achieving further breakthrough improvement [54, 55].

The Kotter model is an example of an empirically based approach to understanding and guiding change management [56]. There are eight steps of change management in the model, which are sequenced to improve performance. The first step is establishing a sense of urgency by creating a "burning platform" that identifies crises, potential crises, or significant opportunities within the organization. Most stakeholders should understand that the status quo is more threatening than change to achieve this feeling state. The second step is building a guiding coalition by establishing a group that has the shared commitment, power, and energy to lead and support a collaborative change effort. While a movement for transformation can start with just one or two people, it must achieve a sufficient mass early on to be successful. Any effort to change can fail if it is simply a grouping of projects and directives, highlighting the third step; there must be an overarching vision that is compelling, clear, and simple enough to communicate at all levels within an organization [56, 57].

According to Kotter's research, organizations attempting to transform often under-communicate by a factor of ten; so, step 4 communicates the vision at every opportunity. Rather than share the vision at a few big meetings and via a few communiques, the vision is embedded into all communication methods, from business trainings to yearly reviews to employee newsletters. Once the vision is communicated, others are empowered to act on the vision, which encourages risk-taking and nontraditional ideas. In step 5, systems or processes that undermine the vision must be changed and any barriers, be they systems, departments, or people, must be removed. The organization must demonstrate successes in the first 12–24 months to build momentum, and step 6 plans for and creates short-term wins. Because success does not simply occur, these short-term wins must be actively planned for and achieved, and participants who carry out these wins should be rewarded and acknowledged publicly.

Once change momentum accelerates, improvements are consolidated, and additional change demonstrated (step 7). It is important not to declare victory too soon, ensuring these short-term wins are seen as only that and not as a final victory, lest the organization celebrate too early, and retreat from the change process. As performance increases, it is essential to institutionalize the new approaches and communicate that the change is due to the transformation (step 8). These changes must be rooted in the culture of the organization. As management turns over, successors must continue to champion the transformation.

Data Management

Data management is an integral part of all quality endeavors with several critical processes. Data are collected to determine a baseline level of performance, identify root causes of underperformance, and then analyzed to decide on the best course of action. The data are then re-measured to ensure that a change results in sustained improvement over time [58].

Collecting Data

A data collecting method should be mapped out in advance of quality improvement initiatives; what will be collected, how often, and by whom. The plan should include the operational definition of each measure, including the numerator, the denominator, and any exclusions to each measure [58]. In considering the QI program from the primary care clinic that was described earlier, the team focused on what percent of patients had their cholesterol tested. Cholesterol levels are not routinely tested in all patients and operational definitions used for the QI program are listed in Table 38.4. The data were collected weekly. The QI team did not have access to an electronic medical record that could automatically collect, aggregate, and report this data from the system so chart audits using manual data collection utilized a sampling methodology, such as auditing 30 randomly chosen charts per week and using those data to estimate overall performance. The development of artificial intelligence and machine learning should help these processes.

Tracking Data

Once measures are identified and defined, they must be tracked. The frequency of tracking data varies depending on the project scope and systems and processes that are actively modified. After the conclusion of a project, outcome data can be monitored less frequently to determine if the change is sustained and performance is stable. However, if new processes are developed to improve a specific quality outcome measure (i.e., A1C), measures should be monitored more frequently to ensure that the new processes are taking hold within the organization. Performance data should be shared with the organizational unit and are commonly displayed as run charts (Fig. 38.3). Other graphs such as pie charts and histograms are also helpful. Dashboards are data displays that show multiple performance graphs. For example, a diabetes dashboard may include two to six different performance graphs.

Statistical process control (SPC) is used in organizations that have adopted the Six Sigma improvement methodology and was developed by Walter Shewhart in the mid-1920s [4]. The goal of SPC is to fully understand the behavior of a particular process to determine whether the process will consistently meet the needs and requirements of the customer. Statistic-based control charts are used in SPC to monitor and control process performance. Similar to run charts, control charts include "control limits" which are mathematically defined, typically a fixed number of standard deviations from the mean [58]. The use of control charts helps organizations to determine when it is necessary to act on a process by differentiating between common and special cause variation.

Table 38.4 Data elements and operational definitions for cholesterol QI program

Data element	Operational definition
Denominator	Patients greater than or equal to 18 years of age who were seen at the practice for an office visit in the last 18 months
Numerator	Patients in the denominator whose Total Cholesterol was tested within the last 365 days of their appointment. This test must have been performed in office or if performed elsewhere results must be documented in the chart noting date performed
Denominator Exclusion	Patients who are receiving only palliative care, as indicated by an applicable diagnosis code on the problem list

Common cause variation is referred to as natural variation within a process. Sometimes data points on a process control chart will fall outside of the control limits signifying changes are far enough from the mean that they cannot be explained by natural variation in the process. Such changes in the process can be attributed to special or assignable causes of variation, which must be identified and removed to ensure outcome goals are achieved.

Analyzing and Interpreting Data

The processes of analyzing and interpreting data are critical in reviewing performance to determine whether goals are being achieved. Interpreting data seeks to draw meaningful conclusions that can be used to evaluate and improve activities, identify gaps, and plan improvement [58]. Returning to the earlier example of cholesterol screening, annotations on the run chart in Fig. 38.3 such as "front desk fidelity" were noted at specific time points and this allowed the QI group to visually track the impact of the intervention and plan future changes. Benchmarking, or comparing results to external references, is another approach to interpreting data and there are many sources that can be used for this purpose.

Acting on Data

The analyzed data allows the study team to engage in the Act phase of the PDSA cycle. Suppose the project is going well and has demonstrated improvement and sustainability. In that case, it may be time to determine how to spread insights to other parts of the healthcare system or work on other metrics within the same organizational unit [58]. If the analyzed data show that progress has been insufficient, steps and course corrections can be taken to remediate the situation. The team would also look to ensure that data are being collected accurately, reanalyze their interpretation to determine if they are addressing the right root causes, re-evaluate their changes to ensure they are being implemented consistently, or increase the rate at which they are making changes.

Many health care institutions have adopted the managing for daily improvement (MDI) concept to embed PDSA-based problem-solving across the organization. The underlying principle of MDI is to engage all staff, from leadership to the front-line, in continuous improvement. MDI consists of four elements, including daily team meetings, information centers, rounding, and daily problem-solving. Information centers offer teams a centralized location to display information and performance data relevant to ongoing improvement work within an organizational unit. Performance data is often displayed using a whiteboard where current performance is compared to targets or goals. During team meetings, staff can discuss challenges in achieving goals and potential ideas to overcome the difficulties identified. In addition to providing a forum for staff to identify and remove barriers to improvement, MDI systems also aid teams in adopting new processes which may require changes in staff behaviors and routines [38].

Disseminating Data

Data can be shared and disseminated in many forms and modes: in graphs and charts, newsletters, emails, bulletin boards, and other communiques. Data are increasingly presented as a digital "dashboard" (e.g., a Microsoft Excel file or charts integrated into the electronic medical record). Dashboards are visual displays of multiple charts showing changes over time, comparisons between different entities, or progress toward a goal. This tool can track and report data at several levels, such as practice-level or provider-level. Figure 38.4 is an example of a provider dashboard for diabetes care.

At the organization or practice level, all metrics that are important should be displayed continuously. Some candidate measures include on-time clinic starts, operating revenue, and the percent of patients who received

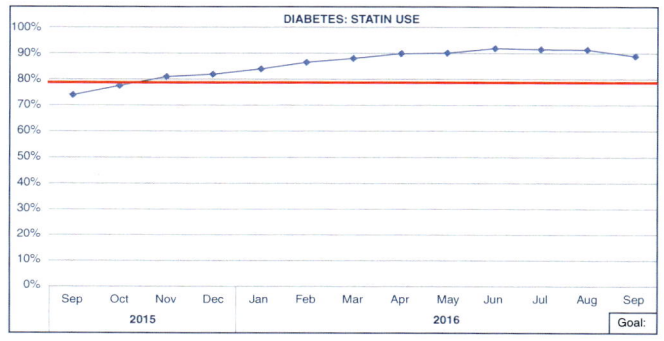

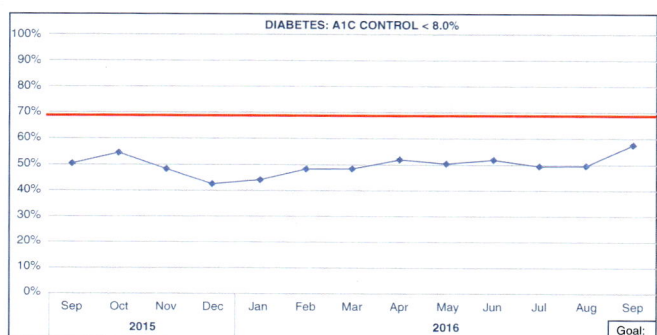

Fig. 38.4 Provider dashboard for diabetes care

indicated preventative services. Data, however, can become overwhelming, and organizations can lose focus on their vision and strategy if changes in metrics repeatedly lead to immediate action. As a result, some organizations have defined core metrics that are most critical to their mission. These *True North Metrics* are vetted and ultimately approved and promoted by the leadership of the respective unit [59].

ThedaCare, for example, uses metrics, such as employee safety, to align their strategic process and determine focal areas of improvement [60]. Other organizations may use a balanced scorecard, which shows a variety of performance data, tied to strategic initiatives. Metrics that are important to their current strategy, for which managers must have an action plan when poor performance is evident, are called *Drive Metrics*. Metrics that are being tracked but do not warrant immediate action despite falling performance are called *Watch Metrics*. Creating a hierarchy of performance indicators helps the organization maintain focus.

Future Directions

Contemporary and future physicians will be expected to provide quality care and engage in continuous quality improvement (QI). Physicians in practice can expect that the quality metrics of their patient panel will be publicly available and that their incentive salary will be tied to these quality outcomes. The importance of ingraining this in physicians is evident in the quality improvement curricula that have become part of medical education [61]. Physician leader positions will be expected to have mastery in QI language, strategies, and tools to help their patients and their organizations achieve better outcomes.

QI will increasingly involve patients since they must be actively engaged in their care to achieve health care goals. In addition to traditional patient engagement methods, some organizations provide patients with a "report card" of their health, identifying recommended health maintenance services. On an organizational level, practices, hospitals, and healthcare systems involve patients directly in the quality improvement process. Many organizations have created patient advisory councils or comparable structures to solicit patient input in clinical operations [62]. These patients, and other engaged stakeholders, can serve on QI teams, providing invaluable information on how to create patient-centered processes.

Health care continues to move away from production-based to value-based reimbursement models for services to decrease cost and increase quality [63]. While these models evolve, organizations will grapple with understanding and defining value, achieving value-based outcomes, and successfully reporting these data for reimbursement [64, 65].

References

1. Toussaint JS. Hospitals can't improve without better management systems. Harv Bus Rev. 2017.
2. Blumenthal D, Dixon J. Health-care reforms in the USA and England: areas for useful learning. Lancet. 2012;380(9850):1352–7.
3. DelliFraine JL, Langabeer JR, Nembhard IM. Assessing the evidence of Six Sigma and Lean in the health care industry. Qual Manage Healthcare. 2010;19(3):211–25.
4. Kubiak TM, Benbow D. The certified Six Sigma black belt handbook. 3rd ed. Milwaukee, WI: ASQ Quality Press; 2017.
5. Furterer S, Wood D. The ASQ certified manager of quality/organizational excellence handbook. 5th ed. Milwaukee, WI: ASQExcellence; 2021.
6. Liker JK, Morgan JM. The Toyota way in services: the case of Lean product development. Acad Manag Perspect. 2006;20(2):5–20.
7. Donaldson MS, Corrigan JM, Kohn LT. To err is human: building a safer health system, vol. 6. National Academies Press; 2000.
8. Richardson WC, Berwick DM, Bisgard JC, Bristow LR, Buck CR, Cassel CK. Crossing the quality chasm: a new health system for the 21st century. Washington, DC: National Academies Press (US); 2001.
9. Viswanathan HN, Salmon JW. Accrediting organizations and quality improvement. Am J Manag Care. 2000;6(10):1117–30.
10. PCMH 2014 scoring: scoring summary. 2017. http://www.ncqa.org/programs/recognition/practices/patient-centered-medical-home-pcmh/pcmh-2014-content-and-scoring-summary.
11. Institute for Healthcare Improvement: about us. 2007. http://www.ihi.org/about/Pages/History.aspx.
12. Berwick DM, Nolan TW, Whittington J. The triple aim: care, health, and cost. Health affairs (Project Hope). 2008;27(3):759–69.
13. Bodenheimer T, Sinsky C. From triple to quadruple aim: care of the patient requires care of the provider. Ann Fam Med. 2014;12(6):573–6.
14. Puffer JC, Borkan J, DeVoe JE, Davis A, Phillips RL Jr, Green LA, et al. Envisioning a new health care system for America. Fam Med. 2015;47(8):598–603.
15. Vockley M. The rise of telehealth: 'triple aim,' innovative technology, and popular demand are spearheading new models of health and wellness care. Biomed Instrum Technol. 2015;49(5):306–20.
16. Berwick DM, Calkins DR, McCannon CJ, Hackbarth AD. The 100 000 lives campaign: setting a goal and a deadline for improving health care quality. JAMA. 2006;295(3):324–7.
17. Barr M, Ginsburg J. The advanced medical home: a patient-centered, physician-guided model of health care. Philadelphia, PA: American College of Physicians; 2006.
18. Physicians AA, of F. Joint principles of the Patient-Centered Medical Home. Del Med J. 2008;80(1):21–2.
19. Hirsch JA, Leslie-Mazwi TM, Nicola GN, Bhargavan-Chatfield M, Seidenwurm DJ, Silva E, et al. PQRS and the MACRA: value-based payments have moved from concept to reality. AJNR Am J Neuroradiol. 2016;37(12):2195–200.
20. Quality Improvement. vol. 2017. U.S. DHHS: Health Resources and Service Administration; 2011. https://www.hrsa.gov/quality/toolbox/methodology/qualityimprovement/index.html.
21. Langley GJ, Moen RD, Nolan KM, Nolan TW, Norman CL, Provost LP. The improvement guide: a practical approach to enhancing organizational performance. Wiley; 2009.
22. Toussaint J, Billi J, Graban M. Lean for Doctors. Catalysis. 2017. https://createvalue.org/white-paper-lean-doctors/.
23. Moen RD, Norman CL. Circling back. Qual Prog. 2010;43(11):22.
24. Tuckman BW. DEVELOPMENTAL SEQUENCE IN SMALL GROUPS. Psychol Bull. 1965;63:384–99.
25. Harry MJ, Schroeder R. Six Sigma: the breakthrough management strategy revolutionizing the world's top corporations. Broadway Business; 2005.

26. Kubiak TM, Benbow DW. The certified Six Sigma black belt handbook. ASQ Quality Press; 2009.
27. George ML. Lean Six Sigma: combining Six Sigma quality with Lean production speed. New York: McGraw-Hill; 2002.
28. Gittner LS, Husaini BA, Hull PC, Emerson JS, Tropez-Sims S, Reece MC, et al. Use of Six Sigma for eliminating missed opportunities for prevention services. J Nurs Care Qual. 2015;30(3):254–60.
29. Paccagnella A, Mauri A, Spinella N. Quality improvement for integrated management of patients with type 2 diabetes (PRIHTA project stage 1). Qual Manag Health Care. 2012;21(3):146–59.
30. Gabow P, Goodman P. The Lean prescription: powerful medicine for our ailing healthcare system. Boca Ranton, FL: CRC Press; 2015.
31. Hung D, Gray C, Martinez M, Schmittdiel J, Harrison MI. Acceptance of Lean redesigns in primary care: a contextual analysis. Health Care Manag Rev. 2017;42(3):203–12.
32. Hung DY, Harrison MI, Martinez MC, Luft HS. Scaling Lean in primary care: impacts on system performance. Am J Manag Care. 2017;23(3):161–8.
33. Virginia Mason Institute. Lean Health Care | Eliminating Waste to Create a Patient-Centered Culture. Virginia Mason Institute. 2018. https://www.virginiamasoninstitute.org/2017/08/lean-health-care/.
34. Dean ML. Lean healthcare deployment and sustainability. New York: McGraw-Hill; 2013.
35. Koenigsaecker G. Leading the Lean enterprise transformation. 2nd ed. New York: CRC Press; 2012.
36. Womack JP, Jones DT. Lean thinking: banish waste and create wealth in your corporation. Simon and Schuster; 2010.
37. Eaton M. The Lean Practitioner's handbook. Kogan Page Publishers; 2013.
38. Graban M, Swartz JE. Healthcare Kaizen: engaging front-line staff in sustainable continuous improvements. CRC Press; 2012.
39. Sobek DK II, Smalley A. Understanding A3 thinking: a critical component of Toyota's PDCA management system. CRC Press; 2011.
40. Hung DY, Harrison MI, Liang S-Y, Truong QA. Contextual conditions and performance improvement in primary care. Qual Manag Health Care. 2019;28(2):70–7.
41. Shortell SM, Blodgett JC, Rundall TG, Kralovec P. Use of Lean and related transformational performance improvement systems in hospitals in the United States: results from a national survey. Jt Comm J Qual Patient Saf. 2018;44(10):574–82.
42. Hung DY, Truong QA, Liang S-Y. Implementing Lean quality improvement in primary care: impact on efficiency in performing common clinical tasks. J Gen Intern Med. 2021;36(2):274–9.
43. Kaltenbrunner M, Bengtsson L, Mathiassen SE, Högberg H, Engström M. Staff perception of Lean, care-giving, thriving and exhaustion: a longitudinal study in primary care. BMC Health Serv Res. 2019;19(1):652.
44. Anderson J. Transforming primary care: redesigning the work for improvement. Community and Family Medicine Grand Rounds. Duke Health; 2017. https://fmch.duke.edu/sites/fmch.duke.edu/files/cfm/CFM-documents/John%20Anderson%20CFM%20Grand%20Rounds.pdf.
45. Wu S, Brown C, Black S, Garcia M, Harrington DW. Using Lean performance improvement for patient-centered medical home transformation at an academic public hospital. J Healthc Qual. 2019;41(6):350–61.
46. Morduchowicz S, Lee JS, Choi L, Kivlahan C, Null D, Smith S, et al. Utilizing Lean leadership principles to build an academic primary care practice of the future. J Gen Intern Med. 2020;35(12):3650–5.
47. Barnas K, Adams E. Beyond heroes: a Lean management system for healthcare. Appleton, WI: ThedaCare Center for Healthcare Value; 2014.
48. Hung DY, Harrison MI, Truong Q, Du X. Experiences of primary care physicians and staff following Lean workflow redesign. BMC Health Serv Res. 2018;18(1):274.
49. Lee P, Pham L, Oakley S, Eng K, Freydin E, Rose T, et al. Using Lean thinking to improve hypertension in a community health centre: a quality improvement report. BMJ Open Qual. 2019;8(1):e000373.
50. Kenney C. Transforming health care: Virginia Mason Medical Center's pursuit of the perfect patient experience. CRC Press; 2012.
51. Toussaint JS, Berry LL. The promise of Lean in health care. 2013;88:74–82.
52. Jha AK, Perlin JB, Kizer KW, Dudley RA. Effect of the transformation of the Veterans Affairs Health Care System on the quality of care. N Engl J Med. 2003;348(22):2218–27.
53. Hung DY, Mujal G, Jin A, Liang S. Patient experiences after implementing Lean primary care redesigns. Health Serv Res. 2020:1475-6773.13605.
54. Kelly S, Hines P. Discreetly embedding the Shingo principles of enterprise excellence at Abbott Diagnostics manufacturing facility in Longford Ireland. Total Qual Manag Bus Excell. 2019;30(11–12):1235–56.
55. Toussaint J, Barnas K. Becoming the change: leadership behavior strategies for continuous improvement for healthcare. New York, NY: McGraw Hill; 2021.
56. Kotter JP. Leading change: why transformation efforts fail. 1995.
57. Kotter JP. Leading change. Harvard Business Press; 1996.
58. Health Resources and Services Administration. Managing data for performance improvement. vol. 2017. U.S. DHHS: Health Resources and Service Administration; 2011. http://www.hrsa.gov/quality/toolbox/methodology/performanceimprovement/index.html.
59. Liker JK. The toyota way. Esensi; 2004.
60. Barnas K. Beyond heroes: a Lean management system for healthcare. ThedaCare Center for Healthcare Value; 2014.
61. Bogetz JF, Rassbach CE, Bereknyei S, Mendoza FS, Sanders LM, Braddock CH. Training health care professionals for 21st-century practice: a systematic review of educational interventions on chronic care. Acad Med. 2015;90(11):1561–72.
62. Newton WP, Atkinson H, Parker DL, Gwynne M. Bringing patients into the patient-centered medical home: lessons learned in a large primary care practice. N C Med J. 2015;76(3):190–3.
63. Tsai TC. Better patient care at high-quality hospitals may save medicare money and bolster episode-based payment models. Health Affairs (Project Hope). 2016;35(9):1681–9.
64. Berwick D. Era 3 for medicine and health care. JAMA. 2016;315(13):1329–30.
65. Ogundeji YK, Bland JM, Sheldon TA. The effectiveness of payment for performance in health care: a meta-analysis and exploration of variation in outcomes. Health Policy. 2016;120(10):1141–50.

Quality of Life and Patient-Centered Outcomes

Maria Gabriela Castro and Margaret C. Wang

Introduction

Patient-centeredness encompasses "providing care that is respectful of and responsive to individual patient preferences, needs, and values and ensuring that patient values guide all clinical decisions" [1]. Although patient-centered care is a major design feature of contemporary health care, actionable strategies are needed to operationalize it in clinical practice [2]. The use of patient-reported outcomes (PRO) promotes patient engagement and supports patient-centered care, particularly among chronically ill patients [3–5]. These data recently started to be systematically recorded and integrated into clinical care planning despite the near universal implementation of electronic health records and the prevalence of personal digital devices in the United States over the past 10 years [6, 7]. In 2021, the rapid onset and ensuing healthcare demands associated with the COVID-19 pandemic accelerated the development of virtual care infrastructures, as this rapidly became the primary form of healthcare delivery [8–11].

This chapter provides an overview to quality of life and associated patient-reported outcomes (PROs). The first section describes commonly used PRO terms and applications of PRO in clinical practice. The next section provides selected examples of the use of PRO and explores the impact of these data on care processes and outcomes. Key milestones in the conceptual development of PRO are provided before the final section outlines current challenges to and future trends in the widespread use of patient-reported outcomes in healthcare.

Defining Patient-Reported Outcomes

The availability of rigorous, research-based questionnaires that solicit information on patients' symptoms, functional status, quality of life, and health behaviors has facilitated the integration of patient-centered information into clinical care and quality improvement. The U.S. Food and Drug Administration (FDA), for example, defines patient-reported

M. G. Castro (✉)
Department of Family Medicine, University of North Carolina at Chapel Hill, Chapel Hill, NC, USA
e-mail: Gabriela_Castro@med.unc.edu

M. C. Wang
Office of the Chief Quality Officer, Stanford Health Care, Palo Alto, CA, USA
e-mail: margaretwang@stanfordhealthcare.org

outcomes as "any report of a patient's (or person's) health condition, health behavior, or experience with healthcare that comes directly from the patient, without interpretation of the patient's response by a clinician or anyone else" [12, 13]. When integrated into clinical care, PRO data can complement clinical indicators and physiological markers obtained through physical examinations, laboratory tests, and imaging studies; improve patient engagement; facilitate shared decision-making between patients and providers; and improve quality of care [3, 14–19]. A Cochrane classification of clinical trial outcomes notes that PROs are among the most important to patients, along with survival (e.g., five-year disease-free rates), morbidity events such as stroke, and caregiver-reported outcomes such as caregiver burden and stress [20].

PRO is an umbrella term and often comprises three concepts: experience, measure, and data [13]. PRO is a first-hand report of patient experiences and perceptions that exist independently from a systematic attempt to measure them; this understanding is characterized by a patient who reports, "I feel better" to a healthcare provider [13, 21]. The second meaning refers to PRO measures (PROM), typically instruments, or scales, that aim to systematically capture subjective patient experiences that cannot be externally measured [13]. The third meaning refers to PRO data as collected by the aforementioned methods, aggregating these data at the level of populations for surveillance from the clinical management perspective or for use as the basis for performance measures within healthcare organizations and systems [13, 22].

PRO components vary across existing classifications. A National Quality Forum report includes domains such as health-related quality of life (HRQoL), which encompasses health and functional status, symptoms and symptom burden (e.g., pain and fatigue), care experiences such as those measured by the Consumer Assessment of Healthcare Providers and Systems (CAHPS) survey, and health behaviors such as adherence, smoking, diet, and physical activity [22]. Other classifications assume that outcomes represent only the effects of care and do not include health behaviors and care experiences which are viewed as patient-reported information from healthcare interactions [23]. It is debatable if reports by proxies, such as caregivers and family members, are considered PRO [13, 20, 23]. Table 39.1 displays the major PRO domains, reflecting the constructs measured, and gives examples of validated tools (questionnaires) utilized at the patient care level.

PRO questionnaires can be generic, disease-specific, or condition-specific. Generic questionnaires are designed for use with any patient population and they address general measures of heath, well-being, and social function [20]. Disease-specific questionnaires assess severity, symptoms, or functional limitations that pertain to a particular disease or diagnostic grouping, such as rheumatoid arthritis or diabetes. Condition-specific questionnaires capture patient symptoms or experiences related to a single condition (e.g., low back pain) or intervention, such as coronary artery bypass surgery.

Table 39.1 Patient-reported outcome domains

Domain	Relevance	Example PRO questionnaires
Symptoms	Quantify and assess impact of symptoms	Patient Health Questionnaire 9 (PHQ-9) General Anxiety Disorder 7-item (GAD-7) [142] Brief Pain Inventory (BPI) [144] The Distress Thermometer [145] Edmonton Symptom Assessment System [140]
Functional status	Ability to engage in activities of daily living	Arthritis impact measurement scales [146] Hip Disability and Osteoarthritis Outcome Score - Physical function Short-form (HOOS-PS) [143]
Health-related quality of life	Impact of condition or treatment on usual or expected physical, emotional, and social well-being	Functional Assessment of Cancer Therapy (FACT) core plus symptom modules [45] European Organization for Research of Cancer Quality of Life Questionnaire Core-30 plus symptom modules [20]
Non-preference	Evaluate functioning relative to minimal and maximal levels of performance for each concept; can be used with any group of individuals	36-item Short Form Survey (SF-36) [17] Patient-Reported Outcomes Measurement Information System (PROMIS) Global Health Short Form [141]
Preference	Assign a relative value or utility to levels of health based on patient preferences	EuroQoL (EQ-5D) [21] Health Utility Index (HUI) [22] Quality of Well-Being scale [23]
Satisfaction with care	Assess satisfaction with received care	Consumer Assessment of Health Plans Surveys (CAHPS) [26]

Modified from: Ahmed S, Berzon RA, Revicki DA, Lenderking WR, Moinpour CM, Basch E et al. The use of patient-reported outcomes (PRO) within comparative effectiveness research: implications for clinical practice and health care policy. Medical care. 2012;50(12):1060–70. doi:10.1097/MLR.0b013e318268aaff

Patient-reported outcomes that are assessed systematically with standardized questionnaires have three key features. They are patient-centric because they capture information that most patients consider important; they are outcomes-oriented, as opposed to assessing processes of care such as screening rates; and they are consistently measured over time, unlike descriptions of symptoms documented in patients' health records [13, 24]. For example, the Short Form (SF-36) Health Survey elicits physical function through questions anchored in activities of daily living, such as lifting heavy objects, climbing stairs and walking; these outcomes are contextualized by self-reported global function and perception of health [25].

Clinical Applications of Patient-Reported Outcomes

One theory-driven taxonomy developed by Greenhalgh describes six applications of PRO in clinical practice and provides evidence of their impact on the processes and outcomes of care [26]. The taxonomy describes applications for two levels at which PRO data are aggregated—individual patients and populations of patients—and whether the application is implemented during patient-provider encounters (see Table 39.2) [27–30].

Individual Level PRO Data

Screening

Screening is a common PRO application, particularly in behavioral health, where it can be used to identify symptoms of depression, anxiety and, more broadly, to assess adverse effects to physical, social, and emotional functioning [31–35]. Validated tools like the Patient-Reported Outcomes Measurement Information System (PROMIS) Scale v1.2 Global Health (Fig. 39.1) elicit symptom self-report and can feasibly be embedded in primary and sub-specialty care workflows to improve detection of common but under-diagnosed conditions like depression [36]. One study reported that over 14% of patients had a positive depression screen, but only 30% of those had a documented mood disorder diagnosis [37, 38]. Primary care patients were 83% less likely to have a "missed" diagnosis with this screening approach, highlighting the importance of detection among patients outside of traditional behavioral health settings [37].

Table 39.2 Taxonomy of PRO applications in clinical practice

Purpose	Used at provider-patient interface	Description
PRO data aggregated at the level of individual patients		
Screening	Yes	Response to PRO measures help identify undetected problems or non-reported symptoms
Monitoring	Yes	Repeated PRO measurements help track progress over time, response to treatment, or both
Facilitating patient-centered care	Yes	Review of PRO data help prioritize patient-provider encounters to address issues and concerns important to the patient
Enabling patient engagement in self-care	No	Feeding back PRO data to the patient enables data-driven self-care management
Facilitating communication within care teams	No	Systematically collected PRO data provide a common language for providers to align patient goals with multidisciplinary team's care management strategies
PRO data aggregated at the level of populations		
Decision aids	Yes	Comparative studies of outcomes, including PROs, from various treatment options provide evidence informing and facilitating shared decision-making between patient and provider
Monitor and manage population health	No	Aggregated PRO data support monitoring and managing populations of patients with specific conditions
Assess and improve quality of care	No	Analyses of aggregated PRO data help identify quality improvement opportunities
Public reporting and pay for performance	No	Organization-level PRO data are reported to external agencies to meet regulatory requirements or for reimbursement or marketing purposes

Adapted from: Greenhalgh J. The applications of PROs in clinical practice: what are they, do they work, and why? *Quality of life research: an international journal of quality of life aspects of treatment, care and rehabilitation.* 2009;18(1):115–23. doi:10.1007/s11136-008-9430-6

Fig. 39.1 Patient Reported Outcomes Measurement Information System (PROMIS)® [141]

PROMIS® Scale v1.2 – Global Health

Global Health

Please respond to each question or statement by marking one box per row.

		Excellent	Very good	Good	Fair	Poor
Global01	In general, would you say your health is:	☐ 5	☐ 4	☐ 3	☐ 2	☐ 1
Global02	In general, would you say your quality of life is:	☐ 5	☐ 4	☐ 3	☐ 2	☐ 1
Global03	In general, how would you rate your physical health?	☐ 5	☐ 4	☐ 3	☐ 2	☐ 1
Global04	In general, how would you rate your mental health, including your mood and your ability to think?	☐ 5	☐ 4	☐ 3	☐ 2	☐ 1
Global05	In general, how would you rate your satisfaction with your social activities and relationships?	☐ 5	☐ 4	☐ 3	☐ 2	☐ 1
Global09r	In general, please rate how well you carry out your usual social activities and roles. (This includes activities at home, at work and in your community, and responsibilities as a parent, child, spouse, employee, friend, etc.)	☐ 5	☐ 4	☐ 3	☐ 2	☐ 1

		Completely	Mostly	Moderately	A little	Not at all
Global06	To what extent are you able to carry out your everyday physical activities such as walking, climbing stairs, carrying groceries, or moving a chair?	☐ 5	☐ 4	☐ 3	☐ 2	☐ 1

In the past 7 days...

		Never	Rarely	Sometimes	Often	Always
Global10r	How often have you been bothered by emotional problems such as feeling anxious, depressed or irritable?	☐ 5	☐ 4	☐ 3	☐ 2	☐ 1

		None	Mild	Moderate	Severe	Very severe
Global08r	How would you rate your fatigue on average?	☐ 5	☐ 4	☐ 3	☐ 2	☐ 1

Global07r	How would you rate your pain on average?	☐ 0 No pain	☐ 1	☐ 2	☐ 3	☐ 4	☐ 5	☐ 6	☐ 7	☐ 8	☐ 9	☐ 10 Worst pain imaginable

Treatment Monitoring

Monitoring is another widely used PRO application. The use of electronic patient-reported outcomes (ePROs) in cancer care can facilitate the timely identification and management of disease and treatment associated symptoms, improve patient satisfaction, quality of life, and even survival [39–41]. Patient reports of treatment side effects complement clinicians' assessment of health status to potentially reduce treatment interruption or discontinuation. For example, a single item from Functional Assessment of Cancer Therapy-General (FACT-G) (i.e., "I am bothered by side effects of treatment") has a significant association with the treating clinician's report of patient adverse effects and self-reported quality of life [42]. When used in pharmaceutical trials and clinical settings, this single item holds promise as an efficient summary measure that reflects the burden of treatment toxicity from the patient's perspective [24].

Facilitating Patient-Centered Care

Primary care clinicians face a myriad, and often unrealistic, set of diagnostic, treatment, and prevention responsibilities and tasks in their clinical workflows [43]. Established protocols, time constraints, quality indices, and organizational priorities direct clinician attention toward biophysical issues and metrics, such as hemoglobin A1c measures for patients with diabetes mellitus, while patients may have other impactful but unaddressed symptoms including disordered sleep, fatigue, and pain. PRO data can assist in identifying and measuring comorbid symptoms, facilitating patient-provider communication, and prioritizing the agenda for the clinical encounter. In this setting PRO data can also promote opportunities for patient activation and engagement, potentially improving adherence to treatment [44]. The SF-36, for example, globally assesses physical, social, and emotional well-being and functional status, and can be incorporated in preventive service planning to personalize priorities, identify goals of care and enhance the care experience [45, 46].

Enhancing Disease Self-Management

Disease self-management is a major component of chronic illness care. Nearly 90% of office-based physicians use electronic health records and more than 40% of households own wearable digital devices including smart watches and fitness trackers, which that have the capacity for data collection and integration [47]. The collection of PRO data with electronic (e.g., wearable) devices and integration into electronic health record (EHR) systems are technically feasible, and patients demonstrate willingness to share personal data [48–50]. In addition, third party payers have promoted PRO data collection through gamification and reward-based programs, such as tracking physical activity, to promote patient awareness of health behaviors [47]. Self-care and self-management applications that collect PROs are found in primary care, rheumatology, cardiology, and post-operative recovery areas [27, 51, 52]. Improved user interfaces and data visualization have increased the accessibility of these applications for a broader audience to engage in self-monitoring and advancing health goals.

The American College of Rheumatology and the European League Against Rheumatism have identified disease activity and health-related quality of life (as measured by SF-36, EQ-5D) as treatment targets, requiring data monitoring tools that can record PROs over time and across primary care and subspecialty settings [53–55]. For example, a smart phone application with a Disease Activity Score (DAS-28) predictive model was concordant with physician assessments in identifying disease severity [53]. During the COVID-19 pandemic, ePROs enabled remote assessment through self-report, a critical adaptation for patients at risk for severe illness due to comorbid chronic illness, or those receiving immunosuppressive treatment [56, 57]. The use of algorithms to triage symptoms and guide treatment is another effective use of PROs and has the potential to integrate with machine-learning programs that can guide individual level or population-level decision-making for care [58, 59].

Facilitating Communication in Multidisciplinary Care Teams

Patients with chronic conditions often receive care from a multidisciplinary team. PRO measures have been advocated as a shared communication platform for multidisciplinary healthcare providers [26, 60]. Data from PRO questionnaires can provide a common platform for collaboratively setting goals with patients, and an approach to gauge treatment effectiveness. Post-stroke care, for example, involves a team including neurologists, primary care providers, physical therapists, speech therapists, social workers, and occupational therapists, who have different scopes of care, responsibilities, and workflow. The Stroke Impact Scale is a PRO tool that can capture important aspects of post-stroke recovery and helps multidisciplinary team members communicate effectively in assessing the patient's health, function, and well-being [61]. In a similar fashion, multidisciplinary teams providing advanced heart failure therapy have used PRO data as the shared communication platform to optimize care [62].

Population-Level PRO Data

Assisting in Decision-Making

Patient-reported outcomes are increasingly used in comparative effectiveness research to assess the impact of treatments on outcomes that are centered on patient preferences and values [29]. In surgical care, pain and functional status outcomes can help patients and providers make informed choices about treatment timing, selection, and adjustment, including decisions about surgery [47, 63, 64]. Population-level normative PRO data can clarify treatment risks and benefits in terms of outcomes such as HRQoL, and the probability that a treatment will deliver patient-preferred outcomes, based on his or her clinical profile. Decision aids incorporating PRO data help engage patients in shared decision-making and improve adherence and self-care by outlining treatment options in terms of outcomes that are most important. This approach can help patients set realistic expectations about treatment effectiveness and post-operative recovery through normative data, [27] a strategy that can improves their health and satisfaction and reduce healthcare costs [63].

Managing Population Health

PRO data at the population level can optimize utilization, inform clinical processes, and establish normative data for patient groups with similar conditions or treatment programs. The AmbuFlex system in Denmark is an example of a program that has effectively collected and managed PRO data in to improving outcomes and cost-effectiveness of care [65]. Fixed interval and patient-initiated telePRO have been used to support self-care, improve quality of care, and reduce utilization in several areas including epilepsy, inflammatory bowel disease and rheumatoid arthritis [65]. Trended over time, aggregate PRO data can also profile the needs of a patient population to guide resource allocations [65–67].

Improving Quality of Care

PRO data collected from individual patients can be aggregated and used to improve the quality of care [68]. At the provider level, academic detailing via sharing successful clinical practices can lead to better outcomes; at the practice level, a quality improvement infrastructure using plan-do-study-act (PDSA) cycles can contextualize currently measured outcomes by correlation with PROs; at the organizational level, data from PRO measures help monitor performance, identify best practices to spread, and direct resources for performance improvement [48]. Using PRO data as part of performance assessment and improvement, coupled with dedicated quality improvement resources, increases the likelihood of improving outcomes [29]. For example, in combination with other HRQoL measures, pain scores can guide the design, implementation, and monitoring of quality improvement efforts to improve the management of pain that affects patients' function, guiding management, resource allocation, and informing program goals [39, 66, 67, 69, 70].

Developmental Milestones in Patient-Reported Outcomes

The conceptual history of PROs can be traced to Donabedian's structure-process-outcome model [71]. Structural attributes of the context in which care occurs, processes of care, and care outcomes are inter-related dimensions by which healthcare quality can be assessed [71, 72]. In this model, outcomes are the effects of healthcare on patients and populations; examples include changes in intermediate outcomes (e.g., blood pressure), adverse events, morbidity, survival, recovery and restoration, and improvements in function and HRQoL. Development, validation, and application of PRO questionnaires and measurement approaches began in the 1940s and by the end of the 1990s, the number of available PRO questionnaires had significantly increased and several key generic measures were developed [73, 74].

The multi-dimensional Medical Outcome Study Short Form (SF-36) Health Survey was developed based on the World Health Organization (WHO) definition of health as a generic measure of HRQoL [46]. Similarly, EuroQol (EQ-5D) was developed through collaboration among five European Union countries to assess key areas including mental health, mobility, activities of daily living (ADLs), self-care, and pain [55]. In the US, PROMIS was developed as part of an initiative funded by the National Institutes of Health as a repository for publicly available PRO questionnaires incorporating computer adaptive testing (CAT) to customize questionnaires as part of the data collection process [75].

The transition from paper-based to electronic health records and the movement to digital health created tremendous opportunity for web-enabled and device-driven PRO data collection [76, 77]. Digital health enables remote electronic assessment of self-reported symptoms, physical function and well-being [78–80]. PRO data can be integrated into clinical decision support and archived for research and analysis, maximizing its applications [81, 82]. Electronic PROMs (ePROMS) offer several advantages in survey completion and data collection time, total program cost and data quality [83–86]. EPROM design can also leverage CAT to further increase efficiency and decrease time burden by selectively queuing questions based on a patients prior responses [87–90].

The proliferation of PRO questionnaires has led a greater integration into research studies. A 2021 comprehensive review of randomized controlled trials funded by the United Kingdom's National Institute for Health Research Programme between 1997 and 2020 reported that 38% of trials used PROs as primary outcomes and 83% used PROs as secondary outcomes with one of the most common tools being the SF-36 [91]. Both the FDA and European Medicines

Agency promote PRO use in guidelines for the approval of pharmacological products and medical devices [12, 92]. For example, a growing number of cancer treatment studies have incorporated PROs to assess symptoms, adverse events, and toxicity in the design of clinical trials and in implementation studies [93–95]. Comparative effectiveness research including PROs has also increased considerably [92, 96, 97]. In addition, PROs are now part of the predictive modeling to forecast resource utilization and post-treatment outcomes, such as total joint arthroplasty [39, 98, 99].

The involvement of patients in the research development of questionnaires continues to expand since providers and researchers cannot authentically represent patients' perspectives and preferences. The active solicitation of patient input during PRO development and implementation in routine practice and clinical trials have become more widely promoted [85, 100]. There is greater awareness that patient-centered care and, by extension, patient-centered research and redesign can benefit from patient partnership. In this paradigm, patients collaborate with researchers to inform research questions and the methods by which they are asked, selecting outcomes that matter, interpreting results, and applying findings [101–103].

In clinical settings, a key development of PRO data has been recognition of technical and ancillary support for integration. There are multiple entry points for PRO data and potential digital outputs that support an array of healthcare delivery system functions and responsibilities (Fig. 39.2) [48]. These include opportunities to report out aggregate data on real-world patient experiences from clinical and research settings, to provide benchmarks for quality of care, to generate feedback for system improvement and to communicate across care settings. Implementation design must address efficient input, timely and accessible outputs and coordination across data collection and interpretation settings [48, 104].

Evidence Base of Patient-Reported Outcomes

The evidence base on the impact of PRO on care processes and outcomes has been mixed due to variability in implementation and methodological issues [24, 104–114]. Although recent analyses report trends of small to moderate improvements in specific outcomes that reflect new developments in PRO use and implementation, the body of evidence regarding implementation and outcomes is still limited and of mixed quality [69, 104, 110, 111]. For example, a review of 116 randomized trials studying the impact of PROM feedback in primary and secondary care settings found moderate evidence for improved quality of life, increased patient-physician communication, diagnosis and notation, and disease control. However, there was minimal difference in general health perceptions, social function and pain, and the effects on physical and mental functioning were uncertain due to low certainty of evidence [104].

A systematic review of 17 studies involving nearly 9000 patients found no evidence to support that routine measurement and feedback using PROMs improves outcomes among patients with common mental health conditions; however, a key limitation was quality and heterogeneity of existing studies [114]. Another systematic review investigating the effect of providing PRO data at the patient and group levels reported weak evidence supporting its use as a screening tool. Studies showing the greatest effect used PRO data as a management tool in outpatient care for specific patient populations [39]. PRO data, when used in isolation,

Fig. 39.2 Illustration of integrated approach of PROMs to meet multiple stakeholder needs. The future of PROMs is in developing an integrated approach to data collection and dissemination that serves the needs of multiple stakeholders, but primarily the patient. Adapted from *Maximising the impact of patient reported outcome assessment for patients and society* (Calvert 2019)

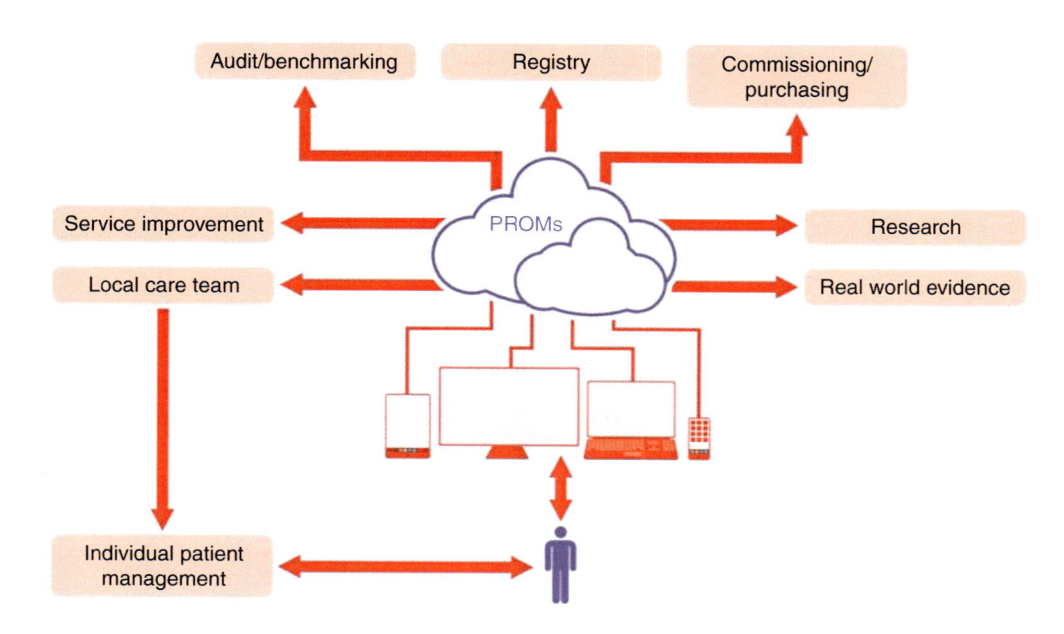

may have a limited effect on outcomes and effective use may be seen part of a comprehensive system of care and follow up.

Santana and Feeny (2014) posit in their conceptual model that the use of PRO improves communication among patients, multidisciplinary providers, and caregivers. Better communication facilitates identifying important issues, patient preferences, and treatment goals, empowering patients to co-create care plans and manage self-care and enhancing shared decision-making. These effects collectively contribute to better outcomes, although the model does not explain how they relate to each other and the relative contribution of each to improved patient outcomes.

Despite heterogeneity in studies about the impact of PROs, it suggests that they do add value to the care of patients with cancer, HIV, arthritis, depression, gastrointestinal disorders, and depression [3]. For example, the Orchestra Project, an innovative approach in which patients and providers partner to manage inflammatory bowel disease, provides evidence that patient outcomes improve when PRO data are used to facilitate ongoing patient-provider learning, shared decision-making, and goal setting and to support patient behavioral change and care management. Disease remission rates increased from 60 to 79% among patients treated at more than 70 pediatric gastroenterology care centers in the ImproveCareNow network [115].

Patient-Reported Outcomes in Chronic Illness Care

Denmark and Sweden have incorporated PRO for individual care and population health into national clinical registries since about 2000 [65, 116, 117]. Central Denmark has programs that leverage ePRO to support clinical decision-making and efficient resource use for patients with chronic conditions at the individual and population level across the region [58]. WestChronic is the supporting system for more than 20 projects across 18 patient groups in a mixed-mode PRO data collection and processing system. The system supports point of care and remote data collection and application using outputs such as on-demand PRO questionnaire distributions to patient groups or tabulations of PRO datasets for research and clinical teams. Key output functions include: (1) data visualizations to support point of care clinical decision-making (2) protocols for automated decision algorithms that compare PRO with normative or historical data, and (3) data sharing to facilitate communication across clinical teams, including teams that did not originate the assessment. The AmbuFlex project, an initiative of ePRO implementation with the WestChronic system, has improved clinical care and resource efficiency for the longitudinal care of patients with chronic conditions [58].

Another AmbuFlex project among patients with epilepsy employed pre-visit questionnaires at preset intervals to assess for symptomatology. This project employed automatic handling to stratify patients by symptoms into three categories—red, yellow, or green. Patients were assigned red status if they had symptoms that prompted assessment, and therefore were automatically scheduled; green status patients had no concerning symptoms and were not scheduled a visit; patients with yellow status were routed for clinician review with decision support [58]. This reduced the need for unnecessary visits and expedited triage and care of patients with potentially concerning symptoms [58].

The Swedish National Quality Registries (NQR) for patient care, quality improvement and research incorporates generic and disease-specific PRO data that can be accessed across healthcare settings [117]. Additionally, annual reporting and feedback on these data from an oversight committee is required for certification to support quality improvement at a systems level. The Swedish NQR has informed perioperative care across several domains including: the Swedish Hip Arthroplasty Register which uses PRO data to adapt pre/post-operative care information for patients with lower educational levels; the Swedish Hernia Register for undetected post-operative patient concerns and as a guide peri-operative counseling; the Swedish National Cataract Register to assess of patient candidacy for surgery. For stroke care, Riksstroke has years of PRO data focusing on patient's perceptions of rehabilitation and return to daily function that guide quality improvement for comprehensive services including community support [117].

Challenges in Using Patient-Reported Outcomes

The challenges associated with collecting and using PRO data in routine clinical practice are well-documented and impact providers, patients, and healthcare systems [118–121]. Providers express concerns that PRO may not significantly improve care outcomes and may increase, not decrease, their workload [52]. In some studies, providers express concerns about the reliability and validity of information that is self-reported by patients [3, 122]. PRO measures are not generalizable across all clinical areas and there are limited comprehensive and clinically relevant measures for geriatrics, palliative care, and complex care [123]. Physicians and other providers may find it challenging to interpret and act on PRO data. For many existing PRO measures, there is limited normative data to help providers identify whether and by how much a patient's reported value is outside of normal limits [123]. Finally, current PRO measures are not always reported in a clinically relevant manner to enhance clinical decision-making or trigger clinical actions [37, 123, 124].

For patients, the burden of completing PRO questionnaires may be excessive due to survey length, functional limitations, and literacy. Patient with limited vision may require questionnaires with larger text. Health literacy impacts patients' ability to complete PRO questionnaires and validated translations may not be available for patients who cannot read English [37, 123]. Considerations of gender identity and sexual orientation are not widely incorporated in the language used in many tools. Most importantly, patients want to understand how the information they provide is used for their benefit and are reluctant to complete PRO questionnaires if unclear [37, 122].

Healthcare organizations may lack incentives or regulatory requirements to systematically collect and use PRO data if the value proposition for use is lacking. The effective integration of PRO into clinical workflows requires several steps: generating buy-in from stakeholders; demonstrating feasibility and value to end users, and; putting infrastructure and processes in place to support workflow integration [48, 125–127]. The latter often includes information technology, building time into clinical workflows for collecting PRO data, using data for shared decision-making discussions and clinical decision-making, and documenting clinical actions related to PRO data [29, 37, 122]. Additionally, the application of PRO data for quality improvement is influenced by patient and facility-level factors, creating potential for misattribution of outcomes to the individual source of clinical practice [24]. Other barriers to the organizational uptake of PROs may include licensure, registration, and associated costs for proprietary instruments (e.g., the EQ-5D FACT) [29, 45, 122].

Future Directions

There are several trends that will inform the future of patient-reported outcomes.

The first reflects increasing efforts across governmental and non-governmental entities to support broader meaningful use of PRO measures. The Center for Medicare and Medicaid Innovation is responsible for innovating payment and healthcare delivery models to improve outcomes supported by $10 billion in funding during its first decade and a renewal for the subsequent one, positioning it to be a primary sponsor for care delivery and payment model innovations that incorporate PROs [128]. Models that have utilized PROs include the Oncology Care Model and the Comprehensive Care for Joint Replacement Model, which includes voluntary reporting of generic and procedure-specific PRO data that link the quality of total hip and knee arthroplasty procedures to hospital payments [129–132]. The Medicare Health Outcomes Survey also collects PROs as a measure of health plan performance among its Medicare Advantage participants, allowing beneficiaries to compare plans by reported functional outcomes [133].

Several non-governmental organizations contribute to the meaningful use of PROs in health care. The National Quality Forum and the National Committee on Quality Assurance endorse PRO measures in their performance measurement sets [46, 122]. The International Consortium for Health Outcomes Measurement, a non-profit advocacy organization, routinely includes PRO measures in recommended standard measurement sets; the standard set for primary and preventive care for older persons includes four PRO measures [102]. An international group of stakeholders outlined several areas of development for future PRO data use in value-based healthcare payment reform: (1) taking intended context of use, patient population, and purpose for collecting data into account when selecting the correct PROM; (2) reducing patient burden and clinician fatigue by standardizing measures to be parsimonious and efficient across settings; (3) addressing the operational data issues, culture change, and financial investments to enable successful PROM implementation and system-level integration; and (4) expanding the potential use of PRO data to monitor and compare provider performance to processes and structural improvements related to healthcare quality [134].

Increased user testing and post-pilot assessments will be needed to ensure that PRO data has value for all users, including providers, patients, caregivers, department administrators, and healthcare executives. Key features of PRO questionnaires that need to be assessed include feasibility, usability, and acceptability. Feasibility refers to how readily a questionnaire can be incorporated into existing clinical workflows [135]. Usability refers to the extent to which an intended user can use the resulting PRO data effectively and satisfactorily to support identified use cases [136]. Acceptability is a function of a questionnaire's perceived accuracy and reliability [74]. Other important factors affecting the implementation of PRO questionnaires in clinical practice are the required level of health literacy and optimal modalities (paper or electronic) for data collection. A typical PRO questionnaire includes 20 or more questions [123], and the feasibility and intended applications of lengthy questionnaires must be established before they are broadly implemented. In addition to the burden they pose to respondents, long questionnaires can overwhelm providers with patient-reported data if they lack specific guidelines for using them.

An important trend will focus on how the integration of PRO questionnaires from research into routine care is considered from the patient perspective. Several issues need to be addressed [122], including the value of using multiple questionnaires and of how much PRO data is required to understand patients' experiences and needs. Patients will become increasingly involved in PRO design and selection. The International Consortium for Health Outcomes

Measurement solicits patients' input on key outcome measures, including PRO, when developing condition-specific standard measurement sets [123]. The PCORI solicits stakeholder input to ensure patient-centeredness in development of research proposals and funding review [101].

Individual patients have a rapidly expanding ability to monitor the outcomes that are most important to them by using devices that track data like caloric intake, daily steps, and sleep patterns. The "democratization of metrics" is modifying patients' expectations about how the effectiveness of healthcare should be assessed. Although the use of standardized PRO measures is a large step in the right direction, providers must also know which outcomes are most important to the patient sitting in the examination room. Many PRO questionnaires are in routine use in clinical practice [122] and as new PRO questionnaires spread from research to clinical settings, the number and complexity of questionnaires that patients, particularly those with multiple conditions, are asked to complete will likely grow. The sustainability of using PRO data as intended will need to be examined and may depend on the value added from the data [137].

The final trend will focus on population-level PRO data that will be used for broad population health improvement. The ongoing movement to more inclusive views of health is embracing broader determinants of health [138]. This shift is exemplified by the IHI 100 Million Healthier Lives initiative, a cross-sectoral collaboration aimed at achieving global health, well-being, and equity [139].

In summary, PRO data has the potential to help healthcare systems align with patient goals for health and quality of life. The advent of digital data collection, analysis and dissemination has transformed the application of PRO across healthcare settings to serve individual and population care needs, creating a common thread of patient centeredness. Most importantly, PRO data provide a common language to organize efforts to improve healthcare-related quality of life. It matters to patients that we ask about their experiences; it matters even more that we use what they tell us to improve their health and well-being.

References

1. Institute of Medicine (US) Committee on Quality of Health Care in America. Improving the 21st-century Health Care System—Crossing the Quality Chasm—NCBI Bookshelf. 2001.
2. Schottenfeld L, Petersen D, Peikes D, Ricciardi R, Burak H, McNellis R, et al. Creating patient-centered team-based primary care. AHRQ Pub. 2016;16(0002-EF). https://www.ahrq.gov/sites/default/files/wysiwyg/ncepcr/tools/PCMH/creating-patient-centered-team-based-primary-care-white-paper.pdf.
3. Lavallee DC, Chenok KE, Love RM, Petersen C, Holve E, Segal CD, et al. Incorporating patient-reported outcomes into health care to engage patients and enhance care. Health Aff (Millwood). 2016;35(4):575–82.
4. Constand MK, MacDermid JC, Dal Bello-Haas V, Law M. Scoping review of patient-centered care approaches in healthcare. BMC Health Serv Res. 2014;14:271.
5. Noonan VK, Lyddiatt A, Ware P, Jaglal SB, Riopelle RJ, Bingham CO, et al. Montreal Accord on Patient-Reported Outcomes (PROs) use series—Paper 3: patient-reported outcomes can facilitate shared decision-making and guide self-management. J Clin Epidemiol. 2017;89:125–35.
6. Dinh-Le C, Chuang R, Chokshi S, Mann D. Wearable health technology and electronic health record integration: scoping review and future directions. JMIR Mhealth Uhealth. 2019;7(9):e12861.
7. Rising CJ, Gaysynsky A, Blake KD, Jensen RE, Oh A. Willingness to share data from wearable health and activity trackers: analysis of the 2019 health information national trends survey data. JMIR Mhealth Uhealth. 2021;9(12):e29190.
8. Bernstein DN, Leonard MS, Hasselberg MJ, Apostolakos MJ, Baumhauer JF. It took a global pandemic to demonstrate the value of using technology to routinely collect and use patient-reported outcomes. J Patient Exp. 2021;8:23743735211054936.
9. Rapid Implementation of an Outpatient Covid-19 Monitoring Program | Catalyst non-issue content. NEJM Catalyst Innovations in Care Delivery.
10. Chevallard M, Belloli L, Ughi N, Adinolfi A, Casu C, Di Cicco M, et al. Use of telemedicine during the COVID-19 pandemic in patients with inflammatory arthritis: a retrospective study on feasibility and impact on patient-reported outcomes in a real-life setting. Rheumatol Int. 2021;41(7):1253–61.
11. Rando HM, Bennett TD, Byrd JB, Bramante C, Callahan TJ, Chute CG, et al. Challenges in defining Long COVID: striking differences across literature, Electronic Health Records, and patient-reported information. medRxiv. 2021.
12. U.S. Department of Health and Human Services FDA Center for Drug Evaluation and Research. Guidance for industry: patient-reported outcome measures: use in medical product development to support labeling claims. Health Qual Life Outcomes. 2009;4:79.
13. NQF: Patient-Reported Outcomes in Performance Measurement. 2022. https://www.qualityforum.org/publications/2012/12/patient-reported_outcomes_in_performance_measurement.aspx.
14. Gutteling JJ, Darlington A-SE, Janssen HLA, Duivenvoorden HJ, Busschbach JJV, de Man RA. Effectiveness of health-related quality-of-life measurement in clinical practice: a prospective, randomized controlled trial in patients with chronic liver disease and their physicians. Qual Life Res. 2008;17(2):195–205.
15. de Wit M, Delemarre-van de Waal HA, Bokma JA, Haasnoot K, Houdijk MC, Gemke RJ, et al. Monitoring and discussing health-related quality of life in adolescents with type 1 diabetes improve psychosocial well-being: a randomized controlled trial. Diabetes Care. 2008;31(8):1521–6.
16. Bingham CO, Noonan VK, Auger C, Feldman DE, Ahmed S, Bartlett SJ. Montreal Accord on Patient-Reported Outcomes (PROs) use series—Paper 4: patient-reported outcomes can inform clinical decision making in chronic care. J Clin Epidemiol. 2017;89:136–41.
17. Griffin SJ, Kinmonth A-L, Veltman MWM, Gillard S, Grant J, Stewart M. Effect on health-related outcomes of interventions to alter the interaction between patients and practitioners: a systematic review of trials. Ann Fam Med. 2004;2(6):595–608.
18. Velikova G, Booth L, Smith AB, Brown PM, Lynch P, Brown JM, et al. Measuring quality of life in routine oncology practice improves communication and patient well-being: a randomized controlled trial. J Clin Oncol. 2004;22(4):714–24.
19. Chapter 18: Patient-reported outcomes | Cochrane Training. 2021. https://training.cochrane.org/handbook/current/chapter-18.

20. Higgins JPT, Thomas J, Chandler J, Cumpston M, Li T, Page MJ, et al., editors. Cochrane handbook for systematic reviews of interventions. Wiley; 2019.
21. Patient-Reported Outcome Measures: Use in Medical Product Development to Support Labeling Claims | FDA. 2022. https://www.fda.gov/regulatory-information/search-fda-guidance-documents/patient-reported-outcome-measures-use-medical-product-development-support-labeling-claims.
22. Keller S, Dy S, Wilson R, Dukhanin V, Snyder C, Wu A. Selecting patient-reported outcome measures to contribute to primary care performance measurement: a mixed methods approach. J Gen Intern Med. 2020;35(9):2687–97.
23. Klose K, Kreimeier S, Tangermann U, Aumann I, Damm K, RHO Group. Patient- and person-reports on healthcare: preferences, outcomes, experiences, and satisfaction—an essay. Health Econ Rev. 2016;6(1):18.
24. Greenhalgh J, Dalkin S, Gibbons E, Wright J, Valderas JM, Meads D, et al. How do aggregated patient-reported outcome measures data stimulate health care improvement? A realist synthesis. J Health Serv Res Policy. 2018;23(1):57–65.
25. 36-Item Short Form Survey Instrument (SF-36) | RAND. 2022. https://www.rand.org/health-care/surveys_tools/mos/36-item-short-form/survey-instrument.html.
26. Greenhalgh J. The applications of PROs in clinical practice: what are they, do they work, and why? Qual Life Res. 2009;18(1):115–23.
27. Bingham CO, Bartlett SJ, Merkel PA, Mielenz TJ, Pilkonis PA, Edmundson L, et al. Using patient-reported outcomes and PROMIS in research and clinical applications: experiences from the PCORI pilot projects. Qual Life Res. 2016;25(8):2109–16.
28. Higginson IJ, Carr AJ. Measuring quality of life: using quality of life measures in the clinical setting. BMJ. 2001;322(7297):1297–300.
29. Wu A. [PDF] Advances in the Use of Patient Reported Outcome Measures in | Semantic Scholar. undefined. 2013.
30. Aaronson N, Elliott TE, Greenhalgh J, Halyard M, Hess R, Miller DM, et al. User's guide to implementing patient-reported outcomes assessment in clinical practice. Undefined. 2016.
31. Gilbody SM, Whitty PM, Grimshaw JM, Thomas RE. Improving the detection and management of depression in primary care. Qual Saf Health Care. 2003;12(2):149–55.
32. Dowrick C. Does testing for depression influence diagnosis or management by general practitioners? Fam Pract. 1995;12(4):461–5.
33. Mazonson PD, Mathias SD, Fifer SK, Buesching DP, Malek P, Patrick DL. The mental health patient profile: does it change primary care physicians' practice patterns? J Am Board Fam Pract. 1996;9(5):336–45.
34. Rubenstein LV, McCoy JM, Cope DW, Barrett PA, Hirsch SH, Messer KS, et al. Improving patient quality of life with feedback to physicians about functional status. J Gen Intern Med. 1995;10(11):607–14.
35. Rubenstein LV, Calkins DR, Young RT, Cleary PD, Fink A, Kosecoff J, et al. Improving patient function: a randomized trial of functional disability screening. Ann Intern Med. 1989;111(10):836–42.
36. Hays RD, Bjorner JB, Revicki DA, Spritzer KL, Cella D. Development of physical and mental health summary scores from the patient-reported outcomes measurement information system (PROMIS) global items. Qual Life Res. 2009;18(7):873–80.
37. Rose M, Bezjak A. Logistics of collecting patient-reported outcomes (PROs) in clinical practice: an overview and practical examples. Qual Life Res. 2009;18(1):125–36.
38. Van Orden KA, Lutz J, Conner KR, Silva C, Hasselberg MJ, Fear K, et al. URMC universal depression screening initiative: patient reported outcome assessments to promote a person-centered biopsychosocial population health management strategy. Front Psych. 2021;12:796499.
39. Snyder C, Hannum SM, White S, Montanari A, Ikejiani D, Smith B, et al. A PRO-cision medicine intervention to personalize cancer care using patient-reported outcomes: intervention development and feasibility-testing. Qual Life Res. 2022;31(8):2341–55.
40. Basch E, Deal AM, Dueck AC, Scher HI, Kris MG, Hudis C, et al. Overall survival results of a trial assessing patient-reported outcomes for symptom monitoring during routine cancer treatment. JAMA. 2017;318(2):197–8.
41. Lizée T, Basch E, Trémolières P, Voog E, Domont J, Peyraga G, et al. Cost-effectiveness of web-based patient-reported outcome surveillance in patients with lung cancer. J Thorac Oncol. 2019;14(6):1012–20.
42. Dharma-Wardene M, Au HJ, Hanson J, Dupere D, Hewitt J, Feeny D. Baseline FACT-G score is a predictor of survival for advanced lung cancer. Qual Life Res. 2004;13(7):1209–16.
43. Bodenheimer T. Primary care—will it survive? N Engl J Med. 2006;355(9):861–4.
44. Ling BS, Klein WM, Dang Q. Relationship of communication and information measures to colorectal cancer screening utilization: results from HINTS. J Health Commun. 2006;11(Suppl 1):181–90.
45. Cella DF, Tulsky DS, Gray G, Sarafian B, Linn E, Bonomi A, et al. The Functional Assessment of Cancer Therapy scale: development and validation of the general measure. J Clin Oncol. 1993;11(3):570–9.
46. Ware JE, Sherbourne CD. The MOS 36-item short-form health survey (SF-36). I. Conceptual framework and item selection. Med Care. 1992;30(6):473–83.
47. Tew M, Dalziel K, Clarke P, Smith A, Choong PF, Dowsey M. Patient-reported outcome measures (PROMs): can they be used to guide patient-centered care and optimize outcomes in total knee replacement? Qual Life Res. 2020;29(12):3273–83.
48. Calvert M, Kyte D, Price G, Valderas JM, Hjollund NH. Maximising the impact of patient reported outcome assessment for patients and society. BMJ. 2019;364:k5267.
49. Tessa Richards: Power to the people—via Paris—The BMJ. 2022. https://blogs-bmj-com.libproxy.lib.unc.edu/bmj/2017/01/20/tessa-richards-power-to-the-people-via-paris/.
50. OECD High-level reflection group on health statistics (July 2017). Recommendations to OECD Ministers from the high-level reflection group on the future of health statistics: Strengthening the international comparison of health system performance through patient-reported indicators. https://www-oecd-org.libproxy.lib.unc.edu/health/paris/. Accessed April 13, 2023.
51. Chiauzzi E, Rodarte C, DasMahapatra P. Patient-centered activity monitoring in the self-management of chronic health conditions. BMC Med. 2015;13:77.
52. Nelson EC, Eftimovska E, Lind C, Hager A, Wasson JH, Lindblad S. Patient reported outcome measures in practice. BMJ. 2015;350:g7818.
53. Shelton J, Casey S, Puhl N, Buckingham J, Yacyshyn E. Electronic patient-reported outcome measures using mobile health technology in rheumatology: a scoping review. PLoS One. 2021;16(7):e0253615.
54. Lopez-Olivo MA, Zogala RJ, Des Bordes J, Zamora NV, Christensen R, Rai D, et al. Outcomes reported in prospective long-term observational studies and registries of patients with rheumatoid arthritis worldwide: an outcome measures in rheumatology systematic review. Arthritis Care Res (Hoboken). 2021;73(5):649–57.
55. Hurst NP, Kind P, Ruta D, Hunter M, Stubbings A. Measuring health-related quality of life in rheumatoid arthritis: valid-

ity, responsiveness and reliability of EuroQol (EQ-5D). Br J Rheumatol. 1997;36(5):551–9.
56. Patient-Reported Indicator Surveys (PaRIS)—OECD. 2022. https://www-oecd-org.libproxy.lib.unc.edu/health/paris/.
57. Kendir, C., et al. "All hands on deck: Co-developing the first international survey of people living with chronic conditions: Stakeholder engagement in the design, development, and field trial implementation of the PaRIS survey", OECD Health Working Papers, No. 149, OECD Publishing, Paris. 2023. https://doi.org/10.1787/8b31022e-en.
58. Hjollund NHI, Larsen LP, Biering K, Johnsen SP, Riiskjær E, Schougaard LM. Use of Patient-Reported Outcome (PRO) measures at group and patient levels: experiences from the generic integrated PRO system, West Chronic. Interact J Med Res. 2014;3(1):e5.
59. Verma D, Bach K, Mork PJ. Application of machine learning methods on patient reported outcome measurements for predicting outcomes: a literature review. Informatics. 2021;8(3):56.
60. Wressle E, Lindstrand J, Neher M, Marcusson J, Henriksson C. The Canadian Occupational Performance Measure as an outcome measure and team tool in a day treatment programme. Disabil Rehabil. 2003;25(10):497–506.
61. Richardson M, Campbell N, Allen L, Meyer M, Teasell R. The stroke impact scale: performance as a quality of life measure in a community-based stroke rehabilitation setting. Disabil Rehabil. 2016;38(14):1425–30.
62. Cedars AM. In heart failure, where you have been may be more important than where you are: a role for patient-reported outcomes. Am J Cardiol. 2017;119(5):813–5.
63. Ayers DC, Li W, Harrold L, Allison J, Franklin PD. Preoperative pain and function profiles reflect consistent TKA patient selection among US surgeons. Clin Orthop Relat Res. 2015;473(1):76–81.
64. Ayers DC, Zheng H, Franklin PD. Integrating patient-reported outcomes into orthopaedic clinical practice: proof of concept from FORCE-TJR. Clin Orthop Relat Res. 2013;471(11):3419–25.
65. Schougaard LMV, Larsen LP, Jessen A, Sidenius P, Dorflinger L, de Thurah A, et al. AmbuFlex: tele-patient-reported outcomes (telePRO) as the basis for follow-up in chronic and malignant diseases. Qual Life Res. 2016;25(3):525–34.
66. Pappot H, Baeksted CW, Nissen A, Knoop A, Mitchell SA, Christensen J, et al. Clinical effects of assessing electronic patient-reported outcomes monitoring symptomatic toxicities during breast cancer therapy: a nationwide and population-based study. Breast Cancer. 2021;28(5):1096–9.
67. Grusdat NP, Stäuber A, Tolkmitt M, Schnabel J, Schubotz B, Wright PR, et al. Cancer treatment regimens and their impact on the patient-reported outcome measures health-related quality of life and perceived cognitive function. J Patient Rep Outcomes. 2022;6(1):16.
68. Snyder CF, Jensen RE, Segal JB, Wu AW. Patient-reported outcomes (PROs): putting the patient perspective in patient-centered outcomes research. Med Care. 2013;51(8 Suppl 3):S73–9.
69. Boehnke JR, Rutherford C. Using feedback tools to enhance the quality and experience of care. Qual Life Res. 2021;30(11):3007–13.
70. Øvretveit J, Zubkoff L, Nelson EC, Frampton S, Knudsen JL, Zimlichman E. Using patient-reported outcome measurement to improve patient care. Int J Qual Health Care. 2017;29(6):874–9.
71. Ayanian JZ, Markel H. Donabedian's lasting framework for health care quality. N Engl J Med. 2016;375(3):205–7.
72. Donabedian A. Evaluating the quality of medical care. Milbank Q. 2005;83(4):691–729.
73. McHorney CA. Health status assessment methods for adults: past accomplishments and future challenges. Annu Rev Public Health. 1999;20:309–35.
74. Greenhalgh J, Meadows K. The effectiveness of the use of patient-based measures of health in routine practice in improving the process and outcomes of patient care: a literature review. J Eval Clin Pract. 1999;5(4):401–16.
75. Riedl D, Rothmund M, Darlington A-S, Sodergren S, Crazzolara R, de Rojas T, et al. Rare use of patient-reported outcomes in childhood cancer clinical trials—a systematic review of clinical trial registries. Eur J Cancer. 2021;152:90–9.
76. Eriksen J, Bertelsen P, Bygholm A. The Digital Transformation of Patient-Reported Outcomes' (PROs) Functionality Within Healthcare. Stud Health Technol Inform. 2020;270:1051–5.
77. Weldring T, Smith SMS. Patient-Reported Outcomes (PROs) and Patient-Reported Outcome Measures (PROMs). Health Serv Insights. 2013;6:61–8.
78. Avery P. Using e-health tools and PROMs to support self-management in patients with inflammatory bowel disease. Br J Nurs. 2021;30(7):394–402.
79. Iivanainen S, Alanko T, Peltola K, Konkola T, Ekström J, Virtanen H, et al. ePROs in the follow-up of cancer patients treated with immune checkpoint inhibitors: a retrospective study. J Cancer Res Clin Oncol. 2019;145(3):765–74.
80. Loo S, Grasso C, Glushkina J, McReynolds J, Lober W, Crane H, et al. Capturing relevant patient data in clinical encounters through integration of an electronic patient-reported outcome system into routine primary care in a Boston Community Health Center: development and implementation study. J Med Internet Res. 2020;22(8):e16778.
81. Haverman L, van Oers HA, van Muilekom MM, Grootenhuis MA. Options for the interpretation of and recommendations for acting on different proms in daily clinical practice using KLIK. Med Care. 2019;57 Suppl 5 Suppl 1:S52–8.
82. Leroux A, Rzasa-Lynn R, Crainiceanu C, Sharma T. Wearable devices: current status and opportunities in pain assessment and management. Digit Biomark. 2021;5(1):89–102.
83. Aiyegbusi OL, Kyte D, Cockwell P, Marshall T, Dutton M, Slade A, et al. Using Patient-Reported Outcome Measures (PROMs) to promote quality of care and safety in the management of patients with Advanced Chronic Kidney disease (PRO-trACK project): a mixed-methods project protocol. BMJ Open. 2017;7(6):e016687.
84. Girgis A, Durcinoska I, Levesque JV, Gerges M, Sandell T, Arnold A, et al. eHealth System for Collecting and Utilizing Patient Reported Outcome Measures for Personalized Treatment and Care (PROMPT-Care) among cancer patients: mixed methods approach to evaluate feasibility and acceptability. J Med Internet Res. 2017;19(10):e330.
85. Knowles SE, Ercia A, Caskey F, Rees M, Farrington K, Van der Veer SN. Participatory co-design and normalisation process theory with staff and patients to implement digital ways of working into routine care: the example of electronic patient-reported outcomes in UK renal services. BMC Health Serv Res. 2021;21(1):706.
86. Meirte J, Hellemans N, Anthonissen M, Denteneer L, Maertens K, Moortgat P, et al. Benefits and disadvantages of electronic patient-reported outcome measures: systematic review. JMIR Perioper Med. 2020;3(1):e15588.
87. White MK, Maher SM, Rizio AA, Bjorner JB. A meta-analytic review of measurement equivalence study findings of the SF-36® and SF-12® Health Surveys across electronic modes compared to paper administration. Qual Life Res. 2018;27(7):1757–67.
88. Jayakumar P, Teunis T, Vranceanu A-M, Lamb S, Williams M, Ring D, et al. Construct validity and precision of different patient-reported outcome measures during recovery after upper extremity fractures. Clin Orthop Relat Res. 2019;477(11):2521–30.
89. Carlozzi NE, Hahn EA, Goodnight SM, Kratz AL, Paulsen JS, Stout JC, et al. Patient-reported outcome measures in Huntington

disease: quality of life in neurological disorders (Neuro-QoL) social functioning measures. Psychol Assess. 2018;30(4):450–8.
90. Bass M, Oncken C, McIntyre AW, Dasilva C, Spuhl J, Rothrock NE. Implementing an application programming interface for PROMIS measures at three medical centers. Appl Clin Inform. 2021;12(5):979–83.
91. Qian Y, Walters SJ, Jacques R, Flight L. Comprehensive review of statistical methods for analysing patient-reported outcomes (PROs) used as primary outcomes in randomised controlled trials (RCTs) published by the UK's Health Technology Assessment (HTA) journal (1997-2020). BMJ Open. 2021;11(9):e051673.
92. Warsame R, D'Souza A. Patient reported outcomes have arrived: a practical overview for clinicians in using patient reported outcomes in oncology. Mayo Clin Proc. 2019;94(11):2291–301.
93. Hilpert F, Du Bois A. Patient-reported outcomes in ovarian cancer: are they key factors for decision making? Expert Rev Anticancer Ther. 2018;18(sup1):3–7.
94. Toumi M, Jarosławski S, Chouhaid C, Fallissard B, Auquier P. Patient-reported outcomes in oncology, beyond randomized controlled trials. Recent Results Cancer Res. 2019;213:57–65.
95. Friese CR, Fauer AJ, Kuisell C, Mendelsohn-Victor K, Wright NC, Griggs JJ, et al. Patient-reported outcomes collected in ambulatory oncology practices: feasibility, patterns, and correlates. Health Serv Res. 2020;55(6):966–72.
96. Nowinski CJ, Miller DM, Cella D. Evolution of patient-reported outcomes and their role in multiple sclerosis clinical trials. Neurotherapeutics. 2017;14(4):934–44.
97. Jevotovsky DS, Thirukumaran CP, Rubery PT. Creating value in spine surgery: using patient reported outcomes to compare the short-term impact of different orthopedic surgical procedures. Spine J. 2019;19(11):1850–7.
98. Plevinsky JM, Gutierrez-Colina AM, Carmody JK, Hommel KA, Crosby LE, McGrady ME, et al. Patient-reported outcomes for pediatric adherence and self-management: a systematic review. J Pediatr Psychol. 2020;45(3):340–57.
99. Sattler LN, Hing WA, Rathbone EN, Vertullo CJ. Which patient factors best predict discharge destination after primary total knee arthroplasty? the ARISE trial. J Arthroplast. 2020;35(10):2852–7.
100. Addario B, Geissler J, Horn MK, Krebs LU, Maskens D, Oliver K, et al. Including the patient voice in the development and implementation of patient-reported outcomes in cancer clinical trials. Health Expect. 2020;23(1):41–51.
101. Selby JV, Beal AC, Frank L. The Patient-Centered Outcomes Research Institute (PCORI) national priorities for research and initial research agenda. JAMA. 2012;307(15):1583–4.
102. ICHOM | Older Person Standard Set | Measuring Outcomes. 2022. https://www.ichom.org/portfolio/older-person/.
103. Vojtila L, Ashfaq I, Ampofo A, Dawson D, Selby P. Engaging a person with lived experience of mental illness in a collaborative care model feasibility study. Res Involv Engagem. 2021;7(1):5.
104. Gibbons C, Porter I, Gonçalves-Bradley DC, Stoilov S, Ricci-Cabello I, Tsangaris E, et al. Routine provision of feedback from patient-reported outcome measurements to healthcare providers and patients in clinical practice. Cochrane Database Syst Rev. 2021;10:CD011589.
105. Rivera SC, Kyte DG, Aiyegbusi OL, Slade AL, McMullan C, Calvert MJ. The impact of patient-reported outcome (PRO) data from clinical trials: a systematic review and critical analysis. Health Qual Life Outcomes. 2019;17(1):156.
106. Carfora L, Foley CM, Hagi-Diakou P, Lesty PJ, Sandstrom ML, Ramsey I, et al. Patients' experiences and perspectives of patient-reported outcome measures in clinical care: a systematic review and qualitative meta-synthesis. PLoS One. 2022;17(4):e0267030.
107. Valderas JM, Kotzeva A, Espallargues M, Guyatt G, Ferrans CE, Halyard MY, et al. The impact of measuring patient-reported outcomes in clinical practice: a systematic review of the literature. Qual Life Res. 2008;17(2):179–93.
108. Anatchkova M, Donelson SM, Skalicky AM, McHorney CA, Jagun D, Whiteley J. Exploring the implementation of patient-reported outcome measures in cancer care: need for more real-world evidence results in the peer reviewed literature. J Patient Rep Outcomes. 2018;2(1):64.
109. Wheat H, Horrell J, Valderas JM, Close J, Fosh B, Lloyd H. Can practitioners use patient reported measures to enhance person centred coordinated care in practice? A qualitative study. Health Qual Life Outcomes. 2018;16(1):223.
110. Skovlund SE, Lichtenberg TH, Hessler D, Ejskjaer N. Can the routine use of patient-reported outcome measures improve the delivery of person-centered diabetes care? A review of recent developments and a case study. Curr Diab Rep. 2019;19(9):84.
111. Ishaque S, Karnon J, Chen G, Nair R, Salter AB. A systematic review of randomised controlled trials evaluating the use of patient-reported outcome measures (PROMs). Qual Life Res. 2019;28(3):567–92.
112. Holmes MM, Lewith G, Newell D, Field J, Bishop FL. The impact of patient-reported outcome measures in clinical practice for pain: a systematic review. Qual Life Res. 2017;26(2):245–57.
113. Gondek D, Edbrooke-Childs J, Fink E, Deighton J, Wolpert M. Feedback from outcome measures and treatment effectiveness, treatment efficiency, and collaborative practice: a systematic review. Admin Pol Ment Health. 2016;43(3):325–43.
114. Kendrick T, El-Gohary M, Stuart B, Gilbody S, Churchill R, Aiken L, et al. Routine use of patient reported outcome measures (PROMs) for improving treatment of common mental health disorders in adults. Cochrane Database Syst Rev. 2016;7:CD011119.
115. Margolis PA, Peterson LE, Seid M. Collaborative Chronic Care Networks (C3Ns) to transform chronic illness care. Pediatrics. 2013;131(Suppl 4):S219–23.
116. Hjollund NHI. Fifteen years' use of patient-reported outcome measures at the group and patient levels: trend analysis. J Med Internet Res. 2019;21(9):e15856.
117. Nilsson E, Orwelius L, Kristenson M. Patient-reported outcomes in the Swedish National Quality Registers. J Intern Med. 2016;279(2):141–53.
118. Philpot LM, Barnes SA, Brown RM, Austin JA, James CS, Stanford RH, et al. Barriers and benefits to the use of patient-reported outcome measures in routine clinical care: a qualitative study. Am J Med Qual. 2018;33(4):359–64.
119. Hsiao C-J, Dymek C, Kim B, Russell B. Advancing the use of patient-reported outcomes in practice: understanding challenges, opportunities, and the potential of health information technology. Qual Life Res. 2019;28(6):1575–83.
120. Agarwal A, Pain T, Levesque J-F, Girgis A, Hoffman A, Karnon J, et al. Patient-reported outcome measures (PROMs) to guide clinical care: recommendations and challenges. Med J Aust. 2022;216(1):9–11.
121. Scholle SH, Morton S, Homco J, Rodriguez K, Anderson D, Hahn E, et al. Implementation of the PROMIS-29 in routine care for people with diabetes: challenges and opportunities. J Ambul Care Manage. 2018;41(4):274–87.
122. Lohr KN, Zebrack BJ. Using patient-reported outcomes in clinical practice: challenges and opportunities. Qual Life Res. 2009;18(1):99–107.
123. Chang C-H. Patient-reported outcomes measurement and management with innovative methodologies and technologies. Qual Life Res. 2007;16(Suppl 1):157–66.
124. Snyder CF, Aaronson NK, Choucair AK, Elliott TE, Greenhalgh J, Halyard MY, et al. Implementing patient-reported outcomes assessment in clinical practice: a review of the options and considerations. Qual Life Res. 2012;21(8):1305–14.

125. Hjollund NHI, Valderas JM, Kyte D, Calvert MJ. Health data processes: a framework for analyzing and discussing efficient use and reuse of health data with a focus on patient-reported outcome measures. J Med Internet Res. 2019;21(5):e12412.
126. Stover AM, Haverman L, van Oers HA, Greenhalgh J, Potter CM, ISOQOL PROMs/PREMs in Clinical Practice Implementation Science Work Group. Using an implementation science approach to implement and evaluate patient-reported outcome measures (PROM) initiatives in routine care settings. Qual Life Res. 2021;30(11):3015–33.
127. Chan EKH, Edwards TC, Haywood K, Mikles SP, Newton L. Implementing patient-reported outcome measures in clinical practice: a companion guide to the ISOQOL user's guide. Qual Life Res. 2019;28(3):621–7.
128. Center for Medicare and Medicaid Innovation. 2020 Report to Congress. 2022. https://innovation.cms.gov/data-and-reports/2021/rtc-2020.
129. McClellan SR, Trombley MJ, Maughan BC, Kahvecioglu DC, Marshall J, Marrufo GM, et al. Patient-reported outcomes among vulnerable populations in the Medicare bundled payments for care improvement initiative. Med Care. 2021;59(11):980–8.
130. Trombley MJ, McClellan SR, Kahvecioglu DC, Gu Q, Hassol A, Creel AH, et al. Association of Medicare's Bundled Payments for Care Improvement initiative with patient-reported outcomes. Health Serv Res. 2019;54(4):793–804.
131. Basch E, Wilfong L, Schrag D. Adding patient-reported outcomes to Medicare's oncology value-based payment model. JAMA. 2020;323(3):213–4.
132. Greene BD, Lange JK, Heng M, Melnic CM, Smith JT. Correlation between patient-reported outcome measures and health insurance provider types in patients with hip osteoarthritis. J Bone Joint Surg Am. 2021;103(16):1521–30.
133. HOS-Modified. 2022. https://www.hosonline.org/en/hos-modified-overview/.
134. Squitieri L, Bozic KJ, Pusic AL. The role of patient-reported outcome measures in value-based payment reform. Value Health. 2017;20(6):834–6.
135. Slover JD, Karia RJ, Hauer C, Gelber Z, Band PA, Graham J. Feasibility of integrating standardized patient-reported outcomes in orthopedic care. Am J Manag Care. 2015;21(8):e494–500.
136. Cox CE, Wysham NG, Kamal AH, Jones DM, Cass B, Tobin M, et al. Usability testing of an electronic patient-reported outcome system for survivors of critical illness. Am J Crit Care. 2016;25(4):340–9.
137. Boyce MB, Browne JP. Does providing feedback on patient-reported outcomes to healthcare professionals result in better outcomes for patients? A systematic review. Qual Life Res. 2013;22(9):2265–78.
138. Kottke TE, Stiefel M, Pronk NP. "Well-being in all policies": promoting cross-sectoral collaboration to improve people's lives. Prev Chronic Dis. 2016;13:E52.
139. 100 Million People Living Healthier Lives Worldwide | IHI—Institute for Healthcare Improvement. 2022. http://www.ihi.org/Engage/Initiatives/100MillionHealthierLives/Pages/default.aspx.
140. Barbera L, Moody L. A decade in review: cancer care Ontario's approach to symptom assessment and management. Med Care. 2019;57 Suppl 5 Suppl 1:S80–4.
141. Cella D, Choi SW, Condon DM, Schalet B, Hays RD, Rothrock NE, et al. PROMIS® adult health profiles: efficient short-form measures of seven health domains. Value Health. 2019;22(5):537–44.
142. Wittchen HU. Generalized anxiety disorder: prevalence, burden, and cost to society. Depress Anxiety. 2002;16(4):162–71. https://doi.org/10.1002/da.10065.
143. Gandek B, Roos EM, Franklin PD, Ware JE Jr. A 12-item short form of the Hip disability and Osteoarthritis Outcome Score (HOOS-12): tests of reliability, validity and responsiveness. Osteoarthr Cartil. 2019;27(5):754–61. https://doi.org/10.1016/j.joca.2018.09.017. Epub 2018 Nov 10
144. Cleeland CS, Ryan KM. Pain assessment: global use of the Brief Pain Inventory. Ann Acad Med Singap. 1994;23(2):129–38.
145. Holland JC. Preliminary guidelines for the treatment of distress. Oncology (Williston Park). 1997;11(11A):109–14; discussion 15–7.
146. Oude Voshaar MA, ten Klooster PM, Taal E, van de Laar MA. Measurement properties of physical function scales validated for use in patients with rheumatoid arthritis: a systematic review of the literature. Health Qual Life Outcomes. 2011;9:99. https://doi.org/10.1186/1477-7525-9-99.

Part V

Social and Environmental Determinants of Chronic Illness

Social Determinants of Health

Robert L. Ferrer

Introduction

Human health is socially produced. The life expectancy gap in 2019 between Japan at 84 years and the Central African Republic at 53 years [1] does not reflect innate differences in human biology, but rather the effects of economic, social, and political forces. The same can be said for the 19-year difference in male life expectancy across counties in the United States (US) or the 15-year gaps across ZIP (postal) codes in the city of San Antonio, Texas. Evidence that health is socially stratified dates back across millennia, a narrative legible in ancient grave sites, where skeletons with taller stature and better bone health lie alongside artifacts suggesting elite status. The "social determinants of health" is a system of ideas for answering questions describing how health is socially patterned and exploring causal pathways between social conditions and human health and illness.

Ancient civilizations were aware that status was linked with longevity [2], but scientific exploration of disparities took hold when public health developed into a data-driven science in the seventeenth century. Pioneers such as John Graunt, Edwin Chadwick, and Friedrich Engels in England, Rudolf Virchow in Germany [3], and Louis-René Villermé in Paris explored the associations between living conditions and mortality rates, observing higher mortality among the less affluent [4–6]. Most of the deaths they tabulated were due to infectious disease. Yet in the epidemiologic transition from infectious to chronic disease that followed—in 1999, for the first time, infectious diseases were no longer the most common cause of death in the world [7]—the role of social factors in shaping health and illness did not diminish. Why does the organization of society have such enduring effects on health and illness? How are the social, cultural, and physical environments that we inhabit become "embodied" [8] in human populations?

The importance of these questions goes well beyond understanding mechanisms. A principal motivation for documenting and explaining inequalities in health status is to understand how they can be alleviated or prevented. In clinical practice and in social services, this means mitigating the effects of social risk factors on individuals; in public health and policy it means creating societies in which opportunities to flourish are widely shared. The most important—and contentious—discussions in these analyses concern accountability and agency. Who is responsible and what should they do? This chapter will define key terms of social determinants, explain why the causes of illness in populations must be thought of differently than the causes in individual patients, review current conceptual frameworks for social determinants, summarize health disparities in chronic disease, and discuss interventions to promote health equity in both health care and population health.

Understanding Social Determinants

Social determinants of health are of interest for two distinct reasons: first, to describe the social *patterning* of illness, and second, to explain the social *causation* of illness [9]. Most studies of social patterning have applied a traditional epidemiological framework, treating "social risk factors" as exposures similar to other hazards [10]. Social risk factors include person-level attributes such as sex and gender identification, race and ethnicity, income and wealth, and educational attainment. These attributes determine an individual's position in hierarchies of power, social status, and economic resources.

A second category of investigation focuses on the circumstances in which people live. These circumstances include availability of healthy food and adequate housing, effective public school systems, community safety, safe employment that pays a living wage, infrastructure for physical activity, diverse transportation options, social and cultural norms for healthy living, social policy that mitigates health or employ-

R. L. Ferrer (✉)
Family & Community Medicine, UT Health San Antonio, San Antonio, TX, USA
e-mail: FerrerR@uthscsa.edu

ment shocks, political inclusion, and many others. This second list captures community-level characteristics. Other than social and cultural norms, each is the product of specific policy decisions, shaped by deliberations about the role of the state in supporting health and well-being, stakeholders' political power, and public financing decisions. Altering these root social causes of ill health is potentially more powerful than subsequently mitigating their effects on individuals. However, addressing root social causes introduces ethical and normative quandaries. Reasoning about root causes requires not just technical expertise but also ethical judgments about what a community or society ought to do in the face of competing interests. How should the free operation of markets be balanced with the distribution of products like tobacco that harm many users? To what extent should the state try to equalize opportunities for well-being?

Social determinants raise complex, multilayered questions that span disciplinary boundaries including molecular biology, physiology, psychology, sociology, economics, ethics, and political science. Combining perspectives from multiple disciplines is necessary to explain paradoxes, such as why the poor spend more than the wealthy on health harming products such as cigarettes [11], or make less use of health protecting resources such as seat belts [12] even when there is no cost. Theories and insights from multiple disciplines also contribute to developing effective interventions. Although chronic diseases such as cancer and heart disease were once considered diseases of affluence, the highest rates are observed in the poorest nations and in the poorest inhabitants of wealthy nations. Once a nation surpasses the annual income threshold of USD $1000 per capita, chronic diseases surpass infections as the leading causes of death. Overall mortality is not fully informative however—we must all die of something—so it may be more instructive to note that about half of chronic disease deaths worldwide occur before age 70 [13].

The definition of social determinants currently in widest use was created by the World Health Organization in 2008 [14]: "The conditions in which people are born, grow, live, work and age. These circumstances are shaped by the distribution of money, power, and resources at global, national and local levels." Table 40.1 defines key concepts that are related to social determinants of health.

An essential understanding about the concept of socioeconomic status is that there is no single underlying "SES" attribute that its indicators measure. Instead, each SES measure has greater relevance in specific circumstances, depending on whether financial resources, knowledge, or social networks offer the most leverage for a specific health problem [20]. It is also worth noting that terms such as "inequality," "disparity," and "inequity," carry different implications when assigning responsibility for unequal outcomes. "Inequality" and "disparity" are often used to document differences in outcomes across social groupings without reference to who or what is generating the differences. A close reading of successive US government reports on population health concludes that their authors adopted "disparities" as a neutral word, referring to between-group differences without assigning responsibility for the differences or even framing the question [21]. Inequities or the structural forces that created them received little attention in the reports.

Table 40.1 Key concepts linked to social determinants of health

Concept	Definition
Social determinants of health	"The conditions in which people are born, grow, live, work and age. These circumstances are shaped by the distribution of money, power and resources at global, national and local levels." (Commission on the Social Determinants of Health:2008tt)
Health inequality	Differences in health outcomes among defined groups, without a judgment about their fairness
Health inequity	Avoidable, unnecessary, and unjust differences in health outcomes among defined groups [15]
Health disparity	Usually a synonym for health inequality; occasionally for health inequity
Social justice	Ethical reasoning about the political processes and structures that govern the distribution of benefits and burdens in society
Social capital	Social networks and their shared norms, values and understandings that enable cooperation within or among groups [16]
Social risk factors	Person-level attributes that place people in socially defined hierarchies. These attributes include race and ethnicity, sex, gender identification, level of education, income and wealth, and occupation
Socioeconomic status (SES)	Measured by education, occupation, or income/wealth
Socioeconomic position (SEP)	Concept of where people stand in relation to one another in social stratification hierarchies
Social class	A tiered structure of economic, social, and cultural power, controlling economically relevant assets, authority, or social relationships [17]
Social epidemiology	The branch of epidemiology that studies the social distribution and social causation of health and illness
Population health	The health outcomes for a defined group, including how outcomes are distributed within the group [18]
Discrimination	Adverse judgments or actions taken against people outside one's social group
Structural racism	Racial inequities normalized in the routine operation of economic, social, or political systems [19]

At the population level, epidemiology's prevailing questions and methods have evolved over the past two centuries in step with changing paradigms of disease causation. Originally deeply concerned with social causation of illness, during the latter half of the twentieth century epidemiology shifted its focus to individuals' risk factors for disease [22]. There were many successes, but even the largest, most rigorous investigations, such as the Framingham Heart Study, explained only about half the variation in risk from person to person. Recognizing the shortcomings of an overly individualistic approach, socially oriented epidemiologists began in the late 1980s and 1990s to urge that epidemiology expand its scope. Of these thinkers, Geoffrey Rose articulated the most coherent and powerful account of disease causation.

Rose emphasized three key principles for population health [23]. First, the determinants of population rates of disease differ from the determinants of individual risks of disease. Asking, "why do some individuals suffer from x?" is different from asking, "why do some populations have high prevalence of x." Within populations, where people tend to share similar environmental exposures ("environment" is defined broadly to include social and cultural forces), genetic variability tends to account for individual cases. Between populations, however, variations in disease prevalence are created by differing social and behavioral exposures. For example, diet explains little variation in cholesterol levels within a population, since basic dietary patterns are shared with minor differences, but much variation between populations, due to major differences in dietary norms.

A series of international comparisons has revealed striking variation in the prevalence of different diseases [24]. For example, many of the major causes of death in industrialized societies range from 5 to 100-fold across different populations [25]. Such marked differences far exceed known genetic variation. Instead, the variation across countries derives from differences in behavior and environmental exposures. Examples include the low incidence of heart disease in Asian societies with little intake of dairy products or fatty meats, and the low incidence of breast cancer in modern hunter-gatherers where puberty occurs late (probably due to nutrition) and pregnancy soon follows, with extended periods of nursing between pregnancies [26]. The individual versus population distinction is supported by many studies documenting that when people emigrate from their country of origin (taking their genetic code with them), they assume the specific disease risks prevalent in their new location [27].

A second critical idea is that almost all exposures and diseases exist in populations as a continuum rather than a dichotomy. Visible morbidity accounts for just one tail of the population distribution. For example, Japan and Finland differ not only in the prevalence of high cholesterol, but also in the distribution of dyslipidemia across their respective populations, which is lower in Japan than in Finland [23]. Entire risk factor distributions can move over time within societies, for example the bell curve of US body mass index during the years of the obesity epidemic [28]. Population prevention is most powerful when it shifts entire population distributions.

Third, a moderate risk applied to a large number of people generates a greater absolute number of cases than a high risk applied to a small number of people. For instance, the many people in Western societies with average cholesterol levels account for more cases of coronary heart disease than the much smaller number with very high cholesterol levels [29]. Rose's alternative to the "high risk" strategy was a "population" strategy seeking population-wide behavioral shifts. Even small shifts in the population distribution of a risk factor such as body weight or blood pressure would sharply reduce the number of people in the high-risk tail. And by changing population norms rather than asking individuals to do what is not "normal" in their society, the population strategy is behaviorally less burdensome.

Social Determinants and Chronic Disease

The relationship between social determinants and chronic disease is well established. To begin, at the population level, higher per capita income is associated with better health. The relationship is robust across many health indicators, including life expectancy, chronic disease burden, and self-rated health status [30]. The association between health and per capita income holds at multiple scales of observation, from neighborhoods to regions to global. Life expectancy and other health status indicators also correlate with educational attainment, occupational status, and social class [31]. Within countries, the relationship is curvilinear, so that life expectancy gains are steepest as income rises from the lowest levels, gradually leveling off at the highest income levels. Chronic disease incidence and deaths are higher among the least affluent residents of wealthy nations [32].

Across countries, life expectancy rises steeply as per capita income increases until annual per capita income reaches about 30,000 USD, after which the curve flattens. Chronic disease deaths occur at higher rates in less affluent countries. The strength of the relationship between social position and chronic disease burden can differ markedly from country to country [32]. Chronic illness in middle age substantially raises the risk of disability [33], creating a cascade of adverse personal and family consequences. This last point is critical for public health and policy because disability reduces earnings and diminishes access to employment-based health insurance, creating further risks for the disabled [34, 35], as well as a cascade that contributes to interpersonal and intergenerational transmission of social class gradients in health [36, 37].

Figure 40.1 displays the relationship between functional status and age, education level, and chronic disease that is derived from 1997–2006 National Health Interview Survey data among 221,195 adults aged 25–64.

In this analysis, functional limitation was defined as severely limited ability to stand, walk, climb steps, stoop, reach, or grasp. Chronic disease was identified by self-report of coronary disease, stroke, diabetes mellitus, chronic obstructive lung disease, or cancer. Disability is strongly predicted at every age by presence of at least one of the five chronic diseases (adjusted OR 3.73 (95% CI 3.59–3.76)).

The relationship between income inequality and health outcomes is more mixed and nuanced. There is heightened interest in the health effects of income inequality—the unequal distribution of income across a population—given the progressive growth in inequality over the last three decades From 1942 to 1982 the share of income going to the top decile of American earners never exceeded 35%. In the years since, however, the top decile's share has climbed steeply, passing 50% in 2012 [38]. Most of those gains went to the top 1% of earners. Incomes continue to diverge; in 1975, the average income of households in the top fifth of income distribution was ten times as large as average household income in the bottom fifth of the distribution; in 2019, average top quintile incomes were 16.6 times as large as those in the bottom quintile.

A 1992 landmark study looked at nine developed countries and reported a significant association between life expectancy and the percentage of income (i.e., income inequality) going to the least wealthy 70% of families [39]. This study launched an avalanche of descriptive and explanatory scholarship on income inequality and health, as well as substantial disagreement about the whether the effect is real or confounded by other variables. The mechanisms through which income inequality harms health have been thoroughly debated, with at least four explanations proposed for why income inequality should influence health. The first is based on simple math. Life expectancy rises steeply as incomes increase from the lowest levels, and then levels off as the top incomes are reached. As a result, when the poor earn a greater share of the wealth, their lives are lengthened more than the lives of the wealthy are shortened when they earn a smaller share of wealth. The result is a net increase in population life expectancy.

A second explanation is that larger gaps in income make the less affluent feel more deprived. Deprivation creates psychological stress that may trigger maladaptive coping mechanisms, such as spending beyond one's means to keep pace with social norms. A third explanation is that societies with greater income inequality also underinvest in human capital, including education, income support, health care, housing, and other critical areas [40]. Underinvestment occurs because income inequality leads to political inequality. A fourth explanation contends that income inequality creates a negative society-wide effect on both rich and poor, metaphorically characterized as social "pollution" that erodes health for everyone. More unequal societies are less cohesive societies [41].

These four explanations are not mutually exclusive and in fact could be operating simultaneously. A 2015 paper sys-

Fig. 40.1 Functional status and age, education level, and chronic disease. (Adapted from reference [38])

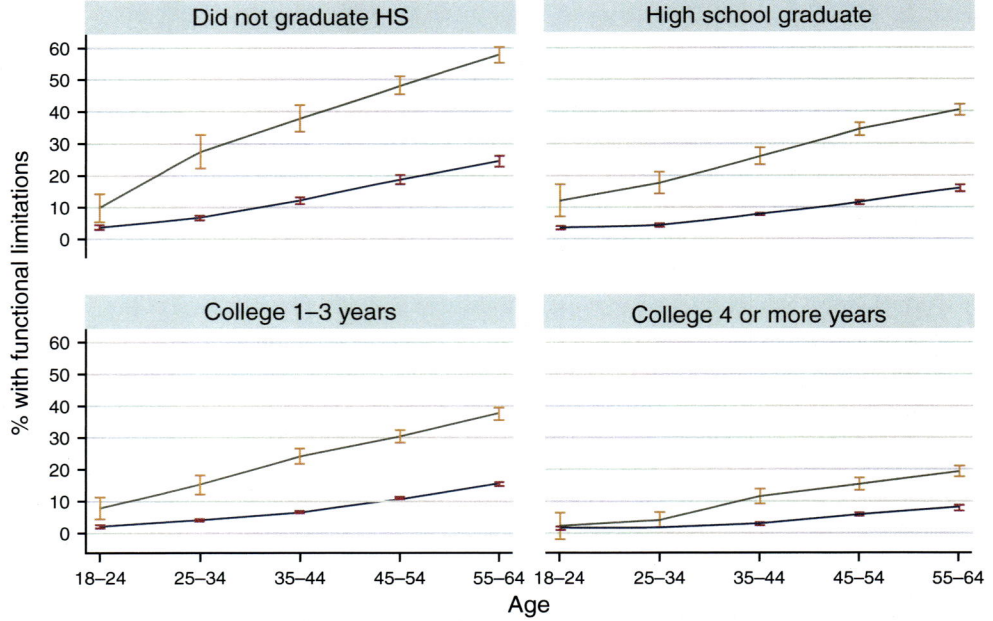

Upper lines: with chronic disease; Lower lines: without chronic disease; 95% CI shown

tematically reviewed the evidence base and concluded that it satisfies epidemiological criteria for causality [41]. A final question about the income inequality hypothesis has to do with its implications, if valid. Presumably, the solution would be to increase income for the least well off, which would also be the solution when poor health is due to low absolute income. Would reducing the incomes of the most affluent also improve health outcomes for the worst off? If the pathway is oversize political and policy influence among the most wealthy, then the answer would be yes.

Race and ethnicity are additional powerful social determinants. Major disparities in mortality by race and ethnicity in the United States appear by middle age, with most of the excess deaths accounted for by common chronic diseases. Income is a major contributor to the disparities [42], but measured income does not have the same meaning among African Americans as it does in non-Hispanic Whites, because at any given income, African Americans' accumulated wealth is substantially lower [42]. Also the link between income and residential environment differs markedly for African Americans. While the great majority of poor non-Hispanic whites live in neighborhoods with low poverty levels, less than 20% of African Americans do. Conversely, only 10% of poor non-Hispanic Whites live in extreme poverty areas. For African Americans, the proportion is 50% [43]. The direction of racial/ethnic disparities sometimes differs by indicator. For example, Hispanics in the United States have longer life expectancy than non-Hispanic Whites but report worse health status [44].

Conceptual and Theoretical Frameworks

Lifestyle

Lifestyle theories focus on unhealthy behaviors because of the direct and powerful effects of behaviors on chronic disease risk. About 80% of chronic disease is linked to 1 of 4 unhealthy behaviors: tobacco use, inadequate physical activity, unhealthy diet, and risky patterns of consuming ethanol [45]. All four behaviors display social patterning, with more smoking, less physical activity, and less healthy diet among socially disadvantaged groups [46], while binge drinking is more common among higher status individuals, although the frequency and intensity of binging is less [47].

Behaviors do not arise is a vacuum. Social norms, availability, convenience, and price play a major role in shaping health behaviors. And those factors are influenced by what is manufactured, marketed, and sold. In turn, markets are governed by policy and regulations enacted through the political process. Nothing better illustrates those forces than the global tobacco epidemic that killed 100 million people in the twentieth century [48], fueled by wide distribution and marketing of tobacco products, social norms encouraging smoking, government subsidies for tobacco growers, and international trade agreements [49]. More recently, tobacco use has diminished in countries that enacted laws restricting smoking in public venues, imposed taxes, and mandated prominent product warnings. Evolving social norms, especially among the more educated, have discouraged smoking. Cigarette manufacturers' organized effort to suppress scientific findings on their products' harms have also come to light [50].

Food production and marketing is subject to many of the same forces as tobacco, with unhealthy products widely distributed and aggressively marketed [51]. Food producers market many foods of low-nutritional quality to low-income and minority consumers [52]. Economic analyses also document how food consumption has increased as the time cost of food preparation has decreased, with fewer meals made at home and more restaurant meals and ready-made foods consumed [53].

The influence of these environmental determinants makes a strong case against focusing on individuals' decontextualized choices as chief determinants of health behaviors. When less than 3% of the US population manages all four of non-smoking status, healthy diet, adequate physical activity, and a normal BMI [54], and only 16% meet 3 of those 4 criteria, it is difficult to argue for a willpower deficiency rather than widespread structural drivers.

Biomedical

Biomedical theories explain how adaptations to socially derived stress activate pathophysiological pathways in neurological, immunological, endocrine, and cardiovascular systems. These mechanisms have been the subject of intense study for several decades. What links social stress to disordered physiology associated with chronic disease is increasingly understood in both animal models and humans. A chain of events beginning in utero creates long term consequences for dysregulation in multiple physiological systems. A detailed treatment is beyond the scope of this chapter [55] but a brief sketch follows.

Large population cohort studies provide evidence for the fetal programming hypothesis [56]. Infants with low birth weight have a higher risk of cardio-metabolic disease as adults, including coronary heart disease and diabetes [56, 57]. The effects are hypothesized to occur through epigenetic changes created by maternal under-nutrition or other stresses [58]. They give rise to a "thrifty phenotype" characterized by insulin resistance, that predisposes to obesity when food is readily available. Early life effects are also evident in the positive associations between achieved height, cognitive test scores, and later occupational attainment [59].

Childhood experiences exert a powerful effect on risk of chronic disease [60]. Critical periods in brain development and its subsequent regulation of endocrine, cardiovascular, and immunological pathways mean that adverse child experiences cast long shadows into adulthood [61]. Longitudinal studies following a Dutch famine in 1944–1945 have documented lower birthweight in the *grandchildren* of women born during the famine [62, 63]. Laboratory experiments with primates demonstrate similar sequelae of adverse rearing conditions [64].

Whether in childhood or later in adult life, repetitive psychosocial stress is distributed along a social gradient. Max Weber [65] theorized that social stratification results in a hierarchy of "life chances," consisting of a set of circumstances, values, and beliefs. In this view, the critical element is the unequal distribution of opportunities in residential area, housing quality, employment, finances, leisure time, access to medical care, and exposure to discrimination and crime.

Evidence for the "life chances" theory has accumulated in several decades of sociological research. Social gradients in stressful circumstances are measured by the number of adverse life events, but even stronger evidence exists for the gradient in chronic strains [66]. Strains result from the mismatch between what one has been socialized to expect (e.g., a good job, happy family life) and one's actual experiences—what Thomas Merton referred to as "anomie." [67] This sociological perspective emphasizes the naturalistic origins of stress arising out of ordinary life pursuits, as opposed to abnormal responses to unusual circumstances [68]. Stress is universal; it is also unevenly distributed.

The consequences of stress are operationalized as "allostatic load." Allostasis refers to the maintenance of stability through change, whereby an organism adapts its physiology to external or internal circumstances in order to protect essential physiological systems [55]. When encountering a dangerous situation, for example, it's advantageous to rapidly increase pulse and blood pressure to fuel the muscles needed to flee. The external to internal link is provided by the brain, which perceives the threat and, through neurological and chemical pathways, sets in motion both the act of running and the changes in the physiological environment that sustain physical activity.

Given an acute danger, allostatic changes in physiology promote resilience—survival—at the expense of stability. Unfortunately, human resilience mechanisms did not evolve in response to the chronic stresses of a modern society, such as demanding jobs that offer little control. Those stresses tend to be frequent, repetitive over long time frames, and differentially distributed by social position [69]. Evidence for allostatic stress responses is strong in both humans and other animals living in social hierarchies [70, 71]. Health consequences of allostatic load include cardiovascular disease, cognitive impairment, and all-cause mortality [72].

Life Course

Childhood experience influences adult health through pathways beyond allostatic load. James Heckman and colleagues have assembled extensive evidence for a "skills" theory of childhood development, and how it shapes educational and occupational attainment, health behaviors, and health outcomes in later life. Parental and social investment in child development builds cognitive and non-cognitive skills (e.g., self-control, patience, risk aversion, delayed gratification, and others). These skills are proposed to be the common origins of later-life socioeconomic status and health outcomes [73].

Given these findings, social gradients in parenting behavior become important policy targets to reduce health disparities in later life [74]. A supportive environment for child rearing has many policy pillars, including adequate parental leave, income support and tax credits for young families, paid time off, early childhood intervention programs, quality day care and early childhood education, and accessible health care.

Fundamental Social Causes

The "fundamental social causes" theory formulated by Link and Phelan [34] is designed to account for the observation that socioeconomic status powerfully influences health even as diverse societies evolve over long time scales, with major changes in the prevailing causes of morbidity and mortality. The SES effect on health endures, the theory says, because higher status bestows advantages including "money, knowledge, prestige, power, and beneficial social connections that protect health no matter what mechanisms are relevant at any given time." Those advantages are deployed to reduce exposure to known risks. The obverse is also important; those with low SES have much less control over their risk exposures. That the advantages—money, knowledge, power, social capital—often come in a bundle is significant, because different risks require different resources.

Link and Phelan's theory would predict that social gradients should appear only when there are effective interventions to reduce or eliminate a health risk [75]. For example, inequalities in rates of sudden infant death syndrome widened following the launch of a campaign educating parents that babies put to sleep on their backs had lower risk [76]. Fundamental social causes theory has at least two limitations. It does not illuminate actionable pathways to mitigating social determinants' impact on specific illnesses. And, while it spotlights the cluster of individual circumstances that shape risk exposures, it does not address what gives rise to those circumstances.

Public Policy

Ultimately, many circumstances of everyday life are shaped by policy on education, poverty reduction, housing, protections against discrimination, labor laws, occupational safety, transportation networks, public health and health care spending, environmental protection, agricultural policy, voting rights, and others [77]. As the preceding sections have shown, these sectors all have health implications. Policy-makers' responsiveness to the needs of citizens across the spectrum of social needs is therefore a key determinant of outcomes. What do we know about that responsiveness?

Using a laboriously constructed data set comprising 1779 public opinion surveys on pending Congressional votes between 1981 and 2002, Martin Gilens [78] disaggregated respondents by income level and compared their preferences with the legislative outcome. He concluded that legislators' votes strongly align with the preferences of the highest income Americans but "bear virtually no resemblance" to the preferences of poor or middle-income Americans. Larry Bartels examined both the US and other high income European and Asian countries and reached similar conclusions [79]. In the words of economist Angus Deaton, "The very rich have no need of national health insurance, of disability or income support schemes, of public education, or of public policy that will limit the inheritance of deprivation from parents to children. They do not wish to pay taxes to support such schemes, and their immense wealth and political influence provides them with a potent weapon to prevent them having to do so" [80].

Social Ecological

A critical insight for social determinants is that phenomena must be understood simultaneously from the macro and micro perspectives because health emerges from the interaction between people and their environment. Studying that interaction defines the field of ecology. Epidemiologists have therefore named this approach "eco-epidemiology" [80] or "ecosocial" theory [8]. Tony McMichael wrote extensively on the relation of human health to different natural and man-made ecosystems, considering the influence of infectious agents, agriculture, urbanization, technological developments, economic systems, and climate [81].

Ecological understanding requires careful attention to history and context. For example, the association of obesity with higher SES in low-income countries reverses as they become more affluent [82]. Monetary and time costs of food and its preparation fall for everyone, making calories more available. Need for manual labor decreases. Norms for healthier diet and leaner body shape evolve more quickly among the affluent as they come to understand and act on the risks of obesity.

Also central to ecology is its use of complexity science, an umbrella term for scientific approaches to study how a system's behavior emerges from the interactions of its parts. When the parts are autonomous and adapting—like humans—systems are subject to non-linear, unpredictable behavior such as epidemics and tipping points. Social environment strongly influences individuals, but human activity creates the social environment [83]. For example, social norms on tolerating (or not) secondhand smoke influence individuals' decision about when and where to smoke which in turn shape the evolution of social norms.

Addressing Social Determinants

Health care settings and providers can neither independently solve the health challenges faced by patients nor ignore them [84]. A 2010 WHO report on the social determinants of health identified 4 leverage points for action [85]: (1) intervene in the healthcare system to reduce consequences of illness among disadvantaged people; (2) reduce the vulnerability of disadvantaged people to health damaging factors; (3) decrease exposure to health damaging factors associated with lower socioeconomic position, and; (4) decrease social stratification.

Promoting Equity as a Value in Health Care

If social disadvantage carries the strong risk of poor health outcomes, what role should health care take in trying to improve those outcomes? Are there specific strategies that practitioners and their health care organizations can apply to better organize themselves to improve the probability of success for patients with social risks? Formulating answers to these questions has become a priority in health care systems around the world as they recognize the powerful influence of social determinants on outcomes and costs.

The notion that health care should take on social determinants is, in a sense, a rediscovery of the past. Sydney Kark, a pioneer for community health centers in South Africa in the 1940s later wrote that, "The main factors that determine a community's health are to be found within the community itself, in its social, biological or cultural features, or in its environment, natural and man-made." [86] By the 1970s the social medicine movement was influential enough to shape the Declaration of Alma Ata (1978), which proposed that primary care would coordinate health-promoting action in education, housing, food, public works, communications, and other sectors [87].

Unfortunately, responsibility for action on social determinants was incompatible with health care's ongoing evolution toward a biomedically specialized workforce with a restricted scope. Today, a renewed focus on social determinants as key drivers of population health is motivating health services to re-expand their field of attention. Among the forces catalyzing this movement in the United States is the changing structure of federal health care payments [88]. Evolving payment mechanisms aim to reward quality care and cost containment while accounting for social risk profiles of health care providers' patient populations. More ambitiously, "accountable care organizations" seek to link together health care and social services to deliver integrated care for defined populations [89].

Collecting Patient Data on Social Risk Factors

As these trends unfold, health care organizations are taking initiative to assess their patient panels for social risk factors and to capture the data in electronic health records.

A report from the National Academy of Medicine [90] recommends broad categories of social and behavioral variables as well as specific measures. The categories include education, race/ethnicity, residential address, neighborhood median household income, patient financial strain, tobacco use, alcohol use, stress, depression, physical activity, social isolation, and intimate partner violence. The committee formulating these recommendations evaluated measures' association with health outcomes; utility for managing individual patients and for policy decisions about populations; availability and validity of existing measures; burden of data collection; potential risks from data disclosure; and data availability from alternative sources.

Currently, such lists can be considered informed hypotheses; the variables could be gathered in different ways at different times, often contingent on the population served. Best practices will emerge as the early experience is analyzed. It is also important to recognize that the International Classification of Diseases (ICD) 10 coding system already contains over 70 "Z" codes (Z55-65) useful for coding adverse social circumstances.

Yet, social risk factor data are but the first step; clinical teams must use the data to systematically intervene. A 2021 NAM report [91] set out a framework describing five activities to address social needs in clinical care: (1) awareness by identify patients' social risks (e.g., does the patient have reliable transport to health services?); (2) adjustment by altering clinical care to account for social risks (e.g., should insulin doses be reduced at the end of the month to avoid hypoglycemia when the patient may be short on funds and skipping meals?); (3) assistance by connecting pts. with resources (e.g., connect with job training opportunities); (4) alignment by organizing and investing in community resources that address social risks (e.g., operate a food pantry), and; (5) advocacy by promoting policies that address social risks (e.g., advocate for community gardens).

Despite the added time and effort necessary for social needs screening in health care, front-line clinicians see potential benefit [92], recognizing that patients' unmet social needs complicate treatment planning, increase care complexity, and contribute to clinician burnout. Scaling up these efforts presents challenges. Health and social service systems almost never have common person identifiers, complicating the development of shared information systems. Some communities are beginning to address this challenge. More problematic is the need for workflows to productively co-manage shared clients.

A caution is that screening for social risk factors could adversely affect patients if poorly implemented. Potential pitfalls include not considering patient perspectives when making referrals for social determinants, inadequate tracking to ensure successful connections to community resources, and failure to focus on family assets as well as deficits [93]. In such efforts, supporting patient dignity is an important outcome in its own right. Evaluation data are illuminating patient perspectives on social risk screening. In a survey of 969 adult patients or parents of pediatric patients at clinic or emergency room visits in nine states, 79% reported screening was very or somewhat appropriate, 14% were neutral, and 7% reported screening was very or somewhat inappropriate [94].

The largest evaluation of social needs screening to date was launched by the Center for Medicaid and Medicare Services (CMMS) in 2017 under their "Accountable Health Communities" initiative [89]. The model is designed to identify patients with social needs, provide navigation to appropriate resources, and create a community structure that ensures adequate capacity, tracking, and performance improvement for the community network [89]. Following the National Academy of Medicine (U.S.) (NAM) social risk factor intervention framework, an "Assistance" track identifies Medicaid and Medicare beneficiaries with health-related social needs and helps navigate them to relevant social services. An "Alignment" track offers patient navigation augmented by community-level efforts to match communities' service capacity with the demand.

Enrollees are labeled high risk if they made at least two emergency department visits in the prior 12 months. Over half of eligible beneficiaries reported multiple social needs. Although 3/4 of eligible beneficiaries participated in navigation, just 14% of those enrolled for a full year reported that their social needs were resolved. During follow-up, beneficiaries receiving assistance did make 9% fewer ER visits than the control group, but there was no effect on hospital admissions or total expenditures per beneficiary [95]. A vexing issue that undercut solutions to other problems was beneficiaries' lack of reliable transportation [95].

Participating health care sites managed the additional screening workload with a combination of existing administrative and clinical personnel, noting that pre- or post-visit telephone contacts were efficient ways to screen, and often preferred by patients. Maintaining up-to-date rosters of community social care resources was challenging, however. And patient acceptance of navigation led to high navigator caseloads, amplified by the fact that 60% of patients accepting navigation had two or more social needs. As a result, many communities' social service agencies were overloaded by the additional referrals, a critical insight that smaller scale studies evaluating social needs screening programs had not uncovered. And the gap in capacity is underestimated because many patients lacked transportation to reach social services.

A study on social needs screening outcomes from a health system in Cleveland, Ohio provides additional insight [96]. Over 5700 patients attending a COVID vaccine clinic were screened to assess food insecurity. Screenings were in-person, by telephone or through an online patient portal. Patients screening positive were referred to community organizations using an electronic referral platform. Seventeen percent screened positive; of those 86% consented to a referral, but just 42% of the consenting group had a referral placed. Of those with a referrral placed, 98% accepted the referral. In the end, however, for just 27% of persons was the food need resolved through connections with food assistance.

The US Preventive Services Task Force added additional perspective in a technical brief reviewing 106 social risk screening studies from health care settings. The most commonly reported outcomes were measures of heath care utilization. The brief concluded that additional randomized trials are needed to document the health outcomes associated with social risk screening [97]. A review [98] of social needs screening in health care provides cautions about the need to better understand the workforce, training, and tools necessary to convert social needs screening into patient benefit. Due to the potentially stigmatizing nature of inquiring about social needs, it must be implemented with sensitivity. Persons who screen positive may not be interested in obtaining help for their social needs [93]. And, like any screening tool, social needs screeners can misclassify respondents [94].

Another practical consideration is that primary health care systems asked to take responsibility for social risk factors are currently absorbing many other obligations including quality improvement and pay for performance programs, transformation to patient-centered medical homes, and adoption of electronic health records. Asking practices to implement yet another complex task adds to change fatigue [99]. Yet, as discussed below, reimbursement is evolving to help support additional personnel and systems. And, ultimately, primary care services are unlikely to be maximally effective without confronting social needs.

Funding for Addressing Social Risk Factors

As data accumulate on the morbidity and expense of chronic conditions linked to social disadvantage [100, 101], funders are recognizing the limitations of reimbursing clinical services without additional support for mitigating individuals' social risk factors. In one example of emerging responses, the US Medicare and Medicaid programs [102] are granting states new legal authority to implement alternative payment models that direct expenditures to patient needs such as housing instability or job training. Many programs also expand the healthcare workforce devoted to identifying needs and interventions, such as nurse care managers or community health workers. Evidence suggests that this workforce can improve health and reduce costs [103].

These new, coordinated social needs screening and intervention programs require support to help underwrite the necessary technology and personnel needed for large-scale impact. In this regard, the high health care costs associated with social risks support a business case for innovation. Pay-for-success models are spreading; many are supported by Medicaid 1115 Waivers that fund health care organizations for initiatives beyond traditional health services. In one expanding model known as "Pathways Hubs," [104] now in 35 communities in the U.S., a coalition of local funders contracts with local agencies, employs community health workers who coach patients toward healthier behaviors while also helping them navigate the local landscape of agencies that address social needs. As patients engage with social services and achieve health care milestones—and lower health care costs—the payor, often Medicaid, triggers a payment to the CHW's agency, closing the financial sustainability loop. In another configuration, insurers are contracting directly with health care systems who themselves employ the additional care coordination personnel [105].

A 2021 systematic review [106] of 35 studies in which health care organizations screened and referred patients with social needs to appropriate resources documented decreased social needs, improvement in health risks (e.g., diet quality, blood cholesterol), and cost-effectiveness. There was also evidence that completed referrals were more common when the referring agency forwarded patients' information to the destination agency, rather than just providing patients with a contact phone number.

Health Care System Performance for Patients with Social Risk Factors

Social risk factors are associated with inequalities in doctor-patient communication, diagnoses, and treatment decisions. Most of this literature has focused on racial and ethnic disparities [107]. At the micro-level of clinician-patient interactions, unintended biases may influence clinical decisions [108]. At the facility level, geographic accessibility, demand for high levels of health literacy, cultural appropriateness, and ability to accommodate multiple languages are important determinants of care quality. At the macro-level of health systems, minority patients are often concentrated in a narrow segment of health care institutions that disproportionately serve socially at-risk patients. However, careful review comparing outcomes within and across institutions that serve populations with different demographics has demonstrated substantial variability in patient outcomes. Within the same hospital, white and minority patients appear to receive the same quality of care [109].And though there are concerns that health care quality at minority-serving institutions is worse than that for hospitals serving more advantaged patients, the evidence is mixed [110]. There is substantial variability across institutions in the quality of care received by socially disadvantaged patients.

Using that variability as a point of departure, it is instructive to ask what strategies high-performing providers use to achieve good outcomes for socially at-risk patients. Even with a large number of care improvement projects in progress, insufficient high-quality evidence is available to answer the question [97]. However, a National Academy of Medicine report [111] characterized several systems practices that show promise in caring for socially at-risk populations. The proposed systems practices were derived from a review of published literature augmented by 60 case studies submitted by stakeholders or gleaned from the gray literature. The systems practices include [111]: (1) committing to health equity by accepting organizational accountability for achieving equitable outcomes across levels of social risk factors; (2) creating data systems and measures to measure equity within the health system; (3) comprehensively assessing needs, seeking to identify unmet clinical and social needs that are driving outcomes; (4) forming collaborative partnerships internally and externally to deliver the new services identified in the needs assessment; (5) planning for care continuity as patients transition across clinical (primary and specialty care, hospital, mental health) and social services, and; (6) engaging patients in their care with assistance tailored to their needs.

Health Literacy

Health literacy is defined as "the degree to which individuals have the capacity to obtain, process, and understand basic information and services needed to make appropriate health decisions" [112]. Because low health literacy correlates with a large number of adverse health outcomes [113], enhancing health literacy is an important strategy to reduce disparities. From a social determinants perspective, universal high-quality education is an essential building block. But health literacy can be approached from two different directions: by enhancing individuals' knowledge or by reducing environmental demands [114]. Both are necessary, but the education component has received much more attention than the demand component. Systems approaches to reducing demand for health literacy both inside and outside of health care might include the following questions, in increasing order of potential efficacy: At what reading level are the written instructions, education materials, web interfaces, and billing correspondence written? In what languages are they available? Is feedback on system features (demand for high literacy) sought by those who lead the systems? Are community members [patients] involved in designing the systems? Goals: Do we measure patients' literacy only or is the demand environment considered? Do we manage the latter? Fundamental beliefs: low health literacy is a problem of educating individuals or also has a strong contribution from the systems we create?

Social Deprivation, Mental Health Disorders, and Comorbid Chronic Disease

Mental and substance use disorders are the leading cause of years lived with disability worldwide, exceeding the burden due to other chronic conditions [115]. This finding is mirrored in individual patient experience, as persons with depression report worse overall health than persons with angina, asthma, arthritis, or diabetes [116]. Not surprisingly, overall health status is rated lower when depression is superimposed on any of those four conditions and lower still with depression and two or more conditions. Concurrent mental illness also appears to account for a large share of the disability reported by persons with chronic disease [117]. And recent declines in U.S. life expectancy among working age adults in the U.S. [118] is attributed in large part to increases in deaths from drug poisoning, ethanol, and suicide.

This unfavorable interaction of mental illness other chronic diseases carries important implications for the care of socially disadvantaged populations because they are more likely to suffer from comorbidity. For example, data from 314 practices in Scotland (covering 1.75 million patients, about 1/3 of the population) described the prevalence and association of chronic disease and mental health comorbidity with an area-level deprivation score [119]: Both mental illness and other chronic diseases share common life course origins such as adverse childhood experiences and stressful life events and environments. They are also linked in potentially reinforcing pathways, as mental disorders predispose to unhealthy behaviors, which lead to chronic diseases associated with pain or functional loss that worsen mental disorders [120]. A trial, in which trained nurses were embedded with primary care practices to coach patients and apply protocol-driven medication adjustments, found that patients reported better quality of life as well as lower depression scores and better control of blood pressure, lipids, and HbA1c levels [121].

Community-Level Action to Identify Social Patterns of Illness and Improve Outcomes

Given the profound impact of social determinants, it is critical to adequately invest in social policies that reduce inequities in living conditions. Attending to health and well-being can, in fact, pay economic dividends. For example, calculations for the Swedish population suggest an inequity "penalty" in the form of health care costs and decreased productivity amounting to 5–6% of GDP [122]. A crucial need to drive progress in preventing chronic disease is to situate accountability. A vision of what broad participation might entail describes an "accountability system" that brings together government, industry, and other interests who agree to benchmark and track progress, sets and enforces incentives or sanctions, and continuously modifies the accountability system in response [123] to how effectively it functions.

An example of such a system is the BIA-Australia Initiative Access to Nutrition Index [123], which tried to engage Australia's largest food and beverage producers to benchmark their obesity prevention and nutrition policies. An independent agency reports publicly every 2 years on corporations' performance in governance, product formulation, marketing, labeling, and other factors. In the 2016 report, 15 of the 22 companies evaluated earned 0% of their global sales on healthy products (or did not disclose the percentage), five earned less than 50%, and two earned more than 50%. The report makes candid assessments: "Many companies, particularly those headquartered in the U.S. (including General Mills, Kraft, Heinz, Kellogg Company and ConAgra), seem systematically to apply lower or no standards and less responsible practices in unregulated markets or those with low levels of regulation." (2016 report, p. 10). Such benchmarking efforts can document progress or make a case for enhancing governments' regulatory oversight [123].

The impact of reports like the Access to Nutrition Index hinges strongly on who is paying attention and their available response levers. Swinburn and colleagues have assembled a taxonomy of different accountability relationships for holding stakeholders to their commitments [124]. They examine the channels of accountability among government, civil society, and private sector stakeholders which is presented in Table 40.2.

Health Policy

Sectors beyond health care substantially influence health. Recognizing this, the 1986 Ottawa Charter declared that, "The prerequisites and prospects for health cannot be ensured by the health sector alone. More importantly, health promotion demands coordinated action by all concerned: by governments, by health and other social and economic sectors, by nongovernmental and voluntary organization, by local authorities, by industry and by the media. People in all walks of life are involved as individuals, families, and communities. Professional and social groups and health personnel have a major responsibility to mediate between differing interests in society for the pursuit of health" [125]. Many jurisdictions are implementing a "health in all policies

Table 40.2 Accountability system stakeholders and responsibilities[a]

	Government > private sector	Civil society > government	Civil society > private sector
Legal	Laws, regulation, monitoring, compliance, procurement	Formal inquiries, litigation	Consumer protections, litigation
Quasi-regulatory	Legislation, oversight of private sector initiatives	Codes of conduct, ethical guidelines, conflict-of-interest, disclosure of interactions	Codes of conduct, ethical guidelines, voluntary commitments
Political	Policy directions, inclusion of civil society in rule-making	Formal advisory committees	Shareholder activism
Market-based	Taxes, subsidies, concessions		Investment, disinvestment, boycotts
Public communications	Feedback to corporations via public media	Advocacy, polls, social media, watchdog organizations, demonstrations	Advocacy, polls, social media, watchdog organizations, demonstrations
Private communications	Private feedback from government officials	Private feedback to government officials	Private feedback from civil society

[a] Table abridged from Swinburn et al. [124] Arrows point away from the party seeking accountability toward the responsible party

(HiAP)" approach to governance [126]. Their objective is not to mandate that health impacts be decisive in policy decisions, but to incorporate health in the set of forecasted consequences. For example, in addition to estimating how much bicycle lanes might reduce traffic congestion, a municipality might project delayed onset of chronic disease among the projected users, as well as the net effect on road injuries. As most municipal functions have consequences for citizen's health, HiAP offers new perspectives when deciding how to allocate resources.

The degree to which governments support poverty reduction, education, public health, environmental protections, active transportation, fair wages, and other determinants influences population health [127]. It is impossible to perform controlled experiments in political and economic regimes, but case studies and comparative longitudinal observations offer important insights. Mortality trends in Russia after the Soviet Union dissolved present a stark example. Life expectancy dropped during 1990–1994, by 6 years for men and 3 years for women [128]. The spike in mortality was not limited to any narrow category of causes, but rather encompassed cardiovascular, infectious, neoplastic, alcohol-related, and violent causes of death.

The principal cause of increased mortality was cardiovascular deaths and hypothesized causal factors included large declines in per capita income, a resurgence in alcohol consumption, increased stress and depression, and the collapse of the health care system. Not surprisingly, the largest mortality increases were seen in the lowest educational groups, but other features were unexpected: persons 25–54 years of age experienced the steepest increase, and mortality increased disproportionately in the most urban and economically developed parts of Russia. A later analysis of mortality trends in 15 European Union nations from 1980–2005 revealed that social welfare spending, other than for healthcare, had the strongest relation with reductions in all-cause, cardiovascular, and alcohol-related deaths [129]. The financial crisis of 2008 demonstrated that economic policy can rapidly and powerfully influence health. In subsequent years, health outcomes were more favorable in the Nordic countries, who chose to invest in social protections, than in Greece and Spain, who implemented austerity measures [130].

Positively Impacting Social Determinants

Given the complexity of social determinants, it's important to seek system transformation commensurate with the challenges. Disadvantage is multidimensional. Economic insecurity, small social networks, and poor control over important life-domains tend to cluster together in families [131]. People who are economically insecure will trade-off their health to maintain their income, through over-work or not making time for health care. Disadvantage complicates decision-making. The many difficulties associated with poverty, such as impending income gaps or deciding which bills to pay when money is scarce, consume people's attention and impose a cognitive burden. In both experimental and field observations, cognitive burden temporarily impairs fluid intelligence and cognitive control [132]. Impaired decision-making and decreased agency stack the deck against realizing one's goals, especially when ingrained habits, prevalent customs, and power interests align to undermine them [133].

Capability: Addressing Social Determinants through Ethics, Measurement, and Action

Given the powerful role of social circumstances in shaping health, and in light of the central importance of health for realizing many other valuable goals—meaningful work, participating in community life, living long enough to nurture future generations, and many others—there is a strong basis for societal attention to health equity. Operationalizing equity by deciding what constitutes a "fair" and ethical allocation of resources has been a principal interest of political philosophers going back to Aristotle [134]. His view was that a just society seeks to provide all with the opportunity to flourish. A modern theory of justice, the Capability Approach (CA), defines flourishing in a person-centered frame: individuals' opportunity to pursue and achieve the outcomes they have reason to value [135]. This account of justice differs from others in which individuals are due a set of primary goods (e.g., income, freedom of speech, association, voting [136]) or fundamental liberties [137].

The core of the CA is that, to thrive, people need more than negative freedoms of the "no one is stopping you from eating healthy food" variety. People require positive freedoms in the form of feasible opportunities. What is feasible depends on individual circumstances. A common set of primary goods won't suffice for people whose disabilities or disempowerment limits their capacity to make use of them. Instead, the CA's chief proponents, Amartya Sen [138] and Martha Nussbaum [139] argue in favor of equitably distributed practical opportunities to live the life one values. Opportunities derive from two pre-conditions: that individuals have adequate resources in the

Fig. 40.2 Capability Approach framework. Abridged from Robeyns I. The Capability Approach: a theoretical survey. *Journal of Human Development.* Routledge; 2005;6(1):93–117

Resource (means to achieve) → Capabilities (opportunity to achieve) → Choice → Achievement

↑

Conversion factors

Abridged from Robeyns I. The Capability Approach: a theoretical survey. *Journal of Human Development.* Routledge; 2005;6(1):93–117.

environment and sufficient agency to take advantage of the resources.

Adequate opportunities allow people to choose from a set of potentially achieved states (the "capabilities" which give the framework its name) to be and do what they value, what Sen calls, "functionings" [138]. Focusing on the preconditions that create substantive opportunities, at both the individual and community levels, is what distinguishes the Capability Approach from other social justice frameworks. It is important to recognize that people's ethical claim in the CA is to feasible opportunities for health rather than health outcomes. With genuine opportunity, however, comes responsibility. To the extent that feasible opportunities are present, people are accountable for their health outcomes [9]. A final, critical point in the CA, is that personal circumstances such as literacy, disability, family support and other factors influence whether an individual can take advantage of available resources. These circumstances are known as "conversion factors."

To illustrate how the Capability Approach applies to chronic disease (Fig. 40.2), consider the practical opportunities necessary to buy and consume healthy food. The capability set of feasible opportunities is influenced by inputs that include relevant goods and services locally available (e.g., fresh produce), community resources (e.g., supermarket), and personal resources available to purchase food. Conversion factors including support for healthy eating within the household and health literacy for food selection and preparation are necessary to turn resources into achievement. In the final step, an individual chooses what to eat from the available opportunities. That choice is influenced by individual preferences, motivation, and social preference formation.

The CA rightly situates choice as contingent on opportunity: the choices one makes depends on the choices one has. How opportunities influence choice is documented in the literature on adaptive preferences, as people lower their aspirations when they see little chance to attain them [140]. At the policy level, the CA focuses on measures that support equitably available opportunities.

Recent studies set out to operationalize the Capability Approach for application in chronic disease prevention. A qualitative study in a disadvantaged neighborhood identified opportunities and constraints for diet and activity resources [141]. Figure 40.3 illustrates the prevalence of the diet and activity resources.

In a second cross-sectional study with 746 patients sampled from seven clinical sites across Texas, path modeling assessed if capability scales were associated with diet and activity intentions (i.e., choices), and three functionings: achieved diet, physical activity, and BMI. Capabilities predicted both behavioral intentions and functionings [142]. In a multiyear follow-up project, health capability assessments were implemented by community health workers in a primary care disease management program [143].

The Capability Approach (CA) offers several strengths as a guide for achieving health equity. First, it lays out a normative ethical framework for what societies should seek to equalize; practical opportunities for people to pursue the goals they value. In this regard, it is notable for focusing not only on the provision of resources but also on the extent people are able to make use of resources. It thus recognizes that both opportunity *and* agency are necessary to achieve outcomes, a perspective that sweeps away the unhelpful polarization of social versus personal responsibility for health. Second, it recognizes that health is both a desirable end in itself and an important resource to achieve other ends.

CA It encourages community deliberation about which capabilities should be prioritized [144]. It can also be operationalized as an evaluative framework to judge whether social justice is being achieved. Many efforts to measure capabilities in important domains have been fielded. These attributes align well with the Ottawa Charter on health promotion: "An individual or group must be able to identify and to realize aspirations, to satisfy needs, and to change or cope with the environment. Health is, therefore, seen as a resource for everyday life, not the sole objective of living. Health is a positive concept emphasizing social and personal resources, as well as physical capacities. Therefore, health promotion is not just the responsibility of the health sector but goes beyond healthy lifestyles to general well-being" [145].

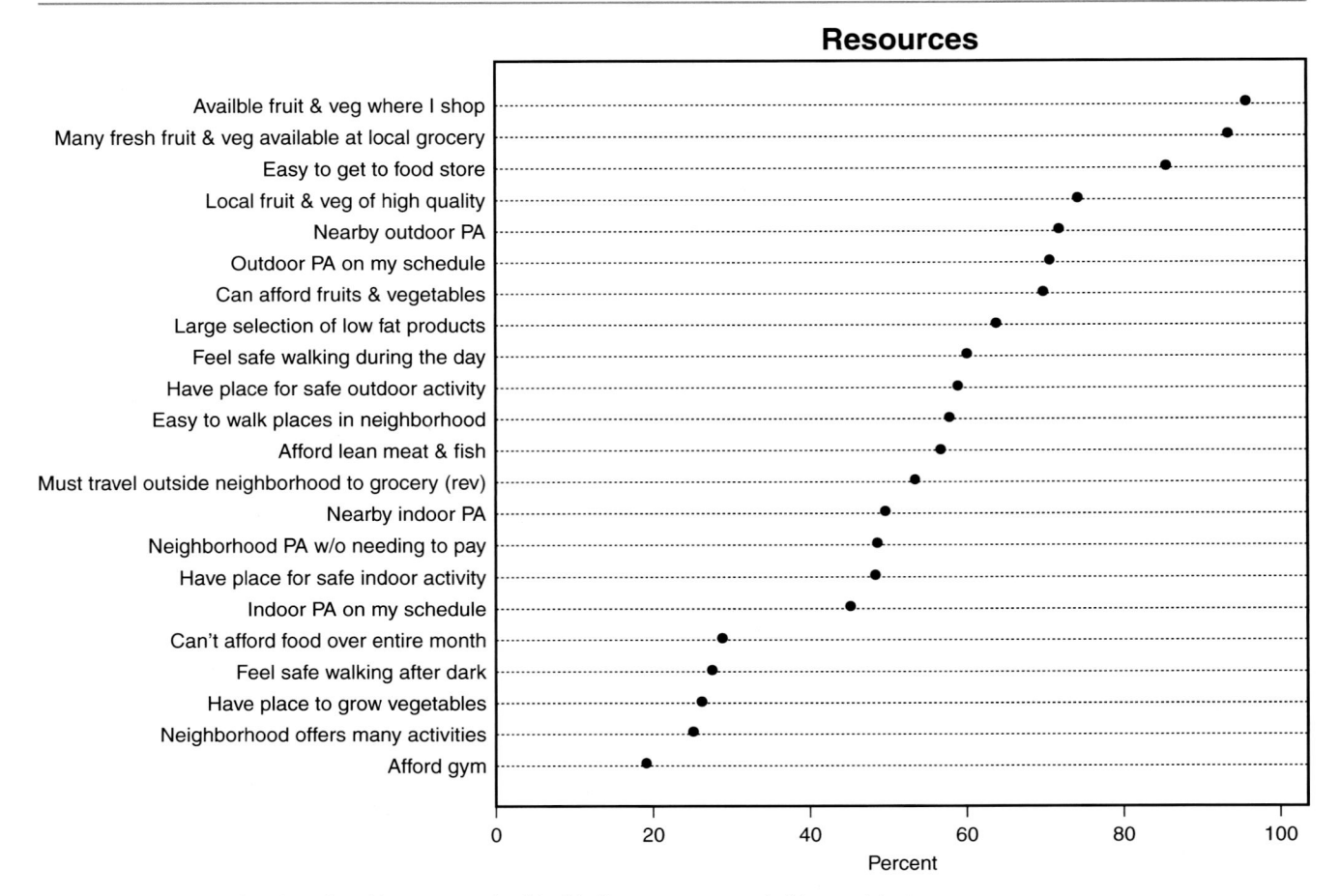

Fig. 40.3 Diet and activity resources in a vulnerable population

Final Comments

A fundamental concept of social determinants is that different health outcomes in different groups do not define inequity. Rather, inequity is judged by the process through which the outcomes are produced. Social, economic, and political forces structure the landscape of behavioral options that are available, affordable, convenient, and widely embraced, the landscape on which individuals with varying resources, constraints, abilities, and attitudes conduct their daily lives. These structured chances generate morbidity and mortality gradients across socially constructed categories including gender, social class, and race/ethnicity.

What we understand much less well, however, is how to move from documenting inequities to achieving equitable health outcomes. In part this has been due to scale mismatch: social determinants generate illness at the population scale while we have often tried to mitigate their behavioral effects in individual persons. Heavy reliance on interventions based on social cognitive models is partly to blame [146]. Often, affluent people enjoy default conditions that favor good outcomes, while the poor do not [147]. But there are other obstacles, including the complexity of sorting through multiple intersecting disadvantages to identify key leverage points. For example, not having access to a grocery store is a disadvantage, but when people from different income levels shop in the same store, the less affluent still tend to purchase less healthy foods [148]. Grocery store access removes one barrier, only to suggest others, such as affordability, nutrition literacy, time demands of food preparation, or susceptibility to marketing.

Progress on identifying effective leverage points calls for rebalancing research strategies. More observational studies documenting associations among social determinants and health outcomes will no longer suffice. In the words of the psychologist Kurt Lewin, "If you truly want to understand something, try to change it." Longitudinal studies and experiments will provide better insights on what works for change.

Table 40.3 Strategic levels for chronic disease prevention

Level	Characteristics	Questions
Components	Actors, physical elements, and subsystems present	What mechanisms do we use to bring about health behavior change?
Feedback	Information flow between actors and system	Who is following health disparities trends in the community? What authority do they have to address inequities?
Structure	Ways in which parts of the system are connected	Are community members involved in designing the systems meant to eliminate inequities?
Goals	Indicators that inform measurement and management	Do we prioritize health literacy or do we address the demand environment as well, for example, the misleading claims in food advertising?
Paradigm	Fundamental beliefs about the system	Is health viewed primarily as an individual or communal responsibility?

Such studies can—and often should—begin as small-scale experiments to ensure fit with local conditions and relationships before scaling up [149].

A critical decision is the extent to which we should seek to address downstream effects or SES itself. Given the difficulty of enacting policies that reduce social inequalities, it can appear more direct to focus on changing health behaviors. But the SES influences on health are so pervasive, that even after accounting for the effects of smoking, inactivity, high alcohol use, diabetes, hypertension, and obesity, employment in a low versus high status occupation is still associated with 26% greater mortality risk [150]. We also have lessons from longitudinal international comparisons demonstrating that increasing spending on social protections is associated with increases in life expectancy [151]. Addressing macro and micro environments is simultaneously necessary. In the U.S. for example, recent assessments estimate that 74% of the variance in life expectancy at birth is attributed to census tracts (which approximate neighborhood scale) rather than larger geographic units [152]. Movements such as Healthy Cities, 100 Million Healthier Lives, and others are diffusing community health improvement models emphasizing cycles of trial, learning, and scaling up.

What unifies the different streams of action on social determinants is the need to honor complexity: the embeddedness of chronic disease determinants in systems shaped by history, social and cultural norms, economic systems, and power hierarchies. Table 40.3 provides a list of strategic levels at which to intervene for chronic disease prevention [153].

Our individual and shared view of health as either a private or commonly held trust is a question that holds the key to success in promoting health, potentially moving us toward a time when the "social determinants of health" are invoked as the foundation of well-being rather than the root of our problems.

References

1. UNDP. Life expectancy at birth, 2019. United Nations Development Program; 2019. www.undp.org. Accessed 8 Aug 2022.
2. Stern BJ. Income and Health. Sci Soc. 1941;5(3):193–206.
3. Mackenbach JP. Politics is nothing but medicine at a larger scale: reflections on public health's biggest idea. J Epidemiol Community Health. 2009;63(3):181–4.
4. Julia C, Valleron AJ. Louis-Rene Villerme (1782-1863), a pioneer in social epidemiology: re-analysis of his data on comparative mortality in Paris in the early 19th century. J Epidemiol Community Health. 2011;65(8):666–70.
5. Acheson ED. Edwin Chadwick and the world we live in. Lancet. 1990;336(8729):1482–5.
6. Engels F. The condition of the working class in England. 1845. Am J Public Health. 2003;93(8):1246–9.
7. Organization), W H O Health. The World Health Report. Published online 1999.
8. Krieger N. Theories for social epidemiology in the 21st century: an ecosocial perspective. Int J Epidemiol. 2001;30:668–77.
9. Venkatapuram S. Health justice: an argument from the capabilities approach. Polity Press; 2011.
10. Krieger N. Epidemiology and the people's health. Oxford University Press; 2011.
11. Current cigarette smoking among U.S. adults aged 18 years and older. Centers for Disease Control and Prevention; 2022. https://www.cdc.gov/tobacco/campaign/tips/resources/data/cigarette-smoking-in-united-states.html.
12. Harper S, Strumpf E, Burris S, Smith GD, Lynch J. Do Mandatory Seat Belt Laws Affect Socioeconomic Inequalities in Seat Belt Use? 2012. https://papers.ssrn.com/abstract=2120120
13. Global Status Report on Noncommunicable Diseases. 2014. https://www.google.com/url?sa=t&rct=j&q=&esrc=s&source=web&cd=&ved=2ahUKEwjkmt7o5MH5AhVAomoFHacaCGUQFnoECBgQAQ&url=https%3A%2F%2Fapps.who.int%2Firis%2Fbitstream%2Fhandle%2F10665%2F148114%2F9789241564854_eng.pdf&usg=AOvVaw3sWrzc0WwwwmzNjBJ6Ahfz.

14. Commission on the Social Determinants of Health. Report of the WHO Commission on Social Determinants of Health; 2008. https://www.who.int/publications/i/item/WHO-IER-CSDH-08.1.
15. Whitehead M. The concepts and principles of equity and health. Int J Health Serv. 1992;31:545–66.
16. Portes A. Social capital: its origins and applications in modern sociology. Annu Rev Sociol. 1998;24:1–24.
17. Savage M, Devine F, Cunningham N, et al. A new model of social class? Findings from the BBC's great British class survey experiment. Sociology. 2013;47(2):219–50.
18. Kindig D, Stoddart G. What is population health? Am J Public Health. 2003;93(3):380–3.
19. Bonilla-Silva E. Rethinking racism: toward a structural interpretation. Am Sociol Rev. 1997;62(3):465–80.
20. Galobardes B. Indicators of socioeconomic position (part 1). J Epidemiol Community Health. 2006;60(1):7–12.
21. Bettez S. The social transformation of health inequities: understanding the discourse on health disparities in the United States. PhD Thesis. University of New Mexico; 2013.
22. Schwartz S, Susser E, Susser M. A future for epidemiology. Annu Rev Public Health. 1999;20:15–33.
23. Rose G. The strategy of preventive medicine. Oxford University Press; 1992.
24. Wu S, Powers S, Zhu W, Hannun YA. Substantial contribution of extrinsic risk factors to cancer development. Nature. 2015;529(7584):43–7.
25. Willett WC. Balancing life-style and genomics research for disease prevention. Science. 2002;296:695–7.
26. Eaton SB, Pike MC, Short RV, Lee NC, Trussell J. Women's reproductive cancers in evolutionary context. Q Rev Biol. 1994 Sep;69(3):353–67.
27. Robertson TL, Kato H, Rhoads GG, et al. Epidemiologic studies of coronary heart disease and stroke in Japanese men living in Japan, Hawaii and California. Am J Cardiol. 1977;39(2):239–43.
28. Flegal KM, Troiano RP. Changes in the distribution of body mass index of adults and children in the US population. Int J Obes Relat Metab Disord. 2000;24(7):807–18.
29. Rose G. Sick individuals and sick populations. Int J Epidemiol. 1985;14:32–8.
30. Marmot M. Social determinants of health inequalities. Lancet. 2005;365(9464):1099–104.
31. Marmot M, Wilkinson RG. Social determinants of health. 2nd ed. Oxford University Press; 2005.
32. Di Cesare M, Khang YH, Asaria P, et al. Inequalities in non-communicable diseases and effective responses. Lancet. 2013;381(9866):585–97.
33. Bauer UE, Bauer UE, Briss PA, et al. Prevention of chronic disease in the 21st century: elimination of the leading preventable causes of premature death and disability in the USA. Lancet. 2014;384(9937):45–52.
34. Link BG, Phelan JC. Social conditions as fundamental causes of disease. J Health Soc Behav. 1995;35:80–94.
35. Baker DW, Sudano JJ, Albert JM, Borawski EA, Dor A. Lack of health insurance and decline in overall health in late middle age. N Engl J Med. 2001;345(15):1106–12.
36. Bowles S, Gintis H. The inheritance of inequality. J Econ Perspect. 2002;16(3):3–30.
37. Haas SA. Health selection and the process of social stratification: the effect of childhood health on socioeconomic attainment. J Health Soc Behav. 2006;47(4):339–54.
38. Saez E. Striking it Richer: the evolution of top incomes in the United States 2018 (book chapter). In Grusky D, Hill J, editors. Inequality in the 21st Century. Routledge; 2018.
39. Wilkinson RG. Income distribution and life expectancy. BMJ. 1992;304(6820):165–8.
40. Lynch JW, Smith GD, Kaplan GA, House JS. Income inequality and mortality: importance to health of individual income, psychosocial environment, or material conditions. BMJ. 2000;320(7243):1200–4.
41. Pickett KE, Wilkinson RG. Income inequality and health: a causal review. Soc Sci Med. 2015;128:316–26.
42. Oliver M, Shapiro T. Black wealth/white wealth. 2nd ed. Routledge; 2006.
43. Sampson RJ, Bean L. Cultural mechanisms and killing fields: a revised theory of community-level racial inequality. In: Peterson RD, Krivo LJ, Hagan J, editors. The many colors of crime: inequalities of race, ethnicity, and crime in America. New York University Press; 2006.
44. Gandhi K, Lim E, Davis J, Chen JJ. Racial-ethnic disparities in self-reported health status among US adults adjusted for sociodemographics and multimorbidities, national health and nutrition examination survey 2011-2014. Ethn Health. 2020;25(1):65–78. https://doi.org/10.1080/13557858.2017.1395812.
45. Mokdad AH, Marks JS, Stroup DF, Geberding JL. Actual causes of death in the United States. JAMA. 2004;291:1238–45.
46. Wang DD, Leung CW, Li Y, et al. Trends in dietary quality among adults in the United States, 1999 through 2010. JAMA Intern Med. 2014;174(10):1587.
47. Centers for Disease Control and Prevention. Morbidity and Mortality Weekly Report. CDC Health Disparities and Inequalities Report, United States, 2013; 2013.
48. World Health Organization. WHO report on the global tobacco epidemic, 2008. 2008: The MPOWER Package.
49. Sud SR, Brenner JE, Shaffer ER. Trading away health: the influence of trade policy on youth tobacco control. J Pediatr. 2015;166(5):1303–7.
50. Brandt AM. Inventing conflicts of interest: a history of tobacco industry tactics. Am J Public Health. 2012;102(1):63–71. https://doi.org/10.2105/AJPH.2011.300292.
51. Mozaffarian D. Book: the politics and science of soda and our health. Lancet. 2016;387:2192–3.
52. Grier SA, Kumanyika SK. The context for choice: health implications of targeted food and beverage marketing to African Americans. Am J Public Health. 2008;98(9):1616–29.
53. Cutler DM, Glaeser EL. Why have Americans become more obese? J Econ Perspect. 2003;17:93–118.
54. Loprinzi PD, Branscum A, Hanks J, Smit E. Healthy lifestyle characteristics and their joint association with cardiovascular disease biomarkers in US adults. Mayo Clin Proc. 2016;91(4):432–42.
55. McEwen BS. Protective and damaging effects of stress mediators. N Engl J Med. 1998;338:171–9.
56. Barker DJP, Osmond C, Forsén TJ, Kajantie E, Eriksson JG. Trajectories of growth among children who have coronary events as adults. N Engl J Med. 2005;353(17):1802–9.
57. Barker D, Osmond C, Winter PD, Margetts B. Weight in infancy and death from ischaemic heart disease. Lancet. 1989;334:577–80.
58. Doblhammer G, Vaupel JW. Lifespan depends on month of birth. Proc Natl Acad Sci U S A. 2001;98(5):2934.
59. Case A, Paxson C. The long reach of childhood health and circumstance: evidence from the Whitehall II study*. Econ J. 2011;121(554):F183–204.
60. Danese A, Moffitt TE, Harrington H, et al. Adverse childhood experiences and adult risk factors for age-related disease: depression, inflammation, and clustering of metabolic risk markers. Arch Pediatr Adolesc Med. 2009;163(12):1135–43.
61. Miller GE, Chen E, Fok AK, Walker H. Low early-life social class leaves a biological residue manifested by decreased glucocorticoid and increased proinflammatory signaling. PNAS. 2009;106:14716–21.

62. Lumey LH, Stein AD. Offspring birth weights after maternal intrauterine undernutrition: a comparison within sibships. Am J Epidemiol. 1997;146(10):810–9.
63. Heijmans BT, Tobi EW, Stein AD, et al. Persistent epigenetic differences associated with prenatal exposure to famine in humans. Proc Natl Acad Sci U S A. 2008;105(44):17046–9.
64. Malter Cohen M, Malter Cohen M, Jing D, et al. Early-life stress has persistent effects on amygdala function and development in mice and humans. Proc Natl Acad Sci U S A. 2013;110(45):18274–8.
65. Weber M. From max weber. In Gerth HH, Mills CW, editors. Routledge; 2009.
66. Turner RJWB, Lloyd DA. The epidemiology of social stress. Am Sociol Rev. 1995;60:104–25.
67. Merton RK. Am Sociol Rev. 1938;3:672–82.
68. Pearlin LI. The sociological study of stress. J Health Soc Behav. 1989;30:241–56.
69. Almeida DM. Resilience and vulnerability to daily stressors assessed via diary methods. Curr Dir Psychol Sci. 2005;14(2):64–8.
70. Sapolsky RM. Why Zebras don't get ulcers. Barnes and Noble Books; 1998.
71. Seeman TE, McEwen BS. Impact of social environment characteristics on neuroendocrine regulation. Psychosom Med. 1996;58:459–71.
72. Bird CE, Seeman T, Escarce JJ, et al. Neighbourhood socioeconomic status and biological "wear and tear" in a nationally representative sample of US adults. J Epidemiol Community Health. 2010;64(10):860–5.
73. Conti G, Heckman J, Urzua S. The education-health gradient. Am Econ Rev. 2010;100(2):234–8.
74. National Research Council. From Neurons to Neighborhoods: the Science of Early Childhood Development; 2000.
75. Phelan JC, Link BG, Diez Roux A, Kawachi I, Levin B. "Fundamental causes" of social inequalities in mortality: a test of the theory. J Health Soc Behav. 2004;45:265–85.
76. Pickett KE, Luo Y, Lauderdale DS. Widening social inequalities in risk for sudden infant death syndrome. Am J Public Health. 2005;95(11):1976–81.
77. Townsend P. Why are the many poor? Int J Health Serv. 1995;16(1):1–32.
78. Gilens M. Inequality and democratic responsiveness. Public Opin Q. 2005;69(5):778.
79. Bartels LM. The social welfare deficit: public opinion, policy responsiveness, and political inequality in affluent democracies. In 22nd Int Conf Eur. https://scholar.google.com/scholar?hl=en&as_sdt=0%2C44&q=bartels+the+social+welfare+deficit&btnG=.
80. Susser M, Susser EY. Choosing a future for epidemiology: II: from black box to Chinese boxes and eco-epidemiology. Am J Public Health. 1996;86:674–7.
81. McMichael AJ. Prisoners of the proximate: loosening the constraints on epidemiology in an age of change. Am J Epidemiol. 1999;149(10):887–97.
82. Pampel FC, Denney JT, Krueger PM. Obesity, SES, and economic development: a test of the reversal hypothesis. Soc Sci Med. 2012;74(7):1073–81.
83. Giddens A. The constitution of society: outline of the theory of structuration. University of California Press; 1984.
84. Nguyen C, Barkin S. Where standardized meets personalized when integrating social determinants of health into the electronic health record. Pediatr Res. 2022;91:1645–6.
85. Irwin A, Scali E. Action on the social determinants of health: learning from previous experiences. World Health Organization; 2010.
86. Kark S. From medicine in the community to community medicine. JAMA. 1974;228:1585–6.
87. World Health Organization Regional Office for Europe. Declaration of Alma-Ata, 1978. https://www.who.int/teams/social-determinants-of-health/declaration-of-alma-ata.
88. Oberlander J, Laugesen MJ. Leap of faith—Medicare's new physician payment system. N Engl J Med. 2015;373(13):1185–7.
89. Alley DE, Asomugha CN, Conway PH, Sanghavi DM. Accountable health communities–addressing social needs through Medicare and Medicaid. N Engl J Med. 2016;374(1):8–11.
90. Committee on Health Literacy, Board on Population Health and Public Health Practice, Board on Health Care Services, Health and Medicine Division, National Academies of Sciences, Engineering, and Medicine. In: Kwan LY, Stratton K, Steinwachs DM, editors. Accounting for social risk factors in Medicare payment. National Academies Press; 2017.
91. Committee on Integrating Social Needs Care into the Delivery of Health Care to Improve the Nation's Health, Board on Health Care Services, Health and Medicine Division, National Academies of Sciences, Engineering, and Medicine. Integrating social care into the delivery of health care. National Academies Press; 2019.
92. Kung A, Cheung T, Knox M, et al. Capacity to address social needs affects primary care clinician burnout. Ann Fam Med. 2019;17(6):487–94.
93. Garg A, Sheldrick RC, Dworkin PH. The inherent fallibility of validated screening tools for social determinants of health. Acad Pediatr. 2018;18(2):123–4.
94. De Marchis EH, Hessler D, Fichtenberg C, et al. Part I: a quantitative study of social risk screening acceptability in patients and caregivers. Am J Prev Med. 2019;57(6, Supplement 1):S25–37.
95. Holcomb J, Highfield L, Ferguson GM, Morgan RO. Association of social needs and healthcare utilization among Medicare and Medicaid beneficiaries in the accountable health communities model. J Gen Intern Med. 2022;37(14):3692–9. https://doi.org/10.1007/s11606-022-07403-w.
96. Chagin K, Choate F, Cook K, Fuehrer S, Misak JE, Sehgal AR. A framework for evaluating social determinants of health screening and referrals for assistance. J Prim Care Community Health. 2021;12:21501327211052204. https://doi.org/10.1177/21501327211052204.
97. Eder M, Henninger M, Durbin S, et al. Screening and interventions for social risk factors: technical brief to support the US Preventive Services Task Force. JAMA. 2021;326(14):1416–28. https://doi.org/10.1001/jama.2021.12825.
98. De Marchis, EH, Brown, E, Aceves, B, et al. State of the Science of Screening in Healthcare Settings. Social Interventions Research and Evaluation Network; 2022. https://sirenetwork.ucsf.edu/tools-resources/resources/state-science-social-screening-healthcare-settings. Accessed 5 Aug 2022.
99. Solberg LI. Theory vs practice: should primary care practice take on social determinants of health now? No Ann Fam Med. 2016;14(2):102–3.
100. Long CL, Franklin SM, Hagan AS, et al. Health-related social needs among older adults enrolled in Medicare advantage. Health Aff (Millwood). 2022;41(4):557–62. https://doi.org/10.1377/hlthaff.2021.01547.
101. Rosenthal TC. The medical home: growing evidence to support a new approach to primary care. J Am Board Fam Med. 2008;21(5):427.
102. Bachrach D, Guyer J, Levin A. Medicaid coverage of social interventions: a road map for states. Milbank Issue Brief. 2016. https://www.milbank.org/publications/medicaid-coverage-social-interventions-road-map-states/.
103. Bachrach D, Pfister H, Wallis K, Lipson M. ADDRESSING PATIENTS' SOCIAL NEEDS; 2014. https://www.commonwealthfund.org/sites/default/files/documents/___media_files_publications_fund_report_2014_may_1749_bachrach_addressing_patients_social_needs_v2.pdf.

104. Redding S, Conrey E, Porter K, Paulson J, Hughes K, Redding M. Pathways community care coordination in low birth weight prevention. Matern Child Health J. 2014;19(3):643–50.
105. Ferrer RL, Gonzalez Schlenker C, Lozano Romero R, et al. Advanced Primary Care in San Antonio: linking practice and community strategies to improve health. J Am Board Fam Med. 2013;26(3):288–98.
106. Escobar ER. Screening and referral care delivery services and unmet health-related social needs: a systematic review. Prev Chronic Dis. 2021:18. https://doi.org/10.5888/pcd18.200569.
107. Smedley BD, Stith AY, Nelson AR, Institute of Medicine. Unequal treatment: confronting racial and ethnic disparities in healthcare. National Academy Press; 2002.
108. Chapman EN, Kaatz A, Carnes M. Physicians and implicit bias: how doctors may unwittingly perpetuate health care disparities. J Gen Intern Med. 2013;28(11):1504–10.
109. Gaskin DJ, Zare H, Haider AH, LaVeist TA. The quality of surgical and pneumonia care in minority-serving and racially integrated hospitals. Health Serv Res. 2016;51(3):910–36.
110. Gaskin DJ, Spencer CS, Richard P, Anderson G, Powe NR, LaVeist TA. Do minority patients use lower quality hospitals? Inquiry. 2011;48(3):209–20.
111. National Academy of Science, Engineering, Medicine. Systems practices for the care of socially at-risk populations. National Academies Press; 2016.
112. AMA Ad Hoc Report on Health Literacy for the Council on Scientific Affairs. JAMA. 1999;281:552–57.
113. DeWalt D, Berkman ND, Sheridan S, Lohr KN, Pignone MP. Literacy and health outcomes: a systematic review of the literature. J Gen Intern Med. 2004;19:1228–39.
114. Institute of Medicine (US) Roundtable on Health Literacy. Measures of health literacy: workshop summary. National Academies Press (US); 2009.
115. Whiteford HA, Degenhardt L, Rehm J, et al. Global burden of disease attributable to mental and substance use disorders: findings from the Global Burden of Disease Study 2010. Lancet. 2013;382(9904):1575–86.
116. Moussavi S, Chatterji S, Verdes E, Tandon A, Patel V, Ustun B. Depression, chronic diseases, and decrements in health: results from the World Health Surveys. Lancet. 2007;370(9590):851–8.
117. Kessler RC, Ormel J, Demler O, Stang PE. Comorbid mental disorders account for the role impairment of commonly occurring chronic physical disorders: results from the national comorbidity survey. J Occup Environ Med. 2003;45(12):1257–66.
118. Harris KM, Woolf SH, Gaskin DJ. High and rising working-age mortality in the US: a report from the National Academies of Sciences, Engineering, and Medicine. JAMA. 2021;325(20):2045–6. https://doi.org/10.1001/jama.2021.4073.
119. Barnett K, Mercer SW, Norbury M, Watt G, Wyke S, Guthrie B. Epidemiology of multimorbidity and implications for health care, research, and medical education: a cross-sectional study. Lancet. 2012;380(9836):37–43.
120. Patel V, Chatterji S. Integrating mental health in care for noncommunicable diseases: an imperative for person-centered care. Health Aff Proj Hope. 2015;34(9):1498–505.
121. Katon WJ, Lin EHB, Von Korff M, et al. Collaborative care for patients with depression and chronic illnesses. N Engl J Med. 2010;363(27):2611–20.
122. Jessop, B. Malmo C for a SS. Malmö's Path towards a Sustainable Future: Health, Welfare and Justice. Socialmedicinsk tidskrift. 2013. https://www.google.com/url?sa=t&rct=j&q=&esrc=s&source=web&cd=&ved=2ahUKEwiAj6GkiML5AhW0mmoFHRmVCYMQFnoECAgQAQ&url=http%3A%2F%2Fsocialmedicinsktidskrift.se%2Findex.php%2Fsmt%2Farticle%2Fdownload%2F1259%2F1050&usg=AOvVaw0h5xhp4Lc07yscBuLlfQs1.
123. Robinson E, Blake MR, Sacks G. Benchmarking food and beverage companies on obesity prevention and nutrition policies: evaluation of the BIA-Obesity Australia Initiative, 2017-2019. Int J Health Policy Manag. 2021;10(Special Issue on Political Economy of Food Systems):857-70. https://doi.org/10.34172/ijhpm.2020.147.
124. Swinburn B, Kraak V, Rutter H, et al. Strengthening of accountability systems to create healthy food environments and reduce global obesity. Lancet. 2015;385(9986):2534–45.
125. WHO. Ottawa Charter for Health Promotion. 1986.
126. Wernham A, Teutsch SM. Health in all policies for big cities. J Public Health Manag Pract. 2015;21:S56–65.
127. Stuckler D, Siegel K. Sick societies: responding to the global challenge of chronic diseases. Oxford University Press; 2011.
128. Leon DA, Chenet L, Shkolnikov VM, et al. Huge variation in Russian mortality rates 1984-94: artefact, alcohol, or what? Lancet. 1997;350:388.
129. Stuckler D, Basu S. The body economic. Basic Books; 2013.
130. Karanikolos M, Mladovsky P, Cylus J, et al. Financial crisis, austerity, and health in Europe. Lancet. 2013;381(9874):1323–31.
131. Wolff J. Disadvantage, risk and the social determinants of health. Public Health Ethics. 2009;2(3):214–23.
132. Mani A, Mullainathan S, Shafir E, Zhao J. Poverty impedes cognitive function. Science. 2013;341(6149):976–80.
133. Zimmerman FJ. Habit, custom, and power: a multi-level theory of population health. Soc Sci Med. 2013;80:47–56.
134. Lord C. Aristotle's "Politics". University of Chicago Press; 2013.
135. Sen A, Hawthorn G. The standard of living. Cambridge University Press; 1988.
136. Rawls J. A theory of justice. Harvard University Press; 2009.
137. Nozick R. Anarchy, State, and Utopia. Basic Books; 1974.
138. Sen A. Inequality reexamined. Oxford University Press; 1992.
139. Nussbaum MC. Creating capabilities. Belknap Press; 2011.
140. Dalton PS, Ghosal S, Mani A. Poverty and aspirations failure. Econ J. 2015;126(590):165–88.
141. Ferrer RL, Cruz I, Burge S, Bayles B, Castilla MI. Measuring capability for healthy diet and physical activity. Ann Fam Med. 2014;12(1):46–56.
142. Ferrer RL, Burge SK, Palmer RF, Cruz I, The RRNeT Investigators. Practical opportunities for healthy diet and physical activity: relationship to intentions, behaviors, and body mass index. Ann Fam Med. 2016;14(2):109–16.
143. Ferrer RL, Gonzalez Schlenker C, Cruz I, et al. Community health workers as trust builders and healers: a cohort study in primary care. Ann Fam Med. 2022;20(5):438–45.
144. Frahsa A, Abel T, Gelius P, Rütten A, the Capital4Health Research Consortium. The capability approach as a bridging framework across health promotion settings: theoretical and empirical considerations. Health Promot Int. 2021;36(2):493–504.
145. WHO.The Ottawa Charter for Health Promotion. 1986.
146. Ogden J. Some problems with social cognition models: a pragmatic and conceptual analysis. Health Psychol. 2003;22(4):424–8.
147. Duflo E. Human values and the design of the fight against poverty. 2012.
148. Handbury J, Rahkovsky I, Schnell M. What drives nutritional disparities? Retail access and food purchases across the socioeconomic spectrum. NBER Working Paper 21126; 2015. http://www.nber.org/papers/w21126

149. Rydin Y, Bleahu A, Davies M, et al. Shaping cities for health: complexity and the planning of urban environments in the 21st century. Lancet. 2012;379(9831):2079–108.
150. Stringhini S, Dugravot A, Shipley M, et al. Health behaviours, socioeconomic status, and mortality: further analyses of the British Whitehall II and the French GAZEL prospective cohorts. PLoS Med. 2011;8(2):e1000419.
151. Beckfield J, Bambra C. Shorter lives in stingier states: social policy shortcomings help explain the US mortality disadvantage. Soc Sci Med. 2016;171:30–8. https://doi.org/10.1016/j.socscimed.2016.10.017.
152. Boing AF, Boing AC, Cordes J, Kim R, Subramanian SV. Quantifying and explaining variation in life expectancy at census tract, county, and state levels in the United States. Proc Natl Acad Sci. 2020;117(30):17688–94. https://doi.org/10.1073/pnas.2003719117.
153. Meadows DH. Thinking in systems: a primer. Chelsea Green Publishing; 2008.

Environmental Determinants of Health

41

Michelle Del Rio and Jacqueline MacDonald Gibson

Introduction

Since the discovery of DNA's structure in 1953, researchers have debated the relative influence of genetic versus environmental factors as determinants of health. Estimates of the environmental contribution to disease have ranged from as low as 13% [1] to as high as 90% [2]. These differences arise in part due to varying definitions of "environment." For example, a recent World Health Organization (WHO) assessment of the environmental contribution to preventable disease defined the environment as including "exposure to pollution and chemicals (e.g., air, water soil products), physical exposures (e.g., noise, radiation), the built environment, other anthropogenic changes (e.g., climate change, vector breeding places), related behaviors and the work environment" [1]. The WHO estimates that 13–32% of the global disease burden is attributable to these environmental determinants. In contrast, thought leaders have suggested that in the extreme, all diseases are environmental because "genetic factors are actually also environmental, but merely on a different time scale" [3]. An intermediate viewpoint defines the environment as all factors external to the genome. However, based in part on prior studies of twins that computed the fraction of diseases attributable to genetic versus non-genetic factors, somewhere between 70 and 90% of disease risks may be attributable to differences in environments [2].

This chapter adopts a perspective of environmental determinants of health consistent with that of the WHO; it focuses on chronic diseases related to pollutants in outdoor air, household indoor air, workplaces, and drinking water and also on diseases potentially affected by climate change. Like the WHO, lead exposure—which can occur through ingestion of dust, soil, air, water, or food—is considered as an environmental determinant. In addition, consistent with the concept of the built environment as a health determinant, the chapter provides evidence of the adverse health impacts that were unintentionally created through automobile-centric urban designs in the post-World War II era. The chapter highlights the environmental factors that are potentially modifiable by individual behaviors or public policies, areas which clinicians may be able to influence.

The chapter begins with an overview of how WHO and others have estimated the burden of chronic diseases attributable to environmental factors. Next, it provides background information on the environmental determinants included in this discussion: outdoor air pollution, household air pollution, water pollution, occupational exposure to hazardous materials, lead exposure, built environments that discourage physical activity, and health outcomes related to climate change. The final section provides guidance for clinicians on identifying and managing environmental determinants in health care practice.

M. Del Rio
Indiana University School of Public Health,
Bloomington, IN, USA
e-mail: midelrio@iu.edu

J. MacDonald Gibson (✉)
Department of Civil, Construction, and Environmental Engineering, North Carolina State University,
Raleigh, USA
e-mail: jmacdon@ncsu.edu

Estimating the Burden of Disease Attributable to Environmental Determinants

In 1990, the World Bank commissioned the first comprehensive study to characterize the contribution of various risk factors to preventable diseases in order to help define intervention approaches and strategies for countries in different development stages [4]. Carried out by the WHO and published in 1996, the study assessed the global and regional disease burden attributable to ten different risk factors, including four environmental determinants: poor water supply and sanitation, air pollution, occupational exposures, and low physical activity [4, 5]. A follow-up burden of disease study, published in 2004, added an additional 16 risk factors [6]. Subsequent updates were published in 2015 and more recently in 2020 by the Institute for Health Metrics and Evaluation (IHME) [7–9]. The IHME's Global Burden of Diseases, Injuries, and Risk Factors Study 2019 (referred to as GBD 2019) identified 87 risk factors, including two new environmental risk factors: high and low, non-optimal temperatures potentially related to climate change [9]. The global studies have led to similar efforts at national and regional scales, such as in Canada [10], the United Arab Emirates [11–13], and Europe [14]. No comprehensive environmental burden of disease study is available for the United States, apart from the estimates included in IHME's report.

Method for Estimating the Environmental Burden of Disease

All global disease projects associated with environmental burden, and their national-level counterparts, have used a similar process that involves combining epidemiologic, environmental, and public health data. Disease burden studies begin by compiling evidence linking exposure to a given risk factor to specific health outcomes. Typically, these risk factor-disease pairs are identified through a comprehensive review of epidemiologic studies. Table 41.1 summarizes the health outcomes linked to risk factors, as determined from a review of previous global burden of disease studies [7, 8, 15].

Table 41.1 Selected environmental determinants of health

Risk Factor	Associated Health Outcomes
Built environment not conducive to walking or cycling for transportation (leading to low physical activity)	breast cancer colorectal cancer diabetes ischemic heart disease ischemic stroke
Outdoor air pollution (particulate matter and ozone)	chronic obstructive pulmonary disease (COPD) ischemic heart disease lower respiratory infections lung cancer stroke
Lead exposure (via corrosive water, soil, dust, and/or food)	intellectual disability (children) high blood pressure (adults) chronic kidney disease (adults)
Household air pollution from second-hand smoke	hemorrhagic stroke ischemic heart disease ischemic stroke lower respiratory infections (children) lung cancer otitis media (children)
Household air pollution from radon	lung cancer
Occupational carcinogens	lung cancer ovarian cancer leukemia nasopharynx cancer
Occupational particulate matter	COPD
Occupational asthmagens	asthma
Waterborne carcinogens	bladder cancer lung/bronchus cancer (arsenic) all cancer (gross alpha radiation)
Waterborne pathogens	diarrheal diseases
High or low non-optimal temperatures	ischemic heart disease stroke hypertensive heart disease diabetes chronic kidney disease lower respiratory infections death

Once risk factor-health outcome relationships are determined, the next step is to estimate a quantity known as the population attributable fraction (*AF*)—the fraction of observed diseases that could be prevented if exposure to a specific risk factor was mitigated. *AF* can be estimated from the following equation [11–13, 16, 17]:

$$AF = \frac{\int_{x=0}^{m} RR(x)P(x)dx - \int_{x=0}^{m} RR(x)P'(x)dx}{\int_{x=0}^{m} RR(x)P(x)dx} \quad (41.1)$$

where x is the pollutant exposure concentration or dose, $RR(x)$ is the relative risk of an adverse health outcome at exposure concentration or dose x, $P(x)$ is the current population exposure distribution, and $P'(x)$ is an alternative (or counterfactual) exposure distribution. When the exposure is eliminated, then $RR(x = 0) = 1$, and the integral on the right side of the numerator reduces to 1. The number of observed cases attributable to the exposure of concern (D_{attrib}) then can be calculated from

$$D_{attrib} = AF \times D_{total} \quad (41.2)$$

where D_{total} is the total number of observed cases. Relative risk functions for each exposure and health outcome are estimated from meta-analyses or systematic reviews of prior epidemiologic studies. The population distribution of exposure is typically estimated from a combination of environmental data collected by state and federal agencies, along with behavioral data from a number of sources, such as the Behavioral Risk Factor Surveillance System [18].

To provide a common metric for comparing disparate health outcomes, such as premature mortality and chronic diabetes, or chronic diabetes and chronic asthma, the WHO developed a concept called the disability-adjusted life year (DALY). The DALY combines two quantities: the years of life lost due to premature mortality (*YLL*) and the years of life lived with "disability" (*YLD*). For each affected population age group, these quantities are calculated as

$$YLD = I \times DW \times L \quad (41.3)$$

$$YLL = N \times L \quad (41.4)$$

where I is the annual number of incident cases, L is the illness duration (for *YLD*) or the remaining life expectancy at the age of death (for *YLL*), and *DW* is the "disability weight," intended to represent the relative level of discomfort and interference with daily activities of life from each disease. The WHO and other organizations have developed standard disability weights for different conditions. The weights are developed from surveys asking health professionals how many imaginary patients with a specific condition they would trade for off 1000 healthy, imaginary people [5]. Table 41.2 shows disability weights for some of the health outcomes discussed in this chapter as used in 2019 Global Burden of Disease Study.

Table 41.2 Selected disability weights used in the GBD 2019 study

Sequela	Disability weight
Mild diarrheal diseases	0.074
Moderate diarrheal diseases	0.188
Severe diarrheal diseases	0.247
Mild idiopathic developmental intellectual disability	0.043
Moderate lower respiratory infections	0.051
Severe lower respiratory infections	0.133
Mild upper respiratory infections	0.006
Moderate upper respiratory infections	0.051
COPD and other mild chronic respiratory problems	0.019
Diagnosis and primary therapy phase of colon and rectum cancers	0.288
Diagnosis and primary therapy phase of lung, bronchus, and trachea cancer	0.288
Diagnosis and primary therapy phase of acute or chronic lymphoid leukemia	0.288
Diabetic foot due to neuropathy due to diabetes mellitus type 1 or type 2	0.15
Uncomplicated diabetes mellitus type 2	0.049
Stage 3 chronic kidney disease and moderate anemia due to hypertension	0.052
Diabetic neuropathy and amputation without treatment due to diabetes mellitus type 1 or type 2	0.282
Blindness due to diabetes mellitus type 1 or type 2 retinopathy	0.187
Moderate angina due to ischemic heart disease	0.08
Severe angina due to ischemic heart disease	0.167
Moderate heart failure due to ischemic heart disease	0.072
Severe heart failure due to ischemic heart disease	0.179
Acute ischemic stroke severity level 1	0.019
Acute ischemic stroke severity level 2	0.07
Acute ischemic stroke severity level 3	0.316
Controlled asthma	0.015
Partially controlled asthma	0.036
Uncontrolled asthma	0.133

Current Estimates of the Environmental Burden of Disease

Globally, the most recent burden of disease estimates attributed 14 million annual deaths (40.1% of total deaths) and 416 million DALYs (34.3% of the global total) in the year 2019 to environmental determinants discussed in this chapter. The published global estimate provides details for 204 countries and territories, including the United States, and compares three time periods (1990, 2010, and 2019). Figure 41.1 combines 2019 IHME estimates of the U.S. burden of disease from non-optimal temperatures, exposure to pollutants in the workplace, outdoor air pollution, household air pollution, built environment factors (through their influence on low physical activity), and environmental lead with recent U.S.-specific estimates of the disease burden from

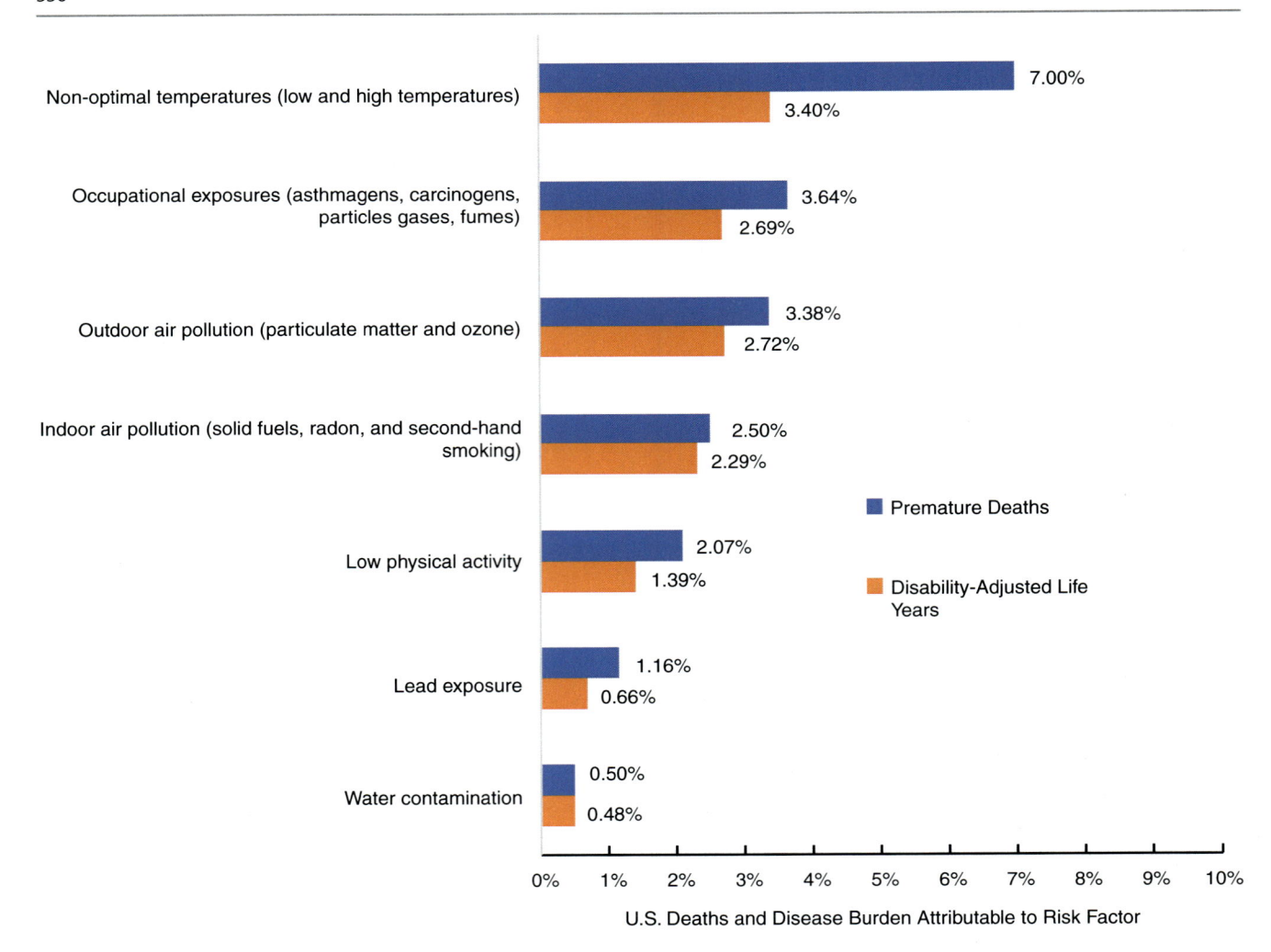

Fig. 41.1 Estimated contribution of environmental determinants to premature deaths and disability-adjusted life years in the United States

water pollution. Using these data, an estimated 363,000 U.S. deaths (20.3% of all deaths) and 7.14 million DALYs (13.6% of the total) are attributable to these determinants. The following sections provide background information on each respective determinant.

Outdoor Air Pollution

Deadly smogs in Donora, Pennsylvania, in 1948 and London in 1952 spurred research to understand the impacts of air pollution on public health in the United States and Europe [19, 20]. In Donora, a smog so thick that daytime was as dark as night sickened about half of the population of 14,000 and led to 20 deaths [19]. In London, a similar smog led to a death toll estimated at the time to be 4000; later reanalysis placed the toll as high as 12,000 [20].

A large body of epidemiological, toxicological, and clinical research since the smogs of the mid-twentieth century has provided strong evidence linking adverse health impacts to exposure to three categories of common air pollutants: particulate matter (PM), ozone (O_3), and nitrogen dioxide (NO_2) [20, 21]. All three pollutants are strong oxidants that can affect health directly through oxidation of lipids and proteins and indirectly through activation of intracellular oxidant pathways [22]. Strong evidence supports causal associations between these pollutants and all-cause mortality, cerebrovascular disease (including stroke), ischemic heart disease, chronic obstructive pulmonary disease (COPD), lower respiratory tract infections, and trachea, bronchus, and lung cancers. Evidence also supports associations with bronchitis in children and adults and with elevated incidence of asthma symptoms in asthmatic children [23]. Today, climate change impacts reflected by wildfires, extreme heat, and longer warm seasons are exacerbating health risks associated with ambient air pollution [24–26].

The GBD 2019 study estimated that more than 4.5 million deaths (12.9% of total deaths) and 124.4 million DALYs

(10.3% of total DALYs) globally were attributable to ambient air pollution [9]. For the United States, GBD 2019 attributed 60,572 deaths (3.4% the total) and 1.4 million DALYs (2.7% of the total) to outdoor air pollution. To avoid double-counting due to the co-occurrence of pollutants, these estimates include only risks from particulate matter and ozone pollution, so estimates should be considered conservative.

According to GBD 2019, there has been little to no progress in the past decade in decreasing health risks associated with ambient air pollution [9]. Globally, risks from particulate matter pollution increased 1.46% (95% confidence interval 0.81–2.10%) per year between 2010 and 2019. Risks from ambient ozone increased 0.15% per year, on average, though this estimate was not statistically significant (95% confidence interval −0.10 to 1.08).

Indoor Air Pollution

Insufficient ventilation has been recognized as dangerous to health since Biblical times. However, until relatively recently, concerns about indoor air quality were driven by the need for odor control and comfort [27, 28]. During the 1980s, however, indoor air pollution rose to prominence, at first due to concerns about radon. Radon pollution of indoor air made national news in 1984 when a worker at the Limerick Nuclear Power Plant in Pennsylvania triggered the radiation monitoring system at the power plant when he arrived at work; tests revealed that the source of his exposure was not occupational but instead the air inside his household, contaminated with radon originating from underlying geologic formations [28, 29]. This incident focused national attention not just on radon but also on other sources of indoor air pollution, including formaldehyde, mold, and, more recently, environmental tobacco smoke. In addition, recent research in the developing world has spotlighted household air pollution arising from combustion of solid fuels indoors for cooking and heating.

In developed countries, recent evidence suggests that the household indoor air pollutants with the largest impacts on chronic disease are environmental tobacco smoke, radon, and mold. A meta-analysis found that children of parents who smoke have twice the risk of hospitalization for serious respiratory infections as those with nonsmoking parents [30]. Similarly, studies have found elevated risks of asthma in children and chronic lymphocytic leukemia, lung cancer, and cardiovascular disease in adults among nonsmokers living with smokers [31–36]. Multiple studies, including several meta-analyses, have found consistent associations between visible mold in the home and the development and exacerbation of asthma in the United States and Europe [37–39]. A meta-analysis of studies from North America and Europe showed consistent associations between the presence of visible mold in the household and the risk of asthma and other respiratory outcomes (such as chronic coughs) in children aged 6–12 [38]. More than 21% of U.S. asthma cases are attributable to mold in the home, according to one study [40].

Recent research also has documented associations between a variety of adverse health effects and indoor emissions of volatile chemicals from modern building materials [41–43]. Among the studied chemicals, evidence is strongest for formaldehyde [41, 42], which has long been known to irritate the eyes and nasal passages in children and adults [42]. Multiple studies have linked development of childhood asthma and asthma exacerbations among those with previously diagnosed asthma to formaldehyde [41, 44]. Although some authors have questioned the strength of this evidence [42], a meta-analysis published in 2010 concluded that, "results indicate a significant positive association between formaldehyde exposure and childhood asthma" [44]. Toxicology research using rats and mice has linked formaldehyde exposure to increased risks of nasopharyngeal cancer, but recent research using molecular methods, in combination with epidemiologic evidence, suggests that these risks are much smaller than suggested by the animal studies of the early 1980s [43, 45].

Formaldehyde can be emitted by a wide variety of indoor sources. Major sources include emissions from composite wood products such as fiber-board, particleboard, and plywood [42]; smoking of electronic and conventional cigarettes; burning of incense, candles, or wood; gas fireplaces; cooking (including cooking with natural gas and cooking or baking fats and fatty foods); oven cleaning; and emissions from carpets and other indoor textiles [46]. Current guidelines suggest that formaldehyde exposure at concentrations less than 0.1 mg/m^3 is unlikely to trigger adverse health effects. Measured mean indoor concentrations are generally lower than this threshold but sometimes are higher. For example, in 2006, formaldehyde exposures in trailers distributed to Hurricane Katrina victims by the U.S. Federal Emergency Management Agency received a great deal of media attention. An independent scientific investigation found that the median formaldehyde concentration measured in four such trailers was 0.54 mg/m^3, and the highest level was 1.1 mg/m^3—more than 5 and 11 times the recommended exposure limit, respectively [47].

The GBD 2019 study attributed 3.7 million deaths (10.6% of total deaths) and more than 130 million DALYs (10.7% of total DALYs) to indoor air pollution [9]. This global estimate includes air pollution due to solid fuels, radon, and secondhand smoke. Most of this burden occurred in the developing world and was associated with indoor use of solid fuels for cooking and heating. For the United States, the GBD 2019 study attributed 44,812 deaths (2.5% of the total) and 1.2 million DALYs (2.3% of the total) to indoor air pollution.

Estimates of deaths and DALYs from mold and formaldehyde were not included in either the global or U.S. studies. However, other burden of disease studies suggest that these two health determinants—especially mold—may pose a substantial disease burden. For example, a study in the United Arab Emirates attributed 12% of adult asthma and 8.6% of child asthma to exposure to mold indoors [13]. In addition, the study attributed 1.4% of children's visits to medical facilities for asthma to formaldehyde exposure.

Occupational Exposure to Environmental Pollutants

Although accidents, such as trips and falls, and ergonomic problems contribute substantially to the occupational disease burden, exposure to chemicals and airborne particulate matter in workplace environments. Physicians have recognized occupational pollutants as an important health determinant since the eighteenth century, when Percival Pott attributed scrotal cancer among young chimney sweeps to their exposure to soot [48]. Previous estimates of disease burden from occupational pollutants have placed these exposures into three categories: (1) occupational asthmagens; (2) occupational particulate matter, gases, and fumes; (3) and occupational carcinogens [43, 44]. For all three categories, the most common resulting diseases overall are respiratory illnesses, including asthma, COPD, and lung cancer [49, 50].

Global estimates have suggested that 11% of asthma is associated with occupational exposures [51]. In 2003, the American Thoracic Society estimated that approximately 15% of asthma is attributable to occupational exposure [47]. A more recent study, published in 2020, estimated that 16.7% of asthma among adult workers and 11.3% of all adult asthma in the United States [52]. Hundreds of biological and chemical agents in workplaces can trigger asthma. Biological agents include grains, flours, plants, wood dusts, and furs and other animal parts. Chemical agents include welding fumes, chlorofluorocarbons, alcohols, and metals and their salts [51]. Prior studies have found that occupational risks for asthma are highest among those employed in mining, manufacturing, service work, agriculture, and transportation. A study in 2007 found that workers most at risk for exposure to airborne contaminants causing new-onset asthma, when compared to exacerbation of pre-existing asthma, include nurses, cleaners, bakers, spray painters, and agricultural workers [53]. In addition to increasing the risk of asthma, exposure to occupational particulate matter can contribute to COPD, silicosis, asbestosis, and coal workers' pneumoconiosis, the latter two of which are essentially exclusively occupational illnesses [51].

Among the hundreds of potential occupational carcinogens, those with the strongest evidence linking occupational exposures to health outcomes, and contributing the most to occupational cancers, are asbestos, diesel engine exhaust, second-hand smoke, and silica [8]. A survey of occupational exposure to 139 carcinogens in European Union workplaces, which is used as the basis for current estimates of the disease burden associated with occupational carcinogens, found that the occupations with highest risk of exposure to these substances are mining, construction, transportation, and manufacturing [54].

The GBD 2019 study estimated that 909,011 deaths (2.6% of total deaths) were attributable to occupational exposures: 350,325 from carcinogens; 524,290 from particulate matter, gases, and fumes; and 34,395 from asthmagens [9]. In addition, 21.4 million DALYs (1.8% of the global total) were attributable to these occupational exposures: 7.7 million, 11.8 million, and 1.9 million to carcinogens; particulate matter, gases, and fumes; and asthmagens respectively. In the United States, the occupational disease burden is higher than that globally as a fraction of the total disease burden, despite having stronger occupational health and safety regulations than in developing countries. GBD 2019 attributed 65,288 U.S. deaths (3.6% of total deaths—1% higher than globally) to occupational exposures. Of these, 46,549; 18,456; and 283 were attributable to carcinogens; particulate matter, gases, and fumes; and asthmagens, respectively. Of total U.S. DALYs, 1.4 million (2.7%) were attributed to occupational exposures, which is about 1% higher than global attributable fraction. Of these, 801,838 were attributable to carcinogens, 498,220 to particulate matter, gases, and fumes; and 106,577 to asthmagens.

While burden of disease analyses are useful indicators of the potential magnitude of risks from environmental exposures, research suggests that the occupational disease burden may be substantially underestimated. Causes of underestimation include the long latency periods between occupational exposures and the onset of some diseases, the multiple potential causative factors for any given disease, and the lack of recognition by primary health care providers that workplace pollutants could have contributed to a patient's health status [55]. A U.S. study designed to assess the impacts of under-reporting of occupational illnesses found that 39% of patients in general medical clinics believed their illness could be "possibly caused by work," and 66% thought it could be "possibly worsened by work," even if not caused by work [56].

Water Pollution

Control of waterborne infectious diseases brought about by the construction of sewer and water treatment systems in cities has been heralded as the greatest public health advance of the twentieth century in the United States. Between 1900 and

1940, U.S. mortality rates declined by 40%, and life expectancy at birth increased from 47 to 63. Nearly half of these gains have been attributed to the reduction in population exposure to waterborne pathogens due to the installation of drinking water chlorination and filtration systems in major U.S. cities [57]. Nonetheless, waterborne disease outbreaks—albeit sporadic—continue to occur in the United States, and some populations are at increased risk, as compared to others.

The vast majority of waterborne disease outbreaks are unreported [58]. Nonetheless, a CDC database including all outbreaks reported since 1971 provides some insights into the nature of waterborne illnesses (Fig. 41.2) and etiologic agents (Fig. 41.3) that continue to pose risks to U.S. population health [59]. The most recent comprehensive assessment of these data analyzed waterborne diseases reported between 1976 and 2006. During that time, there were 766 reported outbreaks attributed to contamination of drinking water from

Fig. 41.2 Illnesses in reported U.S. waterborne disease outbreaks, 1971–2006. Developed from data in [59]

- Acute gastrointestinal illness
- Hepatitis A
- Acute respiratory illness (Legionella)
- Skin conditions
- Neurological illness (Naegleria fowleri)
- Other, unknown, or mixed

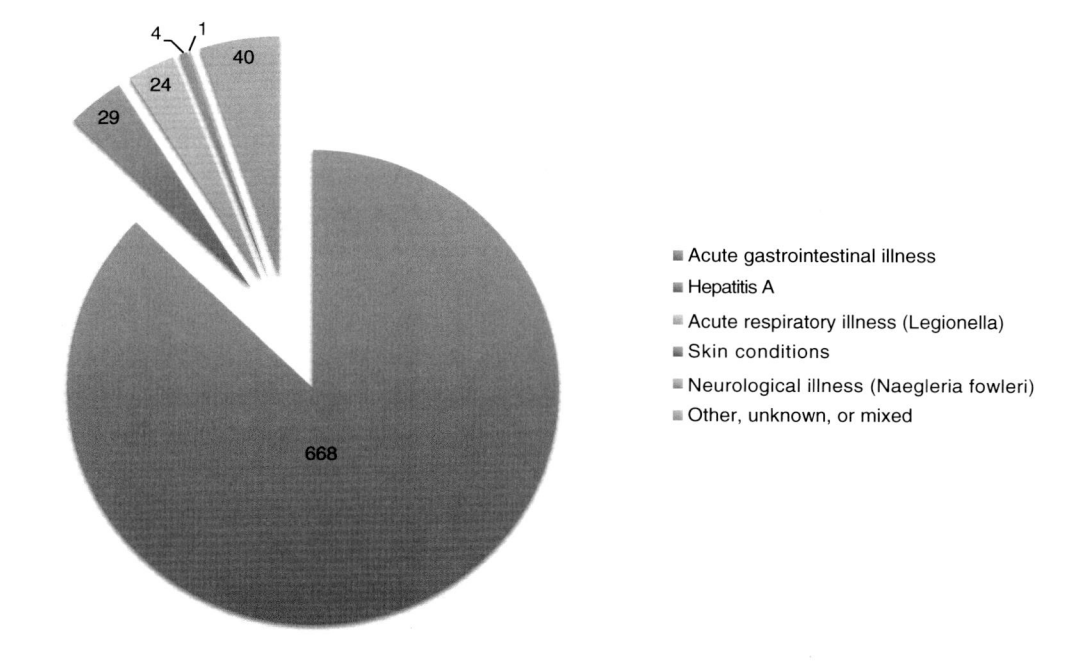

Fig. 41.3 Etiologic agents associated with reported U.S. waterborne disease outbreaks, 1971–2006 (of 456 infectious disease outbreaks with known etiologies). Developed from data in [59]

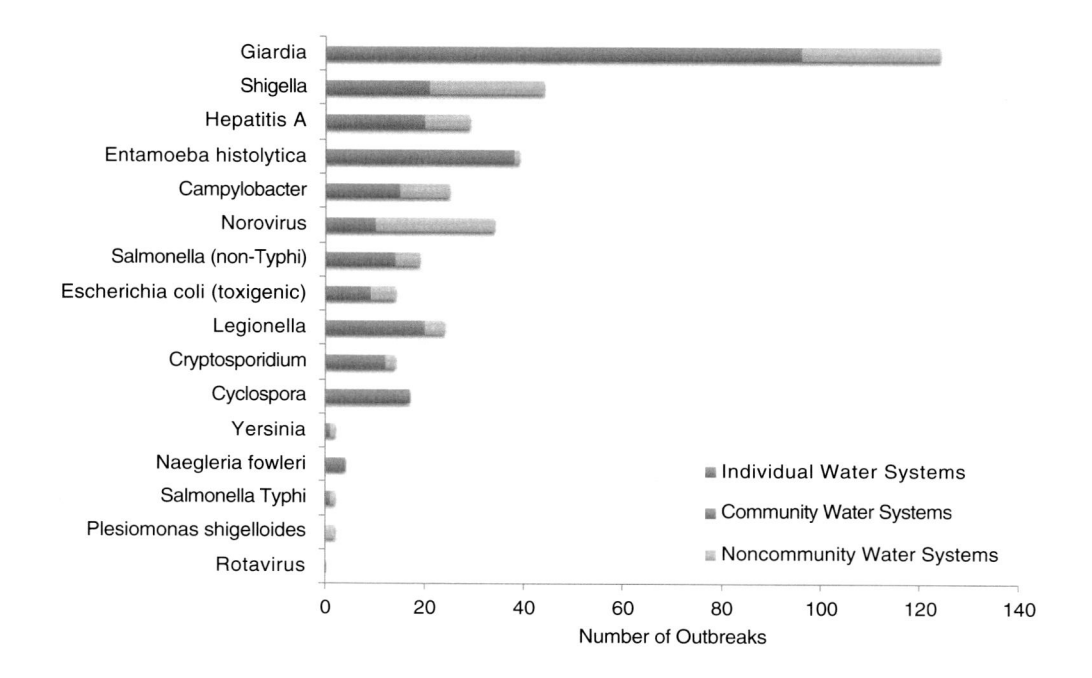

- Individual Water Systems
- Community Water Systems
- Noncommunity Water Systems

public water supplies or individual wells. Among these outbreaks, 88% resulted in acute gastrointestinal illnesses (AGI) caused by a range of intestinal pathogens (Fig. 41.2). Next most common were hepatitis A (4% of outbreaks) and acute respiratory illness caused by *Legionella* (3% of outbreaks).

Outbreak data indicate that the rate of *Legionella* outbreaks is increasing; during the period 2001–2006, *Legionella* caused 29% of reported outbreaks, all from growth and dissemination in premise plumbing, pipes, and storage infrastructure (including two outbreaks in healthcare settings). In addition to outbreaks of AGI, hepatitis A, and *Legionella*, one outbreak of primary amebic meningoencephalitis (caused by *Naegleria fowleri*) occurred, along with several outbreaks of skin rashes. About 11% of outbreaks were caused by chemicals, most commonly copper but also including fluoride, nitrate, arsenic, and other chemicals.

Although AGI arising from waterborne pathogens is usually self-limited, in rare cases these infections can lead to serious chronic or even fatal conditions. For example, *Campylobacter* is associated with Giullain-Barre syndrome; *Salmonella* and *Shigella* with reactive arthritis; *Giardia* with failure to thrive, lactose intolerance, and chronic joint pain; and *E. coli* O157:H7 with hemolytic uremic syndrome [60]. Furthermore, waterborne contaminants associated with self-limiting AGI in healthy populations may lead to severe complications and mortality among sensitive populations, such as the elderly, immunocompromised, pregnant women, and young children. For example, the largest U.S. waterborne disease outbreak in recent history occurred due to contamination of the Milwaukee, Wisconsin, water supply with *Cryptosporidium* for 2 weeks in 1993 [61, 62]. This outbreak sickened more than 400,000 people and caused 50 premature deaths, 85% of them among AIDS patients. Recent evidence suggests that repeated infections with *Cryptosporidium* among infants aged 0–2 can lead to malnutrition, impaired growth, and decreased educational performance during later childhood [63].

While waterborne disease outbreaks are generally rare in large cities, where residents have access to community water and sewer service, breakdowns in these systems occur. In addition to the Milwaukee example, one recent highly publicized example of the failure of a municipal system was the case in Flint, Michigan, where city residents were exposed to elevated levels of lead in their drinking water. The increase in lead exposure was caused by a switch in the city's water supply, from Lake Huron water treated by the City of Detroit to the corrosive water of the Flint River, as part of an effort to save money for the bankrupt city. Recent research has found that the incidence of elevated blood lead levels in children more than doubled (from 2.4 to 4.9%) during this time period [64], placing the exposed children at increased risk of neurocognitive impacts such as reduced IQ and overall life achievement.

About 14% of the U.S. population obtains their drinking water from private wells [65], and in most cases, those with private wells rely on septic or on-site methods to dispose of their domestic wastewater. Private wells are not regulated by the Safe Drinking Water Act, which covers only public water systems—those serving more than 25 people or 15 service connections year-round (community systems) or those regularly serving the public (non-community systems, such as campgrounds, gas stations, and schools, factories, or hospitals with their own water systems). Recent research has shown that those relying on private wells for their drinking water are at increased risk of AGI from waterborne pathogens and that children relying on private wells can be at increased of exposure to lead, compared to those with community water systems. For example, a study in North Carolina found that 7.3% of emergency department visits for AGI could be attributed to microbial contaminants in drinking water; of these visits, 99% were associated with contamination of private wells [66]. These microbial contaminants in some cases can be traced to under-performing septic systems [67, 68]. Multiple studies have documented that lead levels in private well water can be higher than those in community water systems because of uncontrolled corrosion of well components and household plumbing [69], and recent research has linked private well water to an increased risk of elevated blood lead in children [70].

Individuals relying on small or very small water system (e.g., those serving fewer than 3300 people), are also at higher risk of exposure to contamination. These systems lack the economies of scale of larger systems and are more likely to be financially stressed, causing difficulties with appropriate monitoring and maintenance of treatment systems. In a typical year, nearly 90% of violations of the Safe Drinking Water Act occur in small and very small water systems [71–73].

In addition to illnesses tracked in the CDC's waterborne disease surveillance system, contamination of drinking water is associated with other illnesses not easily recognized as waterborne, due to multiple etiologies and a lag between exposure and disease onset. These other illnesses include lead poisoning, such as in the Flint, Michigan case, and cancers. Among carcinogens in drinking water, disinfection byproducts formed by the reaction of disinfectants (such as chlorine) with natural organic compounds in the water (from decayed vegetation and other sources) appear to pose the biggest health impact, followed very distantly by arsenic, which is naturally occurring. Despite the increased cancer risks that may be caused by disinfection byproducts, studies have shown that the benefits of reduced infectious disease risks far outweigh the cancer risks [74].

Arsenic is a naturally occurring chemical concentrated in selected geologic regions. Acute exposure to high levels of arsenic in drinking water causes skin lesions, including

Blackfoot disease, however such acute exposures are generally not observed in the United States. At lower exposure levels, such as those in U.S. groundwater in some geologic regions, chronic exposure to arsenic in drinking water is associated with skin, bladder, kidney, and lung cancer; heart disease; neurological abnormalities; and diabetes [75, 76]. In the United States, health risks from arsenic exposure are likely to be highest in private wells, due to the lack of regulation [77]. Public water systems, in contrast, are required to monitor for arsenic and remove it to very low levels if detected.

The GBD 2019 study attributed 1.23 million deaths (3.5% of the total global deaths) and 65.1 million DALYs (5.4% of the total global DALYs) to unsafe water sources [9]. It attributed another 757,000 deaths (1.34% of the global total) and 41.4 million DALYs (1.63% of the total) to unsafe sanitation. In the United States, these estimates are much lower as a fraction of the total population, with 382 deaths (0.02% of the total U.S. deaths) and 14,500 (0.03% of the total U.S. DALYs) attributed to unsafe drinking water and 682 deaths (0.02% of the total) and 27,200 DALYs (0.02% of the total) to unsafe sanitation. These estimates are based on the fraction of the population in each country with access to improved water and sanitation sources, as defined by the WHO/UNICEF Joint Monitoring Programme for Water Supply and Sanitation (Table 41.3). Those of water and sanitation service levels defined as less than optimal are assumed to be at increased risk of gastrointestinal illnesses, as shown in Table 41.3.

Most U.S. residents have access to safe drinking water sources and sanitation as defined by WHO/UNICEF. For example, private wells and septic systems are considered equivalent to community systems, despite the increased risks described above. As a result, the IHME estimation approach may not provide the most accurate information for U.S. policymaking.

Table 41.3 Water and sanitation service levels and associated relative risks of gastrointestinal illnesses used in global burden of disease calculations

Category	Relative Risk
Drinking water	
Piped, boiled/filtered	1
Piped, solar/chlorinated	1.65
Piped, untreated	2.4
Other improved, boiled/filtered	1.12
Other improved, solar/chlorinated	1.85
Other improved, untreated	2.69
Unimproved or surface, boiled/filtered	1.36
Unimproved or surface, solar/chlorinated	2.25
Unimproved or surface, untreated	3.28
Sanitation	
Sewer or septic	1
Other improved	2.595
Unimproved or open defecation	3.242

We estimated separately the burden of disease in the United States from waterborne pathogens and carcinogens based on recent U.S. studies seeking to characterize this disease burden. To estimate risks of waterborne infectious diseases, we relied on a study published by the CDC in 2021 [78]. That study, based on an analysis of surveillance and administrative data for specific illnesses, attributed 6630 deaths to domestically acquired waterborne infections in the year 2014 (including exposures from contaminated water supplies and contact with contaminants during recreational activities, such as swimming)—more than six times the estimate from the GBD study. In addition, it attributed 2.3 million enteric infections, 96,000 respiratory infections, and 4,670,000 cases of otitis externa to waterborne transmission. (To equate these numbers to DALYs, we used weights shown in Table 41.1 and assumed nearly all infections would be mild.)

To estimate cancer cases attributable to chemical contaminants in drinking water, we applied *AF* estimates from a study quantifying the burden of cancer from drinking water contaminants across North Carolina, which estimated that 0.30% of cancers are attributable to chemical contaminants in drinking water [79]. We multiplied this fraction by GBD 2019 data on deaths and DALYs from all cancers in the United States. Using these data sources, we attribute 8900 deaths (0.5% of total deaths) and 250,000 DALYs (0.48% of the total) to waterborne contaminants. Among the deaths, 2300 are attributable to carcinogens and 6600 to pathogens. Among DALYs, 49,000 are attributable to carcinogens and 201,000 to pathogens. It is important to note that this calculation does not include potentially important adverse effects of chemical contaminants in drinking water, such as elevated blood lead in children, other than cancer, so the actual burden is probably higher than reflected in this estimate.

Lead Exposure

Lead toxicity has been recognized for more than 2000 years. For example, during the first century A.D., Roman scholar and naval commander Pliny, in his *Naturalis Historia*, described poisoning among shipbuilders along with pallor among miners exposed to lead [80, 81]. Nonetheless, until the first cases of childhood lead poisoning were documented in the late nineteenth and early twentieth centuries, lead exposure was thought to occur only in certain high-risk occupations [82]. Recent events in Flint, Michigan, in which lead concentrations in the municipal water supply peaked due to the switch to a corrosive water that leached lead from water pipes, has refocused national attention on health risks of lead exposure [64, 83].

Exposure to lead may occur though ingestion of lead-contaminated dust, water, soil, or food or from inhalation of contaminated air. Until lead was banned from gasoline in progressive stages beginning in 1980, the major source of exposure was ingestion of soil and dust contaminated with airborne lead released by motor vehicles [84]. Dust from lead in household paint is another major source. Lead was banned from household paint in 1978 [85], but homes built before then remain at risk. Even if covered with additional paint layers, household residents (especially children) are at risk of exposure via dust from flaking paint, for example in window casings where friction can erode upper layers and leave a dust residue on windowsills. Consumer products, such as glazed ceramics from certain countries, also can be sources of lead exposure. Lead solder in food cans is a dietary source, although the food industry has collaborated with the Food and Drug Administration over the past three decades to virtually eliminate the use of lead-containing materials in food storage containers manufactured in the United States [86].

As a result of bans on lead in gasoline, household paint, and food cans, U.S. blood lead levels have declined progressively since the 1980s. For example, according to the CDC, the fraction of children with blood lead levels above 10 μg/dL decreased from nearly 8% to less than 0.5% during the time period 1997–2015 [87]. Nonetheless, an estimated 120,000 children under age 5 per year have blood lead levels above 10 μg/dL (the CDC's threshold for elevated blood lead before 2012, when the definition of elevated blood lead changed to 5 μg/dL). In 2012, an estimated 500,000 U.S. children ages 1 through 5 had blood lead levels above 5 μg/dL [88]. This estimate still undercounts the number of children at risk, because it disregards effects that occur beyond age 5 and below 5 μg/dL. Reflecting the scientific consensus that 5 μg/dL is not sufficiently protective, in October 2021, the CDC changed the threshold for elevated blood lead level to 3.5 μg/dL [88].

Over the course of the twentieth century, concern about lead exposure increased as studies demonstrated risks at increasingly lower exposure levels. In the United States, the first documented case of childhood lead poisoning was recorded in 1914 [82]. At the time, the prevailing wisdom was that a child who survived acute poisoning would recover fully. However, in 1943, the first follow-up study of acutely lead poisoned children found that 19 of 20 subjects exhibited cognitive difficulties, including behavioral problems, learning difficulty, and failure in school many years later [82]. In the 1970s, researchers began to document the cognitive effects of lead in children who had been exposed but showed no clinical signs of acute poisoning. As subsequent research has built on these findings [89–92], the CDC has progressively lowered its definition of elevated blood lead concentrations from 60 μg/dL in 1960 to the current 3.5 μg/dL. Adverse impacts, including intellectual disabilities and behavioral problems, can occur even as low as 2.5 μg/dL [82].

At high exposure concentrations, lead can cause acute clinical symptoms in children and adults. The concentration at which acute symptoms occur varies by individual but is generally in the range of 60 μg/dL. In adults, symptoms of acute lead poisoning include peripheral neuropathy with wrist or foot drop, slowed peripheral nerve conduction, colic, clumsiness, clouded thinking, weakness, and paralysis. In addition, acute lead poisoning increases the incidence of stillbirths and female and male infertility. In adults, lead toxicity should be considered in the differential diagnosis of abdominal pain, arthralgia, hypertension, severe headache, increased intracranial pressure, central nervous system dysfunction, anemia, and renal dysfunction. An adult blood lead level above 10 μg/dL should be considered elevated, even though clinical symptoms are rarely seen below 60 μg/dL [82].

Children are more vulnerable to adverse health effects from lead exposure due to their developing central nervous system, increased lead absorption, and more frequent hand-to-mouth behavior. Clinical symptoms of acute exposure, which usually manifest at blood lead levels above 60 μg/dL, may begin with abdominal pain and arthralgia, progress to clumsiness and staggering with headaches and behavioral problems, and in the worst cases lead to encephalopathy (though the latter is rare in the United States). Beginning in the 1970s, researchers began to document associations between permanent IQ loss in children and exposure to lead, even at low exposure levels [89]. Meta-analyses have found a loss of about 1.3 IQ points for every 5 μg/dL increase in blood lead levels in children [93]. Research over the past three decades also shows adverse impacts on social behavior and associated increases in aggression and delinquency later in life. One study of bone lead levels in a juvenile cohort found that 11–38% of delinquent behavior could be attributed to early lead exposure on the basis of bone lead measurements [94]. However, any child with growth failure, abdominal pain, behavior change, hyperactivity, language delay, or anemia should be tested for lead toxicity [82].

When blood lead levels exceed 40 μg/dL, patients should receive chelation therapy, with a five-day course of EDTA (calcium disodium adathamil) or a 19-day course of dimercatosuccinic acid (succimer). A repeated course may be required if blood lead levels do not stabilize. Critically, the source of exposure must be identified through a home inspection (or for workers, work site investigation). Unfortunately, chelation therapy does not eliminate the cognitive damage in children, and the only remedy for low-level lead exposure is therefore primary prevention [82].

WHO and IHME estimates of the burden of disease attributable to lead exposure emphasize the risks of relatively low but widespread exposures, rather than acute exposures [9]. On the basis of the strength of available evidence, they focus on IQ loss leading to mild mental retardation in some children, gastrointestinal effects in children, elevated blood pressure in adults, and anemia in children and adults. Globally, the GBD 2019 study attributed 902,006 deaths (2.6% of the total) and 21.7 million DALYs (1.8% of the total) could be attributed to lead exposure [9]. In the United States, 20,800 deaths (1.2% of the total) and 348,000 DALYs (0.7% of the total) were attributed to lead exposure.

Automobile-Centric Urban Designs

Since World War II, Americans have become much less physically active due to declines in physically active transportation (e.g., walking and biking), occupations, and household activities [85]. Overall, only about 45% of Americans meet the CDC's recommendation of 150 minutes of moderate to vigorous physical activity per week [95]. While about 36% of Americans are aware of the CDC's physical activity guidelines, fewer than 1% could correctly identify the amount of activity the CDC recommends [96]. Failure to meet these guidelines is associated with increased risks of multiple chronic diseases, including breast and colorectal cancers, diabetes, ischemic heart disease, and stroke [9, 97–100].

The decline in physical activity and associated rise in chronic disease rates is in part attributable to automobile-centric urban designs of the post–World War II era, along with increases in automation reducing physical activity at work and home [101–104]. In the United States, highway construction projects and suburban sprawl of the twentieth century in effect eliminated physical activity as a means of transportation for many Americans. For example, only 3.4% of Americans reported walking or biking to work in 2012 [105].

Recent research has shown that U.S. residents who walk to work spend an additional 19.8 min per day walking, when compared to those who drive, and bicycle commuters exercise 32 min a day (28 min due to cycling and 4 due to walking) more than automobile commuters [105]. These results suggest that some Americans could achieve a majority of recommended physical activity by switching from driving to either walking or cycling to work. Similar benefits can be gained by switching from driving to using public transportation. For example, a study in Charlotte, NC, showed that residents who began using a new light rail stop to commute reduced their BMI by 1.18 kg/m², on average, over one year—equivalent to a weight loss of 6.45 lbs. for someone who is 5′5″ tall [106]. Multiple simulation studies have also shown substantial health benefits of reduced chronic diseases, mediated through physical activity, of compact neighborhoods with accessible public transportation, infrastructure (such as sidewalks and bike-share programs) to support walking and cycling, and mixed land uses, in comparison to sprawling suburban neighborhoods lacking in such infrastructure [107–110].

The GBD 2019 study attributed 8321,000 deaths (2.4% of total deaths) and 15.7 million DALYs (1.3% of the total) to low physical [9]. Relative to other environmental determinants, low physical activity risks are much higher in the United States than globally, though these risks have decreased slightly since 2019. In 2019, 37,100 deaths (2.1% of total U.S. deaths) and 726,000 DALYs (1.4% of total U.S. DALYs) were attributed to low physical activity compared to 45,600 (3.0% of total deaths) and 796,000 (1.8% of the total) in 2010. Globally, risks from physical inactivity remained stable between 2010 and 2019.

Climate Change

Over the past several decades, a strong scientific consensus has emerged that human activities have increased and continue to increase global average surface temperatures [111]. On average, the Earth has warmed about 1 °C since preindustrial times, and about 80% of that rise is attributed to human activity [112]. Climate change can trigger cascading events that can exacerbate the illnesses related to environmental determinants. A recent global survey of nearly 4000 healthcare professionals found that 95% agreed climate change is occurring; 77% said it would affect their patients, 81% thought it would affect their communities, and 93% agreed climate change would affect future generations [111]. The majority reported that climate change has already adversely impacted the health of their communities in various ways, ranging from increased illnesses due to air pollution, to physical or mental harm from forest and brush fires, to anxiety, depression, and other mental illnesses.

Climate change occurs through the accumulation of gases that trap heat in the atmosphere, mimicking conditions seen in a greenhouse. The main greenhouse gas is carbon dioxide (CO_2). Once released, CO_2 remains in the atmosphere for a very long time, with an estimated 20% lasting for more than 1000 years [112]. Other, shorter-lived pollutants (including methane and black carbon) also contribute. In 2019, a record high of 36.7 billion metric tons of CO_2 were released globally [113]. The United States is the second-leading emitter, after China, contributing about 11% of the world total. Of the U.S. CO_2 emissions, 92.4% was attributed to energy use in 2019 [114]. The top three U.S. sources of energy use for the same year were transportation (34.6%), electricity and heating (30.6%), and industrial processes (15.6%). Among transportation sources, the largest were passenger cars (40.5%), freight trucks (23.6%), light duty trucks (17.2%), and commercial aircraft (7.2%) [114].

There is substantial evidence that climate change has adverse effects on human health through multiple pathways, although the total magnitude of these impacts is uncertain [115]. The most recent assessment comes from the Intergovernmental Panel on Climate Change Climate (IPCC), the global body charged by the United Nations and World

Meteorological Organization to monitor climate groups health effects. The IPCC has categorized three domains: direct exposures, indirect exposures, and economic and social disruptions [116]. Direct exposures include increases health risks associated with heat stress and with extreme, storm-related weather events. While warming winter climates may decrease deaths attributed to cold weather, the IPCC has concluded that the "increase in heat-related mortality by mid-century will outweigh gains due to fewer cold periods" [116].

Most future climate projections also predict more frequent, intense rainfall events in most parts of the world, with associated increases risks of deaths and injuries due to flooding, especially in small catchments [117]. Climate change also is expected to influence health indirectly by changing natural systems, leading to alterations in exposure to allergens, disease vectors, and water and air pollution. For example, forecasters have estimated an increase in global malaria risks; studies also have predicted increases in risks of waterborne diarrheal diseases in the tropics and subtropics and will magnify the effects of exposure to air pollutants like ozone. Lastly, some forecasters have estimated that climate change could increase malnutrition globally due to effects on the food production system [118].

Characterizing the burden of disease from climate change is challenging because not all disease pathways have been considered in such estimates. The GBD 2019 study was the first to attempt characterizing burden of diseases from non-optimal temperatures. The estimates included the following 12 outcomes: ischemic heart disease, stroke, hypertensive heart disease, diabetes, chronic kidney disease, lower respiratory infection, chronic obstructive pulmonary diseases, homicide, suicide, mechanical injuries, transport-related injuries, and drowning [9]. Globally, the GBD 2019 study estimated that 1.96 million deaths (5.6% of the total) and 37.7 million DALYs (3.1% of the total) could be attributed to non-optimal temperatures [9]. In the United States, 125,489 deaths (7.0% of the total) and 1.8 million DALYs (3.4% of the total) were attributed to non-optimal temperatures in 2019. The WHO estimates that by 2030, approximately 250,000 additional deaths per year world worldwide could be attributable to climate change, due to non-optimal temperatures and because of effects on malnutrition, malaria, and waterborne infectious diseases [115].

Addressing Environmental Risk Factors in Chronic Illness Care

The most prevalent chronic diseases in the United States can be triggered or exacerbated by exposure to pollutants in the ambient, home, or workplace environment. In addition, modern urban designs that discourage physically active transportation (e.g., walking and cycling) in favor of reliance on personal automobiles are now widely recognized as an environmental risk factor affecting chronic disease prevalence [119]. Given the multitude of environmental factors influencing health, untangling the potential role of any one of these factors—or combinations of them—in illnesses presenting to a physician or other health care provider may be daunting. Nonetheless, identifying underlying environmental factors may be critical to effective treatment or management of a patient's disease.

To help clinicians identify potential environmental factors that may be contributing to patients' disease, environmental and occupational medicine specialists have developed systematic approaches to eliciting patient histories and diagnosing environmental or occupational illnesses. Figure 41.4 provides an example, which is adapted from previous questionnaires by the Harvard School of Public Health and Yale University School of Medicine to include questions about risk factors related to the built environment [120, 121]. The approach occurs in three stages, proceeding from the general to the specific. The first stage includes several broad screening questions that elicit information to help the clinician determine whether the patient may have been exposed to pollutants at home or at work. In addition, these screening questions ask whether the patient has observed a temporal relationship between symptoms and exposures (e.g., decreased symptoms during vacations). If such relationships exist, then the suspicion that an underlying environmental risk factor may have triggered or exacerbated health symptoms increases.

The screening stage includes two questions about whether and how much the patient exercises due to evidence regarding the deleterious effects of modern environments on physical activity [119]. Based on the response, the clinician may proceed to a second, more detailed set of items that include job responsibilities, home location, hobbies, and other infrequent activities that could lead to exposure. In patients with symptoms that are associated with low physical activity, clinicians can inquire about potential opportunities to incorporate walking and cycling into the patient's daily routine.

The third step is to characterize health effects of exposures uncovered during the first and second stages. Table 41.1 lists health outcomes associated with risk factors. Clinicians can utilize material safety data sheets—which employers are required to provide to workers or their physicians—reference manuals, occupational safety, and resources from health organization (see Table 41.4), or poison control centers for information about specific hazardous chemicals. Other references include *Dreisbach's Handbook of Poisoning* [122] and *Clinical Toxicology of Commercial Products* [123], available in health science libraries.

The final stage involves identifying treatment options for managing the patient's condition and developing a follow-up

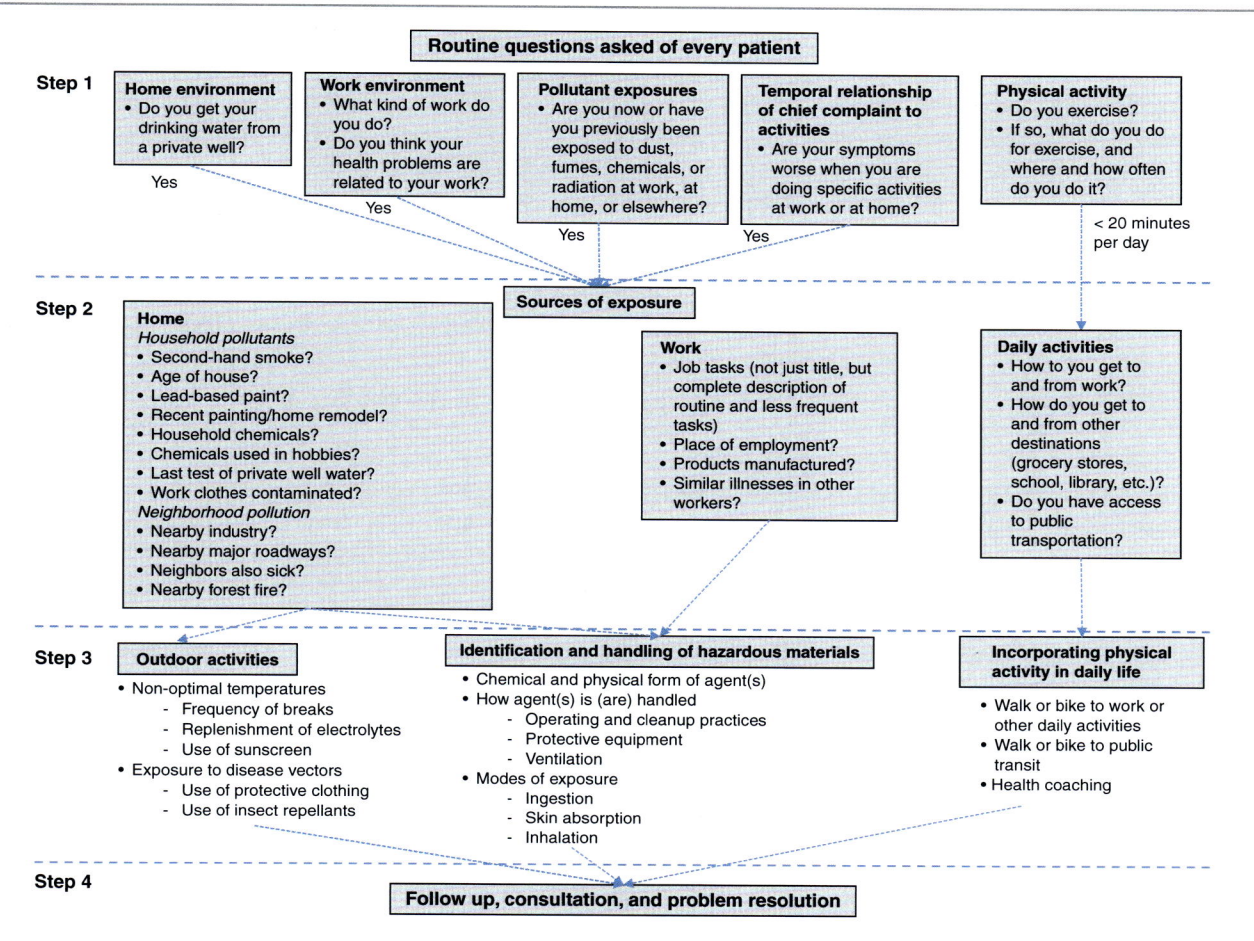

Fig. 41.4 Systematic approach to diagnosing potential environmental contributors to patient health

Table 41.4 Occupational and environmental health organizations in the United States

Organization	Mission	Contact information
Agency for Toxic Substances and Disease Registry	Federal public health agency that provides health information to prevent harmful exposures and diseases related to toxic substances	Telephone: 800-232-4636 Web site: http://www.atsdr.cdc.gov/
American College of Occupational and Environmental Medicine	Organization representing physicians and other health care professionals specializing in the field of occupational and environmental medicine	Telephone: 847-818-1800 Web site: http://www.acoem.org/
Association of Occupational and Environmental Clinics	A nationwide network of more than 60 multidisciplinary clinics and more than 250 occupational and environmental medicine professionals	Telephone: 888-347-2632 Web site: http://www.aoec.org/
National Institute for Occupational Safety and Health	Federal agency responsible for conducting research and making recommendations for the prevention of work-related illness and injury	Telephone: 800-232-4636 Web site: http://www.cdc.gov/niosh/
Pediatric Environmental Health Specialty Units	A national program with experts in the prevention, diagnosis, management, and treatment of health issues related to environmental exposures from preconception through adolescence	Telephone: 888-227-1785 Web site: https://www.pehsu.net/
Occupational Safety and Health Administration (OSHA)	Federal agency responsible for enforcing safety and health legislation. OSHA also offers free on-site consulting to small- and medium-sized businesses. Consultations are separate from enforcement and do not result in penalties	Telephone: 800-321-6742 Web site: http://www.osha.gov/

Source: Re-created with information from [121]

plan. In some cases, eliminating exposure, such as installing a home water treatment system where water contamination is a source of illness, wearing personal protective equipment to guard against occupational exposures, or staying hydrated and taking breaks during extreme heat are solutions. Medical treatment (e.g., chelation therapy for lead exposure) is indicated for some environmental exposures. Clinicians may refer patients to specialists in occupational medicine or other related fields and report suspected environmental and occupational illnesses to public health officials, trade union health specialists, and workplace managers. In the case of exposures in the workplace, physicians can help patients to apply for Workers Compensation to help cover their medical expenses. In some states, workers can claim these benefits even if occupational exposure was not the primary cause if the work environment "precipitated, hastened, aggravated, or contributed to the illness" [120].

Health coaching may be indicated when unhealthy behaviors or lifestyles are potentiated by the modern built environment. Over the past decade, health coaching has emerged as a complimentary approach to mitigating chronic disease [124, 125]. While the functions of health coaching continues to evolve, it may include one-on-one, telephone, or web-based consultations to help patients set and achieve goals for health-promoting behavior changes.

Reporting Requirements for Environmental Diseases

When clinicians suspect that an environmental or occupational factor may have contributed to a clinical condition, it may require reporting to the area health department. These reportable illnesses are designated as infectious and occupational and vary by state (see Table 41.5). In general, reportable occupational conditions are less than those for infectious disease. The Council of State and Territorial Epidemiologists (CSTE) maintains web sites where clinicians can search infectious (http://www.cste.org/?StateReportable) and occupational illness reporting requirements (http://www.cste.org/group/OHWebsites) for their state. Although reporting of suspected environmental or occupational causes of illness to federal agencies is not required, state health departments routinely report selected infectious diseases specified by CSTE and CDC to monitor disease trends and inform national public health policies.

Table 41.5 Reportable conditions in North Carolina and California (as of December 2021)

Condition	State	Condition	State
Acquired immune deficiency syndrome (AIDS)	North Carolina	Lymphogranuloma venereum	North Carolina
Anaplasmosis	California	Malaria	Both
Anthrax	Both	Measles (Rubeola)	Both
Babesiosis	California	Meningitis, pneumococcal	North Carolina
Botulism	Both	Monkeypox	North Carolina
Brucellosis	Both	Mumps	Both
Campylobacteriosis	Both	Nongonococcal urethritis	North Carolina
Chancroid	Both	Novel influenza virus infection	North Carolina
Chickenpox (Varicella) (outbreaks, hospitalizations and deaths)	California	Novel virus infection with pandemic potential	California
Chikungunya virus infection	Both	Paralytic poliomyelitis	North Carolina
Chlamydia trachomatis	North Carolina	Paralytic shellfish poisoning	California
Cholera	Both	Paratyphoid fever	California
Ciguatera fish poisoning	California	Pelvic inflammatory disease	North Carolina
Coccidioidomycosis	California	Pertussis (whooping cough)	California
Creutzfeldt-Jakob disease	Both	Plague	Both
Cryptosporidiosis	Both	Poliovirus infection	California
Cyclosporiasis	Both	Psittacosis	Both
Cysticercosis or taeniasis	California	Q fever	Both
Dengue	Both	Rabies, human	North Carolina

Table 41.5 (continued)

Condition	State	Condition	State
Diphtheria	Both	Rabies, human or animal	California
Domoic acid poisoning (amnesic shellfish poisoning)	California	Relapsing fever	California
Ehrlichiosis	Both	Respiratory syncytial virus-associated deaths in laboratory-confirmed cases <5 years of age	California
Encephalitis, arboviral	North Carolina	Rickettsial diseases, including typhus and typhus-like illnesses	California
Encephalitis, specify etiology: viral, bacterial, fungal, parasitic	California	Rocky Mountain spotted fever	Both
Escherichia coli, Shiga toxin-producing	Both	Rubella (German measles)	Both
Flavivirus infection of undetermined species	California	Rubella congenital syndrome	North Carolina
Foodborne disease	Both	Salmonellosis	Both
Giardiasis	California	Scombroid fish poisoning	California
Gonococcal infections	California	Severe acute respiratory syndrome (SARS)	North Carolina
Gonorrhea	North Carolina	Shiga toxin (detected in feces)	California
Granuloma inguinale	North Carolina	Shigellosis	Both
Haemophilus influenzae, invasive disease	Both	Smallpox	Both
Hantavirus infection	Both	Staphylococcus aureus with reduced susceptibility to vancomycin	North Carolina
Hemolytic uremic syndrome	Both	Streptococcal infection, Group A, invasive disease	North Carolina
Hemorrhagic fever virus infection	North Carolina	Syphilis (for California, all stages, including congenital)	Both
Hepatitis A, acute infection	Both	Tetanus	Both
Hepatitis B (for California, specify acute, chronic, or perinatal)	Both	Toxic shock syndrome	North Carolina
Hepatitis C (for California, specify acute, chronic, or perinatal)	Both	Trichinosis	Both
Hepatitis D	California	Tuberculosis	Both
Hepatitis E	California	Tularemia	Both
Human immunodeficiency virus (HIV) infection confirmed	North Carolina	Typhoid (cases and carriers)	Both
Human immunodeficiency virus (HIV), any stage	California	Typhus, epidemic (louse-borne)	North Carolina
Influenza virus infection causing death	North Carolina	Vaccinia	North Carolina
Influenza, deaths in laboratory-confirmed cases for age 0–64 years	California	Vibrio infections	Both
Influenza due to novel strains (human)	California	Viral hemorrhagic fevers, human or animal (e.g., Crimean-Congo, Ebola, Lassa, and Marburg viruses)	California
Legionellosis	Both	West Nile virus infection	California
Leprosy (Hansen disease)	Both	Whooping cough	North Carolina
Leptospirosis	Both	West Nile virus infection	California
Listeriosis	Both	Whooping cough	North Carolina
Lyme disease	Both	Whooping cough	North Carolina
Meningitis, specify etiology: viral, bacterial, fungal, parasitic	California	Yellow fever	Both
Meningococcal infections	Both	Yersiniosis	California
Middle East respiratory syndrome	Both	Zika virus infection	Both

References

1. Prüss-Ustün A, Wolf J, Corvalán C, Neville T, Bos R, Neira M. Diseases due to unhealthy environments: an updated estimate of the global burden of disease attributable to environmental determinants of health. J Public Health (Bangkok) [Internet]. 2016;1–12. http://jpubhealth.oxfordjournals.org/lookup/doi/10.1093/pubmed/fdw085.
2. Rappaport SM, Smith MT. Environment and disease risks. Science. 2010;330(6003):460–1.
3. Smith KR, Corvalan CF, Kjellstrom T. How much global ill health is attributable to environmental factors? Epidemiology. 1999;10(5):573–84.
4. Lopez AD. The evolution of the global burden of disease framework for disease, injury and risk factor quantification: developing the evidence base for national, regional and global public health action. Global Health [Internet]. 2005 [cited 2014 Aug 14];1(1):5. http://www.pubmedcentral.nih.gov/articlerender.fcgi?artid=1143783&tool=pmcentrez&rendertype=abstract.
5. Murray C, Lopez A. The global burden of disease and injury series, A comprehensive assessment of mortality and disability from diseases, injuries, and risk factors in 1990 and projected to 2020, vol. I. Geneva: World Health Organization; 1996.
6. Ezzati M, Lopez AD, Rodgers A, Murray CJ. Comparative quantification of health risks: global and regional burden of disease attributable to selected major risk factors. Geneva: World Health Organization; 2004.
7. Lim SS, Vos T, Flaxman AD, Danaei G, Shibuya K, Adair-Rohani H, et al. A comparative risk assessment of burden of disease and injury attributable to 67 risk factors and risk factor clusters in 21 regions, 1990–2010: a systematic analysis for the Global Burden of Disease Study 2010. Lancet [Internet]. 2013 [cited 2013 Jan 28];380(9859):2224–60. http://www.ncbi.nlm.nih.gov/pubmed/23245609.
8. Forouzanfar MH, Alexander L, Anderson HR, Bachman VF, Biryukov S, Brauer M, et al. Global, regional, and national comparative risk assessment of 79 behavioural, environmental and occupational, and metabolic risks or clusters of risks in 188 countries, 1990-2013: a systematic analysis for the global burden of disease study 2013. Lancet. 2015;386(10010):2287–323.
9. GBD 2019 Risk Factor Collaborators. Global burden of 87 risk factors in 204 countries and territories, 1990–2019: a systematic analysis for the Global Burden of Disease Study 2019. Lancet. 2020;396(10258):1223–49.
10. Boyd DR, Genuis SJ. The environmental burden of disease in Canada: respiratory disease, cardiovascular disease, cancer, and congenital affliction. Environ Res. 2008;106(2):240–9.
11. MacDonald Gibson J, Farah ZS. Environmental risks to public health in the United Arab Emirates: a quantitative assessment and strategic plan. Environ Health Perspect [Internet]. 2012;120(5):681–686. http://www.pubmedcentral.nih.gov/articlerender.fcgi?artid=3346776&tool=pmcentrez&rendertype=abstract.
12. MacDonald Gibson J, Thomsen J, Launay F, Harder E, DeFelice N. Deaths and medical visits attributable to environmental pollution in the United Arab Emirates. PLoS One [Internet]. 2013 [cited 2013 May 22];8(3):e57536. http://www.pubmedcentral.nih.gov/articlerender.fcgi?artid=3587618&tool=pmcentrez&rendertype=abstract.
13. MacDonald Gibson J, Brammer A, Davidson C, Folley TJ, Launay F, Thomsen J. Environmental burden of disease assessment: a case study in the United Arab Emirates. Dordrecht: Springer; 2013.
14. Hänninen O, Knol AB, Jantunen M, Lim TA, Conrad A, Rappolder M, et al. Environmental burden of disease in Europe: assessing nine risk factors in six countries. Environ Health Perspect. 2014;122(5):439–46.
15. The US Burden of Disease Collaborators. The state of US health, 1990–2016: burden of diseases, injuries, and risk factors among US states. JAMA. 2018;319(14):1444–72.
16. Murray CJL, Ezzati M, Lopez AD, Rodgers A, Van der Hoorn S. Comparative quantification of health risks: conceptual framework and methodological issues. Popul Health Metrics. 2003;1(1):1–20.
17. Ezzati M, Van der Hoorn S, Rodgers A, Lopez AD, Mathers CD, Murray CJ. Estimates of global and regional potential health gains from reducing multiple major risk factors. Lancet. 2003;362(9380):271–80.
18. US Centers for Disease Control and Prevention. Behavioral risk factor surveillance system [Internet]. 2016 [cited 2016 Dec 2]. http://www.cdc.gov/brfss/.
19. Helfand WH, Lazarus J, Theerman P. Donora, Pennsylvania: an environmental disaster of the 20th century. Am J Public Health. 2001;91(4):553.
20. Brunekreef B, Holgate ST. Air pollution and health. Lancet. 2002;360(9341):1233–42.
21. Héroux ME, Anderson HR, Atkinson R, Brunekreef B, Cohen A, Forastiere F, et al. Quantifying the health impacts of ambient air pollutants: recommendations of a WHO/Europe project. Int J Public Health. 2015;60(5):619–27.
22. Brauer M, Hoek G, Van Vliet P, Meliefste K, Fischer P. Estimating long-term average particulate air pollution concentrations: application of traffic indicators and geographic information systems Brunekreef reviewed work (s). Lippincott Williams & Wilkins Stable. http://www.jstor.org/sta. Traffic. 2012.
23. Anenberg SC, Belova A, Brandt J, Fann N, Greco S, Guttikunda S, et al. Survey of ambient air pollution health risk assessment tools. Risk Anal [Internet]. 2016;36(9):1718–1736. http://www.ncbi.nlm.nih.gov/pubmed/26742852.
24. De Sario M, Katsouyanni K, Michelozzi P. Climate change, extreme weather events, air pollution and respiratory health in Europe. Eur Respir J. 2013;42(3):826–43.
25. Grigorieva E, Lukyanets A. Combined effect of hot weather and outdoor air pollution on respiratory health: literature review. Atmosphere. 2021;12(6):1–30.
26. Anenberg SC, Haines S, Wang E, Nassikas N, Kinney PL. Synergistic health effects of air pollution, temperature, and pollen exposure: a systematic review of epidemiological evidence. Environ Health. 2020;19(1):130.
27. Sundell J. On the history of indoor air quality and health. Indoor Air [Internet]. 2004;14(7):51–58. http://www.researchgate.net/profile/Jan_Sundell2/publication/8381109_On_the_history_of_indoor_air_quality_and_health/links/0f3175326668e55d44000000.pdf.
28. Samet JM, Spengler JD. Indoor environments, and health: moving into the 21st century. Am J Public Health. 2003;93(9):1489–93.
29. Skrapits E. Professor recalls "crazy" discovery of radon in berks. The Morning Call. 2015.
30. Li JS, Peat JK, Xuan W, Berry G. Meta-analysis on the association between environmental tobacco smoke (ETS) exposure and the prevalence of lower respiratory tract infection in early childhood. Pediatr Pulmonol [Internet]. 1999;27(1):5–13. http://onlinelibrary.wiley.com/doi/10.1002/(SICI)1099-0496(199901)27:1%3C5::AID-PPUL3%3E3.0.CO;2-5/abstract.
31. Vork KL, Broadwin RL, Blaisdell RJ. Developing asthma in childhood from exposure to secondhand tobacco smoke: insights from a meta-regression. Environ Health Perspect [Internet]. 2007;115(10):1394–1400. http://www.jstor.org/stable/4626929.
32. Kasim K, Levallois P, Abdous B, Auger P, Johnson KC. Environmental tobacco smoke and risk of adult leukemia. Epidemiology [Internet]. 2005;16(5):672–680. http://www.ncbi.nlm.nih.gov/entrez/query.fcgi?cmd=Retrieve&db=PubMed&dopt=Citation&list_uids=16135944.

33. Boffetta P, Nyberg F. Contribution of environmental factors to cancer risk. Br Med Bull. 2003;68:71–94.
34. Cardenas VM, Thun MJ, Austin H, Lally CA, Clark WS, Greenberg RS, et al. Environmental tobacco smoke and lung cancer mortality in the American Cancer Society's cancer prevention study. II. Cancer Causes Control. 1997;8(1):57–64.
35. He J, Whelton PK. Passive cigarette smoking increases risk of coronary heart disease. Eur Heart J [Internet]. 1999;20(24):1764–1765. http://www.ncbi.nlm.nih.gov/pubmed/10581130.
36. Hill SE, Blakely T, Kawachi I, Woodward A. Mortality among lifelong nonsmokers exposed to secondhand smoke at home: cohort data and sensitivity analyses. Am J Epidemiol [Internet]. 2007;165(5):530–540. http://www.ncbi.nlm.nih.gov/pubmed/17172631.
37. Jaakkola MS, Nordman H, Piipari R, Uitti J, Laitinen J, Karjalainen A, et al. Indoor dampness and molds and development of adult-onset asthma: a population-based incident case-control study. Environ Health Perspect [Internet]. 2002;110(5):543–7. http://www.pubmedcentral.nih.gov/articlerender.fcgi?artid=1240846&tool=pmcentrez&rendertype=abstract.
38. Antova T, Pattenden S, Brunekreef B, Heinrich J, Rudnai P, Forastiere F, et al. Exposure to indoor mould and children's respiratory health in the PATY study. J Epidemiol Community Health [Internet]. 2008;62(8):708–714. http://www.ncbi.nlm.nih.gov/pubmed/18621956.
39. Cox-Ganser JM. Indoor dampness and mould health effects—ongoing questions on microbial exposures and allergic versus nonallergic mechanisms. Clin Exp Allergy. 2015;45(10):1478–82.
40. Mudarri D, Fisk WJ. Public health and economic impact of dampness and mold. Indoor Air. 2007;17(3):226–35.
41. Mendell MJ. Indoor residential chemical emissions as risk factors for respiratory and allergic effects in children: a review. Indoor Air. 2007;17(4):259–77.
42. Wolkoff P, Nielsen GD. Non-cancer effects of formaldehyde and relevance for setting an indoor air guideline. Environ Int [Internet]. 2010;36(7):788–799. https://doi.org/10.1016/j.envint.2010.05.012.
43. Golden R. Identifying an indoor air exposure limit for formaldehyde considering both irritation and cancer hazards. Crit Rev Toxicol. 2011;41(8):672–721.
44. McGwin G, Lienert J, Kennedy JI. Formaldehyde exposure and asthma in children: a systematic review. Environ Health Perspect. 2010;118:313–7.
45. Swenberg JA Moeller BC, Lu K, Rager JE, Fry RC, Starr TB. Formaldehyde carcinogenicity research: 30 years and counting for mode of action, epidemiology, and cancer risk assessment. Toxicol Pathol [Internet]. 2012;41(2):181–189. http://tpx.sagepub.com/cgi/doi/10.1177/0192623312466459.
46. Salthammer T. Formaldehyde sources, formaldehyde concentrations and air exchange rates in European housings. Build Environ [Internet]. 2019;150:219–232. https://doi.org/10.1016/j.buildenv.2018.12.042.
47. Maddalena R, Russell M, Sullivan DP, Apte MG. Formaldehyde and other volatile organic chemical emissions in four FEMA temporary housing units. Environ Sci Technol. 2009;43(15):5626–32.
48. Landrigan PJ, Baker DB. The recognition and control of occupational disease. J Am Med Assoc [Internet]. 1991;266(5):676–689. http://www.ncbi.nlm.nih.gov/pubmed/13427395.
49. Leigh JP. Economic burden of occupational injury and illness in the United States. Millbank Q. 2011;89(4):728–72.
50. Kogevinas M, Antó JM, Sunyer J, Tobias A, Kromhout H, Burney P. Occupational asthma in Europe and other industrialised areas: a population-based study. Lancet. 1999;353(9166):1750–4.
51. Driscoll T, Steenland K, Nelson D, Leigh J. Occupational airborne particulates: assessing the environmental burden of disease at national and local levels. Geneva: World Health Organization; 2004.
52. Laditka JN, Laditka SB, Arif AA, Hoyle JN. Work-related asthma in the USA: nationally representative estimates with extended follow-up. Occup Environ Med. 2020;77(9):617–22.
53. Kogevinas M, Zock J, Jarvis D, Kromhout H, Lillienberg L, Plana E, et al. Exposure to substances in the workplace and new-onset asthma: an international prospective population-based study (ECRHS-II). Lancet. 2007;370:336–41.
54. Driscoll T, Steenland K, Pruss-Ustun A, Nelson D, Leigh J. Occupational carcinogens: assessing the environmental burden of disease at national and local levels. Geneva: World Health Organization; 2004.
55. Leigh J, Macaskill P, Kuosma E, Mandryk J. Global burden of disease and injury due to occupational factors. Epidemiology. 1999;10(5):626–31.
56. Harber P, Mullin M, Merz B, Tarazi M. Frequency of occupational health concerns in general clinics. J Occup Environ Med. 2001;43(11):939–45.
57. Cutler DM, Miller G. The role of public health improvements in health advances: the 20th century United States. Demography. 2005;42(1):1–22.
58. Majowicz SE, Edge VL, Fazil A, McNab WB, Doré KA, Sockett PN, et al. Estimating the under-reporting rate for infectious gastrointestinal illness in Ontario. Can J Public Health Rev [Internet]. 96(3):178–81. http://www.ncbi.nlm.nih.gov/pubmed/15913079.
59. Craun GF, Brunkard JM, Yoder JS, Roberts VA, Carpenter J, Wade T, et al. Causes of outbreaks associated with drinking water in the United States from 1971 to 2006. Clin Microbiol Rev [Internet]. 2010 [cited 2013 Aug 21];23(3):507–528. http://www.pubmedcentral.nih.gov/articlerender.fcgi?artid=2901654&tool=pmcentrez&rendertype=abstract.
60. Haas CN, Rose JB, Gerba CP. Quantitative microbial risk assessment [Internet]. Wiley; 1999 [cited 2014 Feb 11]. http://books.google.com/books?hl=en&lr=&id=vjVhhwQh9N8C&pgis=1.
61. Kenzie W Mac, Hoxie N. A massive outbreak in Milwaukee of Cryptosporidium infection transmitted through the public water supply. N Engl J Med [Internet]. 1994 [cited 2013 Aug 16];331(3):161–168. http://www.nejm.org/doi/pdf/10.1056/NEJM199407213310304.
62. Hoxie NJ, Davis JP, Vergeront JM, Nashold RD, Blair KA. Cryptosporidiosis-associated mortality following a massive waterborne outbreak in Milwaukee, Wisconsin. Am J Public Health. 1997;87(12):2032–5.
63. Guerrant RL, Kosek M, Lima AAM, Lorntz B, Guyatt HL. Updating the DALYs for diarrhoeal disease. Trends Parasitol. 2002;18(5):191–3.
64. Hanna-Attisha M, Lachance J, Sadler RC, Schnepp AC. Elevated blood lead levels in children associated with the flint drinking water crisis: a spatial analysis of risk and public health response. Am J Public Health. 2016;106(2):283–90.
65. Dieter C, Maupin M. Public supply and domestic water use in the United States, 2015 [Internet]. U.S. Geological Survey Open-File Report 2017-1131. Reston; 2017. https://doi.org/10.3133/ofr20171131.
66. Stillo FJ, MacDonald Gibson J, Gibson JM. Exposure to contaminated drinking water and health disparities in North Carolina. Am J Public Health. 2017;107(1):180–5.
67. Hunter B, Walker I, Lassiter R, Lassiter V, Gibson JM, Ferguson PL, et al. Evaluation of private well contaminants in an underserved North Carolina community. Sci Total Environ. 2021;789:147823.
68. Arnade LJ. Seasonal correlation of well contamination and septic tank distance. Ground Water. 1999;37(6):920–3.
69. Pieper KJ, Krometis LAH, Gallagher DL, Benham BL, Edwards M. Incidence of waterborne lead in private drinking water systems in Virginia. J Water Health. 2015;13(3):897–908.
70. Gibson JM, Fisher M, Clonch A, MacDonald J, Cook P. Children drinking private well water have higher blood lead than those with city water. Proc Natl Acad Sci U S A. 2020;117(29):16898–907.

71. MacDonald JA, Zander AK, Snoeyink VL. Improving service to small communities. J Am Water Works Assoc. 1997;89(1):58.
72. Rubin SJ. Evaluating violations of drinking water regulations. J Am Water Works Assoc. 2013;105(3):51–2.
73. Dziegielewski B, Bik T. Technical assistance needs and research priorities for small community water systems. J Contemp Water Res Educ [Internet]. 2009;128(1):13–20. http://doi.wiley.com/10.1111/j.1936-704X.2004.mp128001003.x.
74. Havelaar AH, De Hollander AEM, Teunis PFM, Evers EG, Van Kranen HJ, Versteegh JFM, et al. Balancing the risks and benefits of drinking water disinfection: disability adjusted life-years on the scale. Environ Health Perspect. 2013;108(4):315–21.
75. National Research Council. Arsenic in drinking water: 2001 update [Internet]. Washington, DC: National Academy Press; 2001 [cited 2013 May 24]. http://search.lib.unc.edu/search?R=UNCb4104000.
76. Maull EA, Ahsan H, Edwards J, Longnecker MP, Navas-Acien A, Pi J, et al. Evaluation of the association between arsenic and diabetes: a national toxicology program workshop review. Environ Health Perspect. 2012;120(12):1658–70.
77. Kumar A, Adak P, Gurian PL, Lockwood JR. Arsenic exposure in US public and domestic drinking water supplies: a comparative risk assessment. J Exp Sci Environ Epidemiol [Internet]. 2010 [cited 2013 Feb 4];20(3):245–54. http://www.ncbi.nlm.nih.gov/pubmed/19401722.
78. DeFlorio-Barker S, Shrestha A, Dorevitch S. Estimate of burden and direct healthcare cost of infectious waterborne disease in the United States. Emerg Infect Dis. 2021;27:2241–2.
79. DeFelice NB, Leker HG, MacDonald Gibson J. Annual cancer risks from chemicals in North Carolina community water systems. Hum Ecol Risk Assess. 2017;23(5):974–91.
80. Hernberg S. Lead poisoning in a historical perspective. Am J Ind Med. 2000;38(3):244–54.
81. Nriagu JO. Occupational exposure to lead in ancient times. Sci Total Environ [Internet]. 1983;31(2):105–116. http://www.sciencedirect.com/science/article/pii/0048969783900633.
82. Needleman H. Lead poisoning. Annu Rev Med [Internet]. 2004;55:209–222. https://www.nlm.nih.gov/medlineplus/ency/article/002473.htm.
83. Bellinger DC. Lead contamination in Flint—an abject failure to protect public health. N Engl J Med. 2016;374(12):1101–4.
84. Meng Q, Richmond-Bryant J, Davis JA, Cohen J, Svendsgaard D, Brown JS, et al. Contribution of particle-size-fractionated airborne lead to blood lead during the national health and nutrition examination survey, 1999-2008. Environ Sci Technol. 2014;48(2):1263–70.
85. Dixon SL, Gaitens JM, Jacobs DE, Strauss W, Nagaraja J, Pivetz T, et al. Exposure of U.S. children to residential dust lead, 1999-2004: II. The contribution of lead-contaminated dust to children's blood lead levels. Environ Health Perspect. 2009;117(3):468–74.
86. Michael Bolger P, Carrington CD, Capar SG, Adams MA. Reductions in dietary lead exposure in the United States. Chem Speciat Bioavailab. 1991;3(3–4):31–6.
87. U.S. Centers for Disease Control and Prevention. U.S. totals blood lead surveillance [Internet]. 2016 [cited 2016 Dec 9]. https://www.cdc.gov/nceh/lead/data/Chart_Website_StateConfirmedByYear_1997_2015.pdf.
88. Ruckart PZ, Jones RL, Courtney JG, LeBlanc TT, Jackson W, Karwowski MP, et al. Update of the blood Lead reference value—United States, 2021. MMWR Morb Mortal Wkly Rep. 2021;70(43):1509–12.
89. Needleman HL, Landrigan PJ. The health effects of low level exposure to Lead. Annu Rev Public Health [Internet]. 1981;2(1):277–298. http://www.ncbi.nlm.nih.gov/pubmed/7348554, http://www.annualreviews.org/doi/abs/10.1146/annurev.pu.02.050181.001425.
90. Needleman HL, Levitton A, Bellinger D. Lead-associated intellectual deficit. N Engl J Med. 1982;306(6):367.
91. Needleman HL, Schell A, Bellinger D, Leviton A, Allred EN. The long-term effects of exposure to low doses of lead in childhood: an 11-year follow-up report. N Engl J Med. 1990;322(2):83–8.
92. Koller K, Brown T, Spurgeon A, Levy L. Recent developments in low-level lead exposure and intellectual impairment in children. Environ Health Perspect. 2004;112(9):987–94.
93. Fewtrell L, Kaufmann R, Prüss-üstün A. Lead: assessing the environmental burden of disease at national and local levels [Internet]. Geneva; 2003. http://www.who.int/quantifying_ehimpacts/publications/en/leadebd2.pdf.
94. Needleman HL, McFarland CE, Ness R. Bone lead levels in adjudicated delinquency: a case-control study. Neurotoxicol Taratol. 2002;24:11–7.
95. Tucker JM, Welk GJ, Beyler NK. Physical activity in U.S. adults: compliance with the physical activity guidelines for Americans. Am J Prev Med. 2011;40(4):454–61.
96. Kay MC, Carroll DD, Carlson SA, Fulton JE. Awareness and knowledge of the 2008 physical activity guidelines for Americans. J Phys Act Health [Internet]. 2014;11(4):693–698. http://www.ncbi.nlm.nih.gov/pubmed/23493071.
97. Hu G, Sarti C, Jousilahti P, Silventoinen K, Barengo NC, Tuomilehto J. Leisure time, occupational, and commuting physical activity and the risk of stroke. Stroke [Internet]. 2005 [cited 2014 Jan 3];36(9):1994–9. http://www.ncbi.nlm.nih.gov/pubmed/16081862.
98. Hu G, Jousilahti P, Borodulin K, Barengo NC, Lakka TA, Nissinen A, et al. Occupational, commuting and leisure-time physical activity in relation to coronary heart disease among middle-aged Finnish men and women. Atherosclerosis [Internet]. 2007 [cited 2014 Jan 3];194(2):490–497. http://www.ncbi.nlm.nih.gov/pubmed/16979645.
99. Furie GL, Desai MM. Active transportation and cardiovascular disease risk factors in U.S. adults. Am J Prev Med [Internet]. 2012 [cited 2014 Jan 3];43(6):621–8. http://www.ncbi.nlm.nih.gov/pubmed/23159257.
100. Wannamethee SG, Shaper AG, Walker M. Changes in physical activity, mortality, and incidence of coronary heart disease in older men. Lancet [Internet]. 1998;351(9116):1603–1608. http://www.ncbi.nlm.nih.gov/pubmed/9620713.
101. Rodríguez DA, Cho G-H, Evenson KR, Conway TL, Cohen D, Ghosh-Dastidar B, et al. Out and about: association of the built environment with physical activity behaviors of adolescent females. Health Place. 2012;18(1):55–62.
102. Ng SW, Popkin BM. Time use and physical activity: a shift away from movement across the globe. Obes Rev. 2012;13(8):659–80.
103. Jackson RJ. The impact of the built environment on health: an emerging field. Am J Public Health [Internet]. 2003;93(9):1382–1384. http://www.pubmedcentral.nih.gov/articlerender.fcgi?artid=1447976&tool=pmcentrez&rendertype=abstract.
104. Jackson RJ, Dannenberg AL, Frumkin H. Health and the built environment: 10 years after. Am J Public Health [Internet]. 2013;103(9):1542–1544. http://www.ncbi.nlm.nih.gov/pubmed/23865699.
105. Mansfield TJ, MacDonald Gibson J. Estimating active transportation behaviors to support health impact assessment in the United States. Front Public Health. 2016;4(63):1–18.
106. MacDonald JM, Stokes RJ, Cohen DA, Kofner A, Ridgeway GK. The effect of light rail transit on body mass index and physical activity. Am J Prev Med [Internet]. 2010 [cited 2012 Mar 9];39(2):105–12. http://www.pubmedcentral.nih.gov/articlerender.fcgi?artid=2919301&tool=pmcentrez&rendertype=abstract.
107. Woodcock J, Tainio M, Cheshire J, O'Brien O, Goodman A. Health effects of the London bicycle sharing system: health impact modelling study. BMJ [Internet]. 2014 [cited 2014 Aug

108. MacDonald Gibson J, Rodriguez DA, Dennerlein T, Mead J, Hasch T, Meacci G, et al. Predicting urban design effects on physical activity and public health: a case study. Health Place. 2015;35(September):79–84.
109. Mansfield TJ, MacDonald Gibson J. Health impacts of increased physical activity from changes in transportation infrastructure: quantitative estimates for three communities. Biomed Res Int. 2015;2015:812325.
110. Rojas-Rueda D, de Nazelle A, Teixidó O, Nieuwenhuijsen MJ. Replacing car trips by increasing bike and public transport in the greater Barcelona metropolitan area: a health impact assessment study. Environ Int. 2012;49:100–9.
111. Kotcher J, Maibach E, Miller J, Campbell E, Alqodmani L, Maiero M, et al. Views of health professionals on climate change and health: a multinational survey study. Lancet Planet Health [Internet]. 2021;5(5):e316–e323. https://doi.org/10.1016/S2542-5196(21)00053-X.
112. Haines A, Ebi K. The imperative for climate action to protect health. N Engl J Med. 2019;380(3):263–73.
113. Jackson R, Friedlingstein P, Le Quere C, Abernethy S, Andrew R, Canadell J, et al. Global fossil carbon emissions rebound near pre-COVID-19 levels. 2021. https://arxiv.org/abs/2111.02222v1.
114. U.S. Environmental Protection Agency. Inventory of U.S. greenhouse gas emissions and sinks: 1990–2019 [Internet]. Washington, DC; 2021 [cited 2022 Jan 22]. https://www.epa.gov/ghgemissions/inventory-us-greenhouse-gas-emissions-and-sinks-1990-2019.
115. WHO. Quantitative risk assessment of the effects of climate change on selected causes of death, 2030s and 2050s [Internet]. Geneva; 2014. http://www.who.int/globalchange/publications/quantitative-risk-assessment/en/.
116. Smith KR, Woodward A, Campbell-Lendrum D, Chadee DD, Honda Y, Liu Q, et al. Human health: impacts, adaptation, and vulnerability. In: Field CB, Barros VR, Dokken DJ, Mach KJ, Masgtrandrea MD, Bilir TE, editors. Climate change 2014: impacts, adaptation, and vulnerability contribution of working group II to the fifth assessment report of the intergovernmental panel on climate change. Cambridge: Cambridge University Press; 2014. p. 709–54.
117. Sindall R, Mecrow T, Queiroga AC, Boyer C, Koon W, Peden AE. Drowning risk and climate change: a state-of-the-art review. Inj Prev. 2022;injuryprev-2021-044486.
118. Niles MT, Emery BF, Wiltshire S, Brown ME, Fisher B, Ricketts TH. Climate impacts associated with reduced diet diversity in children across nineteen countries. Environ Res Lett. 2021;16(1):015010.
119. Zwald ML, Hipp JA, Corseuil MW, Dodson EA. Correlates of walking for transportation and use of public transportation among adults in St Louis, Missouri, 2012. Prev Chronic Dis. 2014;11(7):1–10.
120. Goldman RH, Peters JM. The occupational and environmental health history. J Am Med Assoc. 1981;246(24):2831–6.
121. Taiwo OA, Mobo BHP, Cantley L. Recognizing occupational illnesses and injuries. Am Fam Physician. 2010;82(2):169–74.
122. True B-L, Dreisbach RH. Dreisbach's handbook of poisoning: prevention, diagnosis, and treatment. 13th ed. Pearl River: Pantheon Publishing Group; 2001.
123. Gosselin RE. Clinical toxicology of commercial products. 5th ed. Baltimore: Williams & Wilkins; 1984.
124. Smith LL, Lake NH, Simmons LA, Perlman A, Wroth S, Wolever RQ. Integrative health coach training: a model for shifting the paradigm toward patient-centricity and meeting new National Prevention Goals. Glob Adv Health Med [Internet]. 2013;2(3):66–74. http://www.pubmedcentral.nih.gov/articlerender.fcgi?artid=3833534&tool=pmcentrez&rendertype=abstract.
125. Kivelä K, Elo S, Kyngäs H, Kääriäinen M. The effects of health coaching on adult patients with chronic diseases: a systematic review. Patient Educ Couns. 2014;97(2):147–57.

Health Inequities and Structural Racism

Dana Iglesias and Alexa Mieses Malchuk

Introduction

Race is not a valid biological concept but is a social construct that gives or denies benefits and privileges [1]. For example, the social inventions of "race" and "whiteness" helped unite white colonists in early American history, dispossessing and marginalizing native people, and permanently enslaving most African-descended people for generations [1]. Racism justified the exploitation of black bodies throughout the history of medicine in the United States. When the practice of hands-on anatomical dissection became popular in medical education in the late eighteenth and early nineteenth centuries, the demand for cadavers exceeded the supply, and grave robbing was a response to this demand [2]. Dr. James Marion Sims, who is considered the father of obstetrics and gynecology and was President of the American Medical Association, conducted research on enslaved black women without informed consent or the use of anesthesia [3]. In 1932, the U.S. Public Health Service Syphilis Study at Tuskegee began research on the natural history of syphilis in black men. Informed consent was not obtained from participants, and many infected men were left untreated even after penicillin became the standard of care for syphilis. This study continued for decades before the Associated Press drew attention to the study and it was halted [4]. Racism and health inequities continue in the present day.

Race is not a genetic construct, as evidenced by a study which reported that 92% of alleles were found in two or more geographic regions; nearly half of the alleles were found in all geographic regions worldwide [5]. A 2019 expert panel noted that the health of African Americans barely improved after emancipation from slavery, owing to the structural challenges that former slaves faced in procuring adequate food, shelter, and clothing [6]. The historical categorization of identifying non-white people and groups as "other" (e.g., African American, indigenous, people of color, etc.) in the US has adversely impacted the health of these groups. Approximately 11% of African Americans are not covered by health insurance, compared to 7% of non-Hispanic whites. Mortality rates for African Americans are higher than for whites for heart diseases, stroke, cancer, asthma, influenza and pneumonia, diabetes, HIV/AIDS, and homicide [7]. African American, indigenous, and other people of color have disproportionately greater morbidity when compared to their white counterparts. Non-Hispanic African-American adults, for example, are more likely to have high blood pressure; Hispanics and non-Hispanic African-American adults are more likely to have obesity and diabe-

D. Iglesias (✉) · A. M. Malchuk
Department of Family Medicine, University of North Carolina at Chapel Hill, Chapel Hill, NC, USA
e-mail: dana_iglesias@med.unc.edu; alexa_mieses_malchuk@med.unc.edu

tes, and non-Hispanic African-American adults report the highest rate of death from heart disease [8].

African Americans have higher mortality rates than all other racial/ethnic groups for many cancer types [9]. Despite comparable incidence rates of breast cancer, African-American women are more likely to die of the disease than white women [9]. Although prostate cancer mortality has substantially declined in recent decades among all men, African-American men are twice as likely as white men to die of prostate cancer and continue to have the highest prostate cancer mortality among all US population groups [9]. Hispanic and African-American women have higher rates of cervical cancer than women of other racial/ethnic groups have, with African-American women having the highest mortality [9]. American Indians/Alaska Natives have higher death rates from kidney cancer than any other racial/ethnic group [9]. Racial disparities also exist in mental health, where African Americans routinely receive poorer quality of care and lack access to culturally competent care [7]. Approximately one third of African Americans who need mental health care receive it, including medication and outpatient services, but report higher utilization of inpatient services [7].

This chapter is a primer to health equity and structural racism. The first section introduces key concepts and is followed by an overview to an organizing framework developed by the National Institute of Minority Health and Health Disparities (NIMHD). Next, the chapter reviews important strategies to reduce and mitigate health disparities, including Community Health Workers (CHW) and Peer Supports as paraprofessionals, trauma-informed care, and educational initiatives. The chapter closes with future directions in the field.

Key Concepts

There are several important concepts that inform an understanding of health inequities. **Ethnicity** is identity ascribed via belonging to a large group of people who have shared customs, faith traditions, places of origin, or related characteristics [10]. **Intersectionality** is the way in which race, class, gender, and other individual characteristics overlap and are intertwined with one another; Kimberlé Crenshaw, who first coined the term, described it as " a lens through which you can see where power comes and collides, where it interlocks and intersects" [11]. **Social Determinants of Health** are the places where people live, learn, work, and play that affect a wide range of health and quality-of life-risks and outcomes [12]. **Health disparities** are preventable differences in the burden of disease, injury, violence, or differences in opportunities to achieve optimal health experienced by socially disadvantaged racial, ethnic, and other population groups, and communities [13].

Structural racism is a system of power which is embedded in norms and laws, and results in structuring opportunity and assigning value that utilizes a social interpretation of personal appearance, including skin color, facial features, and hair texture [14]. Structural racism is recognized as a determinant of equity within a society, contributing to the political, sociocultural, and historical contexts of subgroups of people resulting in disproportionate and unjust differences between their circumstances [15]. Within the context of health and health care, structural and institutional racism is the differential access to health care services and opportunities by race [16]. Structural racism cuts across action and inaction and is most often seen as inaction in the face of need [17].

Cultural humility is a predisposition and perspective that incorporates a lifelong commitment to self-understanding in order to redress the power differential in the provider-patient dynamic [18]. It seeks to develop mutually beneficial and non-paternalistic partnerships with communities on behalf of individuals and defined populations [19]. **Health equity** is the attainment of the highest level of health for all people. Achieving health equity requires valuing everyone equally with focused and ongoing societal efforts to address avoidable inequalities, historical and contemporary injustices, and the elimination of health and health care disparities [20].

Understanding Health Inequities and Disparities

National Institute of Minority Health and Health Disparities (NIMHD) Framework

A research center within the National Institutes of Health (NIH), the National Institute of Minority Health and Health Disparities (NIMHD) offers a multi-faceted conceptual model to promote an understanding of health inequities and disparities across health sectors (Fig. 42.1) [21]. There are domains of influence that project over the life course and include factors across biological, behavioral, physical/built environment, sociocultural environment, and the health care system. Health disparity populations are defined by inequalities of health outcomes due to race/ethnicity, lower socioeconomic status (SES), meaning individuals or communities with lower access to social, educational, and financial resources, (educaton, income and occupation), sexual and gender minority, disability, and geographic region [21]. To address health disparities, the individual, interpersonal, community, and societal levels must be considered [21]. The Kaiser Family Foundation (KFF) offers a visual paradigm for recognizing health disparities in the context of social determinants of health (SDOH) as well (Fig. 42.2). This framework provides an insightful guide on how personal, social, and economic environments via SDOH affect the health and wellbeing of individuals.

National Institute on Minority Health and Health Disparities Research Framework

		Levels of Influence*			
		Individual	**Interpersonal**	**Community**	**Societal**
Domains of Influence (Over the Lifecourse)	**Biological**	Biological Vulnerability and Mechanisms	Caregiver–Child Interaction Family Microbiome	Community Illness Exposure Herd Immunity	Sanitation Immunization Pathogen Exposure
	Behavioral	Health Behaviors Coping Strategies	Family Functioning School/Work Functioning	Community Functioning	Policies and Laws
	Physical/Built Environment	Personal Environment	Household Environment School/Work Environment	Community Environment Community Resources	Societal Structure
	Sociocultural Environment	Sociodemographics Limited English Cultural Identity Response to Discrimination	Social Networks Family/Peer Norms Interpersonal Discrimination	Community Norms Local Structural Discrimination	Social Norms Societal Structural Discrimination
	Health Care System	Insurance Coverage Health Literacy Treatment Preferences	Patient–Clinician Relationship Medical Decision-Making	Availability of Services Safety Net Services	Quality of Care Health Care Policies
Health Outcomes		Individual Health	Family/ Organizational Health	Community Health	Population Health

National Institute on Minority Health and Health Disparities, 2018
*Health Disparity Populations: Race/Ethnicity, Low SES, Rural, Sexual and Gender Minority
Other Fundamental Characteristics: Sex and Gender, Disability, Geographic Region

Fig. 42.1 NIMHD Research Framework

Health Disparities are Driven by Social and Economic Inequities

Economic Stability	Neighborhood and Physical Environment	Education	Food	Community, Safety, & Social Context	Health Care System
		Racism and Discrimination			
Employment Income Expenses Debt Medical bills Support	Housing Transportation Parks Playgrounds Walkability Zip code/ geography	Literacy Language Early childhood education Vocational training Higher education	Food security Access to healthy options	Social integration Support systems Community engagement Stress Exposure to violence/trauma Policing/justice policy	Health coverage Provider & pharmacy availability Access to linguistically and culturally appropriate & respectful care Quality of care

Health and Well-Being: Mortality, Morbidity, Life Expectancy, Health Care Expenditures, Health Status, Functional Limitations

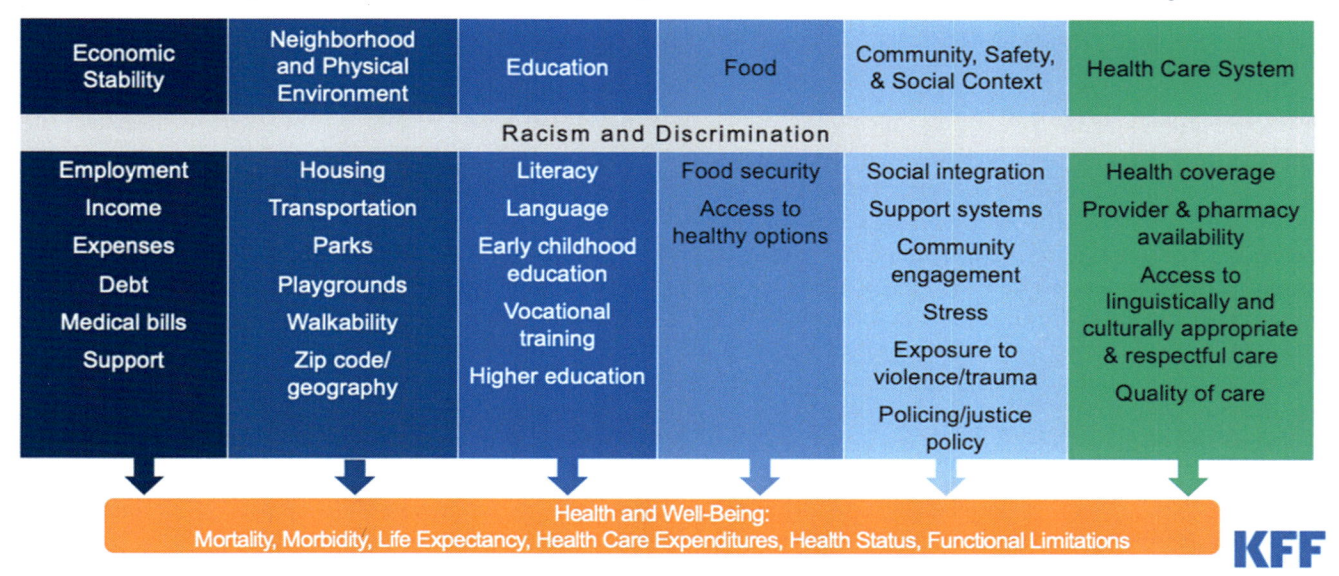

KFF

Fig. 42.2 Kaiser Family Foundation Social Determinants of Health. https://www.kff.org/report-section/disparities-in-health-and-health-care-5-key-questions-and-answers-issue-brief/

Individual Level Factors

Allostatic load describes the effects of frequent stress to the body's adaptive changes in maintaining natural homeostasis [22]. The fight or flight systems reacts to identified threats with a physiological response before returning to baseline once the perceived danger resolves. Continuous negative stimuli cause a momentary rush of cortisol, adrenaline, and norepinephrine that can manifest into a prolonged state of anxiety, resulting in physiologic damage by depleting the regulating balance of the endocrine, immune, and cardiovascular systems [22]. Immune systems that are constantly under duress can trigger the cytokine cascade, making it difficult for the immune system to discern threats and amplify a response, as seen with African-American individuals more adversely affected by Covid-19 with cytokine storm [23]. Allostatic load cumulatively affects all facets of health, changing how the body uses and releases sugar, stores fat, and regulates blood pressure to the brain, heart, and kidneys. This adaptive memory can be passed on to the fetus and the experience of stress in pregnancy can cause changes in fetal brain development [24]. This becomes a predisposition for lifelong stress and emotional dysregulation for populations that experience allostatic burdens [25].

Weathering is the hypothesis that cellular damage due to chronic stress, due to social and economic adversity, microaggression, and political oppression, causes premature deterioration and ageing [26]. All cells have a lifetime or fixed number of divisions permitted which is a progressive physiologic occurrence as the body ages. However, due to increased cellular stress and divisions, those experiencing chronic stress experience premature biological cellular aging. These effects may contribute to higher rates of cancer, shorter life expectancy, and disproportionate disease progression in those experiencing social, structural, and economic marginalization [26].

Interpersonal Factors

Interpersonal factors include adverse childhood events, and social and relational dynamics, particularly bias within health care settings. The landmark Adverse Childhood Events (ACEs) study provides a foundation for relating a person's current health state and behaviors to their childhood experience of maltreatment and family dysfunction [27]. The study observed a direct connection between childhood trauma and adult chronic disease state and created an understanding that linked ACEs to a person's disease state and wellbeing throughout the lifespan. Ten adversities were identified within the family context including: (1) physical abuse, (2) sexual abuse, (3) emotional abuse, (4) physical neglect, (5) emotional neglect, (6) a family member who is depressed or diagnosed with other mental illness, (7) a family member addicted to alcohol or other substance, (8) a family member in prison, (9) witnessed the mother being abused, and (10) losing a parent to separation, divorce, or death [27]. More than half of respondents reported at least one ACE and a fourth reported two or more [27]. A dose-response relationship was identified between increased ACE score risk and subsequent health and social problems, including depression, smoking, alcohol and drug use, physical inactivity, and obesity [27]. Individuals with an ACE score of four or higher were twice as likely to have been diagnosed with cancer and heart disease and four times more likely for emphysema or chronic bronchitis [27]. The CDC's ACE pyramid visually demonstrates the influences of ACEs and of how they affect the health of the individual over their life course (Fig. 42.3).

The Institute of Medicine's report on Unequal Treatment noted that, even when access to care, insurance, family income, and educational status are controlled, racial and ethnic minorities receive inferior health care delivery than their non-minority counterparts and experience worse outcomes [28]. Both explicit and implicit biases are noted as explanatory factors for differences in care, including overt bias, stereotyping, and clinical uncertainty by health care providers [28]. The phenomenon of unconscious or implicit bias is widely studied in social psychology and was initially defined as, "negative unconscious or automatic feelings and beliefs about other people that differ from their voiced and conscious attitudes [29]."

When unconscious bias occurs in health care settings, the mismatch between provider and patient can negatively affect therapeutic relationships. The unconscious assortment of stereotypes and attitudes toward certain groups can influence the diagnosis and treatment of disease, and shared decisions [30]. There are embedded biases based on race, ethnicity, age, gender, sexual orientation, and weight. Provider bias has been described in pain management, chronic disease management, and cancer treatment; preferences are for patients that are white, young, male, heterosexual, and thin [31]. Health care providers have comparable implicit bias as the general population; however, greater bias is associated with poorer care, likely due to unequal treatment recommendations [32]. Negative partiality is "a bias to the acceptance of implicit bias," and can affect uptake and effectiveness of trainings [30].

Racial differences impacting clinical diagnosis, decision-making, and treatment are driven by provider bias, institutional bias, and discrimination [33]. Many information sources and reference materials in medical education use imprecise and incorrect designations for race, ethnicity, and ancestry, which reinforce cultural norms around race, and impedes an understanding of race as a social construct [33]. Racial heuristics, or mental associations and shortcuts for race, apply incorrect descriptors for patients, promoting cognitive errors in clinical diagnosis. For example, labels such as Hispanic, Black, and Asian are often used as synonyms for descriptors such as Mexican, Haitian, or Vietnamese, genetic ancestry, or geographical origin.

Fig. 42.3 The Adverse Childhood Event (ACE) Pyramid. https://www.cdc.gov/violenceprevention/aces/about.html

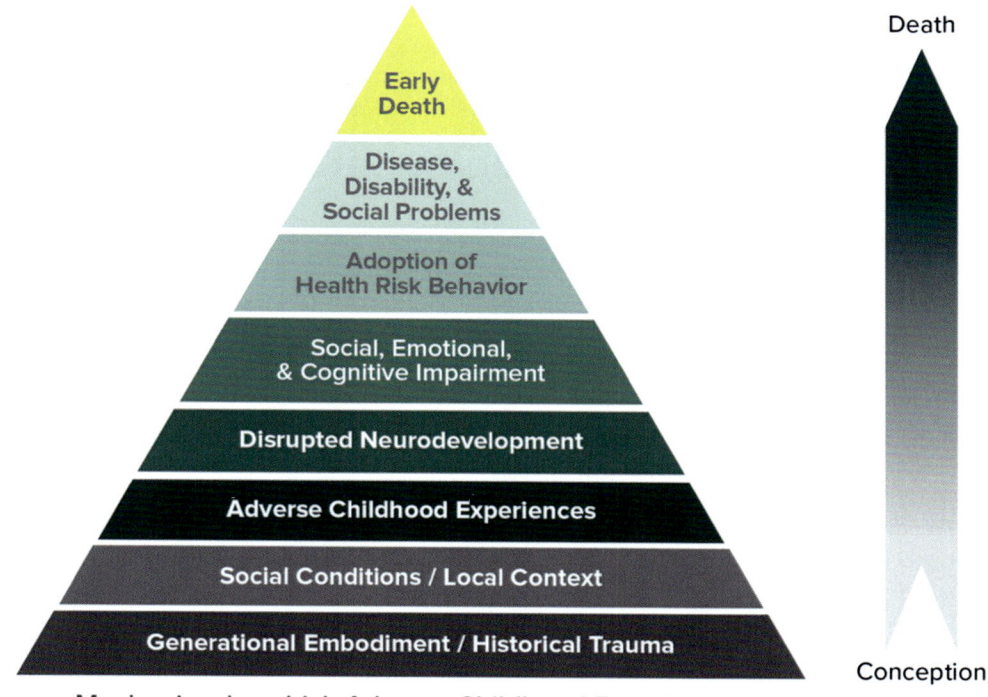

Mechanism by which Adverse Childhood Experiences Influence Health and Well-being Throughout the Lifespan

Race has been used as a surrogate for differences in socioeconomic status, access, and health behaviors. The use of correct racial semantics can help to dissociate these connections [34]. For example, presenting data of racial differences in disease burden without context perpetuates racialized thinking. The highest prevalence of sickle cell disease is in Africa, people of African descent, the Middle East, and areas of the Mediterranean and Asia [34]. African descent includes African Americans and Latin Americans from Central and South America [35]. A misconception that persons who are racialized as black and are uniformly sickle cell disease carriers will result in missed diagnoses or cognitive errors. Generalizing patients' experience of illness based on race also creates treatment errors. The clinical assumptions and attribution error regarding labor pain for Asian patients (e.g., being stoic), Native American patients (e.g., less verbally and non-verbally expressive), Hispanic patients (e.g., laboring or birthing faster) and African-American patients (e.g., higher pain intensity) are unfounded and result in errors in care [32].

Correcting or removing language with racial connotations can interrupt the cycle of negative causal connections and foster better understandings between racial/ethnic groups. Disease designations that use inappropriate geographical or racial terms, such as "Mongolian spot" for congenital dermal melanocytosis and "Red Man syndrome" for vancomycin infusion reaction, should be removed from medical references. The use of race variables in clinical calculators and screening assessments can worsen health disparities if differential risk is assigned for disease conditions based on race [34]. Clinical calculations for glomerular filtration rate (GFR) and spirometry/pulmonary function testing are illustrative examples. GFR guides hypertension and kidney disease treatment and eligibility for renal transplant. Contemporary GFR values adjust for race, reporting higher GFRs for black patients with the same creatinine measurement, which was based on poor quality studies using flawed assumptions of greater muscle mass, higher average creatinine kinase levels, and higher total body potassium and calcium. This bias overestimates GFR and delays access to specialty care [33].

The use of race in spirometry underestimates lung disease prevalence and severity among African-American patients, impacting treatment [33]. Spirometry measurements have historically been based on questionable data from African-American and Asian patients that showed increased estimated lung function capacity [33]. Current guidelines from the American Thoracic Society continue to use race in spirometry calculations [33]. Pulse oximetry often inaccurately measures oxygen saturation in persons with darker skin, which contributes to missing low oxygen levels in African-American patients [36].

Provider-patient concordance occurs when patients perceive personal attributes with their provider [37]. Patients may see themselves as connected or similar to their provider in communication styles, personal beliefs, and values.

Studies of this phenomenon show that providers use of patient-centered communication and the patient's perceived personal similarity predicts patient trust, intent to adhere, and care satisfaction [37]. Concordance can also be observed in culture and language. Although race concordance is the main predictor of perceived ethnic similarity, the use of patient-centered communication is another influencing factor. Enhancing patient-centered communication includes discovering and understanding the patient's disease experience, in verbal and nonverbal messaging, while respecting their beliefs and expectation of care [38]. Training programs can increase provider communication skills and lead to improved outcomes [38].

Community Level Factors

The tangible and intangible resources that are available in communities, such as housing, food, neighborhood safety, and green space, directly impacts a person's capacity to make healthy choices and take actionable steps in wellbeing and managing chronic disease.

Food Insecurity

Food insecurity is the interruption of food by intake or eating patterns due to lacking money or other resources affecting one or more members of the home [39]. In 2020, 38 million people lived in food insecure homes and the problem can be long or short term, influenced by income, employment, race/ethnicity, and disability [40]. Though the national average for food insecurity is 12.3%, prevalence of food insecurity among Hispanic homes is 18.5%, and 22.5% among Black homes [40].

Limited access to full-service grocery stores reduces access to food in urban, rural, and low-income neighborhoods. Food deserts are communities that lack accessible, affordable, and nutritious food choices [39]. Convenience stores, although close, may charge higher prices and offer less choice. Distance and transportation are barriers for patients with chronic disease, disability, and those in rural areas. Programs targeting food insecurity have the potential to influence chronic disease outcomes and health disparities [39].

Housing Stability

Access to housing is a major factor that contributes to health disparities. Redlining, the historical government sponsored practice of facilitating mortgage lenders and insurance providers in restricting services to specified geographic areas based up the applicant's racial characteristic, has resulted in residential segregation [41]. In practice, geographic areas where mixed race or African Americans lived were marked red on maps, and areas desirable for lending were marked in yellow. Conversely, affluent areas marked in blue or green were identified for favorable loans. Low-income families and people of color residing in historically redlined communities have poorer quality housing, higher population density housing in urban areas, and experience higher environmental toxin exposure [42]. From 1934 to 1962, virtually all federal loans were distributed to white Americans [42] and current gentrification practices and policies may represent the second wave of redlining [42].

House quality is the physical condition of the home, and the social and physical environment where the house is located [43]. Factors affecting housing quality include home age and safety, air quality, presence of lead, mold, and asbestos. Poor quality housing is associated with adverse health outcomes associated with chronic disease and mental health [43]. Exposures from hazardous elements like carbon monoxide, allergens, and lead in paint, pipes, and faucets make healthy individuals sick, and worsen underlying conditions. Homes lacking ventilation and proper screens place occupants with diseases such as tuberculosis and COVID-19 at further risk for transmission and poor outcomes [44]. Cold and heat exposure in homes can worsen poor health and mold growth associated with water leaks increases the likelihood of asthma. Overcrowded homes are associated with poor mental health, food insecurity, and increased transmission of infectious disease, such as COVID-19 [43]. Policy efforts can directly impact and improve housing quality, thereby protecting those living in vulnerable public housing [43].

Green Space

The US Environmental Protection Agency describes green spaces as any open land area that enhances the beauty and environmental quality of a neighborhood and is accessible to the public [45]. This land is undeveloped (i.e., no built structures or buildings) and include schoolyards, playgrounds, public plazas and seating areas, vacant lots, parks, community gardens and cemeteries. Local environmental exposure to, and maintenance of, greens space has the capacity to improve health within communities. A systematic review found that green spaces and parks show a protective effect in lower SES populations, suggesting expanding green spaces might be a strategy to improve health equity [45].

Social Connectedness

Social capital is the strength of relationships and camaraderie of members within a defined community [46]. This power of connection can provide support through shared resources of food, clothing, employment, emotional support, and transportation. Social capital within communities is thought to be an important buffer to income equality [46]. The measure of perceived fairness and helpfulness, trust and group membership, lost or gained, is linked with income and mortality [46]. Collective efficacy is a community's ability to create change and exercise informal social control, whether through social norms or other collective action [46]. Communities with collective efficacy have better perceived health, lower neighborhood violence, better access to medical care, healthy food, and places to exercise [46].

Social networks can influence chronic disease and health outcomes, psychologically and through health behaviors [46]. For example, an individual's risk of becoming obese is increased if a friend, sibling, or spouse is also obese, associations that are also observed in tobacco and alcohol use [46]. Alternately, social support is thought to be protective for chronic disease risk [46]. A study of adults of Mexican origin, for example, reported that social support was a buffer against the health effect due to discrimination [46]. Social isolation is decreased personal contact, and with increased age, especially with older adults, adds stress and carries with it negative health behaviors [46]. The highly intersectional nature of community social connections and future health interventions likely needs to occur at multiples levels (individual, interpersonal, and societal). Overall, the data points to the protective effects of social connectedness and potential strategies in reducing disparities [46].

Societal Level Factors

There are several higher level social and environmental factors that influence individual choice and community agency, which ultimately impacts health outcomes, including environmental quality (e.g., clean water and air), policing and mass incarceration, and health care access.

Environment

The World Health Organization identifies climate change as a contributing factor to social and environmental determinants of health, including clean air, safe drinking water, and food and shelter security [47]. Globally, the direct damage and cost to health is predicted to be between two to four billion dollars per year by 2030 [48]. In the US, there were an estimated 300,000 deaths, 11%, attributed to environmental causes in 2012 [47]. Contaminated groundwater for drinking and irrigation increases the risk of adverse health. For example, nearly half of waterborne illnesses, such as Giardia, can be from untreated groundwater with sources of groundwater contamination including agricultural runoff, landfills, septic tanks, and leaking underground storage tanks [47].

Exposure to air pollutants like ozone and fine particulate matter increases risks of lung cancer, cardiovascular disease, and overall mortality, particularly for individuals with asthma and chronic lung disease [47]. Climate change and the associated increased temperatures raises the risk of heat related disease and death, which is reported at higher rates in older adults and for racial and ethnic minorities [47]. Persons who lack temperature regulation and agricultural workers are particularly prone to heat related illness and death [47]. Geographic location influences environmental hazard exposure for individuals residing in rural and urban areas, and disproportionally for racial/ethnic minorities [47]. Individuals who are economically disadvantaged and living in poor housing may be exposed to pests, such as cockroaches and rodents, increasing the risk of disease and negatively impacting quality of life [47].

Carceral System

Incarceration and reimprisonment adversely impact individuals and their communities. Men and women with a history of incarceration have worse mental and physical health, including chronic conditions such as hypertension, asthma, cancer, and infectious disease such as tuberculosis (TB), hepatitis C, and HIV [49]. Imprisoned women are more likely to have experienced ACEs, specifically childhood physical and sexual abuse and carry greater burdens of disease then imprisoned men, with higher rates of hypertension, hepatitis, TB, HIV/AIDS, and sexually transmitted infections compared to imprisoned men [49].

The number of older persons incarcerated, as well as those with chronic disease continues to increase with many receiving inadequate treatment [49]. Reintegration is difficult for those who have spent significant time incarcerated, and families of incarcerated persons are adversely impacted, experiencing stress and loss of income while their family member is away [49]. Securing reliable employment, housing, and healthcare is difficult for formerly incarcerated persons, since prior convictions result in a loss of state and federal benefits such as access to food stamps, driver's license, education assistance, public housing benefits and the right to vote [49]. In consequence, recently released individuals have higher rates of overdose and suicide [49].

Incarcerated individuals are inmates under the jurisdiction of state or federal prisons or individuals who are held in local jails [49]. From 1980 to 2014, the US incarceration rate increased by 220%, with 2.2 million persons were state, federal, or local systems and 4.7 million under community supervision, probation, or parole [49]. The US criminal justice system is oriented to incarceration, a mechanism to punish criminal offenses, as opposed to rehabilitation or restorative justice [49]. The rise of imprisoned persons is directly linked to increases in harsher sentencing rules and unequal policing in poorer and racial/ethnic communities [49]. As a result, racial disparities exist in state and federal carceral systems, with incarcerated persons more likely to be from lower SES education levels and non-white [49]. Although women are imprisoned less often than men are, significant disparities remain [49]. Communities with a greater burden of incarceration report high recidivism, crime rates, poverty, and unemployment [49].

An intersectional approach can promote an understanding of programs and services which would benefit communities that are adversely affected by incarceration. Some policy strategies to mitigate imprisonment would include ending the school to prison pipeline; removing mandatory minimums; decreasing policing; providing alternatives to prison and; reducing penalties for menial and drug offenses [50]. Additionally comprehensive health and reintegration programs will help those recently released to integrate into their communities [50].

Access to Health Services

Access to health care services is influenced by health insurance coverage and by access to primary care and mental health services [51]. Disparities in health insurance coverage promote health inequities, with the most vulnerable delaying or opting out of care due to cost. Lower income Americans are uninsured more often, which adversely affects their health care and outcomes [51]. For example, uninsured adults receive less preventive services for chronic disease, however when insured, patients have improved access to care and better healthcare monitoring [51].

Limited provider availability to primary care and mental health services contribute to poor chronic disease and associated health outcomes [51]. Some Medicaid beneficiaries have difficulty in locating providers due to reduced reimbursement [52] while the lack of transportation and distance to travel is another factor [53]. Hospital closures, especially in rural communities, have reduced access and some have adapted by converting inpatient beds or units into emergency, rehabilitation, or outpatient services at the same physical location [52]. Some communities have health care facilities but lack health care providers due to staffing shortages. The COVID-19 pandemic has worsened these shortages and exposed the racial and health disparities in the workforce [54].

Strategies to Mitigate and Reduce Health Disparities

Trauma-Informed Care

The Diagnostic and Statistical Manual of Mental Disorders (DSM) fifth edition defines traumatic events as exposure to serious injury, sexual violence, or threatened death. Traumatic events are linked to a variety of mental and physical health outcomes [55]. Seventy percent of adults experience at least one traumatic event over their lifetime and 20% progress on to PTSD [55]. Trauma-Informed care recognizes the signs, symptoms and the role trauma have on the individual and staff working in the field of mental and physical health services [56]. Acknowledgment of trauma changes the approach of health care organizations and care teams for its patients and clients to develop a more complete picture of their life circumstances. The goals are to create awareness and educate the clinical and non-clinical workforce, identify and treat trauma, and create a safe environment that builds trust for those who experience trauma. This shifts the paradigm from "What is wrong with the person" to "What has happened to this person [56]?" Various organizations and nonprofits have incorporated Trauma-Informed Care into their organizational policies, practices, and care. The Center for Health Care Strategies has a national initiative focused on understanding and implementing trauma-informed care into health systems [57]. Collaborating centers include Montefiore Medical Group, San Francisco Department of Public Health, and Greater Newark Healthcare Coalition.

The Adverse Childhood Events (ACEs) study and subsequent research is the foundation for screening and implementation of trauma-informed work [57]. For individuals ACE, increasing the quality and frequency of Positive Childhood Experiences (PCEs) can be beneficial in reducing toxic stress and allostatic load since resilience research shows that social support, feelings of control and a sense of meaning are important factors [58]. Examples of PCEs include: (1) the ability to talk to your family about feelings, (2) feeling that your family stood by you during difficult times, (3) enjoyment in participating in community traditions, (4) feeling supported by friends, (5) having two non-parent adults who took genuine interest in you, and (6) feeling safe and protected by an adult in your home [59]. In addition, children who feel a stronger sense of ethnic identity have lower allostatic load. For example, parents of African American, Mexican and Native traditions who discussed the meaning of racial/ethnic identity, socialization, and cultural orientation promoted positive development potentially protected against the negative effects of racial/ethnic discrimination [60].

Team-based care and integrated primary and behavioral health care are care delivery models that can incorporate trauma-informed care principles as ways to address ACEs and reduce health disparities. Twenty-five states have enacted or adopted legislation to address ACEs, toxic stress, and child adversity, and other existing bills have created commissions to address ACEs and implement healthcare workforce training and trauma-informed practices [61]. Consequently, interventions at the family or health service level will need to consider the greater community. Developing life and coping skills without understanding and addressing larger structural forces limits the capacity for meaningful and sustained change, potentially causing a cycle of pathologizing the person instead of the system.

Addressing Unconscious (Implicit) Bias

There are several approaches for addressing implicit bias including: (1) understanding the culture of patients; (2) personalizing and not stereotyping patients; (3) respecting and understanding the power of unconscious bias; (4) recognizing situations that magnify stereotyping and bias such as overloaded, stressful, and time-pressured clinical encounters; (5) being aware of culturally and linguistically appropriate service (CLAS) standards, and; (6) conducting "teach backs" with patients as methods of confirming that the person understands health care instructions [62]. These strategies can promote patient safety, treatment adherence, and quality with evidence-based medicine [62].

The Association of American Medical Colleges (AAMC) offers trainings and resources to understand and address unconscious bias for institutions [63]. These resources provide tools to mitigate bias in the recruitment process, education curriculum, and training [64]. The American Academy of Family Physicians, EveryOne Project, offers Implicit Bias Training and a facilitation guide for health care professionals [65]. The impact of unconscious bias training on disparities is mixed in the literature and points to the need for further study and suggests more comprehensive educational approaches for changing healthcare-provider behaviors in healthcare disparities [66].

More successful programming within medical school education includes longitudinal curriculum, such as the Mayo Clinic Alix School of Medicine. Beginning early in the first few weeks of year 1, the student takes at least two of Implicit Association Tests (IAT), reflects on their results and discusses with peers, read a seminal text on implicit bias, (e.g., *Blindspot*, by Banaji and Greenwald), critically assess case studies, engage in group discussion, and learn strategies to mitigate biases. Year 2 includes 6 months of curricula on cultural humility, health care disparities, racism, and mistrust in health care. Year 3 students examine unconscious biases on diagnostic errors and in year 4, they reflect on this prior training and their ability to provide care to patients as medical professionals in this applied learning format [67].

Community Health Workers

Community health workers (CHWs) are trusted members of a defined community, which enables workers to be linkages between health and social services and the community, facilitating access and improving the quality and cultural competence of services [68].

CHWs have many names: lay health workers, village health workers, community health aides, health advisors, and patient navigators [69]. In addressing health needs, CHWs aim to increase health knowledge and self-sufficiency through outreach, community education, informal counseling, social support, and advocacy [70]. Interventions that employ community health worker models vary by disease process, curricula, population, and outcome. Intervention and studies utilizing CHWs span across health conditions such as diabetes mellitus, cardiovascular disease, HIV/AIDS, asthma, mental health, substance use, maternal and child health, and other chronic conditions. The current body of evidence supports CHW services to improve health care outcomes, including reductions in chronic illness progression, better medication adherence, increased patient involvement, improved overall community health and reduced health care costs [71].

Workforce Education and Training

Medical and health care educational initiatives and training can reinforce bias or encourage new thinking and questioning, potentially mitigating and reducing bias [32]. Although the Institute of Medicine recommended promoting healthcare providers' awareness of disparities and integrating cross-cultural education, this goal has not been achieved [72]. For example, in 2018, most US medical schools did not have documented, standardized, integrated education on health disparities, and only 40% reported content on racial disparity curricula [72].

In recent years, many organizations and institutions have developed strategies to improve Diversity Equity and Inclusion (DEI). The American Medical Association, an organization that excluded black physicians for almost 100 years, has taken steps to reconcile with its history and reorganize as an institution through their Equity Plan strategic plan [73]. The plan includes an open access education tool named Health Equity Education Center, which provides information sources on the history of racism in medicine, and instruction on health equity [73, 74].

Several factors contribute to successful or failed implementation of DEI programs. Unsuccessful programs have focused exclusively on bias training and screening, without substantial organization restructuring that was informed by data [75]. Mandatory diversity trainings and punitive grievance systems were also ineffective, in comparison to voluntary trainings [75]. Successful DEI initiatives were associated with positive, active engagement of the entire organization including senior leadership and data that can gauge an organization's performance in DEI [75]. Organizations may choose to identify a diversity manager, a defined leadership position assigned to develop and direct DEI efforts. Assembling a taskforce is another approach and is successful when leadership and underrepresented staff are partnered together, inclusive of senior, middle, and lower management, in ways that promote inclusivity of diverse staffs and make equity a priority across the entire organizational system [75]. Every organization will require substantial efforts to make measurable change in the education and training of the healthcare workforce [76].

Increasing Workforce Diversity

Increasing the diversity in the healthcare workforce is critical since the majority of US physicians are White (67%), with lesser numbers of Hispanic (6.3%), African American (4.8%), Asian (19.6%), American Indian/Alaska Native (0.1%), and Multiple/Other race (2.1%) [77]. In response, the Health Resource and Service Administration has sponsored multiple scholarship and individual loan repayment programs through National Health Service Corps, Nurse Corps Scholarship and Loan Repayment Program, Faculty Loan Repayment Program, Native Hawaiian Health Scholarship Program [78].

Although the health care workforce is more diverse, the majority of diversity remains at entry level and lower paying positions [79]. Pipeline programs are successful, however many start at the post-secondary level and do not address the needs and attrition at the pipeline sources, primary and secondary education [79]. Initiatives to increase workforce diversity point to the need for comprehensive programs targeting social support, academic support, and financial support [79]. Overall, programing that appears to be successful include an interprofessional approach to increase student diversity interest in healthcare workforce, intra-organization change in admission practices, diversity monitoring, senior leadership buy in, and involves community and university social support for students in order to increase application and admission to programs [80]. For example, there are programs at the University of Cincinnati, Academic Health Center, Associated Medical Schools of New York—The Voice of Medical Education, and University of North Carolina, School of Medicine, Medical Education Development (MED) summer program and Carolina MED EXCEL (Medical Education Development Early eXperience in Clinical Education and Learning) yearlong program [81, 82].

Future Directions

Health information technologies are utilizing artificial intelligence (AI) in clinical algorithms for clinical decision making and managing populations [83]. As these technologies emerge, attention to how constructs of race will be measured and utilized will be critical to prevent further widening of health disparities. There are risks of encoding racial bias in core data inputs, and algorithms must reflect the complexity of its population and health needs, not simplify or narrow them [84]. AI can rely on individual level data of healthcare utilization or other outcomes, and the use of imbalanced data (i.e., does not account for diverse population) results in skewed and bias results. For example, one study reported that an algorithm designed to identify patients with complex needs erroneously allocated the same risks for white and African-American patients [85]. Although healthcare costs were reported less in African-American patients, this was attributed to greater barriers in accessing care [85].

At the practice and policy level, there is an impetus for fundamental change to reduce health inequities. Both the American Medical Association and Agency for Healthcare Research and Quality have adopted policies recognizing race as a social construct with no genetic basis, and encourage medical education and clinical practice to change curriculum and teaching materials to be race conscious and reflective of the context of health disparities [34]. The Affordable Care Act (ACA) helped to reduce health disparities by substantially extending insurance coverage, increasing access for medically vulnerable and lower income patients, and provides protection for patients with pre-existing conditions [86]. Expansion of ACA principles and policies will further the work of reducing disparities.

The problems of structural racism and health disparities are intersectional and complex. It will require the efforts of all cadres of health care workers to fully equip themselves with various tools to navigate these problems. Solutions must come from all sectors of health care to achieve health equity in America.

References

1. Historical Foundations of Race [Internet]. National Museum of African American History and Culture. 2020 [cited 2021 Oct 31]. https://nmaahc.si.edu/learn/talking-about-race/topics/historical-foundations-race.
2. Halperin EC. The poor, the Black, and the marginalized as the source of cadavers in United States anatomical education. Clin Anat. 2007;20(5):489–95.
3. Holland B. The 'Father of Modern Gynecology' performed shocking experiments on enslaved women—HISTORY [Internet]. 2018 [cited 2021 Nov 2]. https://www.history.com/news/the-father-of-modern-gynecology-performed-shocking-experiments-on-slaves.
4. CDC. Tuskegee study—Timeline—CDC—NCHHSTP [Internet]. Centers for Disease Control and Prevention. 2021 [cited 2021 Nov 1]. https://www.cdc.gov/tuskegee/timeline.htm.
5. Rosenberg NA, Pritchard JK, Weber JL, Cann HM, Kidd KK, Zhivotovsky LA, et al. Genetic structure of human populations. Science. 2002;298(5602):2381–5.
6. Milano B. Ramifications of slavery persist in health care inequality [Internet]. Harvard Gazette. 2019 [cited 2021 Nov 2]. https://news.harvard.edu/gazette/story/2019/10/ramifications-of-slavery-persist-in-health-care-inequality/.

7. APA. Mental health, diverse populations and disparities [Internet]. American Psychiatric Association; 2017 [cited 2021 Oct 31]. https://www.psychiatry.org/psychiatrists/cultural-competency/education/mental-health-facts.
8. CDC. Racial and ethnic disparities in heart disease [Internet]. Centers for Disease Control and Prevention. 2019 [cited 2021 Nov 1]. https://www.cdc.gov/nchs/hus/spotlight/HeartDiseaseSpotlight_2019_0404.pdf.
9. National Cancer Institute. Cancer disparities [Internet]. National Cancer Institute. 2020 [cited 2021 Nov 1]. https://www.cancer.gov/about-cancer/understanding/disparities.
10. Ethnic definition & meaning—Merriam-Webster [Internet]. 2021 [cited 2021 Nov 2]. https://www.merriam-webster.com/dictionary/ethnic.
11. Crenshaw K. Kimberlé Crenshaw on intersectionality, more than two decades later [Internet]. News from Columbia Law School. 2017 [cited 2022 May 10]. https://www.law.columbia.edu/news/archive/kimberle-crenshaw-intersectionality-more-two-decades-later.
12. CDC. About Social Determinants of Health (SDOH) [Internet]. Centers for Disease Control and Prevention. 2021 [cited 2021 Nov 1]. https://www.cdc.gov/socialdeterminants/about.html.
13. CDC. Health disparities | healthy aging [Internet]. Centers for Disease Control and Prevention. 2017 [cited 2021 Nov 2]. https://www.cdc.gov/aging/disparities/index.htm.
14. 11 terms you should know to better understand structural racism [Internet]. The Aspen Institute. 2021 [cited 2022 May 11]. https://www.aspeninstitute.org/blog-posts/structural-racism-definition/.
15. Hardeman RR, Homan PA, Chantarat T, Davis BA, Brown TH. Improving the measurement of structural racism to achieve antiracist health policy. Health Aff (Millwood). 2022;41(2):179–86.
16. Jones CP. Confronting institutionalized racism. Phylon. 2002;50(1–2):7.
17. Jones CP. Levels of racism: a theoretic framework and a gardener's tale. Am J Public Health. 2000;90(8):1212–5.
18. Center for Health Equity Advancement—cultural humility [Internet]. Penn Medicine. 2020 [cited 2022 May 11]. https://www.chea.upenn.edu/cultural-humility/.
19. Tervalon M, Murray-García J. Cultural humility versus cultural competence: a critical distinction in defining physician training outcomes in multicultural education. J Health Care Poor Underserved. 1998;9(2):117–25.
20. U.S. DHHS. Disparities | healthy people 2020 [Internet]. Office of Disease Prevention and Health Promotion. 2021 [cited 2022 Jan 29]. https://www.healthypeople.gov/2020/about/foundation-health-measures/Disparities.
21. U.S. DHHS. NIMHD research framework [Internet]. National Institute on Minority Health and Health Disparities. 2021 [cited 2022 Jan 30]. https://www.nimhd.nih.gov/about/overview/research-framework/.
22. McEwen BS. Stressed or stressed out: what is the difference? J Psychiatry Neurosci. 2005;30(5):315–8.
23. Tal Y, Adini A, Eran A, Adini I. Racial disparity in Covid-19 mortality rates—A plausible explanation. Clin Immunol. 2020;217:108481.
24. Coussons-Read ME. Effects of prenatal stress on pregnancy and human development: mechanisms and pathways. Obstet Med. 2013;6(2):52–7.
25. Lu MC, Verbiest S, Dominguez TP. Life course theory: an overview. In: Verbiest S, editor. Moving life course theory into action: making change happen. American Public Health Association; 2018.
26. Geronimus AT, Hicken M, Keene D, Bound J. "Weathering" and age patterns of allostatic load scores among blacks and whites in the United States. Am J Public Health. 2006;96(5):826–33.
27. Felitti VJ, Anda RF, Nordenberg D, Williamson DF, Spitz AM, Edwards V, et al. Relationship of childhood abuse and household dysfunction to many of the leading causes of death in adults. The Adverse Childhood Experiences (ACE) study. Am J Prev Med. 1998;14(4):245–58.
28. Smedley BD, Stith AY, Nelson AR. Unequal treatment: confronting racial and ethnic disparities in health care. Washington, DC: National Academies Press; 2003.
29. Dovidio JF, Gaertner SL. Aversive racism. Elsevier; 2004. p. 1–52.
30. FitzGerald C, Hurst S. Implicit bias in healthcare professionals: a systematic review. BMC Med Ethics. 2017;18(1):19.
31. Nosek BA, Smyth FL, Hansen JJ, Devos T, Lindner NM, Ranganath KA, et al. Pervasiveness and correlates of implicit attitudes and stereotypes. Eur Rev Soc Psychol. 2007;18(1):36–88.
32. Hoffman KM, Trawalter S, Axt JR, Oliver MN. Racial bias in pain assessment and treatment recommendations, and false beliefs about biological differences between blacks and whites. Proc Natl Acad Sci U S A. 2016;113(16):4296–301.
33. Artiga MT, Samantha. Use of race in clinical diagnosis and decision making: overview and implications [Internet]. Kaiser Family Foundation. 2021 [cited 2022 Jan 29]. https://www.kff.org/racial-equity-and-health-policy/issue-brief/use-of-race-in-clinical-diagnosis-and-decision-making-overview-and-implications.
34. Amutah C, Greenidge K, Mante A, Munyikwa M, Surya SL, Higginbotham E, et al. Misrepresenting race—the role of medical schools in propagating physician bias. N Engl J Med. 2021;384(9):872–8.
35. Lopez G, Gonzalez-Barrera A. Afro-Latino: a deeply rooted identity among U.S. Hispanics [Internet]. Pew Research Center. 2016 [cited 2022 May 10]. https://www.pewresearch.org/fact-tank/2016/03/01/afro-latino-a-deeply-rooted-identity-among-u-s-hispanics/.
36. Sjoding MW, Dickson RP, Iwashyna TJ, Gay SE, Valley TS. Racial bias in pulse oximetry measurement. N Engl J Med. 2020;383(25):2477–8.
37. Street RL, O'Malley KJ, Cooper LA, Haidet P. Understanding concordance in patient-physician relationships: personal and ethnic dimensions of shared identity. Ann Fam Med. 2008;6(3):198–205.
38. Hashim MJ. Patient-centered communication: basic skills. Am Fam Physician. 2017;95(1):29–34.
39. U.S. DHHS. Food insecurity | healthy people 2020 [Internet]. 2021 [cited 2022 Jan 29]. https://www.healthypeople.gov/2020/topics-objectives/topic/social-determinants-health/interventions-resources/food-insecurity.
40. Coleman-Jensen A, Rabbitt MP, Hales L, Gregory CA. USDA ERS—key statistics & graphics [Internet]. 2021 [cited 2022 Jan 28]. https://www.ers.usda.gov/topics/food-nutrition-assistance/food-security-in-the-u-s/key-statistics-graphics/.
41. Britannica T. Editors of Encyclopaedia. redlining | discrimination | Britannica [Internet]. 2014 [cited 2022 Jan 28]. https://www.britannica.com/topic/redlining.
42. Garber J. Racist redlining policies still have an impact on health—Lown Institute [Internet]. Lown Institute. 2021 [cited 2022 Jan 28]. https://lowninstitute.org/racist-redlining-policies-still-have-an-impact-on-health/.
43. U.S. DHHS. Quality of housing | healthy people 2020 [Internet]. 2021 [cited 2022 Jan 29]. https://www.healthypeople.gov/2020/topics-objectives/topic/social-determinants-health/interventions-resources/quality-of-housing.
44. Ventilation and Coronavirus (COVID-19) [Internet]. United States Environmental Protection Agency. [cited 2022 May 14]. https://www.epa.gov/coronavirus/ventilation-and-coronavirus-covid-19.
45. Rigolon A, Browning MHEM, McAnirlin O, Yoon HV. Green space and health equity: a systematic review on the potential of green space to reduce health disparities. Int J Environ Res Public Health. 2021;18(5):2563.
46. U.S. DHHS. Social cohesion | healthy people 2020 [Internet]. 2021 [cited 2022 Jan 28]. https://www.healthypeople.gov/2020/topics-objectives/topic/social-determinants-health/interventions-resources/social-cohesion.

47. U.S. DHHS. Environmental conditions | healthy people 2020 [Internet]. 2021 [cited 2022 Jan 29]. https://www.healthypeople.gov/2020/topics-objectives/topic/social-determinants-health/interventions-resources/environmental.
48. Climate change [Internet]. World Health Organization—Health Topics. [cited 2022 May 15]. https://www.who.int/health-topics/climate-change#tab=tab_1.
49. U.S. DHHS. Incarceration | healthy people 2020 [Internet]. 2021 [cited 2022 Jan 29]. https://www.healthypeople.gov/2020/topics-objectives/topic/social-determinants-health/interventions-resources/incarceration.
50. Smit DV. Handbook of basic principles and promising practices on alternatives to imprisonment. 2007.
51. U.S. DHHS. Access to health services | healthy people 2020 [Internet]. 2021 [cited 2022 Jan 29]. https://www.healthypeople.gov/2020/topics-objectives/topic/social-determinants-health/interventions-resources/access-to-health.
52. UNC ShepsCenter. Rural Hospital Closures—Sheps Center [Internet]. The Cecil G. Sheps Center for Health Services Research. 2014 [cited 2022 Jan 29]. https://www.shepscenter.unc.edu/programs-projects/rural-health/rural-hospital-closures/.
53. U.S. DHHS. Access to primary care | healthy people 2020 [Internet]. 2021 [cited 2022 Jan 29]. https://www.healthypeople.gov/2020/topics-objectives/topic/social-determinants-health/interventions-resources/access-to-primary.
54. Wilson V. Inequities exposed: how COVID-19 widened racial inequities in education, health, and the workforce: Testimony before the U.S. House of Representatives Committee on Education and Labor [Internet]. Economic Policy Institute. 2020 [cited 2022 May 15]. https://www.epi.org/publication/covid-19-inequities-wilson-testimony/.
55. Benjet C, Bromet E, Karam EG, Kessler RC, McLaughlin KA, Ruscio AM, et al. The epidemiology of traumatic event exposure worldwide: results from the World Mental Health Survey Consortium. Psychol Med. 2016;46(2):327–43.
56. The Institute on Trauma and Trauma-Informed Care (ITTIC). What is trauma-informed care? [Internet]. University at Buffalo School of Social Work—University at Buffalo. [cited 2022 May 13]. https://socialwork.buffalo.edu/social-research/institutes-centers/institute-on-trauma-and-trauma-informed-care/what-is-trauma-informed-care.html.
57. Menschner C, Maul A. Key ingredients for successful trauma-informed care implementation. Trenton: Center for Health Care Strategies, Incorporated; 2016.
58. American Psychological Association. Task Force on Resilience and Strength in Black Children and Adolescents. Resilience in AfricanAmerican children and adolescents: a vision for optimal development [Internet]. 2008 [cited 2022 Jan 27]. https://www.apa.org/pi/families/resources/resiliencerpt.pdf.
59. Bethell C, Jones J, Gombojav N, Linkenbach J, Sege R. Positive childhood experiences and adult mental and relational health in a statewide sample: associations across adverse childhood experiences levels. JAMA Pediatr. 2019;173(11):e193007.
60. Neblett EW, Rivas-Drake D, Umaña-Taylor AJ. The promise of racial and ethnic protective factors in promoting ethnic minority youth development. Child Dev Perspect. 2012;6(3):295–303.
61. Bradford K. Reducing the effects of adverse childhood experiences [Internet]. National Conference of State Legislatures, vol. 28, no. 29. 2020 [cited 2022 Jan 29]. https://www.ncsl.org/research/health/reducing-the-effects-of-adverse-childhood-experiences.aspx.
62. Seeing patients—Augustus A. White III, MD | Harvard University Press [Internet]. [cited 2022 Jan 30]. https://www.hup.harvard.edu/catalog.php?isbn=9780674049055.
63. Unconscious bias resources for health professionals [Internet]. Association of American Medical Colleges (AAMC), Diversity and Inclusion, Workforce. [cited 2022 May 15]. https://www.aamc.org/what-we-do/equity-diversity-inclusion/unconscious-bias-training.
64. Tool for Assessing Cultural Competence Training (TACCT) [Internet]. Association of American Medical Colleges (AAMC). [cited 2022 May 15]. https://www.aamc.org/what-we-do/equity-diversity-inclusion/tool-for-assessing-cultural-competence-training.
65. Implicit bias resources—The EveryONE project [Internet]. American Academy of Family Physicians (AAFP). [cited 2022 May 15]. https://www.aafp.org/family-physician/patient-care/the-everyone-project/toolkit/implicit-bias.html.
66. Maina IW, Belton TD, Ginzberg S, Singh A, Johnson TJ. A decade of studying implicit racial/ethnic bias in healthcare providers using the implicit association test. Soc Sci Med. 2018;199:219–29.
67. Reddy S, Starr S, Hayes S, Balls-Berry J, Saxon M, Speer M, et al. Implicit bias curricula in medical school: student and faculty perspectives [Internet]. Health Affairs. 2020 [cited 2022 May 15]. https://www.healthaffairs.org/do/10.1377/forefront.20200110.360375/full/.
68. Community Health Workers [Internet]. Association of State and Territorial Health Officials, Medicaid and Public Health Partnership Learning Series. [cited 2021 Nov 28]. https://www.astho.org/Health-Systems-Transformation/Medicaid-and-Public-Health-Partnerships/Learning-Series/Community-Health-Workers/.
69. ILO. International Standard Classification of Occupations—Structure, group definitions and correspondence tables [Internet]. International Labour Organization. 2012 [cited 2021 Nov 22]. https://www.ilo.org/wcmsp5/groups/public/@dgreports/@dcomm/@publ/documents/publication/wcms_172572.pdf.
70. APHA. Support for community health worker leadership in determining workforce standards for training and credentialing [Internet]. Policy statement database. 2014 [cited 2021 Nov 21]. https://www.apha.org/policies-and-advocacy/public-health-policy-statements/policy-database/2015/01/28/14/15/support-for-community-health-worker-leadership.
71. Rosenthal EL, Wiggins N, Ingram M, Mayfield-Johnson S, De Zapien JG. Community health workers then and now: an overview of national studies aimed at defining the field. J Ambul Care Manage. 2011;34(3):247–59.
72. Weiner S. Medical schools overhaul curricula to fight inequities [Internet]. Association of American Medical Colleges (AAMC). 2021 [cited 2022 May 15]. https://www.aamc.org/news-insights/medical-schools-overhaul-curricula-fight-inequities.
73. AMA. The AMA's strategic plan to embed racial justice and advance health equity | American Medical Association [Internet]. 2019 [cited 2022 Jan 28]. https://www.ama-assn.org/about/leadership/ama-s-strategic-plan-embed-racial-justice-and-advance-health-equity.
74. AMA. Home | Health Equity Education Center | AMA Ed Hub [Internet]. 2019 [cited 2022 Jan 28]. https://edhub.ama-assn.org/health-equity-ed-center.
75. Dobbin F, Kalev A. Why diversity programs fail. Harv Bus Rev. 2016.
76. HUD. Diversity and inclusion definitions | HUD.gov / U.S. Department of Housing and Urban Development (HUD) [Internet]. U.S. Department of Housing and Urban Development. [cited 2022 Jan 30]. https://www.hud.gov/program_offices/administration/admabout/diversity_inclusion/definitions.
77. National Center for Health Workforce Analysis. Sex, race, and ethnic diversity of U.S, health occupations (2011–2015) [Internet].

U.S. Department of Health and Human Services, Health Resources and Services Administration. 2017 [cited 2022 May 15]. https://bhw.hrsa.gov/data-research/review-health-workforce-research.

78. Bureau of Health Workforce. Nursing loan repayment, scholarship, and grant programs [Internet]. Health Resources and Services Administration (HRSA) Health Workforce. 2022 [cited 2022 May 15]. https://bhw.hrsa.gov/nursing-programs.

79. Wilbur K, Snyder C, Essary AC, Reddy S, Will KK, Saxon M. Developing workforce diversity in the health professions: a social justice perspective. Health Prof Educ. 2020;6(2):222–9.

80. Glazer G, Tobias B, Mentzel T. Increasing healthcare workforce diversity: urban universities as catalysts for change. J Prof Nurs. 2018;34(4):239–44.

81. Programs & mentorship—equity and inclusion [Internet]. University of Cincinnati, Academic Health Center. [cited 2022 May 15]. https://multisite.uc.edu/ahc/equity-inclusion/programs-mentorship.

82. Diversity programs in New York, the voice of medical education [Internet]. Associated Medical Schools of New York. [cited 2022 May 13]. https://amsny.org/initiatives/diversity-in-medicine/diversity-programs/.

83. Sloane EB, Silva RJ. Artificial intelligence in medical devices and clinical decision support systems. Clinical engineering handbook. Elsevier; 2020. p. 556–568.

84. Igoe KJ. Algorithmic bias in health care exacerbates social inequities—how to prevent it | executive and continuing professional education | Harvard T.H. Chan School of Public Health [Internet]. 2021 [cited 2022 May 15]. https://www.hsph.harvard.edu/ecpe/how-to-prevent-algorithmic-bias-in-health-care/.

85. Johnson CY. Racial bias in a medical algorithm favors white patients over sicker black patients. Ethics of data and analytics. Boca Raton: Auerbach Publications; 2019. p. 10–2.

86. Taylor J, Waldrop T, Bernstein A, Smith-Ramakrishnan V. The ACA improved access to health insurance for marginalized communities, but more work is needed to ensure universal coverage [Internet]. The Century Foundation. 2022 [cited 2022 May 15]. https://tcf.org/content/commentary/the-aca-improved-access-to-health-insurance-for-marginalized-communities-but-more-work-is-needed-to-ensure-universal-coverage/.

Part VI
Health Policy and Chronic Illness Care

Medicare

Jonathan Oberlander

Introduction

Medicare plays a central role in American health care. For over 50 years, it has provided health insurance to older Americans, ensuring their access to medical services and a measure of financial security during retirement. Since 1972, the program has additionally insured persons with permanent disabilities Medicarepermanent disabilities and end-stage renal disease. In 2021, Medicare enrolled over 63 million persons [1], a number that will continue to rise during the next decade as the baby boom generation retires. Medicare has an enormous role in shaping health care payment and delivery since it is the single largest purchaser of medical services in the United States and a major source of income for physicians, hospitals, and other medical providers. The decisions that Medicare makes about how to pay providers, and what types of medical care delivery to promote and experiment with, reverberate across American medicine. The future of payment and delivery reform depends in no small part on their fortunes in Medicare.

When Medicare was enacted in 1965, it emphasized coverage for acute episodes of illness, following the standard insurance model of that time. The needs of persons with chronic conditions received less attention and there were sizable holes in Medicare's benefit package that left many enrollees, who needed ongoing care, vulnerable to high costs and bereft of critical services. Managing chronic disease remains a challenge for Medicare despite the fact that it "is in reality a program serving people with chronic conditions" [2]. This chapter provides an overview of Medicare, its origins, populations served, benefits and financing. It also covers major issues in Medicare reform, including efforts to control program spending, introduce innovations in medical care payment and delivery, the impact of the Affordable Care Act and Covid-19 pandemic, and Medicare for All.

Origins

The United States has a patchwork insurance system, with coverage varying by age, occupation, income, and even the condition of particular organ systems. Why does the United States have a separate government health care program for older Americans and younger persons with permanent disabilities? The answer lies in Medicare's roots in twentieth century debates over national health insurance in the United States. Efforts by reformers to advance national health insurance during the Progressive era (1912–1920) and Franklin Delano Roosevelt's presidency (1933–1945) went nowhere. In 1945, President Harry Truman became the first US president to formally endorse a government health insurance program for all Americans. However, legislation creating such a program did not come close to passing Congress. It failed due to intense opposition from the American Medical Association (AMA), the power in Congress of a de facto conservative coalition comprising Republican and Southern Democratic lawmakers, and fears of socialized medicine that were magnified by rising anti-communist fears and Cold War anxieties [3, 4].

By 1951, Truman administration officials were seeking a new strategy to advance health care reform. Instead of comprehensive universal health insurance for all Americans, they narrowed the goal to enacting a federal insurance program that would cover the costs of hospitalization for elderly

J. Oberlander (✉)
Department of Social Medicine, University of North Carolina at Chapel Hill, Chapel Hill, NC, USA

Department of Health Policy and Management, University of North Carolina at Chapel Hill, Chapel Hill, NC, USA
e-mail: oberland@med.unc.edu

Social Security beneficiaries [3]. The Medicare strategy was born. The strategy was one of incrementalism, shaped by political calculations and constraints. Medicare's architects decided to focus on covering the aged, as they were then called, because older Americans commanded public sympathy and could be seen as deserving of government aid. Moreover, the substantive case for government action was compelling. Before Medicare's enactment, most seniors lacked meaningful health insurance, even though they used many more services than younger Americans do. By connecting Medicare to, and constructing it in, the image of Social Security, reformers hoped to leverage that program's popularity as social insurance and an earned entitlement. And by narrowing coverage to hospital services, Medicare advocates hoped to diminish the AMA's opposition to federal health insurance [3].

That latter goal was not realized—during the 1950s and early 1960s, the AMA campaigned vigorously against Medicare. AMA president David Allman called the proposal to establish federal health insurance for the elderly "nine parts evil to one part sincerity" [5]. In 1961, the AMA hired Ronald Reagan, then an actor who subsequently became governor of California and president of the United States, to make a recording that warned of dire consequences if Medicare became law: "behind it will come other federal programs that will invade every area of freedom we have known in this country. Until one day … we will awake to find that we have socialism" [5]. Meanwhile, the influence of the conservative coalition in Congress—Republicans and Southern Democrats—blocked Medicare's legislative path. The 1964 elections, which President Lyndon Johnson won in a landslide and gave Democrats huge majorities in both the House and Senate, broke the impasse, leading to Medicare's enactment in 1965. Medicaid, a program for certain categories of low-income Americans, was enacted as part of the same legislation as Medicare [3].

Although Medicare was created as a program for the elderly, its advocates believed that was just the start. They saw Medicare as the cornerstone of a national health insurance system. After covering seniors, children were to be next in line for federal health insurance, and its architects envisioned that Medicare would eventually expand to cover all Americans. In 1972, Congress did extend Medicare eligibility to include younger Americans with permanent disabilities who were receiving Social Security Disability Insurance (SSDI) as well as persons with end-stage renal disease. But after 1972, eligibility for Medicare remained largely unchanged, though in 2001 Medicare added automatic coverage for persons with amyotrophic lateral sclerosis, ALS, or Lou Gehrig's disease. Instead, it was Medicaid that followed an expansionary trajectory, including becoming the major government health care program for children. The original vision of Medicare for All has never been realized [6].

Populations Served

Medicare, like Social Security, is an earned entitlement with eligibility established through employment and a social insurance program that covers all eligible Americans regardless of their income, a contrast to welfare programs that are available only to those who earn below a specified income threshold. Medicare insures virtually all Americans age 65 and older, with 54 million older Americans enrolled in the program in 2020 [7]. Older Americans become eligible for Medicare through the Social Security system; persons who qualify for Social Security retirement benefits through either their own work or as dependents qualify for Medicare. Medicare-eligible persons are automatically enrolled into the program when they turn 65 [8, 9]. Notably, Medicare has never charged elderly Americans who have pre-existing conditions higher premiums or refused to cover them, discriminatory practices that were common in the U.S. private insurance market before the 2010 Patient Protection and Affordable Care Act (ACA). Medicare has made insurance accessible and affordable for a population—older Americans—that otherwise would struggle to obtain private coverage [10].

Medicare insures two other populations with complex medical care needs: younger Americans with permanent disabilities and persons with end-stage renal disease (ESRD). While public attention often equates Medicare with older persons, these populations are a significant part of the program. In 2020, there were 8.5 million persons with permanent disabilities under the age of 65 on Medicare, constituting 13.5% of all program enrollees [7]. In 2019, Medicare insured 556,093 persons with ESRD, 47% of whom were younger than age 65. Medicare provides universal insurance for ESRD regardless of age, paying for dialysis and kidney transplants, as well as covered services, for persons with permanent kidney failure [8, 9, 11]. Persons with permanent disabilities who receive Social Security Disability Insurance (SSDI) and are therefore eligible for Medicare must wait for 2 years before their Medicare coverage begins. However, persons with ESRD or ALS who are receiving SSDI do not face a waiting period to enroll in Medicare [8, 9].

The populations that Medicare covers—older Americans, persons with permanent disabilities, and those with end-stage renal disease—have substantial medical needs. Nearly two-thirds of Medicare enrollees have three or more chronic conditions; 32% have a functional impairment in one or more activities of daily living; 25% report they are in fair or poor health, and 22% have five or more chronic conditions [12]. A number of chronic conditions are prevalent in the Medicare population: 59% of Medicare beneficiaries have hypertension, 28% have diabetes and ischemic heart disease, 25% have kidney disease, 14% have heart failure, 12% have chronic obstructive pulmonary disease, and 11% have Alzheimer's or dementia [13]. Many Medicare enrollees also have limited resources, with about half having incomes below $29,650 and one-quarter with savings below $8500 in 2020 [14].

There are substantial racial/ethnic inequities and health disparities among the Medicare population. Black and Hispanic beneficiaries are more likely to be enrolled in the program under age 65 with a permanent disability, while a much larger share of older Black and Hispanic beneficiaries have lower incomes than white beneficiaries [15]. Black and Hispanic enrollees also are more likely than white enrollees to report fair or poor health and to have hypertension and diabetes [15].

Benefits

Medicare is a hybrid program, with a large government insurance plan operating alongside private insurers that enroll an increasingly large share of program beneficiaries. Medicare beneficiaries can choose whether to join the traditional program operated by the federal government (sometimes called Original Medicare) where beneficiaries can generally go to any doctor or hospital that accepts Medicare patients, or instead enroll in a private insurance plan that contracts with the government to provide Medicare benefits (i.e., Medicare Advantage plans) [8, 9]. Private plans in Medicare at first were exclusively health maintenance organizations (HMOs) but now encompass a wider variety of options such as Preferred Provider Organizations (PPOs). Such plans have gained a rapidly growing share of the Medicare population, doubling their enrollment in the past decade. In 2021, 42% of all program beneficiaries were enrolled in a Medicare Advantage plan [16]. Persons with specified chronic conditions such as diabetes or dementia are among the Medicare beneficiaries who are eligible to join Special Needs Plans (SNPs), a type of MA plan [8]. The 2018 CHRONIC Care Act enables MA plans to pay for nonmedical services that address beneficiaries' social needs, including transportation, meals, and pest control [17].

Medicare benefits are divided into four components. Part A (hospital insurance) covers inpatient hospital care, as well as skilled nursing facility, hospice, and home health care. Part B (medical insurance) pays for physicians' services, as well as outpatient care, laboratory services, durable medical equipment, preventive services such as cancer and diabetes screenings, and home health care. Part C comprises the aforementioned Medicare Advantage program that offers Medicare beneficiaries the option to enroll in a private plan as an alternative to traditional Medicare (such plans must cover all Part A and B benefits). Part D provides voluntary coverage for outpatient prescription drugs through private plans that contract with Medicare; MA plans also offer drug coverage [8, 9].

The division of Medicare benefits dates back to the program's 1965 enactment, when insurance for hospital (Part A) and physician services (Part B) were established as separate components [3, 5]. The persistence of these arrangements attests to the enduring influence of policy decisions made over 50 years ago on contemporary Medicare. Yet this separation of service categories, which mirrored practices by some private insurers in 1965, makes little sense today when the aspiration is to integrate medical care across the spectrum of services—an aspiration that is particularly important for persons with chronic illnesses.

Beyond their administrative fragmentation, Medicare benefits are also limited in important ways [8–10]. Medicare does not have a general dental benefit and will not pay for routine dental services. Medicare does not cover hearing aids or routine eye exams. Coverage of skilled nursing care as part of Medicare's home health benefit is limited to part-time or intermittent care. Medicare will not pay for custodial care that provides help with the activities of daily living to persons with chronic illnesses or a disability. Nor does Medicare cover long-term stays in nursing homes, a responsibility that instead falls on Medicaid, although Medicare does cover stays up to 100 days in skilled nursing facilities, including rehabilitation services, after an inpatient hospitalization of at least 3 days. Medicare coverage for care in a psychiatric hospital is limited to 190 days total during a beneficiary's lifetime in the program.

Medicare coverage for hospital stays (part A) requires a sizable deductible ($1556 in 2022) and copayments for prolonged stays; in 2022, $389 per day for days 61–90 and $778 for each lifetime reserve day, of which there are a total of 60 that beneficiaries can draw on during their time on Medicare [8]. Medicare's coverage of hospital care is organized according to benefit periods (i.e., spell of illness) that begin when a patient enters the hospital and end 60 days after a person leaves the hospital. As a result, some Medicare beneficiaries incur multiple deductibles for hospital insurance in one year, which imposes a substantial financial burden on them. There is a separate, more modest deductible ($233 in 2022) for Medicare Part B, which covers physician and outpatient services. Beneficiaries are also responsible for paying 20% of the Medicare-approved amount for physicians' bills and, in 2022, $195 a day for days 21–100 in a skilled nursing facility [8]. Medicare's coverage for outpatient prescription drugs requires substantial cost sharing—including a deductible ($480 for the standard plan in 2022) and coinsurance (25% up to total drug spending of $10,690 of total drug spending, after which beneficiaries pay 5%) [18]. And traditional Medicare has no annual limit on the total amount that enrollees can pay out of their pocket for deductibles, copayments, and coinsurance. Medicare Advantage plans do have such a limit. Relative to typical health plans that large employers offer to their workers, Medicare coverage is somewhat less generous [19].

These limitations in Medicare benefits are longstanding. From its inception, Medicare never covered all of its beneficiaries' medical care costs. Medicare's architects sought to protect older Americans against the most devastating expenses from illness—hospitalization. While physicians' services were included in the 1965 legislation that established Medicare, the program still focused on insuring beneficiaries for acute illness episodes. Policymakers in effect presumed that older Americans' medical care needs were similar to those of younger populations and did not recognize the greater burden of chronic illness among the elderly [20]. While Medicare benefits have expanded in important ways over time, including the addition of outpatient prescription drug coverage in 2003, they still have major limitations that leave program enrollees responsible for paying a substantial portion of their medical bills [20, 21].

As a consequence of gaps in its benefits package, most Medicare beneficiaries carry additional insurance [22]. About 20% of program beneficiaries are so-called "dual eligibles" who receive Medicaid as well as Medicare. Such persons may qualify for Medicare on the basis of age and for Medicaid on the basis of income. For these beneficiaries, Medicaid provides extra benefits and pays the cost sharing that Medicare requires. Another 26% of Medicare beneficiaries have supplemental coverage plans sponsored by their former employer, which commonly cover extra benefits like prescription drugs. About 21% of Medicare beneficiaries purchase their own supplemental insurance policies called Medigap plans that help pay for Medicare cost sharing including deductibles and copayments [22]. The 42% of beneficiaries who receive their Medicare coverage through private Medicare Advantage plans typically receive additional benefits, such as vision and hearing coverage from those plans, which also usually cover prescription drugs, however, such plans often have restricted provider networks [16]. In 2018, 5.6 million Medicare beneficiaries lacked any supplemental coverage, leaving them fully exposed to Medicare's cost-sharing requirements and benefit limitations [22].

Even with most beneficiaries having supplemental sources of coverage, Medicare beneficiaries still play substantial amounts for medical care. In 2016, the Kaiser Family Foundation reported, "the average person with Medicare coverage spent $5,460 out of their own pocket for health care" [23]. Those financial liabilities entail insurance premiums, encompassing both Medicare and private supplemental plans, and payments for medical services. They constitute a substantial burden for low-income enrollees, with out-of-pocket spending also rising with age and for those in poorer health and with chronic conditions. In total, medical care accounted for 12% of all income for beneficiaries in traditional Medicare in 2016 [23].

Expenditures and Financing

Medicare spending totaled $830 billion in 2020, accounting for 20% of all US health care spending and 14% of the federal budget [24]. Medicare is financed by a combination of taxes and beneficiary payments. Medicare hospitalization insurance (Part A) is funded predominantly through payroll taxes that all American workers pay. In 2022, the standard hospitalization insurance payroll tax was 1.45%, with higher-income Americans paying more. Beneficiaries become eligible for Medicare hospital insurance as a result of previously having paid (or their spouses paying) compulsory payroll taxes while they are employed. There is no Part A premium for persons who are eligible because they already contributed taxes to Medicare (10 years of contributions are required). Older Americans who aren't eligible through the Social Security system can pay premiums to join Part A [8, 9].

Medicare Part B—medical insurance—is a voluntary program though persons who don't sign up for the program when first eligible must pay late penalties if they subsequently enroll [8, 9]. It is funded mostly through general revenues, which encompass all the money the federal government collects from individual and corporate income taxes, excise taxes (e.g., tobacco taxes), and other sources. While general revenues fund 75% of Part B spending, the other 25% comes from beneficiary premiums. In 2022, the standard Part B monthly premium was $170 for persons with $91,000 of income or less [8, 9, 12]. Higher-income beneficiaries receive a lower subsidy from the federal government and thus pay higher premiums, with about 7% of Medicare beneficiaries currently paying such income-related premium surcharges. In 2022, for example, Medicare enrollees making between $91,000 and $114,000 paid monthly Part B premiums of $238, with persons with annual incomes between $142,000 and $170,000 paying $442 a month. The funding of Part D prescription drug coverage mirrors the arrangements for Part B, with funding from general revenues and income-related beneficiary premiums. Monthly premiums averaged about $33 in 2022, although there is substantial variation in that cost across plans [16]. Lower-income Medicare beneficiaries are eligible for savings programs that help pay for their premiums for medical (Part B) and prescription drug (Part D) coverage. Beneficiaries who enroll in a Medicare Advantage private plan may pay additional premiums on top of the standard Medicare rates.

Medicare's finances are the subject of much controversy and anxiety. The program is frequently said to be on the verge of bankruptcy. That rhetoric is a direct reflection of Medicare's financing arrangements [5]. Medicare's finances are organized into government trust funds, which are essentially accounting mechanisms to record program revenues and expenditures. Medicare's trust fund for hospital insurance is funded almost entirely from payroll taxes that are specifically earmarked for Medicare. Social Security financing works in a similar fashion. When those payroll taxes aren't sufficient to meet costs, Medicare appears to be running out of money, and is therefore said to be going bankrupt. Trust fund revenues can drop for reasons having nothing to do with changes in Medicare spending, such as a recession that increases unemployment and thereby reduces the amount of taxes that the government collects.

In contrast, most federal programs are financed out of general government revenues; they don't have a specific funding source or earmarked tax that is credited to a trust fund. Federal spending for the military, education, Medicaid, and many other federal programs are paid for through general revenues [5, 10]. No matter how expensive these programs are or how much their costs rise, we usually do not speak of them as going bankrupt. In fact, Medicare's trust fund for Part B (i.e., physicians' services) is similarly funded mostly from general revenues that automatically increase when program costs rise. As a result, it too is immune from bankruptcy talk.

When politicians allege, then, that Medicare is "going bankrupt" they are actually referring to actuarial projections that in some future year the program will not have sufficient funds to pay the entire cost of Medicare hospital insurance. In 2021, for example, actuaries estimated that the Medicare Part A trust fund would become insolvent in 2026, when they said the program would have 91% of the money it needs to pay all costs [7]. Yet the notion that Medicare will ever literally go bankrupt and stop paying for beneficiaries' medical services is misleading [5, 11]. These are projections and policymakers can alter Medicare's future financial circumstances by increasing revenues through higher payroll taxes or decreasing costs by limiting program payments and reforming how Medicare pays for medical services. This has occurred over the past half century-plus of Medicare's operations. Periodically there have been warnings of shortfalls in the hospital insurance trust fund, and each time policymakers have acted to improve Medicare's fiscal condition. There is no chance that politicians would let a program that serves over 50 million (and growing) older Americans ever stop operations. Yet even though bankruptcy rhetoric is misleading, it is nonetheless an important feature of Medicare politics. It is used by reformers and critics alike to push proposals to change Medicare in the name of saving the program [5]. Consequently, major Medicare reforms often happen during periods where the projected date of insolvency for the hospital insurance trust fund is within a decade.

Medicare and the Affordable Care Act

The 2010 Affordable Care Act (ACA, aka Obamacare), which aimed to expand health insurance to America's uninsured population while moderating health care spending growth and reforming medical care delivery, made a number of significant changes to Medicare [25]. The ACA expanded Medicare benefits, providing program beneficiaries with coverage of preventive services such as flu shots and cancer screenings at no cost, enhancing Medicare coverage of outpatient prescription drugs by closing the "doughnut hole" in Part D, and adding coverage for an annual wellness visit. And it raised Medicare taxes on higher-income Americans, including an increase in the hospital insurance payroll tax and a new tax on "unearned" investment income from capital gains, dividends, and other sources for persons making over $200,000 a year.

The ACA also contained substantial reductions in Medicare spending [25, 26]. The ACA's Medicare savings largely reflected reductions in the projected growth in program payments to hospitals and private Medicare Advantage plans. The ACA additionally sought to advance a series of payment and delivery reforms in Medicare, including Accountable Care Organizations (ACOs) and bundled payment, and adopted other initiatives to promote value-based purchasing that reward higher quality care. The ACA also included measures that aimed to improve care for persons with chronic conditions, including: a program that reduces payments to hospitals with high readmission rates for their Medicare patient; the Medicare Community-based Care Transitions Program that funds partnerships between hospitals and community-based organizations to reduce readmissions; and establishment of a new office to improve care coordination for dual persons who are dually eligible for Medicare and Medicaid [25].

The ACA additionally established a new institution—the Center for Medicare & Medicaid Innovation (CMMI)—that could develop, evaluate, and scale up experiments in medical care delivery and payment. And it created an Independent Payment Advisory Board (IPAB) empowered to propose policy changes to restrain Medicare spending if the aforementioned measures didn't work to curb program spending growth, changes that Congress would have to either accept or devise alternatives that would achieve the same amount of savings [27].

Some of the ACA's policies have had substantial impacts on Medicare. The ACA helped produce a slowdown in the rate of growth in Medicare spending that exceeded projections of savings made at the time of the law's enactment. That slowdown reflected, in large part, the ACA's constraints on increases in the prices paid by Medicare to medical providers [28]. Moreover, following ACA payment changes, "unexpected reductions occurred in Medicare hospital days, outpatient visits, skilled nursing facility days, and advanced imaging between 2010 and 2014" [29]. However, other ACA policies have not worked as envisioned. No one has been appointed to the newly created board that was supposed to restrain Medicare spending and Congress repealed IPAB in 2018 amidst intense opposition from the health care industry and partisan polarization that derailed its launch [30]. Meanwhile, the Innovation Center that was established to test and expand new payment and delivery models has had "an underwhelming track record," with these new models producing scant savings [28]. While the ACA was supposed to enable a quicker scaling up of successful demonstration projects in Medicare (and Medicaid), in practice procedural and actuarial barriers, as well as unrealistic expectations about what such projects can achieve within a short time, has meant that the Innovation Center has yet to fulfill its promise [31].

Controlling Medicare Spending

Controlling spending has long been the dominant issue in Medicare policy. When Medicare was enacted in 1965, health care cost control was not a policy issue in the United States. Private insurers at that time often exerted little control over payments to physicians and hospitals. Medicare, which sought to give the elderly access to mainstream medicine, built on that permissive status quo rather than seeking to transform it [3–5]. The 1965 Medicare stature declared that, "nothing in this title shall be construed to authorize any federal officer or employee to exercise any control over the practice of medicine or the manner in which medical services are provided" [5]. The political context of Medicare also shaped its payment policies. Program administrators wanted to ensure a smooth launch for Medicare and secure the medical profession's cooperation. The AMA had fiercely opposed Medicare's enactment and there were fears that doctors would boycott federal health insurance. Medicare's initial payment policies were designed to promote political conciliation rather than fiscal control [32].

Hospitals were reimbursed retrospectively for the services they provided to Medicare beneficiaries on the basis of "reasonable costs," a standard adapted from private plans like Blue Cross [3, 5, 32]. Hospitals received generous capital depreciation allowances and, initially, a 2% bonus on their Medicare charges. Medicare paid physicians retrospectively on a fee-for-service basis, according to their "reasonable charges." Reasonable charges meant that the federal government would pay physicians fees for Medicare patients that reflected their customary charges for similar services to private insurers as well as the prevailing community rate for such services. Medicare did not establish a national fee schedule to limit payments. Instead, the "customary and prevailing" formula gave physicians a strong economic incentive to raise their charges so they could receive higher fees [3, 5, 33]. In sum, Medicare started operations in 1966 without any meaningful limits on program payments to hospitals or physicians.

Medicare's original methods of paying medical care providers were inherently inflationary. Predictably, federal spending on Medicare quickly increased at rates far exceeding the projections that had been made at the time of its enactment. In 1969, only 3 years after the program's beginning, Russell Long, chair of the Senate Finance Committee, declared that Medicare had become a "run-away program" and President Richard Nixon had declared that the US faced a "massive crisis" in medical care [5, 34]. Spending more on medical care, which in earlier decades had been presumed to be a worthwhile investment in the nation's health, was now seen as a fiscal threat [4, 5]. The advent of Medicare and Medicaid transformed the role of the federal government in medical care. Rising health care costs now had a growing claim on the federal budget and Washington consequently had an interest in restraining Medicare spending.

Early efforts to control Medicare spending during the 1970s, including establishing professional standard review organizations to audit inpatient care for inappropriate and unnecessary services, proved largely ineffective [4, 5]. Federal policymakers were reluctant to take on the medical care industry and impose strong payment limits. But as federal spending on Medicare continued to climb in the context of rising government budget deficits, policymakers became more willing to disrupt the status quo. During the 1980s, Congress enacted major reform in both hospital and physician payment. The 1983 Prospective Payment System (PPS) for hospitals was followed in 1989 by the Medicare Fee Schedule (MFS) for physicians [5, 35].

The new arrangements for paying medical care providers amounted to a revolution in Medicare policy. Since the implementation of the PPS and MFS, Medicare has paid doctors and hospitals according to rates prospectively set by the federal government, rather than retrospectively reimbursing costs, as the program initially did. Hospitals are paid on the basis of Diagnosis-Related Groups (DRGs), with Medicare giving hospitals a fixed amount based on a patient's clinical condition and treatment. Physicians are paid according to a preset fee schedule, with the fee for each service calculated on the basis of relative value units (RVUs) that measure the time, effort, skill, intensity, complexity, stress, and practice expenses associated with different medical services. In 1997, Congress extended prospective payment to post-acute care, including home health, skilled nursing facility, and hospital outpatient services. Over time, then, administered pricing has come to play a dominant role in Medicare [35].

The federal government adopted these prospective payment systems to help restrain Medicare spending growth. During 1975–1983, before the implementation of Medicare's hospital PPS, the annual rate of excess growth, defined as growth beyond that attributable to general economic growth and changes in beneficiaries' age composition, was 5.6% [36]. During 1983–1997, as Medicare implemented prospective payment systems, that rate fell to 2.1% and then to 0.5% during 1997–2005 [36]. Federal policymakers have repeatedly used payment reforms to generate Medicare savings. The 2005 Deficit Reduction Act reduced Medicare payments for imaging, durable medical equipment, and home health services [37]. The 2010 ACA cut the growth in Medicare payments to an array of medical providers, with especially large reductions for hospitals and private Medicare Advantage plans. As noted earlier, after the ACA's passage, there was a pronounced slowdown in Medicare spending and the 2011 Budget Control Act led to additional cuts in program payments [24, 29, 37]. In 2009 Medicare per beneficiary spending stood at $10,537; by 2014, it had risen only slightly to $10,809, $1200 lower than predicted in 2010 [38]. Medicare spending in 2014 totaled $580 billion, $126 billion lower than forecast in 2009 [38].

Medicare spending is sometimes portrayed as growing uncontrollably, with cost increases driven inexorably by medical technology and an aging population. Those forces do increase Medicare spending but the record of Medicare spending contradicts the premise that the program is uncontrollable. In fact, Medicare spending growth slowed substantially after the federal government adopted prospective payment systems and used those systems to hold down expenditures. Medicare, in other words, is responsive to policy reform, and its spending is not simply the product of inexorable forces. That does not mean that Medicare's cost problems have been solved and some of Medicare's payment systems have been more effective than others have been. Regulating prices has proven easier than controlling growth in volume and intensity of services, Medicare spending growth has varied across different time periods, and significant fiscal challenges loom in Medicare's future. Still, Medicare's record on cost containment is better than often assumed and federal policymakers have a proven ability to moderate program spending growth.

The impact of prospective payment in Medicare underscores the program's role as an innovator and reform leader in American medical care [39]. DRGs represented an early form of bundled payment that was designed to create incentives for hospitals to economize and control costs [35]. Other payers, including state Medicaid plans, private insurers, and health care systems abroad, also use DRGs. Medicare's RVU-based physician fee schedule is commonly used by private insurers, although they typically do not have as much purchasing power as Medicare so pay higher rates. It also underscores the fact that Medicare's primary cost control strategy has been limiting payments to medical providers through price regulation. On average, commercial insurers pay prices for hospital services that are over double Medicare's payments, and their prices for physician services are 29% higher than Medicare's [40]. During 2013–2018, annual growth in prices paid to medical providers by traditional Medicare averaged 1.3%, compared to 2.7% by commercial insurers; annual per person spending in traditional Medicare rose annually by 1.8%, while spending in commercial insurers increased by 3.2% [40].

Price regulation is an imperfect tool and there is evidence that some services Medicare pays for are mispriced. Additionally, the Medicare Fee Schedule has tilted toward specialists and proceduralists, creating an imbalance that contributes to the undervaluing of primary care in American medicine [33]. Price regulation is nonetheless an important tool, one that has proven effective at slowing down Medicare spending growth.

Payment and Delivery Reform

In recent years, there has been growing enthusiasm in the health policy community and among policymakers for changing how Medicare pays for services. The goal is to create incentives that lead to improved quality and coordination of care, better patient outcomes, and stronger cost control. An array of payment and delivery reforms initiatives are unfolding in Medicare, often under the labels of "value-based purchasing" or "value-based payment" and moving from "volume to value." Such measures are seen in part as a way to overcome: the barriers in traditional Medicare to better management of chronic conditions; fragmentation of responsibility and lack of accountability for persons who receive medical services from multiple providers; the absence of financial incentives to encourage care coordination and discourage unnecessary, duplicative services across multiple settings; and the absence of policies to pay for or incentivize care management as well as inter-provider communication and collaboration [2, 41].

Value-based purchasing comes in many varieties. Under Medicare's Hospital Readmissions Program (HRRP), adopted in 2010 as part of the ACA, the federal government reduces payments to hospitals with excess admissions for targeted conditions such as heart failure, pneumonia, chronic obstructive pulmonary disease (COPD), and persons receiving coronary artery bypass graft surgery [42]. Enactment of HRRP reflected policymakers' concerns with high readmission rates in Medicare. During 2003–2004, about 20% of Medicare beneficiaries who had been discharged from a hospital were re-hospitalized within 30 days, raising questions about the adequacy of discharge planning and follow-up care [43]. By penalizing hospitals financially—an example of so-called pay for performance arrangements—the aim is to reduce readmissions, improve care, and lower costs, though the costs of preventable re-hospitalizations comprise a modest share of total Medicare spending.

Medicare is also experimenting with new forms of bundled payment. Such arrangements pay a group of providers one aggregate, fixed amount for an episode of care or diagnosis rather than separate fees for each service delivered [44]. Bundled payment seeks to create incentives to limit medical spending and improve care coordination; providers who hold down the costs of care under bundled payment do better financially. Doctors and hospitals are at more financial risk in bundled payment than under arrangements where they are reimbursed for costs and services regardless of the volume and intensity of care [45]. Some bundled payment models include post-acute services in the episode of care, thereby incentivizing providers to pay attention to what happens to patients after a hospital stay. Medicare has implemented bundled payment for a number of medical care episodes, including stroke, chronic obstructive pulmonary disease, cardiac procedures, and joint replacement [46]. While participation in such demonstrations was initially voluntary, in 2016 Medicare launched a mandatory bundled payment program for joint replacement.

Accountable Care Organizations (ACOs) embody another effort to transform how Medicare pays for and delivers medical care. ACOs are "networks of physicians and other providers that are held accountable for the cost and quality of the full continuum of care delivered to a group of patients" [47]. Patients typically don't actively enroll in an ACO; instead, they are attributed to it based on where and from which providers they receive medical care. Persons generally can seek services outside of the ACO network, though the ACO is responsible financially for all of their medical care. ACOs operate under spending targets, based on historical spending patterns, for their patient populations. If they hold total costs below that target, they can keep some of the savings; if they exceed the target, they can lose money depending on the model [47]. As a result, ACOs have a financial stake in holding down spending, reversing the traditional incentives of fee-for-service payment that can lead to over-utilization. Many ACOs actually pay providers fee-for-service and then reconcile those payments with the spending target.

ACOs' payments also depend on their ability to meet specified quality of care measures. They may not be eligible for bonuses based on containing spending if quality standards are not met. In Medicare ACOs, examples of these quality measures include patient ratings of providers, depression remission, colorectal cancer, and mammography screening, hemoglobin A1C control in diabetics, hypertension control, statin therapy for cardiovascular disease, and unplanned admissions for patients with multiple chronic conditions [48]. ACOs aim to control spending, improve care coordination and service quality, and enhance population health. In these aims and by making a network of providers accountable for a defined population, ACOs resemble the logic of HMOs that sought to integrate the financing and delivery of medical care within one organization. However, ACOs are looser, less restrictive, and ultimately less organized entities, allowing more beneficiary choice of provider and emphasizing a greater role for physicians and other providers in making care decisions. ACOs are, in effect, HMOs without the parts, such as closed provider networks, that previously proved unpopular and controversial.

Medicare's new formula for updating physician fees also seeks to move beyond paying for the volume of services. Under the Merit-Based Incentive Payment System (MIPS), adopted by Congress in 2015 as part of the Medicare Access and CHIP Reauthorization Act (MACRA), Medicare pays physicians according to their performance on quality, resource use, reporting care information, and clinical practice improvement activities [49]. Physicians who receive a substantial portion of their payments from ACOs, patient-centered medical homes, and other innovative payment models can instead join the Advanced Alternative Payment Models (APM) program. Beginning in 2026, doctors who are in the APM program will receive higher annual fee updates than those participating in MIPS. Many physicians consequently could face new financial incentives to participate in such models [50].

In sum, Medicare's embrace of value-based purchasing through these and other initiatives mark a significant change in federal policy. In 2015, Secretary of Health and Human Services (HHS) Sylvia Burwell declared that "Our goal is to have 85% of all Medicare fee-for-service payments tied to quality or value by 2016, and 90% by 2018 … [and] to have 30% of Medicare payments tied to quality or value through alternative payment models by the end of 2016, and 50% of payments by the end of 2018" [51]. In 2016, HHS announced that it had met the goal of having 30% of Medicare payments to alternative payment models like ACOs [52].

The appeal of value-based purchasing in Medicare, which promises to contain spending while rewarding high quality care and promote better patient outcomes, is understandable. Yet the results of such initiatives have been decidedly mixed. The introduction of the hospital readmissions reduction program initially appeared to be associated with declines in readmission rates for Medicare patients, though some health services researchers argue the program's actual impact has been substantially overstated [53, 54]. The Independence at Home (IAH) Program, which provides primary care services to chronically ill persons in their homes, and enables providers to share in savings if spending and quality targets are met, has not generated a "statistically significant change in overall average annual [Medicare] expenditures" or reduced aggregate use of hospital services, though it has "significantly decreased enrollees' utilization of the emergency department" and "a large majority of patients and their caregivers reported high levels of satisfaction with home-based primary care" [55].

Medicare's Hospital Value-Based Purchasing Program (HVBP), which provides incentive payments to hospitals based on measures of the quality of inpatient care, "did not improve clinical process or patient experience performance in its first year" and a subsequent study found it "has also not reduced mortality" [56]. A demonstration of patient-centered medical homes in Medicare that paid fees to providers for care management, the Multi-Payer Advanced Primary Care Practice, did not produce savings. Separately, in 2015 Medicare implemented a new billing code that allows physicians to receive payment for non-face-to-face services that are part of chronic care management [57]. A review of bundled payment initiatives in Medicare found that "many were associated with little to no reduction in Medicare expenditures, unless large pricing discounts for providers were negotiated in advance" though "initiatives that included post–acute care services were associated with lower expenditures for certain conditions"; and "most initiatives were not associated with significant changes in quality of care, as measured by readmission and mortality rates" [58]. Meanwhile, Medicare's new value-based system for paying physicians, MIPS, has been criticized for its design, complexity, and the limited meaningfulness of its measures and Medicare's Payment Advisory Commission (MedPAC) has recommended eliminating it [59]. It is unclear at this time if MIPS will be fully implemented.

Medicare's much-heralded ACO programs, after taking account of bonuses paid out by the government to high-performing ACOs, have not saved the program much money though some studies conclude they have fared better in improving quality of care [60–62]. Medicare's Shared Savings Program (MSSP)—its primary ACO vehicle—"has been plagued by weak incentives" that have limited its capacity to generate savings and has experienced substantial attrition as a large share of ACOs that initially joined the program have left [63]. Some health services researchers argue that even the limited savings and quality improvements apparently produced by Medicare ACOs are in fact a product of the "nonrandom exit of high-cost clinicians and their patient panels from this voluntary program" [64]. And despite the rhetoric of moving from volume to value, in reality most Medicare payments, as well as those in private insurance, still depend on the volume of services delivered [50].

It is important to distinguish the aspirations of value-based purchasing models from their actual performance. While the goals of such arrangements are laudable, that does not mean they will work well in practice [65]. Indeed, much of the evidence to date regarding value-based purchasing strategies "suggests that incentives for providers do not improve value or lead to better outcomes for patients" [56]. Similarly, the evidence is that "gains from performance-linked payments have generally ranged from absent to modest and have come at great expense, including substantial reporting costs" [66]. In short, based on experiences so far, value-based purchasing seems unlikely to emerge as a panacea for rising Medicare costs. In policymakers' and analysts' desire to find ways to "solve" the multiple challenges facing Medicare, there is, then, a danger of conflating rhetoric with reality, and over-hyping the likely impact of emerging policy alternatives [67]. Much uncertainty remains regarding the ability of payment and delivery reforms to fulfill their promise.

There is also a strong tendency in US health care policy, pervasive in discussions of Medicare reform, to presume the necessity of abandoning fee-for-service payment in order to control health care spending. As noted by Bruce Vladeck, former head of CMS's predecessor, the Health Care Financing Administration, though such a view is "logically powerful," it is also "inconsistent with the facts" [68]. Nations like Canada and Japan that spend much less on medical care than the US actually pay physicians fee-for-service [65, 67, 68]. Simply put, other rich democracies do not rely on value-based purchasing to control costs; they rely on price regulation and budgeting. There are good reasons, such as enhancing coordination and quality of care and curbing overtreatment, to modify or seek alternatives to fee-for-service payment. But international experience demonstrates that jettisoning fee-for-service is not the key to limiting medical care spending.

Medicare and COVID-19

The Covid-19 pandemic that has engulfed the US and much of the world since 2020 has had major implications for Medicare. A number of chronic conditions that are common among Medicare beneficiaries are associated with elevated risk for severe illness and mortality from Covid, as is older age [13, 69]. Covid's initial toll among the Medicare population was devastating. By the end of 2021, data from the Centers for Disease Control and Prevention (CDC) indicated that individuals ages 65 and older had made up only 12% of reported COVID-19 cases, yet they represented 76% of COVID-19 deaths [70]. The burdens of Covid fell unequally in the Medicare population, with disproportionate impacts on persons with end-stage renal disease, who are dually eligible for Medicare and Medicaid, age 85 and older, Black, Hispanic, and American Indian/Alaska Natives [70]. Death rates were especially high among persons in long-term care facilities, accounting by early 2022 for one-quarter of all Covid deaths [71].

Even with the development of effective vaccines, the incidence of long Covid could mean that in coming years Medicare will enroll more persons who already have chronic illness before they join the program. Moreover, for Medicare beneficiaries with chronic conditions the pandemic initially made it difficult to access medical care as many health facilities restricted non-emergent services and many persons delayed such care. However, the pandemic also triggered a shift toward much greater use of telehealth in Medicare, with such visits increasing from about 840,000 in 2019 to 52.7 million in 2020, which could provide an important alternative in coming years for beneficiaries with chronic conditions [72]. Meanwhile, the long-term financial impacts of Covid on Medicare are uncertain [7].

Medicare for All

In recent years, "Medicare for All" has emerged as an aspiration and rallying cry for some health reformers. The 2016 and 2020 campaigns of Vermont Senator Bernie Sanders, who unsuccessfully sought the Democratic nomination for president, helped propel Medicare for All into the political spotlight. This represents a return to the original vision of Medicare's architects in the 1950s and 1960s, who envisioned that Medicare would eventually grow to cover the entire country [6]. While Medicare' designers anticipated that growth would happen incrementally, with different groups joining in stages, contemporary proponents of Medicare for All propose a sweeping transformation that would largely eliminate private insurance in the U.S. as well as Medicaid and enroll the vast majority of Americans, except persons who receive medical services from the Indian Health Services and Veterans' Health Administration, into a new Medicare program within a relatively short time-frame [73]. Medicare for All plans like those proposed by Senator Sanders would also transform Medicare into much more comprehensive coverage, removing all patient copayments, coinsurance, and deductibles, other than limited copays for prescription drugs, and providing insurance for a wide array of medical services, including vision, dental, and long-term care.

The appeal of "Medicare for All" is understandable. After all, over a decade after the ACA's enactment, there are still about 30 million persons in the US who lack any health insurance. Millions of others are underinsured, meaning they are one medical episode away from discovering that their insurance provides inadequate protection against the high costs of care. The US continues to spend far more than other rich democracies on medical care, and American arrangements for health insurance are uniquely inequitable, inefficient, fragmented, complex, and costly [74].

No wonder, then, that some reformers see Medicare for All as an antidote to what ails US health care, a system that could ensure universal coverage, remedy underinsurance, enable reliable cost control, reduce administrative costs, and enhance health security. But the political barriers to enacting Medicare for All are extraordinarily daunting [74–78]. Much of the health care industry, which fears the impact of such a program on their income, fiercely opposes Medicare for All; such proposals' capacity to reduce growth in health care spending may be a substantive advantage but is a political liability. Moreover, Medicare for All would require large visible increases in taxes to replace private financing of health care in a country historically averse to taxation [76]. Many Americans with private, employer-sponsored coverage are satisfied with their current arrangements. Shifting tens of millions of persons from private to government insurance would be a highly controversial form of disruption. While public support for Medicare for All is robust, surveys also show that many Americans don't understand such plans would require them to give up their current insurance [75]. And Medicare for All triggers strong ideological opposition from conservatives who oppose the dramatic expansion of the government's role in health care and raise concerns about its impact on the federal budget. Opponents of such proposals raise the familiar specters of rationing, waitlists, reduced quality of care, and higher taxes.

Furthermore, while Medicare for All is often interpreted as shorthand for government-run insurance, the reality, as noted earlier, is that at present private insurers enroll a substantial portion of program beneficiaries through Medicare Advantage [16]. Thus, a "pure" Medicare for All plan would displace millions of Medicare beneficiaries' current coverage. Alternatively, it could accommodate private insurance within Medicare, which would require a fundamental shift in how many Medicare for All advocates think about that model and the boundaries between government and private insurance.

Whatever its substantive merits, for now Medicare for All remains a political long-shot, more an aspiration than a realistic reform possibility [77]. Even after the Covid-19 pandemic that killed hundreds of thousands of Americans, the legislative prospects of Medicare for All did not improve. Of course, longer-term projections of health policy are inherently uncertain and there is no question that Medicare for All has risen in prominence in recent years. But in order for its enactment to be viable in the future, there would probably have to be an election that produced a transformation of American politics. And in that scenario, there likely would have to be a number of compromises, such as providing less comprehensive benefits and preserving a larger role for private insurance, in the Medicare for All model. Over 50 years after Medicare's enactment, the path to Medicare for All remains elusive.

Reforming Medicare

Although the political prospects of Medicare for All are daunting, there is currently substantial attention among policymakers to reforming the existing Medicare program. Reforms under consideration include making Medicare's outpatient prescription drug coverage more generous to limit beneficiaries' costs; enabling the federal government to regulate payments for prescription drugs used by Medicare beneficiaries; and improving Medicare coverage of dental, hearing, and vision services.

In large part, such proposals represent efforts to fill the myriad gaps in Medicare coverage. Those gaps have major consequences for persons with chronic conditions. For example, among Medicare beneficiaries in traditional Medicare who did not qualify for a low-income subsidy, 30% of prescriptions written for anticancer drugs, 22% for hepatitis C treatments, and more than 50% for disease-modifying therapies for either immune system disorders or hypercholesterolemia were not filled [79]. Forty-seven percent of Medicare beneficiaries lack dental coverage and in 2018, out of pocket spending on hearing care among exceeded $900 [78]. There are also major racial and ethnic disparities in access to such services, with much higher rates of Black (25%) and Hispanic (22%) than White (14%) enrollees reporting they couldn't get dental, hearing, or vision services [80]. Meanwhile, attention to rising prescription drug prices has renewed interest in reforms that would give the federal government the power to set limits on Medicare's payments for prescription drugs, a power currently prohibited by law.

The Biden administration pursued this incrementalist reform agenda in Medicare, backing enactment of new law that established federal regulation of prices of some drugs in Medicare, while also enhancing Medicare benefits to address coverage gaps. The Inflation Reduction Act of 2022 thus marked a milestone in Medicare policy.

The Future of Medicare

In coming years, Medicare faces a series of major fiscal, political, and policy challenges. As the baby boom generation retires, program enrollment is growing substantially. During 2000–2030, the Medicare population is projected to double. While that demographic trend is often portrayed as a fearful prospect, the reality is that the real public policy crisis would be if we did not already have a program, Medicare, that guarantees health insurance to older Americans. Moreover, other rich democracies have older populations than the U.S., yet those nations spend far less on medical care than we do. Demography is not destiny.

Nonetheless, population aging will create financing pressures in Medicare and intensify debates over how to control program spending. As the stakes of Medicare reform grow, Washington will likely see renewed partisan conflict over how to change the program, including controversial proposals to transform Medicare into a modified voucher or "premium support" system that would limit the government's insurance subsidy for program enrollees. At the same time, the aging of the Medicare population will also draw attention to persistent limitations in program benefits, including the absence of long-term care coverage as well as to persistent challenges in caring for chronically ill persons and those with complex medical care needs. Payment and delivery reforms remain a work in progress, and it is unclear if Medicare can successfully rebalance its reimbursement arrangements to reward primary care.

Medicare has been at the center of American medicine for over half a century. In future years, the importance of Medicare and its influence over US health care will only grow, as will its role in serving persons with chronic illness.

References

1. CMS releases latest enrollment figures for Medicare, Medicaid, and Children's Health Insurance Program. https://www.cms.gov/newsroom/news-alert/cms-releases-latest-enrollment-figures-medicare-medicaid-and-childrens-health-insurance-program-chip. Accessed 12 Apr 2022.
2. Berenson RA, Horvath J. Confronting the barriers to chronic care management in Medicare. Health Aff. 2003;Web Exclusive W3-37–53.
3. Marmor TR. The politics of Medicare. Chicago: Aldine Publishing Company; 1973.
4. Starr P. The social transformation of American medicine. New York: Basic Books; 1982.
5. Oberlander J. The political life of Medicare. Chicago: University of Chicago Press; 2003.
6. Oberlander J, Marmor TR. The road not taken: what happened to Medicare for all? In: Cohen AB, Colby DC, Wailoo KA, Zelizer JE. Medicare and Medicaid at 50: America's entitlement programs in the age of affordable care. New York: Oxford University Press; 2015. p. 55–74.
7. The Boards of Trustees, Federal Hospital Insurance and Federal Supplementary Medical Insurance Trust Funds. 2021 annual report of the federal hospital insurance and federal supplementary medical insurance trust funds. https://www.cms.gov/files/document/2021-medicare-trustees-report.pdf. Accessed 12 Apr 2022.
8. Centers for Medicare and Medicaid Services. Medicare & you 2022. https://www.medicare.gov/Pubs/pdf/10050-medicare-and-you.pdf. Accessed 12 Apr 2022.
9. Davis PA, Binder C, Hahn J, Kirchhoff SM, Morgan PC, Villagrana MA, Voorhies P. Medicare primer. Congressional Research Service. https://sgp.fas.org/crs/misc/R40425.pdf. Accessed 22 Apr 2022.
10. Oberlander J. Medicare. In: Beland D, Howard C, Morgan KJ. The Oxford handbook of U.S. social policy. New York: Oxford University Press; 2015. p. 296–314.
11. Henry J. Kaiser Family Foundation. Medicare beneficiaries with end-stage renal disease. https://www.kff.org/state-category/medi-

care/medicare-enrollment-by-eligibility-category/. Accessed 12 Apr 2022.
12. Henry J. Kaiser Family Foundation. An overview of Medicare. https://www.kff.org/medicare/issue-brief/an-overview-of-medicare/. Accessed 20 Apr 2022.
13. Riley KE, Tsai TS, Figueroa JF, Jha AK. Managing Medicare beneficiaries with chronic conditions during the Covid-19 pandemic. https://www.commonwealthfund.org/publications/issue-briefs/2021/mar/managing-medicare-beneficiaries-chronic-conditions-covid#6. Accessed 20 Apr 2022.
14. Koma W, Neuman T, Jacobson G, Smith K. Medicare beneficiaries' financial security before the Coronavirus pandemic. https://www.kff.org/medicare/issue-brief/medicare-beneficiaries-financial-security-before-the-coronavirus-pandemic/. Accessed 12 Apr 2022.
15. Ochieng N, Cubanski J, Neuman T, Artiga S, Damico A. Racial and ethnic health inequities in Medicare. https://files.kff.org/attachment/Report-Racial-and-Ethnic-Health-Inequities-and-Medicare.pdf. Accessed 22 Apr 2022.
16. Freed M, Fuglesten Binek J, Damico A, Neuman T. Medicare advantage in 2021:enrollment update and key trends. https://www.kff.org/medicare/issue-brief/medicare-advantage-in-2021-enrollment-update-and-key-trends/. Accessed 12 Apr 2022.
17. Meyers DJ, Gadbois EA, Brazier J, Tucher E, Thomas KS. Medicare plans' adoption of special supplemental benefits for the chronically ill for enrollees with social needs. JAMA Netw Open. 2020;3(5):e204690. https://doi.org/10.1001/jamanetworkopen.2020.4690.
18. Henry J. Kaiser Family Foundation. An overview of the Medicare Part D prescription drug benefit. https://www.kff.org/medicare/fact-sheet/an-overview-of-the-medicare-part-d-prescription-drug-benefit/. Accessed 12 Apr 2022.
19. Yamomoto D, Neuman T, Kitchman Strollo M. How does the benefit value of Medicare compare to the benefit value of typical large employer plans? A 2012 update. Henry J. Kaiser Family Foundation. https://www.kff.org/health-reform/issue-brief/how-does-the-benefit-value-of-medicare/. Accessed 23 Apr 2022.
20. Schlesinger M, Wetle T. Medicare's coverage of health services. In: Renewing the promise: Medicare and its reform. New York: Oxford University Press; 1988. p. 58–89.
21. Cubanski J, Boccuti C. Medicare coverage, affordability, access. Generations. 2015;39(2):26–34.
22. Koma W, Cubanski J, Neuman T. A snapshot of sources of coverage among Medicare beneficiaries in 2018. https://www.kff.org/medicare/issue-brief/a-snapshot-of-sources-of-coverage-among-medicare-beneficiaries-in-2018/. Accessed 20 Apr 2022.
23. Cubanski J, Koma W, Damico A, Neuman T. How much do Medicare beneficiaries spend out of pocket on health care? https://www.kff.org/medicare/issue-brief/how-much-do-medicare-beneficiaries-spend-out-of-pocket-on-health-care/. Accessed 12 Apr 2022.
24. Center for Medicare and Medicaid Services. NHE fact sheet.https://www.cms.gov/Research-Statistics-Data-and-Systems/Statistics-Trends-and-Reports/NationalHealthExpendData/NHE-Fact-Sheet. Accessed 12 Apr 2022.
25. Davis K, Guterman S, Bandeall F. The affordable care act and Medicare. The Commonwealth Fund. http://www.commonwealthfund.org/~/media/files/publications/fund-report/2015/jun/1821_davis_aca_and_medicare_v2.pdf. Accessed 23 Apr 2022.
26. Cutler DM, Davis K, Stremikis K. The impact of health reform on health system spending. The Commonwealth Fund. https://cdn.americanprogress.org/wp-content/uploads/issues/2010/05/pdf/system_spending.pdf. Accessed 17 July 2017.
27. Oberlander J, Morrison M. Failure to launch? The Independent Payment Advisory Board's uncertain prospects. N Engl J Med. 2013;369(2):105–7.
28. Beeuwkes B, Graves JA. How the ACA dented the cost curve. Health Aff. 2020;39(3):403–12.
29. McMorrow S, Holahan J. The widespread slowdown in health spending growth: implications for future spending projections and the cost of the Affordable Care Act, an update. https://www.rwjf.org/content/dam/farm/reports/issue_briefs/2016/rwjf429930. Accessed 21 Apr 2022.
30. Oberlander J, Spivack S. Technocratic dreams, political realities: the rise and demise of Medicare's Independent Payment Advisory Board. J Health Polit Policy Law. 2018;43(3):483–510.
31. Rocco P, Kelly AS. And engine of change? The affordable care act and shifting politics of demonstration projects. RSF: the Russell Sage Foundation J Soc Sci. 2020;6(2):67–84.
32. Feder JM. Medicare: the politics of federal hospital insurance. Lexington: D.C. Heath; 1977.
33. Laugesen MJ. Fixing Medicare prices: how physicians are paid. Cambridge: Harvard University Press; 2016.
34. Nixon R. Remarks at a briefing on the nation's health system. https://www.presidency.ucsb.edu/documents/remarks-briefing-the-nations-health-system. Accessed 23 Apr 2022.
35. Mayes R, Berenson RA. Medicare prospective payment and the shaping of U.S. health care. Baltimore: Johns Hopkins University Press; 2006.
36. White C. Why did Medicare spending growth slow down? Health Aff. 2008;27(2):793–802.
37. White C, Ginsburg PA. Slower growth in Medicare spending—is this the new normal? N Engl J Med. 2012;366(12):1073–5.
38. White C, Cubanski J, Neuman T. How much of the Medicare slowdown can be explained? Insights and analysis from 2014. Henry J. Kaiser Family Foundation. http://www.kff.org/medicare/issue-brief/how-much-of-the-medicare-spending-slowdown-can-be-explained-insights-and-analysis-from-2014/. Accessed 23 Apr 22.
39. Reinhardt UE. Medicare innovations in the war over the key to the US treasury. In Cohen AB, Colby DC, Wailoo KA, Zelizer JE. Medicare and Medicaid at 50: America's entitlement programs in the age of affordable care. New York: Oxford University Press; 2015. p. 169–189.
40. Congressional Budget Office (CBO). The prices that commercial health insurers and Medicare pay for hospitals' and physicians' services. https://www.cbo.gov/publication/57422. Accessed 21 Apr 2022.
41. A pathway to improving care for Medicare patients with chronic conditions. Hearing before the Committee on Finance, United States Senate. https://www.finance.senate.gov/imo/media/doc/99934.pdf. Accessed 23 Apr 2022.
42. Center for Medicare and Medicaid Services. Readmissions Reduction Program (HRRP). https://www.cms.gov/medicare/medicare-fee-for-service-payment/acuteinpatientpps/readmissions-reduction-program.html. Accessed 22 Apr 2022.
43. Jencks SF, Williams MV, Coleman EA. Rehospitalizations among patients in the Medicare fee-for-service program. N Engl J Med. 2009;360(14):1418–28.
44. Mechanic R. Medicare's bundled payment initiatives: considerations for providers. American Hospital Association. http://www.aha.org/content/16/issbrief-bundledpmt.pdf. Accessed 23 Apr 2022.
45. Bodenheimer T, Grumbach K. Understanding health policy: a clinical approach. 6th ed. New York: McGraw Hill; 2012.
46. Center for Medicare and Medicaid Services. Bundled Payments for Care Improvement (BPCI) initiative: general information. https://innovation.cms.gov/initiatives/bundled-payments/. Accessed 23 Apr 2022.
47. Berenson RA, Burton RA. Next steps for ACOs. Health Affairs Policy Brief. http://healthaffairs.org/healthpolicybriefs/brief_pdfs/healthpolicybrief_61.pdf. Accessed 23 Apr 2022.
48. Centers for Medicare and Medicaid Services. Medicare Shared Savings Program quality measure benchmarks for the 2020/2021 per-

formance years. https://www.cms.gov/files/document/20202021-quality-benchmarks.pdf. Accessed 22 Apr 2022.
49. Rosenthal MB. Physician payment after the SGR-the new meritocracy. N Engl J Med. 2015;373(13):1187–9.
50. Oberlander J, Laugesen MJ. Leap of faith—Medicare's new physician payment system. N Engl J Med. 2015;373(13):1185–7.
51. Burwell SM. Setting value-based payment goals—HHS efforts to improve US health care. N Engl J Med. 2015;372(10):897–9.
52. Radnofsky L. Obama administration hits Medicare payment target early. Wall Street J. 2016.
53. Ody C, Msall L, Dafny LS, Grabowski DC, Cutler DM. Decreases in readmissions credited to Medicare's program to reduce hospital readmissions have been overstated. Health Aff. 2020;38(1):36–43.
54. Joshi S, Nuckols T, Escarere J, Huckfeldt P, Popescu I, Sood N. Regression to the mean in the hospital readmissions reduction program. JAMA Intern Med. 2019;179(9):1167–73.
55. Kimmey L, Anderson M, Cheh V, Li E, McCaulghlin C, et al. Evaluation of the Independence at Home demonstration: an examination of the first four years. https://innovation.cms.gov/files/reports/iah-yr4evalrpt.pdf. Accessed 22 Apr 2022.
56. Doran T, Maurer KA, Ryan AM. Impact of provider incentives on quality and value of health care. Annu Rev Public Health. 2017;38:449–65.
57. Baseman S, Boccuti C, Moon M, Griffin S, Dutta T. Payment and delivery system reform in Medicare: a primer on medical homes, accountable care organizations, and bundled payments. Henry J. Kaiser Family Foundation. http://files.kff.org/attachment/Report-Payment-and-Delivery-System-Reform-in-Medicare.pdf. Accessed 23 Apr 2022.
58. Yee CA, Pizer SD, Frakt A. Medicare's bundled payment initiatives for hospital-initiated episodes: evidence and evolution. Milbank Q. 2020;98(3):908–74.
59. Medicare Payment Advisory Commission (MedPAC). Moving beyond the Merit-based Incentive Payment System. https://www.medpac.gov/wp-content/uploads/import_data/scrape_files/docs/default-source/reports/mar18_medpac_ch15_sec.pdf. Accessed 23 Apr 2022.
60. Song Z, Fisher ES. The ACO experiment in infancy. JAMA. 2016;316(7):705–6.
61. McWilliams JM. Savings from ACOs—building on early success. Ann Intern Med. 2016;165(12):873–5.
62. McWilliams JM, Hatfield LA, Chernew ME, Landon BE, Schwartz AL. Early performance of accountable care organizations in Medicare. N Engl J Med. 2016;374(24):2357–66.
63. McWilliams JM, Chen AJ. Sharpen your pencils. Understanding the latest ACO savings: "curb your enthusiasm" and sharpen your pencils—part 1. https://www.healthaffairs.org/do/10.1377/forefront.20201106.719550/full/. Accessed 22 Apr 2022.
64. Markovitz AA, Hollingsworth JM, Ayanian JZ, Norton EC, Yan PL, Ryan AM. Performance in the Medicare shared savings program after accounting for non-random exit: an instrumental variable analysis. Ann Intern Med. 2019;171(1):27–36.
65. Marmor TR, Oberlander J, White J. The Obama administration's options for health care cost control: hope versus reality. Ann Intern Med. 2009;150(7):485–9.
66. McWilliams JM. Professionalism revealed: rethinking quality improvement in the wake of the pandemic. NEJM Catalyst. 2022;1(5):1–17.
67. Marmor TR, Oberlander J. From HMOs to ACOs: the quest for the holy grail in U.S. health policy. J Gen Intern Med. 2012;27(9):1215–8.
68. Vladeck B. Roundtable on Medicare physician payments: understanding the past so we can envision the future—statement before the Committee on Finance, U.S. Senate. 2012.
69. Centers for Disease Control and Prevention. (CDC). Covid-19: persons with certain medical conditions. https://www.cdc.gov/coronavirus/2019-ncov/need-extra-precautions/people-with-medical-conditions.html. Accessed 23 Apr 2022.
70. Medicare Payment Advisory Commission (MedPAC). Context for Medicare payment policy. https://www.medpac.gov/wp-content/uploads/2022/03/Mar22_MedPAC_ReportToCongress_Ch1_SEC.pdf. Accessed 22 Apr 2022.
71. Chidambaram P. Over 200,000 residents and staff in long-term care facilities have died from Covid-19. https://www.kff.org/policy-watch/over-200000-residents-and-staff-in-long-term-care-facilities-have-died-from-covid-19/. Accessed 22 Apr 2022.
72. Wong Samson L, Tarazi W, Turrini G, Sheingold S. Medicare beneficiaries' use of telehealth in 2020: trends by beneficiary characteristics and location. https://aspe.hhs.gov/sites/default/files/documents/a1d5d810fe3433e18b192be42dbf2351/medicare-telehealth-report.pdf. Accessed 22 Apr 2022.
73. Medicare for All Act of 2019. https://www.sanders.senate.gov/wp-content/uploads/medicare-for-all-act-of-2019.pdf. Accessed 23 Apr 2022.
74. Oberlander J. The virtues and vice of single-payer health care. N Engl J Med. 2016;374(15):1401–3.
75. Oberlander J. Navigating the shifting terrain of US health care reform—Medicare for All, single payer, and the public option. Milbank Q. 2019;97(4):939–53.
76. Oberlander J. Lessons from the long and winding road to Medicare for All. Am J Public Health. 2019;109(11):1497–500.
77. Brown LD. Am J Public Health. 2019;109(11):1506–10.
78. Frakt AB, Oberlander J. Challenges to Medicare for all remain daunting. Health Aff. 2020;39(1):142–5.
79. Dusetzina SB, Huskamp HA, Rothman RL, Pinheiro LC, Roberts AW, Shah ND. Many Medicare beneficiaries do not fill high-price specialty drug prescriptions. Health Aff. 2022;41(4):487–96.
80. Freed M, Cubanski J, Sroczynski N, Ochieng N, Neuman T. Dental, hearing, and vision costs and coverage among Medicare beneficiaries in traditional Medicare and Medicare Advantage. https://www.kff.org/health-costs/issue-brief/dental-hearing-and-vision-costs-and-coverage-among-medicare-beneficiaries-in-traditional-medicare-and-medicare-advantage/. Accessed 23 Apr 2022.

Medicaid

44

Pam Silberman and Ciara Zachary

Introduction

Medicaid is the largest health insurance safety net in the United States, providing health insurance coverage to almost 75 million low-income individuals in March 2021 [1]. The Children's Health Insurance Program (CHIP), which provides coverage to children with incomes that exceed Medicaid eligibility, covered an additional 6.8 million children. Medicaid accounts for approximately 17% of all health care spending in the United States with approximately $632 billion in cost reported for 2019, while CHIP cost an additional almost $19 billion [2].

Medicaid covered more than half (58%) [3] of all nonelderly individuals living in poverty, and almost half (48.5%) of all individuals with incomes up to 200% of the federal poverty level in 2019 [4]. The program paid for almost half of all births (49%) and provided health insurance to more than one-third (38%) of all children in 2017 [5]. Further, Medicaid serves many people with chronic illnesses and disabilities, including approximately 45% of nonelderly adults with a disability, 42% of nonelderly adults living with HIV/AIDS, 19% of Medicare beneficiaries, and 62% of nursing home residents.

Both Medicaid and CHIP are administered and financed jointly by the federal and state governments. The federal government sets broad program parameters, giving states flexibility in how they administer the program. States have some flexibility in eligibility, covered services, provider payments, and delivery system design. In addition, states have the option of operating their CHIP program as an extension of Medicaid (e.g., same services, provider payments, and delivery system), or as a stand-along CHIP program. While there are many similarities between Medicaid and CHIP, there are also distinct differences. Most importantly, Medicaid is an entitlement program, meaning that the state and federal government have to pay for services for any individual who meets the state's eligibility rules. In contrast, the stand-alone CHIP program operates as a block-grant program. States can establish waiting lists if they run through their program budget. This chapter provides an overview of the Medicaid program, as it covers far more people with chronic illnesses—both children and adults—than CHIP. However, some information about the CHIP program is included throughout the chapter.

Historical Developments

Medicaid was created in 1965 as Title XIX of the Social Security Act, but the Act has been amended many times since the program was first established [6, 7]. Many of the changes expanded Medicaid to cover more people or services. Other amendments changed provider payment methodologies and extended states' ability to tailor the overall program structure to meet state needs. Essentially, Congress enacted changes over the years to balance the competing tensions of covering unmet needs (coverage and service expansion), ensuring adequate access and quality, and reducing escalating costs.

When Medicaid was first created, it was limited to families receiving Aid-to-Families with Dependent Children (AFDC) and to older adults and people with disabilities covered under state cash payment programs. The program was optional to the states. But, by 1982, all 50 states and the

P. Silberman · C. Zachary (✉)
Department of Health Policy and Management, Gillings School of Global Public Health, University of North Carolina at Chapel Hill, Chapel Hill, NC, USA
e-mail: pam_silberman@unc.edu; zciara@email.unc.edu

District of Columbia operated a Medicaid program [8]. Congress first amended Medicaid in 1967 when it expanded the program to provide coverage to medically needy individuals: those with substantial medical bills, but who earned too much income to qualify for Medicaid. Congress also directed states to provide comprehensive well-child care, the Early and Periodic Screening, Diagnostic, and Treatment (EPSDT) program—to children under age 21 [6].

Congress created the Supplemental Security Income (SSI) program in 1972, nationalizing the states' old cash payment programs for older adults and people with disabilities. At that time, states were required to provide Medicaid to anyone receiving SSI (or, a state option, to a more limited group of individuals who were elderly or disabled). Amendments in the mid-1980s and early 1990s extended coverage to more pregnant people and children, followed by a larger expansion to children in 1997 with the passage of the Children's Health Insurance Program (CHIP). Like Medicaid, CHIP was also optional to states, but all states chose to adopt the program.

The largest coverage expansion since the inception of Medicaid occurred in 2010, as a result of the passage of the Patient Protection and Affordable Care Act (ACA). The ACA included a mandate that all states expand Medicaid to cover adults up to 138% of the federal poverty level (FPL), even if these adults did not meet eligibility for traditional coverage categories. However, a Supreme Court decision later made the expanded coverage optional to the states.

In addition to the coverage expansion, the Act has been amended over time to try to rein in rising health costs. For example, early in the history of the Medicaid program, hospitals and nursing facilities were reimbursed on a "reasonable cost" basis. This began to change in the 1970s and 1980s. Payments to hospitals and nursing homes were changed from "reasonable costs" to payments that were sufficient to cover the costs of "efficiently and economically operated" facilities. In 1981, states were given more flexibility to reduce program costs by implementing Medicaid managed care and by imposing cost sharing requirements (1982).

Other Medicaid changes aimed to ensure access and quality. To address adequate access, the Medicaid Act was amended in 1989 to "assure that payments [to providers] are consistent with efficiency, economy, and quality of care and are sufficient to enlist enough providers so that care and services are available under the plan at least to the extent that such care and services are available to the general population in the geographic area" (42 USC §1396a(30)(A)). Congress later amended the Medicaid statute in 1990 to ensure that payments to nursing facilities were sufficient to implement the 1987 nursing home quality reforms. Special payment rules were also implemented to protect safety net hospitals—"disproportionate share hospital" payments—federally qualified health centers (FQHCs), and rural health clinics.

Medicaid Eligibility, Covered Services, and Cost Sharing

Eligibility

Historically, to qualify for Medicaid, an individual must have been a citizen or qualified immigrant and the right "type" of person. Their income must have been below a specified income limit, and they could not have too much money in the bank. For example, Medicaid was limited to certain categories of individuals, including pregnant people, children under the age of 19 (or 21 at state option), parents of dependent children, older adults (age 65 or older), or someone living with a disability. The maximum income someone could have and still qualify varied, depending on the different categories of those eligible (Fig. 44.1). Non-disabled, nonelderly adults without dependent children could not qualify, regardless of how poor they were.

The ACA [9] intended to expand Medicaid to adults with incomes below 138% FPL, regardless of whether they fell into one of the coverage categories. However, the US Supreme Court in *National Federation of Independent Business v. Sebelius* [10] overturned the mandate, making Medicaid expansion optional to the states. As of July 2021, 39 states and the District of Columbia expanded their Medicaid program to cover these newly eligible adults (children were already covered through Medicaid or CHIP). The remaining 12 states have chosen not to expand. The American Rescue Plan Act of 2021 included additional financial incentives to encourage the "hold-out" states to adopt Medicaid expansion, but it is unclear whether those incentives will be sufficient to overcome these states' reluctance to extend Medicaid coverage.

In addition to the mandatory coverage groups, states have options of covering other categories of individuals. For example, 34 states operate a "medically needy" program [11]. This allows states to cover individuals who have high medical bills but have too much income to otherwise qualify for Medicaid. In effect, individuals or families must incur medical bills equaling the difference between their countable income and the state's medically needy income limits. This difference operates similarly to a health care deductible for people with private insurance. The individual is responsible for paying this amount, and then Medicaid pays the remainder of the bills over the individual's coverage period.

Congress also gave states the option to expand coverage to women with incomes below 250% FPL if they were diagnosed with breast or cervical cancer. All states provide this coverage, but the number of people covered is generally small. Congress also set up a separate family planning Medicaid program option—providing coverage for family planning services to certain individuals who meet state

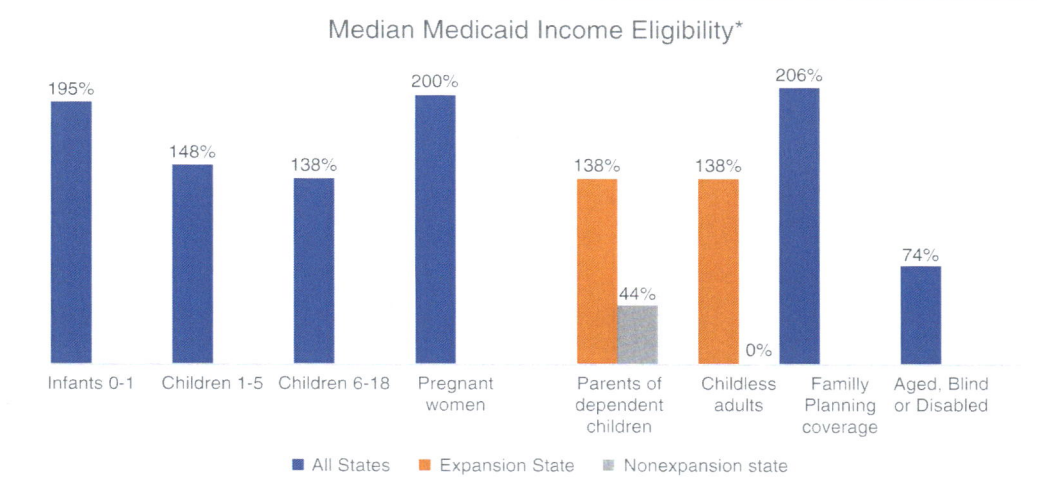

Fig. 44.1 Median Medicaid Income Eligibility by Eligibility Category (As of January 1, 2021). States generally have higher median incomes in their CHIP programs. For example, the median CHIP income limits is: 217% (0–1 year old), 216% (1–5 year old), 155% (6–18 year old), and 262% for pregnant women. (Sources: Brooks T, Gardner A, Tolbert J, Dolan R, Pham O. Medicaid and CHIP Eligibility and Enrollment Policies as of January 2021: Findings from a 50-State Survey. Kaiser Family Foundation. March 8, 2021. Tables 1, 2, 4. https://www.kff.org/report-section/medicaid-and-chip-eligibility-and-enrollment-policies-as-of-january-2021-findings-from-a-50-state-survey-tables/; Medicaid Eligibility through the Aged, Blind and Disabled Pathway (2018 data). State Health Facts. Accessed August 10, 2021. https://www.kff.org/medicaid/state-indicator/medicaid-eligibility-through-the-aged-blind-disabled-pathway/?currentTimeframe=0&sortModel=%7B%22colId%22:%22Location%22,%22sort%22:%22asc%22%7D)

eligibility criteria [12]. States have flexibility in establishing the income limits for this program. As of November 2021, 26 states participated in this Medicaid program [12].

Covered Services

Congress identified certain services that the states must cover in their Medicaid programs ("mandatory services") and other services that are optional to the states ("optional services"). The required services are similar to what most private insurance plans cover, such as inpatient and outpatient hospital services, physician and nurse practitioner visits, family planning, home health, lab and x-ray service. States are also required to cover services provided in rural health clinics and FQHCs (See Fig. 44.2). States must also cover certain services that are not typically covered in private plans, including long-term care services provided in nursing facilities and non-emergency medical transportation. In addition, states must cover Early, Periodic Screening, Diagnosis and Treatment (EPSDT) for children under age 21. EPSDT is similar to well-child care provided by private insurers. But, it also requires states to cover *any Medicaid allowable service*, including optional services that are needed to ameliorate health problems identified in the EPSDT screening.

Of note, states are not mandated to cover prescription drugs ("optional service"), but all states do. In addition, most states provide some coverage of dental, podiatry, and psychological services; physical, occupational, and speech therapy; dentures, prosthetics, eyeglasses, hearing aids, and medical equipment; hospice, personal care services, and PACE (Program of All-Inclusive Care for the Elderly) in their Medicaid programs. A smaller subset of states covers other services such as chiropractic treatment and case management. States are required to cover some specified behavioral health services but have the option to cover a broader array of these services [13]. Nationwide, Medicaid is the largest payor for mental health services in the country, and also a major payor for substance use disorder services [14].

States do not have to provide the same services for adults in the Medicaid expansion population. The ACA mandated that states cover ten essential services that are part of the ACA for the expansion population, such as inpatient and outpatient services, lab and x-ray services, prescription drugs, and behavioral health services. States can cover other Medicaid mandatory or optional services, but are not required to do so. Similarly, stand-alone CHIP need not provide all the same services as does Medicaid. It must provide coverage that is comparable to services covered in commercial health insurance plans and must cover behavioral health and dental services. However, unlike Medicaid, CHIP programs are not required to provide EPSDT services, non-emergency medical transportation, or long-term care services.

Cost Sharing

States may charge some Medicaid enrollees premiums or other out-of-pocket costs. However, certain groups are exempt from any cost sharing, including pregnant people (for preg-

Fig. 44.2 Mandatory and Optional Services for Traditional Medicaid and Medicaid Expansion Populations. (Source: Mandatory and Optional Benefits. Medicaid and CHIP Payment and Access Commission. Accessed August 10, 2021. https://www.macpac.gov/subtopic/mandatory-and-optional-benefits/; Dear State Medicaid Director. Essential Health Benefits in the Medicaid Program. SMDL #12-003, ACA#21. Center for Medicare and Medicaid Services. Nov. 20, 2012. https://www.medicaid.gov/sites/default/files/Federal-Policy-Guidance/downloads/SMD-12-003.pdf)

Mandatory Services	Optional Services		Medicaid Expansion Required Services
• Early, Periodic Screening, Diagnosis and Treatment (EPSDT) • Family planning services • Federally qualified health centers and rural health clinics • Freestanding birth centers • Home health services • Hospital Services, Inpatient and Outpatient • Laboratory and x-ray services • Non-emergency medical transportation • Nursing facility services for individuals over age 21 • Practitioners, including physicians, certified pediatric and family nurse practitioners, and nurse midwives • Tobacco cessation counseling for pregnant women	• Community supported living arrangements • Clinic services • Critical access hospital • Dental services, dentures • Health homes for enrollees with chronic conditions • Homeand community-based services Critical access • Hospice • Institutional services, including inpatient hospital and nursing facility services for individuals 64 or older in an institution for mental diseases, inpatient psychiatric services for individuals under age 21, and intermediate facility services for individuals with intellectual disabilities • Optometry services and eye glasses • Therapy services including physical therapy, occupational therapy, and speech, hearing, and language therapy	• Other diagnostic, screening, preventive, and rehabilitative services, including respiratory care for ventilator dependent individuals • Other licensed practitioner services, including chiropractic • Personal care services • Prescription drugs • Primary care case management services • Private duty nursing services • Program of All Inclusive Care for the Elderly (PACE) services • Prosthetic devises • Services furnished in a religious non medical health care institution • Targeted case management services • Tuberculosis-related services	• Ambulatory patient services • Emergency services • Hospitalization • Pregnancy maternity and newborn care • Mental health and substance use disorder services (in parity with physical health services) • Prescription Drugs • Rehabilitative and habilitative services • Laboratory services • Preventive and wellness services and chronic disease management • Pediatric services including oral and vision care

nancy related services), most children, and those in long-term care nursing facilities. For others, the amount that can be charged depends on the individual's income. Generally, the state can only charge nominal copays for Medicaid enrollees with incomes below 100% FPL [15]. Nominal copays are limited to $4 for most services, or $75 for inpatient hospital services. Those with higher incomes can be charged premiums, copays of up to 20% of the cost of the services, and copays for non-emergency use of the emergency room (if certain other conditions are met). Families with children with CHIP coverage that have incomes above 150% can also be charged premiums or other out-of-pocket costs, as long as total costs do not exceed 5% of family income [16].

Impact of Medicaid Expansion on Health Outcomes

Studies that have looked at the impact of Medicaid expansion on the uninsured have generally found positive associations between expansion and access to health services and health outcomes [17, 18]. For example, studies have shown greater access to care for people with cancer, chronic disease, and other disabilities. Comparably, studies have shown increased access to services for pregnant people, for people living with HIV/AIDS, and for people with mental health or substance use disorder problems. Research has also shown an association between Medicaid expansion and decrease in all-cause mortality, as well as mortality related to specific health conditions including certain types of cancer, cardiovascular disease, or liver disease. Medicaid expansion was also shown to reduce racial, ethnic, and socioeconomic disparities for certain health conditions. Not surprisingly, Medicaid expansion also reduced catastrophic health costs for enrollees, and also helped improve provider payer mixes.

Provider Payments

States have a lot of flexibility in setting provider payment amounts, as long as the payments are designed to promote efficiency, quality and access [19]. The payments should be sufficient to ensure Medicaid enrollees have comparable access to providers to that of others in the same geographic area. Provider payments can vary based on the level of care, underlying condition, and intensity of services. Payments to hospitals, including supplemental payments, are generally comparable to Medicare [20]. However, Medicaid payments to physicians have historically been less than what Medicare pays for similar services. On average, Medicaid reimbursement rates to physicians were only 72% of Medicare rates for 27 common procedures in 2019 [21]. Because of low Medicaid reimbursement rates, approximately 71% of physicians reported that they were willing to accept new Medicaid patients. In contrast 91% of physicians reported willingness to accept new privately insured, and 90% reported a willingness to accept new Medicare patients [22]. Despite lower physician participation rates, Medicaid enrollees report similar ability to access providers as do those with private insurance, and much higher than the uninsured [23].

While states have considerable flexibility in setting provider payments, they are required by statute to have special payment systems for FQHCs and rural health clinics, and for disproportionate share hospitals ("DSH"). States are required to pay FQHCs and rural health clinics using a prospective cost basis, or an alternative payment method which is no less generous [24, 25]. These payments are generally higher than the traditional fee-for-service payments to other physicians and clinics. In addition, states must pay safety net hospitals a supplemental DSH payment to help offset some of the hospitals' uncompensated care costs [26]. States determine the eligibility criteria for DSH hospitals but must target hospitals with a disproportionate number of Medicaid and uninsured patients. The total DSH payments in fiscal year 2019 was $19.7 billion.

Delivery System

When Medicaid was first created, the statute gave enrollees freedom to choose any provider who participated in Medicaid. Individuals could not be "locked into" any particular provider for services. Over the years, Congress has given states more authority to require Medicaid enrollees to obtain care from specific providers, generally through managed care arrangements. There are three primary managed care arrangements: (1) primary care case management, (2) prepaid health plans, and (3) managed care organizations. In primary care case management (PCCM) programs, enrollees select a primary care medical home, which serves to manage and coordinate the patients care. The state generally continues to pay providers on a fee-for-service basis but gives primary care providers an additional case management fee to help pay for care coordination. States can also contract with "prepaid health plans" to provide a subset of services—either outpatient services only, or both outpatient and inpatient care. Typical prepaid ambulatory or inpatient health plans cover services such as transportation, dental, or behavioral health. States can also contract with a managed care organization (MCO) to manage and provide most or all of the Medicaid covered services. This is the most common Medicaid managed care arrangement.

Forty states contracted with MCOs to provide services to some or all of their Medicaid enrollees in 2019 [27]. On average, about 80% of a state's Medicaid population is enrolled in one of the MCOs operating in those states, although the actual percentage varies from 5 to 100%. In addition, 12 states operate a primary care case management program (PCCM), including 5 states that operate both MCOs and PCCM programs. Only 4 states had no managed care arrangements in 2019 (Alaska, Connecticut, Vermont, and Wyoming).

In addition to contracts with MCOs, a number of states have started to move into value-based arrangements with providers. In 2018, there were 10 states with Accountable Care Organization (ACO) arrangements [28]. States with ACOs generally pay these organizations either through a shared savings arrangement, or through global capitation, with requirements that the organizations meet certain quality standards.

Financing

Medicaid is jointly financed between the federal and state government, with the federal government contributing between 50 and 80% of the cost of covered services for eligible individuals. The federal match rate—known as the Federal Medical Assistance Percentage or FMAP—is based on the state's per capita income. States with lower per capita income receive a higher federal match rate. As an example, for federal fiscal year (FFY) 2022, the state's underlying FMAP rate ranged from a low of 50% in 12 states to a high of 78.31% in Mississippi [29]. The FMAP rate for CHIP services is 30% higher than for Medicaid, ranging from 65 to 84.82%.

In addition to the regular FMAP rates for Medicaid and CHIP, the federal government has different match rates for selected covered individuals, services, or program costs. For example, the federal government pays 90% of the costs of those newly made eligible under the ACA (e.g., in Medicaid expansion states). The federal government typically pays 50% for most administrative expenses (such as determining Medicaid eligibility) but pays 90% for certain other administrative expenses such as implementation of a Medicaid information system or a state Medicaid fraud control unit, or for family planning services [30].

Medicaid Expenditures

Overall, Medicaid spending closely tracks enrollment. Program costs go up when more people enroll, and down when there are fewer people on the program. While this relationship generally holds true, the actual costs that a state incurs for its Medicaid program is dependent on many factors including number of enrollees, types of eligibles, covered services, and provider payment amounts. On average, costs for older adults (65 years or older), and people with disabilities is much higher than for other enrollees—about seven times higher than for children and almost five times higher than for parents in FY 2014 [31]. Because of the variation in eligibility, program design, and provider payments, the average cost per full-time eligible individual ranged across the states from a high of $13,611 in North Dakota to a low of $5916 in Nevada in FFY 2018 [32].

Medicaid spending per enrollee has historically grown at a much slower pace than national health expenditures or private insurance (and generally lower than Medicare) (see Fig. 44.3). Between 2016 and 2019, Medicaid spending per enrollee grew an average of 3.4% per year, Medicare grew an average of 3.1%, national health expenditures per capita grew 3.9%. In comparison, private health insurance per enrollee grew 4.8% during this same period [33]. Across the states, Medicaid spending constituted almost 16% of *state-only* spending (e.g., from state general revenues and other state funds). When including the federal Medicaid funds that flow through the states, Medicaid accounts for almost 29% of total state budgets. Paying Medicaid costs can be challenging to states, particularly in economic downturns. Typically, enrollment in the Medicaid program grows during recessions, as more people lose their jobs or cut hours of employment and become eligible. But state revenues generally shrink during economic downturns. This counter-cyclical nature of the Medicaid program creates particular problems for states that must balance their budget every year, unlike the federal government which can operate deficits. If states are required to pay for increased Medicaid costs during an economic downturn, they have less money to pay for other necessary services.

States have responded to economic downturns by instituting policies aimed at reducing Medicaid costs or increasing revenues through provider taxes. For example, states have tried to reduce program costs by freezing provider payments, imposing higher premiums or cost sharing, and incentivizing Medicaid enrollees to participate in wellness initiatives. States have also developed complex care management programs to target high-cost enrollees, employed primary care medical home models, tightened eligibility for long-term care services and expanded home and community-based services, and employed different strategies to rein in rising pharmaceutical costs [34, 35].

The federal and state governments have also taken various actions to address the growing costs of prescription drugs. In 1990 Congress established the Medicaid Drug Rebate Program (MDRP). Drug manufacturers must agree to provide drug

Fig. 44.3 Medicaid Spending Per Enrollee Over Time (2007–2019). (Source: Rudowitz R, Williams E, Hinton E, Garfield R. Medicaid Financing: The Basics. Kaiser Family Foundation. May 7, 2021. Fig. 6. https://www.kff.org/medicaid/issue-brief/medicaid-financing-the-basics/. Datasource: Kaiser Family Foundation estimates based on National health Expenditure Data from the Centers for Medicare and Medicaid Services Office of the Actuary)

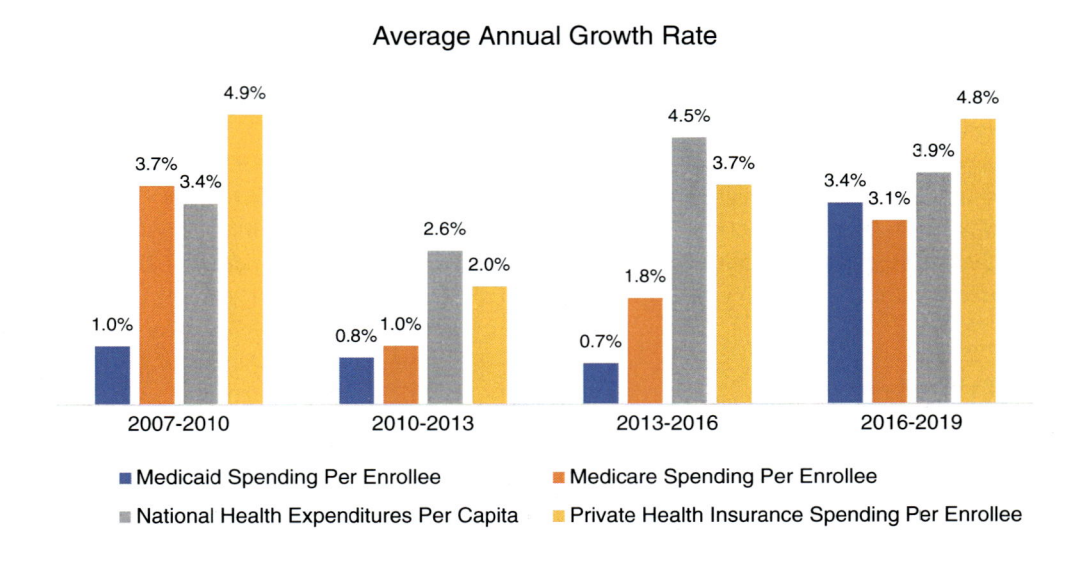

Average Annual Growth Rate

Period	Medicaid Spending Per Enrollee	Medicare Spending Per Enrollee	National Health Expenditures Per Capita	Private Health Insurance Spending Per Enrollee
2007–2010	1.0%	3.7%	3.4%	4.9%
2010–2013	0.8%	1.0%	2.6%	2.0%
2013–2016	0.7%	1.8%	4.5%	3.7%
2016–2019	3.4%	3.1%	3.9%	4.8%

rebates to the state and federal governments for their drugs to be covered in states' Medicaid programs [36]. The rebate amount is determined by many factors such as, whether a drug is generic or has a brand name. Furthermore, the MDRP Act gave Medicaid a "Most Favored Nation" status with regard to pharmaceutical prices. That means that with only a few exceptions, pharmaceutical companies must pass onto to the Medicaid program the lowest cost negotiated with other payors [37]. Some states have gone further to reduce drug costs by limiting dispensing fees to pharmacists, requiring generic substitution unless the prescriber specifies why the brand name drug is medically necessary, or by requiring a supplemental rebate to be listed on the state's preferred drug list [38].

In addition, states have increased revenues to offset the state's share of Medicaid costs through provider taxes and intergovernmental transfers from other governmental entities. In state fiscal year 2019, all states had at least one provider tax, including 43 with hospital taxes, 45 with nursing facility taxes, and 35 with taxes on intermediate care facilities for people with intellectual disabilities [39]. Congress has also stepped up to help the states during recent economic downturns by increasing the federal match rate. For example, as part of the Families First Coronavirus Response Act of 2020, Congress increased the regular FMAP rate to all states by 6.2 percentage points during the COVID-19 public health emergency [33]. In response, states were required to meet certain maintenance of effort requirements, to ensure that people on Medicaid did not lose benefits and to prevent states from restricting eligibility.

Medicaid Waivers

States must generally operate their Medicaid program the same throughout the state (i.e., the "statewideness" requirement). However, Congress gave states the authority to seek waivers of certain program requirements, including statewideness—with permission from the Centers for Medicare Medicaid Services (CMS) [40]. There are three primary Medicaid waivers. Freedom of choice or 1915(b) waivers allow states to implement managed care arrangements and to lock patients into particular primary care providers (42 USC §1915(b)). These are the waivers states have historically used to create primary care case management programs or to contract with managed care organizations.

States can also seek home and community-based services (HCBS) or 1915(c) waivers to enable the state to provide additional home and community-based services to people who would otherwise qualify for institutional care (42 USC §1915(c)). In 2018, 48 states and the District of Columbia operated 265 waivers covering more than 1.8 million people [41]. States can operate more than one waiver, covering different eligibility groups and services (e.g., children with complex medical conditions who would otherwise need long-term hospitalization, people living with HIV/AIDS, people with traumatic brain injury, frail adults or those with disabilities, people with mental illness, or people with intellectual and developmental disabilities).

These waivers must generally be cost neutral to the federal government, which means that the state must demonstrate that the costs of providing home and community-based services are no more than what it would have cost the state to provide institutional care to these individuals. Most states target their 1915(c) waivers to older adults and people with disabilities, or people with intellectual and developmental disabilities. These HCBS offered through 1915(c) waivers do not operate as an entitlement. That means that the state can limit the number of eligible individuals whom it will serve. As a result, there were there are reports that over 800,000 people were on waitlists in 40 states in 2018 [42].

In addition, the state can seek a Section 1115 research and demonstration waiver if they want to test new models of care that promote the objectives of the Medicaid program (42 USC §1115). This waiver is often broader in scope than 1915(b) or (c) waivers. In August 2021, there were 63 approved 1115 waivers operating in 45 states [43]. In addition, 26 states had 30 waivers pending. If the state can demonstrate savings through the new program design, it can use the savings to reduce program costs, or to offer additional services or cover new eligibles.

States have used this authority to expand services or people covered, or to develop targeted managed care systems. For example, in 2021, 18 states have approved 1115 waivers to expand the array of community-based services (e.g., housing, employment or peer support) for people with behavioral health conditions, 32 states cover the costs of substance use disorder services provided in Institutions for Mental Diseases (IMDs), and 13 states have waivers to establish capitation arrangements with managed care providers offering long-term services and supports [43].

States have also sought or obtained waivers intended to limit services or eligibles, or to charge higher costs to enrollees. For example, 12 states have obtained waivers to restrict eligibility or enrollment, including waiving retroactive eligibility—which normally allows Medicaid to cover expenses up to 3 months prior to the enrollee's application date. Other states have sought waivers to lock enrollees out of Medicaid for a specific period of time if they fail to meet certain program rules, including work requirements or paying premiums [43]. Other states have obtained waivers that authorized them to stop covering non-emergency medical transportation, or to charge higher copays above the statutory limits. Some states have also obtained waivers to charge higher premiums than would otherwise be allowed. Federal courts have blocked some of the approved waivers that have restricted coverage or eligibility. However, others are still in effect.

Impact of Medicaid for Persons with Chronic Illnesses

Medicaid enrollees are far more likely to report having one or more chronic illnesses and have more functional limitations than are those with private insurance. For example, children on Medicaid are more likely to have been diagnosed with ADHD/ADD, asthma, or autism, or an intellectual or other developmental disability than those who have private insurance [44]. Nonelderly adults (ages 19–64) on Medicaid are more likely than those with private insurance to have been diagnosed with hypertension, coronary artery disease, heart attack, stroke, diabetes, arthritis, or asthma, and to report limitations with basic or complex activities. They are also more likely to be obese or a current smoker and are more likely to report having a functional limitation.

Medicaid's home and community-based services (HCBS) are especially important for individuals with complex and chronic illnesses. All states are required to provide home health services, which include nursing services, home health aide services, medical equipment and supplies, and often include physical, occupational, or speech therapy services [45]. States can also offer personal care services that help individuals with activities of daily living (such as bathing, dressing, toileting, or transferring), or with instrumental activities of daily living (such as meal preparation, shopping, using the telephone, or medication management) [46]. In FY 2018, 34 states offered personal care services. In addition, states have the option of covering additional HCBS through 1915(c) waivers discussed earlier in the Chapter [47]. In general, HCBS help individuals remain in their homes in the community and reduce the need for institutionalization.

States have also designed other initiatives aimed at those with multiple co-morbidities. For example, some states have established Medicaid health homes to provide more comprehensive care management, transitional services, and referrals to community and social supports for people with multiple chronic illnesses [48]. In 2021, 21 states and the District of Columbia offered at least one Medicaid health home model [49]. States have also instituted complex care management for high-cost Medicaid enrollees (e.g., enrollees with complex health problems and psychosocial needs that have high costs and are high utilizers). Data are mixed on how well these initiatives help improve health outcomes or reduce unnecessary expenditures.

In addition, low-income populations are more likely than others to have unmet social needs that impair health. Studies show that those with unmet social needs are also more likely to have chronic illnesses and experience greater access barriers [50].

Some states have used Medicaid funding to address unmet social needs, such as food or housing insecurity or transportation [51]. For example, North Carolina obtained an 1115 waiver that gave the state the authority to use federal and state Medicaid funds to pay for unmet social needs that affect health [52]. This was the first of its kind—this 1115 waiver authorized the state to use up to $650 million over 5 years in Medicaid funding to pay for selected services to address housing insecurity, food insecurity, non-medical transportation, and interpersonal violence. The pilot program will start serving high-risk individuals who have both underlying health problems and unmet social needs in the spring of 2022.

Final Comments

The Medicaid and CHIP programs provide comprehensive health insurance coverage to some of the most vulnerable people in the United States. On paper, the program covers a wide array of services with limited cost sharing. Further, there is sufficient flexibility in program design to allow states to tailor services to its population. However, it is not a perfect program. In some states, Medicaid enrollees experience difficulties finding treating providers because of low-reimbursement rates. The entitlement nature of the program protects enrollees—but creates challenges to states, particularly during economic downturns. And depending on the leadership at the state and national level, the program acts as a "hot-button" issue for politicians who want to rein in government spending. Nonetheless, studies have shown that the program provides needed health insurance to millions of low-income individuals who could not otherwise afford insurance. The program has been shown to improve access, reduce out-of-pocket spending, and improve health outcomes. And it is a valuable funding source to health care providers, who would otherwise be faced with much larger uncompensated care burdens if the program ceased to exist.

References

1. Total Monthly Medicaid/CHIP Enrollment and Pre-ACA Enrollment. State health facts. Kaiser Family Foundation. 2021. https://www.kff.org/health-reform/state-indicator/total-monthly-medicaid-and-chip-enrollment/?currentTimeframe=0&sortModel=%7B%22colId%22:%22Location%22,%22sort%22:%22asc%22%7D. Accessed 9 Aug 2021.
2. MACStats: Medicaid and CHIP data book. Exhibits 12, 16, 33. 2020. https://www.macpac.gov/wp-content/uploads/2020/12/MACStats-Medicaid-and-CHIP-Data-Book-December-2020.pdf.
3. Health insurance coverage of the nonelderly (0–64) with incomes below 100% Federal Poverty Level (FPL). Timeframe: 2019. State health facts. Kaiser Family Foundation. https://www.kff.org/other/state-indicator/nonelderly-up-to-100-fpl/?currentTimeframe=0&sortModel=%7B%22colId%22:%22Location%22,%22sort%22:%22asc%22%7D. Accessed 9 Aug 2021.

4. Health insurance coverage of the nonelderly (0–64) with incomes below 200% Federal Poverty Level (FPL). Timeframe: 2019. State health facts. Kaiser Family Foundation. https://www.kff.org/other/state-indicator/nonelderly-up-to-200-fpl/?currentTimeframe=0&sortModel=%7B%22colId%22:%22Location%22,%22sort%22:%22asc%22%7D. Accessed 9 Aug 2021.
5. Rudowitz R, Garfield R, Hinton E. 10 things to know about Medicaid: setting the facts straight. Kaiser Family Foundation. Issue Brief. 2019. https://files.kff.org/attachment/Issue-Brief-10-Things-to-Know-about-Medicaid-Setting-the-Facts-Straight.
6. Federal Legislative Milestones in Medicaid and CHIP. Medicaid and CHIP Payment and Access Commission. https://www.macpac.gov/reference-materials/federal-legislative-milestones-in-medicaid-and-chip/. Website accessed 24 Aug 2021.
7. Altman D, Frist W. Medicare and Medicaid at 50 years: perspectives of beneficiaries, health care professionals and institutions, and policy makers. JAMA. 2015;314(4):384–95. file:///C:/Users/psilberm/AppData/Local/Temp/jsc150005.pdf.
8. Paradise J, Lyons B, Rowland D. Medicaid at 50. Kaiser Family Foundation. 2015. https://files.kff.org/attachment/report-medicaid-at-50.
9. Patient protection and affordable care act. Pub Law 111–148 (March 23, 2010), 124 Stat. 119.
10. National Federation of Independent Business v. Sebelius, 567 US 519 (2012).
11. Medicaid Eligibility through the Medically Needy Pathway. 2018. State health facts. Kaiser Family Foundation. https://www.kff.org/other/state-indicator/medicaid-eligibility-through-the-medically-needy-pathway/?currentTimeframe=0&sortModel=%7B%22colId%22:%22Location%22,%22sort%22:%22asc%22%7D. Website accessed 24 Aug 2021.
12. Guttmacher. Medicaid family planning eligibility expansions. As of November 1, 2021. https://www.guttmacher.org/state-policy/explore/medicaid-family-planning-eligibility-expansions. Accessed 15 Nov 2021.
13. Behavioral health services covered under state plan authority. Medicaid and CHIP Payment and Access Commission. https://www.macpac.gov/subtopic/behavioral-health-services-covered-under-state-plan-authority/. Accessed 9 Aug 2021.
14. Behavioral Health Services. Medicaid.gov. Centers for Medicare and Medicaid Services. https://www.medicaid.gov/medicaid/benefits/behavioral-health-services/index.html. Accessed 10 Aug 2021.
15. Federal requirements and state options: premiums and cost sharing. Medicaid and CHIP Payment and Access Commission. 2017. Fact sheet. https://www.macpac.gov/wp-content/uploads/2017/11/Federal-Requirements-and-State-Options-Premiums-and-Cost-Sharing.pdf. 42 CFR §§447.52-447.56.
16. CHIP cost sharing. Medicaid.gov. https://www.medicaid.gov/chip/chip-cost-sharing/index.html. Website accessed 10 Aug 2021.
17. Guth M, Ammula M. Building on the evidence base: studies on the effects of Medicaid expansion, February 2020 to March 2021. Kaiser Family Foundation. 2021. https://files.kff.org/attachment/Report-Building-on-the-Evidence-Base-Studies-on-the-Effects-of-Medicaid-Expansion.pdf.
18. Guth M, Garfield R, Rudowitz R. The effects of Medicaid expansion under the ACA: studies from January 2014 to January 2020. Kaiser Family Foundation. 2020. https://www.kff.org/report-section/the-effects-of-medicaid-expansion-under-the-aca-updated-findings-from-a-literature-review-report/.
19. Rudowitz R. What you need to know about the Medicaid fiscal accountability rule. Kaiser Family Foundation. 2020. https://files.kff.org/attachment/Issue-Brief-What-You-Need-to-Know-About-the-Medicaid-Fiscal-Accountability-Rule.
20. Medicaid hospital payment: a comparison across states and to Medicare. Medicaid and CHIP Payment and Access Commission. Issue Brief. 2017. https://www.macpac.gov/wp-content/uploads/2017/04/Medicaid-Hospital-Payment-A-Comparison-across-States-and-to-Medicare.pdf.
21. Zuckerman S, Skopec L, Aarons J. Medicaid physician fees remained substantially below fees paid by Medicare in 2019. Health Aff. 2021;40(2):343–8. https://www.healthaffairs.org/doi/pdf/10.1377/hlthaff.2020.00611.
22. Holgash K, Heberlein M. Physician acceptance of new Medicaid patients. Medicaid and CHIP Payment and Access Commission. 2019. http://www.macpac.gov/wp-content/uploads/2019/01/Physician-Acceptance-of-New-Medicaid-Patients.pdf. Website accessed 14 Sept 2021.
23. Paradise J. Data note: three findings about access to care and health outcomes in Medicaid. Kaiser Family Foundation. 2017. https://www.kff.org/medicaid/issue-brief/data-note-three-findings-about-access-to-care-and-health-outcomes-in-medicaid/.
24. Medicaid Payment Policy for Federally Qualified Health Centers. Medicaid and Chip Payment and Access Commission. Issue Brief. 2017. https://www.macpac.gov/wp-content/uploads/2017/12/Medicaid-Payment-Policy-for-Federally-Qualified-Health-Centers.pdf.
25. Rural Health Clinics (RHCs). Rural health information hub. https://www.ruralhealthinfo.org/topics/rural-health-clinics#medicaid. Website accessed 23 Aug 2021.
26. Disproportionate share hospital payments. Medicaid and Chip Payment and Access Commission. https://www.macpac.gov/subtopic/disproportionate-share-hospital-payments/. Website accessed 23 Aug 2021.
27. Share of Medicaid population covered under different delivery systems. As of July 1, 2019. State health facts. Kaiser Family Foundation. https://www.kff.org/medicaid/state-indicator/share-of-medicaid-population-covered-under-different-delivery-systems/?currentTimeframe=0&sortModel=%7B%22colId%22:%22Location%22,%22sort%22:%22asc%22%7D. Website accessed 10 Aug 2021.
28. Medicaid accountable care organizations: state Update. Center for Health Care Strategies. 2018. https://www.chcs.org/media/ACO-Fact-Sheet-02-27-2018-1.pdf.
29. Federal Financial Participation in State Assistance Expenditures; Federal Matching Shares for Medicaid, the Children's Health Insurance Program, and Aid to Needy Aged, Blind, or Disabled Persons for October 1, 2021 through September 30, 2022. 85 Fed. Reg. 76586-76589 (November 30, 2020). https://www.govinfo.gov/content/pkg/FR-2020-11-30/pdf/2020-26387.pdf.
30. Federal Match Rates for Medicaid Administrative Activities. Medicaid and Chip Payment and Access Commission. https://www.macpac.gov/federal-match-rates-for-medicaid-administrative-activities/. Website accessed 11 Aug 2021.
31. Medicaid spending per full-benefit enrollees: FY 2014. State health facts. https://www.kff.org/medicaid/state-indicator/medicaid-spending-per-full-benefit-enrollee/?currentTimeframe=0&sortModel=%7B%22colId%22:%22All%20Full-Benefit%20Enrollees%22,%22sort%22:%22desc%22%7D. Website accessed 11 Aug 2021.
32. MACStats: Medicaid and CHIP Chart Book. Medicaid and CHIP Payment and Access Commission. 2020. Exhibit 22. https://www.macpac.gov/wp-content/uploads/2020/12/MACStats-Medicaid-and-CHIP-Data-Book-December-2020.pdf.
33. Rudowitz R, Williams E, Hinton E, Garfield R. Medicaid financing: the basics. Kaiser Family Foundation. 2021. https://www.kff.org/medicaid/issue-brief/medicaid-financing-the-basics/.
34. Wiender J, Romaire M, Thach N, Collins A, Kim K, Pan H, Chiri G, Sommers A, Haber S, Musumeci MB, Paradise J. Strategies to reduce Medicaid spending: findings from a literature review. Kaiser Family Foundation. 2017. https://

www.kff.org/medicaid/issue-brief/strategies-to-reduce-medicaid-spending-findings-from-a-literature-review/view/print/.
35. Garfield R, Dolan R, Williams E. Costs and savings under federal policy approaches to address Medicaid prescription drug spending. Kaiser Family Foundation. 2021. https://www.kff.org/medicaid/issue-brief/costs-and-savings-under-federal-policy-approaches-to-address-medicaid-prescription-drug-spending/.
36. Dolan R. Understanding the Medicaid prescription drug rebate program. Kff.org. 2019. https://www.kff.org/medicaid/issue-brief/understanding-the-medicaid-prescription-drug-rebate-program/. Accessed 27 Sept 2021.
37. Institute for Health Policy. The Medicaid drug rebate program and the impact of "best Price" rule. Kaiser Permanente; 2020. https://www.kpihp.org/wp-content/uploads/2020/10/Best_Price_101.pdf.
38. Dolan R, Tian M. Pricing and payment for Medicaid prescription drugs. Kaiser Family Foundation. 2020. https://www.kff.org/medicaid/issue-brief/pricing-and-payment-for-medicaid-prescription-drugs/.
39. State Health Facts. Medicaid provider taxes or fees. Kaiser Family Foundation. https://www.kff.org/state-category/medicaid-chip/medicaid-policy-action-trends/medicaid-provider-taxes-or-fees/. Website accessed 9 Sept 2021.
40. Waivers. Medicaid and CHIP Payment and Access Commission. https://www.macpac.gov/medicaid-101/waivers/. Website accessed 12 Aug 2021.
41. Total number of Medicaid section 1915(c) home and community-based services waivers: 2018. State health facts. Kaiser Family Foundation. https://www.kff.org/health-reform/state-indicator/total-number-of-medicaid-section-1915c-home-and-community-based-services-waivers/?currentTimeframe=0&sortModel=%7B%22colId%22:%22Location%22,%22sort%22:%22asc%22%7D. Website accessed 12 Aug 2021.
42. Musumeci MB, O'Malley Watts M, Chidambaram P. Key state policy choices about medicaid home and community-based services. Appendix Table 9: Medicaid HCBS waiver waiting list enrollment, by target population and state, FY 2018. Kaiser Family Foundation. 2020. https://www.kff.org/report-section/key-state-policy-choices-about-medicaid-home-and-community-based-services-appendix-tables/.
43. Medicaid waiver tracker: approved and pending section 1115 waivers by state. Kaiser Family Foundation. 2021. https://www.kff.org/medicaid/issue-brief/medicaid-waiver-tracker-approved-and-pending-section-1115-waivers-by-state/#Map1. Website accessed 19 Aug 2021.
44. MACStats: Medicaid and CHIP chart book. Medicaid and CHIP Payment and Access Commission. 2020. Exhibits 39, 43. https://www.macpac.gov/wp-content/uploads/2020/12/MACStats-Medicaid-and-CHIP-Data-Book-December-2020.pdf.
45. Musumeci MB, O'Malley Watts M, Chidambaram P. Key state policy choices about Medicaid home and community-based services. Kaiser Family Foundation. 2020. https://www.kff.org/report-section/key-state-policy-choices-about-medicaid-home-and-community-based-services-issue-brief/.
46. U.S. Centers for Medicare & Medicaid Services. Home- and community-based services. CMS.gov. 2020. https://www.cms.gov/Outreach-and-Education/American-Indian-Alaska-Native/AIAN/LTSS-TA-Center/info/hcbs. Accessed 13 Oct 2021.
47. Malley Watts M, Musumeci M, Chidambaram P. Medicaid home and community-based services enrollment and spending. 2020. https://files.kff.org/attachment/Issue-Brief-Medicaid-Home-and-Community-Based-Services-Enrollment-and-Spending.
48. Health Homes. Medicaid.gov. https://www.medicaid.gov/medicaid/long-term-services-supports/health-homes/index.html. Website accessed 14 Sept 2021.
49. Approved Medicaid health home state plan amendments. 2021. https://www.medicaid.gov/state-resource-center/medicaid-state-technical-assistance/health-home-information-resource-center/downloads/hh-map.pdf. Website accessed 14 Sept 2021.
50. Cole M, Nguyen K. Unmet social needs among low-income adults in the United States: associations with health care access and quality. Health Serv Res. 2020;55(Suppl. 2):873–82. https://onlinelibrary.wiley.com/doi/epdf/10.1111/1475-6773.13555.
51. Hinton E, Stolyar L. Medicaid Authorities and Options to Address Social Determinants of Health (SDOH). Kaiser Family Foundation. 2021. Issue Brief. https://www.kff.org/medicaid/issue-brief/medicaid-authorities-and-options-to-address-social-determinants-of-health-sdoh/.
52. Wortman Z, Tilson EC, Cohen MK. Buying health for north Carolinians: addressing nonmedical drivers of health at scale. Health Aff. 2020;39(4):649–54. https://www.healthaffairs.org/doi/pdf/10.1377/hlthaff.2019.01583.

Value-Based Care

Mark Gwynne

Introduction

Value-based care and associated value-based payment models are part of the health care landscape in the United States (US) and are defined by clinical quality outcomes and the costs of care across defined populations. The patient experience of care and the provider experience are other value components in what has been termed the "Quadruple Aim" [1]. High value care can be characterized by high quality outcomes and low total cost costs of care for a population; low value care denotes poor quality and high cost. Payment models have been developed to incentivize providers and provider organizations to align with high value care. This chapter provides an overview to value-based care. The first section reviews the historical developments that contributed to value-based care becoming a central feature of US health care. The subsequent section outlines several organizational programs and payment models, such as accountable care organizations, that are associated with value-based care. The chapter closes with future directions in this area.

Historical Developments

The movement to align payment models with high value care began in the early 2000s as health care costs in the United States dramatically escalated and reached unsustainable levels. The largest burden to both cost and quality outcomes has been attributed to chronic disease, since six in ten Americans report a chronic disease, and four in ten have multimorbidity [2]. The cost of managing chronic disease accounts for 85% of total health care spending and has increased by $7–9 billion annually over the past decade, reaching $4.1 trillion in 2020 [3]. Health care accounts for 19.7% of the US GDP in 2020 and a per capita cost of $12,530, which is 38% more than the next highest cost industrialized nation, Switzerland, whose per capita cost is $7138 [4, 5]. Unfortunately, this spending has not resulted in the most effective, safe, and high quality healthcare. The US ranks last of 11 economically developed countries across 71 measures and 5 key domains of healthcare access, care processes, administrative efficiency, equity, and health care outcomes [4, 5].

Between 1996 and 2013, healthcare costs increased by almost $1 trillion and these costs disproportionately increased more than the utilization of healthcare services [6]. For example, the relative costs due to ambulatory service utilization increased, while those for inpatient utilization have decreased. Costs that are attributable to population growth, aging, and greater disease prevalence have also increased, however more than half of the increased cost was due to price and service intensity. In other words, each episode of care has resulted in more services, and the unit cost of those services has been higher. These trends have led to discussion about the appropriate utilization of healthcare services, including overutilization and underutilization, as well as reducing unwarranted variation in care, which may account for $20 M–$30 M (per $1 B in revenue) in unnecessary costs for a typical healthcare organization [7–9].

The increasing financial burden of healthcare is increasingly being passed on to patients and families. Even among employed Americans who receive employer-based healthcare benefits, rising costs are unsustainable. For example, the Affordability Index, a measure that captures the healthcare cost burden for employed Americans has shown a dramatic increase in the proportion of wages spent on healthcare, reaching more than 30% by 2016 [11]. Many Americans are increasingly worried about accessing affordable healthcare and paying for key healthcare services. In 2021, 37 million Americans reported more difficulty paying for healthcare services, while 20% of households reported delaying care due to cost, even among higher income households [12].

The Institute of Medicine's (IOM) 2001 release of *Crossing the Quality Chasm* called for healthcare reform that would create a more accessible, equitable, and high quality

M. Gwynne (✉)
Department of Family Medicine and UNC Health Alliance,
University of North Carolina at Chapel Hill, Chapel Hill, NC, USA
e-mail: Mark.Gwynne@unchealth.unc.edu

system of care [13]. This seminal publication articulated a framework to overhaul the US healthcare system and create a safe, effective, patient-centered, timely, efficient, and equitable system that would address quality shortcomings and inequitable access to care, especially for those without health insurance. Strategies focused on clinical quality and safety, including investment in broad based quality improvement infrastructure across health care systems. Several years later, federal legislation, such as the Health Information Technology for Economic and Clinical Health Act (HITECH), focused on the prioritization of electronic and digital data and information infrastructure that would be necessary to support high quality care, an important structural component to redesigning care and managing populations [14].

Although the IOM report called for aligning payment policies to catalyze quality improvement, it would take nearly a decade before the passage of The Patient Protection and Affordable Care Act of 2008 (ACA), which outlined the transformation of healthcare financing from fee for volume, to fee for value and outcomes [15]. The ACA was a catalyst in transformation that focused on three domains: (1) testing new models of health care delivery; (2) shifting from a reimbursement system based on the volume of services provided to one based on the value of care and, (3) investing in resources for system-wide improvement.

Payment model reform was at the center of the ACA by providing a foundation to shift from fee for service (FFS), or payment to providers based on the type and quantity of services provided, to a payment system that incentivized value outcomes, such a high quality care. Paying for the volume of services offered, which is the foundation of FFS, is commonly thought to be a key driver in escalating healthcare costs. ACA legislation also funded the Center for Medicare and Medicaid Innovation (CMMI), as a catalyst to develop, implement, and test new innovative payment and delivery models that would promote value-based care. Payment models from CMMI were developed to address hospital care, primary care, networks of providers as well as specific specialties.

The Patient Centered Medical Home (PCMH) model provided a framework to redesign processes within primary care with a focus on the personal physician, who coordinates whole person care and enhanced access [16]. The Centers for Medicare and Medicaid Services (CMS) as well as several commercial insurers provided supplemental payment models for practices and systems that promoted adoption of PCMH changes, including enhanced fee for service rates and per member per month (PMPM) supplemental payments [17, 18]. Concurrently, CMS provided financial incentives or penalties to hospitals based on how well or poorly patients transitioned between care settings, such as from hospital discharge to home and how often they were readmitted to a hospital within the next 30 days. These programs re-aligned financial incentives with efforts to redesign care with measurable outcomes of improved clinical quality and reduced costs.

Programs and Payment Models

Hospital Quality and Value Programs

CMS recognized that a significant proportion of the cost of care occurs in acute care settings, such as hospitals, and promoted financial incentive and penalty models addressing hospital care. The Hospital Readmission Reduction Program (HRRP) penalizes hospitals with the highest rates of 30-day unplanned hospital readmissions for six key clinical conditions [19]. To adapt, many hospitals and health care systems redesigned care at the time of hospital discharge to reduce adverse events and prevent readmissions. Through this work, transitional care emerged, such as Coleman's Care Transitions Program and Project RED [20, 21]. Common elements among these programs included targeted medication management, ensuring adequate hospital follow-up with the appropriate provider, proactively managing condition specific symptoms after discharge, and coordinating care and information exchange through electronic health records. The overall impact of these approaches on overall hospital readmissions has been mixed, however the focus on patient transitions resulted in many health care systems linking acute and ambulatory care more closely.

The Hospital-Acquired Conditions Reduction Program (HACRP) implemented financial penalties for preventable events during hospitalizations, such as catheter acquired urinary tract infections among others. CMS also implemented the Hospital Value-Based Purchasing Program (HVBPP) which adjusts hospital payments based on specific clinical outcomes, patient and community engagement, safety, efficiency, and cost reduction measures. These payment models, based on penalties and changes to FFS have not had appreciable effects on quality outcomes and mortality [22–24]. However, focusing on measurable quality outcomes encouraged many hospitals and health systems to create the data infrastructure to actively measure and implement care redesign initiatives intended to improve quality outcomes.

Alternative Payment Models (APM's)

CMMI launched the Health Care Payment Learning & Action Network (HCP-LAN) in 2015 to provide foundational elements of alternative payment models, and to align payment models across the public and private sectors that would catalyze the transition from volume to value. Through this work, HCP-LAN created a new Alternate Payment Model (APM) Framework (Fig. 45.1) that described a pro-

Category 1
FEE FOR SERVICE – NO LINK TO QUALITY & VALUE

Category 2
FEE FOR SERVICE – LINK TO QUALITY & VALUE

A Foundational Payments for Infrastructure & Operations (e.g., care coordination fees and payments for HIT investments)

B Pay for Reporting (e.g., bonuses for reporting data or penalties for not reporting data)

C Pay-for-Performance (e.g., bonuses for quality performance)

Category 3
APMS BUILT ON FEE-FOR-SERVICE ARCHITECTURE

A APMs with Shared Savings (e.g., shared savings with upside risk only)

B APMs with Shared Savings and Downside Risk (e.g., episode-based payments for procedures and comprehensive payments with upside and downside risk)

3N Risk Based Payments NOT Linked to Quality

Category 4
POPULATION – BASED PAYMENT

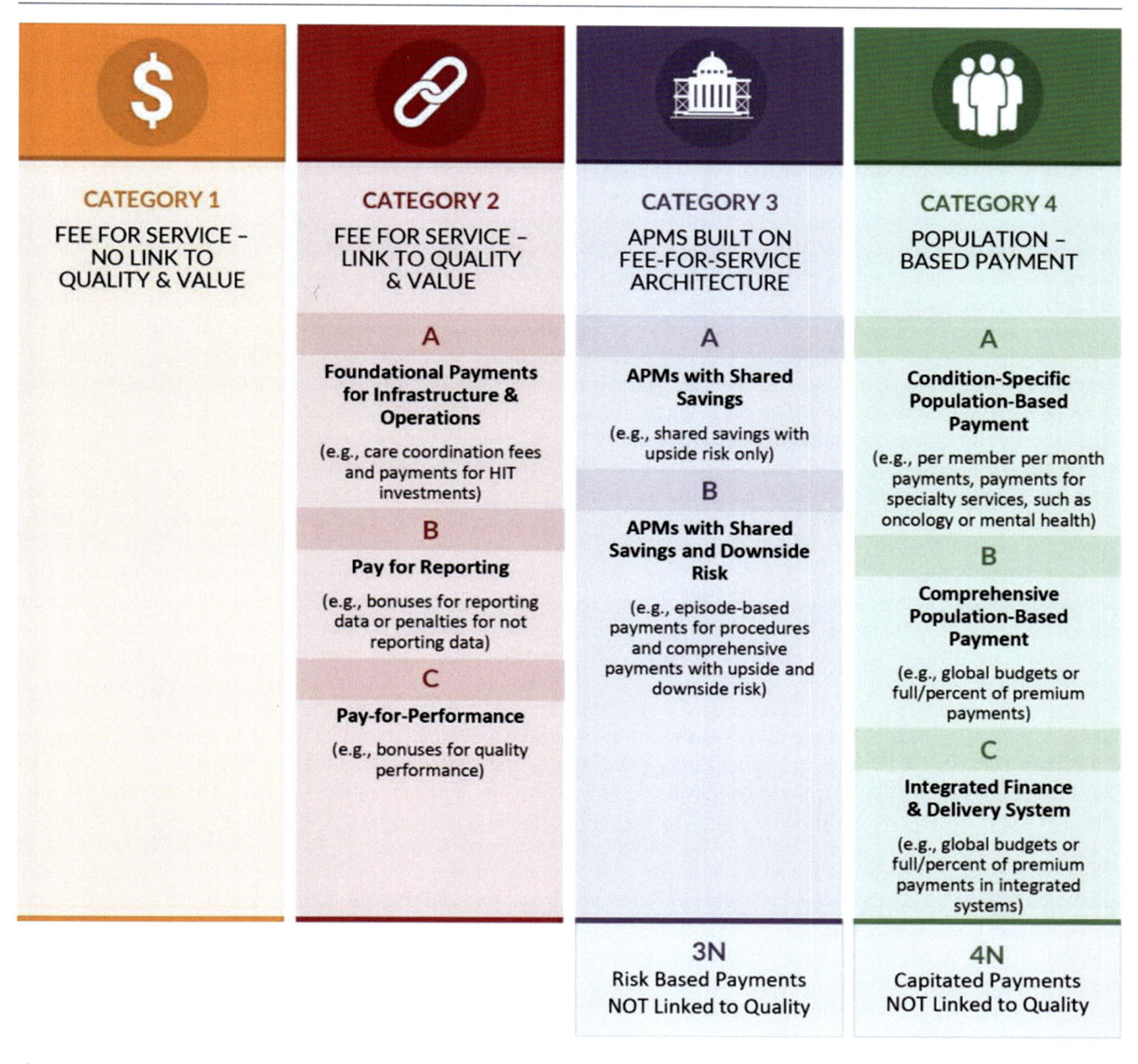

A Condition-Specific Population-Based Payment (e.g., per member per month payments, payments for specialty services, such as oncology or mental health)

B Comprehensive Population-Based Payment (e.g., global budgets or full/percent of premium payments)

C Integrated Finance & Delivery System (e.g., global budgets or full/percent of premium payments in integrated systems)

4N Capitated Payments NOT Linked to Quality

Fig. 45.1 HCP-LAN Alternative Payment Model (APM) Framework (from reference [25])

gression of alternative payment models with each category moving further away from fee for service alone (category 1), and closer to population-based payment models (category 4) [25]. Category 1, or fee for service, reimburses providers for the quantity of services provided, regardless of quality. This model incents volume of services instead of value, and has been considered one of the key drivers of the escalating costs of healthcare in the US. Models in category 2 retain fee for service however introduce positive financial rewards for achieving defined clinical quality outcomes. These quality targets are often tied to preventative services, such as cancer screenings, or clinical outcomes for chronic disease, such as glycemic (e.g., HbA1c) control in patients with diabetes mellitus. These models are often referred to as Pay for Performance (P4P) and incent providers to measure and improve performance in managing chronic disease.

Category 3 models have roots in the FFS architecture but begin to introduce total cost of care financial benchmarks. Providers can be rewarded if they provide care at a cost better than benchmark, and they may incur financial risk for performance worse than the total cost of care (TCOC) benchmark. Category 4, or population-based payments, move away from FFS and pay providers proactively for the expected cost of providing care for a defined population.

Providers are at full financial risk if they provide care for more than the proactive payments. Some Category 4 models are referred to as capitation, or capitated payment models, while others are referred to as bundled payment models, or episodic payment models.

Category 4 introduces the most financial risk but also provides the most flexibility for providers and systems to redesign care that can achieve high quality outcomes while reducing unnecessary utilization of care, reducing unwarranted variations in care, and ultimately reducing the total cost of care. Category 3 and 4 models are considered Advanced Alternative Payment Models (Fig. 45.1). An important provision within the Medicare Access and CHIP Reauthorization Act (MACRA) of 2015 incented providers to adopt advanced APM's by providing a 5% bonus on all Medicare part B reimbursement through 2025 [26]. APM's have four core components, which can vary depending on the model: patient attribution, clinical quality model, total cost of care benchmarking, and the financial model.

Patient Attribution

The population being managed must be clearly defined in order to estimate an expected cost of health care services. Patients are typically attributed, or linked, to providers who participate in the Accountable Care Organization (ACO) or Clinically Integrated Network (CIN) through which the APM is managed [27]. The Federal Trade Commission (FTC) has defined a CIN as a "structured collaboration between physicians and hospitals to develop clinical initiatives designed to improve the quality and efficiency of healthcare services" [34]. CIN's differ from ACO's in that CIN's can incorporate several ACO's and ACO contracts and are focused on integrating care across different providers and care settings.

Most APM's are designed for primary care, however several models attribute patients to medical specialists such as oncology, cardiology, nephrology, or through procedural specialists such as orthopedic surgeons. Understanding how patients are attributed to APM's allows ACO's to gather data, engage providers, and develop initiatives that coordinate care directly for patients with greater health care needs. Patients are attributed to an ACO prospectively, before the performance year starts, or retrospectively, at the end of a performance year. More advanced APM's utilize prospective patient attribution so that ACO's can understand their population and coordinate care early in a performance year.

Quality Model

Each APM incorporates a set of quality measures that are relevant to the population served. It is important to balance any cost reduction strategy with relevant quality outcomes to promote high quality care. Quality measures are often subsets of larger national measure sets and performance standards which account for clinical quality, health service utilization, and patient experience. Examples include measures developed by the National Committee for Quality Assurance (NCQA) or American Heart Association (AHA) for clinical quality, National Quality Forum (NQF) for utilization, and the Consumer Assessment of Healthcare Providers and Systems (CAHPS) for patient experience [28–30]. To ensure the balance of cost and quality, APM's often structure models so that performance in the quality measure sets adjusts financial performance proportionally. Higher quality can allow maximum financial incentive while lower quality can reduce financial incentives.

Total Cost of Care Benchmarking

To manage the cost of care for a population, it is important to understand the expected cost of care for that population. The total cost of care benchmark is the expected cost a population would incur given the population demographics, disease burden, and other factors. The four key components in building a valid benchmark are the historic cost for the defined population, the expected medical cost trend over the performance year, an applied risk adjustment to account for the medical and psychosocial complexity of the population, and a regional adjustment to account for the marked regional variations in health services utilization and cost across the US [31]. The relative risk of a Medicare population is captured using CMS's Hierarchical Condition Categories—Risk Adjustment Factor (HCC-RAF), which assigns a numerical value to clinical conditions, or combinations of conditions, to account for the risk of those conditions to an individual, and the likely cost of managing those conditions [32]. For example, a patient with Diabetes Mellitus (DM) as well as Congestive Heart Failure (CHF) and End Stage Renal Disease (ESRD) would have a higher HCC-RAF score than a patient with Diabetes alone.

Financial Model

Each APM includes a framework for providers to share in either the benefits of decreasing total costs of care (i.e., shared savings or gainshare), or the risks of exceeding total cost of care benchmarks (i.e., shared risk). Models are structured as 'upside only' if there are only positive financial incentives, or shared savings. Two-sided risk models, which include both upside and downside risk, allow for both gainshare as well as payment from providers back to payers, including CMS, if the cost of care exceeds the total cost benchmark. Many APM's provide a pathway to downside risk, usually with one or more years

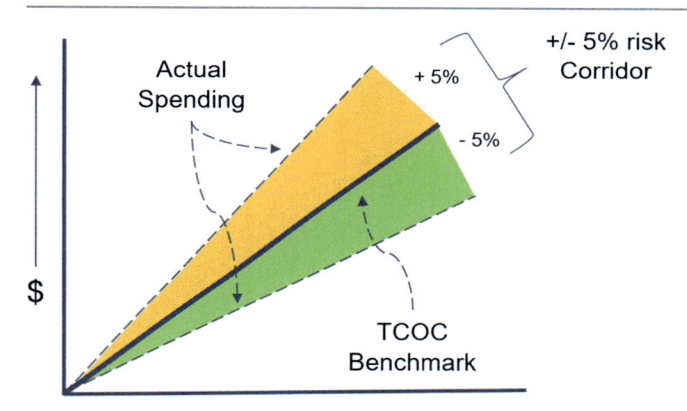

Fig. 45.2 Illustrative example of APM Total Cost of Care Benchmark and risk corridors. Subsequent Shared savings and Shared Losses can be any proportion of performance above or below TCOC benchmark

of upside gainshare only, followed by two-sided risk. CMS has provided pathways for providers to increasingly take on downside risk, as their capabilities for managing populations expands. In most APM's providers can choose "risk corridors," or percentages of upside and downside risk that they are comfortable managing (Fig. 45.2). Each model also offers sharing rates of both gainshare and risk, for example 50/50 sharing of any savings better than TCOC benchmark, or 75/25 sharing of any risk payments for financial performance worse than TCOC benchmark.

Accountable Care Organizations (ACOs)

The ACA outlined several paths to redesign care across providers and communities. One model, the Accountable Care Organization (ACO), is defined as a legal entity through which groups of doctors, hospitals, and other healthcare providers can voluntarily assume responsibility for a defined population and provide coordinated, high quality and low-cost care to patients. ACO's can then contract together for Alternative Payment Models (APM's) [33]. ACO's are based on the concept that coordinating care for patients, especially those with chronic illness and psychosocial complexity, will lead to better outcomes at less overall cost. When an ACO succeeds both in delivering high quality care and in spending health care dollars more efficiently, the ACO shares in the savings generated with the payer.

ACOs must meet regulatory requirements, including having the legal authority and administrative organization to contract with payers, being governed by the participating providers, being responsible for the care of a defined population, and demonstrating that they can effectively measure the quality and efficiency of care delivery while aligning payment with the quality and efficiency of care delivered [34]. Structurally, ACO's must have the administrative capabilities to manage APM's, a network of providers, and a data infrastructure to identify and support patients at risk. These requirements often result in developing core ACO services such as advanced analytics and reporting, patient risk stratification, population segmentation, electronic health record solutions, quality improvement initiatives, and a clinical care model tailored to meet the needs of the population. Population health services often include care management capabilities, targeted interventions around chronic disease management and, increasingly, home based care and community engagement initiatives.

ACO's develop these capabilities internally or may partner with Clinically Integrated Networks and Population Health Service Organizations (PHSO) to leverage resources and capacity. PHSO's are emerging within the healthcare landscape as companies that provide core population management capabilities, such as care management, data and analytics and patient outreach services, to health systems or practice networks to facilitate their entry into value-based care and contracting. The ACO model has been broadly adopted and in 2021, there were almost 1200 ACO's nationally with contracts covering over 36 million lives. Participation plateaued between 2018–2021, a trend likely due to a CMS policy change in 2018 requiring ACO's to have a clear path for taking on downside financial risk (Fig. 45.3) [35]. The COVID-19 pandemic also created significant financial instability within provider networks at the same time, which impacted providers and health systems willingness to take on downside financial risk.

ACO's often organize around specific payment models that are targeted to specific populations, such as primary care, however many have evolved to manage multiple APM's across populations and specialties. CMS has advanced a series of Primary Care APM's since 2010 (Fig. 45.4) [10]. The largest model, the Medicare Shared Savings Program (MSSP), included 447 ACO's in 2021, covering 10.7 million Medicare patients. Participation in this program, rebranded as Pathways to Success, peaked in 2018 with 561 participating ACO's. Other models, such as Comprehensive Primary Care (CPC), and the Next Generation ACO (NextGen) catalyzed the ACO to the center of the value-based care transformation. CPC included over 500 practices and resulted in improved care management for high-risk patients, enhanced access, improved coordination of care transitions, and associated decreased emergency department utilization, although limited reduction in Medicare spending [36, 37]. The NextGen model, with 41 participating ACO's, markedly reduced Medicare spending, including reduced costs within post-acute providers and increased routine care for patients [38].

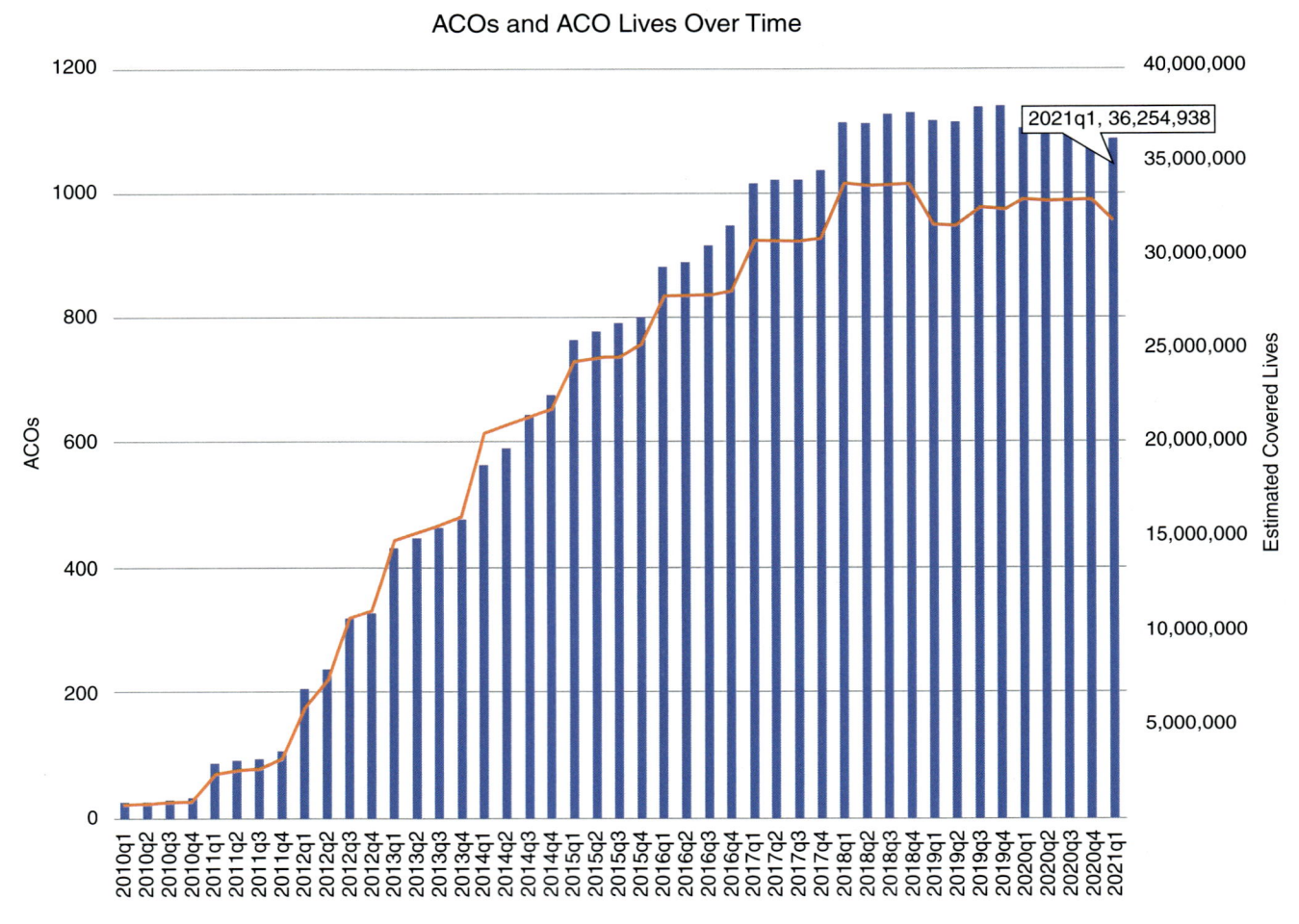

Fig. 45.3 Number of ACOs and ACO-covered lives 2010 to Q1 2021 (from reference [35])

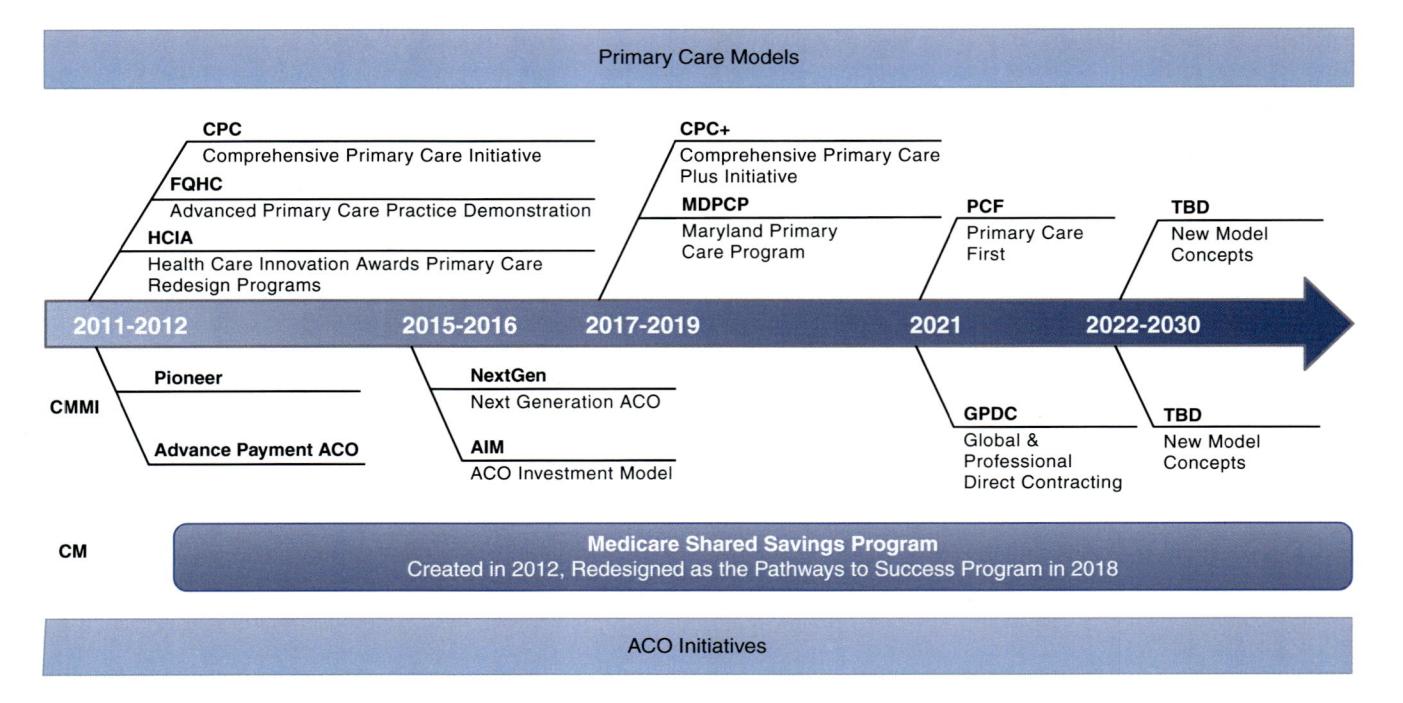

Fig. 45.4 CMS and CMMI Primary Care Alternative Payment Model 2012–2022 (from reference [10])

Table 45.1 CMS sponsored bundle payment models

Model name	Model dates	# Participants	Bundled payment structure	Types of bundles
BPCI 1	4/2013–12/2016	24 hospitals	Retrospective acute care hospital stay only	Inpatient conditions and procedures
BPCI 2	10/2013–9/2018	422 hospitals 277 physician groups	Retrospective acute care hospital stay and 30, 60, or 90 days post-acute	48 inpatient and chronic disease
BPCI 3	10/2013–9/2018	873 SNF's 116 HH agencies 9 inpatient rehab facilities 1 long term care facility 144 provider groups	Retrospective acute care hospital stay and 30, 60, or 90 days post-acute	48 inpatient and chronic disease
BPCI 4	10/2013–9/2018	23 hospitals	Prospective acute inpatient and all readmission related services through 30 days post-discharge	48 inpatient and chronic disease
CJR	4/2016–12/2021	800 hospitals in year 1–2 465 hospitals in Year3–5	Retrospective inpatient stay and up to 90 days post-acute	Lower joint replacement
OCM	7/2016–6/2021	175 providers	Monthly enhanced payments plus retrospective 6 month episode starting with chemotherapy	Chemotherapy for cancer
BPCI advanced	10/2018–12/2023	1299 groups	Retrospective inpatient, post-acute and ambulatory with 90 day duration	29 inpatient 3 outpatient
CEC/ESCO	10/2015–3/2021	37 dialysis organizations	Retrospective, yearly part A and part B related to dialysis and ESRD costs	ESRD and dialysis
KCF	1/2022	85 participants		CKD stages 4–5 and ESRD

Episode-Based Payment Models

Since 2013, CMS and CMMI have developed a series of specialty, procedure, and condition specific alternative payment models, often referred to as episode-based, or bundled payment models [39] (Table 45.1). Conditions and procedures were chosen based on their overall contribution to the cost and quality of care for Medicare beneficiaries, such as musculoskeletal care and orthopedic surgery, advanced kidney disease, cancer, as well as longitudinal chronic disease like congestive heart failure. Financially, these models continue to pay fees for services (FFS) delivered within the defined episode. The total cost of care for both inpatient and outpatient services bundled within the defined episode are then retrospectively compared to previously calculated benchmark cost targets. If costs are less than projected, providers receive a share of those savings, and if costs are higher, providers pay back the difference to CMS if the model has shared risk.

Like other APM's, performance is also assessed based on quality outcomes, which are often specialty or condition specific. CMS and CMMI sponsored episode-based payment models have included Bundled Payments for Care Improvement (BPCI) Models, the Comprehensive Care for Joint Replacement (CJR) Model, the Oncology Care Model (OCM), the BPCI Advanced Model and the Comprehensive ESRD Care Model (CEC, ESCO) [39]. In 2020, CMMI also launched the Kidney Care First model to address cost and quality among patients with advanced kidney disease (Table 45.1). The BPCI programs reduced Medicare per-episode payments, and those programs designed for surgical conditions were more successful than for medical conditions [40]. Evaluation of CMSs episodic payment models over time has shown mixed results, with some studies showing reductions in utilization of services with preserved quality outcomes. However, even though some episodic payment models resulted in decreased utilization and lower costs, they have not demonstrated net savings to Medicare [40].

Current State of Accountable Care

The ACO model has been widely adopted as a mechanism to advance value-based care and a vehicle for healthcare transformation. Between 2012 and 2021, there was a six-fold proliferation of ACO's nationally [35]. Originally, ACOs were based in hospitals, physician practices, or physician networks. However, the rapid evolution of value-based care has attracted new entrants into the market. Private equity backed provider groups such as Landmark Health, ChenMed, and VillageMD are creating value-based provider organizations to contract directly with payers for full risk, or 100%

two-sided risk, to manage complex Medicare patients in specific locations. These new provider organizations have developed comprehensive care models that include care management, behavioral health services, home based care, data systems, and outreach efforts that improve the manner in which care is coordinated for medically and psychosocially complex patients. Other new primary care organizations such as CityBlock Health have adopted similar comprehensive patient care models with targeted focus on high-risk populations such as those enrolling in Medicaid.

Clinically Integrated Networks (CIN's) have also evolved rapidly and grown to have broad regional presence, sometimes spanning several states. Some CIN's, such as Aledade, have acted as conveners of providers, including independent primary care, or nephrologists. CIN's need to build or purchase key capabilities to facilitate integrated care and population health, like advanced analytics and population health services. This has generated a dramatic expansion of companies offering these services, and investment in this market. In 2020, for example, venture capital investment increased 57% from 2019, a previous record year, to almost $17 billion [41]. Much of this investment has focused specifically on Healthcare Information Technology (HIT), a key facilitator of clinical integration.

Organizations with a more specific clinical focus have also emerged and are seeking value contracts directly with payers, or value-based relationships with CIN's. These organizations manage specific, complex, and high-cost populations, such as behavioral health or end stage renal disease (ESRD). Cricket Health, for example, utilizes care managers trained to the specific needs of patients with ESRD, directly engages providers caring for patients with ESRD in hospital transitions, and coordinates specific high-cost aspects of patient care, such as hemodialysis [42]. These providers often offer virtual care or in-home care capabilities.

Since high functioning ACO's and CIN's rely on trained personnel, workflows, and technologies to successfully coordinate care across populations and regions, there has been rapid growth of technologic solutions to help scale effective interventions. Enhancing care in the home, through remote patient monitoring (RPM), for example, has become a mainstay for managing complex patients [43]. These systems monitor vital signs and other biometric data at home and can detect early changes and alert providers to intervene before patients decompensate and require more expensive hospital level care. Chatbot technology is increasingly used to engage patients through their electronic devices to manage chronic disease and transitions of care. Although this technology can scale population health interventions, and is showing promise to improve outcomes, further study is needed [44, 45].

Data systems are also evolving that can analyze inputs from multiple different sources to help identify patients at risk for adverse outcomes. Data needs to be visualized, easily accessible, and facilitate action. Often, data visualization is facilitated through Electronic Health Record (EHR) systems through which providers can identify opportunities to intervene at the point of care as well as across a population. Given the emergence of robust data and analytics, patterns of care may be more easily identified, including variations in how care is delivered, as well as outcomes across and between healthcare systems and across and between providers [8, 9].

Health care settings do not solely account for variations in health service utilization, which points to the influence of how providers make decisions within system workflows [46]. An understanding of these factors has allowed ACO's and CIN's to explore why variations exist, and whether they lead to similar or disparate health outcomes. In response, initiatives have focused on redesigning care using data driven, point of care tools to enhance clinical decisions and improve outcomes [47]. Often, improving clinical outcomes through supporting providers and redesigning care pathways leads to a more efficient and a less costly healthcare system.

Future Directions

The past two decades provided a foundation for transforming the US healthcare system with a focus on value and improving health outcomes. The pace of change will continue to increase. CMS, under the HCP-LAN, has an aspirational goal that 50% of Medicaid and 100% of Medicare payments will be tied to improved outcomes and Value by 2025 [48]. There is also increasing effort to design value-based payment models across payers, including Medicare, Medicaid, Medicare Advantage, and commercial insurers, often called an All-Payer Model [49]. Most physicians and health systems are more engaged and successful in implementing improvement efforts when they apply to all patients in a clinical setting, and not those defined by payor source. For example, the Maryland All-Payer model has successfully reduced overall healthcare spending [50] and there are increasing calls to expand this model more broadly [51].

Large, multistate employers like Walmart and Amazon are increasingly seeking value focused provider partners to improve the health outcomes of their employees, or are developing health care options themselves, such as Amazon Care and Walmart Health. Employers like these are the largest purchasers of health care and are responsible for providing healthcare coverage for their employees, with a vested interest in accessing high quality, cost-effective care. The pace of change is significant and the COVID-19 pandemic highlighted the need to focus on improving outcomes, particularly for vulnerable populations as they typically suffer the most from inequitable access to high quality care [52].

Years of population health interventions have demonstrated that simply offering prevention and chronic disease management is not enough to improve health [53]. Poor health outcomes are more often rooted in the Social Determinants of Health (SDOH), or the socioeconomic barriers to accessing equitable care. The US Department of Health and Human Services define the Social Determinants of Health as "the conditions in the environment where people are born, live, learn, work, play, worship and age that affect a wide range of health, functioning and quality-of-life outcomes and risks." [54].

SDOH can be described within domains of economic stability, education access and quality, health care access and quality, neighborhood and built environment and social and community context. ACO's and Population Health Service Organizations are increasingly identifying these SDOH barriers and implementing solutions, particularly to address lack of transportation, food insecurity, housing insecurity and language barriers [55]. ACO's and health systems are also increasingly seeking partnerships with community organizations focused on addressing the SDOH to effectively engage patients and families who face significant barriers and are at risk for poor outcomes.

CMS and others have proposed frameworks to facilitate partnership between healthcare providers and community-based organizations to collectively address health related social needs of populations. CMS proposed the Accountable Health Communities Model, which supports healthcare providers in screening populations for unmet social needs, referring to community services able to address social needs and helping patients navigate the system to ensure they receive those community-based services [56]. Aligning clinical and community services holds promise in meeting the social needs of populations at risk. For example, The North Carolina Institute of Medicine (NCIOM) has also proposed Accountable Care Communities, partnerships between health care systems and community agencies, similarly positioned to address unmet social needs while reducing overall healthcare spending. The NCIOM report, Partnering to Improve Health: A guide to Starting an Accountable Care Community outlined the core components and partnerships needed within communities to achieve these goals [57].

Health equity is an increasing focus in population health, with long neglected attention given to disparate outcomes by race, ethnicity, sexual orientation, and gender identity. Many ACO's and population health service organizations with developed data systems can identify disparities in outcomes for disease prevention, chronic disease management, and access to services by gender, age, race, home zip code and other demographic characteristics. The root causes of health disparities are structural and complex, and will require innovative partnerships between providers, health systems, community organizations, government agencies, payers, and other healthcare delivery stakeholders. A focus on value-based care may be a vehicle through which health care systems can effectively address health disparities by developing effective interventions to promote equitable access to high quality care.

The movement to value-based care has also ushered in renewed interventions and investment to provide care in patient's homes and communities. These services are beginning to span the spectrum of home based care, from peer support and community health workers to remote patient monitoring, home based primary and palliative care, as well as more advanced service such as Hospital at Home [58]. CMS's Hospital Without Walls waiver enacted in 2020 paved the way for health systems to provide enhanced services in patient homes, including those with higher acuity needs previously cared for in a hospital [59]. Home and community-based services are often a lower cost alternative than bricks and mortar healthcare facilities. The trend toward increasing care in the home is expected to continue, especially with increased investment from commercial payers in home based care providers, such as Humana's acquisition of Kindred at Home and Heal and UnitedHealth Group's purchase of LHC [60].

Enhanced access to care has also expanded digital and virtual care. Although virtual care options existed prior to 2020, the COVID pandemic catalyzed virtual care offerings across geographies and specialties. Medicare recipients increased utilization of telehealth services from 840,000 visits in 2019 to 52.7 million in 2020, a 63-fold increase [61]. Also in 2020, one third of Behavioral Health visits among Medicare beneficiaries were virtual, a marked and rapid increase [61]. This trend is likely to continue, as virtual and digital care has become a mainstay of population health management.

The evolution of alternative payment models has catalyzed significant change in how providers and health systems deliver care. Increased accountability to deliver high quality outcomes at a lower total cost of care shows promise in making healthcare more accessible, affordable, and equitable for all Americans. To sustain progress, however, health systems, insurers, and government agencies will need to continue investment in enhanced care teams to support health care providers, interoperable data systems, solutions to address Social Determinants of Health, and promote home and community-based interventions. Coordinating care across the healthcare continuum for patients with complex illness and significant barriers to care is at the center of value and will require continued innovation and collaboration within the medical community ecosystem.

References

1. Berwick DM, Nolan TW, Whittington J. The triple aim: care, health, and cost. Health Aff (Millwood). 2008;27(3):759–69.
2. https://www.cdc.gov/chronicdisease/index.htm. Accessed January 2022.
3. Hartman M, Martin AB, Washington B, Catlin A, The National Health Expenditure Accounts Team. National health care

spending in 2020: growth driven by federal spending in response to the COVID-19 pandemic. Health Aff (Millwood). 2022;41(1):13–25.
4. Schneider E, Shah A, Doty M, Tikkanen R, Fields K, Williams II R. Mirror, mirror 2021 reflecting poorly: health care in the U.S. compared to other high-income countries. The Commonwealth Fund. 2021. https://www.commonwealthfund.org/sites/default/files/2021-08/Schneider_Mirror_Mirror_2021.pdf.
5. https://data.oecd.org/healthres/health-spending.htm. Accessed February 2022.
6. Dieleman JL, Squires E, Bui AL, et al. Factors associated with increases in US health care spending, 1996-2013. JAMA. 2017;318(17):1668–78.
7. hcita-unwarranted-variations-in-care.pdf (advisory.com). Accessed January 2022.
8. Song Z, Kannan S, Gambrel RJ, et al. Physician practice pattern variations in common clinical scenarios within 5 US metropolitan areas. JAMA Health Forum. 2022;3(1):e214698.
9. Fisher ES, Wennberg DE, Stukel TA, Gottlieb DJ, Lucas FL, Pinder EL. The implications of regional variations in medicare spending. Part 1: the content, quality, and accessibility of care. Ann Intern Med. 2003;138(4):273–87.
10. https://innovation.cms.gov/strategic-direction-whitepaper. Accessed January 2022.
11. Emanuel EJ, Glickman A, Johnson D. Measuring the burden of health care costs on US families: the affordability index. JAMA. 2017;318(19):1863–4.
12. West Health-Gallup 2021 Healthcare in America report. https://s8637.pcdn.co/wp-content/uploads/2021/12/2021-Healthcare-In-America_West-Health-and-Gallup.pdf. Accessed January 2022.
13. Institute of Medicine. Crossing the quality chasm: a new health system for the 21st century. Washington, DC: The National Academies Press; 2001.
14. https://www.hhs.gov/hipaa/for-professionals/special-topics/hitech-act-enforcement-interim-final-rule/index.html. Accessed January 2022.
15. https://www.healthcare.gov/glossary/patient-protection-and-affordable-care-act. Accessed January 2022.
16. Gwynne MD, Daaleman TP. Patient-centered medical home. In: Daaleman T, Helton M, editors. Chronic illness care. Cham: Springer; 2018.
17. https://medicaid.ncdhhs.gov/blog/2022/08/05/enhanced-medical-home-payments-advanced-medical-homes-serving-members-eligible-tailored-care Accessed July 2022.
18. https://www.pcpcc.org/sites/default/files/media/paymentreform-pub.pdf. Accessed July 2022.
19. https://www.cms.gov/Medicare/Medicare-Fee-for-Service-Payment/AcuteInpatientPPS/Readmissions-Reduction-Program. Accessed January 2022.
20. https://caretransitions.org/ Coleman. Accessed January 2022.
21. https://www.bu.edu/fammed/projectred/. Accessed January 2022.
22. Sankaran R, Sukul D, Nuliyalu U, Gulseren B, Engler TA, Arntson E, et al. Changes in hospital safety following penalties in the US hospital acquired condition reduction program: retrospective cohort study. BMJ. 2019;366:l4109.
23. Figueroa JF, Tsugawa Y, Zheng J, Orav EJ, Jha AK. Association between the value-based purchasing pay for performance program and patient mortality in US hospitals; observational study. BMJ. 2016;353:i2214.
24. Papanicolas I, Figueroa JF, Orav EJ, Jha AK. Patient hospital experience improved modestly, but no evidence medicare incentives promoted meaningful gains. Health Aff (Millwood). 2017;36(1):133–40. https://doi.org/10.1377/hlthaff.2016.0808. PMID: 28069856.
25. Alternative payment model APM framework. hcp-lan.org. Accessed January 2022.
26. https://www.cms.gov/Medicare/Quality-Initiatives-Patient-Assessment-Instruments/Value-Based-Programs/MACRA-MIPS-and-APMs/MACRA-MIPS-and-APMs. Accessed January 2022.
27. Lewis VA, McClurg AB, Smith J, Fisher ES, Bynum JP. Attributing patients to accountable care organizations: performance year approach aligns stakeholders' interests. Health Aff (Millwood). 2013;32(3):587–95.
28. https://www.ncqa.org. Accessed July 2022.
29. https://www.qualityforum.org/Home. Accessed July 2022.
30. https://www.ahrq.gov/cahps/index.html. Accessed July 2022.
31. https://www.dartmouthatlas.org. Accessed January 2022.
32. Pope GC, John Kautter MS, Ingber MJ, Freeman S, Sekar R, Cordon Newhart MA. Evaluation of the CMS-HCC risk adjustment model, RTI International CMS contract no. HHSM-500-2005-00029I TO 0006. 2011.
33. https://www.cms.gov/Medicare/Medicare-Fee-for-Service-Payment/ACO.
34. https://www.ftc.gov/terms/clinical-integration. Accessed January 2022.
35. Muhlestein D, Bleser WK, Saunders RS, McClellan MB. All-payer spread of ACOs and value-based payment models in 2021: the crossroads and future of value-based care. Health Affairs Blog; 2021.
36. Peikes D, Dale S, Ghosh A, Taylor EF, Swankoski K, O'Malley AS, Day TJ, Duda N, Singh P, Anglin G, Sessums LL, Brown RS. The comprehensive primary care initiative: effects on spending, quality, patients, and physicians. Health Aff (Millwood). 2018;37(6):890–9.
37. Smith B, Phil M. CMS innovation center at 10 years—Progress and lessons learned. N Engl J Med. 2021;384:759–64.
38. Second evaluation report next generation accountable care organization model evaluation. NORC at the University of Chicago. https://innovation.cms.gov/files/reports/nextgenaco-secondevalrpt.pdf. Accessed January 2022.
39. https://innovation.cms.gov/files/reports/episode-payment-models-wp.pdf. Accessed January 2022.
40. Joynt Maddox KE, Oray EJ, Zheng J, Epstein AM. Evaluation of medicare's bundled payments initiative for medical conditions. N Engl J Med. 2018;379:260–9.
41. https://www.svb.com/trends-insights/reports/healthcare-investments-and-exits/q1-2021-annual. Accessed February 2022.
42. https://www.crickethealth.com. Accessed July 2022.
43. Farias FAC, Dagostini CM, Bicca YA, Falavigna VF, Falavigna A. Remote patient monitoring: a systematic review. Telemed J E Health. 2020;26(5):576–83.
44. Schachner T, Keller R, von Wangenheim F. Artificial intelligence-based conversational agents for chronic conditions: systematic literature review. J Med Internet Res. 2020;22(9):e20701.
45. Milne-Ives M, de Cock C, Lim E, Shehadeh MH, de Pennington N, Mole G, Normando E, Meinert E. The effectiveness of artificial intelligence conversational agents in health care: systematic review. J Med Internet Res. 2020;22(10):e20346.
46. Newhouse JP, Garber AM, Graham RP, McCoy MA, Mancher M, Kibria A, editors. Variation in health care spending: target decision making, not geography. The National Academies Press; 2013.
47. Cliff BQ, Avancena ALV, Hirth RA, Lee SYD. The impact of choosing wisely interventions on low-value medical services: a systematic review. Milbank Q. 99(4):1024–58.
48. https://hcp-lan.org. Accessed February 2022.
49. Muhlestein D, Bleser WK, Saunders RS, McClellan MB. All-payer spread of ACO's and value-based payment models in 2021: the crossroads and future of value-based care. Health Affairs Blog. 2021;
50. Haber S, Beil H, Morrison M, et al. Evaluation of the Maryland all-payer model, vol. 1: final report. Waltham: RTI International; 2019. https://downloads.cms.gov/files/md-allpayer-finalevalrpt.pdf. Accessed February 2022.

51. Emanuel EJ, Johnson DW, Guido M, Goozner M. Meaningful value-based payment reform, part 2: expanding the Maryland model to other states. Health Affairs Forefront. 2022.
52. 2021 National Healthcare Quality and Disparities Report. Rockville: Agency for Healthcare Research and Quality. https://www.ahrq.gov/research/findings/nhqrdr/nhqdr21/index.html. Accessed July 2022.
53. SDOH reference.
54. https://health.gov/healthypeople/priority-areas/social-determinants-health. Accessed February 2022.
55. Murray GF, Rodriguez HP, Lewis VA. Upstream with a small paddle: how ACO's are working against the current to meet patients' social needs. Health Aff. 2020;39(2):199–206. https://doi.org/10.1377/hlthaff.2019.01266.
56. https://innovation.cms.gov/innovation-models/ahcm. Accessed February 2022.
57. https://nciom.org/nc-health-data/guide-to-accountable-care-communities. Accessed July 2022.
58. https://www.johnshopkinssolutions.com/solution/hospital-at-home. Accessed February 2022.
59. https://qualitynet.cms.gov/acute-hospital-care-at-home, https://www.cms.gov/newsroom/press-releases/cms-announces-comprehensive-strategy-enhance-hospital-capacity-amid-covid-19-surge. Accessed July 2022.
60. https://www.beckerspayer.com/payer/5-recent-payer-investments-in-home-care-services.html. Accessed July 2022.
61. Samson LW, Tarazi W, Turrini G, Sheingold S. Medicare beneficiaries' use of telehealth in 2020: trends by beneficiary characteristics and location. Office of Health Policy, US Department of Health and Human Service. https://aspe.hhs.gov/sites/default/files/documents/medicare-telehealth-report.pdf. Accessed March 2022.

46

Health Care Workforce

Erin Fraher, Bruce Fried, and Brianna Lombardi

Introduction

Ensuring that the health workforce is equipped to care for patients with chronic conditions is increasingly important to employers struggling to keep pace with the growing demands placed on the United States (US) health care system by an aging population. Eighty-six percent of healthcare spending in the US is for patients with one or more chronic conditions [1]. It is estimated as many as three in five individuals have a chronic health condition with 33% having two or more chronic diseases [2]. Labor costs are a significant expenditure for employers; approximately 50% of a hospital's bottom line is spent on wages [3]. US health care spending is rising, growing by 9.7%, reaching $4.1 trillion or 19.7% of gross domestic product [4]. With the costs of caring for patients with chronic illness consuming an ever-increasing percentage of state and federal budgets, policy makers are seeking ways to bend the cost curve, including implementing new payment models that shift from rewarding volume to incentivizing value. New payment models will require transforming the workforce from one predominantly trained to treat episodic illnesses to one prepared to prevent and manage chronic disease and improve population health. Such a transformation will require recruiting, retaining, and managing a workforce that is prepared to provide chronic care on interprofessional teams and is adequately distributed in needed geographies, specialties, and care settings.

Defining the Health Care Workforce

The health care workforce frequently cares for patients with multiple chronic conditions including hypertension, hyperlipidemia, arthritis, diabetes, coronary artery disease, chronic obstructive pulmonary disease, chronic kidney disease, and Alzheimer's Disease/dementia [5]. Individuals with chronic health conditions are at risk for comorbid behavioral health disorders, including depression and substance use disorders that worsen physical health outcomes and impede healthy behaviors. Characterizing the chronic care workforce is challenging because this workforce consists of a range of licensed and unlicensed providers who working in inpatient, outpatient, long-term, community, and home-based settings. Table 46.1 shows the numbers of workers in traditional health care occupations.

The largest licensed health professional group in the US is nursing, with close to three million registered nurses (RNs) employed in health care, more than three times the number of physicians. The majority of nurses (61%) are employed in hospitals [6]. Licensed practical nurses (LPNs) make up an additional 676,000 health professionals. About half of LPNs work in long-term care with three out of four of these LPNs employed in skilled nursing facilities [7].

There are about 939,000 physicians in active clinical practice in the US. Per capita physician supply has increased steadily over time, from 17 physicians per 10,000 population in 1980 to 29 physicians per 10,000 in 2019 [8]. However, growth among specialties has not been equal. Proceduralist specialties, such as vascular & interventional radiology and interventional cardiology are growing rapidly, with the workforce expanding by 98% and 129% respectively between 2010 and 2020. By contrast, primary care specialties and those who manage the health care of patients with chronic conditions in the community have grown more slowly. The number of internists increased by only 5.3%, and

E. Fraher (✉) · B. Lombardi
Department of Family Medicine, University of North Carolina at Chapel Hill, Chapel Hill, NC, USA

Cecil G. Sheps Center for Health Services Research, University of North Carolina at Chapel Hill, Chapel Hill, USA
e-mail: fraher@email.unc.edu; brianna_lombardi@med.unc.edu

B. Fried
Department of Health Policy and Management, University of North Carolina at Chapel Hill, Chapel Hill, NC, USA
e-mail: Bruce_Fried@unc.edu

Table 46.1 Number of Health Care Workers, Select Occupations, United States, 2020

	Number of workers
Physicians and Surgeons[a]	938,980
Family physicians	118,198
General internists	120,171
Geriatricians	5974
Other specialties	694,637
Physician assistants	125,280
Nurse practitioners	211,280
Registered nurses	2,986,500
Licensed practical and vocational nurses	676,440
Nursing assistants	1,371,050
Medical assistants	710,200
Dentists [b]	201,117
Dental hygienists & dental assistants	506,970
Pharmacists	315,470
Pharmacy technicians	415,310
Optometrists	36,690
Chiropractors	34,760
Podiatrists	9710
Occupational therapists	126,610
Occupational therapists and aides	48,380
Physical therapists	220,870
Physical therapist assistants and aides	138,520
Respiratory therapists	131,890
Speech-language pathologists	148,450
Audiologists	13,300
Social workers [c]	292,890
Community health workers	58,670
Home health and personal care aids	3,211,590

Source: May 2020. Bureau of Labor Statistics, https://www.bls.gov/oes/current/oes_nat.htm#29-0000

[a] AAMC 2020 Physician Specialty Data Report, https://www.aamc.org/data-reports/workforce/interactive-data/active-physicians-largest-specialties-2019

[b] 2020 ADA https://www.ada.org/en/science-research/health-policy-institute/data-center/supply-and-profile-of-dentists

[c] Social Workers = Healthcare and Mental Health Social Workers

family physicians grew by just 6.2% over the same period. The Association of American Medical Colleges has projected that the US will be short between 17,800 and 48,000 primary care physicians by 2034 [9].

In addition to family physicians and internists, geriatricians play an important role in caring for older patients with multiple chronic conditions. Table 46.2 displays the distribution and change of physician subspecialties over a 10-year timeframe. The number of geriatricians in active practice in the US increased 14% between 2015 and 2020; however, this growth rate is deceiving because the total number of geriatricians is small. In 2020, there were 5974 geriatricians in practice, representing just 2.4% of primary care providers. Despite increased demand and potential shortages, family medicine, general internal medicine and geriatrics have not been popular career choices due to perceived low prestige and low remuneration compared to other specialties [10–12].

Other Healthcare Practitioners

In addition to physicians and nurses, many other health care practitioners are needed to care for patients with chronic disease. Therapists make up the next largest group with nearly 625,000 occupational, physical, speech (speech and language pathologists) and respiratory therapists in practice in the US. Therapists are sometimes overlooked in health workforce planning discussions despite the critical and increasingly important role they play in addressing the health care needs of patients with chronic disease in acute and community-based settings. For example, as Medicare has moved away from paying for individual procedures toward providing single payments for episodes of care for conditions like hip fractures and joint replacement, health systems are increasingly focused on ways to deploy physical and

Table 46.2 Percentage change in the number of active physicians by specialty, United States, 2010–2020

	2010	2020	% growth 2010–2020
Interventional cardiology	1923	4407	129.17
Vascular & interventional radiology	1990	3943	98.14
Critical care medicine	7101	13,093	84.38
Pain medicine & pain management	3224	5871	82.10
Neuroradiology	2345	4089	74.37
Pediatric hematology/oncology	1981	3079	55.43
Pediatric cardiology	2012	2966	47.42
Internal medicine/pediatrics	3844	5509	43.31
Geriatric medicine	4278	5974	39.64
Vascular surgery	2853	3943	38.21
Nephrology	8362	11,407	36.41
Endocrinology, diabetes & metabolism	5891	7994	35.70
Infectious disease	7149	9687	35.50
Neonatal-perinatal medicine	4404	5919	34.40

Table 46.2 (continued)

	2010	2020	% growth 2010–2020
Emergency medicine	33,984	45,202	33.01
Hematology & oncology	12,743	16,274	27.71
Rheumatology	4917	6265	27.42
Child & adolescent psychiatry	7706	9787	27.00
Gastroenterology	12,852	15,469	20.36
Radiation oncology	4459	5306	19.00
All specialties	*799,501*	*938,980*	*17.45*
Dermatology	10,820	12,516	15.67
Physical medicine & rehabilitation	8502	9767	14.88
Neurological surgery	5047	5748	13.89
Allergy & immunology	4325	4900	13.29
Family medicine/general practice	106,549	118,198	10.93
Internal medicine	109,048	120,171	10.20
Neurology	12,916	14,146	9.52
Pediatrics	55,509	60,618	9.20
Ophthalmology	17,943	19,312	7.63
Plastic surgery	6822	7317	7.26
Otolaryngology	9232	9777	5.90
Obstetrics & gynecology	40,377	42,720	5.80
Anesthesiology	40,123	42,267	5.34
Urology	9826	10,201	3.82
Cardiovascular disease	21,819	22,521	3.22
Psychiatry	38,289	38,792	1.31
Radiology & diagnostic radiology	27,986	28,025	0.14
Preventive medicine	6824	6675	−2.18
General surgery	26,314	25,564	−2.85
Orthopedic surgery	19,822	19,069	−3.80
Thoracic surgery	4682	4479	−4.34
Anatomic/clinical pathology	14,975	12,643	−15.57
Pulmonary disease	6077	5106	−15.98

Source: Association of American Medical Colleges, https://www.aamc.org/data/workforce/reports/458514/1-9-chart.html

occupational therapists to improve patients' functional status and reduce the risk of costly hospital readmissions and support patients remaining safely in the community.

Workforce Planning for Chronic Care

Ensuring an adequate overall supply of providers is just one of many challenges facing the chronic care workforce. The US also faces a persistent misdistribution of health care providers. Nearly 62 million Americans representing 20% of the US population live in rural areas, where only 11.4% of the nation's physicians practice [13]. The Department of Health and Human Services uses a ratio of one primary care physician per 3500 population as the standard for designating primary care health professional shortage areas (HPSAs). More than 25 million Americans live in a rural area that has been designation as a primary care HPSA, and it would take more than 4000 practitioners to eliminate these shortage designations [14]. In primary care shortage areas, patients with chronic disease may have difficulty accessing care, which often leads to fewer visits for routine and preventive services needed to avoid hospitalization, particularly for persons with ambulatory sensitive conditions such as asthma, diabetes, COPD, heart failure, and hypertension [15]. The National Health Service Corps (NHSC) places an interprofessional workforce in vulnerable rural and urban communities including physicians, nurses, behavioral health, and substance use disorder care providers. Desire to serve in the NHSC has historically exceeded available slots due to insufficient funding [16]. However, funding has increased dramatically with recent investments from the American Rescue Plan. The field strength of the NHSC stands at nearly 12,000 providers practicing in underserved tribal, rural, and urban communities.

The lack of racial and ethnic diversity of the workforce remains a significant problem. For example, fewer than 6% of all physicians in the US identify as Latino/a, 5% as Black, and 0.3% as American Indian or Alaskan Native [17]. The workforce of the NHSC is more diverse than the general health care workforce is [16].

There is an increasing demand not only for primary care physicians, but also for specialists including vascular surgeons, cardiologists, general surgeons, nephrologists, and pulmonologists who can meet the needs of the growing number of patients with diabetes, heart failure, COPD, and asthma [18]. Workforce projections suggest that the future number and distribution of primary care and specialty physicians will not be adequate to meet the growing burden of chronic disease.

Team-Based Care

To address these shortages, care is increasingly being delivered by interprofessional teams of health care providers who, by working in the highest roles and functions allowed by their training, free up physicians to care for patients with the most complex health care needs [19]. Using three different scenarios regarding the amount of preventive and chronic care that could be delegated to non-physician providers (77%, 60% and 50% of preventive care, and 47%, 30% and 25% of chronic care), it is estimated that a primary care team could effectively care for a panel of 1947, 1532 or 1397 patients respectively [20]. Team-based models that expand physician panels have the potential to increase the capacity of the primary care workforce to serve the needs of an aging population. This change in the structure of primary care practice will require retraining physicians and other providers to practice in team-based models of care, remapping of workflows, developing standing orders that empower non-clinicians to share more responsibilities, educating patients, and instituting primary care payment reform that supports team-based care [20].

Team-based models of care are an effective strategy to address the physical, behavioral, and social needs of individuals with chronic health conditions. The standard 15-min visit with a physician is poorly suited for chronic disease management. Some practices have addressed this challenge by employing nurse practitioners, physician assistants, pharmacists, registered nurses, medical assistants, social workers, and other health professionals. A physician may pair with a non-physician team member who assists patients with tasks such as paperwork, authorizations, scheduling tests, coordinating referrals to specialists, and connecting to community-based resources [21].

Nurse Practitioners

Individual states determine the scope of practice legally allowed for health professionals and there is considerable variation between states. In most states in the western region of the US, nurse practitioners (NPs) can evaluate and diagnose patients, order and interpret tests, and initiate and manage treatments, including prescribing medications. In other states, including many states in the American south, a NP's scope of practice is limited and their practice must be supervised by a physician. Health workforce experts warn that the current state-based system for health professions regulation is problematic and they have urged policy reforms to redesign scope-of-practice laws and regulations to better support the transformation of the workforce that will be necessary to effectively care for the population [22]. Scope of practice reform and competitive salaries can support the increasingly important role of NPs in long-term care where they work with physicians in a collaborative model to care for increasingly complex chronically ill older adults [23].

Medical Assistants

The use of medical assistants (MAs) on teams is rapidly growing. There are over 700,000 MAs in practice in the US and their numbers are expected to increase by 20% between 2020 and 2030 [24]. MAs are not licensed but certification is available through national organizations such as the Association of American Medical Assistants (AAMA) although certification is often not required for employment. MA training is highly variable in length and rigor with programs ranging from 6 months to 2 years. Some MAs enter the workforce with a high school degree and receive on-the-job training [25]. The legal requirements governing the types of services MAs can provide vary considerably between states.

As the population of patients with chronic disease has grown, the roles of many MAs have expanded beyond the traditional tasks of rooming patients and taking vital signs. In some primary care practices, MAs take patient histories, give immunizations, provide preventative care services, act as health coaches, and serve as scribes to document clinical encounters [25–27]. MAs follow standing orders and algorithm-based protocols that do not require the direct involvement of the physician or other providers [28]. MAs also manage patient panels by using patient registries or data from electronic health records to identify and contact patients who are overdue for services, visits, and other needs [23, 29, 30]. As care delivery models change, placing more emphasis on prevention and between-visit care, MAs will take on even more roles in population health and panel management, patient education, coaching, and patient counseling.

Nursing Assistants

Nursing assistants, or certified nursing assistants (CNAs), are a large and growing workforce that works under the supervision of a Registered Nurse or Licensed Practical

Nurse. CNAs are certified by their state and fulfill direct care roles that vary based on their setting. CNAs most often support patient care related to activities of daily living and monitoring vital signs. This workforce plays a significant role in long-term care settings, providing an estimated 80–90% of the care to older adults in nursing homes, a patient population that often has multiple chronic conditions and cognitive impairment [31]. CNAs are largely a female workforce with a high proportion from diverse racial, ethnic, and international backgrounds. Although CNAs report being satisfied with their work, turnover rates among CNAs are high and CNAs often do not feel respected or valued by other health professionals and administrators [32]. Increasing CNA compensation, improving their employment benefits, providing career mobility opportunities, enhancing opportunities for CNAs to take on new responsibilities on the care team and increased training for CNA supervisors have been suggested as ways to strengthen the workforce, decrease turnover, and improve health outcomes for the patients they serve [33].

Registered Nurses

About 40% of registered nurses (RNs) work outside of acute care [6]. RNs have a significant and yet largely untapped potential to increase access to primary care by managing the needs of patients with a wide range of chronic medical and mental health conditions, including substance use. Many RNs who are employed in primary care spend much of their time triaging patients. While it is important and essential to determine which patients need immediate care, RNs who function in this capacity are limited from taking on a range of other direct patient care responsibilities. Innovative primary care practices are optimizing and reconfiguring the RN role to include care coordination, management of aging and chronically ill patients, enhancement of patients' self-management skills for chronic physical and behavioral health conditions, and provision of transitional care and wellness services [34]. Other high functioning primary care practices use RNs for same day appointments or group visits, and deploy nurses to conduct health risk appraisals, depression screens, health promotion, and disease prevention services [28, 35]. The migration of foreign-born to the United States nurses is critical to help address nursing shortages in the US, especially in long-term care facilities [36].

Pharmacists

The use of pharmacotherapy to treat and manage chronic disease has broadened the role of the pharmacist. Traditionally, pharmacists were employed in retail pharmacies and mostly focused on dispensing medications. In recent years, pharmacists have taken on increasing patient care roles, including coordinating drug therapies, developing medication management plans, educating patients, promoting medication compliance, and performing medication reconciliation to reduce medication interactions and duplication [37]. California, Montana, New Mexico and North Carolina have created advanced practice pharmacy designations that expand pharmacists' scope of practice to include direct patient care, however since most pharmacists are employed in retail settings and paid based by dispensing fees, reimbursement for direct patient care services remains limited [38].

Addressing Social and Behavioral Health Needs

Social determinants of health such as safe housing, transportation, educational and job opportunities, access to nutritious foods, racism, discrimination, and violence adversely impact patients' physical and mental health [39]. Social needs and chronic health conditions are closely connected as the stress associated with social needs contributes to a patient's inability to focus on healthy behaviors. Individuals with chronic disease often face challenges that impede their ability to work and pay health care bills which further exacerbates social needs. Health systems are increasingly aware that addressing social needs is an important component of treating chronic health conditions, enhancing the quality of care, and reducing costs [40]. As such, health systems are increasingly incorporating social care interventions, sometimes as part of chronic disease care management models within primary care settings [41]. Teams that address social and behavioral health needs include professionals and paraprofessionals such as social workers, community health workers, and patient navigators who have not traditionally been considered part of the health care workforce but are increasingly serving important roles in settings caring for patients with chronic disease.

Social Workers

Social workers play an increasingly important role on teams, helping chronic care patients address social, behavioral health and substance abuse care needs in acute, primary care practices, home-based care, and community settings. They have capacity to work alongside nurses to provide in-home visits, psychosocial assessments, patient education, referral to community resources, and regular check-ins for chronically ill older adults. Team care that pairs geriatricians with social workers lowers costs and reduces hospital days in chronically ill older men who are frequent users of health services, due to social workers' help with financial resources, psychosocial problems, and improved discharge planning

[42]. Social workers improve both the behavioral and physical health of patients without increasing overall costs for populations, including those with chronic illness and behavioral health needs [43]. Social workers integrate behavioral health into standard care by addressing mental health and substance abuse problems. They serve as care managers for patients with chronic conditions, monitor treatment plans and adherence, consult with primary care providers, and perform behavioral health interventions.

Public Health Workers

In addition to the traditional roles of managing infectious disease outbreaks, promoting vaccines, and tracking community illness, the public health workforce faces the challenge of caring for an aging population with an increased prevalence of chronic disease. Public health measures that address obesity, tobacco use, poor nutrition, and inactivity can reduce the risk factors that contribute to chronic illness. While the potential role of public health in preventing and managing chronic disease is significant, health care systems and public health services in the US have largely operated in separate spheres. Adequately funding the nation's public health infrastructure and better coordinating care between health care settings and public health systems can address chronic illness and the fragmentation of care [44, 45].

Community Health Workers

Community Health Workers (CHWs) are trusted, lay members from a community who work as volunteers or are employed by health systems to deliver a range of services to individuals with chronic illness including peer support, health promotion and patient education, and care navigation [46]. CHWs often reflect the race/ethnicity, languages spoken, socioeconomic status and lived experience of the communities they serve. Evidence suggests that when CHWs are deployed on teams, they increase access to care, improve understanding between community members and the health care system, increase adherence to care plans and reduce health disparities for marginalized and under resourced communities [47]. Recognizing these benefits, 21 state Medicaid programs or Medicaid Managed Care Organizations in 2022 reimburse CHWs or consider CHWs "allowable staff" [48].

Innovative Models

Community paramedicine (CP) is a relatively new and evolving healthcare model. It allows paramedics and emergency medical technicians (EMTs) to operate in expanded roles to provide primary care services, and integrate patient services between local public health agencies, home health agencies and providers. Community paramedics can administer injections, care for wounds, manage medications, educate patients, and provide other in-home services to patients. CPs can also provide follow-up care after hospitalization and a range of other services to older adults with chronic conditions with the aim of reducing readmissions [49, 50]. The concept behind CP is to provide a community-based model of healthcare that fills gaps in the healthcare infrastructure and decreases costs by reducing emergency transports and readmissions to the hospital [51]. There is growing interest in CP programs, particularly in rural communities where residents have reduced access to healthcare and poorer health outcomes than their urban counterparts.

Another model is The Community Aging in Place, Advancing Better Living for Elders (CAPABLE) program, a community-based model of care that serves dually eligible older adults (low-income seniors on both Medicare and Medicaid). This innovative program addresses the health care needs of enrollees by providing assistive devices and modifying the home to make ambulation and navigation easier and safer [52]. These services are delivered by an occupational therapist with support from nurses and handymen, who install equipment and make necessary home modifications. Improving the ability to perform the activities of daily living improves medication management and reduces depression in chronically ill patients.

Health Care Financing for Chronic Care

Health care financing is evolving from fee-for-service to value-based care payment models. Value-based care reimburses health care professionals based on the quality of care they provide, in contrast to fee-for-service payment models that reimburse based on the volume of services delivered [53]. Under value-based care, practices and providers contract with payers such as Medicare, Medicaid, and third-party insurance companies to provide care for a defined population of patients. The amount paid to providers to care for that patient population is risk-adjusted to account, for example, for the higher costs of caring for older patients and patients with multiple chronic diseases.

Physicians and practices can receive financial incentives for meeting specific quality metrics and performance measures that are tied to better outcomes for patients, including lower emergency room use and lower rates of hospital readmissions. They can also be penalized if these performance measures are not achieved. Performance measures often include quality metrics regarding the delivery of routine and preventive care services such as colon cancer screening and mammography, and chronic disease management services including controlling a diabetic patient's blood sugar and blood pressure [54].

Health care practices can also receive payment for care for Medicare wellness visits and chronic care management [55]. This reimbursement stream has accelerated the use of care coordinators to reduce care fragmentation and address the service gaps often confronted by patients with chronic disease. Nurses often fill this coordination role, arranging referrals between primary care and specialty physicians and acting as case managers for complex patients. This coordination role is critical for lowering costs and improving care quality because patients with multiple chronic conditions and complex therapeutic regimens are at particularly high risk for hospital readmission in the days and weeks following discharge. When done effectively, transitional care intervention after hospitalization delivered by nurses, social workers or other clinicians can increase the length of time between the hospital discharge and readmission or death while also decreasing costs, particularly in vulnerable populations such as older adults hospitalized with heart failure [56].

In 2020, about 39% of health care dollars were fee-for-service payments, 20% were based on pay-for-performance contracts or care coordination fees, and the remaining 41% were from value-based care arrangements [57]. Because they focus on prevention and managing the "upstream" factors that contribute to health, value-based care models and care coordination payments have expanded the boundaries of many traditional roles in the health care system [58]. These new roles focus on meeting patients' health care needs across the continuum from home to community and between acute and long-term care settings. New payment models are requiring health system planners to adopt a broader definition of who is in the workforce and shift from thinking of a "health workforce" to a "workforce for health" [59]. This broader definition will highlight the important roles that social workers, patient navigators, community health workers, paramedics, public health professionals and other community-based workers play in keeping patients healthy in their homes and communities.

Gaps in Training the Chronic Care Workforce

The healthcare workforce needs to manage a growing population of patients with chronic diseases, yet many health professional students feel they lack basic chronic care competencies [60, 61]. Learners may also lack exposure to the wide range of other health and community-based workers with whom they will practice as they manage patients' chronic health and psychosocial needs across a continuum of different settings. More robust interprofessional training and practice opportunities are needed to bring together traditional health care providers and non-traditional workforce members such as social workers, community health workers, public health professionals and other community-based and social service workers. These interprofessional teamwork competencies must be taught to students but also to the workforce already employed. Certification organizations and education institutions need to ensure that health care professionals who care for patients with chronic disease have opportunities to access affordable, convenient, and evidence-based continuing education.

Training Mismatch

The future practice patterns of health care professionals are influenced by the settings in which they train. Most chronic illness care is provided in primary care outpatient settings [19], yet most health professions students, including those training to be physicians, nurses, and therapists, receive most of their clinical training in acute care settings, such as hospitals [62, 63]. More training in well-performing primary care practices that have redesigned workflows and reallocated tasks to deliver care efficiently and effectively to patients with chronic disease is needed to provide trainees with the skills they will require for practice.

The physician workforce is similarly not being prepared to meet the needs of an aging population with complex care needs. Obstacles to expanding the physician workforce include the perceived low prestige of primary care, the perceived futility of care for chronically ill people, and low remuneration [11]. Physicians in training report frustration regarding the lack of time available in ambulatory care visits that restrict the capacity to address the complex health care needs of patients with chronic illness, although they acknowledge satisfaction with this kind of practice [64].

As of 2020, federal and state support for graduate medical education (GME) in the US totaled $19 billion annually, funding nearly 140,000 residency training positions in 1657 teaching hospitals [65, 66]. Given the substantial investment of public funding in GME training, the National Academy of Medicine, General Accounting Office and others have called for greater social accountability for these funds to train a workforce that matches the population health needs, including an increased focus on training more primary care physicians prepared to provide care to chronically ill people in ambulatory and community-based settings [67].

Although most primary care is provided by family physicians and general internists, more geriatricians are needed in teaching and practice settings. The number of new geriatricians has increased slightly since 2016 due to an increase in the number of internal medicine physicians becoming board certified in geriatrics (Fig. 46.1) [68]. About two-thirds of board certified geriatricians are internists and the remaining third are family physicians.

Fig. 46.1 American Board of Medical Specialties Certifications in Geriatrics, 2010–2019. Source: American Board of Medical Specialties Certification Report 2019–2020. 2021

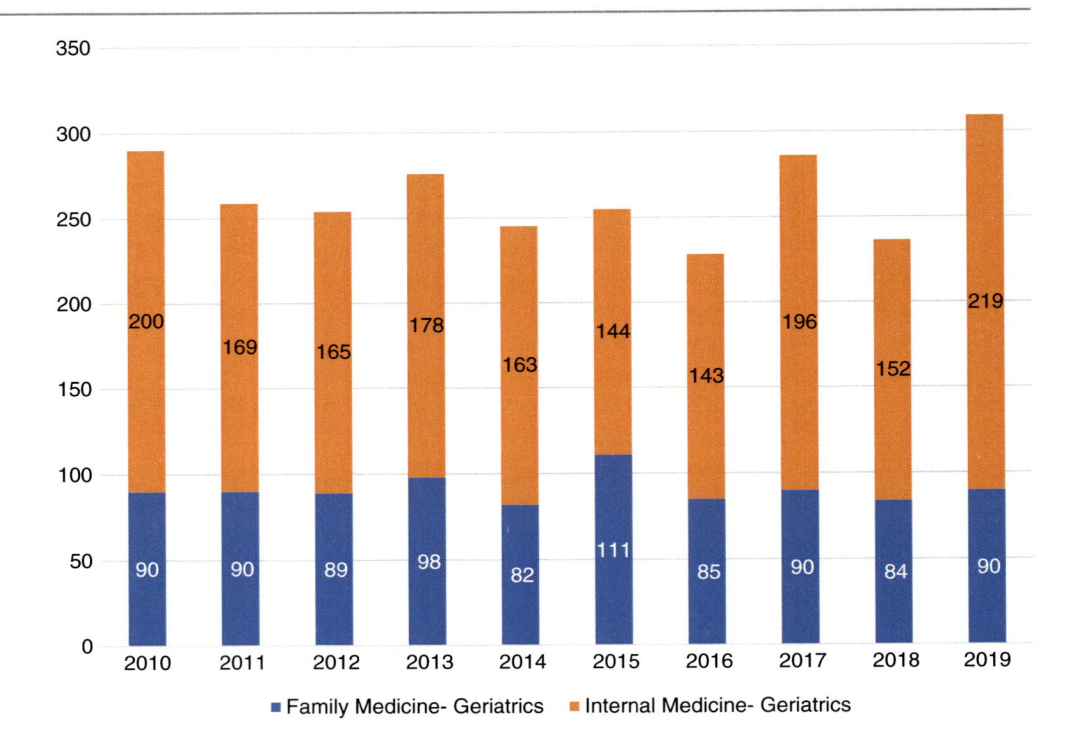

Year	Family Medicine- Geriatrics	Internal Medicine- Geriatrics
2010	90	200
2011	90	169
2012	89	165
2013	98	178
2014	82	163
2015	111	144
2016	85	143
2017	90	196
2018	84	152
2019	90	219

Table 46.3 Average annual physician salaries in the United States (2017)

Primary care physicians		Specialty physicians	
Obstetrics/Gynecology	$286,000	Orthopedics	$489,000
Internal medicine	$225,000	Cardiology	$410,000
Geriatrician (median)	$186,174	Gastroenterology	$391,000
Family medicine	$209,000	General surgery	$362,000
Pediatrics	$202,000	Nephrology	$280,000
Primary care physicians overall	$217,000	Specialty physicians overall	$316,000

Sources: Grisham S., 2017; "Physician—geriatrics salaries." Salary.com: http://www1.salary.com/Physician-Geriatrics-Salary.html

The Role of Compensation

Salary is an important factor in recruiting and retaining healthcare workers, but other factors are also important, including autonomy, the ability to provide high quality care, positive relationships with supervisors and peers, a supportive organization, good working conditions with a reasonable workload, and the ability to maintain work/life balance [69]. Given the important role that primary care clinicians play in providing continuous and longitudinal care to a growing population of chronically ill patients and the increasing demand for such clinicians, one might expect that the labor market would place a high value on these professionals, resulting in substantial increases in compensation. However, this has not been the case and as recently as 2017 the average physician salary of a cardiologist, gastroenterologist, or general surgeon was nearly twice that of a family physician, general internist, geriatrician, or pediatrician (Table 46.3) [70, 71]. Compensation for primary care physicians increased 5.3% on average between 2018 and 2020, while compensation for advanced practice providers (e.g., nurse practitioners and physician assistants) increased 3.4% during the same time period. The salaries of specialists decreased 3–5%; however, this decrease was attributed to the COVID-19 pandemic and likely to fully recover [72]. Physician compensation is complex with many contributing factors. The effect of evolving payment models, including the transition to value-based payment models which emphasize the role of prevention and primary care, make the long-term trends in compensation unclear. While there is a dire shortage of geriatricians, the number of trainees choosing this field has either decreased or been flat in recent years, causing some medical educators to give up on training geriatricians as primary care providers and prepare them to serve as consultants to generalist physicians who treat older patients [73].

The salary differential between geriatricians and primary care providers and other, better paid, physician specialties is a contributing factor to the relatively slow growth in their supply. The future supply of primary care physicians and geriatricians is not likely to keep pace with demand and much of chronic care is likely to shift to nurse practitioners

(NPs). There has been a rapid growth in the supply of nurse practitioners and increasing evidence that the quality of care and patient satisfaction is comparable to physicians for certain conditions [74]. The cost of NPs providing primary care for Medicare beneficiaries is 29% lower than for patients assigned to physicians. Coupling these cost of care trends with the growing supply of NPs incentivizes the shift in chronic care from physicians to NPs [75]. Future health care models are likely to see NPs and physicians working in teams, with physicians using their more advanced training to oversee, consult, and advise on the management of the more medically complex patients.

In contrast with the comparatively low salaries earned by geriatricians, NPs specializing in geriatrics earn more than the average NP salary, which ranges from $72,420 to $140,930 [76]. In 2017, the median salary for non-specialized nurse practitioners was $90,600 while the salary for geriatric NPs and palliative care NPs was $92,000 and $96,126 respectively suggesting that NPs are paid slightly more for working in chronic care [77].

Workforce Staffing Challenges

Staffing shortages in chronic care occur across the health care spectrum; from low-wage positions like home health aides to high income professions such as physicians, nurses, and therapists [78, 79]. Healthcare organizations struggle to maintain the salaries, benefits, and work environment that attracts and retains a chronic care work force. As previously noted, provider salaries tend to be lower in primary care and some health care workers find work with chronically ill people less professionally rewarding than work in acute care. Turnover is also a common problem, and burnout within the health workforce is at an all-time high. Health care employers will need to focus on multiple strategies to recruit health care workers, increase worker engagement, address burnout, and support employees to practice in chronic care [80–82].

Organizational Staff Retention and Turnover

Staff turnover is a pervasive concern in healthcare and there are five factors that contribute to turnover: inadequate management and supervisory practices; excessive workload; poor compensation and benefits; feelings of disrespect and lack of recognition; and poor employee engagement strategies [83]. For example, low levels of compensation, particularly when workload pressures increase, may result in employees feeling that they are not recognized and valued for their efforts. Similarly, lack of positive and constructive supervision is likely to lead to employees feeling emotionally disengaged from the organization.

The COVID-19 pandemic brought these retention and turnover issues to the forefront. Job demands and pressures increased in unparalleled ways, the personal health risks faced by healthcare workers, and employees' concern about the well-being of loved ones, created a perfect storm of factors that have resulted in health care workers leaving the workforce at unprecedented rates [79]. The pandemic created an even greater need for effective management practices, but many health organizations, and in particular long-term care facilities, had a less than satisfactory history of employee engagement [79].

Employee engagement is a term that is used frequently among healthcare leaders and is key to employee retention [84]. Engagement is associated with employees' sense of the fairness of an organization's policies and procedures, often referred to as procedural justice. Engaged employees identify with the organization, and their identification with the organization enables employees "to view, and internalize, an organization's success as his/her personal success" [84]. Because they feel emotionally connected to the organization, highly engaged employees can remain effective contributors even when they face personal crises and difficult work situations.

Engagement is different from job satisfaction, which is considered as a necessary but insufficient prerequisite for employee engagement [85]. An employee can, for example, be very satisfied with their compensation, but be willing to move to another organization for a marginally higher salary. Engagement results from broader aspects of an organization's culture including respectful treatment of all employees at all levels; fair and equitable compensation; trust between employees and senior management; job security; and opportunities for employees to use their skills and abilities in their work [85]. The presence of these factors collectively increases the probability that employees will not only feel a sense of job satisfaction, but also feel emotionally attached and committed to the organization.

Organizations should monitor turnover trends including the types of employees who are leaving and where they are going, and then design evidence-based retention strategies [86]. Although exit interviews with employees yield useful data, a recent and promising innovation is the use of "stay interviews" [87] that ask current employees to describe why they remain in the organization. These surveys ask short and targeted questionnaires that can provide quick information to assist in the development and continuation of valued supports for the current workforce. Since compensation is often an issue, organizations can institute reward systems that may include incentive pay. There is no shortage of suggestions to reduce turnover and ongoing research will help establish the strategies that work [88, 89].

Burnout

Burnout has always been a concern in the health care workforce and has worsened during the COVID-19 pandemic.

Burnout not only affects the individual provider's health and well-being but also has negative impact on the system including increased turnover and medical errors. During the COVID-19 pandemic, close to 50% of health workers reported burnout and many also experienced depression, sleep difficulties, and thoughts of suicide [82, 90]. Health systems have generally aimed to address burnout through individual-level stress-mitigation strategies (e.g., meditation and self-care trainings) [91]. However, organizational-level efforts like ensuring time for rest, decreasing workload, providing essential resources, and supporting team-building initiatives may be more effective strategies to reduce provider burnout [91]. In the wake of the COVID-19 pandemic, ongoing interventions at the organizational level will need to buffer the effects of difficult working conditions and support the current workforce to prevent worker turnover across the health care sector.

Future Directions

The growing, aging US population is driving an increased demand for workers in occupations that provide care to patients with chronic illness. Home health and personal care aides, certified nursing assistants, registered nurses, licensed practical nurses and medical assistant jobs are projected to grow significantly between 2020 and 2030 (Table 46.4) [76]. Despite these increases, supply may not keep pace with demand.

The staffing requirements for working in chronic care include not only relevant education and skills, but also less easily measured competencies such as empathy and communication skills, and the ability to work effectively with patients and families, often in a relatively autonomous manner. Finding the right fit between an employee, the organization, and the patient population is an important predictor of job satisfaction and organizational commitment [92]. Evaluating candidates may involve cognitive tests, assessments of physical abilities that are relevant to the job, personality tests, reference checks, and interviews, though even the best processes may not accurately predict future performance or longevity with the organization. Organizations may face constraints by a limited pool of qualified candidates in which case they may prefer employees who show a willingness to learn.

Table 46.4 Estimated growth rates for health care workers between 2020 and 2030 [76]

Home health aides and personal care aides	33%
Nursing assistants	8%
Medical assistants	18%
Licensed practical and licensed vocational nurses	9%
Registered nurses	9%

Source: U.S. Bureau of Labor Statistics: US Department of Labor; 2021. https://www.bls.gov/ooh/healthcar

The larger challenges facing the chronic care workforce will include meeting the needs of an aging population that will require multiple types of chronic care services, in addition to behavioral health and social needs of the population. The workforce will need to be comprised of a broad range of disciplines that can provide patients with medical care, rehabilitation, care coordination, discharge planning, community resources, personal care services, nutritional services, and social and emotional support, as well as support for family members. These services will be provided in a variety of settings including outpatient clinics, rehabilitation facilities, hospitals, assisted living and skilled nursing facilities, hospices, and patients' homes. Care transitions across these locations must be integrated with well communicated plans.

The workforce of the future will be more likely to provide chronic illness care at home, rather than in traditional health care settings; they will leverage safe and effective electronic monitoring technologies that will, in some cases, reduce the need for scarce and expensive human resources. The use of remote patient monitoring technology will allow health care workers to focus on care responsibilities and workflows where technology cannot offer a substitute. To augment the supply of needed health care workers in areas where they are not available, the local health system may rely on the concept of plasticity, which suggests that there are multiple configurations of professionals in a community that can meet the needs of the population [93]. For example, not every community will have access to a geriatrician or physician skilled in chronic illness care, but through training and task shifting, other health care providers may effectively provide care. The World Health Organization recommends that task-shifting arrangements may be more efficient than traditional models but must also be safe, effective, equitable, and sustainable [94].

Successful healthcare teams are likely to transform from the traditional care delivery model, with fixed members (e.g., physicians, nurses), to alternatives where teams are quickly assembled and are responsive to specific and time limited care needs. This approach will require developed competencies from care disciplines that are flexible and nimble (e.g., scaffolding), so that team performance will not be dependent on team-building techniques (i.e., teaming) [95, 96]. These ideas all allow greater flexibility and fluidity in the provision of team care that is required to meet the needs of the chronic care population.

References

1. Gerteis J ID, Deitz D, LeRoy L, Ricciardi R, Miller T, Basu J. Multiple chronic conditions chartbook: 2010 Medical Expenditure Panel Survey Data. 2014.
2. Centers for Disease Control and Prevention. About chronic disease. 2021 [updated April 28, 2021]. https://www.cdc.gov/chronicdisease/about/index.htm.

3. Dunn L. Getting a handle on hospital costs 2015. http://www.hhnmag.com/articles/3614-getting-a-handle-on-hospital-workforce-costs.
4. Centers for Medicare and Medicaid Services. National Health Expenditure Data Historical. 2021. https://www.cms.gov/Research-Statistics-Data-and-Systems/Statistics-Trends-and-Reports/NationalHealthExpendData/NationalHealthAccountsHistorical.
5. Centers for Medicare and Medicaid Services. Chronic condition charts. 2018.
6. Bureau of Labor Statistics. Occupational outlook handbook registered nurses work environment. 2021. https://www.bls.gov/ooh/healthcare/registered-nurses.htm#tab-3.
7. Coffman JM, Chan K, Bates T. Profile of the licensed practical nurse/licensed vocational nurse workforce, 2008 and 2013. UCSF Health Workforce Research Center on long-term care; 2015.
8. Association of American Medical Colleges. 2020 physician specialty data report. 2020.
9. IHS Markit Ltd. The complexities of physician supply and demand: projections from 2019 to 2034. Washington, DC: AAMC; 2021.
10. Golden AG, Silverman MA, Issenberg SB. Addressing the shortage of geriatricians: what medical educators can learn from the nurse practitioner training model. Acad Med. 2015;90(9):1236–40.
11. Golden AG, Silverman MA, Mintzer MJ. Is geriatric medicine terminally ill? Ann Intern Med. 2012;156(9):654–6.
12. Bodenheimer T, Grumbach K, Berenson RA. A lifeline for primary care. N Engl J Med. 2009;360(26):2693–6.
13. National Rural Health Association. Health care workforce distribution and shortage issues in rural America. 2012.
14. Bureau of Health Workforce, Health Resources and Services Administration (HRSA), U.S. Department of Health & Human Services. Designated health professional shortage areas statistics 2021. https://data.hrsa.gov/topics/health-workforce/shortage-areas.
15. Bindman AB, Grumbach K, Osmond D, Komaromy M, Vranizan K, Lurie N, et al. Preventable hospitalizations and access to health care. JAMA. 1995;274(4):305–11.
16. Billings AN, Jabbarpour Y, Westfall J. The National Health Service corps at 50 years. Am Fam Physician. 2022;105(2):129–30.
17. Association of American Medical Colleges. Diversity in medicine: facts and figures 2019. 2019.
18. Dall TM, Gallo PD, Chakrabarti R, West T, Semilla AP, Storm MV. An aging population and growing disease burden will require a large and specialized health care workforce by 2025. Health Aff (Millwood). 2013;32(11):2013–20.
19. Bodenheimer T, Chen E, Bennett HD. Confronting the growing burden of chronic disease: can the U.S. health care workforce do the job? Health Aff (Millwood). 2009;28(1):64–74.
20. Altschuler J, Margolius D, Bodenheimer T, Grumbach K. Estimating a reasonable patient panel size for primary care physicians with team-based task delegation. Ann Fam Med. 2012;10(5):396–400.
21. Bodenheimer T, Ghorob A, Willard-Grace R, Grumbach K. The 10 building blocks of high-performing primary care. Ann Fam Med. 2014;12(2):166–71.
22. Frogner BK, Fraher EP, Spetz J, Pittman P, Moore J, Beck AJ, et al. Modernizing scope-of-practice regulations—time to prioritize patients. N Engl J Med. 2020;382(7):591–3.
23. McGilton KS, Bowers BJ, Resnick B. The future includes nurse practitioner models of care in the long-term care sector. J Am Med Dir Assoc. 2022;23(2):197–200.
24. Bureau of Labor Statistics. Occupational outlook handbook medical assistants job outlook 2021.
25. Chapman SA, Marks A, Dower C. Positioning medical assistants for a greater role in the era of health reform. Acad Med. 2015;90(10):1347–52.
26. Bodenheimer TS, Smith MD. Primary care: proposed solutions to the physician shortage without training more physicians. Health Aff (Millwood). 2013;32(11):1881–6.
27. Bodenheimer T, Willard-Grace R, Ghorob A. Expanding the roles of medical assistants: who does what in primary care? JAMA Intern Med. 2014;174(7):1025–6.
28. Bodenheimer T. Lessons from the trenches—a high-functioning primary care clinic. N Engl J Med. 2011;365(1):5–8.
29. Ghorob A, Bodenheimer T. Share the care: building teams in primary care practices. J Am Board Fam Med. 2012;25(2):143–5.
30. Fraher EP, Cummings A, Neutze D. The evolving role of medical assistants in primary care practice: divergent and concordant perspectives from MAs and family physicians. Med Care Res Rev. 2021;78(1_suppl):7S–17S.
31. Riggs CJ, Rantz MJ. A model of staff support to improve retention in long-term care. Nurs Adm Q. 2001;25(2):43–54.
32. Pennington K, Scott J, Magilvy K. The role of certified nursing assistants in nursing homes. J Nurs Adm. 2003;33(11):578–84.
33. Scales K. Transforming direct care jobs, reimagining long-term services and supports. J Am Med Dir Assoc. 2022;23(2):207–13.
34. Bodenheimer T, Mason D. Registered nurses: partners in transforming care. 2017.
35. Mastal M, Levine J. The value of registered nurses in ambulatory care settings: a survey. Nurs Econ. 2012;30(5):295–304.
36. Thompson RA, Corazzini KN, Konrad TR, Cary MP, Silva SG, McConnell ES. Registered nurse migration to the United States and the impact on long-term care. J Am Med Dir Assoc. 2022;23(2):315–7.
37. Sandberg SF, Erikson C, Owen R, Vickery KD, Shimotsu ST, Linzer M, et al. Hennepin health: a safety-net accountable care organization for the expanded Medicaid population. Health Aff (Millwood). 2014;33(11):1975–84.
38. Isasi F, KI. The expanding role of pharmacists in a transformed health care system. 2015.
39. Commission on Social Determinants of Health, World Health Organization. Closing the gap in a generation: health equity through action on the social determinants of health: Commission on Social Determinants of Health final report: World Health Organization; 2008.
40. McQueen A, Li L, Herrick CJ, Verdecias N, Brown DS, Broussard DJ, et al. Social needs, chronic conditions, and health care utilization among Medicaid beneficiaries. Popul Health Manag. 2021;24(6):681–90.
41. National Academies of Sciences, Engineering, and Medicine. Integrating social care into the delivery of health care: moving upstream to improve the nation's health. 2019.
42. Sommers LS, Marton KI, Barbaccia JC, Randolph J. Physician, nurse, and social worker collaboration in primary care for chronically ill seniors. Arch Intern Med. 2000;160(12):1825–33.
43. Fraser MW, Lombardi BM, Wu S, de Saxe Zerden L, Richman EI, Fraher EP. Social work in integrated primary care: a systematic review. 2016.
44. Ogden LL, Richards CL, Shenson D. Clinical preventive services for older adults: the interface between personal health care and public health services. Am J Public Health. 2012;102(3):419–25.
45. Elliott L, McBride TD, Allen P, Jacob RR, Jones E, Kerner J. Health care system collaboration to address chronic diseases: a nationwide snapshot from state public health practitioners. Prev Chronic Dis. 2014;11:E152.
46. Sabo S, Allen CG, Sutkowi K, Wennerstrom A. Community health workers in the United States: challenges in identifying, surveying, and supporting the workforce. Am J Public Health. 2017;107(12):1964–9.
47. Rosenthal EL, Brownstein JN, Rush CH, Hirsch GR, Willaert AM, Scott JR, et al. Community health workers: part of the solution. Health Aff. 2010;29(7):1338–42.

48. National Academy for State Health Policy. State community health worker models 2021. https://www.nashp.org/state-community-health-worker-models/#tab-id-2.
49. Goodwin J. Community paramedicine mobile integrated healthcare 2013. http://www.emsworld.com/article/10957645/community-paramedicine-mobile-integrated-healthcare.
50. McGinnis K. Rural and frontier emergency medicine services: agenda for the future. National Rural Health Association; 2004.
51. Choi BY, Blumberg C, Williams K. Mobile integrated health care and community paramedicine: an emerging emergency medical services concept. Ann Emerg Med. 2016;67(3):361–6.
52. Szanton SL, Leff B, Wolff JL, Roberts L, Gitlin LN. Home-based care program reduces disability and promotes aging in place. Health Aff (Millwood). 2016;35(9):1558–63.
53. Modica C. The value transformation framework: an approach to value-based care in federally qualified health centers. J Healthc Qual. 2020;42(2):106–12.
54. Aledade. A comprehensive guide to value based care for primary care. 2021.
55. Edwards ST, Landon BE. Medicare's chronic care management payment—payment reform for primary care. N Engl J Med. 2014;371(22):2049–51.
56. Naylor MD, Brooten DA, Campbell RL, Maislin G, McCauley KM, Schwartz JS. Transitional care of older adults hospitalized with heart failure: a randomized, controlled trial. J Am Geriatr Soc. 2004;52(5):675–84.
57. Health Care Payment Learning and Action Network. APM measurement progress of alternate payment models. 2021.
58. Fraher EP, Ricketts TC 3rd. Building a value-based workforce in North Carolina. N C Med J. 2016;77(2):94–8.
59. Fraher E. Workforce planning in a rapidly changing healthcare system 2017. http://www.shepscenter.unc.edu/wp-content/uploads/2017/02/FraherSCHA_SCIOMFeb13.pdf.
60. Darer JD, Hwang W, Pham HH, Bass EB, Anderson G. More training needed in chronic care: a survey of US physicians. Acad Med. 2004;79(6):541–8.
61. Pham HH, Simonson L, Elnicki DM, Fried LP, Goroll AH, Bass EB. Training U.S. medical students to care for the chronically ill. Acad Med. 2004;79(1):32–40.
62. Blanchard J, Petterson S, Bazemore A, Watkins K, Mullan F. Characteristics and distribution of graduate medical education training sites: are we missing opportunities to meet US health workforce needs? Acad Med. 2016;91(10):1416–22.
63. Fraher E, Spetz J, Naylor MD. Nursing in a transformed health care system: new roles, new rules. Robert Wood Johnson Foundation Interdisciplinary Nursing Quality Research Initiative. 2015.
64. Thomas DC, Kessler C, Sachdev N, Fromme HB, Schwartz A, Harris I. Residents' perspectives on rewards and challenges of caring for ambulatory care patients living with chronic illness: findings from three academic health centers. Acad Med. 2015;90(12):1684–90.
65. Office. USGA. Physician workforce: HHS needs better information to comprehensively evaluate graduate medical education funding. https://www-gao-gov.proxy.lib.umich.edu/assets/700/690854.pdf.2018.
66. Eden J, Berwick DM, Wilensky GR. Graduate medical education that meets the nation's health needs. Washington: National Academies Press; 2014.
67. Phillips RL Jr, George BC, Holmboe ES, Bazemore AW, Westfall JM, Bitton A. Measuring graduate medical education outcomes to honor the social contract. Acad Med. 2022;97:643.
68. American Board of Medical Specialties. ABMS Board Certification Report 2019–2020. 2021.
69. White K, Clement D. Healthcare professionals. In: Fottler M, Fried B, editors. Human resources in healthcare: managing for success. Chicago: Health Administration Press; Association of University Programs in Health Administration; 2015.
70. Medscape Physician Compensation Report. In: Grisham S, editor. 2017.
71. Physician-geriatrics salaries 2017 [cited 2017. Salary.com]. http://www1.salary.com/Physician-Geriatrics-Salary.html.
72. Medical Group Management Association. Datadive provider compensation. Provider pay and the pandemic. 2021.
73. Span P. Even fewer geriatricians in training. New York Times. 2013.
74. Stanik-Hutt J, Newhouse RP, White KM, Johantgen M, Bass EB, Zangaro G, et al. The quality and effectiveness of care provided by nurse practitioners. J Nurse Pract. 2013;9(8):492–500.
75. Bodenheimer T, Bauer L. Rethinking the primary care workforce—an expanded role for nurses. N Engl J Med. 2016;375(11):1015–7.
76. U.S. Bureau of Labor Statistics: US Department of Labor; 2017 [Occupations with the most job growth, 2014 and projected 24]. https://www.bls.gov/emp/ep_table_104.htm.
77. PayScale.com Seattle: PayScale; 2017 [Nurse Practitioner salary]. http://www.payscale.com/research/US/Job=Nurse_Practitioner_(NP)/Salary.
78. Becker's Hospital Review. Staffing shortages by state. https://www.beckershospitalreview.com/workforce/13-states-experiencing-workforce-shortages-in-at-least-25-of-hospitals-23-anticipate-it.html2022. https://www.beckershospitalreview.com/workforce/13-states-experiencing-workforce-shortages-in-at-least-25-of-hospitals-23-anticipate-it.html.
79. Frogner BK, Dill JS. Tracking turnover among health care workers during the COVID-19 pandemic: a cross-sectional study. JAMA Health Forum. 2022;3(4):e220371.
80. Rangachari P, Woods JL. Preserving organizational resilience, patient safety, and staff retention during COVID-19 requires a holistic consideration of the psychological safety of healthcare workers. Int J Environ Res Public Health. 2020;17(12):4267.
81. Raffoul M, Bartlett-Esquilant G, Phillips RL Jr. Recruiting and training a health professions workforce to meet the needs of tomorrow's health care system. Acad Med. 2019;94(5):651–5.
82. Prasad K, McLoughlin C, Stillman M, Poplau S, Goelz E, Taylor S, et al. Prevalence and correlates of stress and burnout among US healthcare workers during the COVID-19 pandemic: a national cross-sectional survey study. EClinicalMedicine. 2021;35:100879.
83. DR. Retention. In: CJS, BJF, editors. Human resources in healthcare: managing for success, 5th ed. Chicago: Health Administration; 2021.
84. He H, Zhu W, Zheng X. Procedural justice and employee engagement: roles of organizational identification and moral identity centrality. J Bus Ethics. 2014;122(4):681–95.
85. Society for Human Resource Management. 2017 employee job satisfaction and engagement: the doors of opportunity are open: executive summary. 2017.
86. Fleshner I. On shift [Internet] 2015. [cited 2017]. blog.onshift.com/perfect-storm-high-turnover-coupled-increasing-demand-ltc-workers.
87. Finnegan RP. The power of stay interviews for engagement and retention: Society for Human Resource Management; 2018.
88. Smikle J. Why they stay: retention strategies for long term care. Provider (Washington, DC). 2015;41(11):39–40, 2.
89. Barbera E. The keys to reducing turnover in long-term care. McKnight's [Internet]. 2014. http://www.mcknights.com/the-world-according-to-dr-el/the-keys-to-reducing-turnover-in-long-term-care/article/333071/.
90. Chor WPD, Ng WM, Cheng L, Situ W, Chong JW, Ng LYA, et al. Burnout amongst emergency healthcare workers during the COVID-19 pandemic: a multi-center study. Am J Emerg Med. 2021;46:700–2.

91. West CP, Dyrbye LN, Erwin PJ, Shanafelt TD. Interventions to prevent and reduce physician burnout: a systematic review and meta-analysis. Lancet. 2016;388(10057):2272–81.
92. Kristof-Brown AL, Zimmerman RD, Johnson EC. Consequences of individuals' fit at work: a meta-analysis of person-job, person-organization, person-group, and person-supervisor fit. Pers Psychol. 2005;58(2):281–342.
93. Holmes GM, Morrison M, Pathman DE, Fraher E. The contribution of "plasticity" to modeling how a community's need for health care services can be met by different configurations of physicians. Acad Med. 2013;88(12):1877–82.
94. World Health Organization. Task shifting: rational redistribution of tasks among health workforce teams: global recommendations and guidelines. Geneva: World Health Organization; 2007.
95. Edmondson A. Teaming: how organizations learn, innovate, and compete in the knowledge economy. In: Schein EH, editor. San Francisco: Wiley; 2012.
96. Valentine M, Edmondson A. Team scaffolds: how mesolevel structures enable role-based coordination in temporary groups. Organ Sci. 2014;26(2):405–22.

Index

A

Abdominal injury, 104
Aberrant Behavior Checklist-Community (ABC-C), 327
Abuse Focused Cognitive Behavioral Therapy (AF-CBT), 107
Academic-community partnerships, 116
Access to Care, 322
Access to Nutrition Index, 537
Accountability system, 537
Accountable Care Organizations (ACOs), 140, 215, 270, 464, 534, 587, 590, 601, 611
Accountable Health Communities, 140, 534
    model, 615
    program, 465
Accreditation Council for Graduate Medical Education (ACGME), 287
ACHIEVE project, 449
Activities of daily living (ADLs), 257, 269
Act phase, 507
Acute care, 246
Acute COVID-19, 382
Acute dystonia, 340
Acute hospital care
    admission
        admitting orders, 233
        anticipated length of stay, 235
        care level, 233
        discharge care needs, 235
        iatrogenic errors, 233, 234
        laboratory and diagnostic testing, 234
        medication management, 234, 235
        nosocomial infections, 233, 234
    advance care planning, 232, 237, 238
    antibiotic and medication stewardship, 235, 236
    behavioral health, 240
    care teams, 237
    collateral information, 232
    coordinating care, 241
    COVID-19 pandemic, 240
    discharge planning
        discharge summary, 239, 240
        medication reconciliation, 239
        patient education, 239
        post-discharge location, 238, 239
        transitional care, 240
    history and physical examination, 232
    medication reconciliation, 232
    mortality, cost, and length of stay, 231
    patient capacity, 240, 241
    patient status changes, 236
Acute inpatient rehabilitation (AIR), 256, 257
Acute pain management, 252
Acute rehabilitation, 256

Addressing unconscious (implicit) bias, 575
Adherence, 116
Administration for Children and Families (ACF), 133
Administration for Community Living (ACL), 132, 133
Adult day services (ADS) centers, 273, 274
Adult foster care, 276, 277
Advance care planning (ACP), 314, 324
Advance Practice Provider (APPs), 454
Advanced Cardiovascular Life Support (ACLS), 214
Advanced Emergency Medical Technician (AEMT), 246
Advancing Care Together (ACT) program, 438
Adverse Childhood Events (ACEs), 570, 571, 574
Adverse drug reactions, 3
Affordability Index, 607
Affordable Care Act (ACA), 118, 120, 121, 258, 270, 271, 305, 493, 501, 576, 587, 588, 598, 608
Age-Friendly Health Systems, 317
Ageism, 311, 312
Agency for Healthcare Research and Quality (AHRQ), 276, 464, 465
Agent Orange, 412
Ages and Stages Questionnaire, 439
Aging, 29
Aid-to-Families with Dependent Children (AFDC), 597
Airborne hazard, 412
Alcohol use disorder, see Substance use disorder (SUD)
Alcohol Use Disorders Identification Test (AUDIT), 409, 410, 436, 439
Alcohol Use Disorders Identification Test-Consumption (AUDIT-C), 419, 436
Alcoholics Anonymous (AA), 78, 114
Algorithmovigilence, 476
"Alignment" track, 534
Allostasis, 532
Allostatic load, 532
All-Payer Model, 614
Alternative payment models (APM), 215, 608–612
Alzheimer's Association, 136
Alzheimer's disease, 619
AmbuFlex project, 518
AmbuFlex system, 516
Ambulatory care
    access and time challenges, 214
    COVID-19 pandemic, 216
    definition, 209
    payment models and financing
        capitation, 215
        direct primary care, 215
        fee for service, 215
        telehealth services, 215, 216
        value-based payments, 215
    payment reform, 216
    teaching and training, 216

Ambulatory primary care
    Barbara Starfield's 4 C's model, 211
    chronic disease care quality, 210, 211
    definition, 209
    DPC, 212
    PCMH, 211
    research, 216
    team-based care, 212
    Wagner's chronic care model, 211
American Association on Intellectual and Developmental Disabilities (AAIDD), 322
American Cancer Society (ACS), 135
American College of Emergency Physicians (ACEP), 251
American Correctional Association, 364
American Diabetes Association (ADA), 135
American Geriatric Society (AGS), 251, 314
American Heart Association (AHA), 135, 610
American Medical Association (AMA), 583
American Medical Directors Association (AMDA), 262
American Recovery and Reinvestment Act (ARRA), 223, 232, 484
Amyotrophic lateral sclerosis, 392
Analyzing and interpreting data, 507
Angiotensin-converting enzyme 2 (ACE2), 20, 381
Anti-inflammatory nutritional supplements, 386
Anti-psychotic medications, 259, 328
Antipsychotics, 259
Antiretroviral therapy (ART), 419
Anxiety disorders, 117
Area Deprivation Index (ADI), 475
Artificial intelligence (AI), 469–472, 576
Asplenia, 164
Assertive Community Treatment (ACT) teams, 341
"Assistance" track, 534
Assisted living, 276
Association for Supervision and Curriculum Development, 303
Association of American Medical Colleges (AAMC), 575
Asthma, 47
Asymptomatic carotid artery stenosis, 151
Atenolol, 389
Attention deficit and hyperactivity disorder (ADHD), 327
Attributable fraction (*AF*), 549
Auditory dysfunction, 411, 412
Autoimmune diseases, 5

B
Balancing measures, 501
Basic Life Support (BLS), 214
Bayes net algorithms, 472
Behavioral counseling, 51
Behavioral health, 117, 614
Behavioral health consultant (BHC), 435
Behavioral health disorders, 432
Behavioral health integration models, 434
Behavioral health professionals (BHPs), 432, 434, 439, 440
Behavioral health services, 432–435
Behavioral issues, 259
Behavior change, 115
Benzodiazepines, 340
Biomedical theories, 531, 532
Bipolar disorder, 336, 340
Bisoprolol, 389
Black Americans, 262
Black and Latino/Hispanic older adults, 312
Black box computational approaches, 472
Blackfoot disease, 555

Borg Rate of Perceived Exertion (RPE) scale, 385
Brain Injury Screening Questionnaire (BISQ) screens, 409
Breast cancer, 568
    implementation, 150, 151
    overview, 150
    potential benefits, 150
    potential harms, 150
Breathing difficulties, 387
Bruises, 103, 104
BUILD Health Challenge, 140
Bundled Payments for Care Improvement (BPCI) Models, 613
Bundle payment models, 613
The Bureau of Health Workforce, 133
Bureau of Primary Health Care, 133
Burnout, 627

C
Cancer
    definition, 5, 6
    screening, 325
    smoking cessation, 47
Cancer survivors
    acute, 395
    advancing survivorship care
        chronic illness care models, 400
        self-management, peer, and family support, 401
    cancer organization guidelines, 399, 400
    chronic, 395
    conceptual framework, 399
    cured, 395
    effectiveness of, 395
    epidemiology
        functional status and quality of life, 397, 398
        mortality, 397
        multimorbidity, 398
        prevalence, 396, 397
        syndromes, 398
    gaps in clinical practice, 400
    health care systems, 402
    long-term effects, 395
    models and guidelines, 399
Capability approach (CA), 538, 539
CAPABLE program, 278
Capitated and value-based reimbursement model, 465
Carceral system, 573–574
Cardiac disorders, 325
Cardiac magnetic resonance imaging (MRI), 388
Cardiopulmonary exercise testing (CPET), 387
Cardiovascular disease (CVD), 8, 9, 30, 337, 419, 420
    in children, 169
    physical activity, 31, 32
    secondary prevention, 151
    smoking cessation, 45, 47
Caregivers
    caregiver assessment guidelines, 92
    chronically ill children, 89, 90
    COVID-19 pandemic, 91
    cultural aspects, 94, 95
    dementia, 90
    demographics of, 87, 88
    effects of caregiving
        caregiver burden, 88
        financial consequences, 89
        physical consequences, 88
        positive effects, 88

    psychological consequences, 88, 89
    end-of-life care, 91, 92
    informal caregiving, 92
    interventions, 92, 93
    mental health disorders, 90, 91
    physical disability, 91
    public policy, 93–94
Care management, 463, 465
    definition, 461
    functions, 462
    implementation, 462–464
CARES Act, 423
Care Transitions Intervention (CTI), 448
Cash-only care, 212
Catechol-O-methyltransferase (COMT), 8
Centennial Care initiative, 120
Center for Development and Disability (CDD), 330
Center for Medicare and Medicaid Innovation (CMMI), 278, 519, 587, 608
Centers for Disease Control (CDC), 372, 382
Centers for Disease Control and Prevention, 99, 131, 132, 303
Centers for Medicare and Medicaid Services (CMS), 130, 131, 246, 248, 258, 290, 303, 330, 608
Cerebrovascular disease, 550
Certified electronic health record technology, 464
Certified nursing assistants (CNAs), 622
Cervical cancer screening, 325, 353
Change management, 505
Chat-based hotlines, 66
Chemical agents, 552
Chemobrain, 398
ChenMed, 613
Child abuse and neglect
    abdominal injury, 104
    emotional neglect, 105
    factors, 102, 103
    family social support system, 103
    fractures, 104
    guidelines, 100, 101
    head trauma, 104, 105
    health care needs, 107
    high-stress situations, 103
    individual characteristics, 102
    management approach, 107
    mandated reporting, 106
    medical neglect, 105
    morbidity and mortality, 101
    opportunity, 108
    parent characteristics, 102
    physical abuse, 103, 104
    physical neglect, 105
    poverty and unemployment, 102
    prevention, 108
    screening, 101, 102
    sexual abuse, 105
    skin injuries, 103, 104
    stress, 101
    trauma informed care, 106
Child Abuse Prevention and Treatment Act, 99
Childhood trauma, 336
Child Nutrition Programs, 134
Children's Health Insurance Program (CHIP), 130, 304, 597, 598
Children's Health Insurance Program Reauthorization Act (CHIPRA), 304
Children, with chronic illness
    community, 303, 304
    COVID-19 and, 304
    education, 306
    family role and socialization, 306
    growth and development, 305
    health disparities in care and research, 304
    home care, 302, 303
    hospitals, 302
    medicaid and financing, 304, 305
    outpatient medical home, 302
    psychological consequences, 306
    quality of care and population health, 304
    schools, 303
    transition to adulthood, 306, 307
Chinese immigrant community, 274
Chlamydia screening, 147
Chronic Care Model (CCM), 62, 118, 119, 460
    comprehensive approach, 48
    emotional support, 49
    family and social support, 49
    public health interventions, 49
    team-based care, 48
Chronic care workforce, 628
Chronic disease (illness), 362
    community applications, 475
    definition, 473
    health care provider applications, 473, 474
    health policy applications, 475
    home applications, 473
    individual patient applications, 473
    practice applications, 474
    in US adults, 473
Chronic disease, in older adults
    advance care planning (ACP), 314
    COVID-19, 312
    epidemiology of, 311
    geriatric syndromes, 315
    life expectancy and prognosis, 314
    organization of care
        care transitions, 316
        hospital, 315, 316
        nursing home care, 316
        outpatient and community care, 316
        telehealth, 317
    physical function, 313
    quality of life, 313
    social determinants of health (SDOH), 312
        access to food, 313
        elder abuse, 313
        health disparities, 313
        health literacy, 312
        social support and community resources, 312, 313
    systems of support, 314
Chronic disease management, 362
Chronic disease prevention, 541
Chronic fatiguing illnesses, 383
Chronic hepatitis C infection, 6, 376
Chronic illness care, 400, 558–560
    emerging payment models, 270
    financing community-based long-term care, 269, 270
    home-based clinical care (*see* Home-based clinical care)
    nonresidential community-based care (*see* Non-residential community-based care)
    telehealth and virtual care, 273
Chronic kidney disease (CKD), 166, 167, 558
Chronic lymphocytic leukemia, 551
Chronic obstructive pulmonary disease (COPD), 550, 558
    physical activity, 32
    smoking cessation, 47

Chronic pain, 8, 408–411
Cisgender/heterosexual peers, 349, 351
Classification task, 470
Climate change, 557, 558
Clinical algorithms, 248
Clinical decision support (CDS), 10, 11, 472, 474, 486–490, 493, 494
Clinical Pharmacogenetics Implementation Consortium (CPIC), 10, 11
Clinical policies, 349
Clinical quality measures (CQMs), 490
Clinically Integrated Network (CIN), 610, 614
Clonidine, 389
CMS TCM payment codes, 450
Cochrane reviews, 322
Cognitive behavioral therapy (CBT), 341
Cognitive challenges, 321
Cognitive effects, 389
Cognitive impairment, 420
Collaborative Assessment and Management of Suicidality (CAMS), 352
Collaborative care management model (CoCM), 436–438, 441
Co-located behavioral health, 431–441
Co-located care management, 302
Colon cancer, 325
Colorectal cancer (CRC) screening, 146
Committee on the Quality of Care in Nursing Homes, 263
Common chronic diseases, 301
Common medical comorbidities, 384
Communication and patient planning (CAPP), 237
Community, 303
Community Aging in Place, Advancing Better Living for Elders (CAPABLE) program, 272, 624
Community applications, 475
Community-based care
 administrative and regulatory issues, 278
 adult foster care, 276, 277
 assisted living, 276
 Continuing Care Retirement Communities (CCRCs), 277
 disparities in access, 279
 Green House Model, 277
 and health equity, 278
 medical foster home care, 277
 quality of care in long-term care, 279, 280
 senior housing, 276
Community-Based Care Transition Programs, 271
Community-based programs, 108
Community-based services, 603, 615
Community Care of North Carolina (CCNC), 67
Community-centered health home (CCHH), 139
Community engagement, 138, 139
Community health workers (CHWs), 116–118, 365, 575, 624
Community immunity, 158, 159
Community Mental Health Act, 342
Community mental health centers (CMHC's), 342
Community organizations
 Accountable Health Communities, 140
 ACOs, 140
 BUILD Health Challenge, 140
 CCHH, 139
 Culture of Health initiative, 139
 Medicaid managed care plans, 140
 Medicare Advantage Health Plans, 140
 primary care practices, 137–139
 REACH, 138
 Section 1115 waivers, 140
Community paramedicine (CP), 624

Community partnerships, 140, 141
 Accountable Health Communities, 140
 ACOs, 140
 BUILD Health Challenge, 140
 CCHH, 139
 Culture of Health initiative, 139
 Medicaid managed care plans, 140
 Medicare Advantage Health Plans, 140
 REACH, 138
 Section 1115 waivers, 140
Community programs, 359
Compensated work therapy, 422
Comprehensive Addiction Recovery Act (CARA) in 2016, 79
Comprehensive Care for Joint Replacement (CJR) Model, 519, 613
Comprehensive ESRD Care Model, 613
Comprehensive medication review, 183, 184
Comprehensive Primary Care (CPC), 611
Computed tomography (CT), 387
Computer adaptive testing (CAT), 516
Concussion, 409
Condition-specific questionnaires, 512
Conflict management, 201, 203, 294
Consumer Assessment of Healthcare Providers and Systems (CAHPS), 512
Continuing Care Retirement Communities (CCRCs), 277
Continuous quality improvement, 440
Continuum of Care (CoC) program, 422
Conversion therapy, 351
Coordinated social needs screening, 535
Coordination of care, 252
Coronary artery disease (CAD), 31, 32
Cough, 388
COVID-19, 20, 21, 61, 67, 91, 108, 109, 134, 166, 203, 209, 210, 216, 247, 258, 269, 273, 292, 304, 312, 322, 325, 327, 329, 381, 388, 423–425, 465, 535, 591, 592, 614, 615, 627
Criminal legal system, 359
Critical time intervention strategies, 421
Cryptosporidium, 554
Cultural competence, 199
Cultural Formulation Interview (CFI), 378
Cultural humility, 199, 568
Culturally and linguistically appropriate service (CLAS), 575
Culture of Health initiative, 139
Cut down, Annoyance, Guilt, and Eye-Opener (CAGE) questions, 409, 410, 439

D

Data collecting method, 506
Data management
 Act phase, 507
 analyzing and interpreting data, 507
 collection, 506
 disseminating data, 507, 508
 tracking, 506, 507
Data systems, 614
Decision aids, 288
De facto mental health system, 432
Dementia, 90, 259, 292, 293, 619
Deming cycle, 499–501
Democratization of metrics, 520
Demography, 593
DePaul Symptom Questionnaire (DSQ), 384
Depression, 117, 256, 410–412
Depressive disorders, 302
Developmental disabilities, 321

Diabetes, 47, 558
Diabetes mellitus, 9, 31, 166
Diagnostic and Statistical Manual of Mental Disorders (DSM), 574
DIAMOND program, 437
Diffusing capacity of lung for carbon monoxide (DLCO), 387
Digital divide, 226
Digital health, 120, 190, 402
Dimercatosuccinic acid, 556
Direct primary care (DPC), 212
Disability adjusted life year (DALY), 549
Discrimination, 351, 528
Disease-specific questionnaires, 512
Disparities, 359
Disposition, 248
Disproportionate share hospitals (DSH), 601
Disseminating data, 507, 508
Diversity Equity and Inclusion (DEI), 575
Drive Metrics, 508
Drowning, 558
Drug Abuse Screening Test (DAST), 409, 410, 419, 436, 439
Drug-related problem, 182, 183
Drug use disorder, *see* Substance use disorder
Durable medical equipment (DME), 451, 452, 454
Durable Powers of Attorney for Health Care (DPAHC), 249
Dutch Pharmacogenetics Working Group (DPWG), 11

E
Early and Periodic Screening, Diagnostic, and Treatment (EPSDT) program, 130, 598
Eating disorders, 352
Eco-epidmiology/ecosocial theory, 533
Ecology of medical care, 209, 210
Edinburgh Postnatal Depression Scale, 439
ED observation unit (EDOU), 248
Effective care coordination, 402
eHealth Enhanced Chronic Care Model, 460
Elder abuse, 313
Elder mistreatment
  guidelines, 102
  management approach, 108
  opportunity, 108
  patient evaluation, 105, 106
  prevention, 108
Electronic health records (EHRs), 349, 351, 352, 440, 472, 481–494, 614
Electronic health tools, 66
Electronic medical record (EMR), 248, 288
Electronic patient-reported outcomes (ePROs), 515
Electronic PROMs (ePROMS), 516
Embedded care managers (ECM), 462
Emergency care
  arrival at emergency department, 247, 248
  assessment and treatment, 248
  definition, 245
  disposition, 248, 249
  field/pre-arrival, 247
  public and private organizations and agencies, 245
  quality of care, 249
  special consideration
    older adults, 250, 251
    pain management, 251, 252
Emergency Care Designations, 246
Emergency department (ED), 245, 246, 249, 251
Emergency Medical Responder (EMR), 246
Emergency medical services (EMS), 245, 246
Emergency medical technicians (EMTs), 624
Emergency medicine (EM), 245
Emergency medicine physicians, 245
Emergency Medicine Technician-Basic (EMT-B), 246
Emergency Medicine Treatment & Labor Act (EMTALA), 246
Emergency Nurses Association (ENA), 251
Emergency Severity Index (ESI) score, 247
Employee engagement, 627
Empowerment, 62, 63
Endocrine Society, 354
End of life care
  advance care planning, 288
  children, 294, 295
  chronic disease and changes, 285
  decisions and communication, 287, 288
  dementia, 292, 293
  financial reimbursement and cost savings, 290
  intellectual disabilities or mental illness, 293, 294
  modern hospice and palliative care movement, 286, 287
  palliative sedation, 289
  physician assisted death, 289
  provision and place of end-of-life care, 290–292
  quality of care, 289, 290
  racial disparities and cultural diversity, 295
  value-based payment models, 295
  withdrawing, withholding, and refusing care, 289
  workforce and wellbeing, 295
End stage renal disease (ESRD), 584, 614
Energy expenditure, 30
Enhancelink Initiative and Transitional Care Coordination Model, 363
Environmental determinants, 531
  anthropogenic changes, 547
  built environment, 547
  chronic illness care, 558–560
  estimates burden of disease, 548–549
    automobile-centric urban designs, 557
    climate change, 557, 558
    household air pollution, 549
    indoor air pollution, 551–552
    lead toxicity, 555, 556
    nonoptimal temperatures, 549
    occupational exposure, 552
    outdoor air pollution, 549–551
    water pollution, 552–555
  etiologic agents, 553
  exposure to pollution and chemicals, 547
  genetic vs. non-genetic factors, 547
  household air pollution, 547
  outdoor air pollution, 547
  physical exposures, 547
  reporting requirements, 560–562
  water pollution, 547
Epidermal growth factor receptor (*EGFR*) mutations, 5
Epilepsy, 324
ePrognosis, 314
Equitable COVID-19 Homelessness Response project, 424
Ethnicity, 568
EuroQol (EQ-5D), 516
Evidence-based guideline driven care, 351
Evidence-based medicine, 473
Exclusive language, 350
Exercise, 29, 34
Expanded Chronic Care Model, 460, 461
Exposure-related injuries, 420

F

Faith-based organizations, 136, 137
Family medicine, 620
Family role and socialization, 306
Fecal immunochemical test (FIT), 146
Fecal occult blood testing (FBT), 146
Federal Affordable Care Act, 449
Federal agencies, *see* U.S. Department of Health and Human Services (HHS)
Federal criminal legal system, 360
Federally qualified health center (FQHC), 120, 349
Fee-for-service payment models, 67
Financial empowerment approaches, 422
Financial model, 610–611
Financial risk, 610
5 As approach, 436
Five-Star Quality Rating System, 259
Food insecurity, 572
Formaldehyde, 551
Forming stage, 500
Fractures, 104
Frailty, 29, 398
Freestanding emergency departments (FSEDs), 246
Front desk fidelity, 507
Functional Assessment of Cancer Therapy-General (FACT-G), 515
Functional Assessment of Cancer Treatment (FACT), 519
Fundamental social causes theory, 532

G

Gastaut syndrome, 7
Gastrointestinal problems, 324
Gender affirming hormone treatment, 354
Gender affirming therapy, 354
Gender identity, 347
Gender spectrum, 354
Gene-drug pairs
    autoimmune diseases, 5
    cancer, 5, 6
    cardiovascular disease, 8, 9
    chronic pain, 8
    diabetes mellitus, 9
    infectious diseases, 5–7
    psychiatric and neurologic conditions, 7, 8
General internal medicine, 620
Generalized Anxiety Disorder-7 (GAD-7), 351, 378, 384, 437, 439, 440
Generic questionnaires, 512
Genetics, role of, 3, 4
Geneva Convention, 371
The Geriatric Resources for Assessment and Care of Elders (GRACE) model, 278
Geriatric syndromes, 315
Germline polymorphisms, 5
Gilbert syndrome, 6
Giullain-Barre syndrome, 554
Glomerular filtration rate (GFR), 571
Gonorrhea screening, 147
Governmental cash assistance, 373
Graduate medical education (GME), 625
Green House model, 277
Green space, 572
Guided Care model, 278

H

Harm reduction interventions, 419
Harvard Trauma Questionnaire, 378
HCP-LAN alternative payment model (APM) framework, 609
Head trauma, 104, 105
Health and social service systems, 534
Health behaviors, 115
Healthcare disparities, 433
Healthcare Effectiveness Data and Information Set (HEDIS) metrics, 498
Health care financing, 624, 625
Healthcare Information Technology (HIT), 614
Health care organization (HCO), 463
Healthcare providers, 349, 473, 474
Health care reform, 118
Health care services, 362, 574
Health care systems, 329, 349, 400–402, 417
The Healthcare Systems Bureau, 134
Health care workforce
    burnout, 628
    CHWs, 624
    CNAs, 623
    community paramedicine, 624
    defining, 619, 620
    health care financing, 624, 625
    healthcare practitioners, 620–621
    medical assistants, 622
    nurse practitioners, 622
    pharmacists, 623
    public health workers, 624
    racial and ethnic diversity, 621
    registered nurses, 623
    remote patient monitoring technology, 628
    role of compensation, 626–627
    social determinants, 623
    social workers, 623
    staff turnover, 627
    staffing requirements, 628
    staffing shortages, 627
    team-based care, 622
    team-building techniques, 628
    training mismatch, 625–627
Health disparities, 528, 568
    addressing unconscious (implicit) bias, 575
    CHWs, 575
    increasing workforce diversity, 576
    trauma informed care, 574
    workforce education and training, 575–576
Health equity, 476, 477, 568, 615
Health in all policies (HiAP) approach, 538
Health inequities and disparities, 472, 528
    community level factors, 572–573
    individual level factors, 570
    interpersonal factors, 570–572
    NIMHD framework, 568
    societal level factors, 573–574
Health information exchange (HIE), 248, 491, 492
Health information technology (HIT), 120, 121, 203, 204, 330, 481
Health Information Technology for Economic and Clinical Health Act (HITECH), 484, 486, 608
Health insurance, 245
Health Insurance Portability and Accountability Act (HIPAA), 361
Health IT, 481, 483–486, 488, 489, 491–493

Health literacy (HL), 63, 64, 186, 187, 536, 539, 541
Health policy, 475, 537, 538
Health-related quality of life (HRQoL), 512, 516
Health Resources and Services Administration (HRSA), 133, 134, 422
Health systems, 349
Healthy Outcomes Medical Excellence (HOME) project, 329
Hearing loss and tinnitus, 411
Heart Rhythm Society, 388
Heath care utilization, 535
Hematopoietic Stem Cell Transplant (HSCT) Recipients, 164, 165
Hepatitis A vaccines, 168
Hepatitis B vaccines
    chronic liver disease, 168
    CKD, 167
    diabetes mellitus, 166
Hepatitis C vaccines, 364, 573
Herd immunity, 158, 159
Hip fractures, 256
HITS, 100
HIV, *see* Human immunodeficiency virus
The HIV/AIDS Bureau, 134
Home and community-based services (HCBS), 130, 131, 269–270, 603
Home applications, 473
Home-based clinical care
    aging in place and villages movement, 275
    consultative visits and specialty care, 271
    evaluation and assessment, 272
    home-based medical care (HBMC), 271
    home-based primary care (HBPC), 271
    home health agencies (HHA), 270
    hospital-at-home model, 272
    palliative care, 272
    smart home and robotic technologies, 275
Home-based end-of-life care, 291
Home based medical care, 271
Home-based primary care (HBPC), 271, 316
Home health agencies (HHA), 270, 271
Homeless Management Information System (HMIS), 422
Homelessness, 410, 412, 413, 417, 418
Homelessness Screening Clinical Reminder (HSCR), 420
Home safety assessments, 272
Homicide, 558
Hospital-Acquired Conditions Reduction Program (HACRP), 608
Hospital-at-home (HaH) model, 272, 315
Hospitalizations, 272, 291
Hospital Outpatient Quality Reporting Program (Hospital OQR), 249
Hospital Readmissions Reduction Program (HRRP), 258, 449, 608
Hospital Value-Based Purchasing Program (HVBPP), 608
House quality, 572
Housing First, 421–423
Housing stability, 572
Human papillomavirus (HPV) vaccination, 353
Human immunodeficiency virus (HIV), 5, 47, 163, 164, 363, 573
Human leukocyte antigen B (HLA-B), 6
Human Rights Campaign, 347
Huntington's disease, 7
Hypertension, 32
Hypertensive heart disease, 558
Hypothalamic-pituitary-adrenal axis, 349

I

Imminent risk of homelessness, 418
Inactivated influenza vaccine (IIV), 162
Incarceration
    clinical service, 362
    hepatitis C, 364
    human immunodeficiency virus (HIV), 363
    legal precedents, 360
    mental health, 362, 363
    organization of care, 360, 361
    post release and reentry, 364, 365
    pregnancy, 364
    reentry programs, 365, 366
    substance use disorders, 363
    transgender persons, 359
Inclusive language, 350
Income assistance interventions, 422
Income inequality, 530, 531
Individual patient applications, 473
Inequity, 528, 537, 540
Influenza vaccines, 166
    chronic liver disease, 168
    CKD, 166, 167
    pulmonary disease, 167
Information technology (IT), 190, 225, 401, 464
Informed consent, 361
Informed hypotheses, 534
Institute for Healthcare Improvement (IHI), 183, 498–500, 503, 520
Institute of Medicine (IOM), 383, 607
Institutional Special Needs Plans (I-SNPs), 316
Institutions for Mental Diseases (IMDs), 603
Instrumental activities of daily living (IADLs), 269
Integrated behavioral health (IBH)
    access, 433
    collaborative care management model, 436–438
    co-located behavioral health, 434
    continuity of care, 433
    costs, 433
    emotional and physical health, 432, 433
    healthcare disparities, 433
    implementation strategies & considerations
        communication, 440
        mission & vision, 438
        practice improvement, 440
        schedules, 440
        staffing & training, 438, 439
        workflow, 439
        workspace design, 439
    primary care behavioral health, 435
    SBIRT, 435, 436
    stigma, mental health, 433
Integrated behavioral health care, 433
Integrating resiliency models, 441
Integration Playbook, 438
Integration Workforce Study (IWS), 438
Intellectual and developmental disabilities (IDD)
    acute problem behaviors, 327, 328
    clinical assessment and management, 322–325
    COVID-19 on Individuals with, 329
    functional domains for adults with, 323
    multiple causes of, 321
    organization and health care services, 329, 330
    preventive services, 325, 326
    Psychiatric Conditions and Mental Health Disorders, 326, 327
    psychotropic medications, 328, 329
Intellectual disability, 293
Intensive case management (ICM), 341
Interactive Systems Framework for Dissemination and Implementation, 425
Interdisciplinary care team (IDT), 131

Interdisciplinary health care, 329
International Children's Palliative Care Network (ICPCN), 294
International Classification of Diseases (ICD) 10 coding system, 534
International Organization of Migration (IOM), 372
International Red Cross, 374
International Review of Research in Developmental Disabilities, 322
Interpersonal violence, 351
Intersectionality, 347, 568
Intervention programs, 532, 535
Interventions to Reduce Acute Care Transfers (INTERACT) program, 258, 316
Intestinal parasites, 377
Intimate partner violence (IPV)
    approach to, 107
    definition, 99
    fractures, 104
    guidelines, 100
    morbidity and mortality, 101
    opportunity, 108
    patient evaluation, 102
    prevention, 108
    sexual abuse, 105
    stress, 101
Invasive fungal infections, 6, 7
Involuntary civil commitment (IVC), 241
Ischemic heart disease, 550, 558
Ivabradine, 389

J
Joint Commission, 360
Juran Trilogy, 497

K
Kaiser Family Foundation (KFF), 568
Kidney Care First model, 613
Kotter model, 505

L
Laboratory testing, 385
Landmark Health, 613
Lay health advisors, 138
Lead toxicity, 555, 556
Lean, 501–505
Learning Health Systems (LHS), 474
Legal Services Corporation (LSC), 136
Lesbian, gay, bisexual, or transgender (LGBT), 348
Lesbian, gay, bisexual, transgender, or queer (LGBTQ+), 94, 95, 279
LGBTQIA+, 347
Licensed practical nurses (LPNs), 619
"Life chances" theory, 532
Life course, 532
Lifestyle theories, 531
Lifetime disparities, 355
Limerick Nuclear Power Plant, 551
Link and Phelan's theory, 532
Literally homeless, 418
Lithium, 340
Live-attenuated vaccines, 156
Living Healthy course, 66
Living Wills (LW), 249
Local public health departments (LHD), 135
Long-acting injectable medications (LAI's), 340
Long-stay residents, 255
Long-term acute care hospitals (LTACHs), 257
Long-term care diagnosis-related groups (LTC-DRGs), 260
Lower respiratory infection, 558
Lung cancer, 149, 150, 551

M
Machine learning (ML), 469–473
Major depressive disorder, 7, 410
Malignant neoplasms, 294
Managed care organizations (MCOs), 120, 601
Managing for daily improvement (MDI), 507
Mass incarceration, 359
Maternal and Child Health Bureau's (MCHG) programs, 134
Meaningful use (MU), 464, 481, 484, 486–493
Mean life expectancy, 314
Mechanical injuries, 558
Medicaid, 130, 269, 274, 305
    beneficiaries, 574
    CHIP program, 597, 604
    chronic illnesses and disabilities, 597
    cost sharing, 599–600
    covered services, 599
    delivery system, 601
    eligibility, 598–599
    expansion on health outcomes, 600–601
    expenditures, 602–603
    financing, 601–602
    funding, 604
    payment, 262
    persons with chronic illnesses, 604
    provider payments, 601
    reasonable costs, 598
    spending, 602
    substantial medical bills, 598
    waivers, 603
Medicaid Act, 598
Medicaid Drug Rebate Program (MDRP), 602
Medicaid's home and community-based services (HCBS), 604
Medical assistants (MAs), 622
Medical comorbidities, 382
Medical complications, 256
Medical discharge planning, 365
Medical insurance, 586
Medical respite and recuperative care programs (MRPs), 422
Medicare, 130, 269
    ACA, 587, 588
    beneficiaries, 585, 586
    benefits, 585–586
    controlling spending, 588, 589
    coverage of hospital care, 585
    covid-19 pandemic, 591, 592
    dual eligibles, 586
    enactment, 592
    end-stage renal disease, 583
    expenditures and financing, 586–587
    health disparities, 585
    limitations in, 586
    "Medicare for All", 592
    origins, 583–584
    payment and delivery reform, 295, 589–591
    permanent disabilities, 583
    policy, 588
    reforming medicare, 593
    social security, 584
    standard insurance model, 583

Medicare Access and CHIP Reauthorization Act (MACRA), 499, 590
Medicare for All model, 592
Medicare Health Outcomes Survey (HOS), 519
Medicare per-episode payments, 613
Medicare's Hospital Value-Based Purchasing Program (HVBP), 591
Medicare's new formula, 590
Medicare's Shared Savings Program (MSSP), 591
Medication for opioid use disorder (MOUD), 365
Medication management
    communication strategies, 187, 188, 190
    comprehensive medication review, 183, 184
    health literacy, 186, 187
    medication reconciliation, 183
    MRP, 182, 183
    nonadherence, 185, 186
    in outpatient settings, 181
    patient counseling, 184, 185
    therapeutic outcomes, 182
    treatment adherence strategies, 190, 191
Medication related problems (MRPs), 182, 183
Medicine, 575
Meningococcal conjugate vaccines (MCV), 164, 165
Mental and substance use disorders, 536
Mental health, 90, 91, 362, 363
Mental health screenings, 363
Mental health/substance use problem, 48
Mental illness, 293, 431–433
Metabolic disorders, 325
Metabolic surgery, 24
Metoprolol, 389
MFH program, 277
mHealth, 222
Mild cognitive delays, 306
Mild traumatic brain injury (mTBI), 409
Military sexual trauma (MST), 411
Mini-Mental State Examination, 420
Minimum Data Set (MDS), 258
Minority stress, 349, 351
Mitigation methods, 476
Mobile messaging, 66
Moderate fatigue, 385
Modified Checklist for Autism in Toddlers-Revised (M-CHAT-R), 439
Modified Medical Research Council (mMRC) scale, 387
Mongolian spot, 571
Montreal Cognitive Assessment (MoCA©), 389
Moral injury, 410
Motivational interviewing, 50, 51
Multi-dimensional Medical Outcome Study Short Form (SF-36) Health Survey, 516
Multi-disciplinary rounding (MDR), 237
Multimorbidity, 301
Musculoskeletal disorders, 324
Musculoskeletal injuries, 408, 409

N

NAM social risk factor intervention framework, 534
Narcotics Anonymous (NA), 78
National Academy of Medicine (NAM), 383
National Alliance on Mental Illness (NAMI), 136
National Assessment of Adult Literacy, 312
National Association of Professional Geriatric Care Managers, 271
National Center for Chronic Disease Prevention and Health Promotion (NCCDPHP), 132
National Commission on Correctional Healthcare (NCCHC), 364
National Committee for Quality Assurance (NCQA), 498, 519, 610
National Health and Nutrition Examination Survey, 312
National Health Service Corps (NHSC), 621
National Institute for Health and Care Excellence in the UK (NICE), 148, 149
National Institute of Minority Health and Health Disparities (NIMHD), 568
National Quality Forum, 512, 519
Natural language processing (NLP), 469–473, 475, 476
Negative predictive value (NPV), 145, 146
Neurodegenerative and neuromuscular diseases, 170
Neuropsychology testing, 389
Next Generation ACO (NextGen), 611
NIMHD research framework, 569
Non-Communicating Adults Pain Checklist, 323
Nondiscrimination, 322
Non-emergent services, 362
Nongovernmental organizations
    ACS, 135
    ADA, 135
    AHA, 135
    Alzheimer's Association, 136
    faith-based organizations, 136, 137
    LSC, 136
    NAMI, 136
    United Way, 136
Non-pharmaceutical behavioral approaches, 327
Non-pharmaceutical interventions, 259
Non-pharmacologic treatments, 252, 388
Non-profit organizations, 274
Non-residential community-based care
    adult day services (ADS) centers, 273, 274
    area agencies on aging and senior centers, 273
    home-based personal care services, 273
    programs of all-inclusive care for the elderly (PACE), 274, 275
Normalization process theory (NPT), 464
Norming stage, 500
Nurse practitioners (NPs), 622, 626–627
Nurses Improving Care for Healthsystem Elders (NICHE) program, 315
Nursing assistants, 622
Nursing home care, 255

O

Obesity, 169, 170
    approach to patient, 21, 22
    co-morbidities, 20
    COVID-19 infection, 20, 21
    definition, 19, 20
    health disparities, 21
    Lifestyle Medicine, 21
    long-term outcomes, 25
    metabolic surgery, 24
    nutrition and dietary treatments, 22
    physical activity, 22, 30
    physiologic basis, 20
    prevalence, 19
    public health and economic burdens, 21
    weight loss medications, 22–24
Occupational exposures, 552
    Agent Orange, 412
    airborne hazard, 412
    hearing loss and tinnitus, 411
Office for American Indian, Alaska Natives and Native Hawaiian Programs, 133
Office of Elder Justice and Adult Protective Services, 133

Postural orthostatic tachycardia syndrome (POTS), 388
Poverty and unemployment, 102
Practice applications, 474
Precision medicine, 11
Precision oncology, 5
Pre-exposure prophylaxis (PrEp) agents, 353
Preferred Provider Organizations (PPOs), 585
Pregnancy, 101, 168, 169, 364
Premier HealthCare, 330
Prenatal care, 364
Pressure ulcers, 259
Prevalence, definition of, 145, 146
Preventive services, 149
Primary Care Behavioral Health (PCBH), 435
Primary care case management (PCCM) programs, 601
Primary care provider (PCP), 213
Primary Care Transformation, 278
Primary psychosis, 335
Private long-term care insurance, 269
Proceduralist specialties, 619
Process map, 499
Process measures, 501
Programs of all-inclusive care for the elderly (PACE), 131, 269, 274, 275, 316
Project Better Outcomes by Optimizing Safe Transitions (BOOST), 448
Project Extension for Community Healthcare Outcomes (ECHO), 302
Project Reengineering Discharge (RED), 448
Prolonged/frequent hospitalizations, 302
Prostate cancer screening, 146
Prostate specific antigen (PSA) test, 146
Protein-conjugated vaccines, 156
Psychiatric emergencies, 341
Psychiatric hospitals, 342
Psychological distress, 306
Psychosis, 335
Psychosocial needs, 351
Psychotherapy counseling services, 384
Psychotic disorders, 335
Psychotropic medications, 328
Public health workers, 624
Public policy, 93–94, 533
Pulmonary function tests (PFTs), 387
Pulmonary rehabilitation, 387
Pyridostigmine, 389

Q

Quadruple Aim, 607
Qualitative data, 499
Quality Assurance Performance Improvement (QAPI), 258
Quality control, 497, 501
Quality improvement (QI), 53, 364
 change management, 505, 506
 data management, 506
  Act phase, 507
  analyzing and interpreting data, 507
  collection, 506
  disseminating data, 507, 508
  tracking, 506, 507
 federal government, 499
 innovation and launched federal initiatives, 498
 Institute for Healthcare Improvement, 498–499
 metrics, 304
 models and frameworks
  Deming Cycle/PDSA, 499–501
  Lean, 501–503
  Six Sigma, 501
 patient-centered medical home, 498
 practice level, 503
 principles, 499
 quality patient care, 498
 system level QI and transformation, 504, 505
 variation, 497
Quality of care, 249, 258, 289, 290, 364
Quality patient care, 498
Quality planning, 497
Quantitative data, 499
Queer/transgender persons of color (QTPOC), 348

R

Race, 304, 567
Racial and Ethnic Approaches to Community Health (REACH), 138
Racial disparities, 359
Racism, 567
Radiation monitoring system, 551
Readmission, 450–451
Rebalancing research strategies, 540
Recommended immunizations, 377
Recovery Management Checkups (RMC), 78
Red Man syndrome, 571
Reforming medicare, 593
Refugee Convention, 371
Refugee Health Screener-15 (RHS-15), 378
Refugee medical assistance (RMA), 373
Refugees and asylum seeker, in U.S.
 causes and social determinants of mental disorders, 378
 and chronic disease, 375
 chronic hepatitis and HIV, 376, 377
 cultural factors, 378
 defined, 371
 domestic medical examination (DME), 372, 373
 infectious disease, 376
 international policies and governing bodies, 372
 intestinal parasites, 377
 mental health issues, 377, 378
 mental health screening, 378
 refugee primary care, 379, 381
 social and community issues
  family structure, 375
  health and health literacy, 375
  poverty and limited resources, 375
  stages of migration, 374
 status and citizenship trajectory, 373
 treatment consideration, 378, 379
 tuberculosis, 376
 U.S. refugee resettlement processes, 372
 vaccine-preventable diseases, 377
Registered nurses (RNs), 619, 623
Regression, 470, 473
Remote patient monitoring (RPM), 221, 222, 614
Rental assistance, 422
Residential care, 255
Residential settings, 329
Respiratory therapists, 387
Robotic technologies, 275
Rule of Tens, 385

S

Schizophrenia, 114, 117, 336

Index

School-based health centers, 303
Schools, 303
Screening
    asymptomatic carotid artery stenosis, 151
    benefits, 147, 148
    breast cancer
        implementation, 150, 151
        overview, 150
        potential benefits, 150
        potential harms, 150
    clinical practice, 148
    community-based settings, 148
    disease prevalence, 145, 146
    engagement in, 148
    evidence gaps, 148
    individual screening, 146, 147
    lung cancer
        evidence, 149
        implementation, 150
        potential benefits, 150
        potential harms, 150
    NICE, 149
    NPV, 145, 146
    opportunistic screening, 147
    overdiagnosis, 147
    population based screening, 146
    PPV, 145, 146
    recommendations, 146
    risks of, 147
    sensitivity, 145
    specificity, 145
    USPSTF, 149
Screening, Brief Intervention, and Referral to Treatment (SBIRT), 352, 435, 436
Secondary prevention, 151
Secondhand smoke (SHS), 45
Self-Determination Act, 286
Self-management, 114–117
    case management/population health services, 66, 67
    CCM, 62
    chronic disease management at home, 64, 65
    empowerment, 62, 63
    health literacy, 63, 64
    historical development, 61
    peer support, 66
    physician-directed care, limitations, 61
    SDM, 63
    technological advancements, 64, 66
Senior housing, 276
Serious and persistent mental illness (SMI), 418
Serious mental illness (SMI)
    bipolar disorder, 336, 340
    defined, 335
    healthcare models and programs, 341
        alcohol and substance use disorder, 339
        Assertive Community Treatment (ACT) teams, 341
        Community mental health centers (CMHC's), 342
        dementia and cognitive impairment, 339
        emerging service models, 343
        intellectual and developmental disability, 339
        metabolic disorders, 337, 338
        peer support specialists (PSS), 342
        psychiatric hospitals, 342
        psychiatric residential treatment facilities, 342
        tobacco use disorder, 338
        traumatic brain injury (TBI), 339
    medical comorbidities, 337–339
    nonpharmacologic management strategies, 340
    prevalence of, 335
    psychiatric emergencies, 341
    schizophrenia, 336, 340
Severe Acute Respiratory Syndrome Coronavirus-2 (SARS-CoV-2), 157, 381
Severe fatigue, 385
Severe mental illness (SMI), 366
Sexual abuse, 105
Sexual and gender minority (SGM)
    cancer screening, 353
    clinics and practices considerations, 349, 350
    community, 352
    cultural humility and inclusive practices, 350, 351
    gender affirming therapy, 354
    health care system considerations, 349
    inclusive chronic care, 349
    mental health, 351, 352
    older adults, 354, 355
    patient care for chronic conditions, 351
    psychosocial factors, 351
    stigma, discrimination and minority stress, 348, 349
    substance use disorders, 352, 353
    suicide, 352
    youth and emerging adults, 354
Sexual assault, 351
Sexual orientation, 348
Sexual orientation and gender identity data (SOGI), 95, 347, 351
Sexuality, 326
Sexually transmitted infections (STIs), 101
Shanghai integration model (SIM), 117, 118
Shanghai Sixth People's Hospital (S6PH), 117, 118
SHARE program, 198
Shared Decision-Making (SDM), 63
Short Form (SF-36) Health Survey, 512, 513, 515, 516
Short stay care, 255
Sickle cell diseases, 164
Signature wounds, 409
Six Minute Walk Test (6MWT), 387
Six Sigma, 501, 506
Skilled nursing facility (SNF), 239, 256, 257, 447, 454, 455
Skilled physical therapy, 257
Skin injuries, 103, 104
Small water system, 554
Social and peer support, 341
Social capital, 528, 572
Social causation of illness, 529
Social class, 528
Social cognitive models, 540
Social connectedness, 572–573
Social determinants of health (SDOH), 101, 102, 116, 136, 140, 151, 248, 312, 360, 420, 465, 475, 528, 568, 569, 615
    accountability system, 537
    benchmarking efforts, 537
    capability approach, 538, 539
    chronic disease, 527–531, 536–539, 541
    community-level characteristics, 528
    comorbid chronic disease, 536
    conceptual and theoretical frameworks
        biomedical theories, 531, 532
        eco-epidmiology/ecosocial theory, 533
        "fundamental social causes" theory, 532
        life course, 532
        lifestyle theories, 531
        public policy, 533

Social determinants of health (SDOH) (cont.)
  definition, 528
  diet and activity resources, 540
  functional limitation, 530
  health literacy, 536
  health policy, 537, 538
  income inequality, 530, 531
  mental and substance use disorders, 536
  patient data collection, 534, 535
  promoting equity, 533
  racial/ethnic disparities, 531
  social causation of illness, 527
  social deprivation, 536
  social patterning of illness, 527
  social risk factors, 535
  substantial variability, 536
  systems practices, 536
Social Enterprise Interventions (SEI), 422
Social epidemiology, 528, 529
Social isolation, 115, 312, 573
Social issues
  health disparities, 412
  homelessness, 412
  non-health care benefits, 413
Social justice, 528
Social loneliness, 312
Social media, 54
Social minority stress, 352
Social networks, 573
Social risk factors, 527, 528, 534–536
Social security, 584
Social Security Act, 131, 246
Social Security Disability Insurance (SSDI), 584
Social service agencies, 135
Social support, 115
Social Vulnerability Index (SVI), 475
Social workers, 271, 623
Society for Academic Emergency Medicine (SAEM), 251
Socioeconomic position (SEP), 528
Socioeconomic status (SES), 528, 532, 533, 541
Socio-technical system, 474
Solid organ transplant (SOT) recipients, 165
Special Needs Plans (SNPs), 585
Special Supplemental Nutrition Program for Women, Infants, and Children (WIC), 134
Specific, measurable, attainable, relevant, and time-bound (SMART), 501
Speech language pathologists, 387
SPIKES algorithm, 201, 203
Staffing shortages, 627
Staff turnover, 627
Standardized questionnaires, 384
State health agencies, 135
Statistical methods, 470
Statistical process control (SPC), 506
Stereotypes and bias, 331
Stigma, mental health, 432, 433
STOP-BANG for sleep apnea, 384
Storming stage, 500
Stroke, 256, 558
Stroke Impact Scale, 515
Structural racism, 199, 528, 568, 576
Study to Understand Prognoses and Preferences for Outcomes and Risks of Treatment (SUPPORT), 289
Subacute nursing facility (SNF), 248
Substance Abuse and Mental Health Services Administration (SAMHSA), 134, 341, 434
Substance use disorder (SUD), 378, 409, 410, 417–422
  definition, 71, 72
  screening, 72, 73
  treatment
    barriers, 74–76
    harm reduction, 75, 76
    integration, 79
    intensive residential treatment, 74, 75
    interventions, 73
    monitoring effectiveness, 78, 79
    patient-centered approach, 73
    peer-based recovery, 78
    pharmacotherapy, 76, 77
    psychosocial interventions, 77, 78
    specialty treatment settings, 73, 74
    Telehealth, 79
Suicide, 66, 363, 409–412, 558
Supplemental Nutrition Assistance Program (SNAP), 134, 375
Sutter Health, 504, 505
Swallowing difficulties, 324
Swedish National Quality Registries (NQR), 518
Systemic racism, 262

T

Team, 498–501, 503, 505–507
Team-based care, 574
Team-based models, 622
TeamSTEPPS approach, 453
Teamwork, 499, 500
Technical expert, 500
Technological advancements, 64, 66
Technological developments, 121
Telehealth, 53, 79, 273, 330
  acute hospital care, 225
  asynchronous communication, 221
  barriers, 223
  challenges, 226, 227
  COVID-19 pandemic impact, 223
  digital divide, 226
  direct patient care, 222
  E-consults, 221
  electronic health records, 223
  E-visits, 221
  factors, 223, 224
  health chatbots, 222
  in-person visits, 222
  IT infrastructure, 225
  legal and compliance considerations, 226
  limitations, 222, 224
  medical information exchange, 222, 223
  mHealth, 222
  patient location, 224
  post-acute virtual care, 225
  primary care, 224
  RPM, 221, 222
  services, 223
  specialty care, 224
  synchronous communication, 221
  system oversight and workflows, 225, 226
  urgent care, 224
Telemedicine, 247
Telemedicine consultation, 247
Temporary Assistance for Needy Families (TANF), 375, 422
ThedaCare, 505, 508
Theoretical or empirically based model, 460
2,3,7,8-tetrachlorodibenzo-p-dioxin (TCDD), 412

Index

Thiopurine methyltransferase (TPMT), 5
Thirdhand smoke (THS), 45
Three Component Model (TCM), 462, 463
Thrifty phenotype, 531
Tinnitus, 411–412
Tobacco cessation counseling, 66
Tobacco use, 169
    addiction criteria, 42, 44
    adolescents and young adults, 54
    behavioral counseling, 42
    behavioral therapies, 54
    CCM
        comprehensive approach, 48
        emotional support, 49
        family and social support, 49
        public health interventions, 49
        team-based care, 48
    cessation benefits
        asthma, 47
        asymptomatic patients and disease prevention, 45–47
        cancer, 47
        cardiovascular disease, 45, 47
        COPD, 47
        diabetes, 47
        HIV, 47
        inpatient setting, 48
        mental health/substance use problem, 48
    e-cigarettes, 44, 45, 54
    education to health care team members, 55
    5As model, 49–53
    genetics, 54
    heated tobacco products, 45
    impact on, 42, 43
    interventions, 42
    nicotine vaccines and galenic formulations, 54
    physiologic changes, 42
    population health and health care system, 53, 54
    prenatal treatment, 55
    recommendations, 42
    SHS, 45
    smoked tobacco, 43, 44
    smokeless tobacco, 44
    social media, mHealth, and eHealth, 54
    THS, 45
Topiramate, 325
Total cost of care (TCOC) benchmark, 609
Total joint arthroplasty, 256
Toxoid vaccines, 156
Toyota Production System, 497, 502, 504–505
Tracking data, 506, 507
Traditional medicaid, 600
TRANSFoRm project, 474
Transitional care, 213
Transitional Care Management (TCM), 448–450, 452–455
Transitions Clinic Network (TCN), 365
Transitions of care
    advance care planning, 453
    anticipating and preventing reasons for readmission, 450, 451
    bridging components, 453
    CMS TCM payment codes, 450
    CPT codes, 449
    definition, 447
    disparities, 455
    effective, 448, 450
    history, 447
    interprofessional approach
        family and patient role, 455
        medical assistant role, 454
        nurse role, 454
        pharmacist role, 454
        physical and occupational therapist role, 454
        physicians and APPs, 454
        social worker role, 454
    pre-discharge planning, 451
        discharge summary, 451
        durable medical equipment, 452
        follow-up visits, 452, 453
        medications, 451
        patient education, 451
        phone calls, 452
        transportation, 452
    programs, 448
Transport-related injuries, 558
Trauma-Focused Cognitive Behavioral Therapy (TF-CBT), 107
Trauma informed care, 106, 350, 351, 420, 574
Traumatic brain injury (TBI), 339, 409–412
Treatment techniques, 389
The Trevor Project for youth, 352
True North Metrics, 508
Tuberculosis (TB), 376, 573
2010 Affordable Care Act (ACA), 54, 258

U

UCare Complete, 330
Unbiased and non-judgmental communication approach, 326
United Nations Convention on Rights of Persons with Disabilities, 322
United Nations High Commissioner for Refugees (UNHCR), 371, 372, 374
United States (US) health care system, 619
United States Preventive Services Task Force (USPSTF), 100
United Way, 136
Universal screening, 436
Universal suicide screening, 352
University of California at San Francisco (UCSF), 354
Unsupervised machine learning, 470
Urgent care
    acute illness, 212, 213
    chronic disease metrics, 213
    definition, 209
    organization, 214
    overview, 212
    PCP, 213
    research, 216
    selection, 213
    transitional care, 213
Uridine diphosphate glucuronosyltransferase (UGT) 1A1, 6
Urinary incontinence, 259
US-based voluntary resettlement agencies, 372
US Center for Medicare and Medicaid Services (CMS), 288
US, Child Protective Service (CPS) agencies, 99, 101
US criminal legal system, 359
US Department of Agriculture (USDA), 134
U.S. Department of Health and Human Services (HHS)
    ACF, 133
    ACL, 132, 133
    CDC, 131, 132
    CMS, 130, 131
    HRSA, 133, 134
    mission of, 130
    SAMHSA, 134
    strategic plan, 130
US Department of Housing and Urban Development (HUD), 276
US Environmental Protection Agency, 572

US health care spending, 619
US healthcare system, 608
US Interagency Council on Homelessness, 423
US Preventive Services Task Force (USPSTF), 149, 353, 535
US refugee resettlement processes, 373

V

Vaccine-preventable diseases (VPDs), 157, 159
Vaccines
  cardiovascular disease, in children, 169
  chronic liver disease, 167, 168
  CKD, 166, 167
  cocooning, 157, 158
  communication approach, 170, 171
  community immunity, 158, 159
  data-informed feedback, 171
  diabetes mellitus, 166
  evidence-based approaches, 170
  immunization guidelines, 160
  immunization recommendations
    European Union, 159
    in low- and middle-income countries, 160
    in United Kingdom, 159, 160
    in United States, 159
  immunocompromised host
    asplenia, 164
    chemotherapy, 164
    chronic illness, 165, 166
    high-level immunosuppression, 163
    HIV, 163, 164
    HSCT recipients, 164, 165
    low-level immunosuppression, 163
    patients on immunosuppressive therapy, 163
    primary immunodeficiencies, 162, 163
    principles, 162
    sickle cell diseases, 164
    SOT recipients, 165
  inactivated vaccines
    polysaccharide vaccines, 156
    protein-conjugated vaccines, 156
    protein subunit vaccines, 156
    SARS-CoV-2 vaccines, 157
    toxoids, 156
    VLP vaccines, 156
    whole cell/killed antigen vaccines, 156
  live-attenuated vaccines, 156
  missed opportunities, 171
  neurodegenerative and neuromuscular diseases, 170
  obesity, 169, 170
  passive immunization, 157
  patient reminders and recall systems, 171
  pregnancy, 168, 169
  provider reminders, 171
  pulmonary disease, 167
  recommendations, 171
  tobacco use disorder, 169
Vaccines for Children (VFC) program, 159
Value based care, 624
  ACA, 608
  ACO, 611, 613, 614
  alternative payment model, 612
  APM's, 608–611
  chronic disease management, 614–615
  CMS, 608
  community-based services, 615
  cost and quality outcomes, 607
  HCP-LAN, 614
  health equity, 615
  hospital quality and value programs, 608
  overutilization and underutilization, 607
  PCMH, 608
  SDOH, 615
  TCOC benchmark, 611
  value-based payment models, 607
Value-based payment models, 441
Value-based purchasing, 589
Venous thromboembolism (VTE), 233
Veteran, 407
Veteran care
  chronic health issues
    chronic pain, 411
    depression, 410
    military sexual trauma, 411
    moral injury, 410
    musculoskeletal injuries, 408, 409
    PTSD, 410
    substance abuse disorder, 410
    suicide, 410, 411
    TBI, 409
    Women's Health Care, 411
  cost, 408
  eligibility, 408
  history, 408
  occupational exposures
    agent orange, 412
    airborne hazard, 412
    hearing loss and tinnitus, 411, 412
  social issues
    health disparities, 412
    homelessness, 412
    non-health care benefits, 413
  validated screening tools, 409
  Veterans Health Administration, 408
Veteran population, 408, 410–412
Veterans Health Administration (VHA), 408
VillageMD, 613
Virtual care, 79
Virus-like particle (VLP) vaccines, 156
Vision and hearing impairments, 326

W

Watch Metrics, 508
Well-informed theory, 460
Well-integrated health care teams, 421
WestChronic system, 518
"Whole community" approach, 423
Whole School, Whole Community, Whole Child (WSCC) educational model, 303, 306
Woman Abuse Screening Tool (WAST), 100
Women's Health Care, 411
Women's Initiative Supporting Health, 365
World Health Organization (WHO), 160, 312, 376, 381, 547
World Professional Association for Transgender Health (WPATH), 354

Y

YMCAs, 137

Z

"Z" codes (Z55-65), 534
Zero harm, 502

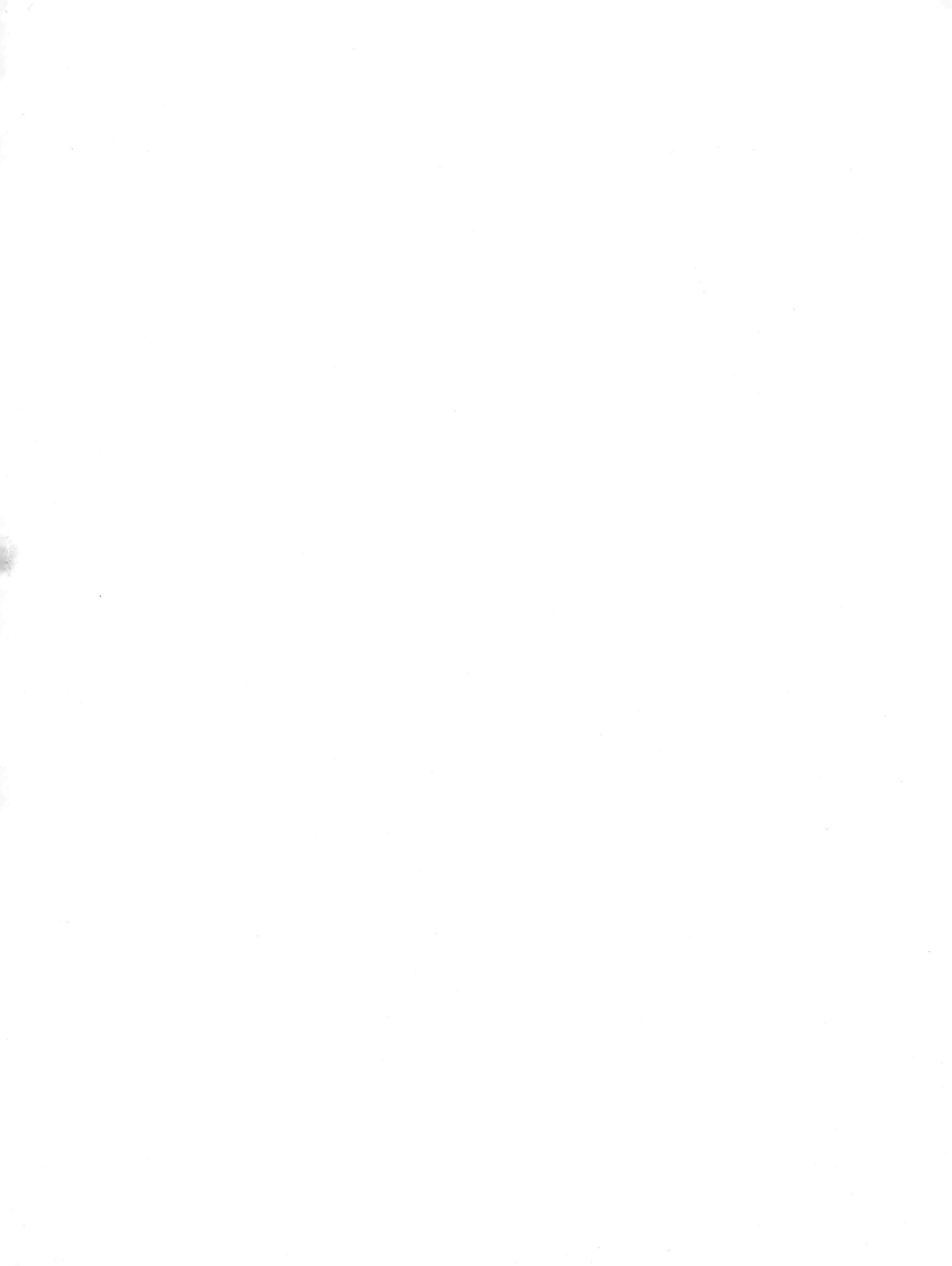

Printed in the United States
by Baker & Taylor Publisher Services